Recommended Dietary Allowances (RDA) and Adequate Intakes (AI) for Vitamins

Age (yr)	Thiamin RDA (mg/day)	Riboflavin RDA (mg/day)	Niacin RDA (mg/day)[a]	Biotin AI (µg/day)	Pantothenic acid AI (mg/day)	Vitamin B_6 RDA (mg/day)	Folate RDA (µg/day)[b]	Vitamin B_{12} RDA (µg/day)	Choline AI (mg/day)	Vitamin C RDA (mg/day)	Vitamin A RDA (µg/day)[c]	Vitamin D RDA (IU/day)[d]	Vitamin E RDA (mg/day)[e]	Vitamin K AI (µg/day)
Infants														
0–0.5	0.2	0.3	2	5	1.7	0.1	65	0.4	125	40	400	400 (10 µg)	4	2.0
0.5–1	0.3	0.4	4	6	1.8	0.3	80	0.5	150	50	500	400 (10 µg)	5	2.5
Children														
1–3	0.5	0.5	6	8	2	0.5	150	0.9	200	15	300	600 (15 µg)	6	30
4–8	0.6	0.6	8	12	3	0.6	200	1.2	250	25	400	600 (15 µg)	7	55
Males														
9–13	0.9	0.9	12	20	4	1.0	300	1.8	375	45	600	600 (15 µg)	11	60
14–18	1.2	1.3	16	25	5	1.3	400	2.4	550	75	900	600 (15 µg)	15	75
19–30	1.2	1.3	16	30	5	1.3	400	2.4	550	90	900	600 (15 µg)	15	120
31–50	1.2	1.3	16	30	5	1.3	400	2.4	550	90	900	600 (15 µg)	15	120
51–70	1.2	1.3	16	30	5	1.7	400	2.4	550	90	900	600 (15 µg)	15	120
>70	1.2	1.3	16	30	5	1.7	400	2.4	550	90	900	800 (20 µg)	15	120
Females														
9–13	0.9	0.9	12	20	4	1.0	300	1.8	375	45	600	600 (15 µg)	11	60
14–18	1.0	1.0	14	25	5	1.2	400	2.4	400	65	700	600 (15 µg)	15	75
19–30	1.1	1.1	14	30	5	1.3	400	2.4	425	75	700	600 (15 µg)	15	90
31–50	1.1	1.1	14	30	5	1.3	400	2.4	425	75	700	600 (15 µg)	15	90
51–70	1.1	1.1	14	30	5	1.5	400	2.4	425	75	700	600 (15 µg)	15	90
>70	1.1	1.1	14	30	5	1.5	400	2.4	425	75	700	800 (20 µg)	15	90
Pregnancy														
≤18	1.4	1.4	18	30	6	1.9	600	2.6	450	80	750	600 (15 µg)	15	75
19–30	1.4	1.4	18	30	6	1.9	600	2.6	450	85	770	600 (15 µg)	15	90
31–50	1.4	1.4	18	30	6	1.9	600	2.6	450	85	770	600 (15 µg)	15	90
Lactation														
≤18	1.4	1.6	17	35	7	2.0	500	2.8	550	115	1200	600 (15 µg)	19	75
19–30	1.4	1.6	17	35	7	2.0	500	2.8	550	120	1300	600 (15 µg)	19	90
31–50	1.4	1.6	17	35	7	2.0	500	2.8	550	120	1300	600 (15 µg)	19	90

NOTE: For all nutrients, values for infants are AI.

[a]Niacin recommendations are expressed as niacin equivalents (NE), except for recommendations for infants younger than 6 months, which are expressed as preformed niacin.

[b]Folate recommendations are expressed as dietary folate equivalents (DFE).

[c]Vitamin A recommendations are expressed as retinol activity equivalents (RAE).

[d]Vitamin D recommendations are expressed as cholecalciferol and assume an absence of adequate exposure to sunlight.

[e]Vitamin E recommendations are expressed as α-tocopherol.

Recommended Dietary Allowances (RDA) and Adequate Intakes (AI) for Minerals

Age (yr)	Sodium AI (mg/day)	Chloride AI (mg/day)	Potassium AI (mg/day)	Calcium RDA (mg/day)	Phosphorus RDA (mg/day)	Magnesium RDA (mg/day)	Iron RDA (mg/day)	Zinc RDA (mg/day)	Iodine RDA (µg/day)	Selenium RDA (µg/day)	Copper RDA (µg/day)	Manganese AI (mg/day)	Fluoride AI (mg/day)	Chromium AI (µg/day)	Molybdenum RDA (µg/day)
Infants															
0–0.5	120	180	400	200	100	30	0.27	2	110	15	200	0.003	0.01	0.2	2
0.5–1	370	570	700	260	275	75	11	3	130	20	220	0.6	0.5	5.5	3
Children															
1–3	1000	1500	3000	700	460	80	7	3	90	20	340	1.2	0.7	11	17
4–8	1200	1900	3800	1000	500	130	10	5	90	30	440	1.5	1.0	15	22
Males															
9–13	1500	2300	4500	1300	1250	240	8	8	120	40	700	1.9	2	25	34
14–18	1500	2300	4700	1300	1250	410	11	11	150	55	890	2.2	3	35	43
19–30	1500	2300	4700	1000	700	400	8	11	150	55	900	2.3	4	35	45
31–50	1500	2300	4700	1000	700	420	8	11	150	55	900	2.3	4	35	45
51–70	1300	2000	4700	1000	700	420	8	11	150	55	900	2.3	4	30	45
>70	1200	1800	4700	1200	700	420	8	11	150	55	900	2.3	4	30	45
Females															
9–13	1500	2300	4500	1300	1250	240	8	8	120	40	700	1.6	2	21	34
14–18	1500	2300	4700	1300	1250	360	15	9	150	55	890	1.6	3	24	43
19–30	1500	2300	4700	1000	700	310	18	8	150	55	900	1.8	3	25	45
31–50	1500	2300	4700	1000	700	320	18	8	150	55	900	1.8	3	25	45
51–70	1300	2000	4700	1200	700	320	8	8	150	55	900	1.8	3	20	45
>70	1200	1800	4700	1200	700	320	8	8	150	55	900	1.8	3	20	45
Pregnancy															
≤18	1500	2300	4700	1300	1250	400	27	12	220	60	1000	2.0	3	29	50
19–30	1500	2300	4700	1000	700	350	27	11	220	60	1000	2.0	3	30	50
31–50	1500	2300	4700	1000	700	360	27	11	220	60	1000	2.0	3	30	50
Lactation															
≤18	1500	2300	5100	1300	1250	360	10	13	290	70	1300	2.6	3	44	50
19–30	1500	2300	5100	1000	700	310	9	12	290	70	1300	2.6	3	45	50
31–50	1500	2300	5100	1000	700	320	9	12	290	70	1300	2.6	3	45	50

NOTE: For all nutrients, values for infants are AI.

Tolerable Upper Intake Levels (UL) for Vitamins

Age (yr)	Niacin (mg/day)[a]	Vitamin B6 (mg/day)	Folate (µg/day)[a]	Choline (mg/day)	Vitamin C (mg/day)	Vitamin A (µg/day)[b]	Vitamin D (IU/day)	Vitamin E (mg/day)[c]
Infants								
0–0.5	—	—	—	—	—	600	1000 (25 µg)	—
0.5–1	—	—	—	—	—	600	1500 (38 µg)	—
Children								
1–3	10	30	300	1000	400	600	2500 (63 µg)	200
4–8	15	40	400	1000	650	900	3000 (75 µg)	300
9–13	20	60	600	2000	1200	1700	4000 (100 µg)	600
Adolescents								
14–18	30	80	800	3000	1800	2800	4000 (100 µg)	800
Adults								
19–70	35	100	1000	3500	2000	3000	4000 (100 µg)	1000
>70	35	100	1000	3500	2000	3000	4000 (100 µg)	1000
Pregnancy								
≤18	30	80	800	3000	1800	2800	4000 (100 µg)	800
19–50	35	100	1000	3500	2000	3000	4000 (100 µg)	1000
Lactation								
≤18	30	80	800	3000	1800	2800	4000 (100 µg)	800
19–50	35	100	1000	3500	2000	3000	4000 (100 µg)	1000

[a]The UL for niacin and folate apply to synthetic forms obtained from supplements, fortified foods, or a combination of the two.

[b]The UL for vitamin A applies to the preformed vitamin only.

[c]The UL for vitamin E applies to any form of supplemental α-tocopherol, fortified foods, or a combination of the two.

Tolerable Upper Intake Levels (UL) for Minerals

Age (yr)	Sodium (mg/day)	Chloride (mg/day)	Calcium (mg/day)	Phosphorus (mg/day)	Magnesium (mg/day)[d]	Iron (mg/day)	Zinc (mg/day)	Iodine (µg/day)	Selenium (µg/day)	Copper (µg/day)	Manganese (mg/day)	Fluoride (mg/day)	Molybdenum (µg/day)	Boron (mg/day)	Nickel (mg/day)	Vanadium (mg/day)
Infants																
0–0.5	—	—	1000	—	—	40	4	—	45	—	—	0.7	—	—	—	—
0.5–1	—	—	1500	—	—	40	5	—	60	—	—	0.9	—	—	—	—
Children																
1–3	1500	2300	2500	3000	65	40	7	200	90	1000	2	1.3	300	3	0.2	—
4–8	1900	2900	2500	3000	110	40	12	300	150	3000	3	2.2	600	6	0.3	—
9–13	2200	3400	3000	4000	350	40	23	600	280	5000	6	10	1100	11	0.6	—
Adolescents																
14–18	2300	3600	3000	4000	350	45	34	900	400	8000	9	10	1700	17	1.0	—
Adults																
19–50	2300	3600	2500	4000	350	45	40	1100	400	10,000	11	10	2000	20	1.0	1.8
51–70	2300	3600	2000	4000	350	45	40	1100	400	10,000	11	10	2000	20	1.0	1.8
>70	2300	3600	2000	3000	350	45	40	1100	400	10,000	11	10	2000	20	1.0	1.8
Pregnancy																
≤18	2300	3600	3000	3500	350	45	34	900	400	8000	9	10	1700	17	1.0	—
19–50	2300	3600	2500	3500	350	45	40	1100	400	10,000	11	10	2000	20	1.0	—
Lactation																
≤18	2300	3600	3000	4000	350	45	34	900	400	8000	9	10	1700	17	1.0	—
19–50	2300	3600	2500	4000	350	45	40	1100	400	10,000	11	10	2000	20	1.0	—

[d]The UL for magnesium applies to synthetic forms obtained from supplements or drugs only.

NOTE: An Upper Limit was not established for vitamins and minerals not listed and for those age groups listed with a dash (—) because of a lack of data, not because these nutrients are safe to consume at any level of intake. All nutrients can have adverse effects when intakes are excessive.

SOURCE: Adapted with permission from the *Dietary Reference Intakes* series, National Academies Press. Copyright 1997, 1998, 2000, 2001, 2002, 2005, 2011 by the National Academies of Sciences.

ADVANCED NUTRITION AND HUMAN METABOLISM

SIXTH EDITION

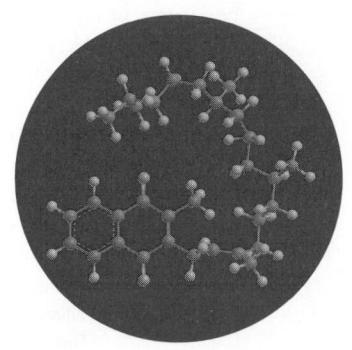

ADVANCED NUTRITION AND HUMAN METABOLISM

SIXTH EDITION

Sareen S. Gropper

AUBURN UNIVERSITY

Jack L. Smith

UNIVERSITY OF DELAWARE

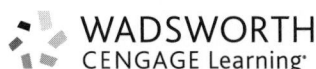

WADSWORTH
CENGAGE Learning·

Australia · Brazil · Japan · Korea · Mexico · Singapore · Spain · United Kingdom · United States

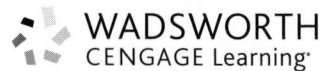
WADSWORTH
CENGAGE Learning·

Advanced Nutrition and Human Metabolism, Sixth Edition
Sareen S. Gropper and Jack L. Smith

Publisher: Yolanda Cossio

Senior Acquiring Sponsoring Editor:
 Peggy Williams

Development Editor: Elesha Feldman

Editorial Assistant: Sean Cronin

Media Editor: Miriam Myers

Marketing Manager: Janet del Mundo

Marketing Coordinator: Jing Hu

Marketing Communications Manager:
 Mary Anne Payumo

Manufacturing Planner: Karen Hunt

Rights Acquisitions Specialist- Img and Txt:
 Don Schlotman

Art and Cover Direction, Production Management,
 and Composition: PreMediaGlobal

Cover Designer: Norman Baugher

Cover Image: © Natalia Karpova/Shutterstock

© 2013, 2009, 2005 Wadsworth, Cengage Learning

ALL RIGHTS RESERVED. No part of this work covered by the copyright herein may be reproduced, transmitted, stored, or used in any form or by any means graphic, electronic, or mechanical, including but not limited to photocopying, recording, scanning, digitizing, taping, Web distribution, information networks, or information storage and retrieval systems, except as permitted under Section 107 or 108 of the 1976 United States Copyright Act, without the prior written permission of the publisher.

For product information and technology assistance, contact us at
Cengage Learning Customer & Sales Support, 1-800-354-9706

For permission to use material from this text or product,
submit all requests online at **www.cengage.com/permissions**.
Further permissions questions can be emailed to
permissionrequest@cengage.com.

Library of Congress Control Number: 2012935123

ISBN-13: 978-1-133-10405-6

ISBN-10: 1-133-10405-3

Wadsworth
20 Davis Drive
Belmont, CA 94002-3098
USA

Cengage Learning is a leading provider of customized learning solutions with office locations around the globe, including Singapore, the United Kingdom, Australia, Mexico, Brazil and Japan. Locate your local office at **www.cengage.com/global.**

Cengage Learning products are represented in Canada by Nelson Education, Ltd.

To learn more about Wadsworth, visit **www.cengage.com/wadsworth**

Purchase any of our products at your local college store or at our preferred online store **www.cengagebrain.com**.

Printed in the United States of America
4 5 6 7 19 18 17 16 15

*To my children Michelle and Michael, and to my husband, Daniel,
for their ongoing encouragement, support, faith, and love.*

Sareen Gropper

*To my wife, Carol, for her continued support, constant inspiration, and
assistance in the preparation of this book.*

Jack Smith

BRIEF CONTENTS

CONTENTS

PREFACE

Since the first edition was published in 1990, much has changed in the science of nutrition. But the purpose of the text—to provide thorough coverage of normal metabolism for upper-division nutrition students—remains the same. We continue to strive for a level of detail and scope of material that satisfy the needs of both instructors and students. With each succeeding edition, we have responded to suggestions from instructors, content reviewers, and students that have improved the text by enhancing the clarity of the material and by ensuring accuracy. In addition, we have included the latest and most pertinent nutrition science available to provide future nutrition professionals with the fundamental information vital to their careers and to provide the basis for assimilating new scientific discoveries as they happen.

Just as the body of information on nutrition science has increased, so has the team of authors working on this text. Dr. James Groff and Dr. Sara Hunt coauthored the first edition. In subsequent editions, Dr. Sareen Gropper became a coauthor as Dr. Hunt entered retirement. In the fourth edition, Dr. Jack L. Smith joined the author team. Drs. Gropper and Smith have continued to devote their efforts and time in coauthoring this sixth edition.

NEW TO THIS EDITION

All chapters of the sixth edition have been thoroughly updated with new references, and many feature new or enhanced illustrations. The presentation of the minerals has been reorganized to centralize coverage of the electrolytes with the discussion of fluid balance and to separate essential from nonessential trace minerals. Scientific research methodologies are now addressed in context within the nutrient chapters.

Chapter 1 The Cell: A Microcosm of Life

- added a new section on control of gene expression that introduces level of control at the translational, processing, and transcription stages
- expanded discussion of cell structure to include types of cell membrane receptors and their role in the control of cellular function and the action of hormones
- new Perspective feature on nutritional genomics

Chapter 2 The Digestive System: Mechanism for Nourishing the Body

- expanded coverage of prebiotics and probiotics
- expanded discussion of disorders causing malfunction of the gastrointestinal tract

Chapter 3 Carbohydrates

- added a new Perspective on the health implications of high-fructose corn syrup
- expanded coverage of hexokinase and hexokinase 4 (glucokinase) and provided a new accompanying table illustrating the different properties of the isozymes
- added information on facilitated transport of glucose, GLUT isoforms, and transport of other substances across cell membranes
- expanded coverage on the regulation, metabolic control, and interrelation of metabolic pathways for carbohydrate

Chapter 4 Fiber

- expanded examples of food sources of different types of fibers
- added information on the soluble and insoluble dietary fiber contents of foods
- added a new Perspective on prebiotics and health

Chapter 5 Lipids

- expanded coverage of fatty acid, diacylglycerol, and cholesterol absorption
- expanded coverage of *trans* fatty acids
- expanded coverage of essential fatty acids, including the opposing effects of n-3 and n-6 eicosanoids and created a new table outlining the differences

Chapter 6 Protein

- to facilitate student learning, reorganized the chapter to first emphasize amino acid classification and sources and then the processes of digestion, absorption, and metabolism; intestinal cell amino acid metabolism is now discussed in the context of interorgan flow of amino acids and organ-specific amino acid metabolism

- expanded the coverage of protein synthesis to include a discussion of translation
- added a section on changes in body composition with aging, which includes a discussion of sarcopenia
- added the indicator amino acid oxidation technique to the discussion of adequacy of protein and amino acid intakes
- added a discussion of the impact of low-grade inflammation on protein metabolism to the Perspective

Chapter 7 Integration and Regulation of Metabolism and the Impact of Exercise and Sport

- added a new Perspective on metabolic syndrome
- expanded coverage of insulin signaling and signaling receptors
- expanded coverage of energy homeostasis, including the role of AMP-activated protein kinase and malonyl-CoA

Chapter 8 Body Composition, Energy Expenditure, and Energy Balance

- added a new reference table for calculation of energy expenditure from various activities
- added several new photographs illustrating methods of assessing body composition and energy expenditure, as well as a new obesity prevalence graph
- expanded coverage of body mass index and body adiposity index
- extended coverage of the hormonal influences on body weight regulation and created a new table summarizing the roles of the regulating agents

Chapter 9 Water-Soluble Vitamins

- provided more thorough coverage of the water-soluble vitamin contents of foods
- expanded coverage of the metabolic roles of vitamin C, folate, and biotin
- updated and expanded coverage of the relationships between some of the water-soluble vitamins and various diseases including, for example, vitamin C and colds, cancer, heart disease, and eye health; folate and dementia, heart disease, cancer, and neural tube defects; and vitamin B_{12} and heart disease and neural tube defects

Chapter 10 Fat-Soluble Vitamins

- provided more thorough coverage of the fat-soluble vitamin contents of foods
- expanded the discussion of the roles of vitamin E in gene expression and vitamin D in muscle function
- expanded the figures illustrating the metabolism of vitamin A
- added a new figure providing an overview of the blood clotting process
- updated and expanded the coverage of the relationships between the fat-soluble vitamins and diseases including, for example, carotenoids and eye health, heart disease, and cancer; vitamin E and dementia, heart disease, eye health, and cancer; and vitamin K and bone health
- included the latest dietary intake recommendations for vitamin D

Chapter 11 Major Minerals

- provided more thorough coverage of the major mineral contents of foods
- expanded the discussion of calcium absorption as well as bone formation and resorption
- updated the discussion of the associations between sodium, calcium, and magnesium and hypertension in the Perspective
- added coverage of the roles of phosphorus in the body
- added new figures depicting calcium's intracellular actions and mechanisms for maintaining cytosolic calcium concentrations; also added the structures of important phosphorus-containing compounds
- included the latest dietary intake recommendations for calcium

Chapter 12 Water and Electrolytes

- expanded the discussion of the role of vasopressin (ADH) in the reabsorption of water and sodium and the excretion of potassium
- expanded coverage of the role of the renin-angiotensin II-aldosterone system in the reabsorption of water and sodium and the excretion of potassium
- expanded coverage of natriuretic peptides, which promote sodium and water excretion

Chapter 13 Essential Trace and Ultratrace Minerals

- provided more thorough coverage of the trace and ultratrace mineral contents of foods

- expanded coverage of the mechanisms involved in trace mineral absorption
- added more subheads to help students better recognize the functions of the trace minerals
- updated the discussion of the associations between selenium and cancer, molybdenum and cancer, and chromium and diabetes
- added a new biochemical function of molybdenum and expanded the discussion of the proposed functions of chromium in cells
- added new figures illustrating the digestion, absorption, enterocyte use, and transport of iron, zinc, and copper; iron uptake and storage; zinc's role in gene expression; copper use and excretion; and selenium metabolism

Chapter 14 Nonessential Trace and Ultratrace Minerals

- expanded the discussion of the metabolism of arsenic in the body and added a new accompanying figure
- updated the discussion of the role of vanadium in the treatment of diabetes mellitus
- added a new Perspective on identifying bogus claims associated with dietary supplements

PRESENTATION

The presentation of the text is designed to make the book easy for the reader to use. The second color draws attention to important elements in the text, tables, and figures and helps generate reader interest. The Perspectives provide applications of the information in the chapter text.

Because this book focuses on normal human nutrition and physiological function, it is an effective resource for students majoring in either nutrition sciences or dietetics. Intended for a course in advanced nutrition, the text presumes a sound background in the biological sciences. At the same time, however, it provides a review of the basic sciences—particularly biochemistry and physiology, which are important to understanding the material. This text applies biochemistry to nutrient use from consumption through digestion, absorption, distribution, and cellular metabolism, making it a valuable reference for health care workers. Health practitioners may use it as a resource to refresh their memories with regard to metabolic and physiological interrelationships and to obtain a concise update on current concepts related to human nutrition.

We continue to present nutrition as the science that integrates life processes from the molecular to the cellular level and on through the multisystem operation of the whole organism. Our primary goal is to give a comprehensive picture of cell reactions at the tissue, organ, and system levels. Subject matter has been selected for its relevance to meeting this goal.

ORGANIZATION

Each of the 14 chapters begins with a topic outline, followed by a brief introduction to the chapter's subject matter. These features are followed in order by the chapter text, a brief summary that ties together the ideas presented in the chapter (in Chapters 1–8 and 12), a reference list, and a Perspective (or two) with its own reference list.

The text is divided into three sections. Section I (Chapters 1 and 2) focuses on cell structure, gastrointestinal tract anatomy, and function with respect to digestion and absorption. The chapter on the cell (Chapter 1) also opens the discussion of energy transformation and of the role of gene expression in the regulation of metabolic processes.

Section II (Chapters 3–8) discusses metabolism of the macronutrients. This section reviews primary metabolic pathways for carbohydrates, lipids, and proteins, emphasizing those reactions particularly relevant to issues of health. Since most of the body's energy production is associated with glycolysis or the tricarboxylic acid cycle by the way of the electron transport chain and oxidative phosphorylation, the carbohydrates chapter (Chapter 3) covers these aspects of energy transformation. We include a separate chapter (Chapter 4) on fiber. The metabolism of alcohol, which contributes to the caloric intake of many people, is discussed within the lipids chapter (Chapter 5). Alcohol's chemical structure more closely resembles that of carbohydrates, but its metabolism is more similar to that of lipids. Chapter 7 discusses the interrelationships among the metabolic pathways that are common to the macronutrients. This chapter also includes a discussion of the regulation of the metabolic pathways and a description of the metabolic dynamics of the fed-fast cycle, along with a presentation of the effects of physical exertion on the body's metabolic pathways. The chapter on body composition (Chapter 8) emphasizes energy balance and the influence of energy balance on the various body compartments. This chapter also includes a brief discussion of hormonal control of food intake, the prevalence of obesity, and the regulation of body weight.

Section III (Chapters 9–14) concerns those nutrients considered regulatory in nature: the water- and fat-soluble vitamins and the minerals, including the major minerals, trace minerals, and ultratrace minerals. These chapters cover nutrient features such as digestion, absorption, transport, function, metabolism, excretion, deficiency, toxicity, and assessment of nutriture, as well as the latest Recommended Dietary Allowances or Adequate Intakes for each nutrient. Information about the major minerals has been split into two chapters: Chapter 11 addresses calcium, phosphorus, and magnesium, and Chapter 12 discusses sodium, potassium, and chloride. Chapter 12 integrates coverage of the maintenance of the body's homeostatic environment—including discussions of body fluids, electrolyte balance, and pH maintenance—with the presentation of the electrolytes.

SUPPLEMENTARY MATERIAL

To enhance teaching and learning from the textbook, a Power Lecture CD-ROM is available. This multimedia collection of visual resources provides instructors with a collection of figures from the textbook. Instructors may use illustrations to create custom classroom presentations, visually based tests and quizzes, or classroom support materials. In addition, a robust test bank is available both electronically (on the CD-ROM and as a Web site download) and in printed form. Students will find study tools and online practice tests for each chapter on the book's Course Mate Web site.

ACKNOWLEDGMENTS

Although this textbook represents countless hours of work by the authors, it is also the work of many other hardworking individuals. We cannot possibly list everyone who has helped, but we would like to call attention to a few individuals who have played particularly important roles. We thank our undergraduate and graduate nutrition students for their ongoing feedback. We thank the acquisitions editor, Peggy Williams; our developmental editor, Elesha Feldman; our art director, John Walker; our marketing manager, Janet del Mundo; our content project manager for editorial production, Kailash Rawat; and our permissions editor, Don Schlotman. We extend special thanks to our production team and our copy editor, Sarah Wales-McGrath.

We thank two additional contributors, who also worked with us on the sixth edition of the text: Ruth M. DeBusk, Ph.D., R.D., for writing the Perspective "Nutritional Genomics: A New Perspective on Food," and Rita M. Johnson, Ph.D., R.D., F.A.D.A., for the Perspective "Genetics and Nutrition: The Effect on Folic Acid Needs and Risk of Chronic Disease."

We are indebted to the efforts of Carole A. Conn (University of New Mexico), who was lead author for the test bank; and Rita M. Johnson (Indiana University of Pennsylvania), Kevin Schalinske (Iowa State University), and Mary Jacob (California State University, Long Beach), who contributed to the test bank.

We owe special thanks to the reviewers whose thoughtful comments, criticisms, and suggestions were indispensable in shaping this text.

Sixth Edition Reviewers

Jodee L. Dorsey, Florida State University
Jennifer Hemphill, Florida State University
Elizabeth A. Kirk, Bastyr University and University of Washington
Steven E. Nizielski, Grand Valley State University
Scott K. Reaves, California Polytechnic State University
Karla P. Shelnutt, University of Florida

Fifth Edition Reviewers

Richard C. Baybutt, Kansas State University
Patricia B. Brevard, James Madison University
Marie A. Caudill, California State Polytechnic University, Pomona
Prithiva Chanmugam, Louisiana State University
Michele M. Doucette, Georgia State University
Michael A. Dunn, University of Hawaii at Mānoa
Steve Hertzler, Ohio State University
Steven Nizielski, Grand Valley State University
Kimberli Pike, Ball State University
William R. Proulx, SUNY Oneonta
Scott K. Reaves, California State University, San Luis Obispo
Donato F. Romagnolo, University of Arizona, Tucson
James H. Swain, Case Western Reserve University

1

THE CELL: A MICROCOSM OF LIFE

CELLS ARE THE VERY ESSENCE OF LIFE. Cells may be defined as the basic living, structural, and functional units of the human body. They vary greatly in size, chemical composition, and function, but each one is a remarkable miniaturization of human life. Cells move, grow, ingest food and excrete wastes, react to their environment, and even reproduce. This chapter provides a brief review of the basics of a cell, including cellular components, communication, energy, and transport. An overview of the natural life span of a typical cell is provided because of its importance in nutrition and disease.

Cells of all multicellular organisms are called **eukaryotic cells** (from the Greek *eu,* meaning "true," and *karyon,* "nucleus"). Eukaryotic cells evolved from simpler, more primitive cells called **prokaryotic cells** (from the Greek meaning "before nucleus").The major distinguishing feature between the two cell types is that eukaryotic cells possess a defined nucleus, whereas prokaryotic cells do not. Also, eukaryotic cells are larger and much more complex structurally and functionally than their ancestors. Because this text addresses human metabolism and nutrition, all descriptions of cellular structure and function in this and subsequent chapters pertain to eukaryotic cells.

Specialization among cells is a necessity for the living, breathing human, but cells in general have certain basic similarities. All human cells have a plasma membrane and a nucleus (or have had a nucleus), and most contain an endoplasmic reticulum, Golgi apparatus, and mitochondria. For convenience of discussion, this book considers a "typical cell" to enable us to identify the various organelles and their functions, which characterize cellular life. Considering the relationship between the normal functioning of a typical cell and the health of the total organism—the human being—brings to mind the old rule: "A chain is only as strong as its weakest link."

Figure 1.1 shows the fine structure of a typical animal cell. A similar view of a typical animal absorptive cell (such as an intestinal epithelial cell) is included in the discussion of digestion in Chapter 2.

Our discussion begins with the plasma membrane, which forms the outer boundary of the cell, and then moves inward to examine the organelles held within this membrane. This chapter covers the information about molecules in the cell that is needed to understand cell structure and function. The chemical structures of the molecules are described later in the appropriate chapters.

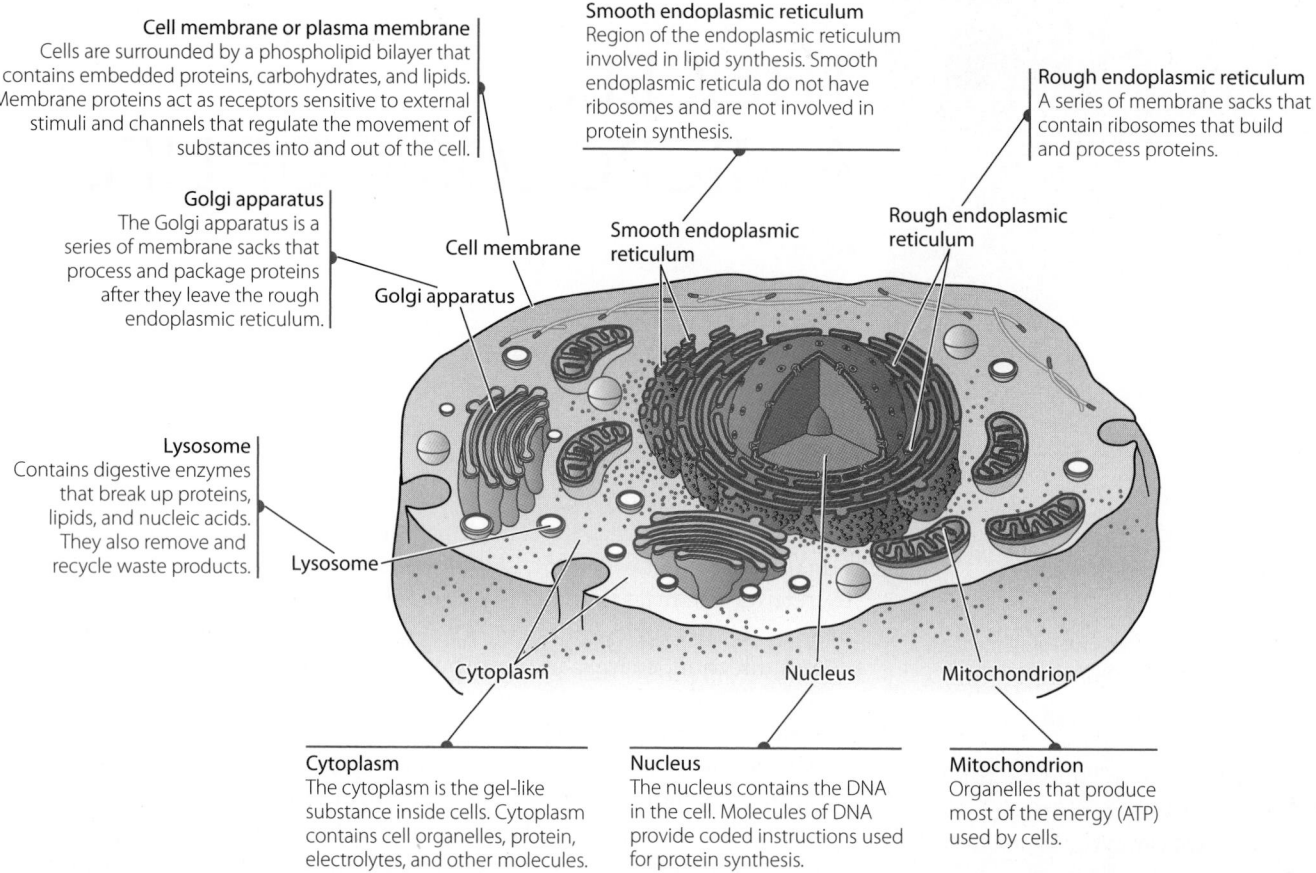

Cell membrane or plasma membrane
Cells are surrounded by a phospholipid bilayer that contains embedded proteins, carbohydrates, and lipids. Membrane proteins act as receptors sensitive to external stimuli and channels that regulate the movement of substances into and out of the cell.

Smooth endoplasmic reticulum
Region of the endoplasmic reticulum involved in lipid synthesis. Smooth endoplasmic reticula do not have ribosomes and are not involved in protein synthesis.

Rough endoplasmic reticulum
A series of membrane sacks that contain ribosomes that build and process proteins.

Golgi apparatus
The Golgi apparatus is a series of membrane sacks that process and package proteins after they leave the rough endoplasmic reticulum.

Lysosome
Contains digestive enzymes that break up proteins, lipids, and nucleic acids. They also remove and recycle waste products.

Cell membrane
Golgi apparatus
Smooth endoplasmic reticulum
Rough endoplasmic reticulum
Lysosome
Cytoplasm
Nucleus
Mitochondrion

Cytoplasm
The cytoplasm is the gel-like substance inside cells. Cytoplasm contains cell organelles, protein, electrolytes, and other molecules.

Nucleus
The nucleus contains the DNA in the cell. Molecules of DNA provide coded instructions used for protein synthesis.

Mitochondrion
Organelles that produce most of the energy (ATP) used by cells.

Figure 1.1 Typical animal cell.
Source: Beerman/McGuire, Nutritional Sciences, 1/e. © Cengage Learning.

COMPONENTS OF TYPICAL CELLS

Plasma Membrane

The plasma membrane is the membrane that encapsulates and surrounds the cell, allowing it to become a distinct unit. The plasma membrane, like other membranes found within the cell, has distinct functions and structural characteristics. Nevertheless, all membranes share some common attributes:

• Membranes are sheet-like structures composed primarily of phospholipids and proteins held together by noncovalent interactions.

• Membrane phospholipids have both a hydrophobic and a hydrophilic moiety. This structural property of phospholipids allows them to spontaneously form bimolecular sheets in water, called lipid bilayers. Figure 1.2 depicts the cellular membrane as it would surround a cell. Figure 1.3 shows a close-up of the cell membrane that illustrates several of its functions. Note the phospholipid bilayer and the proteins in the cell membrane, and the intracellular space inside the cell and extracellular space outside the cell. The core of the bilayer is hydrophobic, which inhibits many water-soluble compounds from passing into and out of the cell. The

integral transport protein shown in Figure 1.3 is part of a transport system that enables essential water-soluble substances to cross the plasma membrane. The hydrophobic core of the bilayer also helps to retain essential water-soluble substances within the cell.

• Phosphoglycerides and phosphingolipids (phosphate-containing sphingolipids) comprise most of the membrane phospholipids. Chemical structures and properties of the phospholipids in the cellular membrane are described more fully in Chapter 5. Of the phosphoglycerides, phosphatidylcholine and phosphatidylethanolamine are particularly abundant in humans and higher animals. Another important membrane lipid is cholesterol, which is found in the hydrophobic portion of the bilayer in amounts that vary considerably from membrane to membrane. Membranes with higher levels of cholesterol are less fluid.

• Membrane proteins give biological membranes their functions: They serve as pumps, gates, receptors, energy transducers, and enzymes. These functions are represented in Figure 1.3. Many of these proteins have either lipid or carbohydrate attachments.

• Membranes are asymmetrical. The inside and outside faces of the membrane are different.

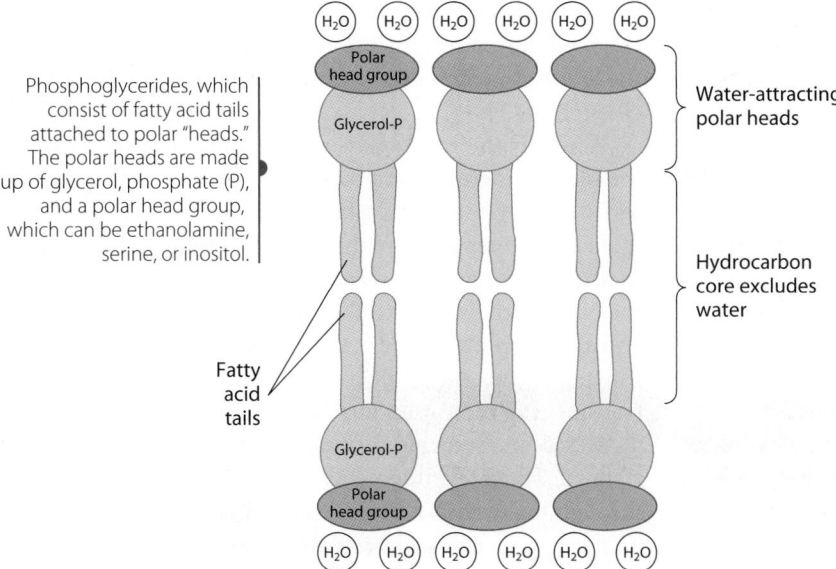

Phosphoglycerides, which consist of fatty acid tails attached to polar "heads." The polar heads are made up of glycerol, phosphate (P), and a polar head group, which can be ethanolamine, serine, or inositol.

Figure 1.2 Lipid bilayer structure of biological membranes.

- Membranes are not static but are fluid structures. The lipid and protein molecules within them move laterally with ease and rapidity.

Membranes are not structurally distinct from the aqueous compartments of the cell they surround. For example, the **cytosol** (or **cytoplasm**), which is a gel-like, aqueous, transparent substance that fills the cell, connects the various membranes of the cell. This interconnection creates a structure that makes it possible for a signal generated at one part of the cell to be transmitted quickly and efficiently to other regions of the cell.

The plasma membrane protects the cellular components while at the same time allowing them sufficient exposure

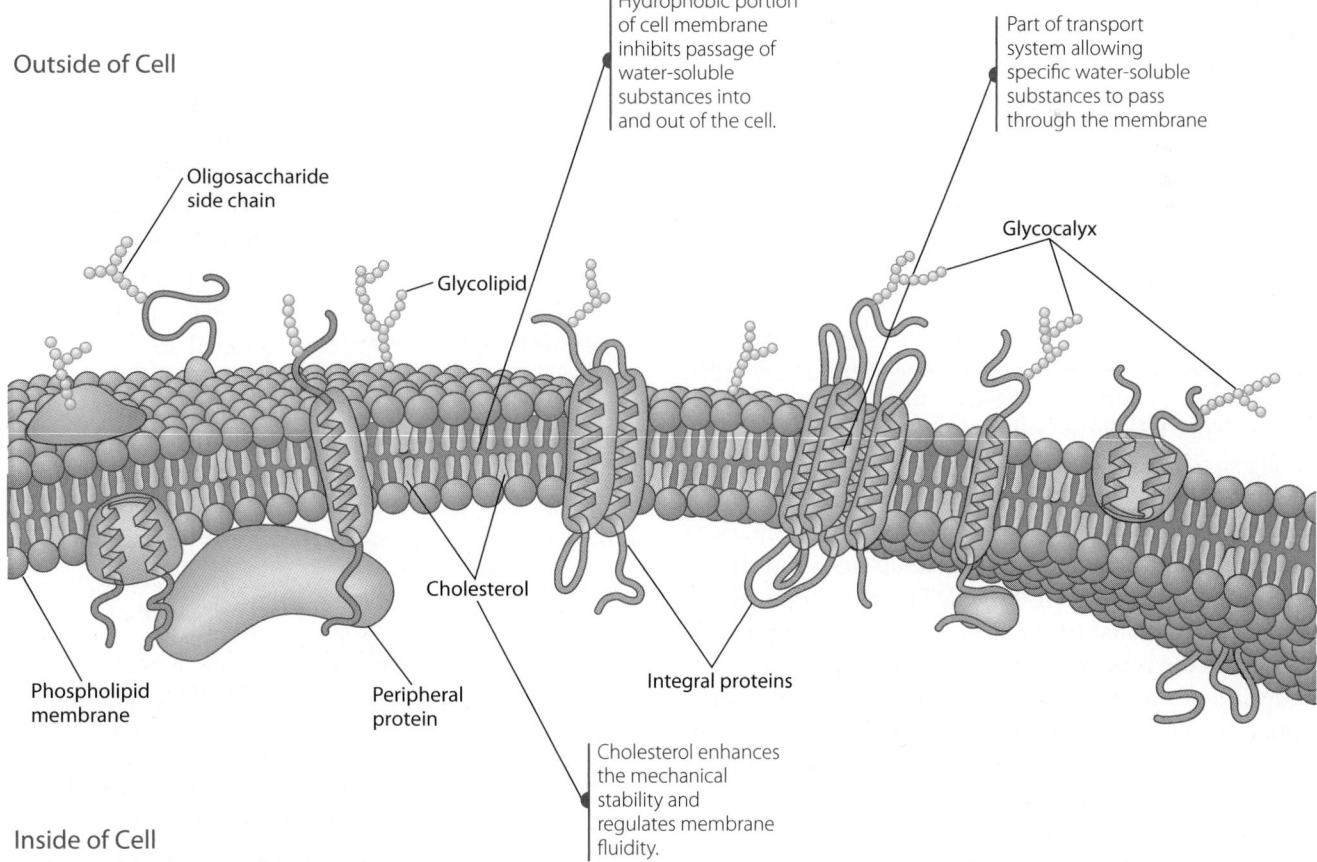

Figure 1.3 Fluid model of cell membrane. Lipids and proteins are mobile. They can move laterally in the membrane.

to their environment for stimulation, nourishment, and removal of wastes. Plasma membranes are chemically distinct from other membranes. Plasma membranes have:

- Greater carbohydrate content, due to the presence of glycolipids and glycoproteins. Some carbohydrate is found in all membranes, but most of the glycolipids and glycoproteins of the cell are associated with the plasma membrane.
- Greater cholesterol content. Cholesterol enhances the mechanical stability of the membrane and regulates its fluidity.

Figure 1.3 illustrates the position of a cholesterol molecule between two phospholipid molecules. The hydrocarbon side chain of the cholesterol molecule associates with the hydrocarbon fatty acid tails of the phospholipids, creating a hydrophobic region. The hydroxyl groups of the cholesterol are positioned close to the polar head groups of the phospholipid molecules, resulting in a more hydrophilic region [1,2]. This layering of polar and nonpolar regions has led to the concept of the lipid bilayer to describe the plasma membrane structure. The cholesterol's rigid planar steroid rings are positioned so as to interact with and stabilize those regions of the hydrocarbon chains closest to the polar head groups. The rest of the hydrocarbon chain remains flexible and fluid. Cholesterol, by regulating fluidity of the membrane, regulates membrane permeability, thereby exercising some control over what may pass into and out of the cell. The fluidity of the membrane also appears to affect the structure and function of the proteins embedded in the lipid membrane.

The carbohydrate moiety of the glycoproteins and the glycolipids in membranes helps maintain the asymmetry of the membrane because the oligosaccharide side chains are located exclusively on the membrane layer facing away from the cytoplasmic matrix. In plasma membranes, therefore, the sugar residues are all exposed to the outside of the cell, forming what is called the **glycocalyx,** the layer of carbohydrate on the cell's outer surface. On the membranes of the organelles, however, the oligosaccharides are directed inward, into the lumen of the membrane-bound compartment. Figure 1.3 illustrates the glycocalyx and the location of oligosaccharide side chains in the plasma membrane.

Although the exact function of the sugar residues is unknown, they are believed to act as specificity markers for the cell and as "antennae" to pick up signals for transmission of substances in the cell. The membrane glycoproteins are crucial to the life of the cell, very possibly serving as the receptors for hormones, certain nutrients, and various other substances that influence cellular function. Glycoproteins also may help regulate the intracellular communication necessary for cell growth and tissue formation. Intracellular communication occurs through pathways that convert information from one part of a cell to another in response to external stimuli. Generally, it involves the passage of chemical messengers from organelle

to organelle or within the lipid bilayers of membranes. Intracellular communication is examined more closely in the "Receptors and Intracellular Signaling" section of this chapter.

Whereas the lipid bilayer determines the structure of the plasma membrane, proteins are primarily responsible for the many membrane functions. The membrane proteins are interspersed within the lipid bilayer, where they mediate information transfer (as receptors), transport ions and molecules (as channels, carriers, and pumps), and speed up metabolic activities (as enzymes). Figure 1.3 illustrates the integral proteins, which are involved in transporting molecules into and out of the cell.

Membrane proteins are classified as either integral or peripheral. The integral proteins are attached to the membrane through hydrophobic interactions and are embedded in the membrane. Peripheral proteins, in contrast, are associated with membranes through ionic interactions and are located on or near the membrane surface (Figure 1.3). Peripheral proteins are believed to be attached to integral membrane proteins either directly or through intermediate proteins [1,2].

Most receptor and carrier proteins are integral proteins, whereas the glycoproteins of the cell recognition complex are peripheral proteins [1]. Functions of membrane proteins, as well as functions of proteins located intracellularly, are described later in this chapter.

Cytoplasmic Matrix

Modern techniques have greatly increased our knowledge of the structure, function, and molecular makeup of the cytoplasmic matrix, a structure within the cytosol that makes up the cytoskeleton, which offers support for other organelles. The advent of the electron microscope provided static images of the cytoskeleton of eukaryotic cells. More recent techniques have provided considerable information about the dynamics and molecular structure of the cytoskeleton in living cells.

The cytoskeleton is made up of three distinct, well-defined components: **microtubules, microfilaments,** and **intermediate filaments** (Figure 1.4). Cells are in continuous motion, and the components of the cytoplasmic skeleton are dynamic and capable of reorganization as the needs of the cell change. The cytoskeleton provides cells with:

- structural support, which defines the cell's shape
- a framework for positioning of the various organelles (such as microvilli, which are extensions of intestinal cells)
- a network to direct the movement of materials and organelles within the cells
- a means of independent locomotion for specialized cells (such as sperm, white blood cells, and fibroblasts)

Recent research [3] suggests the cytoskeleton might even be an important pathway for intercellular communication

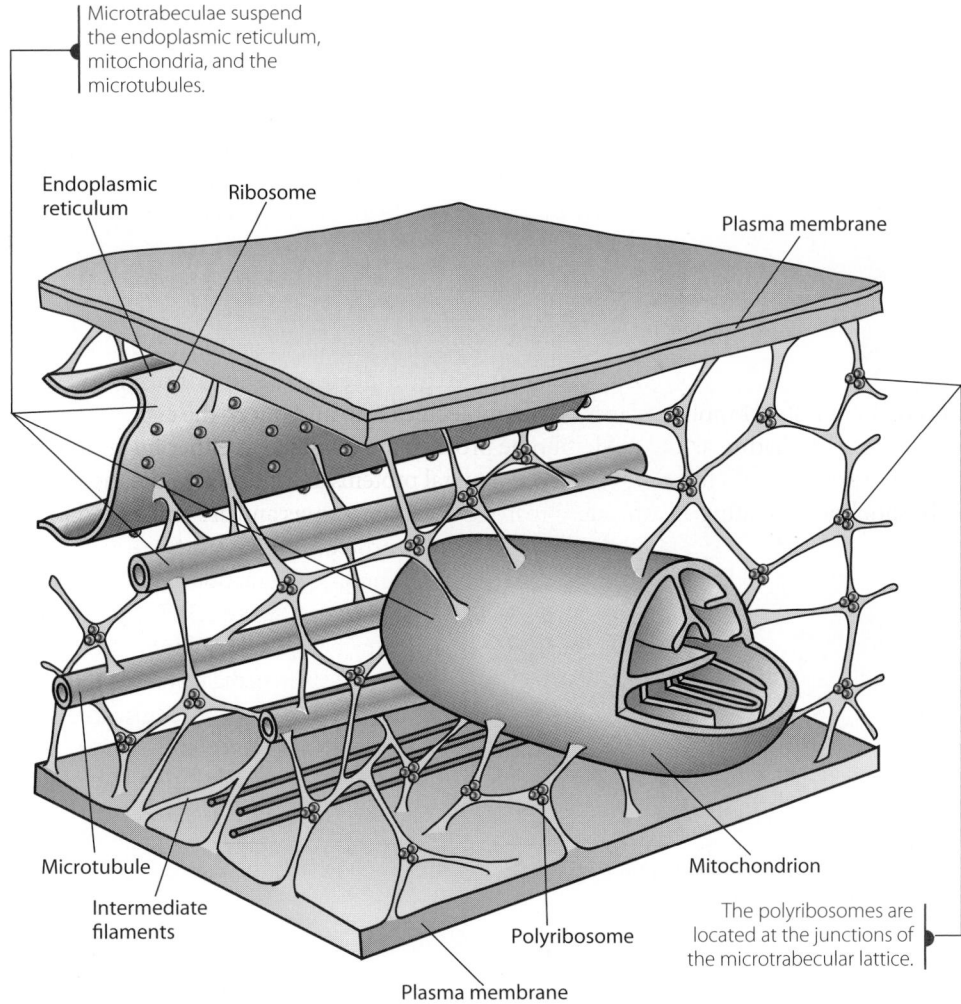

Microtrabeculae suspend the endoplasmic reticulum, mitochondria, and the microtubules.

Endoplasmic reticulum

Ribosome

Plasma membrane

Microtubule

Intermediate filaments

Polyribosome

Mitochondrion

The polyribosomes are located at the junctions of the microtrabecular lattice.

Plasma membrane

Figure 1.4 The cytokeleton (microtrabecular lattice) provides a structure for cell organelles, microvillae (as found in intestinal mucosa cells), and large molecules. The cytoplast is shown at about 300,000 times its actual size and was derived from hundreds of images of cultured cells viewed in a high-voltage electron microscope.
Source: Adapted from Porter and Tucker, "The Ground Substance of the Cell," 1981, 'Scientific American.' Used by permission of Nelson Prentiss.

and the transfer of RNA and DNA. If this suggestion is verified, it will have a major impact on how diseases are treated.

Microtubules

Microtubules, which occur in nearly every eukaryotic cell, are hollow, relatively rigid tubular structures. Flagella, cilia, and dividing cells are all dependent upon microtubules. They are made up of two types of globular tubulin subunits, which are organized linearly. Microtubules are rigid enough to provide mechanical support for the cell and help determine its shape. The internal organization of cells is also influenced by their microtubules.

Microfilaments

Microfilaments are made up of globular subunits of the protein actin, which form a flexible, helical filament in the presence of adenosine triphosphate (ATP). Depending on the type of cell and its function, microfilaments can be organized into highly ordered arrays; loose, ill-defined networks; or tightly anchored bundles. The subunits of actin have an electrical charge. The polymer of the actin subunits has a different charge than the subunits and therefore a different structure and function at each end.

Monomers are continually added at one end and removed at the other to form a steady state. Based on conditions within the cell, the microfilaments can be either "assembled" or "disassembled." This reorganization is required for cell locomotion, changes in cell shape, phagocytosis, and other dynamic processes.

Intermediate Filaments

Intermediate filaments (IFs) are unbranched and found only in animal cells. Intermediate filaments provide mechanical strength to cells that are subjected to physical stress such as neurons, muscle cells, and epithelial cells that line body cavities. IFs form filaments similar to those of microtubules and microfilaments, but IFs are chemically different in that they are not made up of a single protein. Instead they are chemically a heterogeneous group of structures. IFs are also dynamic and undergo constant assembly and disassembly controlled by phosphorylation or dephosphorylation.

The fluid portion of the cytoplasmic matrix not associated with the microtubules contains small molecules such as glucose, amino acids, oxygen, and carbon dioxide. This arrangement of the polymeric and fluid portions apparently gives the cytosol its gel-like consistency.

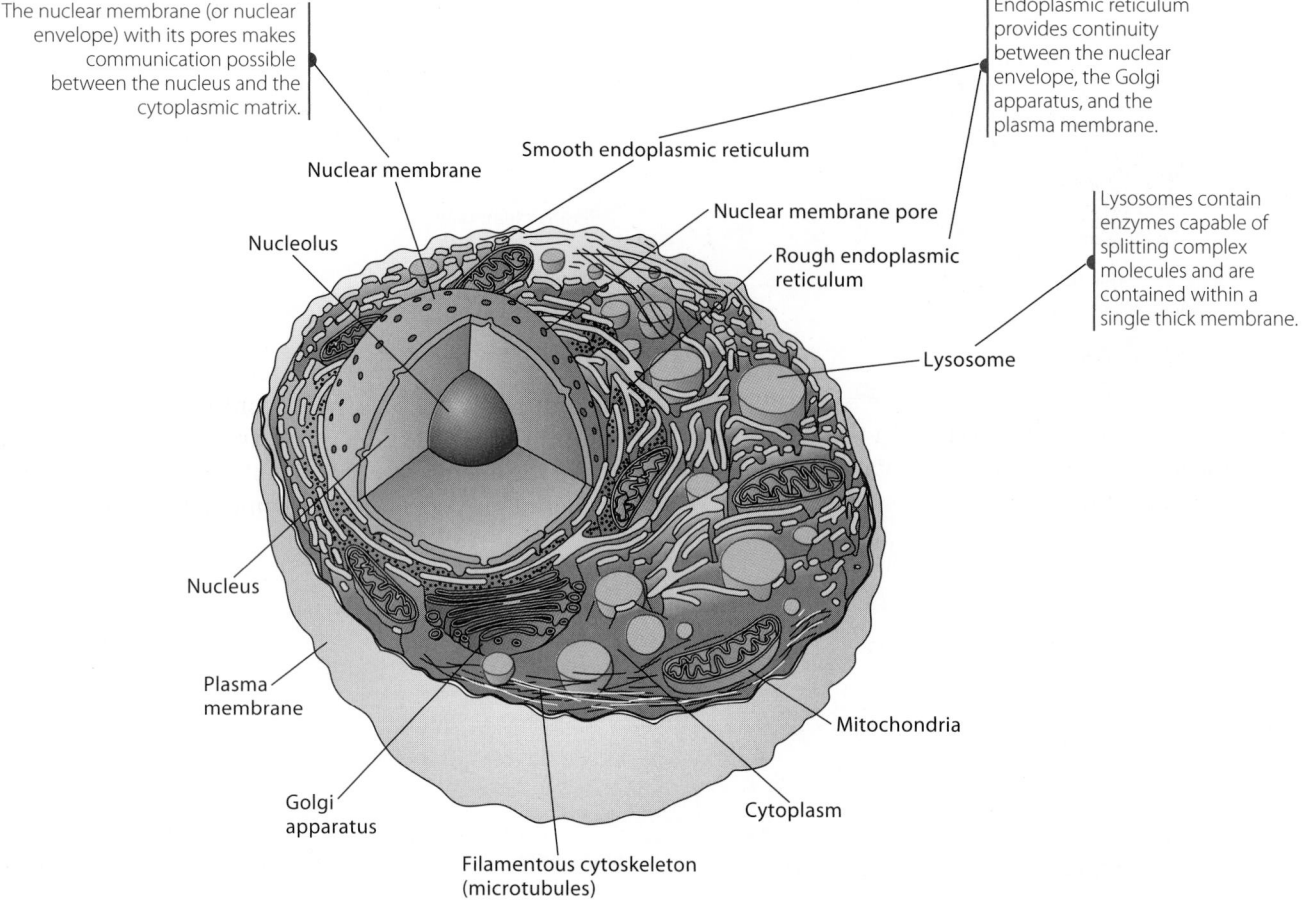

The nuclear membrane (or nuclear envelope) with its pores makes communication possible between the nucleus and the cytoplasmic matrix.

Endoplasmic reticulum provides continuity between the nuclear envelope, the Golgi apparatus, and the plasma membrane.

Lysosomes contain enzymes capable of splitting complex molecules and are contained within a single thick membrane.

Nuclear membrane

Smooth endoplasmic reticulum

Nuclear membrane pore

Nucleolus

Rough endoplasmic reticulum

Lysosome

Nucleus

Plasma membrane

Mitochondria

Golgi apparatus

Cytoplasm

Filamentous cytoskeleton (microtubules)

Figure 1.5 Three-dimensional depiction of a typical mammalian liver cell.

Figure 1.5 summarizes the structures of a cell in a three-dimensional model. Because the aqueous part of the cell contacts with the cytoskeleton over a very broad surface area, enzymes that are associated with the polymeric lattice are brought into close proximity to their substrate molecules in the aqueous portion, thereby facilitating reactions (see the "Catalytic Proteins (Enzymes)" section of this chapter). Furthermore, if enzymes that catalyze the reactions of a metabolic pathway are oriented sequentially, so that the product of one reaction is released in close proximity to the next enzyme for which it is a substrate, the velocity of the overall pathway will be greatly enhanced. Evidence indicates that such an arrangement does in fact exist among the enzymes that participate in glycolysis.

Possibly all metabolic pathways occurring in the cytoplasmic matrix are influenced by its structural arrangement. The separation or association of metabolic pathways (or both) is important in regulating metabolism. This topic is covered more fully in Chapter 7. Metabolic pathways of particular significance that occur in the cytoplasmic matrix and that might be affected by its structure include:

- glycolysis
- hexose monophosphate shunt (pentose phosphate pathway)
- glycogenesis and glycogenolysis
- fatty acid synthesis, including the production of nonessential, unsaturated fatty acids

Normal intracellular communication among all cellular components is vital for cell activation and survival. The importance of the microtubular network is evidenced by its function to support and interconnect cellular components. The network also helps components communicate.

The cytoplasmic matrix of eukaryotic cells contains a number of organelles, enclosed in bilayer membranes. Each of these components is described briefly in the following sections. Figures 1.1 and 1.5 show these organelles. (For more detailed information about the structure and function of the cell matrix, consult a textbook in cell biology such as [4].)

Mitochondrion

The **mitochondria** are the primary sites of oxygen use in the cell and are responsible for most of the metabolic energy (adenosine triphosphate, or ATP) produced in cells. The size and shape of the mitochondria in different tissues vary according to the function of the tissue. In muscle tissue, for example, the mitochondria are held tightly among

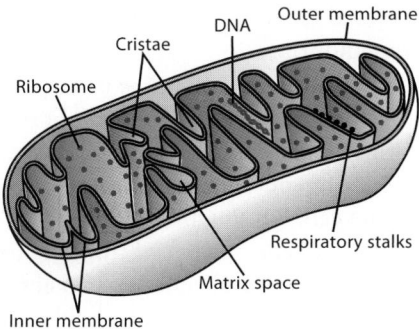

Figure 1.6 The mitochondrion.

the fibers of the contractile system. In the liver, however, the mitochondria have fewer restraints, appear spherical, and move freely through the cytoplasmic matrix.

Mitochondrial Membrane

The mitochondrion consists of a matrix or interior space surrounded by a double membrane (Figures 1.6 and 1.7). The mitochondrial outer membrane is relatively porous, whereas the inner membrane is selectively permeable, serving as a barrier between the cytoplasmic matrix and the mitochondrial matrix. The inner membrane has many invaginations, called the cristae, which increase its surface area, and all the components of the electron transport chain are embedded within it.

The electron transport (respiratory) chain is central to the process of **oxidative phosphorylation,** the mechanism by which most cellular ATP is produced. The components of the electron transport chain carry electrons and hydrogens during catalytic oxidation of nutrient molecules by enzymes in the mitochondrial matrix. The details of this process are described more fully in Chapter 3. Briefly, the mitochondria carry out the flow of electrons through the electron transport chain. This electron flow is strongly exothermic, and the energy released is used in part for ATP synthesis, an endothermic process. Molecular oxygen is ultimately, but indirectly, the oxidizing agent in these reactions. The function of the **electron transport chain** is to couple the energy released by nutrient oxidation to the formation of ATP. The chain components are precisely positioned within the inner mitochondrial membrane, an important feature of the mitochondria, because it brings the oxidizable products released in the matrix into close proximity with molecular oxygen. Figure 1.7 shows the flow of major reactants into and out of the mitochondrion.

Mitochondrial Matrix

Among the metabolic enzyme systems functioning in the mitochondrial matrix are those that catalyze the reactions of the tricarboxylic cycle (TCA cycle; Chapter 3) and fatty

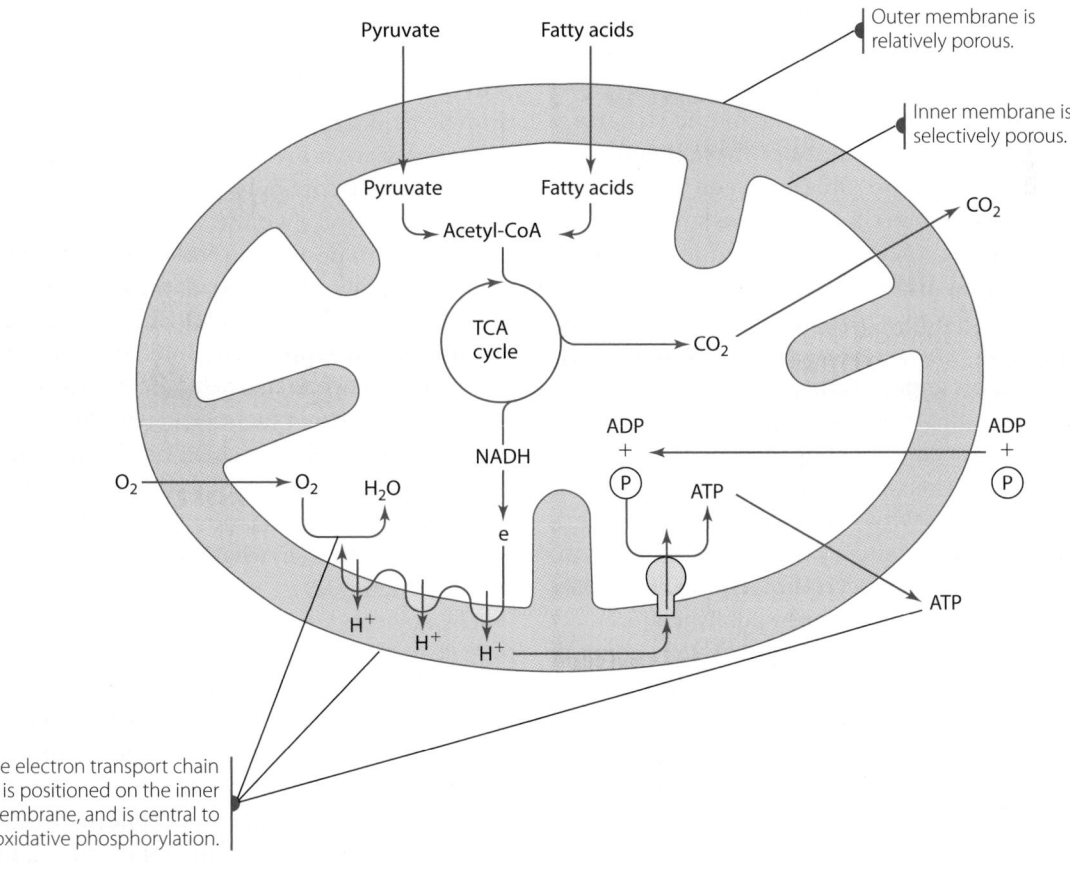

Figure 1.7 Overview of a cross section of the mitochondria.

acid oxidation (Chapter 5).Other enzymes are involved in the oxidative decarboxylation and carboxylation of pyruvate (Chapter 3) and in certain reactions of amino acid metabolism (Chapter 6).

Mitochondria are capable of both fission and fusion, depending upon the needs of the cell. They reproduce by dividing in two. Although the nucleus contains most of the cell's deoxyribonucleic acid (DNA), the mitochondrial matrix contains a small amount of DNA and a few ribosomes, so limited protein synthesis occurs within the mitochondrion. The genes contained in mitochondrial DNA, unlike those in the nucleus, are inherited only from the mother [5]. The primary function of mitochondrial genes is to code for proteins vital to producing ATP [2]. Most of the enzymes operating in the mitochondrion, however, are coded by nuclear DNA and synthesized on the rough endoplasmic reticulum (RER) in the cytosol. The enzymes are then incorporated into existing mitochondria.

All cells in the body, with the exception of the erythrocyte, possess mitochondria. The erythrocyte disposes of its mitochondria and nucleus during the maturation process and then must depend solely on the energy produced through anaerobic mechanisms, primarily glycolysis.

Nucleus

The nucleus is the largest of the organelles within the cell.Because of its DNA content, the nucleus initiates and regulates most cellular activities. Surrounding the nucleus is the **nuclear envelope.** The nuclear envelope is composed of two bilayer membranes (an inner and an outer membrane) that are dynamic structures (Figure 1.5). The dynamic nature of these membranes makes communication possible between the nucleus and the cytoplasmic matrix and allows a continuous channel between the nucleus and the endoplasmic reticulum. At various intervals the two membranes of the nuclear envelope fuse, creating pores in the envelope (Figure 1.5). The nucleus and the microtubules of the cytoskeleton appear to be interdependent. The polymerization and the intracellular distribution of the microtubules are controlled by nucleus-based activities. Clusters of proteins on the outer nuclear membrane are centers of these activities. These clusters, called microtubule organization centers (MTOCs), begin polymerizing and organizing the microtubules during mitosis. A review of MTOC activity has been published [6,7].

The matrix held within the nuclear envelope contains molecules of DNA that encode the cell's genetic information plus all the enzymes needed for its duplication. The nuclear matrix also contains the minerals necessary for the activity of the nucleus. Condensed regions of the chromatin within the nuclear envelope, called **nucleoli,** contain not only DNA and its associated alkaline proteins (histones) but also considerable amounts of RNA (ribonucleic acid). This particular RNA is believed to give rise

to the microsomal RNA (i.e., RNA associated with the endoplasmic reticulum).

Encoded within the nuclear DNA of the cell are thousands of genes that direct the synthesis of proteins. Each gene codes for a single specific protein. The cell **genome** is the entire set of genetic information, that is, all of the DNA within the cell. Barring mutations that may arise in the DNA, daughter cells, produced from a parent cell by mitosis, possess the identical genomic makeup of the parent. The process of DNA replication enables the DNA to be precisely copied at the time of mitosis.

After the cell receives a signal that protein synthesis is needed, protein biosynthesis occurs in phases called transcription, translation, and elongation (Figure 1.8). Each phase requires DNA activity, RNA activity, or both. These phases, together with replication, are reviewed briefly in this chapter, but the scope of this subject is large; interested readers should consult a current cell biology text or comprehensive biochemistry text for a more thorough treatment of protein biosynthesis [4,8].

Nucleic Acids

Nucleic acids (DNA and RNA) are macromolecules formed from repeating units called **nucleotides,** sometimes referred to as nucleotide bases or just bases. Structurally, they consist of a nitrogenous core (either purine or pyrimidine), a pentose sugar (ribose in RNA, deoxyribose in DNA), and phosphate. Five different nucleotides are contained in the structures of nucleic acids: Adenylic acid and guanylic acid are purines, and cytidylic acid, uridylic acid, and thymidylic acid are pyrimidines. The nucleotides are more commonly referred to by their nitrogenous base core only—namely, adenine, guanine, cytosine, uracil, and thymine, respectively. For convenience, particularly in describing the sequence of the polymeric nucleotides in a nucleic acid, the single-letter abbreviations are most often used. Adenine (A), guanine (G), and cytosine (C) are common to both DNA and RNA, whereas uracil (U) is unique to RNA, and thymine (T) is found only in DNA. When two strands of nucleic acids interact with each other, as occurs in replication, transcription, and translation, bases in one strand pair specifically with bases in the second strand: A always pairs with T or U, and G pairs with C, in what is called **complementary base pairing** (Figure 1.9).

The nucleotides are connected by phosphates esterified to hydroxyl groups on the pentose—that is, deoxyribose or ribose—component of the nucleotide. The carbon atoms of the pentoses are assigned prime (′) numbers for identification. The phosphate group connects the 3′ carbon of one nucleotide with the 5′ carbon of the next nucleotide in the sequence. The 3′ carbon of the latter nucleotide in turn is connected to the 5′ carbon of the next nucleotide in the sequence, and so on. Therefore, nucleotides are attached to each other by 3′, 5′ diester bonds. The ends of a nucleic acid

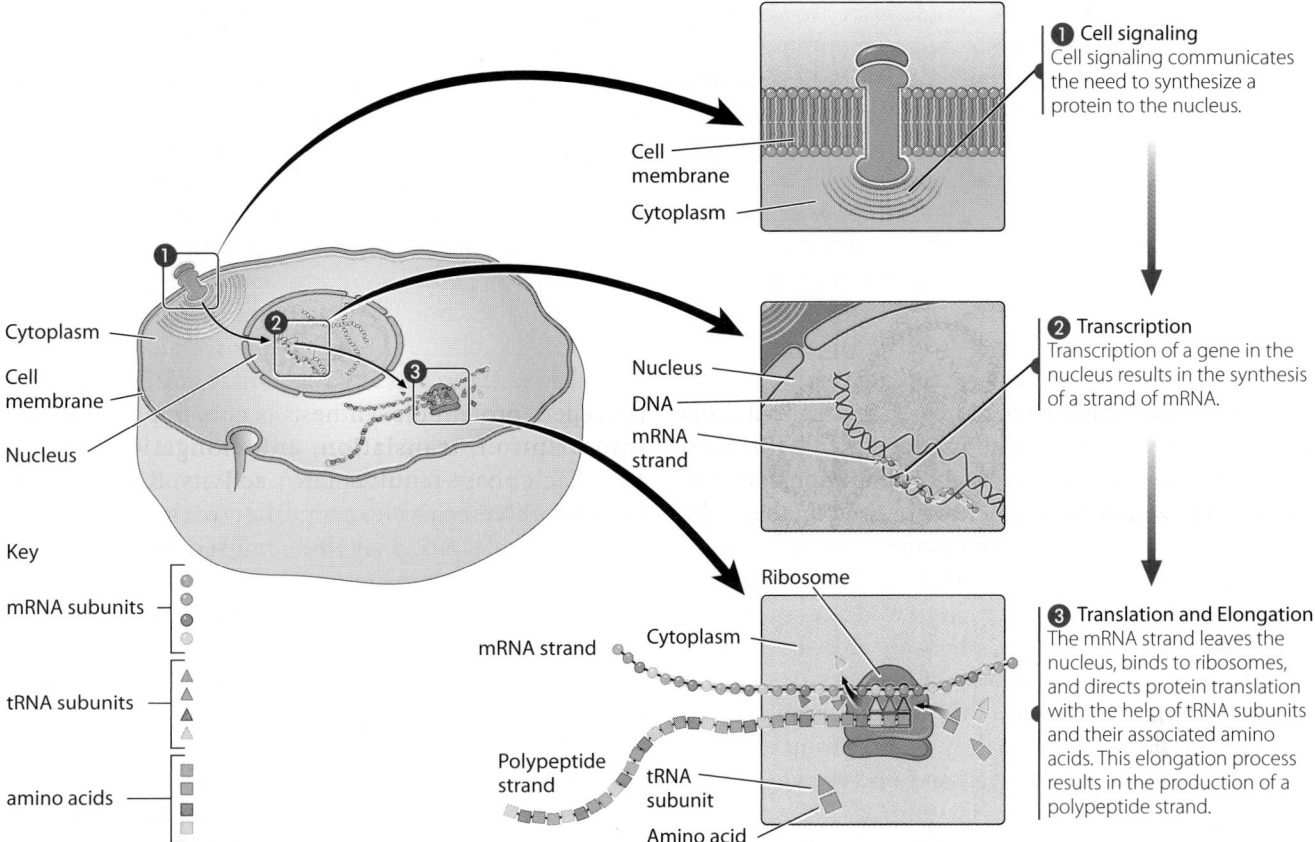

1 Cell signaling
Cell signaling communicates the need to synthesize a protein to the nucleus.

2 Transcription
Transcription of a gene in the nucleus results in the synthesis of a strand of mRNA.

3 Translation and Elongation
The mRNA strand leaves the nucleus, binds to ribosomes, and directs protein translation with the help of tRNA subunits and their associated amino acids. This elongation process results in the production of a polypeptide strand.

Cell membrane
Cytoplasm

Nucleus
DNA
mRNA strand

Ribosome
Cytoplasm
mRNA strand
Polypeptide strand
tRNA subunit
Amino acid

Cytoplasm
Cell membrane
Nucleus

Key
mRNA subunits
tRNA subunits
amino acids

Figure 1.8 Steps of protein synthesis. 1. Signals that protein synthesis needs to occur. 2. Transcription: The DNA molecule (gene) synthesizes the corresponding mRNA. 3. Translation: The corresponding mRNA molecule binds to a ribosome and directs protein synthesis based on the codon for each amino acid and the appropriate tRNA.

Source: Beerman/McGuire, Nutritional Sciences, 1/e. © Cengage Learning.

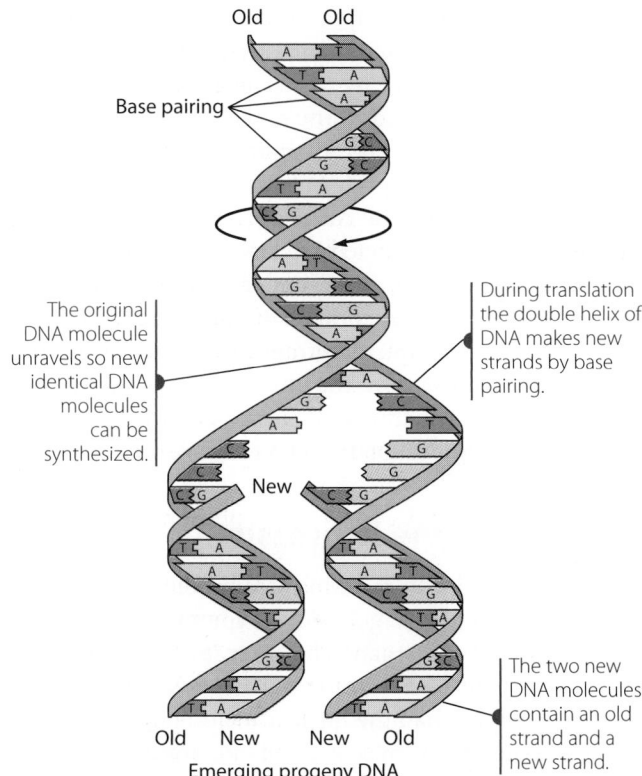

Old   Old

Base pairing

The original DNA molecule unravels so new identical DNA molecules can be synthesized.

During translation the double helix of DNA makes new strands by base pairing.

New

The two new DNA molecules contain an old strand and a new strand.

Old   New   New   Old
Emerging progeny DNA

Figure 1.9 DNA replication.

chain are called either the free 3′ end or the free 5′ end, meaning that the hydroxyl groups at those positions are not attached by phosphate to another nucleotide.

Cell Replication

Cell replication involves the synthesis of daughter DNA molecules that are identical to the parental DNA. At cell division, the cell must copy its genome with a high degree of fidelity. Each strand of the DNA molecule acts as a template for synthesizing a new strand. Figures 1.8 and 1.9 illustrate replication by base pairing and show the formation of the two new strands. The DNA molecule consists of two large strands of nucleic acid that are intertwined to form a double helix. During cell division the two unravel, with each forming a template for synthesizing a new strand through complementary base pairing. Incoming nucleotide bases first pair with their complementary bases in the template and then are connected through phosphate diester bonds by the enzyme DNA polymerase. The end result of the **replication** process is two new DNA chains that join with the two chains from the parent molecule to produce two new DNA molecules. Each new DNA molecule is therefore identical in base sequence to the parent, and each new cell of a tissue consequently carries within its nucleus identical information to direct its functioning.

The two strands in the DNA double helix are antiparallel, which means that the free 5′ end of one strand is connected to the free 3′ end of the other. With this process, a cell is able to copy or replicate its genes before it passes them on to the daughter cell. Although errors sometimes occur during replication, mechanisms exist that correct or repair mismatched or damaged DNA. Refer to a biochemistry text [8] for details.

Transcription

Transcription is the process by which the genetic information (through the sequence of base pairs) in a single strand of DNA makes a specific sequence of bases in a messenger RNA(mRNA) chain (Figure 1.8). A single strand of DNA can make many copies of the corresponding mRNA, which become multiple templates for the assembly of a specific protein molecule. This process multiplies the information contained in the DNA to produce many corresponding protein molecules. Transcription requires **transcription factors,** which are proteins involved in each aspect of the transcription process.

Transcription proceeds continuously throughout the entire life cycle of the cell. In the process, various sections of the DNA molecule unravel, and one strand—called the **sense strand**—serves as the template for synthesizing mRNA. The genetic code (gene) of the DNA is transcribed into mRNA through complementary base pairing, as in DNA replication, except that the purine adenine (A) pairs with the pyrimidine uracil (U) instead of with thymine (T). **Genes** are composed of critically sequenced base pairs along the entire length of the DNA strand that is being transcribed. A gene, on average, is just over 1,000 base pairs in length, compared with the nearly 5 million (5×10^6) base pair length of typical chromosomal DNA chains. Although these figures provide a rough estimate of the number of genes per transcribed DNA chain, not all the base pairs of a gene are transcribed into functional mRNA.

Many genes for specific proteins are located on regions of the DNA nucleotide sequences that are not adjacent to each other. Those regions that are part of the gene but do not code for a protein product are called **introns** (intervening sequences).They have to be removed from the mRNA before it is translated into protein (see the "Translation" section of this chapter). Enzymes excise the introns from the newly formed mRNA, and the ends of the functional, active mRNA segments are spliced together in a process called posttranscriptional processing. The gene segments that get both transcribed and translated into the protein product, called **exons** (expressed sequences), require no posttranscriptional processing.

Translation

Translation is the process by which genetic information in an mRNA molecule specifies the sequence of amino acids in the protein product. After the mRNA is synthesized in the nucleus (Figure 1.8), the mRNA is exported into the cytoplasmic matrix, where it is attached to ribosomal RNA (rRNA) of the ribosomes of the rough endoplasmic reticulum (RER) or to the freestanding polyribosomes (or polysomes; Figure 1.4). On the ribosomes, the transcribed genetic code is used to bring amino acids into a specific sequence that produces a protein with a clearly delineated function.

The genetic code for specifying the amino acid sequence of a protein resides in the mRNA in the form of three-base sequences called **codons.** Each codon codes for a single amino acid. Although a given amino acid may have several codons (e.g., the codons CUU, CUC, CUA, and CUG all code for the amino acid leucine), codons can code for only one amino acid. Each amino acid has one or more transfer RNAs (tRNAs), which deliver the amino acid to the mRNA for peptide synthesis. The three-base sequences of the tRNA attach to the codons by complementary base pairing.

Amino acids are first activated by ATP at their carboxyl end and then transferred to their specific tRNAs that bear the anticodon complementary to each amino acid's codon. For example, because codons that code for leucine are sequenced CUU, CUC, CUA, or CUG, the only tRNAs to which an activated leucine can be attached would need to have the anticodon sequence GAA, GAG, GAU, or GAC. The tRNAs then bring the amino acids to the mRNA situated at the protein synthesis site on the ribosomes. After the amino acids are positioned according to codon-anticodon association, peptide bonds are formed between the aligned amino acids in a process called **elongation** (Figure 1.8). Elongation extends the polypeptide chain of the protein product by translation. Each incoming amino acid is connected to the end of the growing peptide chain with a free carboxyl group (C-terminal end) by formation of further peptide bonds. New amino acids are incorporated until all the codons (corresponding to one completed protein or polypeptide chain) of the mRNA have been translated. At this point, the process stops abruptly, signaled by a "nonsense" codon that does not code for any amino acid. The completed protein dissociates from the mRNA. After translation, the newly synthesized protein may require some chemical, structural, or spatial (three-dimensional) modification to attain its active form.

Control of Gene Expression

Each cell in the body contains a complete set of genes. Only a portion of the genes are expressed in specialized cells of a given organ. This concept has been demonstrated by the cloning of sheep from an unfertilized sheep egg cell that had the nuclear material removed and a cell from the sheep's mammary gland. The regulation of gene expression occurs primarily at three different levels.

(1) Transcription-level control mechanisms determine if a particular gene can be transcribed. Transcriptional control is accomplished by large numbers of proteins (called transcriptional factors) that can bind to the DNA at a site other than the one involved in serving as a template for the mRNA. These transcriptional factors can enhance, inhibit, or, in some cases, alter the frequency (number of times transcription occurs within a specified time span) of the gene's transcription. Several hormones such as insulin, thyroid hormone, glucagon, and glucocorticoids and other compounds can alter the transcription of DNA by binding with receptors in the nucleus [4,9,10]. (2) Processing-level control mechanisms determine the path by which mRNA can be translated into a polypeptide. This mechanism of regulating gene expression is based upon the splicing of RNA molecules, thus making it possible for one gene to code for two associated proteins. (3) Translation-level control mechanisms determine whether a particular mRNA is actually translated and, if so, how often and for how long. Translation-level control mechanisms generally operate through interactions between specific mRNAs and various small RNA strands present within the cytosol. The translation-level control mechanism can involve the localization of the mRNA in a particular part of the cell or organ. The control of gene expression is vastly more complex than has been stated here. For more detailed information on the subject refer to a recent textbook on molecular biology and biochemistry or cell biology [4,8].

Experimental Tools: Blotting

Sophisticated methods have been used to study DNA transcription, translation, and protein synthesis. One such technique introduced in the mid-1970s was used for identifying specific DNA sequences and is called Southern blotting after the researcher who developed it. The DNA is denatured, which breaks it into many smaller fragments with differing numbers of base pairs. This mixture is then placed on a gel electrophoretic plate to separate the DNA fragments based on size. The original technique used polyacrylamide gels, which can separate fragments that have between 25 and 2,000 base pairs. For larger fragments with more base pairs, Agarose is used. The rate of a fragment's movement in the gel is based upon its molecular weight; thus, fragments with fewer base pairs move faster than those with a larger number. After the electrophoretic separation the fragments are transferred to a filter (either nitrocellulose or nylon) by passing a salt solution through the gel and converted to single-stranded DNA (by treatment with NaOH). The filter is then dried, which tightly fixes the DNA to the filter (blotting), and then incubated with a "probe." For Southern blotting, the probe is a purified single-stranded DNA that has been labeled with either a radioactive tracer (such as ^{32}P) or a fluorescent marker so that it can be identified. The corresponding base pairs in the probe will hybridize with the separated single-stranded DNA. For a radioactive marker the filter is placed on X-ray film; after it is developed, the separated DNA shows up as a black band. The fluorescent probe is identified by the emitted light.

The Southern blotting technique has been extended for both specific RNA sequences and proteins. If a specific RNA is separated and a hybridizing probe is used, the technique is called Northern blotting. Specific proteins can be separated by a similar electrophoretic technique and transferred to a filter. The probe in this case is specific, labeled antibodies that will identify the protein of interest. This technique is called Western blotting [8].

Endoplasmic Reticulum and Golgi Apparatus

The **endoplasmic reticulum (ER)** is a network of membranous channels pervading the cytosol and providing continuity among the nuclear envelope, the Golgi apparatus, and the plasma membrane. This structure, therefore, is a mechanism for communication from the innermost part of the cell to its exterior (Figures 1.1 and 1.5). The channel between the two membranes of the ER is different than the cytosol and is isolated from it.

The ER cannot be separated from the cell as an isolated entity in the laboratory. During mechanical homogenization, the structure of the ER is disrupted and reforms into small spherical particles called microsomes. The ER is classified as either rough (granular) or smooth (agranular). The granularity or lack of granularity is determined by the presence or absence of ribosomes. Rough endoplasmic reticulum (RER), so named because it is studded with ribosomes, abounds in cells where protein synthesis is a primary function. Smooth endoplasmic reticulum (SER) is found in most cells; however, because it is the site of synthesis for a variety of lipids, it is more abundant in cells that synthesize steroid hormones (e.g., within the adrenal cortex and gonads) and in liver cells, which synthesize fat transport molecules (the lipoproteins). In skeletal muscle, the smooth endoplasmic reticulum is called **sarcoplasmic reticulum** and is the site of the calcium ion pump, a necessity for the contractile process.

Ribosomes associated with RER are composed of ribosomal RNA (rRNA) and structural protein. All proteins to be secreted (or excreted) from the cell or destined to be incorporated into an organelle membrane in the cell are synthesized on the RER. The clusters of ribosomes (i.e., polyribosomes or polysomes) that are freestanding in the cytosol are also the synthesis site for some proteins. All proteins synthesized in polyribosomes in the cytosol remain within the cytoplasmic matrix or are incorporated into an organelle.

Located on the RER of liver cells is a system of enzymes important in detoxifying and metabolizing many different drugs. This enzyme complex consists of a family of cytochromes called the P450 system that functions along with other enzymes. The P450 system is particularly active in oxidizing drugs, but because its action results in the simultaneous oxidation of other compounds as well, the system is collectively referred to as the mixed-function oxidase system. Lipophilic substances—for example, the steroid hormones and numerous drugs—can be made hydrophilic by oxidation, reduction, or hydrolysis, thereby enabling them to be excreted easily in the bile or urine. This system is discussed further in Chapter 5.

The **Golgi apparatus** functions closely with the ER in trafficking and sorting proteins synthesized in the cell, and is particularly prominent in neurons and secretory cells. It consists of four to eight membrane-enclosed, flattened cisternae that are stacked in parallel (Figures 1.1 and 1.5). The Golgi cisternae are often referred to as "stacks" because of this arrangement. Tubular networks have been identified at either end of the Golgi stacks:

- The *cis*-Golgi network is a compartment that accepts newly synthesized proteins coming from the ER.
- The *trans*-Golgi network is the exit site of the Golgi apparatus. It sorts proteins for delivery to their next destination [11].

Proteins (polypeptides) destined for the Golgi apparatus form within the RER. Once they are transferred to the Golgi apparatus, additional molecules (such as carbohydrates or lipids) can be added to them there. The Golgi apparatus is the site for membrane differentiation and the development of surface specificity. For example, the polysaccharide moieties of mucopolysaccharides and of the membrane glycoproteins are synthesized and attached to the polypeptide during its passage through the Golgi apparatus. Such an arrangement allows for the continual replacement of cellular membranes, including the plasma membrane.

The ER is a quality-control organelle in that it prevents proteins that have not achieved normal tertiary or quaternary structure from reaching the cell surface. The ER can retrieve or retain proteins destined for residency within the ER, or it can target proteins for delivery to the *cis*-Golgi compartment. Retrieved or exported protein "cargo" is coated with protein complexes called coatomers, abbreviated COPs (coat proteins). Some coatomers are structurally similar to the clathrin coat of endocytic vesicles and are described later in this chapter. The choice of what is retrieved or retained by the ER and what is exported to the Golgi apparatus is mediated by signals that are inherent in the terminal amino acid sequences of the proteins in question. Certain amino acid sequences of cargo proteins are thought to interact specifically with certain coatomers [12].

The membrane-bound compartments of the ER and the Golgi apparatus are interconnected by transport vesicles, in which cargo proteins are moved from compartment to compartment. The vesicles leaving a compartment are formed by a budding and pinching off of the compartment membrane, and the vesicles then fuse with the membrane of the target compartment. The specificity of vesicle-membrane interactions has been the focus of considerable research [12].

Secretion of products such as proteins from the cell can be either constitutive or regulated. If secretion follows a constitutive course, the secretion rate remains relatively constant, uninfluenced by external regulation. Regulated secretion, as the name implies, is affected by regulatory factors, and therefore its rate is changeable.

Lysosomes and Peroxisomes

Lysosomes and **peroxisomes** are cell organelles packed with enzymes. Whereas the lysosomes serve as the cell's digestive system, the peroxisomes perform some specific oxidative catabolic reactions. Lysosomes are particularly large and abundant in cells that perform digestive functions—for example, the macrophages and leukocytes. Approximately 36 powerful enzymes capable of splitting complex substances such as proteins, polysaccharides, nucleic acids, and phospholipids are held within the confines of a single thick membrane. The lysosome, just like a protein synthesized for excretion, is believed to develop through the combined activities of the ER and the Golgi apparatus. The result is a carefully packaged group of lytic enzymes (Figures 1.1 and 1.5).

The membrane surrounding these catabolic enzymes has the capacity for selective fusion with other vesicles so that **catabolism** (or digestion) may occur as necessary. Wastes produced by this process can be removed from the cells by exocytosis. Important catabolic activities performed by the lysosomes include participation in **phagocytosis**, in which foreign substances taken up by the cell are digested or rendered harmless. An example of digestion by lysosomes is their action in the proximal tubules of the kidney. Lysosomes of the proximal tubule cells are believed to digest the albumin absorbed by endocytosis from the glomerular filtrate. Lysosomal phagocytosis protects against invading bacteria and is part of the normal repair process following a wound or an infection.

A second catabolic activity of lysosomes is **autolysis,** in which intracellular components, including organelles, are digested following degeneration or cellular injury. Autolysis also can serve as a survival mechanism for the cell as a whole. Digesting dispensable intracellular components can provide the cell with nutrients necessary to fuel functions essential to life. The mitochondrion is an example of an organelle whose degeneration requires autolysis. It is estimated that the mitochondria of liver cells must be renewed approximately every 10 days.

Another catabolic activity of the lysosomes is bone resorption, an essential process in the normal modeling of bone. Lysosomes of the osteoclasts promote mineral dissolution and collagen digestion, both of which are necessary actions in bone resorption and in regulating calcium and phosphorus homeostasis. Lysosomes, with their special membrane and numerous catabolic enzymes, also function in hormone secretion and regulation. Their role in the secretion of the thyroid hormones is particularly important (see Chapter 13).

In the early 1960s, the peroxisomes were first recognized as separate intracellular organelles. These small bodies are believed to originate by "budding" from the SER. The peroxisomes are similar to the lysosomes in that they are bundles of enzymes surrounded by a single membrane. Rather than having digestive action, however, the enzymes within the peroxisomes are catabolic oxidative enzymes. Although the mitochondrial matrix is the major site where fatty acids are oxidized, very–long-chain fatty acids are oxidized in peroxisomes. Peroxisomes are also the site for certain reactions of amino acid catabolism. Some oxidative enzymes involved in these pathways catalyze the release of hydrogen peroxide (H_2O_2) as an oxidation product. Because H_2O_2 is a very reactive chemical that could cause cellular damage if not promptly removed or converted, H_2O_2–releasing reactions are segregated within these organelles. The enzyme catalase, present in large quantities in the peroxisomes, degrades the potentially harmful H_2O_2 into water and molecular oxygen. Other enzymes in the peroxisomes are important in detoxifying reactions. Particularly important is the oxidation of ethanol to acetaldehyde.

CELLULAR PROTEINS

Proteins synthesized on the cell's free polyribosomes remain within the cell to perform their specific structural, digestive, regulatory, or other functions. Among the more interesting areas of biomolecular research has been determining how newly synthesized protein finds its way from the ribosomes to its intended destination. At the time of synthesis, signal sequences direct proteins to their appropriate target compartment. These targeting sequences, located at the N-terminus of the protein, are generally cleaved (though not always) when the protein reaches its destination. Interaction between the signal sequences and specific receptors located on the various membranes permits the protein to enter its designated membrane or become incorporated into the designated organelle.

A long list of metabolic diseases is attributed to a deficiency of, or the inactivity of, certain enzymes (protein catalysts). Tay-Sachs disease, phenylketonuria, maple syrup urine disease, and the lipid and glycogen storage diseases are a few well-known examples. As a result of research on certain mitochondrial proteins, it is believed that in at least some cases the enzymes are not necessarily inactive or deficient but rather fail to reach their correct destination [13–15].

Several cellular proteins are of particular interest to the health science student:

- **receptors,** proteins that modify the cell's response to its environment
- **transport proteins,** proteins that regulate the flow of nutrients into and out of the cell
- **enzymes,** the catalysts for the hundreds of biochemical reactions taking place in the cell

Receptors and Intracellular Signaling

Receptors are highly specific proteins located in the plasma membrane and facing the exterior of the cell. Bound to the outer surface of these specific proteins are oligosaccharide chains, which are believed to act as recognition markers. Membrane receptors act as attachment sites for specific external stimuli such as hormones, growth factors, antibodies, lipoproteins, and certain nutrients (examples are shown in Figures 1.10 and 1.11). These molecular stimuli, which bind specifically to receptors, are called **ligands.** Receptors are also located on the membranes of cell organelles; less is known about these receptors, but they appear to be glycoproteins necessary for correctly positioning newly synthesized cellular proteins.

Although most receptor proteins are probably integral membrane proteins, some may be peripheral. In addition, receptor proteins can vary widely in their composition and mechanism of action. Although the composition and mechanism of action of many receptors have not yet been determined, at least three distinct types of receptors are known to exist:

- those that bind the ligand stimulus and convert it into an internal signal that alters behavior of the affected cell
- those that function as ion channels
- those that internalize their stimulus intact

Examples of these three types of receptors follow.

Receptors That Produce Internal Chemical Signals

The internal chemical signal most often produced by a stimulus-receptor interaction is $3'$, $5'$-cyclic adenosine monophosphate (cyclic adenosine monophosphate [AMP], or cAMP). It is formed from adenosine triphosphate (ATP) by the enzyme adenyl cyclase. Cyclic AMP is frequently referred to as the second messenger in the stimulation of target cells by hormones. Figure 1.10 presents a model for the ligand-binding action of receptors, which leads to production of the internal signal cAMP. As shown in the figure, the stimulated receptor reacts with guanosine triphosphate (GTP)–binding protein (G-protein), which activates adenylcyclase, triggering production of cAMP from ATP. G-protein is a trimer with three subunits (designated α, β, and γ). The α-subunit binds with GDP or GTP

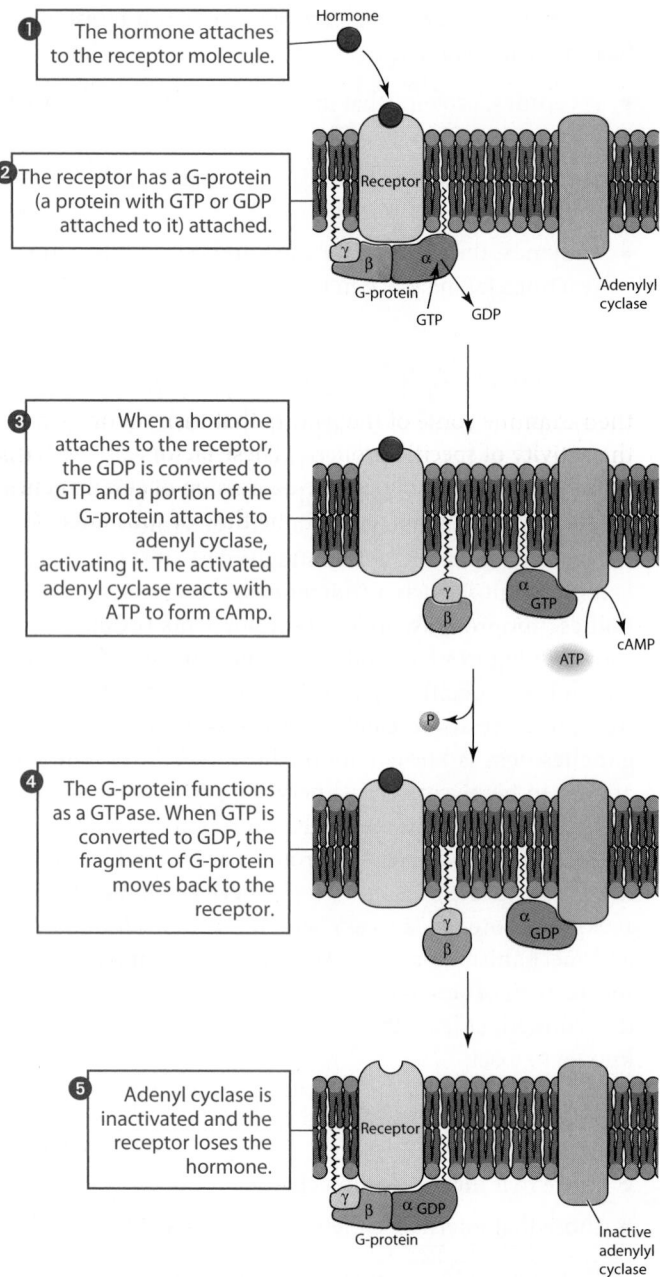

Figure 1.10 An example of an internal chemical signal by a second messenger.

two subunits are bound in such a way that the catalytic portion of the molecule is inhibited sterically by the presence of the regulatory subunit. Phosphorylation of the enzyme by cAMP causes the subunits to dissociate, thereby freeing the catalytic subunit, which regains its full catalytic capacity.

Many intracellular chemical messengers are known other than those cited as examples in this section [16]. Listed here, along with cAMP, are several additional examples:

- cyclic AMP (cAMP)
- cyclic GMP (cGMP)
- Ca^{+2}
- inositol triphosphate
- diacyl glycerol
- fructose-2,6-bisphosphate

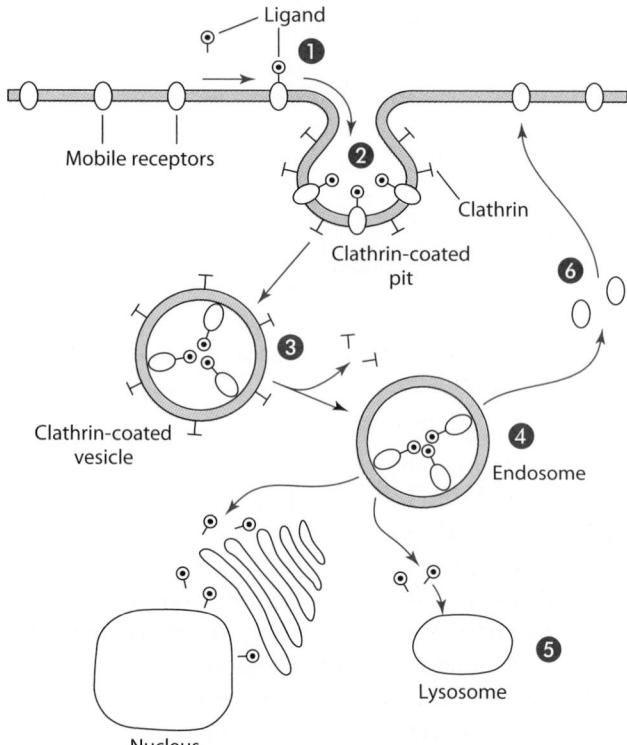

and has GTPase activity. Attachment of a hormone to the receptor stimulates the exchange of GDP for GTP. The GTP binding causes the trimers to disassociate and the α unit to associate with an effector protein, adenylyl cyclase. A single hormone-binding site can produce many cAMP molecules.

The mechanism of action of cAMP signaling within the cell is complex, but it can be viewed briefly as follows: cAMP is an activator of protein kinases. **Protein kinases** are enzymes that phosphorylate (add phosphate groups to) other enzymes and, in doing so, convert the enzymes from inactive forms into active forms. In some cases, the phosphorylated enzyme is the inactive form. Protein kinases that can be activated by cAMP contain two subunits: a catalytic and a regulatory subunit. In the inactive form of the kinase, the

1️⃣ Ligand binds with its receptor on the cell membrane.

2️⃣ Ligand and receptor move into a clathrin-coated pit.

3️⃣ Pit closes off and forms a clathrin-coated vesicle.

4️⃣ The vesicle forms an endosome.

5️⃣ Ligand can be used by the cell or undergo lysosomal degradation.

6️⃣ Receptor is recycled to the surface of the cell membrane.

Figure 1.11 Internalization of a stimulus into a cell via its receptor.

Receptors That Act as Ion Channels

Receptors can also act as ion channels in stimulating a cell. In some cases, the binding of the ligand to its receptor causes a voltage change, which then becomes the signal for an appropriate cellular response. Such is the case when the neurotransmitter acetylcholine is the stimulus. The receptor for acetylcholine appears to function as an ion channel in response to voltage change. Stimulation by acetylcholine signals the channels to open, allowing sodium (Na) ions to pass through an otherwise impermeable membrane [17].

Receptors That Internalize Stimuli

The internalization of a stimulus into a fibroblast by way of its receptor is illustrated in Figure 1.11. Receptors that perform in such a manner exist for a variety of biologically active molecules, including the hormones insulin and tri-iodothyronine. Low-density lipoproteins (LDLs) are taken up by certain cells in much the same fashion (see Chapter 5), except that their receptors, rather than being mobile, are already clustered in coated pits. These pits, vesicles formed from the plasma membrane, are coated with several proteins, among which clathrin is primary. (Phosphatidyl inositol also plays an important role in these vesicles; this will be discussed more fully in Chapter 7.) A coated pit containing the receptor with its ligand soon loses the clathrin coating and forms a smooth-walled vesicle. This vesicle delivers the ligand into the depths of the cell and then is recycled, along with the receptor, into the plasma membrane. If the endocytotic process is for scavenging, the ligand (perhaps a protein) is not used by the cell but instead undergoes lysosomal degradation, as shown in Figure 1.11 and exemplified by the endocytosis of LDL.

Receptors' Role in Homeostasis

The cells of every organ in the body have specialized receptors that respond to changes in external conditions. The reaction of a fibroblast to changes in blood glucose levels is a good example of cellular adjustment to the existing environment that is made possible through receptor proteins. When blood glucose levels are low, muscular activity leads to release of the hormone epinephrine by the adrenal medulla. Epinephrine becomes attached to its receptor protein on the fibroblast, thereby activating the receptor and causing it to stimulate G-protein and adenyl cyclase, which catalyzes the formation of cAMP from ATP. Then cAMP initiates a series of enzyme phosphorylation modifications, as described earlier in this section, which result in the phosphorolysis of glycogen to glucose-1-phosphate for use by the fibroblast.

In contrast, when blood glucose levels are elevated, the hormone insulin, secreted by the β-cells of the pancreas, reacts with its receptors on the fibroblast and is transported into the cell by receptor-mediated endocytosis. Insulin allows diffusion of glucose into the cell by increasing the number of glucose receptors in the cell membrane, which in turn promote diffusion of glucose by its transport protein. (Glucose transporters are covered in Chapter 3.) The hormone itself is degraded within the cell [1]. More examples will be cited in subsequent chapters.

Transport Proteins

The cell produces many different types of proteins. So far, this chapter has covered the synthesis of structural proteins. We will now focus on the functional proteins, which include transport proteins and catalytic proteins. We will then examine some of the factors that turn on or turn off the activity of specific proteins. These factors are the basis for nutritional control over the expression of certain genes.

Transport proteins regulate the flow of substances (including nutrients) into and out of the cell. Transport proteins may function by acting as carriers (or pumps), or they may provide protein-lined passages (pores) through which water-soluble materials of small molecular weight may diffuse. Figure 1.3 shows the integral and peripheral proteins of the cell membrane that function as transport proteins.

The active transport protein that has been studied most is the sodium (Na^+) pump. The Na^+ pump is essential not only to maintain ionic and electrical balance but also for intestinal and renal absorption of certain key nutrients (e.g., glucose and certain amino acids). These nutrients move into the epithelial cell of the small intestine against a concentration gradient, necessitating both a carrier and a source of energy, both of which are provided by the Na^+ pump. (This topic is covered in Chapter 3.)

The process of facilitated (non–energy dependent) transport is also an important mechanism for regulating the flow of nutrients into the cell. It is used broadly across a wide range of cell types. Proteins involved in this function are often called transporters; probably the most thoroughly studied of these are the glucose transporters, discussed in Chapter 3.

Catalytic Proteins (Enzymes)

Enzymes are proteins that are distributed throughout all cellular compartments. Enzymes are catalysts that take part in a reaction but are not part of the final product of that reaction, and are essentially regenerated. Enzymes have an "active site" where they bind with a substrate. Often, biologically metabolic pathways involve a number of enzymatic reactions that are associated with each other. Enzymes that are components of the cellular membranes are usually found on the inner surface of the membranes; the exceptions are enzymes that function externally. Examples are the digestive enzymes: isomaltase, the disaccharidases (lactase, sucrase, and maltase), and certain peptidases located on the brush border of the epithelial cells lining the small intestine. Membrane-associated enzymes are found distributed throughout the cell organelles, with the greatest concentration found in the mitochondria. As mentioned earlier, the enzymes of the electron transport chain, where energy transformation occurs, are located within the inner membrane of the mitochondria.

Metabolic processes occurring in the cells are governed by enzymes that have been synthesized on the cell's RER under the direction of mRNA that was produced from nuclear DNA. The functional activity of most enzymes, however, depends not only on the protein portion of the molecule but also on a nonprotein prosthetic group or co-enzyme. If the nonprotein group is an organic compound, it may contain a chemically modified B-complex vitamin. Commonly, however, the prosthetic group is inorganic (i.e., metal ions such as Mg, Zn, Cu, Mn, or Fe).

Enzymes have an active center that possesses a high specificity. This means that a substrate must "fit" perfectly into the specific contours of the enzyme's active site so that the reacting parts of the substrate are in close proximity to the reacting parts of the enzyme. The most common analogy used to describe this is a lock and key. The concept of interlocking pieces of a puzzle has also been used to convey that the substrate and enzyme must fit. The enzyme's specificity can come from the reactive groups of its amino acids as part of the amino acid sequence or primary structure. The specificity may also originate from the three-dimensional or tertiary structure of the enzyme.

The velocity of an enzyme-catalyzed reaction (the number of molecules of substrate reacted on in a specified time) increases if all of the active sites on all of the enzyme molecules are "filled" with substrate. As the concentration of the substrate increases, the number of molecules of substrate available to the enzyme increases. This increases the number of substrate molecules acted on by the enzyme-catalyzed reaction and is said to increase the rate of the reaction. However, this relationship applies only to a concentration of substrate that is less than the concentration that "saturates" the enzyme. At saturation levels of substrate, the enzyme molecule functions at its maximum velocity (V_{max}), and the occurrence of a still higher concentration of substrate cannot increase the velocity further.

The velocity of a chemical reaction is defined by an equilibrium constant. For enzyme-catalyzed reactions this equilibrium constant is known as K_m, or the Michaelis constant. K_m is a useful parameter that aids in establishing how enzymes react in the living cell. K_m represents the concentration of a substrate that is found in an occurring reaction when the reaction is at one-half its maximum velocity. If an enzyme has a high K_m value, then an abundance of substrate must be present to raise the rate of reaction to half its maximum velocity; in other words, the enzyme has a low affinity for its substrate and it takes more substrate to react with the active site of the enzyme. An example of an enzyme with a high K_m is glucokinase, an enzyme operating in the liver cells. Because glucose can

diffuse freely into the liver, the fact that glucokinase has a high K_m is very important to blood glucose regulation. If glucokinase had a high affinity for glucose, too much glucose would be removed from the blood during periods of fasting. Glucokinase (with its high K_m) can still convert excess glucose to glucose phosphate when the glucose load is high—for example, following a high-carbohydrate meal. The liver glucokinase does not function at its maximum velocity when glucose levels are in the normal range. The enzyme therefore can be thought of as a protection against high cellular concentrations of glucose.

The nature of enzyme catalysis can be described by the following reactions:

$$\text{Enzyme (E)} + \text{substrate (S)} \longleftrightarrow \text{E-S complex}$$

(reversible reaction)

The substrate activated by combination with the enzyme is converted into an enzyme-product (E-P) complex through rearrangement of the substrate's ions and atoms:

$$\text{E-S} \longleftrightarrow \text{E-P}$$
$$\text{E-P} \longrightarrow \text{E} + \text{P}$$

The product is released, and the enzyme is free to react with more of the substrate.

Reversibility

Most biochemical reactions are reversible, meaning that the same enzyme can catalyze a reaction in both directions. The extent to which a reaction can proceed in a reverse direction depends on several factors, the most important of which are the relative concentrations of substrate (reactant) and product and the differences in energy content between reactant and product. In instances when a large disparity in either energy content or concentration exists between reactant and product, the reaction can proceed in only one direction. Such a reaction is unidirectional rather than reversible. This topic is discussed later in this chapter. In unidirectional reactions, the same enzyme cannot catalyze in both directions. Instead, a different enzyme is required to catalyze the reverse direction of the reaction. Comparing glycolysis (the oxidation of glucose) with gluconeogenesis (the synthesis of glucose) allows us to see how unidirectional reactions may be reversed by introducing a different enzyme.

Simultaneous reactions, catalyzed by various multi-enzyme systems or pathways, constitute cellular metabolism. Enzymes are compartmentalized within the cell and function in sequential chains. A good example of a multienzyme system is the tricarboxylic acid cycle (TCA cycle) located in the mitochondrial matrix. Each sequential reaction is catalyzed by a different enzyme, and some reactions are reversible, whereas others are unidirectional. Although some reactions in almost any pathway are reversible, it is important to understand that removal of one of the products (by that product reacting to produce the next compound in the pathway) drives the reaction toward forming more of that product. Removing (or using) the product, then, becomes the driving force that causes reactions to proceed primarily in the desired direction.

Regulation

An important aspect of nutritional biochemistry is the regulation of metabolic pathways. Anabolic (synthetic) and catabolic (oxidative) reactions must be kept in a balance appropriate for life (and perhaps growth) of the organism. Regulation primarily involves the adjustment of the catalytic activity of certain participating enzymes. This enzyme regulation occurs through three major mechanisms:

- covalent modification of enzymes through hormone stimulation
- modulation of allosteric enzymes
- increase in enzyme concentration by induction (synthesis of more enzyme)

Covalent Modification With the first of these mechanisms, covalent modification, the enzyme is inactive until a modification is made. This is usually achieved by the addition or hydrolytic removal of phosphate groups to or from the enzyme. This is the mechanism involving cAMP and protein kinase activation covered in the "Receptors That Produce Internal Chemical Signals" section of this chapter. An example of covalent modification of enzymes is the regulation of glycogenesis (synthesis of glycogen from glucose units) and glycogenolysis (breakdown of glycogen to glucose units). Some enzymes are synthesized as inactive precursors. Examples are the proteolytic enzymes that are secreted into the stomach or intestine as a proenzyme. A portion of the peptide is removed by hydrolysis to make a fully active enzyme.

Allosteric Enzyme Modulation The second important regulatory mechanism is that exerted by certain unique enzymes called allosteric enzymes. The term *allosteric* refers to the fact that these enzymes possess an allosteric or specific "other" site besides the catalytic site. Specific compounds, called modulators, can bind to these allosteric sites and profoundly influence the activity of these regulatory enzymes. Modulators may be positive (i.e., causing an increase in enzyme activity), or they may exert a negative effect (i.e., inhibit activity). Modulating substances are believed to alter the activity of the allosteric enzyme by changing the conformation (three-dimensional structure) of the polypeptide chain or chains of the enzyme, thereby altering the binding of its catalytic site with the intended substrate. Negative modulators are often the end products of a sequence of reactions. As an end product accumulates above a certain critical concentration, it can inhibit, through an allosteric enzyme, its own further production.

An excellent example of an allosteric enzyme is phosphofructokinase in the glycolytic pathway. Glycolysis gives rise to pyruvate, which is decarboxylated and oxidized to acetyl-CoA, which enters the mitochondrion and is further oxidized by the TCA cycle by combining with oxaloacetate to form citrate. Citrate is a negative modulator of phosphofructokinase. Therefore, an accumulation of citrate in the cell matrix causes the glycolytic pathway to be inhibited by regulating phosphofructokinase. In contrast, an accumulation of AMP or adenosine diphosphate (ADP), which indicates that ATP is depleted, signals the need for additional energy in the cell in the form of ATP. AMP or ADP therefore modulates phosphofructokinase positively. The result is an active glycolytic pathway that ultimately leads to the formation of more ATP through the TCA cycle–electron transport chain connection.

Allosteric mechanisms of regulation are considered to be of one of two types. In one type, the K series, the K_m is affected, which alters the binding of the substrate to the enzyme. If the allosteric effect is positive, the enzyme can become "saturated" at a lower concentration. The other type of allosteric regulation, called the V series, increases the maximum velocity of the enzymatic reaction. If the allosteric effector is an inhibitor, the maximum velocity (V_m) of the reaction will be decreased.

Induction The third mechanism of enzyme regulation, *enzyme induction,* creates changes in the concentration of certain inducible enzymes by increasing enzyme synthesis. Inducible enzymes are adaptive, meaning that they are synthesized at rates dictated by cellular circumstances. In contrast, constitutive enzymes, which are synthesized at a relatively constant rate, are uninfluenced by external stimuli. Induction usually occurs through the action of certain hormones, such as the steroid hormones and the thyroid hormones, and is exerted through changes in the expression of genes encoding the enzymes. Dietary changes can elicit the induction of enzymes necessary to cope with the changing nutrient load. This regulatory mechanism is relatively slow, however, compared to the first two mechanisms discussed, which exert their effects in terms of seconds or minutes.

The reverse of induction is the blockage of enzyme synthesis by blocking the formation of the mRNA of specific enzymes. This regulation of translation is one of the means by which small molecules, reacting with cellular proteins, can exert their effect on enzyme concentration and the activity of metabolic pathways.

Specific examples of enzyme regulation are described in subsequent chapters that deal with metabolism of the major nutrients. It should be noted at this point, however, that *enzymes targeted for regulation essentially catalyze unidirectional reactions.* In every metabolic pathway, at least one reaction is essentially irreversible, exergonic, and enzyme limited. That is, the rate of the reaction is limited only by the activity of the enzyme catalyzing it. Such enzymes are frequently called the regulatory enzymes, capable of being stimulated or suppressed by one of the mechanisms described. Logically, an enzyme catalyzing a reaction reversibly at near equilibrium in the cell cannot be a regulatory enzyme because its up or down regulation would affect its forward and reverse activities equally. This effect, in turn, would not accomplish the purpose of regulation, which is to stimulate the rate of the metabolic pathway in one direction to exceed the rate of the pathway in the reverse direction.

Examples of Enzyme Types

Enzymes participating in cellular reactions are located throughout the cell in both the cytoplasmic matrix (cytoplast) and the various organelles. The location of specific enzymes depends on the site of the metabolic pathways or metabolic reactions in which those enzymes participate. Enzyme classification, therefore, is based on the type of reaction catalyzed by the various enzymes. Enzymes fall within six general classifications:

- **Oxidoreductases** (dehydrogenases, reductases, oxidases, peroxidases, hydroxylases, and oxygenases) are enzymes that catalyze all reactions in which one compound is oxidized and another is reduced. Examples of oxidoreductases are the enzymes found in the electron transport chain located on the inner membrane of the mitochondria. Other examples are the cytochrome P450 enzymes located on the ER of liver cells.

- **Transferases** are enzymes that catalyze reactions not involving oxidation and reduction in which a functional group is transferred from one substrate to another. Included in this group of enzymes are transketolase, transaldolase, transmethylase, and the transaminases. The transaminases (α-amino transferases), which figure so prominently in protein metabolism, are located primarily in the mitochondrial matrix.

- **Hydrolases** (esterases, amidases, peptidases, phosphatases, and glycosidases) are enzymes that catalyze cleavage of bonds between carbon atoms and some other kind of atom by adding water. Digestive enzymes fall within this classification, as do those enzymes contained within the lysosome of the cell.

- **Lyases** (decarboxylases, aldolases, synthetases, cleavage enzymes, deaminases, nucleotide cyclases, hydrases or hydratases, and dehydratases) are enzymes that catalyze cleavage of carbon-carbon, carbon-sulfur, and certain carbon-nitrogen bonds (peptide bonds excluded) without hydrolysis or oxidation-reduction. Citrate lyase, which frees acetyl-CoA for fatty acid synthesis in the cytoplast, is a good example of an enzyme belonging to this classification.

- **Isomerases** (isomerases, racemases, epimerases, and mutases) are enzymes that catalyze the interconversion of optical or geometric isomers. Phosphohexose isomerase, which converts glucose-6-phosphate to fructose-6-phosphate in glycolysis (occurring in the cytoplast), exemplifies this particular class of enzyme.

- **Ligases** are enzymes that catalyze the formation of bonds between carbon and a variety of other atoms, including oxygen, sulfur, and nitrogen. Forming bonds catalyzed by ligases requires energy that usually is provided by hydrolysis of ATP. A good example of a ligase is acetyl-CoA carboxylase, which is necessary to initiate fatty acid synthesis in the cytoplast. Through the action of acetyl-CoA carboxylase, a bicarbonate ion (HCO_3^-) is attached to acetyl-CoA to form malonyl-CoA, the initial compound in starting fatty acid synthesis.

Clinical Applications of Cellular Enzymes

All of the hundreds of enzymes present in the human body are synthesized intracellularly, and most of them function within the cell in which they were formed. These are the enzymes responsible for catalyzing the myriad of metabolic reactions occurring in each cell. Some are secreted in an inactive form and are rendered active in the extracellular fluids where they function. Those that function in the bloodstream are called plasma-specific enzymes.

Diagnostic enzymology focuses on intracellular enzymes, which, because of a problem within the cell structure, escape from the cell and ultimately express their activity in the serum. By measuring the serum activity of the released enzymes, both the site and the extent of the cellular damage may be determined. If the site of the damage is to be determined with reasonable accuracy, the enzyme being measured must exhibit a relatively high degree of organ or tissue specificity. For instance, lactate dehydrohenase (LDH) is an enzyme that is widely distributed among cells of the heart, liver, skeletal muscle, and lymph nodes; erythrocytes; and platelets. Elevated serum levels of LDH do not have diagnostic value until the enzyme is separated into its five different isozyme forms and each is measured individually. Each isozyme is organ specific. The amount of elevation of the isozyme from the heart is an indication of the extent of tissue damage following an infarction (which causes ischemia to a portion of the heart muscle following a blood clot in a cardiac artery).

Intracellular enzymes normally are retained within the cell where they are produced by the plasma membrane. The plasma membrane is metabolically active, and its integrity depends on the cell's energy consumption and therefore its nutritive status. Any process that impairs the cell's use of nutrients can compromise the structural integrity of the plasma membrane. Membrane failure can also arise from mechanical disruption, such as would be caused by a viral attack on the cell. Damage to the plasma membrane is manifested as leakiness and eventual cell death, allowing unimpeded passage of substances, including enzymes, from intracellular to extracellular compartments.

Factors contributing to cellular damage and resulting in abnormal egress of cellular enzymes include the following events: tissue ischemia (**ischemia** refers to an impairment of blood flow to a tissue or part of a tissue; it deprives affected cells of oxygen and oxidizable nutrients), tissue necrosis, viral attack on specific cells, damage from organic chemicals such as alcohol and organophosphorus pesticide, and hypoxia (inadequate intake of oxygen).

Increases in blood serum concentrations of cellular enzymes can be good indicators of even minor cellular damage because the intracellular concentration of enzymes is hundreds or thousands of times greater than in blood and also because enzyme assays are extremely sensitive.

Conditions for Diagnostic Suitability

Not all intracellular enzymes are valuable in diagnosing damage to the cells in which they are contained. Several conditions must be met for the enzyme to be suitably diagnostic:

- The enzyme must have a sufficiently high degree of organ or tissue specificity.
- A steep concentration gradient of enzyme activity must exist between the interior and exterior of the cells under normal conditions. This makes small increases in serum activity detectable.
- The enzyme must function in the cytoplasmic compartment of the cell so that it leaks out whenever the plasma membrane suffers significant damage.
- The enzyme must be stable for a reasonable period of time in the vascular compartment.

Increased Production Factors

The most common cause of increased production of an enzyme that results in a spike in its serum concentration is malignant disease (cancer). Substances that occur in body fluids as a result of malignant disease are called tumor markers. A tumor marker may be produced by the tumor itself or by the host, in response to a tumor.

In addition to enzymes and isoenzymes, other forms of tumor markers include hormones, oncofetal protein antigens such as carcinoembryonic antigen (CEA), and products of oncogenes. **Oncogenes** are mutated genes that encode abnormal, mitosis-signaling proteins that cause unchecked cell division.

APOPTOSIS

Dying is said to be a normal part of living. So it is with the cell. Like every living thing, a cell has a well-defined life span, after which its structural and functional integrity diminishes and it is removed by other cells through phagocytosis.

Cells are constantly turned over in the body. For instance, 10^{10} neutrophils (a type white blood cell) die and are replaced each day [18]. As cells die, they are replaced by new cells that are continuously being formed through cell mitosis. However, both daughter cells formed in the mitotic process do not always enjoy the full life span of the parent. If they did, the number of cells, and consequently tissue mass, could increase inordinately. Therefore, one of the two cells produced by mitosis generally is programmed to die before its sister. In fact, most dying cells are already doomed at the time they are formed. Those targeted for death are usually smaller than their surviving sisters, and their phagocytosis begins even before the mitosis generating them is complete. The processes of cell division and cell death must be carefully regulated to generate the proper number of cells during development. Once cells mature, the appropriate number of cells must be maintained. The mechanism by which naturally occurring cell death arises has been subjected to intense research in recent years [18–23]. The mechanisms involved in cell death and those reactions that control them are important in the growth and development of the fertilized egg as well as the development of certain cancers and in immunological reactions.

Programmed Death

Many terms have been used to describe naturally occurring cell death. It is now most commonly referred to as *programmed cell death,* to distinguish it from pathological cell death, which is not part of any normal physiological process. The term describing programmed cell death is **apoptosis,** a word borrowed from the Greek meaning to "fall out."

Potential Mechanisms

Apoptotic cell death (and cell survival) is brought about by several mechanisms. This is an area of active research, and much has been learned about those factors that initiate the process and those that inhibit it. Additional details of the cell biology and biochemistry of apoptosis can be found in several excellent reviews and in textbooks of cell biology and biochemistry [18–23]. During embryological development, apoptosis is one mechanism used by the body to control neurons innervating target organs. Apoptosis is thought to be important in the development of several neurological degenerative diseases such as Alzheimer's disease, Parkinson's disease [24], and Huntington's disease.

In mammalian cells, apoptosis can be triggered by both intra- and extracellular pathways. The intracellular pathway can be triggered by several different stimuli such as irreparable DNA damage, lack of oxygen, or abnormally high levels of Ca^{+2} [20]. (Ionic calcium is generally membrane bound.) The damage caused by these stimuli results in a release of proapoptotic factors from the mitochondria into the cytoplasm by increasing the permeability of the outer mitochondrial membrane. The release of factors from the mitochondria can be antagonized by proteins originating from specific genes. One of the proteins released from mitochondria that promotes apoptosis is cytochrome c [25]. This protein activates a group of cysteine protease enzymes called **caspases.** Caspases are normally inactive in the cell and must be converted to an active form. The caspases are released as inactive procaspases, which can be activated by the binding of two of the proenzyme's molecules: one molecule of the caspases activates the other. These proteolytic enzymes are called caspases because they contain the amino acid cysteine in their catalytic site and are responsible for most of the changes that occur in the apoptotic process. For instance, one of the caspases activated by cytochrome c is a potent DNAase that cleaves the genome of the cell into fragments of approximately 180 base pairs. This irreversible damage to the genome is one of the triggers that leads to apoptosis.

As stated previously, the intracellular mechanism of apoptosis involves the release of cytochrome c from the intermitochondrial space into the cytoplasmic matrix. Once cytochrome c has translocated to the cytoplasmic matrix, it activates the caspases. A family of proteins designated Bcl-2 (B-cell lymphoma gene product) is synthesized. Bcl-2 proteins are integral membrane proteins on the outer membrane of the mitochondrion. Some of the Bcl-2 proteins are proapoptotic while others block the process and prevent the release of mitochondrial cytochrome c. Genetic over-expression of Bcl-2 prevents cells from undergoing apoptosis in response to various stimuli. In these situations the role of Bcl-2 in preventing apoptosis is to block release of cytochrome c from the mitochondrion [25].

The extracellular pathway for apoptosis is initiated by the extracellular hormones or agonists that belong to the **tumor necrosis factor** (TNF) family. TNFs are **cytokines** that are important in regulating metabolism. These compounds are discussed in Chapter 7. TNFs recognize and activate their corresponding receptors. Through a series of protein-protein interactions, they recruit specific adaptor proteins. TNFs trigger a cascade of reactions transforming procaspases into active caspases, resulting in cell death and producing proteins that function as inhibitors or anti-apoptotic factors that inhibit the release of cytochrome c into the cytosol.

Cell death appears to be activated by specific genes in dying cells. Genes designated *Casp-9* and *Apaf-1* must be expressed within dying cells for cell death to occur. The *Casp-9* and *Apaf-1* genes encode proteins that activate cytotoxic activity. The expression of these genes therefore must be tightly controlled to avoid damage to the wrong cells. A major control factor is a third gene that produces the group of Bcl-2 proteins already discussed. Mutations to the gene that controls the Bcl-2 proteins have been shown to kill an animal under study by causing the death of cells otherwise intended to survive [18–23].

Interestingly, many of the proteins released in the process of apoptosis are found in the mitochondria or in its outer membrane space. Most have a specific role there. Only when they are released into the cytosol do they have a role in apoptosis. If cell death is prevented, a transformed cell can continue to grow rather than be destroyed, creating a tumor.

Apoptosis initiates an internal and external destruction of the cell. Dead cells are removed by phagocytosis and their contents are never released into the extracellular fluid or circulation—the phagocytic process prevents any of the cell's contents from escaping into the extracellular space. Therefore, apoptosis does not trigger any autoimmunity. Other mechanisms for cell death, on the other hand, can release cellular contents into the extracellular space. Animal experiments and the study of human patients show that a defect in the apoptotic process appears to make an individual prone to autoimmune diseases. Studies in humans are on-going to determine if specific human autoimmune diseases are related to a defect in the apoptotic process.

Recent research has shown that retinoic acid (RA) is involved in the regulation of apoptosis through gene expression [26]. (RA is further discussed in Chapter 10.) The involvement of RA in apoptosis is cell specific. RA can either enhance the apoptotic process or, in some cases, enhance cell survival. In specific cancers, RA has been used as a therapeutic agent to kill cancerous cells. As more is learned about the specific mechanisms that determine RA's activity, its use in oncology is likely to increase.

The active form of vitamin D (1, 25-dihydroxyvitamin D) is involved in cell death and survival pathways. Depending upon the tissue involved, the vitamin metabolite has been used in the protection of cells (enhancing survival) or in killing tumor cells in conjugation with the appropriate chemotherapeutic agent [27].

Other mechanisms of cell death exist. One such mechanism is termed **oncosis.** Oncosis (from *onksos,* meaning "swelling") is defined as a prelethal pathway leading to cell death accompanied by cellular swelling, organelle swelling, and increased membrane permeability. The process of oncosis results in the depletion of cellular energy stores. Oncosis may result from toxic substances or pathogens that interfere with ATP generation. This form of cell death differs from apoptosis, which causes cell death without any inflammation process.

As stated earlier, the investigation into the mechanism of apoptosis is active. The study of how cell death can be controlled has important disease implications. Investigating the death of cells in the heart following a myocardial infarction, the relationship between preventing apoptosis and oncogenesis, and cell death caused by pathological organisms may lead to future breakthroughs.

BIOLOGICAL ENERGY

The previous sections of this chapter provide some descriptive insight into the makeup of a cell, how it reproduces, and how large and small molecules are synthesized within a cell or move in or out of a cell. All of these activities require energy. The cell obtains this energy from small molecules transformed (oxidized) to provide heat and chemical energy. The small molecules that are constantly required are supplied by the nutrients in food. The next section covers some basics of energy needs in the cell.

Most of the processes that sustain life involve energy. Some processes use energy, and others release it. The term *energy* conjures an image of physical "vim and vigor," the fast runner or the weight lifter straining to lift hundreds of pounds. This notion of energy is accurate insofar as the contraction of muscle fibers associated with mechanical work is an energy-demanding process, requiring adenosine triphosphate (ATP), the major storage form of molecular energy in the cell. Beyond the ATP required for physical exertion the living body has other, equally important, requirements for energy, including:

- the biosynthetic (anabolic) systems by which substances can be formed from simpler precursors
- active transport systems by which compounds or ions can be moved across membranes against a concentration gradient
- the transfer of genetic information

This section addresses the key role of energy transformation and heat production in using nutrients and sustaining life.

Energy Release and Consumption in Chemical Reactions

Energy used by the body is ultimately derived from the energy contained in the **macronutrients**—carbohydrate, fat, and protein (and alcohol). If this energy is released, it may simply be expressed as heat, as would occur in the combustion of flammable substances, or be preserved in the form of other chemical energy. Energy cannot be created or destroyed; it can only be transformed.

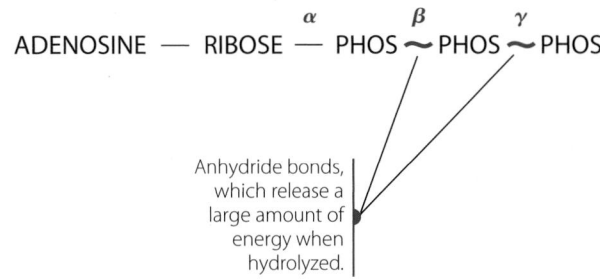

Figure 1.12 Adenosine triphosphate (ATP).

Burning a molecule of glucose outside the body liberates heat, along with CO_2 and H_2O as products of combustion, as shown:

$$C_6H_{12}O_6 + 6O_2 \longrightarrow 6CO_2 + 6H_2O + heat$$

The metabolism of glucose to the same CO_2 and H_2O within the cell is nearly identical to that of simple combustion. The difference is that in metabolic oxidation a significant portion of the released energy is salvaged as chemical energy in the form of new, high-energy bonds. These bonds represent a usable source of energy for driving energy-requiring processes. Such stored energy is generally contained in phosphate anhydride bonds, chiefly those of ATP (Figure 1.12). The analogy between the combustion and the metabolic oxidation of a typical nutrient (palmitic acid) is illustrated in Figure 1.13. The metabolic oxidation illustrated releases 59% of the heat produced by the combustion and conserves about 40% of the chemical energy.

Expressions of Energy

Units of Energy

The unit of energy used throughout this text is the calorie, abbreviated cal. In the expression of the higher caloric values encountered in nutrition, the unit kilocalories (kcal) is often used: 1 kcal = 1,000 cal. The international scientific

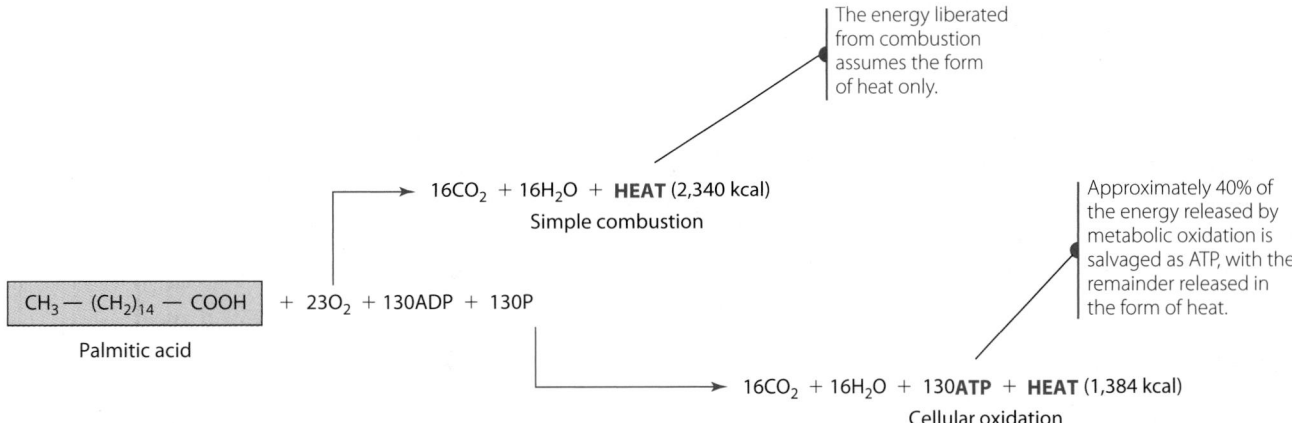

Figure 1.13 A comparison of the simple combustion and the metabolic oxidation of the fatty acid palmitate.

community and many scientific journals use another unit of energy, called the joule (J) or the kilojoule (kJ). Calories can easily be converted to joules by the factor 4.18:

$$1 \text{ cal} = 4.18 \text{ J, or } 1 \text{ kcal} = 4.18 \text{ kJ}$$

To help you become familiar with both terms, this text primarily uses *calories* or *kilocalories,* followed by the corresponding values in joules or kilojoules in parentheses. Nutrition and the calorie have been closely linked over the years. However, although you may be more comfortable with the calorie and kilocalorie units, as a student of nutrition you should become familiar with joules and kilojoules because they are used in most scientific publications.

Free Energy

The potential energy inherent in the chemical bonds of nutrients is released if the molecules undergo oxidation either through combustion or through oxidation within the cell. This energy is defined as **free energy** if, on its release, it is capable of doing work at constant temperature and pressure—a condition that is met within the cell. In equations, G is used as an abbreviation for free energy and ΔG for the change in free energy.

CO_2 and H_2O are the products of the complete oxidation of organic molecules containing only carbon, hydrogen, and oxygen, and they have an inherent free energy. The energy released in the course of oxidation of the organic molecules is in the form of either heat or chemical energy. The products have less free energy than do the original reactants. Because energy is neither created nor lost during the reaction, the total energy remains constant. Thus, the difference between the free energy in the products and that in the reactants in a given chemical reaction is a useful parameter for estimating the tendency for that reaction to occur. This difference is symbolized as follows:

$$G_{\text{products}} - G_{\text{reactants}} = \Delta G \text{ of the reaction}$$

where G is free energy and Δ is a symbol signifying change.

Exothermic and Endothermic Reactions

If the G value of the reactants is greater than the G value of the products, as in the case of the oxidation reaction, the reaction is said to be **exothermic,** or energy releasing, and the change in G (ΔG) is negative. In contrast, a positive ΔG indicates that the G value of the products is greater than that of the reactants, indicating that energy must be supplied to the system to convert the reactants into the higher-energy products. Such a reaction is called **endothermic,** or energy requiring.

Exothermic and endothermic reactions are sometimes referred to as downhill and uphill reactions, respectively, terms that help create an image of energy input and release. The free energy levels of reactants and products in a typical exothermic, or downhill, reaction can be likened to a boulder on a hillside that can occupy two positions, A and B, as illustrated in Figure 1.14. As the boulder descends to level B from level A, energy capable of doing work is liberated, and the change in free energy is a negative value. The reverse reaction, moving the boulder uphill to level A from level B, necessitates an input of energy, or an endothermic process, and the change is a positive value. The quantity of energy released in the downhill reaction is precisely the same as the quantity of energy required for the reverse (uphill) reaction—only the sign of ΔG changes.

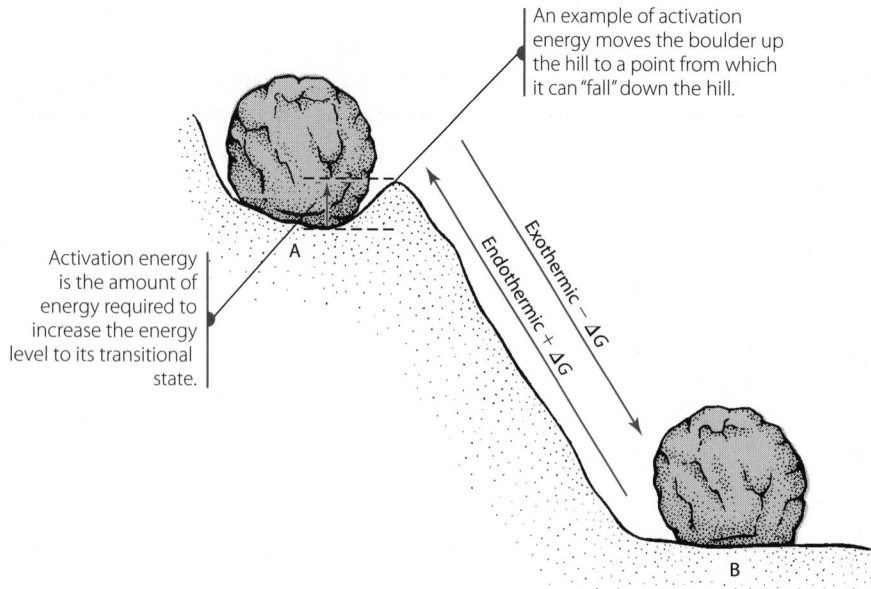

Figure 1.14 The uphill-downhill concept illustrating energy-releasing and energy-demanding processes.

Activation Energy

Although exothermic reactions are favored over endothermic reactions in that they require no external energy input, they do not occur spontaneously. If they did, no energy-producing nutrients or fuels would exist throughout the universe because they would all have transformed spontaneously to their lower energy level. A certain amount of energy must be introduced into reactant molecules to activate them to their **transition state,** a higher energy level or barrier at which the exothermic conversion to products can indeed take place. The energy that must be imposed on the system to raise the reactants to their transition state is called the **activation energy.** Refer again to the boulder-and-hillside analogy in Figure 1.14. The boulder does not spontaneously descend until the required activation energy can dislodge it from its resting place to the brink of the slope.

Cellular Energy

The cell derives its energy from a series of chemical reactions, each of which exhibits a free energy change. The reactions occur sequentially as nutrients are systematically oxidized ultimately to CO_2 and H_2O. Nearly all the reactions in the cell are catalyzed by enzymes. Within a given catabolic pathway—for example, the oxidation of glucose to CO_2 and H_2O—some reactions may be energy consuming (have a $+\Delta G$ for the reaction). However, energy-releasing (those with a $-\Delta G$) reactions are favored, so the net energy transformation for the entire pathway has a $-\Delta G$ and is exothermic.

Reversibility of Chemical Reactions

Most cellular reactions are reversible, meaning that an enzyme (E) that can catalyze the conversion of hypothetical substance A into substance B can also catalyze the reverse reaction, as shown:

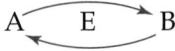

Using the A, B interconversion as an example, let us review the concept of reversibility of a chemical reaction. In the presence of the specific enzyme E, substance A is converted to substance B. Initially, the reaction is unidirectional because only A is present. However, because the enzyme is also capable of converting substance B to substance A, the reverse reaction becomes significant as the concentration of B increases. From the moment the reaction is initiated, the amount of A decreases, while the amount of B increases to the point at which the rate of the two reactions becomes equal. At that point, the concentrations of A and B no longer change, and the system is said to be in equilibrium. Enzymes are only catalysts and do not change the equilibrium of the reaction. This concept is discussed more fully later. Whether the A ⟶ B reaction or the B ⟶ A reaction is energetically favored is indicated by the relative concentrations of A and B at equilibrium.

The equilibrium between reactants and products can be defined in mathematical terms and is called the equilibrium constant (K_{eq}). K_{eq} is simply the ratio of the equilibrium concentration of product B to that of reactant A: $K_{eq} = [B]/[A]$. The [] signify the concentration. If the denominator ([A]) is very small, dividing it into a much larger number results in K_{eq} being large. [A] will be small if most of A (the reactant) is converted to the product B. In other words, K_{eq} increases in value when the concentration of A decreases and that of B increases. If K_{eq} has a value greater than 1, substance B is formed from substance A, whereas a value of K_{eq} less than 1 indicates that at equilibrium A will be formed from B. An equilibrium constant equal to 1 indicates that no bias exists for either reaction. The K_{eq} of a reaction can be used to calculate the standard free energy change of the reaction.

Standard Free Energy Change

To compare the energy released or consumed in different reactions, it is convenient to define the free energy at standard conditions. Standard conditions are defined precisely: a temperature of 25°C (298 K); a pressure of 1.0 atm (atmosphere); and the presence of both the reactants and the products at their standard concentrations, namely 1.0 mol/L. The standard free energy change (ΔG^0) (the superscript zero designates standard conditions) for a chemical reaction is a constant for that particular reaction. The ΔG^0 is defined as the difference between the free energy content of the reactants and the free energy content of the products under standard conditions. Under such conditions, ΔG^0 is mathematically related to K_{eq} by the equation

$$\Delta G^0 = -2.3 \, RT \log K_{eq}$$

where R is the gas constant (1.987 cal/mol) and T is the absolute temperature, 298 K in this case. The factors 2.3, R, and T are constants, and their product is equal to $-2.3(1.987)(298)$, or $-1,362$ cal/mol. The equation therefore simplifies to

$$\Delta G^0 = -1,362 \log K_{eq}$$

This topic is important in understanding the energetics of metabolic pathways, but you should refer to a biochemistry textbook [8] for additional information on this subject.

Equilibrium Constant and Standard Free Energy Change

The equilibrium constant of a reaction determines the sign and magnitude of the standard free energy change. For example, referring once again to the A ⟶ B reaction, the logarithm of a K_{eq} value greater than 1.0 will be positive, and because it is multiplied by a negative number, the sign of ΔG^0 will be negative. We have established that the reaction A ⟶ B is energetically favored if ΔG^0 is negative. Conversely, the log of a K_{eq} value less than 1.0 would be negative, and when multiplied by a negative number the sign of ΔG^0 would be positive. The ΔG^0 in this case indicates that the formation of A from B (B ⟶ A) is favored in the equilibrium.

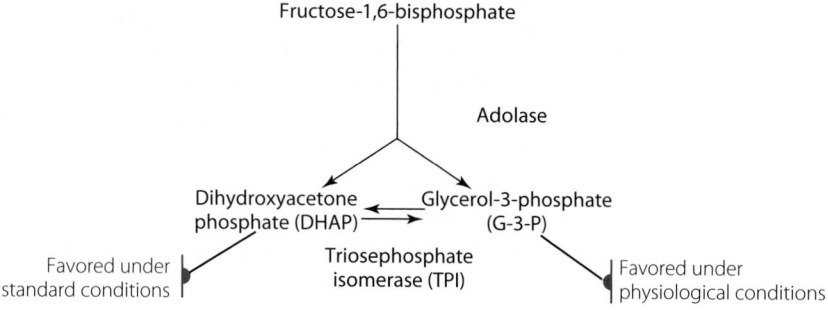

Figure 1.15 Example of a shift in the equilibrium by changing from standard conditions to physiological conditions.

Standard pH

For most compartments in the body, the pH is near neutral; for biochemical reactions, a standard pH value of 7 is adopted by convention. For human nutrition, the standard free energy change of reactions is designated $\Delta G^{0'}$. This book uses this notation.

Nonstandard Physiological Conditions

Physiologically standard conditions do not often exist. The difference between standard conditions and nonstandard conditions can explain why a reaction having a positive $\Delta G^{0'}$ can proceed exothermically ($-\Delta G^0$) in the cell. For example, consider the reaction catalyzed by the enzyme triosephosphate isomerase (TPI) shown in Figure 1.15. This particular reaction occurs in the glycolytic pathway through which glucose is converted to pyruvate. (The chemical structures and the pathway are discussed in detail in Chapter 3). In the glycolytic pathway, the enzyme aldolase produces 1 mol each of dihydroxyacetone phosphate (DHAP) and glyceraldehyde-3-phosphate (G-3-P) from 1mol of fructose-1,6-bisphosphate. Let us focus on the reaction that TPI catalyzes, which is an isomerization between the two products of the aldolase reaction. As explained in Chapter 3, only the G-3-P is further degraded in the subsequent reactions of glycolysis. This circumstance results in a substantially lower concentration of the G-3-P metabolite than of DHAP.

For this reaction, two important conditions within the cell deviate from "standard conditions": namely, the temperature is the temperature of the body, ~37°C (310 K), and neither the G-3-P nor DAHP are at 1.0 mol/L concentrations. The value of $\Delta G^{0'}$ for the reaction DHAP (reactant) $\longrightarrow$ G-3-P (product) is +1,830 cal/mol (+7,657 J/mol), indicating that under standard conditions the formation of DHAP is preferred over the formation of G-3-P. If we assume that the cellular concentration of DHAP is 50 times that of G-3-P because G-3-P is further metabolized, ΔG^0 for the reaction is calculated to be equal to −577 cal/mol (−2,414 J/mol). The negative ΔG^0 shows that the reaction to form G-3-P is favored, as shown, despite the positive $\Delta G^{0'}$ for this reaction.

The Role of High-Energy Phosphate in Energy Storage

The preceding section addressed the fundamental principle of free energy changes in chemical reactions and the fact that the cell obtains this chemical free energy through the catabolism of nutrient molecules. It also stated that this energy must somehow be used to drive the various energy-requiring processes and anabolic reactions so important in normal cell function. This section explains how ATP can be used as a universal source of energy to drive reactions. Examples of very high-energy phosphate compounds are shown in Figure 1.16.

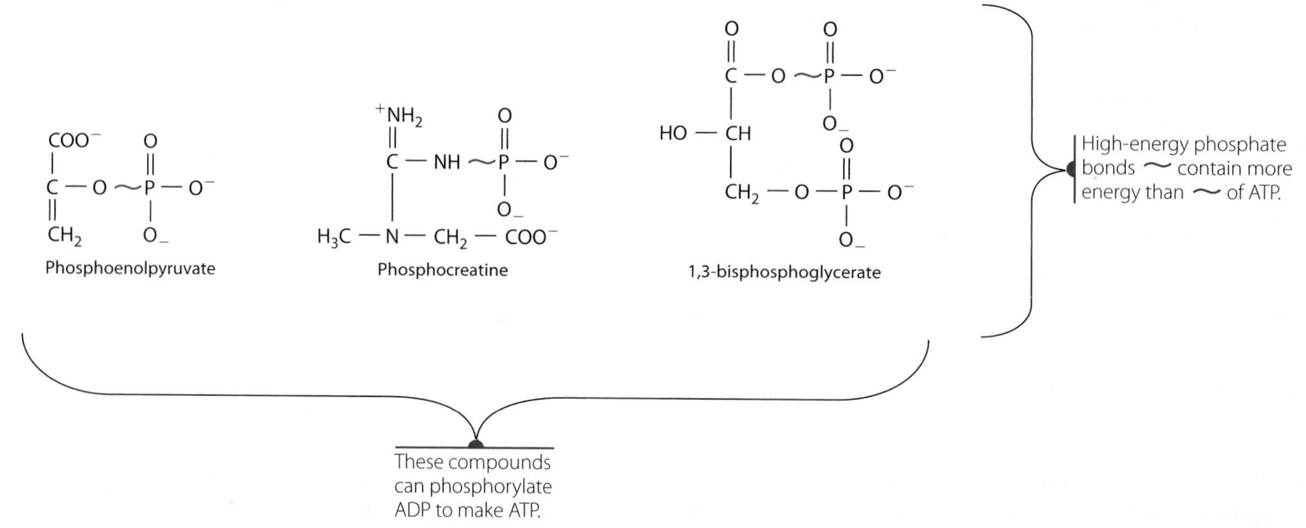

Figure 1.16 Examples of very high-energy phosphate compounds.

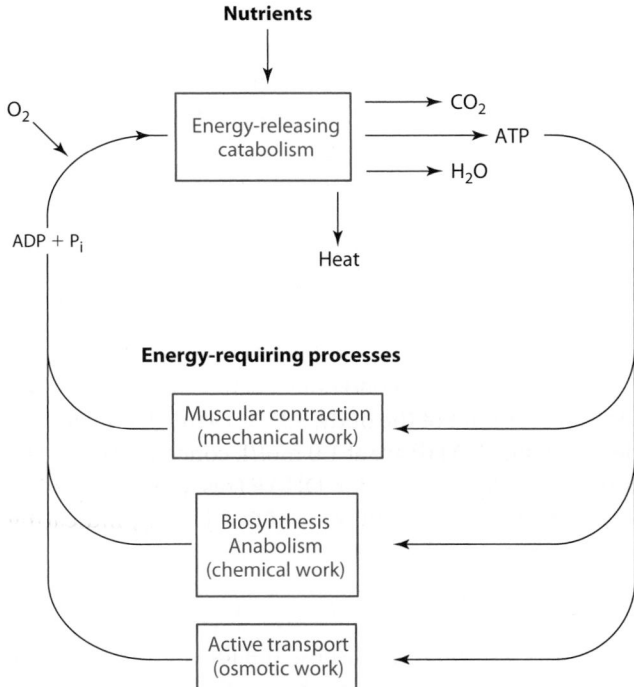

Figure 1.17 An illustration of how ATP is generated from the coupling of ADP and phosphate through the oxidative catabolism of nutrients and how it in turn is used for energy-requiring processes.

Phosphoenolpyruvate and 1,3-diphosphoglycerate are components of the oxidative pathway of glucose (Chapter 3), and phosphocreatine is a storage form of high-energy phosphate available to replenish ATP in muscle. The hydrolysis of the phosphate anhydride bonds of ATP can liberate the stored chemical energy when needed. ATP thus can be thought of as an energy reservoir, serving as the major linking intermediate between energy-releasing and energy-demanding chemical reactions in the cell. In nearly all cases, the energy stored in ATP is released by the enzymatic hydrolysis of the anhydride bond connecting the β- and γ-phosphates in the molecule (Figure 1.12). The products of this hydrolysis are adenosine diphosphate (ADP) and inorganic phosphate (P_i). In certain instances, the free phosphate group is transferred to various acceptors, a reaction that activates the acceptors to higher energy levels. The involvement of ATP as a link between the energy-releasing and energy-requiring cellular reactions and processes is summarized in Figure 1.17.

Coupled Reactions in the Transfer of Energy

Some reactions require energy, and others yield energy. The coupling of these reactions makes it possible for a pathway to continue. The oxidation of glucose in the glycolysis pathway demonstrates the importance of coupled reactions in metabolism. An understanding of how chemical energy is transformed from macronutrients (the carbohydrate, protein, fat, and alcohol in food) to storage forms (such as ATP), and how the stored energy is used to synthesize needed compounds for the body, is fundamental to the study of human nutrition. These topics are covered in this section as well as throughout this book. The $\Delta G^{0'}$ value for the phosphate bond hydrolysis of ATP is intermediate between those of certain high-energy phosphate compounds and compounds that possess relatively low-energy phosphate esters. ATP's central position on the energy scale lets it serve as an intermediate carrier of phosphate groups. ADP can accept the phosphate groups from high-energy phosphate donor molecules and then, as ATP, transfer them to lower-energy receptor molecules. Two examples of this transfer are shown in Figure 1.18. By receiving the phosphate groups, the acceptor molecules become activated to a higher energy level, from which they can undergo subsequent reactions such as entering the glycolysis pathway. The end result is the transfer of chemical energy from donor molecules through ATP to receptor molecules. The second example is the transfer of a P_i group from creatine phosphate to ADP. Creatine phosphate serves as a ready reservoir to renew ATP levels quickly, particularly in muscle.

If a given quantity of energy is released in an exothermic reaction, the same amount of energy must be added to the system for that reaction to be driven in the reverse direction. For example, hydrolysis of the phosphate ester bond of glucose-6-phosphate liberates 3,300 cal/mol (13.8 kJ/mol) of energy, and the reverse reaction, in which the phosphate is added to glucose to form glucose-6-phosphate, necessitates the input of 3,300 cal/mol (13.8 kJ/mol). These reactions can be expressed in terms of their

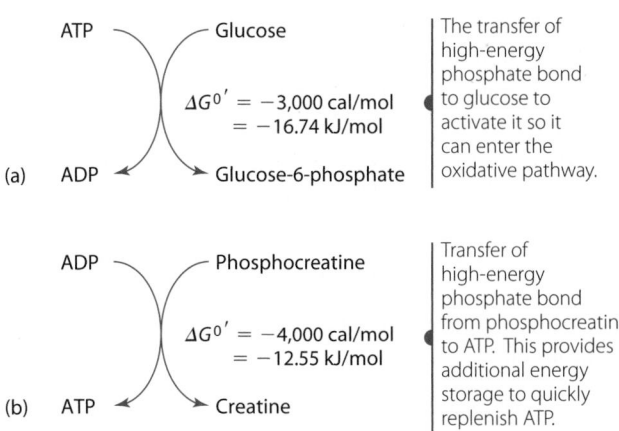

Figure 1.18 Examples of high-energy phosphate bonds being transferred.

G-6-P $\xrightarrow[\Delta G^{0'} = -3,300 \text{ cal/mol} (-13.8 \text{ kJ/mol})]{}$ Glucose + P_i

G-6-P $\xleftarrow[\Delta G^{0'} = +3,300 \text{ cal/mol} (+13.8 \text{ kJ/mol})]{}$ Glucose + P_i

Forward reaction favored

The hydrolysis of glucose-6-phosphate (G-6-P) to glucose and P_i has a negative $\Delta G^{0'}$ and is favored. The reverse reaction is not energetically favored.

ATP $\xrightarrow[\Delta G^{0'} = -7,300 \text{ cal/mol} (-30.54 \text{ kJ/mol})]{}$ ADP + P_i

ATP $\xleftarrow[\Delta G^{0'} = +7,300 \text{ cal/mol} (+30.54 \text{ kJ/mol})]{}$ ADP + P_i

The hydrolysis of ATP to ADP and P_i has a large negative $\Delta G^{0'}$ and is favored. The reverse reaction occurs with the electron transport chain to provide the energy needed.

Glucose + ATP $\xrightarrow[\Delta G^{0'} = -4,000 \text{ cal/mol} (-16.7 \text{ kJ/mol})]{}$ G-6-P + ADP

Coupled reaction favored

The coupled reaction phosphorylating glucose and hydrolyzing ATP is energetically favored, with a negative $\Delta G^{0'}$ of 4,000 cal/mol.

Figure 1.19 Exothermic reactions.

standard free energy changes as shown in Figure 1.19. To phosphorylate glucose, the reaction must be coupled with the hydrolysis of ATP, which provides the necessary energy. The additional energy from the reaction is dissipated as heat.

The addition of phosphate to a molecule is called a phosphorylation reaction. It generally is accomplished by the enzymatic transfer of the terminal phosphate group of ATP to the molecule, rather than by the addition of free phosphate as suggested in Figure 1.19. The reverse reaction is hypothetical, designed only to illustrate the energy requirement for phosphorylation of the glucose molecule. In fact, the enzymatic phosphorylation of glucose by ATP is the first reaction glucose undergoes upon entering the cell. This reaction promotes glucose to a higher energy level, from which it may be indirectly incorporated into glycogen as stored carbohydrate or systematically oxidized for energy. Phosphorylation therefore can be viewed as occurring in two reaction steps:

1 hydrolysis of ATP to ADP and phosphate

2 addition of the phosphate to the substrate (glucose) molecule

A net energy change for the two reactions coupled together is shown in Figure 1.19. The net $\Delta G^{0'}$ for the coupled reaction is –4,000 cal/mol (16.7 kJ/mol).

The significance of these coupled reactions cannot be overstated. They show that even though energy is consumed in the endothermic formation of glucose-6-phosphate from glucose and phosphate, the energy released by the ATP hydrolysis is sufficient to force (or drive) the endothermic reaction that "costs" only 3,300 cal/mol. The coupled reactions result in 4,000 cal/mol (16.7 kJ/mol) left over. The reaction is catalyzed by the enzyme hexokinase or glucokinase, both of which hydrolyze the ATP and transfer the phosphate group to glucose. The enzyme brings the ATP and the glucose into close proximity, reducing the activation energy of the reactants and facilitating the phosphate group transfer. The overall reaction, which results in activating glucose at the expense of ATP, is energetically favorable, as evidenced by its high, negative standard free energy change.

Reduction Potentials

As we will see when we discuss the formation of ATP in Chapter 3, ATP is formed in the electron transport chain after the macronutrients are oxidized. To better understand these oxidations and reductions, you need to understand reduction potentials. The energy to synthesize ATP becomes available following a sequence of individual reduction-oxidation (redox) reactions along the electron transport chain, with each component having a characteristic ability to donate and accept electrons. The released energy is used in part to synthesize ATP from ADP and phosphate. The tendency of a compound to donate and to receive electrons is expressed in terms of its **standard reduction potential,** $E_{0'}$. The more negative the values of $E_{0'}$ are, the greater the ability of the compound to donate electrons, whereas increasingly positive values signify an increasing tendency to accept electrons. The reducing capacity of a compound (its tendency to donate H^+ and electrons) can be expressed by the $E_{0'}$ value of its half-reaction, also called the compound's electromotive potential.

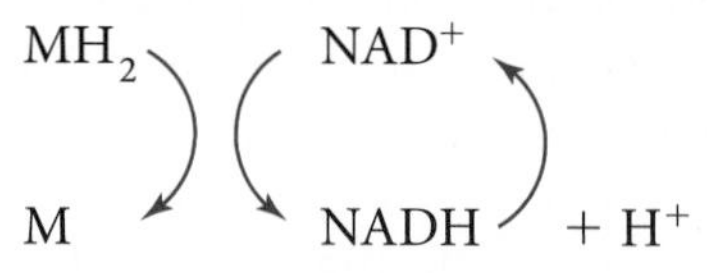

$$MH_2 \quad \rangle \langle \quad NAD^+$$
$$M \qquad NADH + H^+$$

Free energy changes accompany the transfer of electrons between electron donor–acceptor pairs of compounds and are related to the measurable electromotive force of the electron flow. Remember that *in electron transfer, an electron donor reduces the acceptor, and in the process the electron donor becomes oxidized. Consequently, the acceptor, as it is reduced, oxidizes the donor.* The quantity of energy released is directly proportional to the difference in the standard reduction potentials, $\Delta E_{0'}$, between the partners of the redox pair. The free energy of a redox reaction and the $\Delta E_{0'}$ of the interacting compounds are related by the expression

$$\Delta G^{0'} = -nF\Delta E_{0'}$$

where $\Delta G^{0'}$ is the standard free energy change in calories, n is the number of electrons transferred, and F is a constant called the Faraday (23,062 cal absolute volt equivalent).

An example of a reduction-oxidation reaction that occurs within the electron transport system is the transfer of hydrogen atoms and electrons from NADH through the flavin mononucleotide (FMN)–linked enzyme NADH dehydrogenase to oxidized coenzyme Q (CoQ). The half-reactions and $E_{0'}$ values for each of these reactions follow:

$$NADH + H^+ \longrightarrow NAD^+ + 2H^+ + 2e^-$$

$$E_{0'} = -0.32 \text{ volt}$$

$$CoQH_2 \longrightarrow CoQ + 2H^+ + 2e^-$$

$$E_{0'} = +0.04 \text{ volt}$$

Because the NAD^+ system has a relatively more negative $E_{0'}$ value than the CoQ system, NAD^+ has a greater reducing potential than the CoQ system because electrons tend to flow toward the system with the more positive $E_{0'}$. The reduction of CoQ by NADH therefore is predictable, and the coupled reaction, linked by the FMN of NADH dehydrogenase, can be written as follows:

NADH + H$^+$ FMN   CoQH$_2$

$E_0' = -0.32$ volt $E_0' = +0.04$ volt

NAD$^+$ FMNH$_2$ CoQ

$$\Delta E_{0'} = 0.36 \text{ volt}$$

Inserting this value for $\Delta E_{0'}$ into the energy equation gives

$$\Delta G^{0'} = -2(23{,}062)(0.36) = -16{,}604 \text{ cal/mol}$$

The amount of energy liberated from this single reduction-oxidation reaction within the electron transport chain therefore is more than enough to phosphorylate ADP to ATP, which, as you will recall, requires approximately 7,300 cal/mol (35.7 kJ).

SUMMARY

This brief walk through the cell—beginning with its outer surface, the plasma membrane, and moving into its innermost part, where the nucleus is located—provides a view of how this living entity functions. Characteristics of the cell that seem particularly notable are these:

- The flexibility of the plasma membrane in adjusting or reacting to its environment while protecting the rest of the cell as it monitors what may pass into or out of the cell. Prominent in the membrane's reaction to its environment are the receptor proteins, which are synthesized on the rough endoplasmic reticulum and moved through the Golgi apparatus to their intended site on the plasma membrane.

- The communication among the various components of the cell made possible through the cytoplast, with its microtrabecular network, and also through the endoplasmic reticulum and Golgi apparatus. The networking is such that communications flow not only among components within the cell but also between the nucleus and the plasma membrane.

- The efficient division of labor among the cell components (organelles). Each component has its own specific functions to perform, with little overlap. Furthermore, much evidence is accumulating to support the concept of an "assembly line" not only in oxidative phosphorylation on the inner membrane of the mitochondrion but also in almost all operations, wherever they occur.

- The superb management exercised by the nucleus to ensure that all the proteins needed for smooth operation are synthesized. The proteins needed as recognition markers, receptors, transport vehicles, and catalysts (enzymes) are available and located in the appropriate place in the cell as needed.

- The fact that, like all living things, cells must die a natural death. This programmed process is called apoptosis, a particularly attractive focus of current research. The removal of a dead cell's contents without any contents escaping into the extracellular fluid is an important role of the apoptotic process.

Despite the efficiency of the cell, it is still not a totally self-sufficient unit. Its continued operation is contingent on receiving appropriate and sufficient nutrients. Nutrients needed include not only those that can be used to produce immediate metabolic energy (ATP) but also those stored as chemical energy. Most of the stored chemical energy is needed to maintain normal body temperature (released as heat energy). About 40% of the stored energy is conserved in the form of high-energy phosphate bonds, principally ATP. The ATP can, in turn, activate various substrates by phosphorylation to higher energy levels from which they can undergo metabolism by specific enzymes. The exothermic hydrolysis of the ATP phosphate is sufficient to drive the endothermic phosphorylation, thereby completing the energy transfer from nutrient to metabolite. The oxidative pathways for the macronutrients (carbohydrate, fat, protein, and alcohol) provide a continuous flow of energy for maintaining heat and replenishing ATP. The cell also needs nutrients required as building blocks for structural macromolecules. In addition, the cell must have an adequate supply of the so-called regulatory nutrients (i.e., vitamins, minerals, and water).

With a view of the structure of the "typical cell," the division of labor among cellular component parts, and the location within the cell where many of the key metabolic reactions necessary to continue life take place, we can now consider in subsequent chapters how the cell receives its nourishment and how the nutrients are metabolized.

References Cited

1. Berdanier CD. Role of membrane lipids in metabolic regulation. Nutr Rev. 1988; 46:145–49.
2. Edlin M. The state of lipid rafts: from model cell membranes. Annu Rev Biophys Biomol Structure. 2003; 32:257–83.
3. Belting M, Wittrup A. Nanotubes, exosomes, and nucleic acid-binding peptides provide novel mechanisms of intercellular communication in eukaryotic cells: implications in health and disease. J Cell Biol. 2008; 183:1187–91.
4. Karp G. Cell and Molecular Biology: Concepts and Experiments. 6th ed. New York: John Wiley & Sons, Inc. 2010.
5. Young P. Mom's mitochondria may hold mutation. Sci News. 1988; 134:706.
6. Baluska F, Volkmann D, Barlow P. Nuclear components with microtubule-organizing properties in multicellular eukaryotes: functional and evolutionary considerations. Int Rev Cytol. 1997; 175:91–135.
7. Nogales E. Structural insights into microtubule function. Annu Rev Biochem. 2000; 69:277–302.
8. Garrett R, Grisham C. Biochemistry, 4th ed. Boston: Brooks/Cole. 2010.
9. Chakravarty K, Cassutoh H, Reshef L, Hanson R W. Factors that control the tissue-specific transcription of the gene for phosphoenolpyruvate carboxykinase-C. Crit Rev Biochem Molec Biol. 2005; 40:129–54.
10. Yabaluri N, Bashyam MD. Hormonal regulation of gluconeogenic gene transcription in the liver. J Biosci. 2010; 35:473–84.
11. Griffiths G, Simons K. The trans Golgi network: sorting at the exit site of the Golgi complex. Science. 1986; 234:438–43.
12. Teasdale R, Jackson M. Signal-mediated sorting of membrane proteins between the endoplasmic reticulum and the Golgi apparatus. Annu Rev Cell Dev Biol. 1996; 12:27–54.
13. Mihara K. Cell biology: moving inside membranes. Nature. 2003; 424:505–6.
14. Neupert W. Protein import into mitochondria. Annu Rev Biochem. 1997; 66:863–917.
15. Wickner WT, Lodish JT. Multiple mechanisms of protein insertion into and across membranes. Science. 1985; 230:400–07.
16. Barritt GJ. Networks of extracellular and intracellular signals. In: Communication within Animal Cells. Oxford, England: Oxford University Press. 1992 pp. 1–19.
17. Marx JL. A potpourri of membrane receptors.Science. 1985; 230:649–51.
18. Nagata, S. Apoptosis and autoimmune disease. Ann NY Acad Sci. 2010; 10–16.
19. Liu J, Lin M, Yu J, et al. Targeting apoptotic and autophagic pathways for cancer therapeutics. J Canlet. 2011; 300:105–14.
20. Seo AY, Joseph AM, Dutta D, et al. New insights into the role of mitochondria in aging: mitochondrial dynamics and more. J Cell Sci. 2010; 123:2533–42.
21. Mevorach D, Trahtemberg U, Krispin A, et al. What do we mean when we write "senescence," "apoptosis," "necrosis," or "clearance of dying cells"? Ann NY Acad Sci. 2010; 1209:1–9.
22. Harr MW, Distelhorst CW. Apoptosis and autophagy: decoding calcium signals that mediate life or death. Cold Spring Harb Perspect Biol. 2010; 2a005579:1–18.
23. Yan N, Shi Y. Mechanisms of apoptosis through structural biology. Annu Rev Cell Dev Biol. 2005; 21:35–56.
24. Bueler H. Mitochondrial dynamics, cell death and the pathogenesis of Parkinson's disease. Apopotosis. 2010; 15:1336–53.
25. Jiang X, Wang X. Cytochrome c-mediated apoptosis. Annu Rev Biochem. 2004; 73:87–106.
26. Noy N. Between death and survival: retinoic acid in regulation of apoptosis. Ann Rev Nutr. 2010; 30:201–17.
27. Diker-Cohen T, Koren R, Ravid A. Programed cell death of stressed keratinocytes and its inhibition by vitamin D: the role of death and survival signaling pathways. Apoptosis. 2006; 11:519–34.

Suggested Readings

Barritt GJ. Networks of extracellular and intracellular signals. In: Communication within Animal Cells. Oxford, England: Oxford University Press. 1992 pp. 1–19.
Karp G. Cell and Molecular Biology: Concepts and Experiments. 6th ed. New York: John Wiley & Sons, Inc. 2010. *An update text providing much additional detail on subjects covered in the chapter.*
Masters C, Crane D. The Peroxisome: A Vital Organelle. Cambridge, England: Cambridge University Press. 1995. *A clearly written overview of the multifaceted functions of this important organelle.*

Web Sites

www.nlm.nih.gov
National Library of Medicine: MEDLINE
www.nmsociety.org
The Nutrition and Metabolism Society is a growing organization dedicated to the science of nutrition and metabolism.
www.clinchem.org
Clinical Chemistry; Journal of the American Association for Clinical Chemistry.

NUTRITIONAL GENOMICS: A NEW PERSPECTIVE ON FOOD, BY RUTH DEBUSK, PhD, RD

Nutritional genomics is concerned with gene-environment interactions. This emerging discipline uses genetic technology to study the mechanisms by which genes and environmental factors communicate and the functional consequences of such interactions. A major focus of current research is the influence of these interactions on human health. Among the anticipated successes that will flow from nutritional genomics research is the ability to identify effective approaches for the management and prevention of diet-related disease.

One fundamental biological principle underlying gene-environment interactions is critically important to the functional ability, and thereby health, of living organisms: The information contained within a gene, when translated into the amino acid sequence of a protein, is directly related to the functional capacity of the organism. For example, the gene *INS* encodes the information needed to make the protein hormone insulin. Once synthesized, insulin plays a key role in the entry of glucose into muscle cells, where it can supply cellular energy. In the absence of insulin or in the presence of an insulin protein whose function is impaired, glucose is not able to enter cells as needed and diabetes results.

In a second example, the enzyme 5,10-methylene-tetrahydrofolate reductase catalyzes the conversion of 5,10-methylenetetrahydrofolate to 5-methyltetrahydrofolate, the active form of the B vitamin folate. This enzyme is encoded by the *MTHFR* gene. In individuals with a variation in this gene, the activity of the enzyme is impaired and the dietary requirement for folate is elevated as compared with the Dietary Reference Intake level typically recommended. By supplying higher levels of folate in the diet, food is able to "rescue" an individual from his or her genetic limitation in the *MTHFR* gene. Thus food, in addition to providing gustatory and social pleasure, is a powerful environmental factor in terms of communicating with the genetic material and influencing biological responses.

NUTRIGENETICS, NUTRIGENOMICS, AND NUTRITIONAL EPIGENETICS

Nutritional genomics encompasses the subdisciplines of nutrigenetics, nutrigenomics, and nutritional epigenetics. The previously mentioned *INS* and *MTHFR* examples describe the biological outcomes of a change in the deoxyribonucleic acid (DNA) (a "gene variant") and are examples of nutrigenetics. This subdiscipline is concerned with detecting gene variants within an individual, discovering their effect on function, and identifying which environmental factors interact with those variants to trigger dysfunction or disease. The expectation is that, as was seen with the *INS* and *MTHFR* gene variants, the presence of a variant potentially alters the individual's goodness-of-fit with his or her environment compared with someone who does not have the variant. This information can provide the clinician with clues as to the individual's genetic susceptibilities that increase the risk of disease and which foods and other environmental factors to avoid.

Examples abound of gene variants that convey a latent genetic susceptibility to developing a disease state that manifests only upon exposure to a specific food. Food allergies, intolerances, and sensitivities provide interesting examples. Immunoglobulin E (IgE)—mediated food allergy is one such example in which a genetic susceptibility lies dormant until triggered by the interaction with an offending food. With appropriate nutrigenetic testing, it is possible to know in advance that a person is at risk of potentially deadly anaphylaxis from certain foods. Nutrigenetics can also help to eliminate the trial-and-error aspects of food intolerances. Lactose intolerance is a case in point. Whether the production of lactase, the enzyme responsible for digesting the milk sugar lactose, persists beyond childhood is genetically determined and varies by population. For Caucasians of northern European descent, lactase persistence and lifelong lactose tolerance is the norm and results from a single nucleotide change in the lactase (*LCT*) gene[1]. It is presumed that other food intolerances are also genetically based and that their early detection will enable diets to be tailored to the individual's metabolic capabilities.

Celiac disease is similarly genetically determined but environmentally triggered, can manifest at any stage in the life cycle, and is characterized by gastrointestinal inflammation in response to the gluten component in wheat, barley, and rye. This disorder is estimated to occur at a frequency of 1 in 133–200 individuals, depending upon the study population [2–5]. Of the gene variants associated with the development of celiac disease, changes in the *HLA-DQ2* and *HLA-DQ8* genes have been identified as being necessary but not sufficient for the development of the disorder [6]. Being able to detect these variants prenatally or at least early in the postnatal period can prevent the infant from developing the disease. Failure to recognize celiac susceptibility and prevent its occurrence through lifelong adherence to a gluten-free diet can result in severe digestive tract inflammation, intestinal tract malignancies, malabsorption and, ultimately, severe malnutrition.

Nutrigenomics is another subdiscipline of nutritional genomics. This subdiscipline is concerned with identifying environmental factors that have an effect on the expression of genes, identifying which genes respond to which environmental factors, defining the mechanisms involved, and determining useful health-related applications of these interactions. Nutrigenomics is of interest from a diet-disease perspective because it holds the promise of using food in a targeted fashion, beyond food's ability to supply the raw materials for cellular function. If, for example, an individual has a susceptibility to chronic inflammation, the clinician may recommend that he eat a diet that supplies sufficient omega-3 fats to reduce the expression of genes that code for inflammatory cytokines, thereby blunting the inflammatory response.

The *GST* gene that encodes glutathione-S-tranferase, an enzyme that functions in the Phase II biotransformation of lipid-soluble toxins into water-soluble forms that can be excreted, exemplifies both nutrigenetics and nutrigenomics. Individuals whose genome includes a variant in the *GST* gene will be impaired in their ability to protect against toxins and their detrimental effects. The *GST* variant is an example of nutrigenetics, in that it illustrates the effect of having an impaired Phase II enzyme and its consequences to biotransformation. Impaired biotransformation can lead to disease for an individual regularly exposed to an environment with an elevated level of toxic chemicals.

The *GST* example also serves as an example of nutrigenomics. In humans there are two additional *GST* genes that encode similar enzymes that can compensate for the faulty gene. The expression of these additional *GST* genes can be switched on by glucosinolates, sulfur-containing metabolites formed from the digestion of cruciferous vegetables such as broccoli and other members of the cabbage family. Nutrigenomics researchers are interested in identifying environmental factors that can increase the expression of other genes that can circumvent the limitation caused by a particular gene variant, such as those seen with the faulty *GST* gene. In this case, food is the environmental factor and glucosinolates are the bioactive components within food that can communicate with the genetic material and influence gene expression. Similarly Suhr and colleagues [7] have identified several phytonutrients from food that confer chemoprotection by controlling gene expression. Additional discussion of the role of bioactives in influencing gene expression can be found in the "Bioactive Food Components" section.

A third subdiscipline of nutritional genomics is nutritional epigenetics, which represents yet another mechanism for regulating gene expression. Epigenetics is the study of changes in gene expression that do not involve changes in the nucleotide sequence of DNA. Instead, chemical "tags" that can affect gene expression are added (to the DNA or to the histone proteins associated with DNA). One common type of epigenetic regulation of gene expression involves opening and closing DNA to control its accessibility to being transcribed. DNA that is tightly compacted is not available to be transcribed and, thus, expressed. The addition and removal of acetyl groups from the histone proteins that aid DNA in condensing and decondensing is a common mechanism for controlling gene expression. A second mechanism, the addition and removal of methyl groups to cytosine-containing nucleotides within the DNA sequence, can similarly control gene expression. The presence of methyl groups typically silences gene expression. In both instances, the ultimate source of these tags—that is, the acetyl and methyl groups—is the diet. The end result is the regulation of gene expression, which makes nutritional epigenetics yet another mechanism for fine-tuning the control of this process. Nutritional epigenetics is particularly important during development, during cellular differentiation, and in maintaining the distinct pattern of gene expression that characterizes the myocyte in contrast to the hepatocyte, for example.

Further, a cell's pattern of tags is heritable and can be passed to subsequent generations. From the work of Wolff and colleagues [8], Waterland and Jirtle [9], and Waterland [10], it is clear that diet plays a major role in epigenetic patterning. Although there are currently more questions than answers concerning epigenetics and its associated mechanisms and consequences, nutrition can be expected to factor prominently and will be an important determinant in the ability to reach one's genetic potential and optimal health [11,12].

Nutritional genomics is an emerging field and considerable research is needed to generate well-documented associations among genes, diseases, and food before this field will fully make its impact. Once the research foundation is in place, the expectation is that nutritional genomics will be the source of effective therapeutic approaches to diet-related disease.

GENETIC VARIATION AND FUNCTION

As described previously, faulty *INS* and *MTHFR* genes have functional consequences for the individual. These detrimental variations in the *INS* and *MTHFR* genes come about through changes (mutations) in the nucleotide sequence of the DNA over evolutionary time and are called gene variants. The vast majority of gene variants result from a change in one nucleotide subunit of DNA. When a change in a single nucleotide occurs frequently in a population, it is referred to as a "single nucleotide polymorphism" or "SNP" (pronounced "snip").

It is estimated that SNPs comprise approximately 10% of the human genome. SNPs are the basis for the uniqueness of each individual, and some result in differences in observable traits, such as hair color, eye color, or stature. The majority influence metabolic processes critical to the workings of the trillions of cells that comprise the human body and provide its functional abilities. When a SNP in the DNA results in a

change in the amino acid structure of the encoded protein such that the folding of the protein is altered in a way that negatively influences its function, the potential exists for dysfunction or disease to result. Although such changes are technically mutations (any change in the DNA sequence is a mutation), the term *gene variant* is typically used for those mutations whose impact on function is not sufficiently detrimental to cause disease by themselves. Such mutations are "silent" in their effect on function until they interact with one or more environmental factors. Thus it is not the existence of a change in the DNA but the impact of that change on function that is consequential.

Once a person's variants are known, a well-documented association has been demonstrated between the variant and a disease, and the mechanism by which the dysfunction is triggered has been identified, then developing a therapeutic strategy for countering the negative effect on function becomes possible. For example, the *VDR* gene codes for the vitamin D receptor that is needed for cells to absorb vitamin D. If one has a variant in the *VDR* gene that impairs the absorption of vitamin D, a therapeutic intervention might include increased exposure to sunlight, increased intake of vitamin D–containing foods, a vitamin D dietary supplement, or a combination of these approaches. Clinicians then have an effective approach for countering the genetic limitations of that individual to prevent or at least limit the severity of the dysfunction associated with particular gene variants.

Gene variants are detected using well-established genetic technology. Because each cell with a nucleus contains a full complement of the individual's genetic material, multiple sources of DNA samples exist, from white blood cells to secretions to swabs taken from the inside of the cheek. Swabbing the cheek is a noninvasive method that is increasingly used to obtain DNA for genetic testing. In the laboratory the DNA is extracted and amplified, and specific "probe" sequences with fluorescent dye attached are used to query whether a sample from an individual contains a particular gene variant. If it does, the fluorescent probe will bind to the sample DNA and can then be detected.

BIOACTIVE FOOD COMPONENTS

Bioactive food components were introduced in the discussion of nutrigenomics. Of keen interest to researchers are the mechanisms by which food influences gene expression. Lipophilic, small–molecular-weight molecules such as essential fatty acids, vitamin A, and steroid molecules are able to traverse the cellular and nuclear membranes. They subsequently interact with DNA by means of transcription factors, specialized proteins that bind to DNA in one region of the protein and in a second region are able to bind small–molecular-weight ligands. Many of these ligands originate with the diet and are capable of binding to one or more transcription factors and influencing gene expression. Expression may be activated or silenced fully or partially to meet the ever-changing needs of the cells.

Bioactives that are either too large or too hydrophilic to pass through the lipid bilayer of the cellular and nuclear

membranes communicate with the cell by interacting with cell surface receptors. Binding to the receptors triggers signal transduction, a cascade of events that typically leads to the translocation of a transcription factor to the nucleus, where it can then bind DNA and turn gene expression on or off, as appropriate.

The identification and isolation of bioactive food components is an active area of study within nutrigenomics. Bioactives may be traditional nutrients, such as vitamins or essential fatty acids, or nontraditional nutrients, such as the phytonutrients epigallocatechin-3-O-gallate from green tea, lycopene from tomatoes, and resveratrol from purple grape juice. Bioactive food components may also be potential toxins that enter the food supply inadvertently. In addition to the example of glucosinolates in cruciferous vegetables discussed previously, another bioactive food component that has positive implications for many inflammatory disease states is derived from linolenic acid, an essential fatty acid of the omega-3 class. This bioactive can modulate the expression of genes that promote inflammation, such as the *PPARG* (peroxisome proliferator-activated receptor gamma), *IL1* (interleukin 1), *IL6* (interleukin 6), and *COX2* (cyclooxygenase-2) genes [13,14].

The communication between bioactive food components and the genetic material is an intricate web of events by which cells adjust to the state of their environment. As the fund of knowledge about which bioactives affect which genes and influence which functions accumulates, diet therapy is expected to become increasingly effective because it will become possible to select specific foods to target particular mechanisms. Further, expect to see a movement away from general nutrient recommendations intended for the "average" person and toward recommendations personalized for the individual.

References Cited

1. Enattah NS, Sahi T, Savilahti E, et al. Identification of a variant associated with adult-type hypolactasia. Nat Genet. 2002; 30:233–37.

2. Fasano A, Berti I, Gerarduzzi T, et al. Prevalence of celiac disease in at-risk and not-at-risk groups in the United States: a large multicenter study. Arch Intern Med. 2003; 163:286–92.

3. Sollid LM, Lie BA. Celiac disease genetics: current concepts and practical applications. Clin Gastroenterol Hepatol. 2005; 3:843–51.

4. Ludvigsson JF, Montgomery SM, Ekbom A, et al. Small-intestinal histopathology and mortality risk in celiac disease. JAMA. 2009; 302:1171–78.

5. Rubio-Tapia A, Kyle RA, Kaplan EL, et al. Increased prevalence and mortality in undiagnosed celiac disease. Gastroenterology. 2009;137:88–93.

6. Romanos J, van Diemen CC, Nolte IM, et al. Analysis of HLA and non-HLA alleles can identify individuals at highrisk for celiac disease. Gastroenterology. 2009; 137:834–40.

7. SurhYJ, KunduJK, Na HK. Nrf2 as a master redox switch in turning on the cellular signaling involved in the induction of cytoprotective genes by some chemopreventive phytochemicals. Planta Med. 2008; 74:1526–39.

8. Cooney CA, Dave AA, Wolff GL. Maternal methyl supplements in mice affect epigenetic variation and DNA methylation of offspring. J Nutr. 2002; 197(suppl):S2392–S2400.

9. Waterland RA, Jirtlem RL. Early nutrition, epigenetic changes at transposons and imprinted genes, and enhanced susceptibility to adult chronic diseases. Nutrition. 2004; 20:63–68.

10. Waterland RA. Early environmental effects on epigenetic regulation in humans. Epigenetics. 2009; 4:523–25.

11. McKay JA, Mathers JC. Diet induced epigenetic changes and their implications for health. Acta Physiol (Oxf). 2011; 202:103–18.

12. Stover PJ, Caudill MA. Genetic and epigenetic contributions to human nutrition and health: managing genome-diet interactions. J Am Diet Assoc. 2008; 108:1480–87.

13. Massaro M, Scoditti E, Carluccio MA, et al. Omega-3 fatty acids, inflammation and angiogenesis: nutrigenomics effects as an explanation for anti-atherogenic and anti-inflammatory effects of fish and fish oils. J Nutrigenet Nutrigenomics. 2008; 1:4–23.

14. Wall R, Ross RP, Fitzgerald GF, et al. Fatty acids from fish: the anti-inflammatory potential of long-chain omega-3 fatty acids. Nutr Rev. 2010; 68:280–89.

Suggested Readings

Corella D, Ordovas JM. Nutrigenomics in cardiovascular medicine.Circ Cardiovasc Genet. 2009; 2:637–51.

Fenech M, El-Sohemy A, Cahill L, et al. Nutrigenetics and nutrigenomics: viewpoints on the current status and applications in nutrition research and practice. Nutrigenet Nutrigenomics. 2011; 4:69-89.

Kussmann M, Krause L, Siffert W. Nutrigenomics: where are we with genetic and epigenetic markers for disposition and susceptibility? Nutr Rev. 2010 Nov; 68(suppl 1):S38–47.

McKay JA, Mathers JC. Diet induced epigenetic changes and their implications for health. Acta Physiol (Oxf). 2011; 202:103–18.

Ordovás JM, Robertson R, Cléirigh EN. Gene-gene and gene-environment interactions defining lipid-related traits. Curr Opin Lipidol. 2011 Apr; 22:129–36.

Ordovás JM, Smith CE. Epigenetics and cardiovascular disease. Nat Rev Cardiol. 2010; 7:510–9.

Simopoulos AP: Nutrigenetics/nutrigenomics. Annu Rev Public Health. 2010; 31:53–68.

Smith CE, Ordovás JM. Fatty acid interactions with genetic polymorphisms for cardiovascular disease. Curr Opin Clin Nutr Metab Care. 2010; 13:139–44.

2

THE DIGESTIVE SYSTEM: MECHANISM FOR NOURISHING THE BODY

NUTRITION IS THE SCIENCE OF NOURISHMENT. Ingestion of foods and beverages provides the body with at least one, if not more, of the nutrients needed to nourish the body. The body needs six classes of nutrients: carbohydrate, lipid, protein, vitamins, minerals, and water. For the body to use the carbohydrate, lipid, protein, and some vitamins and minerals found in foods, the food must first be digested—in other words, the food first must be broken down mechanically and chemically. This process of digestion occurs in the digestive tract and, once complete, yields nutrients ready for absorption and use by the body.

THE STRUCTURES OF THE DIGESTIVE TRACT AND THE DIGESTIVE AND ABSORPTIVE PROCESSES

The digestive tract, approximately 16 feet in length, includes organs that comprise the gastrointestinal (GI) tract (also called the alimentary canal or gut) as well as certain accessory organs. The main structures of the digestive tract include the oral cavity, esophagus, and stomach (collectively referred to as the upper digestive tract), and the small and large intestines (called the lower digestive tract). The accessory organs include the pancreas, liver, and gallbladder. The accessory organs provide or store secretions that ultimately are delivered to the lumen of the digestive tract and aid in the digestive and absorptive processes. Figure 2.1 illustrates the digestive tract and accessory organs. Figure 2.2 provides a cross-sectional view of the gastrointestinal tract that shows the lumen (interior passageway) and the four main tunics, or layers, of the gastrointestinal tract:

- the mucosa
- the submucosa
- the muscularis externa
- the serosa, or adventitia

Some of these layers contain sublayers. The mucosa, the innermost layer, is made of three sublayers: the epithelium or epithelial lining, the lamina propria, and the muscularis mucosa. The mucosal epithelium, which lines the lumen of the gastrointestinal tract, is the surface that is in contact with nutrients in the food we eat. Exocrine and endocrine cells also are found among the epithelial cells of the mucosa. The exocrine cells secrete a variety of substances, such as enzymes and juices, into the lumen of the gastrointestinal tract, and the endocrine cells secrete various hormones into the blood. The lamina propria

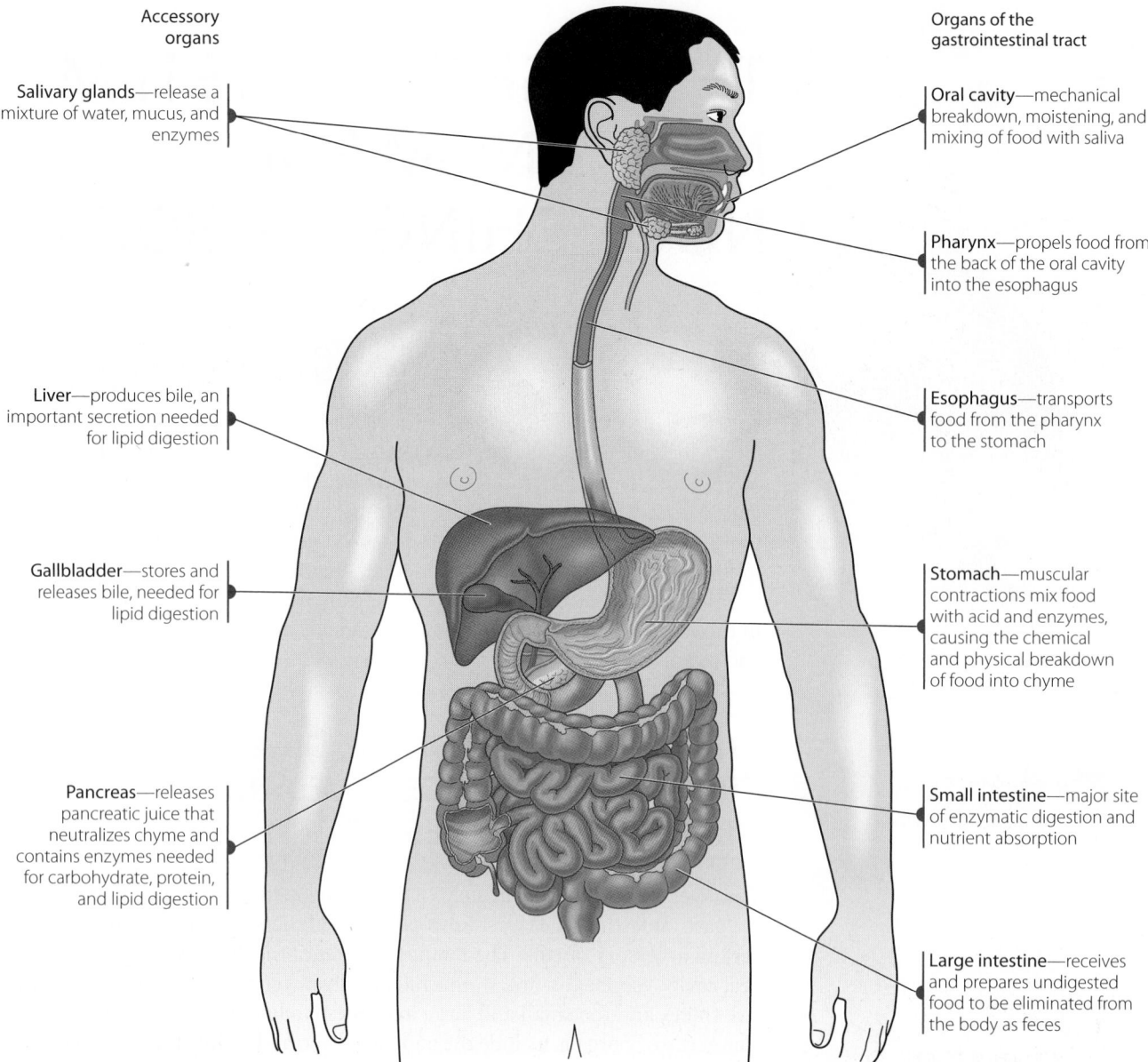

Accessory organs

Salivary glands—release a mixture of water, mucus, and enzymes

Liver—produces bile, an important secretion needed for lipid digestion

Gallbladder—stores and releases bile, needed for lipid digestion

Pancreas—releases pancreatic juice that neutralizes chyme and contains enzymes needed for carbohydrate, protein, and lipid digestion

Organs of the gastrointestinal tract

Oral cavity—mechanical breakdown, moistening, and mixing of food with saliva

Pharynx—propels food from the back of the oral cavity into the esophagus

Esophagus—transports food from the pharynx to the stomach

Stomach—muscular contractions mix food with acid and enzymes, causing the chemical and physical breakdown of food into chyme

Small intestine—major site of enzymatic digestion and nutrient absorption

Large intestine—receives and prepares undigested food to be eliminated from the body as feces

Figure 2.1 The digestive tract and its accessory organs.
Source: Beerman/McGuire, Nutritional Sciences, 1/e. © Cengage Learning.

lies below the epithelium and consists of connective tissue and small blood and lymphatic vessels. Lymphoid tissue is also found within the lamina propria. This lymphoid tissue contains a number of white blood cells, especially macrophages and lymphocytes, which provide protection against ingested microorganisms. The third sublayer of the mucosa, the muscularis mucosa, consists of a thin layer of smooth muscle.

Next to the mucosa is the submucosa. The submucosa, the second tunic or layer, is made up of connective tissue and more lymphoid tissue, and contains a network of nerves called the submucosal plexus, or plexus of Meissner. This plexus controls, in part, secretions from the mucosal glands and helps regulate mucosal movements and blood flow. The lymphoid tissue in the submucosa is similar to that found in the mucosa and protects the body against

foreign substances. The submucosa binds the first mucosal layer of the gastrointestinal tract to the muscularis externa, or third layer of the gastrointestinal tract.

The muscularis externa contains both circular and longitudinal smooth muscle, important for peristalsis, as well as the myenteric plexus, or plexus of Auerbach. This plexus controls the frequency and strength of contractions of the muscularis to regulate gastrointestinal motility.

The outermost layer, the serosa or adventitia, consists of connective tissue and the visceral peritoneum. The peritoneum is a membrane that surrounds the organs of the abdominal and pelvic cavities. In the abdominal cavity, the visceral peritoneum surrounds the stomach and intestine, and the parietal peritoneum lines the cavity walls. Their arrangement creates a double-layered membrane within the abdominal cavity. These membranes are

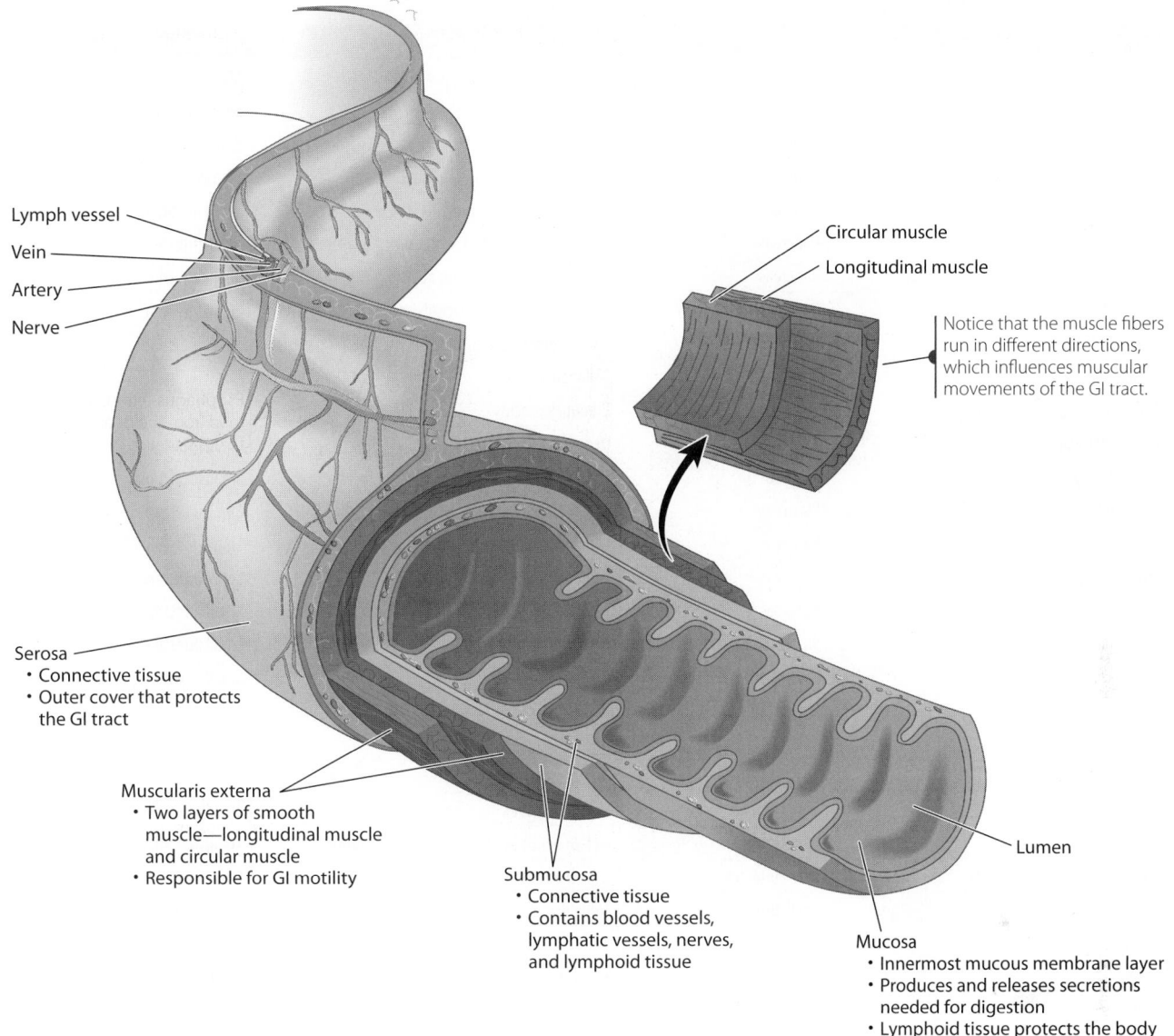

Figure 2.2 The sublayers of the small intestine.

Source: Beerman/McGuire, Nutritional Sciences, 1/e. © Cengage Learning.

somewhat permeable and highly vascularized. Between the two membranes is the peritoneal cavity. The selective permeability and the rich blood supply of peritoneal membranes allow the peritoneal cavity to be used in dialysis, an ultrafiltration process used to treat kidney failure.

The digestive process begins in the oral cavity and proceeds sequentially through the esophagus, stomach, small intestine, and finally into the colon (large intestine). The next subsections of this chapter describe the structures and digestive processes that occur in each of these parts of the digestive tract. Other sections include information on the structures and roles of the pancreas, liver, and gallbladder and the roles of a variety of enzymes. Table 2.1 provides an overview of some of the enzymes and zymogens (proenzymes or inactive enzymes, which must be chemically altered to function as an enzyme) that participate in digesting the nutrients in foods.

The Oral Cavity

The mouth and pharynx (or throat) constitute the oral cavity and provide the entryway to the digestive tract. On entering the mouth, food is chewed by the actions of the teeth and jaw muscles and is made ready for swallowing by mixing with secretions (saliva) released from the salivary glands. Three pairs of small, bilateral saliva-secreting salivary glands—the parotid, the submandibular, and the sublingual—are distributed throughout the lining of the oral cavity, along the jaw from the base of the ear to the chin (Figure 2.3). These glands are affected by the actions of the parasympathetic and sympathetic nervous systems. Secretions (about 1 L/day) from these glands constitute saliva. Specifically, the parotid glands secrete water, electrolytes (sodium, potassium, chloride), and enzymes. The submandibular and sublingual glands secrete

Table 2.1 Digestive Enzymes and Their Actions

Enzyme or Zymogen/Enzyme	Site of Secretion	Preferred Substrate(s)	Primary Site of Action
Salivary α amylase	Mouth	α (1-4) bonds in starch, dextrins	Mouth
Lingual lipase	Mouth	Triacylglycerol	Stomach, small intestine
Pepsinogen/pepsin	Stomach	Carboxyl end of phe, tyr, trp, met, leu, glu, asp	Stomach
Gastric lipase	Stomach	Triacylglycerol (mostly medium chain)	Stomach
Trypsinogen/trypsin	Pancreas	Carboxyl end of lys, arg	Small intestine
Chymotrypsinogen/chymotrypsin	Pancreas	Carboxyl end of phe, tyr, trp, met, asn, his	Small intestine
Procarboxypeptidase/carboxypeptidase A	Pancreas	C-terminal neutral amino acids	Small intestine
Carboxypeptidase B	Pancreas	C-terminal basic amino acids	Small intestine
Proelastase/elastase	Pancreas	Fibrous proteins	Small intestine
Collagenase	Pancreas	Collagen	Small intestine
Ribonuclease	Pancreas	Ribonucleic acids	Small intestine
Deoxyribonuclease	Pancreas	Deoxyribonucleic acids	Small intestine
Pancreatic α amylase	Pancreas	α (1-4) bonds, in starch, maltotriose	Small intestine
Pancreatic lipase and colipase	Pancreas	Triacylglycerol	Small intestine
Phospholipase	Pancreas	Lecithin and other phospholipids	Small intestine
Cholesterol esterase	Pancreas	Cholesterol esters	Small intestine
Retinyl ester hydrolase	Pancreas	Retinyl esters	Small intestine
Amino peptidases	Small intestine	N-terminal amino acids	Small intestine
Dipeptidases	Small intestine	Dipeptides	Small intestine
Nucleotidase	Small intestine	Nucleotides	Small intestine
Nucleosidase	Small intestine	Nucleosides	Small intestine
Alkaline phosphatase	Small intestine	Organic phosphates	Small intestine
Monoglyceride lipase	Small intestine	Monoglycerides	Small intestine
Alpha dextrinase or isomaltase	Small intestine	α (1-6) bonds in dextrins, oligosaccharides	Small intestine
Glucoamylase, glucosidase, and sucrase	Small intestine	α (1-4) bonds in maltose, maltotriose	Small intestine
Trehalase	Small intestine	Trehalose	Small intestine
Disaccharidases	Small intestine		Small intestine
Sucrase		Sucrose	
Maltase		Maltose	
Lactase		Lactose	

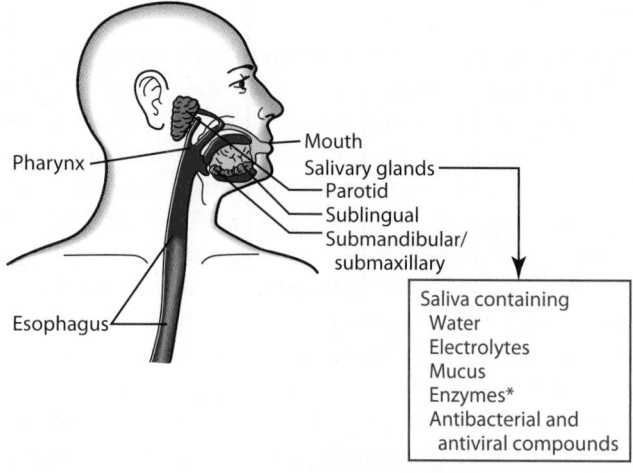

*Main enzyme in saliva is salivary amylase, which hydrolyzes α (1-4) bonds in starch.

Figure 2.3 Secretions of the oral cavity.

water, electrolytes, enzymes, and mucus. Saliva is primarily (99.5%) water, which helps dissolve foods. The principal enzyme of saliva is α amylase (also called ptyalin; Table 2.1). This enzyme hydrolyzes internal α (1-4) bonds within starch. A second digestive enzyme, lingual lipase, is produced by lingual serous glands on the tongue and in the back of the mouth. This enzyme hydrolyzes dietary triacylglycerols (triglycerides) in the stomach, but its activity both diminishes with age and is limited by the coalescing of the fats within the stomach. Activity of lingual lipase in infants against triacylglycerols in milk improves digestion of dietary fats. Mucus secretions found in saliva contain glycoproteins (compounds consisting of both carbohydrates and proteins). Mucus lubricates food and coats and protects the oral mucosa. Antibacterial and antiviral compounds, one example being the antibody IgA (immunoglobulin A), along with trace amounts of organic substances (such as urea) and other solutes (e.g., phosphates, bicarbonate), are also found in saliva.

The Esophagus

From the mouth, food, now mixed with saliva and called a bolus, is passed through the pharynx into the esophagus. The esophagus is about 10 inches long (Figure 2.1). The passage of the bolus of food from the oral cavity into the esophagus constitutes swallowing. Swallowing, which can be divided into several stages—voluntary, pharyngeal, and esophageal—is a reflex response initiated by a voluntary action and regulated by the swallowing center in the medulla of the brain. To swallow food, the esophageal sphincter relaxes, allowing the esophagus to open. Food then passes into the esophagus. Simultaneously, the larynx (part of the respiratory tract) moves upward, inducing the epiglottis to shift over the glottis. The closure of the glottis is important in keeping food from entering the trachea, which leads to the lungs. Once food is in the esophagus, the larynx shifts downward to allow the glottis to reopen.

When the bolus of food moves into and down the esophagus, both the striated (voluntary) muscle of the upper portion of the esophagus and the smooth (involuntary) muscle of the distal portion are stimulated by cholinergic (parasympathetic) nerves. The result is peristalsis, a progressive wavelike motion that moves the bolus through the esophagus into the stomach. The process usually takes less than 10 seconds.

At the lower (distal) end of the esophagus, just above the juncture with the stomach, lies the gastroesophageal sphincter, also called the lower esophageal sphincter (Figure 2.4). Calling it a sphincter may be a misnomer because no consensus exists about whether this particular muscle area is

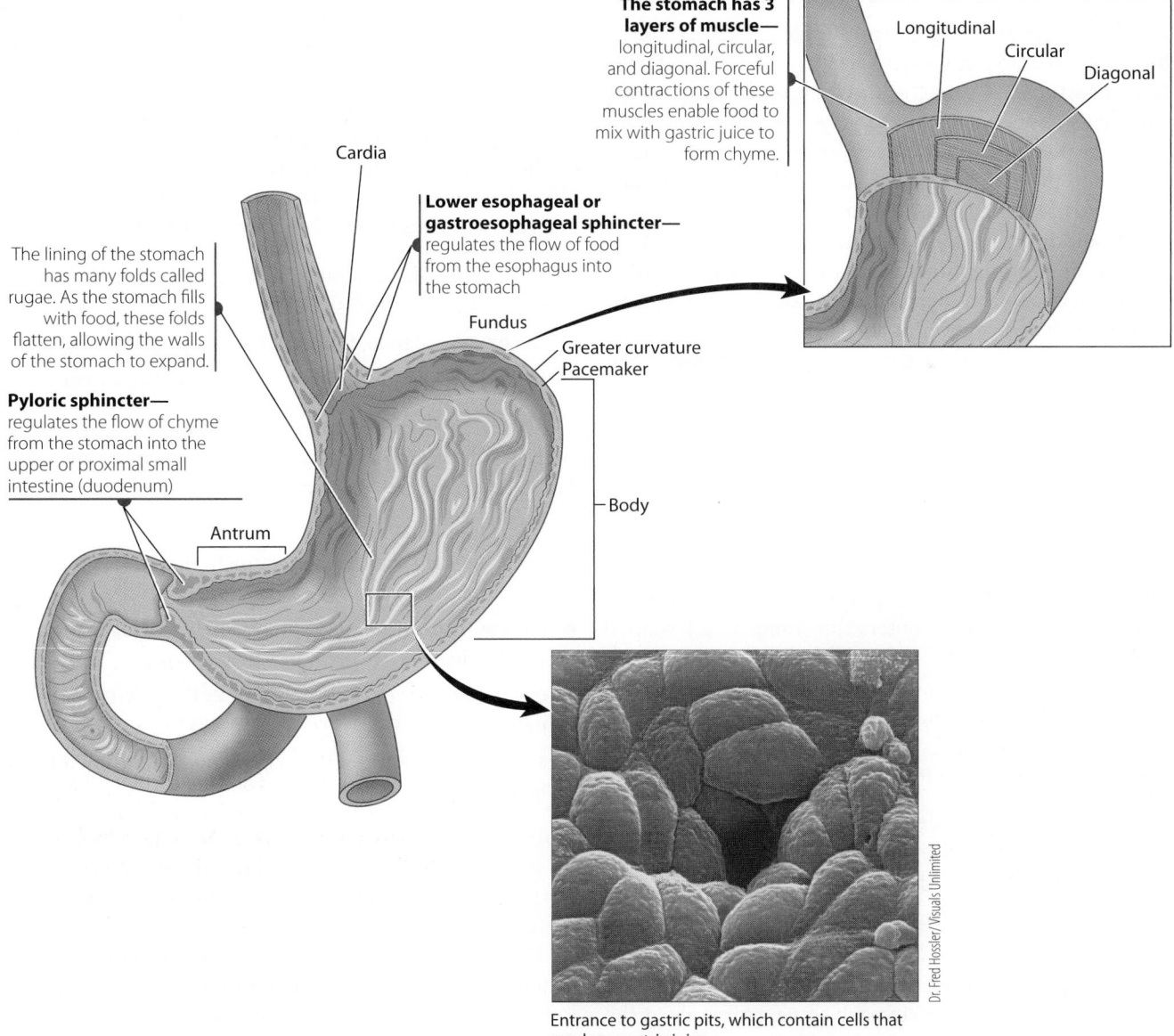

The stomach has 3 layers of muscle—longitudinal, circular, and diagonal. Forceful contractions of these muscles enable food to mix with gastric juice to form chyme.

Longitudinal

Circular

Diagonal

Cardia

Lower esophageal or gastroesophageal sphincter—regulates the flow of food from the esophagus into the stomach

Fundus

Greater curvature
Pacemaker

Body

The lining of the stomach has many folds called rugae. As the stomach fills with food, these folds flatten, allowing the walls of the stomach to expand.

Pyloric sphincter—regulates the flow of chyme from the stomach into the upper or proximal small intestine (duodenum)

Antrum

Dr. Fred Hossler/Visuals Unlimited

Entrance to gastric pits, which contain cells that produce gastric juice

Figure 2.4 Structure of the stomach.
Source: Beerman/McGuire, Nutritional Sciences, 1/e. © Cengage Learning.

sufficiently hypertrophied to constitute a true sphincter. Several sphincters or valves, which are circular muscles, are located throughout the digestive tract; these sphincters allow food to pass from one section of the gastrointestinal tract to another. On swallowing, the gastroesophageal sphincter pressure drops. This drop in gastroesophageal sphincter pressure relaxes the sphincter so that food may pass from the esophagus into the stomach.

Multiple mechanisms, including neural and hormonal, regulate gastroesophageal sphincter pressure. The musculature of the gastroesophageal sphincter has a tonic pressure that is normally higher than the intragastric pressure (the pressure within the stomach). This high tonic pressure at the gastroesophageal sphincter keeps the sphincter closed. Keeping this sphincter closed is important because it prevents gastroesophageal reflux, the movement of substances from the stomach back into the esophagus.

Selected Diseases and Conditions of the Esophagus

A person experiencing gastroesophageal reflux feels a burning sensation in the midchest, a condition referred to as heartburn. Gastric acid, when refluxed from the stomach and present in the esophagus, is an irritant to the esophageal mucosa. Repeated exposure of the esophageal mucosa to this gastric acid can irritate the esophagus and lead to esophagitis, or inflammation of the esophagus. Foods and food-related substances can indirectly affect gastroesophageal sphincter pressure and cause reflux. Smoking, chocolate, high-fat foods, alcohol, and carminatives such as peppermint and spearmint, for example, promote relaxation of the gastroesophageal sphincter and increase the likelihood of acid reflux into the esophagus. Gastroesophageal reflux disease, reflux esophagitis, and treatments for these conditions are described in the Perspective at the end of this chapter.

The Stomach

Once the bolus of food has passed through the gastroesophageal sphincter, it enters the stomach, a J-shaped organ located on the left side of the abdomen under the diaphragm. The stomach extends from the gastroesophageal sphincter to the duodenum, the upper or proximal section of the small intestine. The stomach contains four main regions (shown in Figure 2.4):

- The cardia region lies below the gastroesophageal sphincter and receives the swallowed food from the esophagus.
- The fundus lies adjacent or lateral to and above the cardia.
- The large central region of the stomach is called the body. The body of the stomach serves primarily as the reservoir for swallowed food and is the main production site for gastric juice.
- The antrum or distal pyloric portion of the stomach consists of the lower or distal one-third of the stomach.

The antrum grinds and mixes food with the gastric juices, thus forming chyme (a thick, semiliquid mass of partially digested food). The antrum also provides strong peristalsis for gastric emptying through the pyloric sphincter into the duodenum. The pyloric sphincter is found at the juncture of the stomach and duodenum.

The stomach begins mixing the food with gastric juices and enzymes using its circular, longitudinal, and oblique smooth muscles. It holds the partially digested chyme before releasing it in small quantities, at regular intervals, into the duodenum. The volume of the stomach when empty (resting) is about 50 mL (~2 oz), but on being filled it can expand to accommodate from 1 L to approximately 1.5 L (~37–52 oz) or more. When the stomach is empty, folds (called rugae, see Figure 2.4) present in all but the antrum section of the stomach are visible; however, when the stomach is full, the rugae disappear.

The digestive process is facilitated by gastric juices, which are produced in significant quantities by glands in the body of the stomach. Gastric juice is produced by three functionally different gastric glands, found within the gastric mucosa and submucosa of the stomach:

- the cardiac glands, found in a narrow rim at the juncture of the esophagus and the stomach
- the oxyntic glands, found in the body of the stomach
- the pyloric glands, located primarily in the antrum

Several cell types, which secrete different substances, may be found within a gastric gland, as shown in Figure 2.5. For example, some of the cells found in a gastric oxyntic gland include:

- neck (mucus) cells, located close to the surface mucosa, which secrete bicarbonate and mucus
- parietal (oxyntic) cells, which secrete hydrochloric acid and intrinsic factor
- chief (peptic or zymogenic) cells, which secrete pepsinogens
- enteroendocrine cells, which secrete a variety of hormones

Unlike the oxyntic glands, the cardiac glands contain no parietal cells. The pyloric glands contain mucus and parietal cells, as well as enteroendocrine cells called G-cells.

The main constituents of gastric juice produced by the different cells of the gastric glands include water, electrolytes, hydrochloric acid, enzymes, mucus, and intrinsic factor. The next section describes some of these constituents: hydrochloric acid, enzymes, and mucus.

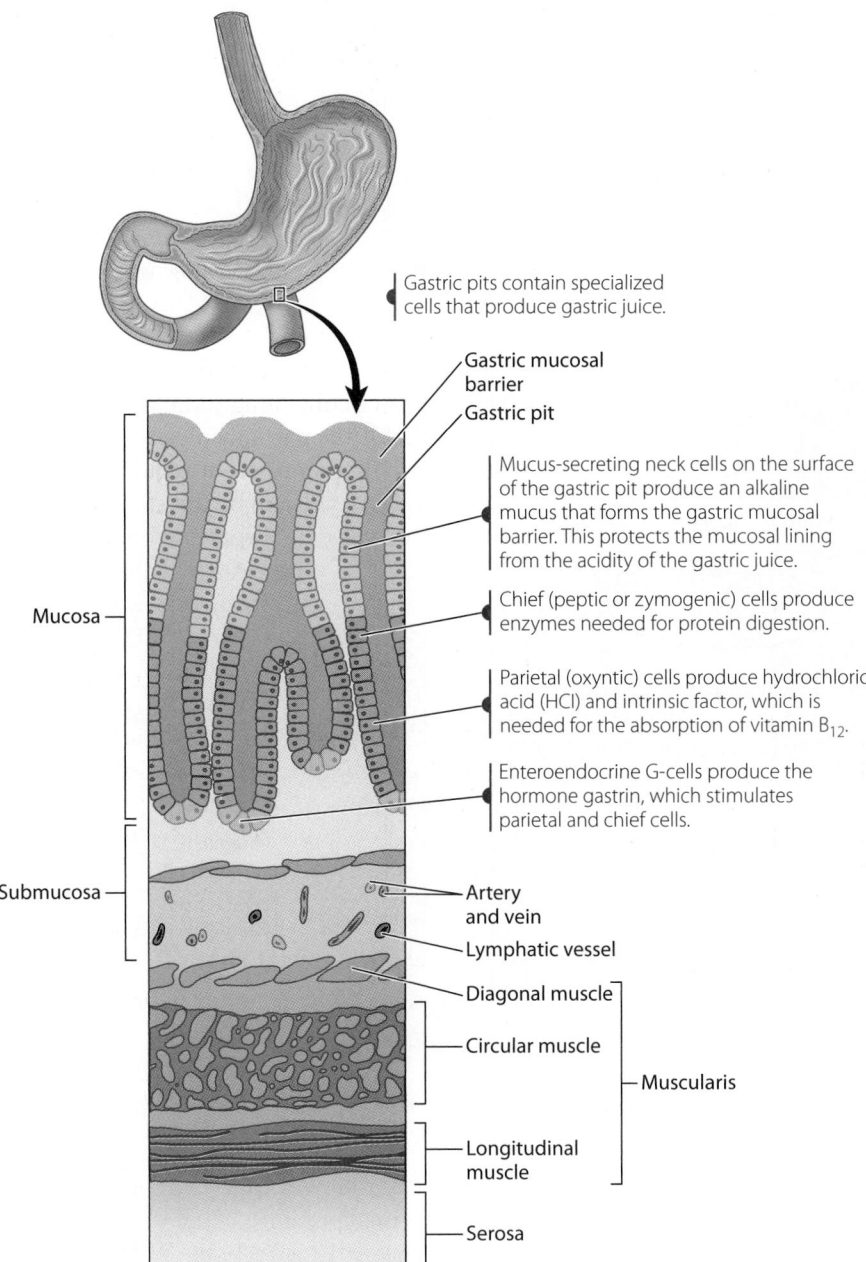

Gastric pits contain specialized cells that produce gastric juice.

Gastric mucosal barrier

Gastric pit

Mucus-secreting neck cells on the surface of the gastric pit produce an alkaline mucus that forms the gastric mucosal barrier. This protects the mucosal lining from the acidity of the gastric juice.

Chief (peptic or zymogenic) cells produce enzymes needed for protein digestion.

Parietal (oxyntic) cells produce hydrochloric acid (HCl) and intrinsic factor, which is needed for the absorption of vitamin B_{12}.

Enteroendocrine G-cells produce the hormone gastrin, which stimulates parietal and chief cells.

Mucosa

Submucosa

Artery and vein

Lymphatic vessel

Diagonal muscle

Circular muscle

Longitudinal muscle

Muscularis

Serosa

Figure 2.5 A gastric gland and its secretions.
Source: Beerman/McGuire, Nutritional Sciences, 1/e. © Cengage Learning.

Gastric Juice

Gastric juice contains an abundance of hydrochloric acid secreted from gastric parietal cells (Figure 2.6). Parietal cells contain both a potassium chloride transport system and a hydrogen (proton) potassium ATPase exchange system. The potassium chloride system transports both ions into the gastric lumen. The hydrogen potassium ATPase system (H^+, K^+-ATPase), also referred to as a proton pump, allows the exchange of two potassium ions for two hydrogens (protons) with each ATP molecule hydrolyzed. Some diffusion of chloride into and out of the parietal cell and some diffusion of potassium into gastric juice also have been proposed. Nonetheless, the net effect is that hydrogen and chloride (i.e., hydrochloric acid) are secreted into the gastric lumen as part of gastric juice. Hydrochloric acid has several functions in gastric juice, including:

- converting or activating the zymogen pepsinogen to form pepsin
- denaturing proteins, which results in the destruction of the tertiary and secondary protein structure and thereby opens interior bonds to the proteolytic effect of the enzyme pepsin
- releasing various nutrients from organic complexes
- acting as bactericide agent, killing many bacteria ingested along with food

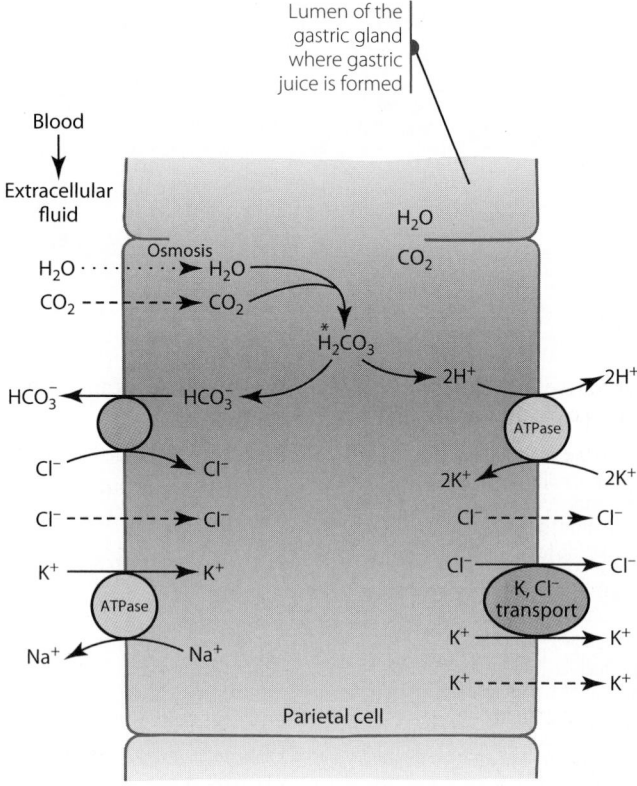

*In parietal cells, the enzyme carbonic anhydrase catalyzes this formation of carbonic acid, which dissociates to yield hydrogen ions needed for hydrochloric acid formation. This same enzyme functions in the pancreas to produce bicarbonate found in pancreatic juice.

Figure 2.6 A proposed mechanism by which hydrochloric acid (HCl) is secreted into the stomach by parietal cells. Dashed line indicates diffusion. An empty circle indicates non-energy dependent transport.

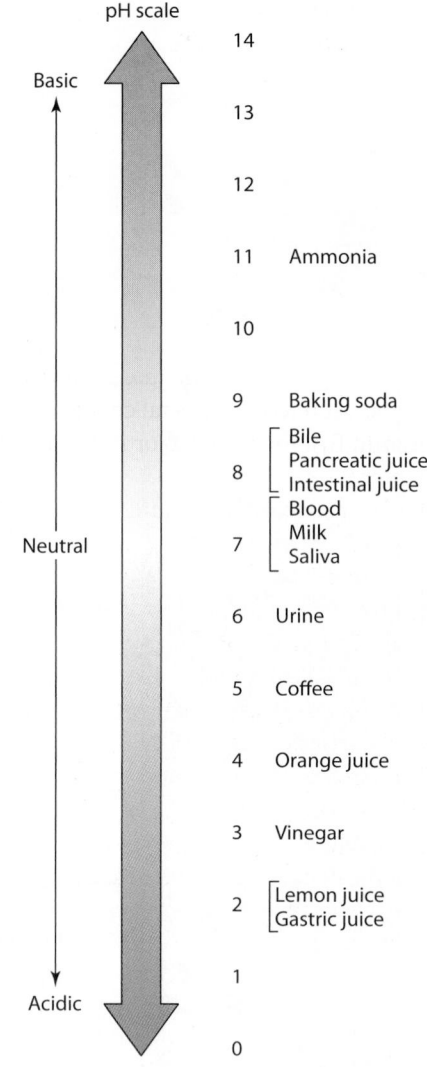

Figure 2.7 Approximate pHs of selected body fluids, compounds, and beverages.

The high concentration of hydrochloric acid in the gastric juice is responsible for its low pH, about 2. The pH value is the negative logarithm of the hydrogen ion concentration. The lower the pH is, the more acidic the solution is. Figure 2.7 shows the approximate pH values of body fluids and, for comparison, some other compounds and beverages. Notice that the pH of orange juice (and typically of all fruit juices) is higher than that of gastric juice. Thus, drinking such juices cannot lower the gastric pH.

Three enzymes (Table 2.1) are found in gastric juice. The main enzyme, pepsin, is made by the chief cells and functions as the principal proteolytic enzyme in the stomach. Pepsin is derived from either of two pepsinogens, I or II. Pepsinogen I is found primarily in the body of the stomach, where most hydrochloric acid is secreted. Pepsinogen II is found in both the body and the antrum of the stomach. The distinction between the two groups of pepsinogens has no known implications for digestion; however, higher concentrations of pepsinogen I correlate positively with acid secretion and have been associated with an increased incidence of peptic ulcers. Pepsinogens are secreted in granules into the gastric lumen by chief cells when they are stimulated by acetylcholine, acid, or both. Pepsinogens can be converted to pepsin, an active

enzyme, in an acid environment (pH < ~5) or in the presence of previously formed pepsin.

$$\text{Pepsinogen} \xrightarrow{\text{Acid or pepsin}} \text{Pepsin}$$

Pepsin functions as a protease, an enzyme that hydrolyzes proteins. Specifically, pepsin is an endopeptidase, meaning that it hydrolyzes interior peptide bonds within proteins. Optimal pepsin activity occurs at about pH 3.5. Another enzyme present in the gastric juice is α amylase, which originates from the salivary glands in the mouth. This enzyme, which hydrolyzes starch, retains some activity in the stomach until it is inactivated by the low pH of gastric juice. The third enzyme found in gastric juice is gastric lipase, which is made by chief cells. Gastric lipase hydrolyzes primarily short- and medium-chain triacylglycerols and is thought to be responsible for up to about 20% of lipid digestion in humans. Additional information about pepsin and amylase can be found in Chapters 6 and 3, respectively. Gastric lipase is discussed further in Chapter 5.

Gastric juice also contains mucus, which is secreted by gastric neck or mucus cells. Secretion of mucus is stimulated by various prostaglandins and by nitric oxide. Mucus, which consists of a network of glycoproteins (mucin), glycolipids, water, and bicarbonate (HCO_3^-), lubricates the ingested gastrointestinal contents and coats and protects the gastric mucosa from mechanical and chemical damage. Mucus forms a layer about 2 mm thick on top of the gastric mucosa. Tight junctions between gastric cells also help prevent H^+ from penetrating into the gastric mucosa and initiating peptic ulcer formation.

Another constituent of gastric juice is intrinsic factor. Intrinsic factor is secreted by parietal cells and is necessary to absorb vitamin B_{12}. Intrinsic factor is discussed in more detail in Chapter 9.

In summary, gastric juice contains several important compounds that aid in the digestive process. However, little chemical digestion of nutrients occurs in the stomach except for the initiation of protein hydrolysis by the protease pepsin and the limited continuation of starch hydrolysis by salivary α-amylase. The only absorption that occurs in the stomach is that of water, alcohol, a few fat-soluble drugs such as aspirin, and a few minerals. The hydrochloric acid and intrinsic factor generated in the stomach are important for absorbing nutrients such as iron and essential for absorption of vitamin B_{12}, respectively. Nourishment and survival are possible without the stomach as long as a person receives injections of vitamin B_{12}. Nevertheless, a healthy stomach makes attaining adequate nourishment much easier.

Regulation of Gastric Secretions

Gastric secretions are regulated by multiple mechanisms including various hormones and peptides. Several of these hormones and peptides and their actions are shown in Figure 2.8. Hormones that inhibit gastric secretions include peptide YY, enterogastrone, glucose-dependent insulinotropic peptide (formerly called gastric inhibitory peptide—GIP), and secretin. Somatostatin, synthesized by pancreatic and intestinal cells, acts in a paracrine fashion by entering gastric juice, and inhibits gastric secretions. The release of gastric secretions also is inhibited by the neuropeptides vasoactive intestinal polypeptide (VIP) and substance powder (P), some prostaglandins, and nitric oxide.

In contrast, other hormones and neuropeptides stimulate gastric secretions. Gastrin-releasing peptide (GRP), also called bombesin, is released from enteric nerves and stimulates gastrin and hydrocholoric acid release. Gastrin, synthesized primarily by enteroendocrine G-cells in the stomach and proximal small intestine, acts on parietal cells directly to stimulate hydrochloric acid release as well as on chief cells to stimulate pepsinogen release. Gastrin also stimulates gastric motility and the cellular growth of (i.e., has trophic action on) the stomach. Gastrin release occurs in response to vagal stimulation, gastric distention, and hydrochloric acid in contact with gastric mucosa, as well as gastrin-releasing peptide, epinephrine, and ingestion of specific substances or nutrients such as coffee, alcohol, calcium, amino acids, and peptides. The role of gastrin in acid secretion is especially evident in people

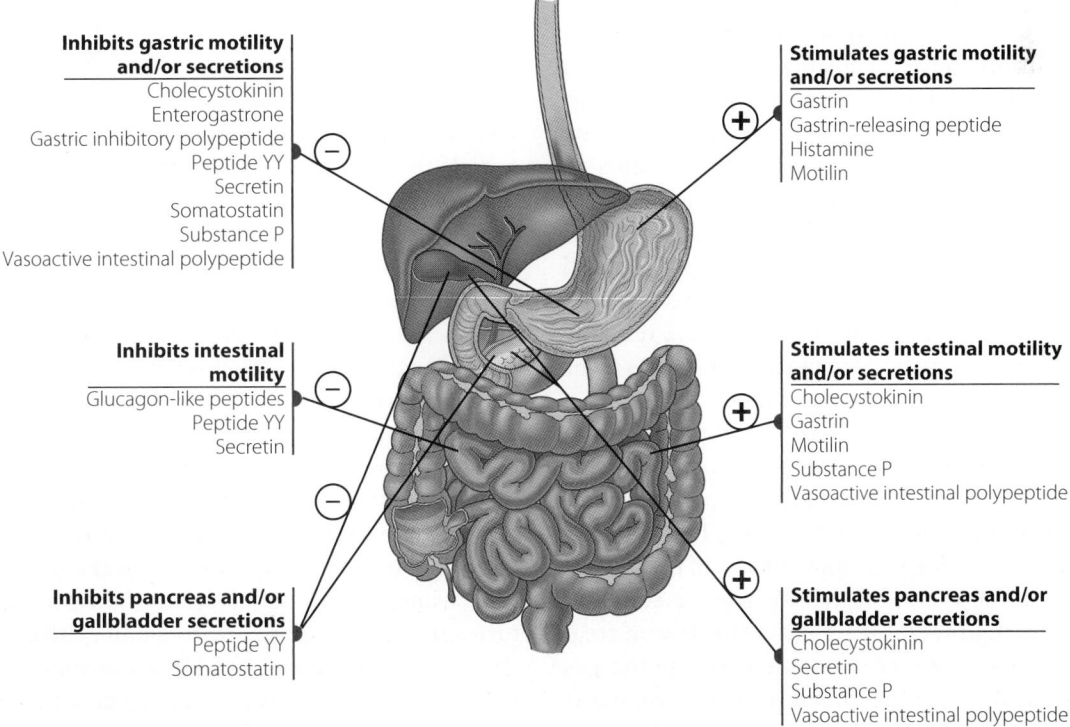

Inhibits gastric motility and/or secretions
Cholecystokinin
Enterogastrone
Gastric inhibitory polypeptide
Peptide YY
Secretin
Somatostatin
Substance P
Vasoactive intestinal polypeptide

Stimulates gastric motility and/or secretions
Gastrin
Gastrin-releasing peptide
Histamine
Motilin

Inhibits intestinal motility
Glucagon-like peptides
Peptide YY
Secretin

Stimulates intestinal motility and/or secretions
Cholecystokinin
Gastrin
Motilin
Substance P
Vasoactive intestinal polypeptide

Inhibits pancreas and/or gallbladder secretions
Peptide YY
Somatostatin

Stimulates pancreas and/or gallbladder secretions
Cholecystokinin
Secretin
Substance P
Vasoactive intestinal polypeptide

Figure 2.8 The effects of selected gastrointestinal hormones/peptides on gastrointestinal tract secretions and motility.

with Zollinger-Ellison syndrome. This condition, usually caused by a tumor, is characterized by extremely copious secretion of gastrin into the blood, which produces higher than normal blood concentrations of gastrin (referred to as hypergastrinemia). Hypergastrinemia leads to gastric hypersecretion and the formation of multiple ulcers in the stomach, duodenum, and sometimes even the jejunum.

In addition to being stimulated by gastrin, acid release into the stomach is also stimulated by other means. For example, the vagus nerve releases acetylcholine and stimulates the release of histamine. Both acetylcholine and histamine stimulate acid secretion. Moreover, gastrin also stimulates histamine release. Thus, direct mediators or potent secretogogues (compounds that stimulate secretion) of hydrochloric acid release by the parietal cells include:

- gastrin, which acts on parietal cells in the stomach
- acetylcholine, released from the vagus nerve for action on parietal cells
- histamine, released from gastrointestinal tract mast (enterochromaffin) cells, which binds to H_2 receptors on parietal cells

Selected Diseases and Conditions of the Stomach

Understanding how hydrochloric acid is produced in the body and what stimulates its release is essential to understanding the treatment of peptic ulcers. Peptic ulcers typically result when the normal defense and repair systems that protect the mucosa of the gastrointestinal tract are disrupted. The most common cause of peptic ulcers is the bacterium *Helicobacter pylori*; however, chronic use of many substances, including aspirin, alcohol, and nonsteroidal anti-inflammatory drugs (NSAID) like ibuprofen, can disrupt the mucus-rich and bicarbonate-rich barriers that protect the mucosa and deeper layers of the gastrointestinal tract and can promote the development of ulcers. Several drugs used to treat peptic ulcers, known as H_2 receptor blockers—Tagamet (cimetidine), Zantac (ranitidine), Pepcid (famotidine), and Axid (nizatidine)—bind to the H_2 receptors on the parietal cells. When histamine is released, it cannot bind to the H_2 receptor (the drug blocks histamine's ability to bind), and acid release from the parietal cell is diminished. Other drugs (referred to as proton pump inhibitors) used to treat ulcers—Prilosec (omeprazole), Nexium (esomeprazole), Protonix (pantoprazole), and Aciphex (rabeprazole)—work by binding to the ATPase/proton pump (Figure 2.6) at the secretory surface of the parietal cell and thus directly inhibit hydrogen release into the gastric juice. Drug therapies are quite effective in treating peptic ulcers; however, foods that irritate the gastric mucosa also must be avoided during acute peptic ulcer episodes. If a peptic ulcer results in bleeding into the gastrointestinal tract, further medical nutrition therapy may require increased consumption of nutrients such as protein and iron.

Regulation of Gut Motility and Gastric Emptying

When food is swallowed, the proximal portion of the stomach relaxes to accommodate the ingested food. The relaxation, considered to be a reflex, is controlled by two processes mediated by the vagus nerve: receptive relaxation and gastric accommodation. Signals for antral contraction (necessary for gastric emptying) occur at regular intervals and begin in the proximal stomach at a point along the greater curvature. The signals then migrate distally toward the pyloric sphincter at the juncture of the stomach and the small intestine. The pacemaker, located between the fundus and body of the stomach (Figure 2.4), signals the antrum. The pacemaker determines the frequency of the contractions that occur. As the food moves into the antrum, the rate of contractions increases so that in the distal portion of the stomach food is liquefied into chyme. The rate of contractions is about 3 per minute in the stomach and increases to about 8 to 12 per minute in the proximal small intestine. The rate per minute decreases slightly to about 7 per minute in the distal small intestine.

The migrating motility or myoelectric complex, a series of contractions with several phases, moves distally like a wave down the gastrointestinal tract, but mainly in the stomach and intestine. The migrating motility complex waves occur approximately every 80 to 120 minutes during interdigestive periods, but their frequency changes during digestive periods. The migrating motility complex sweeps out gastrointestinal (especially gastric and intestinal) contents and prevents bacterial overgrowth in the intestine. Its activity is influenced by a variety of factors, including hormones and peptides. For example, the peptide motilin, secreted by cells of the duodenum, causes intestinal smooth muscle to contract and may be involved in inducing and regulating different phases of the migrating motility complex. Ghrelin also appears to increase migrating motility complex activity, especially within the intestine.

Gastric emptying is also influenced by several other factors. Receptors in the duodenal bulb (the first few centimeters of the proximal duodenum) are sensitive to the volume of chyme and to the osmolarity of the chyme present in the duodenum. Large volumes of chyme, for example, result in increased pressure within the stomach and promote gastric emptying. The presence of hypertonic/hyperosmolar (very concentrated) or hypotonic/hyposmolar (very dilute) chyme in the duodenum activates osmoreceptors. Activation of the osmoreceptors in turn slows gastric emptying to facilitate the formation of chyme that is isotonic. In addition to volume and osmolarity, the chemical composition of the chyme also affects gastric emptying. Carbohydrate-rich and protein-rich foods appear to empty at about the same rate from the stomach; high-fat foods, however, slow gastric emptying into the duodenum. Salts and monosaccharides also slow gastric emptying, as do many free amino acids, such as tryptophan and phenylalanine, and complex carbohydrates, especially soluble fiber. The presence of acid in the duodenum stimulates the secretion of hormones and regulatory peptides that, along with some reflexes, also influence gastric emptying. For example, hormones such as secretin, glucose-dependent insulinotropic peptide (GIP), somatostatin, peptide YY, and enterogastrone decrease or inhibit gastric motility, as does the ileogastric reflex.

Although contractions within the stomach promote physical disintegration of solid foods into liquid form, complete liquefaction is not necessary for the stomach contents to empty through the pyloric sphincter into the duodenum. Particles as large as 3 mm in diameter (~ 1/8 inch) can be emptied from the stomach through the sphincter, but solid particles are usually emptied with fluids when they have been degraded to a diameter of about 2 mm or less. Approximately 1 to 5 mL (~ up to 1 tsp) of chyme enters the duodenum about twice per minute. Contraction of the pylorus and proximal duodenum is thought to be coordinated with contraction of the antrum to facilitate gastric emptying. Gastric emptying following a meal usually takes between 2 and 6 hours; however, in those who are critically ill, gastric emptying is often delayed, resulting in high gastric residual volumes.

The Small Intestine

Once through the pyloric sphincter, chyme enters the small intestine. The small intestine (Figure 2.9), which represents the main site for nutrient digestion and absorption, is composed of the duodenum (slightly less than 1 foot long) and the jejunum and ileum (which together are approximately 9 feet long). Microscopy is generally needed to identify where one of these sections of the small intestine ends and the other begins. However, the Treitz ligament, a suspensory ligament, is found at about the site where the duodenum and jejunum meet. The lumen of the jejunum is generally larger than that of the ileum.

Structural Aspects, Secretions, and Digestive Processes of the Small Intestine

Although the structure of the small intestine consists of the same layers identified in Figure 2.2, the epithelial lining or mucosa of the small intestine is structured to maximize surface area and thus its ability to absorb nutrients. The small intestine has a surface area of approximately 300 m^2, an area about equal to a 3-foot-wide sidewalk more than three football fields in length. Several structures, shown in Figure 2.10, that contribute to this enormous surface area include:

- large circular folds of mucosa, called the folds of Kerckring, that protrude into the lumen of the small intestine

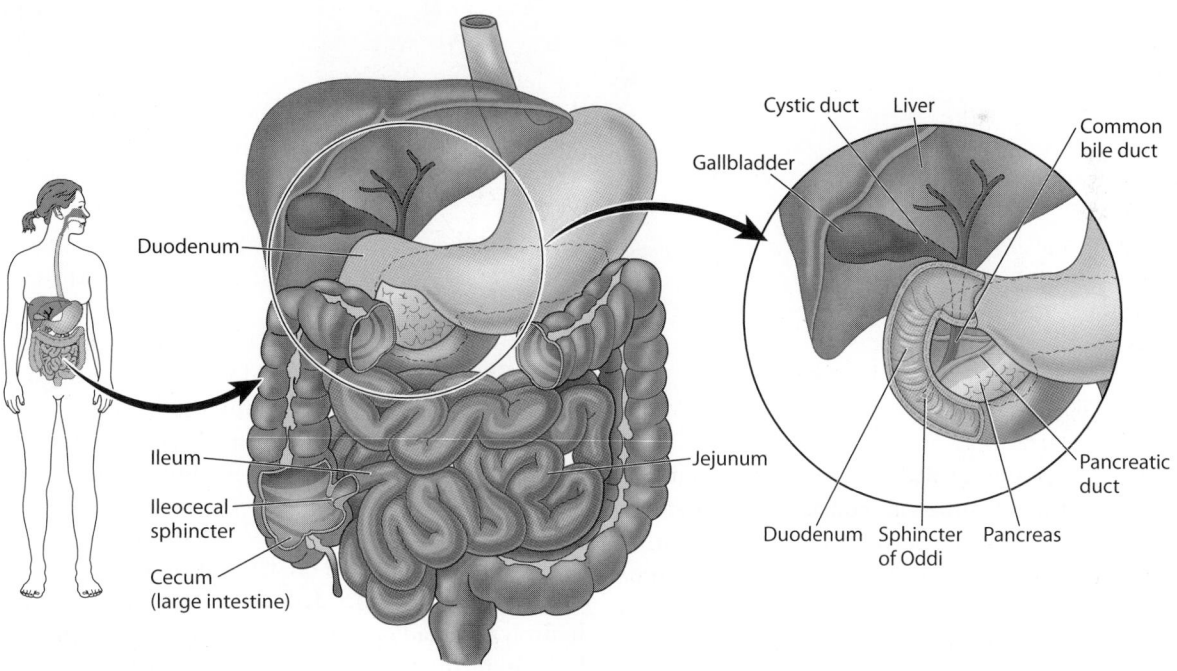

The small intestine is divided into 3 regions: the duodenum, jejunum, and ileum. The ileocecal sphincter regulates the flow of material from the ileum, the last segment of the small intestine, into the cecum, the first portion of the large intestine.

The duodenum receives secretions from the gallbladder via the common bile duct. The pancreas releases its secretions into the pancreatic duct, which eventually joins the common bile duct. The sphincter of Oddi regulates the flow of these secretions into the duodenum.

Figure 2.9 The small intestine.

Source: Beerman/McGuire, Nutritional Sciences, 1/e. © Cengage Learning.

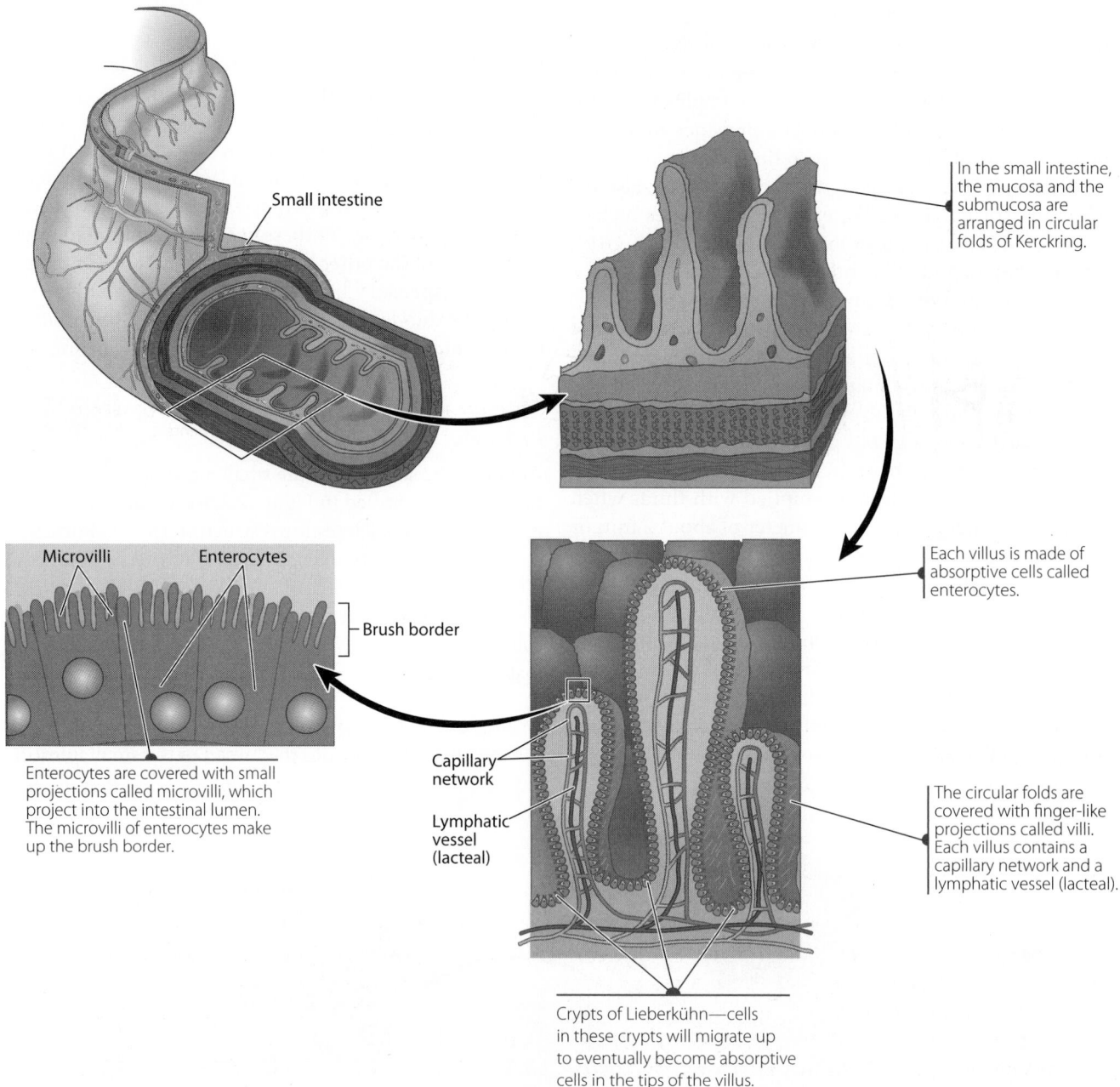

In the small intestine, the mucosa and the submucosa are arranged in circular folds of Kerckring.

Each villus is made of absorptive cells called enterocytes.

The circular folds are covered with finger-like projections called villi. Each villus contains a capillary network and a lymphatic vessel (lacteal).

Microvilli   Enterocytes

Brush border

Enterocytes are covered with small projections called microvilli, which project into the intestinal lumen. The microvilli of enterocytes make up the brush border.

Capillary network

Lymphatic vessel (lacteal)

Crypts of Lieberkühn—cells in these crypts will migrate up to eventually become absorptive cells in the tips of the villus.

Figure 2.10 The structure of the small intestine.
Source: Beerman/McGuire, Nutritional Sciences, 1/e. © Cengage Learning.

- finger-like projections, called villi, that project out into the lumen of the intestine and consist of hundreds of intestinal cells called **enterocytes** (or absorptive epithelial or mucosal cells) along with blood capillaries and a central lacteal (lymphatic vessel) for transport of nutrients out of the enterocytes

- microvilli, hair-like extensions of the plasma membrane of the enterocytes that make up the villi

The microvilli possess a surface coat, or glycocalyx, as shown in Figure 2.11; together, these make up the brush border of the enterocytes. Covering the brush border (the side of the enterocyte that borders the lumen) is an unstirred water (fluid) layer. That is, the unstirred water layer lies between the brush border membrane of the intestine and the intestinal lumen. Its presence can significantly affect lipid absorption, as discussed in Chapter 5.

Most of the digestive enzymes produced by the enterocytes are found embedded in the brush border, and they hydrolyze already partially digested nutrients, mainly carbohydrate and protein (Table 2.1). Structurally, the digestive enzymes are glycoproteins. The carbohydrate (glyco) portion of these glycoprotein enzymes may in part make up the glycocalyx. The glycocalyx, which lines the luminal side of the intestine, is thought to consist of numerous fine filaments that extend almost perpendicular from the microvillus membrane to which it is attached. Digestion of nutrients is usually completed on the brush border but may

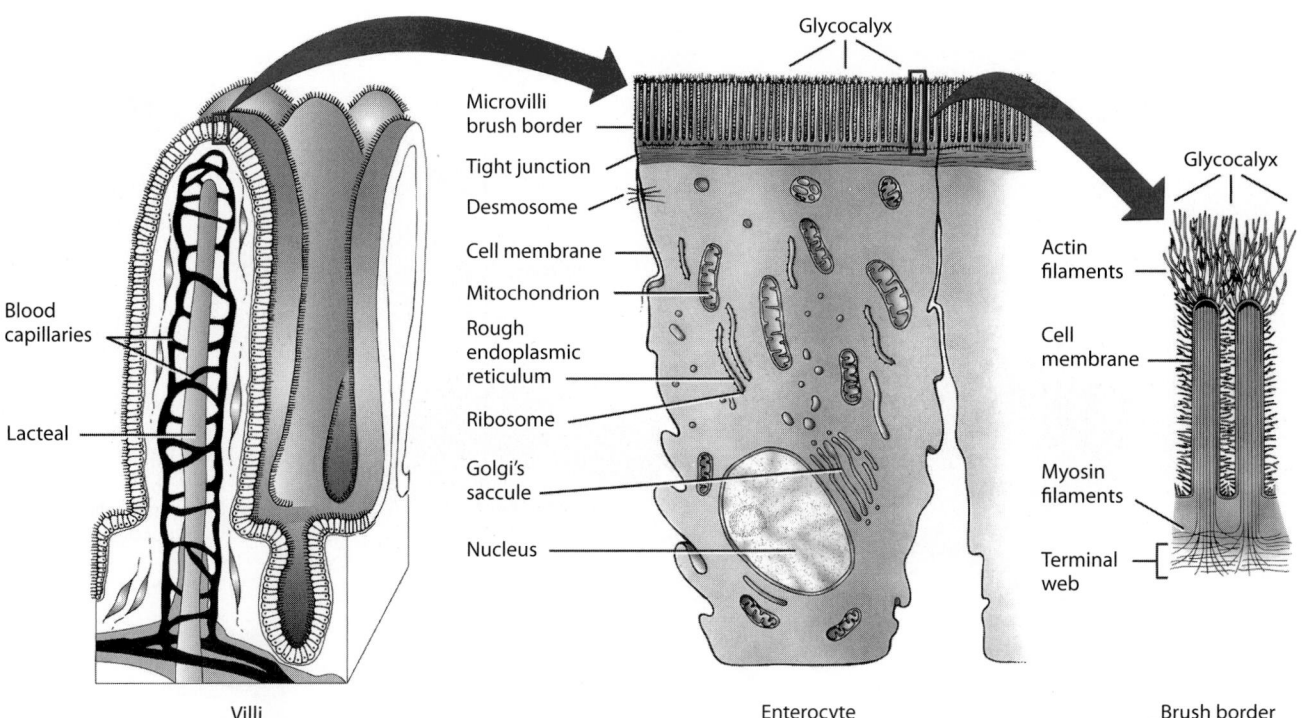

Figure 2.11 Structure of the absorptive cell of the small intestine.

be completed within the cytosol (cytoplasm) of the entero-cytes. More detailed information on carbohydrate, fat, and protein digestion is provided in Chapters 3, 5, and 6.

The small intestine also contains small pits or pockets called crypts of Lieberkühn (Figure 2.10) that lie between the villi. Epithelial cells in these crypts continuously undergo mitosis. The new cells gradually migrate upward and out of the crypts toward the tips of the villi. Toward the tip, many former crypt cells function as absorptive enterocytes. Ultimately, the enterocytes are sloughed off into the intestinal lumen and excreted in the feces. Enterocyte turnover is rapid, approximately every 3 to 5 days. Cells in the crypts include Paneth cells that secrete antimicrobial peptides (called defensins) with broad activity, mast (enterochromaffin) cells with endocrine functions, and goblet cells that secrete both small cysteine-rich proteins with antifungal activity and mucus. Mucus adheres to the mucosa and acts as a barrier to protect the epithelial mucosal cell surface from the acidic chyme. Cells and glands in the crypts of Lieberkühn also secrete large volumes of intestinal juices and electrolytes into the lumen of the small intestine to facilitate nutrient digestion. Much of this fluid is typically reabsorbed by the villi.

Chyme moves through the small intestine, propelled by various contractions (Figure 2.12) influenced by the nervous system. Contractions of longitudinal smooth muscles, often called sleeve contractions, mix the intestinal contents with the digestive juices. Standing contractions of circular smooth muscles, called segmentation, produce bidirectional flow of the intestinal contents, occur many times per minute, and mix and churn the chyme with digestive secretions in the small intestine. Peristaltic waves, or progressive contractions, also accomplished primarily through action of the circular muscles, move the chyme distally along the intestinal mucosa toward the ileocecal valve.

Chyme moving from the stomach into the duodenum initially has a pH of about 2 because of its gastric acid content. The duodenum is protected against this gastric acidity by secretions from the Brunner's glands and from the pancreas. The Brunner's glands are located in the mucosa and submucosa of the first few centimeters of the duodenum (duodenal bulb). Their mucus-containing secretions are viscous and alkaline, with a pH of approximately 8.2 to 9.3. The mucus itself is rich in glycoproteins and helps protect the epithelial mucosa from damage. The pancreatic secretions released into the duodenum are rich in bicarbonate, which helps to neutralize the acid released from the stomach. Disruptions or inadequate release of these alkaline-rich secretions or excessive gastric acid secretion into the duodenum can precipitate the development of duodenal ulcers, which typically form around the duodenal bulb. As with gastric peptic ulcers, medications to suppress acid production are helpful in treating duodenal ulcers.

Regulation of Intestinal Secretions and Motility

Several hormones and peptides influence the release of intestinal secretions as well as intestinal motility. For example, vasoactive intestinal polypeptide (VIP), present in neurons within the gut, has been shown to stimulate intestinal secretions and relax most gastrointestinal sphincters.

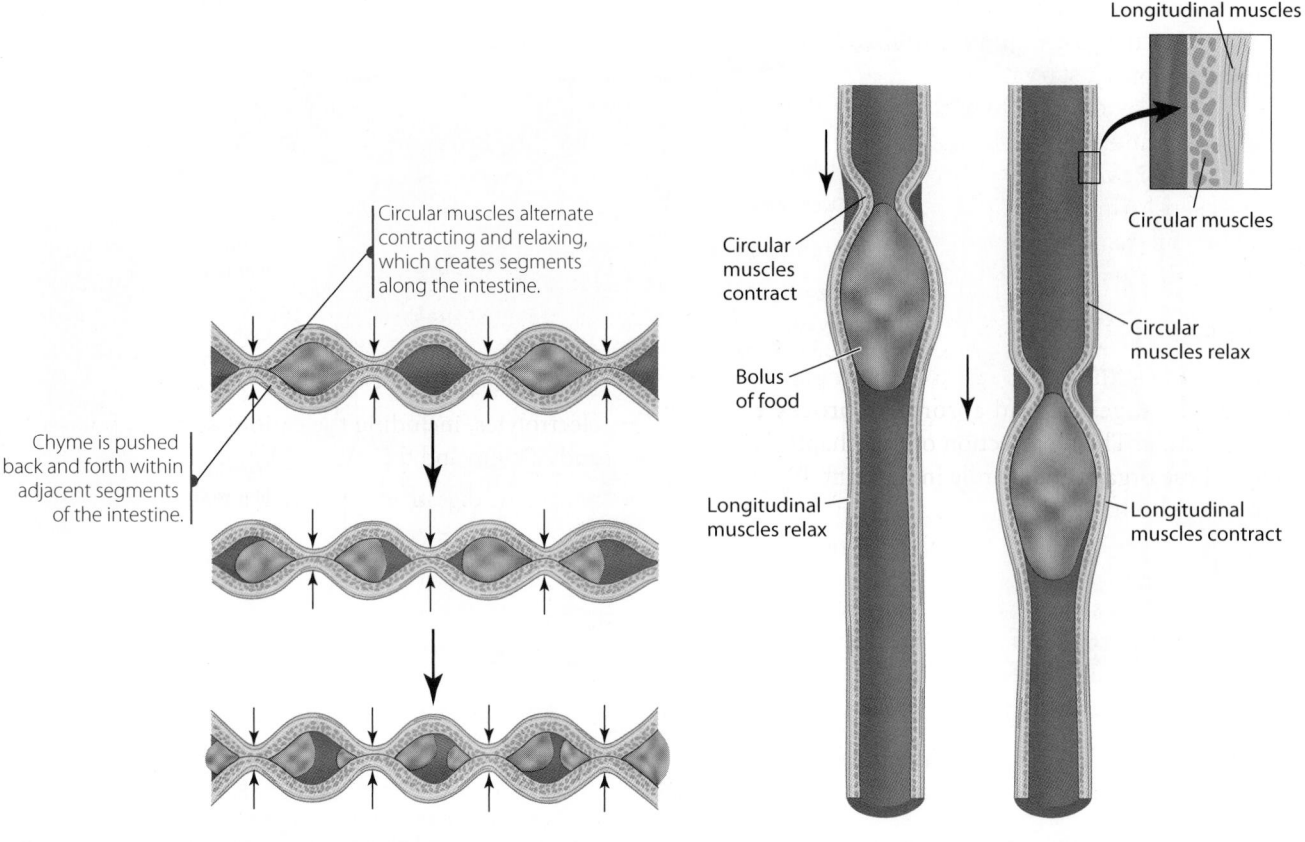

Segmentation. Segmentation mixes food in the GI tract by moving the food mass back and forth. The circular muscles contract and relax, which creates a "chopping" motion.

Peristalsis. Peristalsis consists of a series of wavelike rhythmic contractions and relaxation involving both the circular and longitudinal muscles. This action propels food forward through the GI tract.

Figure 2.12 Movement of chyme in the gastrointestinal tract.
Source: Beerman/McGuire, Nutritional Sciences, 1/e. © Cengage Learning.

The neuropeptide substance P, the peptide motilin, and, to a lesser extent, the hormone cholecystokinin (CCK, also called CCK-pancreozymen and abbreviated CCK-PZ) increase intestinal motility. Conversely, motility of the intestine is inhibited or diminished by peptide YY, secretin, and glucagon-like peptides.

Immune System Protection of the Gastrointestinal Tract

A variety of immune system cells and lymphoid tissue protect the digestive tract. These cells and tissues are found throughout the GI tract but are present in especially high concentrations in the small intestine. The lymphoid tissue is found primarily in the mucosa (especially the lamina propria) and submucosa and is called mucosa-associated lymphoid tissue (MALT) or, if found in the nonmucosal layer of the gastrointestinal tract, gut-associated lymphoid tissue (GALT). Both MALT and GALT are composed of multiple types of cells including leukocytes, especially T- and B-lymphocytes; plasma cells; natural killer (NK) cells; and macrophages, among others. The leukocytes

tend to be located between the intestinal epithelial cells and make up approximately 15% of the epithelial mucosa. The majority of the body's plasma cells are found in the lamina propria. The plasma cells produce secretory IgA, which binds antigens ingested with foods, inhibits the growth of pathogenic bacteria, and inhibits bacterial translocation. In addition to these cells, microfold (M)-cells are associated with some lymphocytes and cover or overlie, usually in a single layer, Peyer's patches. Peyer's patches are aggregates of lymphoid tissue that also are located in the mucosa and submucosa. The M-cells are antigen-presenting cells; these M-cells pass or transport foreign antigens to the Peyer's patches or MALT lymphocytes, which in turn mount an immune response. After processing the foreign antigens, some of these lymphocytes are released from the Peyer's patches and enter circulation to augment the immune response. Dendritic cells, a type of macrophage, also are found in the gastrointestinal tract. They destroy foreign antigens and stimulate lymphocytes to destroy antigens.

Although the gastrointestinal tract provides a defense against bacteria and other foreign substances that may have been ingested with consumed food, this barrier can be easily destroyed. Atrophy of the mucosal and submu- cosal layers of the gastrointestinal tract, which may occur with illness, injury, starvation, or extended periods with little food intake, can lead to bacterial translocation. Bac- terial translocation (the presence of gastrointestinal tract– derived bacteria or their toxins in the blood or lymph) can result in sepsis (infection) and, potentially, multiple sys- tem organ failure.

The Accessory Organs

Three organs—the pancreas, liver, and gallbladder— facilitate the digestive and absorptive processes in the small intestine. The next section of this chapter describes each of these organs and its role in nutrient digestion, ab- sorption, or both.

The Pancreas

The pancreas is a slender, elongated organ that ranges in length from about 6 to 9 inches. The pancreas is found be- hind the greater curvature of the stomach, lying between the stomach and the duodenum (Figures 2.1 and 2.13). Two types of active cells are found in the pancreas (Figure 2.13b):

- ductless endocrine cells that secrete hormones into the blood
- acinar exocrine cells that produce the digestive juice and enzymes

The endocrine cells are found among the 1 to 2 mil- lion cells that make up the islets of Langerhan, located primarily in the tail region of the pancreas. While these cells make up less than 5% of the gland's volume, they are responsible for the secretion of several important hor- mones. The A or α-cells secrete glucagon. The B or β-cells secrete insulin, and the D or δ-cells secrete somatostatin.

The exocrine cells package digestive enzymes in secre- tory structures called granules and release them by exocy- tosis into pancreatic juice. Pancreatic juice, produced by the acinar cells, contains:

- bicarbonate, important for neutralizing the acidic chyme passing into the duodenum from the stom- ach and for maximizing enzyme activity within the duodenum
- electrolytes, including the cations sodium, potassium, and calcium and the anion chloride
- pancreatic digestive enzymes in a watery solution

To facilitate the release of pancreatic juice, the acinar cells of the pancreas are arranged in a circular pattern and are attached to small ducts. The pancreatic juice is secreted into the small ducts within the pancreas. These small ducts coalesce to form a large main pancreatic duct (Wirsung duct), which later joins with the common bile duct at the greater duodenal papilla, also called the am- pulla of Vater, to form the bile pancreatic duct. The bile pancreatic duct empties into the duodenum through the sphincter of Oddi (Figure 2.13a). Blockage of this duct, as may occur with gallstones from the gallbladder, may im- pair the release of pancreatic juice out of the pancreas and can lead to acute pancreatitis (inflammation of the pan- creas), a potentially life-threatening condition. Pancreati- tis is described in the Perspective at the end of this chapter.

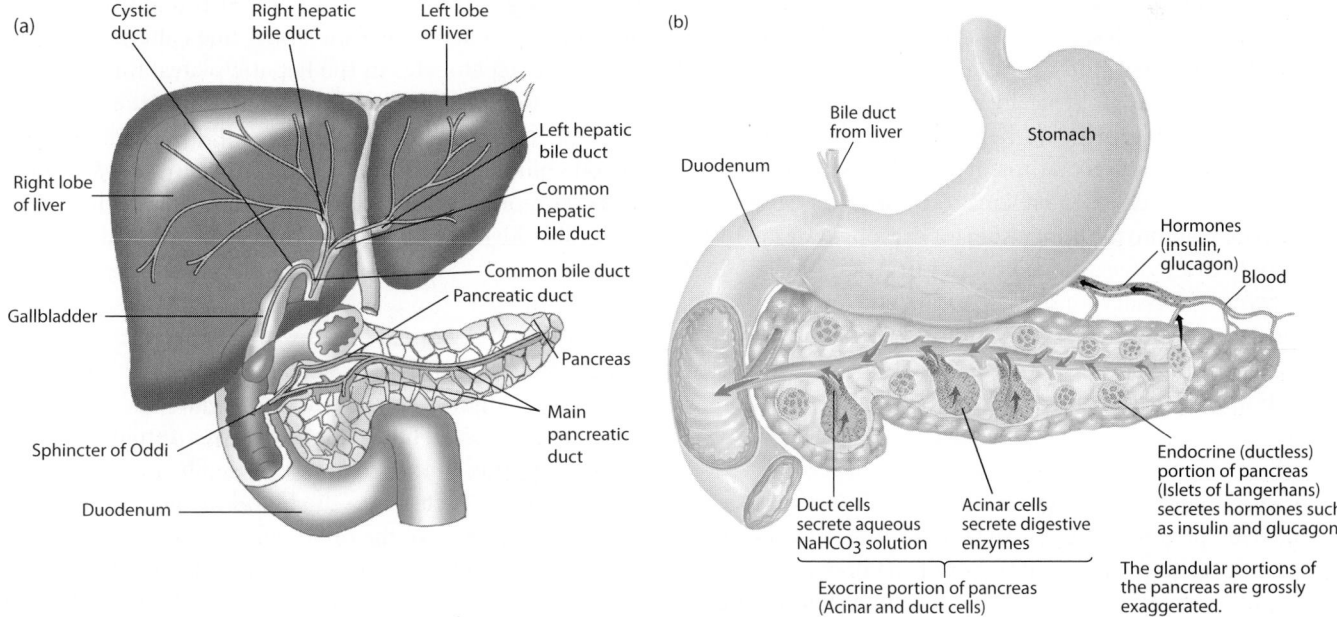

Figure 2.13   (a) The ducts of the gallbladder, liver, and pancreas. (b) Schematic representation of the exocrine and endocrine portions of the pancreas.

Source: From Understanding Human Anatomy and Physiology, 1st edition, by Stalheim-Smith/Fitch, 1993, Brooks/Cole. © Cengage Learning.

Regulation of Pancreatic Secretions Pancreatic juice is released when the pancreatic acinar cells are stimulated by hormones and the parasympathetic nervous system. The hormone secretin, secreted into the blood by enteroendocrine S-cells found in the mucosa of the proximal small intestine, is secreted in response to the release of acidic chyme into the duodenum. Secretin stimulates the pancreas to secrete water, bicarbonate, and pancreatic enzymes. In addition to secretin, cholecystokinin (secreted by enteroendocrine I-cells of the proximal small intestine and enteric nerves) and the neuropeptide substance P stimulate the secretion of pancreatic juices and enzymes into the duodenum. Similarly, vasoactive intestinal polypeptide (VIP), present in neurons within the gut, also stimulates pancreatic bicarbonate release into the small intestine. In contrast, somatostatin, which works in a paracrine fashion, inhibits pancreatic exocrine secretions. A variety of other gastrointestinal-derived hormones and peptides affect pancreatic insulin release including amylin, galanin, and somatostatin (inhibitory) and glucose-dependent insulinotropic polypeptide and glucagon-like peptide (stimulatory).

Pancreatic Digestive Enzymes The enzymes released by the pancreas, listed in Table 2.1, digest approximately half of all ingested carbohydrates, half (50%) of all proteins, and almost all (80–90%) of ingested fat. Proteases—enzymes that digest proteins—found in pancreatic juice and secreted into the duodenum include trypsinogen, chymotrypsinogen, procarboxypeptidases, proelastase, and collagenase. As a group, proteases hydrolyze peptide bonds, either internally or from the ends, and the net result of their collective actions is the production of polypeptides shorter in length than the original polypeptide or protein, oligopeptides (typically 4–10 amino acids in length), tripeptides, dipeptides, and free amino acids. The latter three may be absorbed into the enterocyte. Oligopeptides and some tripeptides are typically further hydrolyzed by brush border aminopeptidases before being absorbed. More detailed information on protein digestion is given in Chapter 6. Only one enzyme, pancreatic α-amylase, is secreted by the pancreas into the duodenum for carbohydrate digestion; carbohydrate digestion is covered in detail in Chapter 3. Enzymes necessary for lipid digestion and produced by the pancreas include pancreatic lipase, which is the major fat-digesting enzyme, and colipase. These enzymes and fat digestion are described in detail in Chapter 5.

The Liver

Another accessory organ to the gastrointestinal tract is the liver, pictured in Figures 2.1, 2.13, and 2.14. The liver, the largest single internal organ of the body, is made up of two lobes, the right lobe and left lobe. These lobes in turn contain functional units called lobules. The lobules (Figure 2.14) are made up of plates or sheets of hepatocytes (liver cells). The plates of cells are arranged so that

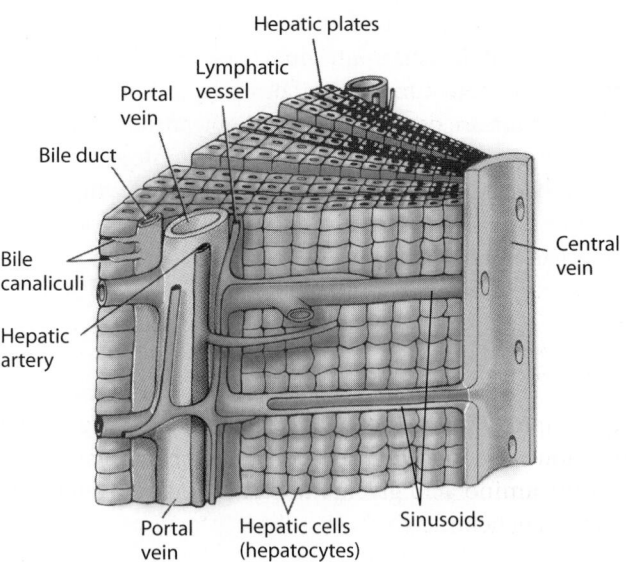

Figure 2.14 Structure of a liver lobule.

they radiate out from central veins. Thus, the liver has multiple plates of cells radiating from multiple central veins. The central veins direct blood from the liver into general circulation through hepatic veins and then ultimately into the inferior vena cava. Blood passes between the plates of liver cells by way of sinusoids, which function like a channel and arise from branches of the hepatic artery and from the portal vein. The portal vein brings blood rich in nutrients from the digestive tract and pancreas to the liver. Sinusoids allow blood from these two blood vessels (the portal vein and the hepatic artery) to mix and also enable uptake of nutrients through the endothelial cells that line the sinusoids. Sinusoids also contain macrophages called Kupffer's cells, which phagocytize bacteria and other foreign substances and thus serve to protect the body. Bile canaliculi lie between the hepatocytes in the hepatic plates. Bile, covered in the section on the gallbladder, drains from the canaliculi into bile ducts. As shown in Figure 2.13, the right and left hepatic bile ducts join to form the common hepatic duct. The common hepatic duct unites with the cystic duct from the gallbladder to form the common hepatic bile duct.

The Gallbladder

The gallbladder, a small organ with a capacity of approximately 40 to 50 mL (1.4–1.8 oz), is located on the surface of the liver (Figures 2.9 and 2.13). The gallbladder concentrates and stores the bile made in the liver until it is needed for fat digestion in the small intestine. The hormone cholecystokinin, secreted into the blood by enteroendocrine cells (called I-cells) of the proximal small intestine, stimulates the gallbladder to contract and release bile into the duodenum. In contrast, somatostatin, which works in a paracrine fashion, inhibits gallbladder contraction. Bile flow into the duodenum is regulated by the intraduodenal segment of the common hepatic bile duct and the sphincter of Oddi, located at the junction of the common hepatic bile duct and the duodenum (Figure 2.13). Bile synthesis, storage, function in fat digestion, recirculation, and excretion are described in the next sections.

Bile Synthesis   Bile is a greenish-yellow fluid composed mainly of bile acids and salts but also cholesterol, phospholipids, and bile pigments (bilirubin and biliverdin) dissolved in an alkaline solution. The bile acids are synthesized in the hepatocytes from cholesterol, which in a series of reactions is oxidized to chenodeoxycholic acid and cholic acid, the two principal or primary bile acids (see Chapter 5 for further details). Chenodeoxycholic acid and cholic acid, once formed, conjugate primarily (~75%) with the amino acid glycine to form the conjugated bile acids glycochenodeoxycholic acid (glycochenodeoxycholate) and glycocholic acid (glycocholate), respectively.

Bile Acid		Amino Acid		Conjugated Bile Acid
Cholic acid	+	glycine	⟶	Glycocholic acid
Chenodeoxycholic acid	+	glycine	⟶	Glycochenodeoxycholic acid

Alternately and to a lesser (25%) extent, chenodeoxycholic acid and cholic acid conjugate with the amino acid taurine to form two additional primary conjugated bile acids.

Bile Acid		Amino Acid		Conjugated Bile Acid
Cholic acid	+	taurine	⟶	Taurocholic acid
Chenodeoxycholic acid	+	taurine	⟶	Taurochenodeoxycholic acid

Conjugation of the bile acids with these amino acids results in better ionization and thus in improved ability to form micelles. The formation and role of micelles in fat digestion are discussed in Chapter 5. Chenodeoxycholic acid and cholic acid are primary bile acids and make up 80% of the body's total bile acids. The remaining 20% of the bile acids is made up of secondary products produced in the large intestine from bacterial action on chenodeoxycholic acid to form lithocholic acid and on cholic acid to form deoxycholic acid. In addition to being conjugated to amino acids, most conjugated bile acids are present in bile as bile salts owing to bile's pH (~7.6–8.6). Sodium is the predominant biliary cation, although potassium and calcium bile salts may also be found in the alkaline bile solution.

Although bile acids and salts make up a large portion of bile, other substances are also found in bile. These other substances include both cholesterol and phospholipids, especially lecithin, and make up what is referred to as the bile acid–dependent fraction of bile. In addition, water, electrolytes, bicarbonate, and glucuronic acid conjugated bile pigments (mainly bilirubin, biliverdin, or both—waste end products of hemoglobin degradation that are excreted in bile

and give bile its color) are secreted into bile by hepatocytes. This alkaline-rich fraction of the bile is referred to as bile acid independent. The bile components must remain in the proper ratio to prevent gallstone formation (cholelithiasis), although other factors influence gallstone production.

Selected Conditions/Diseases of the Gallbladder   Gallstones are thought to form when bile becomes supersaturated with cholesterol. Cholesterol precipitates out of solution and provides a crystalline-like structure within which calcium, bilirubin, phospholipids, and other compounds deposit, ultimately forming a "stone." Gallstones may reside silently in the gallbladder; irritate the organ, causing cholecystitis (inflammation of the gallbladder); or lodge in the common bile duct, blocking the flow of bile (choledocholithiasis) into the duodenum. Gallstones also may block the pancreatic duct, causing pancreatitis (inflammation of the pancreas), as described in the Perspective at the end of this chapter.

Bile Storage   During the interdigestive periods, bile is sent from the liver to the gallbladder, where it is concentrated and stored. The gallbladder concentrates the bile so that as much as 90% of the water, along with some of the electrolytes, is reabsorbed by the gallbladder mucosa. The fluid reabsorption thus leaves the remaining bile constituents (i.e., bile acids and salts, cholesterol, lecithin, bilirubin, and biliverdin) in a less dilute form. Concentration of the bile permits the gallbladder to store more of the bile produced by the liver between periods of food ingestion. Cholecystokinin, released in response to chyme entering the duodenum, stimulates gallbladder contraction. Bile is secreted into the duodenum through the sphincter of Oddi.

The Function of Bile   Bile acids and bile salts act as detergents to emulsify lipids, that is, to break down large fat globules into small (about 1 mm diameter) fat droplets. Bile acids and salts, along with phospholipids, help to absorb lipids by forming small (<10 nm) spherical, cylindrical, or disklike complexes called micelles. Micelles can contain as many as 40 bile salt molecules. More thorough coverage of the functions of bile is found in Chapter 5.

The Recirculation and Excretion of Bile   The human body has a total bile acid pool of about 2.5 to 5.0 g. Greater than 90% of the bile acids and salts secreted into the duodenum are reabsorbed by active transport in the ileum. Small amounts of the bile may be passively reabsorbed in the jejunum and the colon. About half of the cholesterol contained within the bile is taken up by the jejunum and used in forming chylomicrons (see Chapter 5). The remainder of the cholesterol is excreted. Bile that is absorbed in the ileum enters the portal vein and is transported, attached to the plasma protein albumin in the blood, back to the liver. Once in the liver, the reabsorbed bile acids are reconjugated to amino acids if necessary and secreted into bile along with the newly

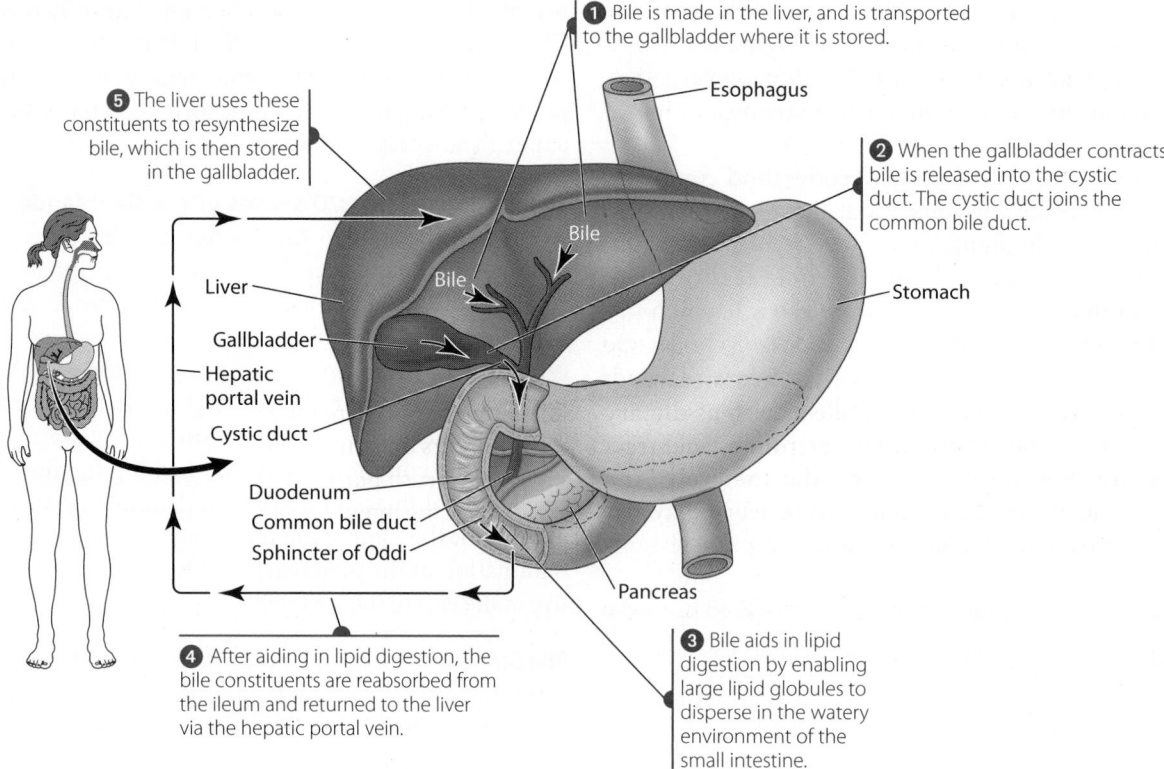

1 Bile is made in the liver, and is transported to the gallbladder where it is stored.

5 The liver uses these constituents to resynthesize bile, which is then stored in the gallbladder.

2 When the gallbladder contracts, bile is released into the cystic duct. The cystic duct joins the common bile duct.

3 Bile aids in lipid digestion by enabling large lipid globules to disperse in the watery environment of the small intestine.

4 After aiding in lipid digestion, the bile constituents are reabsorbed from the ileum and returned to the liver via the hepatic portal vein.

Figure 2.15 Enterohepatic circulation of bile.

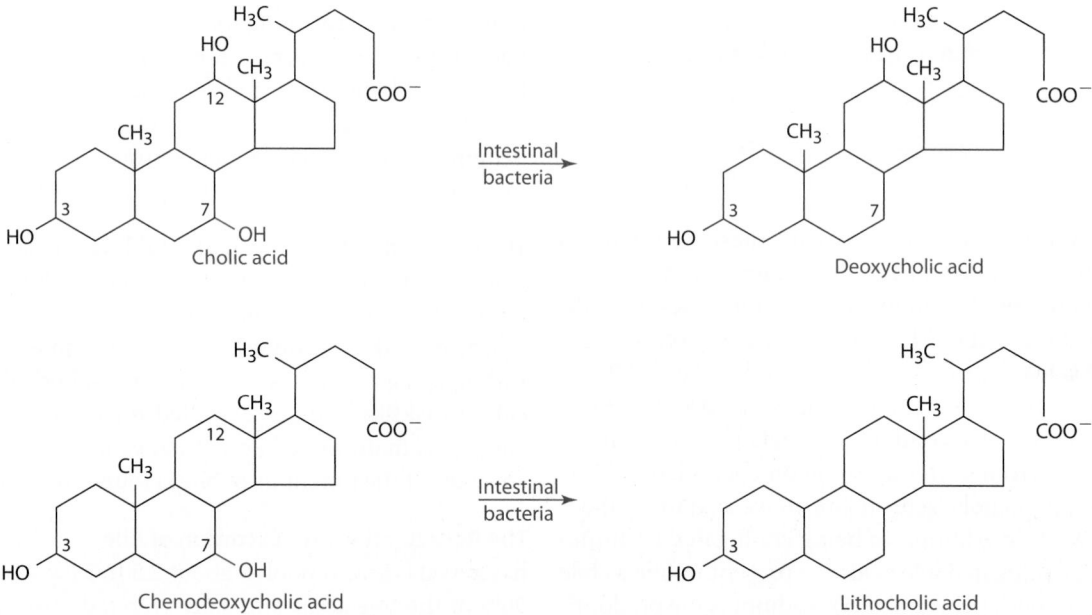

Figure 2.16 The synthesis of secondary bile acids by intestinal bacteria.
Source: Beerman/McGuire, Nutritional Sciences, 1/e. © Cengage Learning.

synthesized bile acids. New bile acids typically are synthesized in amounts about equal to those lost in the feces. New bile, mixed with recirculated bile, is sent through the cystic duct to be stored in the gallbladder. The circulation of bile, termed enterohepatic circulation, is pictured in Figure 2.15. The pool of bile is thought to recycle at least twice per meal.

Some of the bile acids that are not reabsorbed in the ileum may be deconjugated by bacteria in the colon and possibly the terminal ileum to form secondary bile acids (Figure 2.16). For example, cholic acid, a primary bile acid, is converted to the secondary bile acid deoxycholic acid, which can be reabsorbed. Chenodeoxycholic acid is converted to the secondary bile acid lithocholic acid, which, unlike deoxycholic acid, is typically excreted in the feces. About 0.5 g of bile salts are lost daily in the feces.

Bile Circulation and Hypercholesterolemia Knowing how bile is recirculated and excreted helps in understanding the mechanisms by which various drug therapies and functional foods help to treat high blood cholesterol concentrations (hypercholesterolemia). People with hypercholesterolemia are often given certain medications—specifically, resins such as cholestyramine (Questran)—that bind bile in the gastrointestinal tract and enhance its fecal excretion from the body. In addition, some food manufacturers add plant (phyto-) stanols and sterols to foods such as margarines, orange juice, and granola bars. These phytostanols and phytosterols (as well as some dietary fibers) bind bile as well as dietary and endogenous cholesterol in the gastrointestinal tract and enhance their fecal excretion from the body. The increased fecal excretion of the bile, decreased recirculation of the bile, and decreased absorption of cholesterol require the body to use cholesterol to synthesize new bile acids. The increased use of cholesterol to make more bile diminishes the body's cholesterol concentrations. Thus, the goal of using such medications and functional foods is to lower blood cholesterol concentrations and reduce risk of cardiovascular disease. Health claims on the labels of some of the products containing phytosterols state that "Plant sterols, eaten twice a day with food for a total of 1.3 g daily total, may reduce heart disease risk in a diet low in saturated fat and cholesterol." Daily consumption of plant sterols has been shown to decrease total and low-density lipoprotein (LDL) plasma cholesterol concentrations in people with normal or high blood lipid concentrations.

The Digestive and Absorptive Processes

Most nutrients must be digested—that is, broken down into smaller pieces—before they can be absorbed. Nutrient digestion occurs both in the lumen of the gastrointestinal tract and on the brush border, and is accomplished through enzymes from the mouth, stomach, pancreas, and small intestine and with the help of bile from the liver. Once digested, nutrients must move into the cells of the gastrointestinal tract by a process known as absorption. Although some nutrient absorption may occur in the stomach, the absorption of most nutrients begins in the duodenum and continues throughout the jejunum and ileum, as shown in Figure 2.17.

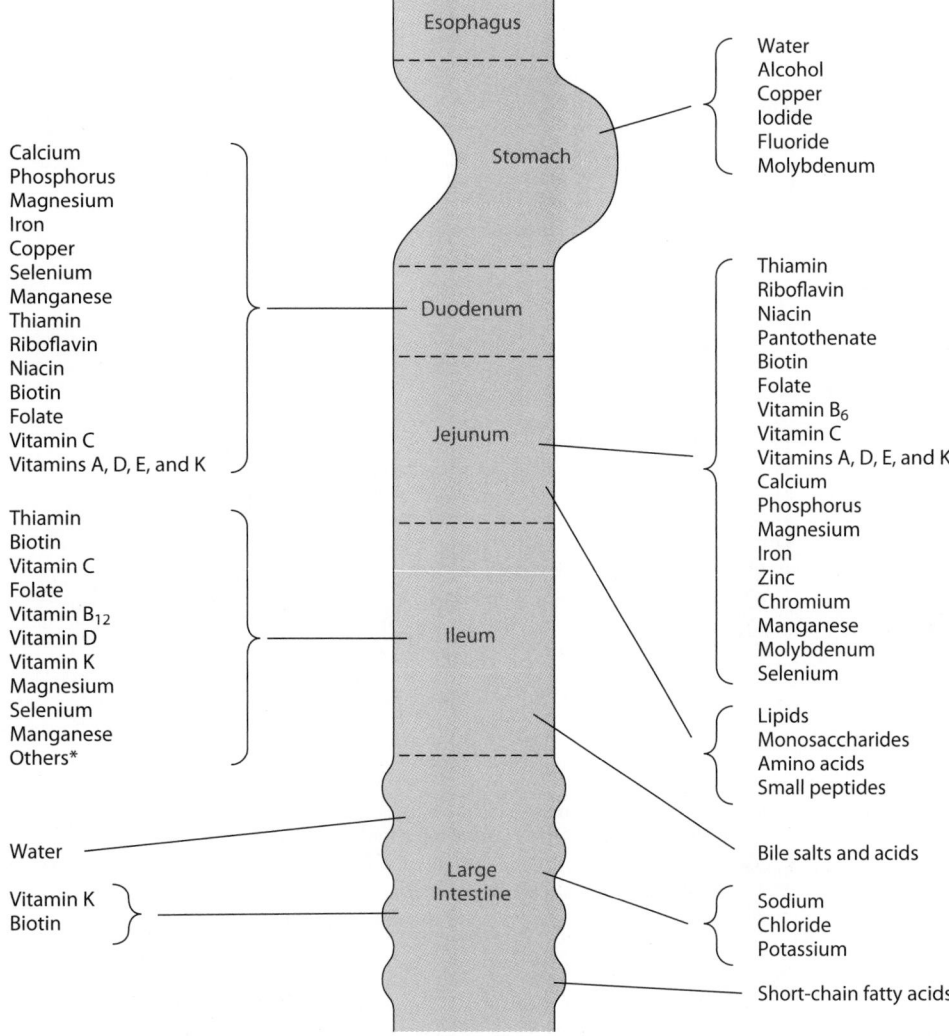

Figure 2.17 Sites of nutrient absorption in the gastrointestinal tract.

*Many additional nutrients may be absorbed from the ileum depending on transit time.

Generally, most absorption occurs in the proximal (upper) portion of the small intestine.

The digestion and absorption of nutrients within the small intestine are rapid, with most of the carbohydrate, protein, and fat being absorbed within 30 minutes after chyme has reached the small intestine. The presence of unabsorbed food in the ileum may increase the amount of time material remains in the small intestine and therefore may increase nutrient absorption.

Nutrients may be absorbed into enterocytes by diffusion, facilitated diffusion, active transport, or, occasionally, pinocytosis or endocytosis (Figure 2.18). In addition, a few nutrients may be absorbed by a paracellular (between cells) route. The mechanism of absorption for a nutrient depends on several factors:

- solubility (fat versus water) of the nutrient
- concentration or electrical gradient
- size of the molecule to be absorbed

The absorption and transport of amino acids, peptides, monosaccharides, fatty acids, monoacylglycerols, and glycerol—that is, the end products of macronutrient digestion—are considered in depth in Chapters 3, 5, and 6.

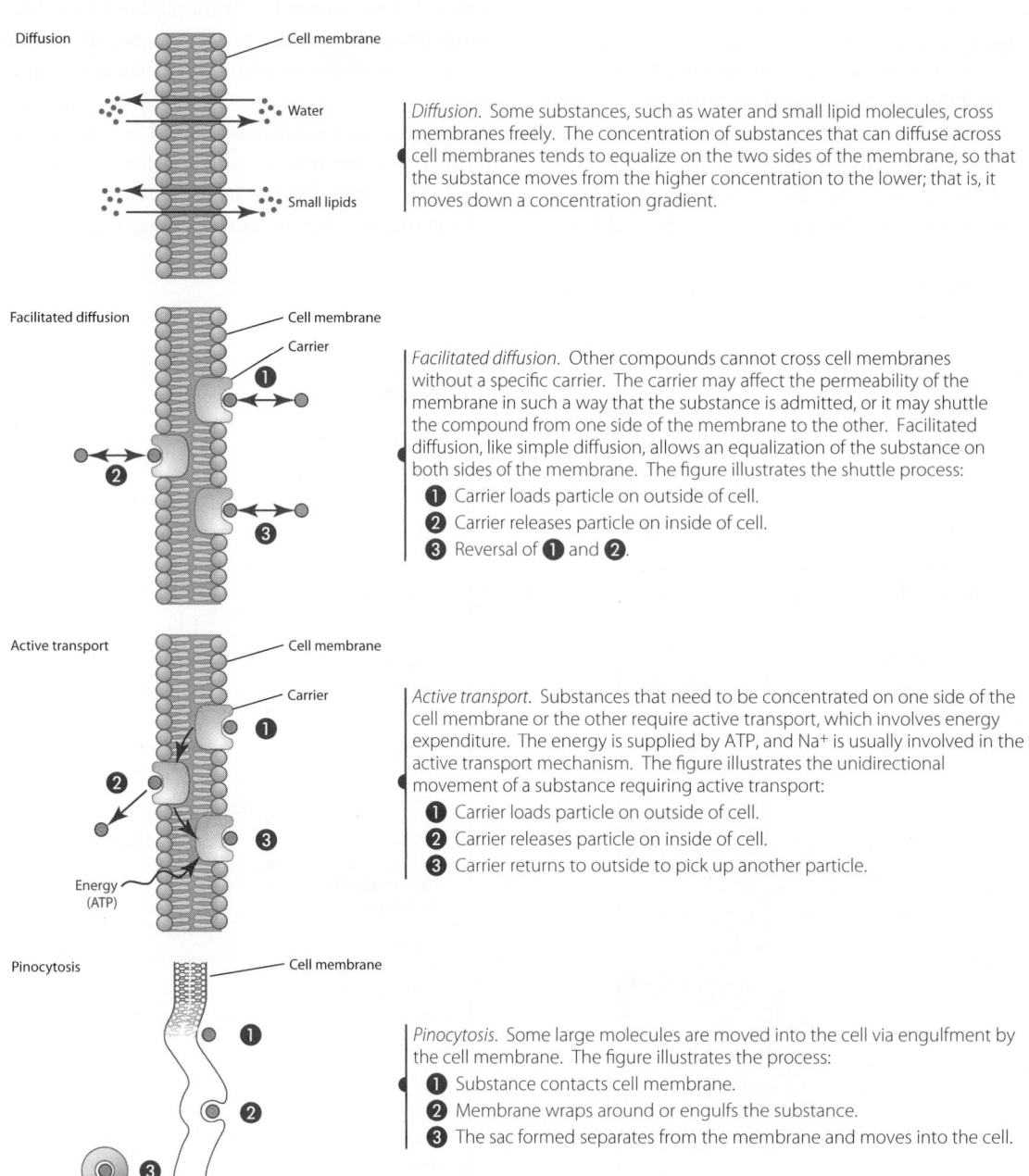

Diffusion. Some substances, such as water and small lipid molecules, cross membranes freely. The concentration of substances that can diffuse across cell membranes tends to equalize on the two sides of the membrane, so that the substance moves from the higher concentration to the lower; that is, it moves down a concentration gradient.

Facilitated diffusion. Other compounds cannot cross cell membranes without a specific carrier. The carrier may affect the permeability of the membrane in such a way that the substance is admitted, or it may shuttle the compound from one side of the membrane to the other. Facilitated diffusion, like simple diffusion, allows an equalization of the substance on both sides of the membrane. The figure illustrates the shuttle process:
- ❶ Carrier loads particle on outside of cell.
- ❷ Carrier releases particle on inside of cell.
- ❸ Reversal of ❶ and ❷.

Active transport. Substances that need to be concentrated on one side of the cell membrane or the other require active transport, which involves energy expenditure. The energy is supplied by ATP, and Na+ is usually involved in the active transport mechanism. The figure illustrates the unidirectional movement of a substance requiring active transport:
- ❶ Carrier loads particle on outside of cell.
- ❷ Carrier releases particle on inside of cell.
- ❸ Carrier returns to outside to pick up another particle.

Pinocytosis. Some large molecules are moved into the cell via engulfment by the cell membrane. The figure illustrates the process:
- ❶ Substance contacts cell membrane.
- ❷ Membrane wraps around or engulfs the substance.
- ❸ The sac formed separates from the membrane and moves into the cell.

Figure 2.18 Primary mechanisms for nutrient absorption.

The digestion and mechanisms of absorption for each of the vitamins and minerals are described in detail in Chapters 9 to 14; the general sites of absorption are shown in Figure 2.17.

Unabsorbed intestinal contents are passed from the ileum through the ileocecal sphincter into the colon, although some may serve as substrates for bacteria that inhabit the small intestine. Bacterial counts in the small intestine range up to about 10^3 per gram of intestinal contents; counts may be even higher near the ileocecal sphincter. Examples of some of the bacteria that may be found in the small intestine include bacteroides, enterobacteria, lactobacilli, streptococci, and staphylococci.

The Colon (Large Intestine)

From the ileum (which is the distal or terminal section of the small intestine), unabsorbed materials empty through the ileocecal sphincter into the cecum, the right side of the colon (large intestine). From the cecum, materials move sequentially through the ascending, transverse, descending, and sigmoid sections of the colon (Figure 2.19). The colon in its entirety is almost 5 feet long and is larger in diameter than the small intestine, thus explaining the terminology distinction (large versus small) between the two intestines.

Rather than being a part of the entire wall of the digestive tract, as it is in the upper digestive tract, the longitudinal muscle in the colon is gathered into three muscular bands or strips called teniae (also spelled taenia or teneae) coli that extend throughout most of the colon. Contraction of a strip of longitudinal muscle, along with contraction of circular muscle, causes the uncontracted portions of the colon to bulge outward, creating pouches (haustra). Contractions typically occur in one area of the colon and then move to a different, nearby area.

On initially entering the colon, the intestinal material is still quite fluid. Contraction of the musculature of the large intestine is coordinated so as to mix the intestinal contents gently and to keep material in the proximal (ascending) colon a sufficient length of time to allow nutrients to be absorbed.

The proximal colonic epithelia absorb sodium, chloride, and water more effectively than does the small intestinal mucosa. For example, about 90% to 95% of the water and sodium entering the colon each day is absorbed. Colonic absorption of sodium is influenced by a number of factors, including hormones. Antidiuretic hormone (also called vasopressin) secreted from the pituitary gland, for example, decreases sodium absorption, whereas glucocorticoids like cortisol secreted from the adrenal gland and mineralocorticoids such as aldosterone secreted from the adrenal gland increase sodium absorption in the colon.

Secretions into the lumen of the colon are few, but present. Goblet cells secrete mucus. Mucus protects the colonic mucosa and acts as a lubricant for fecal matter. Potassium is secreted, possibly through an active secretory pathway, into the colon. Bicarbonate is also secreted in exchange for chloride absorption. Bicarbonate provides an alkaline environment that helps neutralize acids produced by colonic anaerobic bacteria. Sodium and hydrogen ion exchanges also occur, permitting electrolyte absorption.

The end result of the passage of material through the colon, which usually takes about 12 to 70 hours, is that the unabsorbed materials are progressively dehydrated. Typically, the approximately 1 L of chyme that enters the large intestine each day is reduced to less than about 200 g of defecated material containing sloughed gastrointestinal cells, inorganic matter, water, small amounts of unabsorbed nutrients and food residue, constituents of digestive juices, and bacteria.

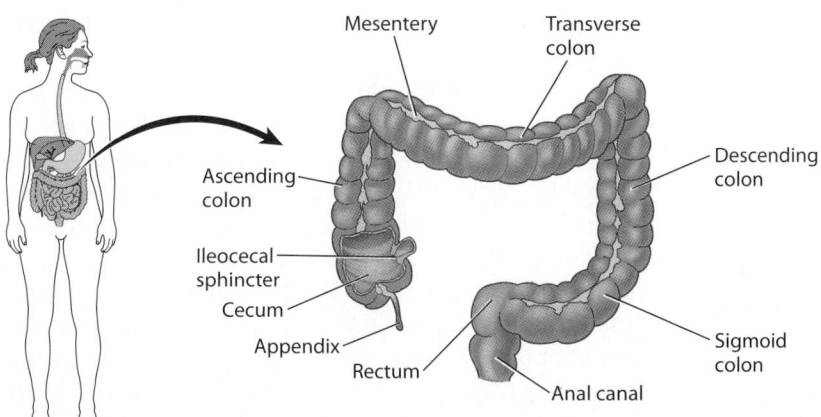

Figure 2.19 The colon.
Source: Beerman/McGuire, Nutritional Sciences, 1/e. © Cengage Learning.

Intestinal Bacteria (Microflora), Probiotics, and Disease

Both gram-negative and gram-positive bacterial strains, representing over 400 species of at least 40 genera, have been isolated from human feces. Although intestinal bacterial counts in the large intestine have been reported to be as high as 10^{12} per gram of gastrointestinal tract contents, bacteria are found throughout the gastrointestinal tract. The mouth contains mostly anaerobic bacteria. The stomach contains few bacteria because of its low pH, but some more acid-resistant bacteria that are present include *Lactobacillus* and *Streptococcus*. The proximal small intestine contains both aerobes and facultative anaerobes. Most bacteria found in the ileum and large intestine are anaerobes, including bacteroides, lactobacilli, and clostridia. Other examples of intestinal microflora (bacteria adapted to living in a specific environment) that inhabit the large intestine are bifidobacteria, methanogens, eubacteria, and streptococci. Anaerobic species are thought to outnumber aerobic species by at least 10 fold, but the exact composition of the microflora is affected by a variety of factors such as substrate availability, pH, medications, and diet, among others.

Bacteria gain nutrients for their own growth from undigested and/or unabsorbed food residues in the intestines. Enzymes synthesized by the bacteria but lacking in humans allow for the digestion of many nutrients. Bacteria use primarily dietary carbohydrate such as plant polysaccharides and other sugars, and to a lesser extent amino acids and undigested protein, as substrates necessary for their growth. For example, starch that has not undergone hydrolysis by pancreatic amylase may be used by gram-negative bacteroides and by gram-positive bifidobacteria or eubacteria. Glycoproteins (mainly mucins) found in mucus secretions of the gastrointestinal tract may be broken down and used by bacteria such as bacteroides, bifidobacteria, and clostridia. In addition, sugar alcohols such as sorbitol and xylitol; disaccharides such as lactose; and some fibers such as some hemicelluloses, fructooligosaccharides, pectins, and gums may be degraded by selected bacteria found in the colon. Digestive enzymes themselves may even serve as substrates for bacteria such as bacteroides and clostridia. The breakdown of carbohydrate and protein by bacteria is an anaerobic process referred to as **fermentation**.

The fermentation of carbohydrates by intestinal bacteria has been associated with some of the symptoms of functional gut or gastrointestinal disorders such as irritable bowel syndrome. Classic symptoms of these gut disorders include bloating, gas (flatulence), abdominal cramping, and diarrhea. Fermentable short-chain carbohydrates, including the oligosaccharides fructans and galactans, the disaccharide lactose, and the monosaccharide fructose, as well as polyols (sugar alcohols) such as sorbitol, xylitol, maltitol, mannitol, and isomalt, have received the most attention as causative agents and have been coined FODMAP—*f*ermentable, *o*ligo-, *d*i-, *m*onosaccharides *a*nd *p*olyols. Restriction of foods rich in these carbohydrates is thought to help alleviate symptoms but results in an extensive list of foods to avoid. For example, to minimize fructose consumption, one must limit foods with added high-fructose corn syrup, which include many sauces and condiments (barbeque sauce, ketchup, syrups), fruit drinks, agave, honey, and some whole fruits. Fructans that need to be limited are found in many vegetables, such as asparagus, broccoli, artichoke, cabbage, garlic, onions, shallots, leek, and snow peas. To avoid galactans, one must minimize intakes of soy products, broccoli, lentils, kidney beans, and chickpeas. Lactose is found primarily in dairy products; polyols, in a number of gums and mints as well as in some fruits like apples, watermelon, plums, peaches, and pears, to name a few. The effectiveness of such dietary restrictions in treating functional gut disorders has not been established.

As described previously, bacteria degrade mostly carbohydrate but also some amino acids and protein to produce the energy and substances, such as carbon atoms, necessary for bacterial growth and maintenance. Acids are one of the principal end products of bacterial carbohydrate fermentation in the large intestine. Specifically, lactic acid and various short-chain fatty acids—acetic acid, butyric acid, and propionic acid—are generated from bacterial action. These short-chain fatty acids, formerly called volatile fatty acids, serve many purposes. They, especially butyric acid, are thought to stimulate gastrointestinal cell proliferation and help maintain the integrity of the intestinal epithelial cells. Further, the presence of the acids lowers the luminal pH in the colon to effect changes in nutrient absorption and in the growth of certain species of bacteria. In addition, these acids provide substrates for body cell use. Butyric acid, for example, may be absorbed by a Na^+/H^+ or a K^+/H^+ exchange system in the colon, where it is a preferred energy source for colonic epithelial cells. Butyric acid also may regulate gene expression and cell growth. Propionic and lactic acids are absorbed in the colon and taken up for use by liver cells. Acetic acid is absorbed and used by muscle and brain cells. Absorption of these acids appears to be concentration dependent.

In addition to the short-chain fatty acids, bacteria generate a number of other substances. For example, vitamins such as biotin and vitamin K are produced by intestinal bacteria and may be absorbed to varying degrees by the body. Several different gases also are produced by colonic bacteria, including methane (CH_4), hydrogen (H_2), hydrogen sulfide (H_2S), and carbon dioxide (CO_2). One estimate suggests that colonic bacterial fermentation of about 10 g of carbohydrate can generate several liters of hydrogen gas. Much of the hydrogen and other gases that are generated can be used by other bacteria in the colon. Gases not used are excreted. Measurement of the hydrogen gas produced by bacteria is used as a basis to diagnose *lactose intolerance,* a condition in which the enzyme lactase is not made in sufficient quantities and thus is not available to digest the disaccharide lactose. Lactose intolerance is fairly common among adults, especially those of African American, American Indian, and Asian heritage. When someone with lactose intolerance ingests the sugar lactose (e.g., by drinking milk), the lactose cannot be digested in the small intestine and enters the colon undigested. In the colon, the undigested lactose is fermented by colonic bacteria. These colonic bacteria, upon fermenting large quantities of lactose, in turn produce a lot more hydrogen gas than usual. Much of the hydrogen gas made by the bacteria is absorbed by the body and then exhaled in the breath. To diagnose lactose intolerance, a person usually is asked to consume about 50 g of lactose, and their breath is analyzed for hydrogen gas for the next several hours. Generally, if the person is lactose intolerant, hydrogen gas excretion in the breath increases for about 1 to 1½ hours after lactose is consumed. An absence of an increase in breath hydrogen gas concentrations suggests adequate lactose digestion. Symptoms of lactose intolerance include bloating, gas, and abdominal pain.

Amino acids also are degraded by bacteria. For example, bacterial degradation of the branched-chain amino acids generates branched-chain fatty acids such as isobutyric acid and isovaleric acid. Deamination (removal of the amino group) of aromatic amino acids yields phenolic compounds. Amines such as histamine result from bacterial decarboxylation of amino acids such as histidine. Ammonia is generated by bacterial deamination of amino acids as well as by bacterial urease action on urea (secreted into the gastrointestinal tract from the blood). The ammonia can be reabsorbed by the colon and recirculated to the liver, where it can be reused to synthesize urea or amino acids. About 25%, or 8 g, of the body's urea may be handled in this fashion. This process must be controlled in people with *liver disease.* High amounts of ammonia in the blood are thought to contribute to the development of hepatic encephalopathy and coma in people with liver disease (cirrhosis). Thus, diets that do not contain excessive amounts of protein are commonly recommended for people with advanced liver disease. Uric acid and creatinine may also be released into the digestive tract and metabolized by colonic bacteria.

Probiotics (*pro* means "life" in Greek)—foods that contain live/active cultures of specific strains of bacteria—are of interest in the health field. The intent of consuming probiotics is for the bacteria to survive the passage through the upper digestive tract and then establish themselves in (colonize) the lower gastrointestinal tract, primarily the colon, and exert beneficial effects on the person's health. At present, probiotics are mostly consumed as yogurt with live cultures or in fermented milk. To be considered a probiotic, the product must contain 100 million live active bacteria per gram. In the United States, yogurt is often fermented by *Lactobacillus bulgaricus* and *Streptococcus thermophilus*, and milk is usually fermented by *L. acidophilus* and *L. casei*. Other bacteria used to manufacture dairy products include *Leuconostoc esntheroides*, *L. mesenteroides*, and *Lactococcus lactis*. The most common probiotic bacteria are lactic acid bacteria such as bifidobacteria and lactobacilli. Other food sources of probiotics include miso, tempeh, and some soy beverages.

In addition to probiotics, **prebiotics** are also of importance. Prebiotics are food ingredients that are not digested by human digestive enzymes but can benefit the host by acting as substrate for the growth and/or activity of one or more selected species of bacteria in the colon, and thus improve the health of the host. For example, consuming various types of fiber such as fructooligosaccharides appears to effectively increase selected microbial populations, especially bifidobacteria and lactobacilli. The increased presence of these health-promoting bacteria in turn helps to inhibit the growth of other, pathogenic bacteria. Prebiotics and their uses are discussed in more detail in the Perspective for Chapter 4.

Probiotics appear to be beneficial in preventing and treating several conditions. Some of these conditions include diarrhea, inflammatory bowel diseases (Crohn's disease and ulcerative colitis), colon cancer, infected pancreatic necrosis, and post–liver transplant infections; however, with the exception of certain types of diarrheal illnesses, data are not sufficient to support routine probiotic use [1-6].

The mechanisms by which probiotics exert their effects are not clear, but some of the several hypotheses include both immunological and nonimmunological roles. Probiotics are generally thought to:

- enhance the host's immune defense system by increasing secretory IgA production, tightening the mucosal barrier, enhancing lymphocyte cytokine responses, enhancing phagocytic activity, and enhancing intestinal cell mucin production and secretion (to enhance the mucus layer), among other actions

- displace, exclude, or antagonize pathogenic bacteria from colonizing, for example, by competing for attachment sites on the intestinal mucosa or by strengthening the mucosal barrier to normalize intestinal permeability and to prevent pathogenic bacterial translocation

- acidify the colonic pH by producing fermentation products such as short-chain fatty acids

- transform and promote excretion of toxic substances such as bile acids, nitrosamines, heterocyclic amines, and mutagenic compounds
- enhance fecal bulk production, which may decrease (speed up) transit time and thereby lower the colon's exposure time to toxic substances [1-6].

Studies examining the effectiveness of probiotics typically provided at least 1 to 10 billion colony-forming units (CFU) per dose. Doses are given once or twice daily or sometimes a few times per week. Tolerance is typically satisfactory; however, bacterial sepsis (infection) is possible, especially in those with impaired immune function (immunosuppression), intestinal tract dysfunction (characterized by increased gastrointestinal permeability or a defective barrier), or other chronic health conditions such as diabetes mellitus, cancer, abscesses, and organ transplant.

COORDINATION AND REGULATION OF THE DIGESTIVE PROCESS

Neural Regulation

The sympathetic and parasympathetic nervous systems, as well as the enteric nervous system, mediate gastrointestinal activities. Sympathetic nervous system fibers, arising in the thoracic and lumbar regions of the spinal cord, innervate all areas of the gastrointestinal tract. Generally, norepinephrine, released from the nerve endings, acts on smooth muscle of the digestive tract to inhibit activity. Sympathetic efferent neurons, for example, decrease muscle contractions and constrict sphincters to diminish gastrointestinal motility. In contrast, the parasympathetic nervous system typically stimulates the digestive tract, promoting motility (peristalsis), gastrointestinal reflexes, and secretions. For example, the facial and glossopharyngeal nerves stimulate saliva production, and the vagus nerve, which innervates the esophagus, stomach, pancreas, and proximal colon, stimulates gastric acid secretion, among other processes.

The nervous system of the gastrointestinal tract is referred to as the enteric (relating to the intestine) nervous system. The system includes millions of neurons and their processes embedded in the wall of the gastrointestinal tract beginning in the esophagus and extending to the anus. The enteric nervous system, which is connected to the central nervous system largely through the vagus nerve and other pathways out of the spinal cord, can be divided into two neuronal networks, or plexuses: the myenteric plexus (or plexus of Auerbach) and the submucosal plexus (or plexus of Meissner). The location and actions of these two plexuses are given here:

Myenteric Plexus	Submucosal Plexus
Lies in the muscularis externa between longitudinal and circular muscles of the muscularis propria	Lies in the submucosa (mostly in the intestines)
Controls peristaltic activity and gastrointestinal motility	Controls mainly gastrointestinal secretions and local blood flow

Impulses, either stimulatory or inhibitory, are sent from the enteric nervous system to the smooth circular and longitudinal muscles of the gastrointestinal tract. The myenteric plexus controls peristalsis, and when this plexus is stimulated, gastrointestinal activity generally increases. The submucosal plexus typically controls secretion release, receiving information from stretch receptors and gastrointestinal epithelial cells in the intestinal wall. Also under control by the enteric nervous system is the regulation of gut motility by the migrating myoelectric or motility complex, described in the "Regulation of Gut Motility and Gastric Emptying" section of this chapter.

The enteric nervous system also affects gastrointestinal reflexes, called enterogastric reflexes. Reflexes are an involuntary response to stimuli and in the gastrointestinal tract affect secretions, blood flow, and peristalsis as well as other processes involved in digestion. Two examples of enterogastric reflexes are the ileogastric reflex and the gastroileal reflex. With the ileogastric reflex, gastric motility is inhibited when the ileum becomes distended. With the gastroileal reflex, ileal motility is stimulated when gastric motility and secretions increase. Other reflexes affect the small and large intestines. For example, the colonoileal reflex from the colon inhibits the emptying of the contents of the ileum into the colon. The intestinointestinal reflex diminishes intestinal motility when a segment of the intestine is overdistended.

Regulatory Peptides

Factors influencing digestion and absorption are coordinated, in part, by a group of gastrointestinal tract molecules called regulatory peptides or, more specifically, gastrointestinal hormones and neuropeptides. Regulatory peptides affect a variety of digestive functions, including gastrointestinal motility, intestinal absorption, cell growth, and the secretion of digestive enzymes, electrolytes, water, and other hormones.

Some of the regulatory peptides—such as gastrin, cholecystokinin, secretin, glucose-dependent insulinotropic peptide (GIP), and motilin—are considered hormones. In fact, many of the hormones can be categorized together (and called families) based on their amino acid sequences.

Some regulatory peptides are termed paracrines and neurocrines. When released by endocrine cells, paracrines diffuse through extracellular spaces to their target tissues rather than being secreted into the blood (like hormones) for transport to target tissues. Some paracrines affecting the gastrointestinal tract include somatostatin, glucagon-like peptides, and insulin-like growth factor.

The functions of regulatory peptides with respect to the gastrointestinal tract and the digestive process are numerous and have been addressed to varying degrees in the sections on regulation of gastric and intestinal secretions and motility. Most, but not all, hormones and peptides have multiple actions; some are strictly inhibitory or stimulatory, whereas some mediate both types of responses. More than 100 regulatory peptides are thought to affect gastrointestinal functions. Table 2.2 summarizes some of the functions of a few of these peptides, while more detailed information is provided hereafter.

- Gastrin, secreted into the blood primarily by enteroendocrine G-cells in the antrum of the stomach and proximal small intestine, acts mainly in the stomach. Gastrin release occurs in response to vagal stimulation, ingestion of specific substances or nutrients, gastric distention, hydrochloric acid in contact with gastric mucosa, and the effects of local and circulating hormones. Gastrin principally stimulates the release of hydrochloric acid, but it also stimulates gastric and intestinal motility and pepsinogen release. Gastrin also stimulates the cellular growth of (i.e., has trophic action on) the stomach and both the small and large intestines. Gastrin also stimulates the release of the hormone glucagon by the pancreas.

- Cholecystokinin (CCK), secreted into the blood by enteroendocrine I-cells of the proximal small intestine and

by enteric nerves in the ileum and colon, principally stimulates secretion of pancreatic juice and enzymes into the duodenum. It also stimulates gallbladder contraction, which facilitates the release of bile into the duodenum, and to a limited extent, it inhibits gastric emptying and motility. Cholecystokinin also stimulates the release of glucagon by the pancreas. Further, the hormone is found in neurons in the brain, where it influences the perception of appetite, among other processes.

- Secretin is secreted into the blood by enteroendocrine S-cells found in the proximal small intestine in response to the release of acidic chyme into the duodenum. Secretin acts primarily on pancreatic acinar cells to stimulate the release of pancreatic juice and enzymes into the intestine. Secretin is thought to stimulate pepsinogen release but inhibit gastric acid secretion. It may also inhibit motility of most of the gastrointestinal tract, especially the stomach and proximal small intestine.

- Motilin, a peptide secreted by enteroendocrine M-cells of the duodenum and jejunum, stimulates gastric and duodenal motility, gastric and pancreatic secretions, and gallbladder contraction.

- Glucose-dependent insulinotropic peptide (GIP), previously called gastric inhibitory peptide, is produced by enteroendocrine K-cells of the duodenum and jejunum and primarily stimulates insulin secretion, but also inhibits gastric secretions and motility.

- Peptide YY (PYY), secreted by enteroendocrine cells of the ileum, inhibits gastric acid and pancreatic juice secretions and inhibits gastric and intestinal motility.

- Enterogastrone, secreted by the ileum, inhibits to a minor extent gastric and pancreatic secretions.

- Amylin, secreted by the pancreatic, gastric, and intestinal endocrine cells, delays gastric emptying and inhibits postprandial glucagon secretion.

Table 2.2 Selected Regulatory Hormones/Peptides of the Gastrointestinal Tract, Their Production Site, and Selected Functions

Hormone/Peptide	Production Sites	Some Selected Function(s)
Gastrin	Stomach and small intestine	Stimulates motility and gastric acid release
Cholecystokinin	Small intestine	Stimulates gall bladder contraction and pancreatic secretions
Secretin	Small intestine	Stimulates pancreas juice and enzyme secretion and inhibits gastrointestinal motility
Motilin	Small intestine	Stimulates gastric and intestinal motility
Glucose-dependent insulinotropic peptide	Small intestine	Stimulates insulin secretion and inhibits gastric secretions and motility
Peptide YY	Small intestine	Inhibits motility and gastric and pancreatic secretions
Enterogastrone	Small intestine	Inhibits gastric secretions
Amylin	Pancreas, stomach, small intestine	Inhibits gastric emptying
Somatostatin	Pancreas and small intestine	Inhibits gastric secretions and motility, and pancreatic (exocrine) and gall bladder secretions
Glucagon-like peptides	Small and large intestines	Inhibits gastrointestinal tract motility
Substance P	Neurons and small intestine	Inhibits gastric secretions and stimulates intestinal motility

Paracrine-acting substances usually work by entering secretions. Three examples of paracrine-acting peptides are:

- Somatostatin, synthesized by pancreatic δ (D)-cells and intestinal cells, appears to mediate the inhibition of gastrin release as well as the release of GIP, secretin, vasoactive intestinal polypeptide, and motilin and thus inhibits gastric acid, gastric motility, pancreatic exocrine secretions, and gallbladder contraction.
- Glucagon-like peptides are secreted by enteroendocrine L-cells of the ileum and colon and by the nervous system. These peptides decrease gastrointestinal motility and increase proliferation of the gastrointestinal tract; they also influence glucagon and insulin secretion.
- Insulin-like growth factors, also secreted by endocrine cells of the gastrointestinal tract, increase proliferation of the gastrointestinal tract.

Four examples of neurocrine peptides are:

- Vasoactive intestinal polypeptide (VIP) is present in central and peripheral neurons. It is not thought to be present in intestinal endocrine cells. VIP is thought to stimulate intestinal secretions, relax most gastrointestinal sphincters, inhibit gastric acid secretion, and stimulate the release of pancreatic secretions.
- Gastrin-releasing peptide (GRP), also called bombesin, released from enteric nerves, stimulates gastrin release as well as other peptides like cholecystokinin, glucagon-like peptides, and somatostatin.
- Neurotensin, produced by neurons and N-cells of the small intestine mucosa (especially the ileum), may inhibit motility but its exact physiological role in the digestive process at normal circulating concentrations is unclear. Neurotensin has multiple actions in the brain.
- Substance powder (P), found in nerve and endocrine cells in the gastrointestinal tract, increases blood flow to the gastrointestinal tract, inhibits acid secretion, increases motility of the small intestine, and binds to pancreatic acinar cells associated with enzyme secretion.

In addition to effects on gastrointestinal tract secretions and motility, many hormones and neuropeptides influence food intake. Ghrelin, for example, a peptide secreted primarily from endocrine cells of the stomach and small intestine, acts on the hypothalamus to stimulate food intake. Plasma concentrations of ghrelin typically rise before eating (e.g., a fasting situation) and decrease immediately after eating, especially carbohydrates. Ghrelin also stimulates expression of neuropeptide Y (NPY). Neuropeptide Y also stimulates eating but inhibits secretion of gastric ghrelin and insulin. Neuropeptide Y is typically effective as long as leptin concentrations are relatively low. Leptin is secreted mainly by white adipose tissue, and the amount secreted is proportional to fat stores. Leptin suppresses food intake and inhibits neurons from releasing neuropeptide Y and the appetite-stimulating neuropeptide agouti-related protein (AGRP). Thus, the net effect is the suppression of the appetite-stimulating peptides neuropeptide Y and agouti-related protein. Leptin is known to work in conjunction with α-melanocyte-stimulating hormone (α-MSH). Specifically, leptin's ability to inhibit food intake is based, at least in part, on α-MSH's stimulation of MC_4 receptors, primarily in the hypothalamus. Corticotropin-releasing hormone (CRH) also suppresses food intake and appears to work in conjunction with leptin. Other hormones suppressing food intake (or serving as satiety factors) include cholecystokinin, enterostatin, serotonin, and glucagon-like peptide. Thus, the various mediators of the digestive process work in concert to stimulate and inhibit food intake and to break down and absorb the nutrients.

SUMMARY

Examining the various mechanisms in the gastrointestinal tract that allow food to be ingested, digested, and absorbed, and its residue to then be excreted, reveals the complexity of the digestion and absorption processes. Normal digestion and absorption of nutrients depend not only on a healthy digestive tract but also on integration of the digestive system with the nervous, endocrine, and circulatory systems.

The many factors that influence digestion and absorption—including dispersion and mixing of ingested food, quantity and composition of gastrointestinal secretions, enterocyte integrity, the expanse of intestinal absorptive area, and the transit time of intestinal contents—must be coordinated so that the body can be nourished without disrupting the homeostasis of body fluids. Much of the coordination required is provided by regulatory peptides, some of which are provided by the nervous system as well as by the endocrine cells of the gastrointestinal tract.

Although the basic structure of the digestive tract, which consists of the mucosa, submucosa, muscularis externa, and serosa, remains the same throughout, structural modifications enable various segments of the gastrointestinal tract to perform more specific functions. Gastric glands that underlie the gastric mucosa secrete fluids and compounds necessary for the stomach's digestive functions. Other particularly noteworthy features are the folds of Kerckring, the villi, and the microvilli, all of which dramatically increase the surface area exposed to the contents of the intestinal lumen. This enlarged surface area helps maximize absorption, not only of ingested nutrients but also of endogenous secretions released into the gastrointestinal tract.

Study of the digestive system makes abundantly clear the fact that a person's adequate nourishment, and therefore his or her health, depends in large measure on a normally functioning gastrointestinal tract. Particularly crucial to nourishment and health is a normally functioning small intestine because that is where the greatest amount of digestion and absorption occurs. Later chapters of this book expand on digestion and absorption of individual nutrients.

References Cited

1. Quigley EMM. Prebiotics and probiotics: modifying and mining the microbiota. Pharmacol Res. 2010; 61:213–18.
2. Douglas LC, Sanders ME. Probiotics and prebiotics in dietetics practice. J Am Diet Assoc. 2008; 108:510–21.
3. Predidis GA, Versalovic J. Targeting the human microbiome with antibiotics, probiotics, and prebiotics: gastroenterology enters the metagenomics era. Gastroenterology. 2009; 136:2015–31.
4. Whelan K, Myers CE. Safety of probiotics in patients receiving nutrition support: a systematic review of case reports, randomized controlled trials, and nonrandomized trials. Am J Clin Nutr. 2010; 91:687–703.
5. Williams NT. Probiotics. Am J Health-Syst Pharm. 2010; 67:449–58.
6. Ohland CL, MacNaughton WK. Probiotic bacteria and intestinal epithelial barrier function. Am J Physiol Gastrointest Liver Physiol. 2010; 298:G807–19.

AN OVERVIEW OF SELECTED DIGESTIVE SYSTEM DISORDERS WITH IMPLICATIONS FOR NOURISHING THE BODY

In Chapter 2, digestion is defined as a process by which food is broken down mechanically and chemically in the gastrointestinal (GI) tract. Digestion ultimately provides nutrients ready for absorption into the body through the cells of the GI tract, principally the cells (enterocytes) of the small intestine. Secretions required to digest nutrients are produced by multiple organs of the GI tract. These secretions include primarily enzymes, but also hydrochloric acid important for gastric digestion, and bicarbonate and bile important for digestion and absorption in the intestine. If one or more organs malfunctions because of disease, fewer secretions may be synthesized and released into the GI tract. Without secretions, or with less than normal amounts of secretions, nutrient digestion may be impaired, resulting in nutrient malabsorption.

Many conditions or diseases alter the function of organs of the GI tract and thus affect digestion. For example, some GI tract diseases may cause decreased synthesis and release of secretions needed for nutrient digestion. Other conditions or diseases that affect the GI tract—for example, malfunction of sphincters—can alter motility or clearing of the GI contents through the organs of the GI tract. Clearing problems may cause back fluxes (refluxes) of secretions from, for example, the stomach into the esophagus (remember, normally the contents of the GI tract move from the esophagus to the stomach, and not vice versa). Conditions in which the GI mucosa is inflamed or damaged, as well as conditions that increase transit time or speed up the movement of GI contents (food and nutrients) through the GI tract, typically result in nutrient malabsorption because the body does not have enough time to digest and absorb nutrients.

An understanding of the physiology of the GI tract and its accessory organs, and of the diseases affecting the GI tract, is essential to understanding how to modify a person's diet from the standard dietary recommendations for healthy populations of the United States. This perspective addresses, in a general fashion, four disorders that affect the gastrointestinal tract and outlines the implications of these conditions for nourishing the body.

GASTROESOPHAGEAL REFLUX DISEASE

Gastroesophageal reflux disease (GERD) is a disorder marked by reflux or backward flow of gastric contents (acidic chyme) from the stomach to the esophagus. After food is chewed and swallowed, the food enters the esophagus and then passes through the gastroesophageal sphincter into the stomach. Normally, the gastroesophageal sphincter displays a relatively high pressure that prevents the reflux of stomach contents into the esophagus. However, changes or decreases in the gastroesophageal sphincter pressure, sometimes called lower esophageal sphincter incompetence, can ultimately result in GERD. Increases in abdominal pressure, such as may occur with overeating, bending, lifting, lying down, vomiting, or coughing, also can increase reflux and cause GERD.

Recurrent reflux of gastric contents, including hydrochloric acid, into the esophagus from the stomach can damage and inflame the esophageal mucosa and result in reflux esophagitis (inflammation of the esophagus caused by the refluxed gastric contents). The severity of the esophagitis depends in part on the volume and acidity of the gastric contents that are refluxed and on the length of time the gastric contents are in contact with the esophageal mucosa. The more acidic the contents, and the longer the contents are in contact with the mucosa, the more damage results. Weak peristalsis and delays in gastric emptying are likely to prolong contact time and increase damage. The resistance of the esophageal mucosa also affects the severity of the damage. Repeated bouts of GERD resulting in reflux esophagitis cause, to varying degrees, esophageal edema (swelling); esophageal tissue damage, including erosion and ulceration; blood vessel (usually capillary) damage; spasms; and fibrotic tissue formation, which can cause a narrowing (stricture) within the esophagus.

A person experiencing GERD or reflux esophagitis typically complains of heartburn, that is, a burning sensation in the midchest region, but may also complain of excessive belching and/or coughing. The symptoms usually occur within an hour of eating and worsen if the person lies down soon after eating.

To address nutrition implications of this condition, we first need to reexamine some of the foods, nutrients, or substances in foods that influence gastroesophageal sphincter pressure, that may promote increased acid production, and that may irritate an inflamed esophagus. Several substances decrease gastroesophageal sphincter pressure, including high-fat foods, chocolate, nicotine, alcohol, and carminatives. Carminatives are volatile oil extracts of plants, most often oils of spearmint and peppermint. Other substances increase gastric secretions, especially acid production. Alcohol, calcium, decaffeinated and caffeinated coffee, and tea (specifically, methylxanthines) stimulate gastric secretions, including hydrochloric acid. Citrus products and other acidic foods or beverages, as well as some spices, are known to directly irritate an inflamed esophagus. Ingesting these substances or foods is likely to aggravate irritated esophageal mucosa.

Based on this knowledge, some of the recommendations for the patient with GERD or reflux esophagitis include:

- avoiding substances that can further decrease gastroesophageal sphincter pressure, which is already low because of the condition
- avoiding substances that may promote the secretion of acid, which would be present in higher concentrations than normal if refluxed
- avoiding foods or substances that may irritate an inflamed esophagus

To implement these recommendations, people with GERD or reflux esophagitis must be told which foods or substances to avoid, such as high-fat foods or meals, chocolate, coffee, tea, alcohol, carminatives such as peppermint and spearmint, citrus products, acidic foods, and spices such as red and black pepper, nutmeg, cloves, and chili powder.

In addition to avoiding substances that reduce gastroesophageal sphincter pressure, that promote the secretion of acid, and that can irritate an inflamed esophagus, recommendations can also include increasing the intake of foods or nutrients that increase gastroesophageal sphincter pressure. Protein is a nutrient that increases gastroesophageal sphincter pressure. Consequently, a higher than normal protein intake is encouraged; however, excessive protein intakes, especially from foods high in calcium such as dairy products, are not recommended. The reason for avoiding excessively high intakes of dairy foods relates to the fact that the amino acids and peptides (generated by digesting the protein in the dairy products) and calcium in dairy products are known to stimulate gastrin release. Although gastrin increases gastroesophageal sphincter pressure, it is also a potent stimulator of hydrochloric acid secretion.

In addition to noting the previously stated nutrition recommendations, remember that reflux is more likely to occur with increased gastric volume (i.e., eating large meals), increased gastric pressure (e.g., from obesity), and placement of gastric contents near the sphincter (i.e., bending, lying down, or assuming a recumbent position). Thus, recommendations for people with GERD or reflux esophagitis should include:

- eating smaller meals (and avoiding large ones)
- drinking fluids between meals, instead of with a meal, to help minimize large increases in gastric volume

- losing weight, if the person is overweight or obese
- avoiding tight-fitting clothes
- avoiding lying down, lifting, or bending for at least 2 hours after eating

INFLAMMATORY BOWEL DISEASES

Inflammatory bowel diseases (IBDs) include ulcerative colitis and Crohn's disease and are characterized by acute, relapsing, or chronic inflammation of various segments of the GI tract, especially the intestines. Although the causes of IBDs are unclear, nutrient malabsorption is a significant problem for several reasons. First, because of the disease-associated inflammation of the mucosa, brush border disaccharidase and peptidase activities are diminished, and thus nutrient digestion is impaired. Second, nutrient transit time is typically decreased—that is, GI tract contents move through the GI tract more quickly than usual and thus leave little time for absorption. Third, malabsorption occurs because of direct damage to the absorptive mucosa cells (enterocytes). Exacerbating the poor nutrient absorption is poor food intake, which is especially common during acute attacks.

Manifestations of IBDs include excessive diarrhea and steatorrhea (large amounts of fat in the feces), which may occur up to 20 times per day. Diarrhea is associated with increased losses of fluid and electrolytes (especially potassium) from the body. Fluid and electrolyte imbalance or even dehydration can result. Blood is often present in the feces, especially if deeper areas of the GI mucosa are severely inflamed or ulcerated. Loss of blood impairs the body's protein and mineral (especially iron) status. If IBD has affected the ileum (as is common with Crohn's disease), vitamin B_{12} absorption may be impaired (this vitamin is absorbed in the ileum), reabsorption of bile salts from the ileum may be diminished, and fat malabsorption may occur. Although pancreatic lipase is available to hydrolyze dietary triacylglycerols, the lack of sufficient bile or diminished bile function caused by bacterial alteration of bile can decrease micelle formation and thus decrease absorption of fatty acids and fat-soluble vitamins into the enterocyte. Unabsorbed fatty acids bind to calcium and magnesium in the lumen of the intestine; the resulting insoluble complex, sometimes called a soap, is excreted in the feces.

Dietary recommendations for people with IBD are aimed at replacing nutrient losses, correcting nutrient imbalances, and improving nutrition status. Some of these dietary recommendations include:

- increasing iron intake above the Recommended Dietary Allowance (RDA) because of increased iron losses with the bloody diarrhea and decreased absorption
- following a low-fat diet because fat absorption is impaired
- increasing calcium and magnesium intake because absorption of these nutrients is diminished by soap formation and overall malabsorption with diarrhea

- consuming a higher amount of protein than normal because protein is lost from the blood into the feces with bloody diarrhea and malabsorption of amino acids
- taking fat-soluble vitamin supplements, possibly in a water-miscible form to improve absorption
- increasing fluid and electrolyte intakes to rehydrate and restore electrolyte balance
- increasing overall intake of nutrients to meet energy and nutrient needs

Easily digestible, carbohydrate-rich foods that are low in fiber, high-protein low-fat foods, and lactose-free foods should provide the bulk of the person's energy needs if oral intake is deemed appropriate. Medium-chain triacylglycerol (MCT) oil, which is absorbed directly into portal blood and does not need bile for absorption, may be added in small amounts to different foods throughout the day to increase energy intake. Sometimes, however, complete rest of the GI tract is needed, and a person with IBD may need to be fed intravenously (by parenteral nutrition).

CELIAC DISEASE

Celiac disease, also called gluten- or gliadin-sensitive enteropathy or celiac sprue, results from an intolerance to gluten. Gluten is the general name for storage proteins, also called prolamins, in grains. Grains vary in their storage proteins, however, and in people with celiac disease, three storage proteins—secalin in rye, hordein in barley, and gliadin in wheat—appear to elicit or trigger the problems.

Consuming any of these grains alone, or foods made with any of these grains, triggers both immune and inflammatory responses in a person with celiac disease. Although the severity of the condition varies, the small intestine of someone with celiac disease becomes inflamed; lymphocytes and other immune system cells and the cytokines produced by the cells invade and attack the mucosa. The villi typically become atrophied or blunted, with corresponding changes in the crypt to villous height ratio. Because of the villi destruction, digestion and absorption become severely impaired. Manifestations of celiac disease include diarrhea, abdominal pain, malabsorption, and weight loss. Over time and if untreated, an infant or child with celiac disease may even exhibit signs of protein-energy malnutrition characterized by poor somatic muscle mass, hypotonia, abdominal distension, peripheral edema, depleted subcutaneous fat stores, and poor growth. Older children also may complain of constipation, nausea, reflux, and vomiting. This disorder affects other parts of the body as well as the intestines. Extraintestinal symptoms often include skin rashes, and muscle and joint pain. Fertility problems, especially in women with celiac disease, have been noted, along with bone problems including delayed bone growth and development and ultimately osteoporosis.

The cause of celiac disease is not clear, but it is thought to have a genetic component. The condition has been linked to the presence of several specific human leukocyte antigens. Diagnosis of celiac disease is based on the presence of a combination of serum antibody markers and biopsy of the small intestine.

Treatment of celiac disease requires lifelong exclusion of any form of any product that contains rye, barley, or wheat. However, because many foods contain combinations of grains, the list of foods to exclude is extensive. For example, grains such as triticale, which is a combination of rye and wheat, and malt, which is a partial hydrolysate of barley, cannot be consumed. A list of all the foods allowed and not allowed with celiac disease is beyond the scope of this perspective. Fortunately, food labels now must state if products contain wheat, and products that are gluten free often advertise this on the label. Further, the tremendous increase in the availability of gluten-free products in grocery stores has made living with celiac disease a little easier.

CHRONIC PANCREATITIS

Pancreatitis, or inflammation of the pancreas, provides an excellent example of the nutritional ramifications of a condition affecting an accessory organ of the GI tract. Remember that the exocrine portion of the pancreas produces several enzymes needed to digest all nutrients. *Chronic* refers to an ongoing or long-lasting situation.

Chronic pancreatitis can result from long-term excessive use of alcohol, gallstones, liver disease, viral infections, and use of certain medications, among other factors. With time, sections of pancreatic tissue become dysfunctional. Acinar cells, for example, can ultimately fail to produce sufficient digestive enzymes and juices. Consequently, a person with chronic pancreatitis experiences pain, especially with eating, as well as nausea, vomiting, and diarrhea. The diarrhea results in part from the maldigestion, with resulting malabsorption of several nutrients.

Diminished secretion of pancreatic lipase into the duodenum, caused by the chronic pancreatitis, results in maldigestion of fat and thus malabsorption of fat and fat-soluble vitamins. Fat is malabsorbed because not enough pancreatic lipase is available to hydrolyze the fatty acids from the triacylglycerols. This hydrolysis is necessary for fatty acids and monoacylglycerols to form micelles, the form in which the fatty acids are carried into the enterocyte for absorption. Thus, with pancreatitis, the insufficiency of enzymes available for fat hydrolysis necessitates a low-fat diet.

In addition to insufficient pancreatic lipase secretion, bicarbonate secretion into the duodenum is also diminished with pancreatitis. Bicarbonate, in part, increases the pH of the small intestine. Intestinal enzymes function best at an alkaline pH, which is provided by the release of bicarbonate into the intestine.

Oral supplements of pancreatic enzymes may be needed to replace the diminished output of these enzymes by the malfunctioning, inflamed pancreas. Medications such as antacids, H_2 receptor blockers, or proton pump inhibitors may also be needed. The medications are taken to diminish acid production and thus increase intestinal pH. In effect, they replace the bicarbonate and thus help maintain an appropriate pH for enzyme function. Exogenous insulin may also have to be administered if insulin is no longer produced in sufficient quantities by the damaged pancreatic endocrine cells.

These four conditions illustrate how diseases that affect the GI tract—malfunction of a sphincter (GERD and reflux esophagitis); destruction of enterocyte function (IBD), especially destruction of the enterocyte absorptive surface (celiac disease); and chronic malfunction of a GI tract accessory organ that provides secretions needed for nutrient digestion (pancreatitis)—affect the body's ability to digest and absorb nutrients. Furthermore, these conditions illustrate how nutrient intakes must deviate from recommended levels—in some cases to lower levels, and in other cases to higher levels—depending on the condition. Such dietary modifications are typical of many conditions that affect not only the gastrointestinal tract but also other organ systems.

3 CARBOHYDRATES

THE MAJOR SOURCE OF ENERGY FUEL in the average human diet is carbohydrate, supplying half or more of the total caloric intake. Roughly half of dietary carbohydrate is in the form of polysaccharides such as starches and dextrins, derived largely from cereal grains and vegetables. The remaining half is supplied as simple sugars, the most important of which include sucrose, lactose, and, to a lesser extent, maltose, glucose, and fructose.

OVERVIEW OF STRUCTURAL FEATURES

Carbohydrates are polyhydroxy aldehydes or ketones, or substances that produce these compounds when hydrolyzed. They are constructed from carbon, oxygen, and hydrogen atoms that occur in a proportion that approximates that of a "hydrate of carbon," CH_2O, accounting for the term *carbohydrate*. Carbohydrates comprise two major classes: simple carbohydrates and complex carbohydrates. Simple carbohydrates include monosaccharides and disaccharides. Complex carbohydrates include oligosaccharides containing 3 to 10 saccharide units and polysaccharides containing more than 10 units (Figure 3.1).

Simple Carbohydrates

- **Monosaccharides** are structurally the simplest form of carbohydrate in that they cannot be reduced in size to smaller carbohydrate units by hydrolysis. Monosaccharides are called simple sugars and are sometimes referred to as monosaccharide units or residues. The most abundant monosaccharide in nature—and certainly the most important nutritionally—is the six-carbon sugar glucose.

- **Disaccharides** consist of two monosaccharide units joined by covalent bonds. Within this group, sucrose, consisting of one glucose and one fructose residue, is nutritionally the most significant, furnishing approximately one-third of total dietary carbohydrate in an average diet.

Complex Carbohydrates

- **Oligosaccharides** consist of short chains of monosaccharide units that are also joined by covalent bonds. The number of units is designated by a prefix (*tri-, tetra-, penta-*, and so on), followed by the word *saccharide*. Among the oligosaccharides, trisaccharides occur most frequently in nature.

- **Polysaccharides** are long chains of monosaccharide units that may number from several into the hundreds or even thousands. The major polysaccharides of interest in nutrition are glycogen, found in certain animal tissues, and starch and cellulose, both of plant origin. All these polysaccharides consist of only glucose units.

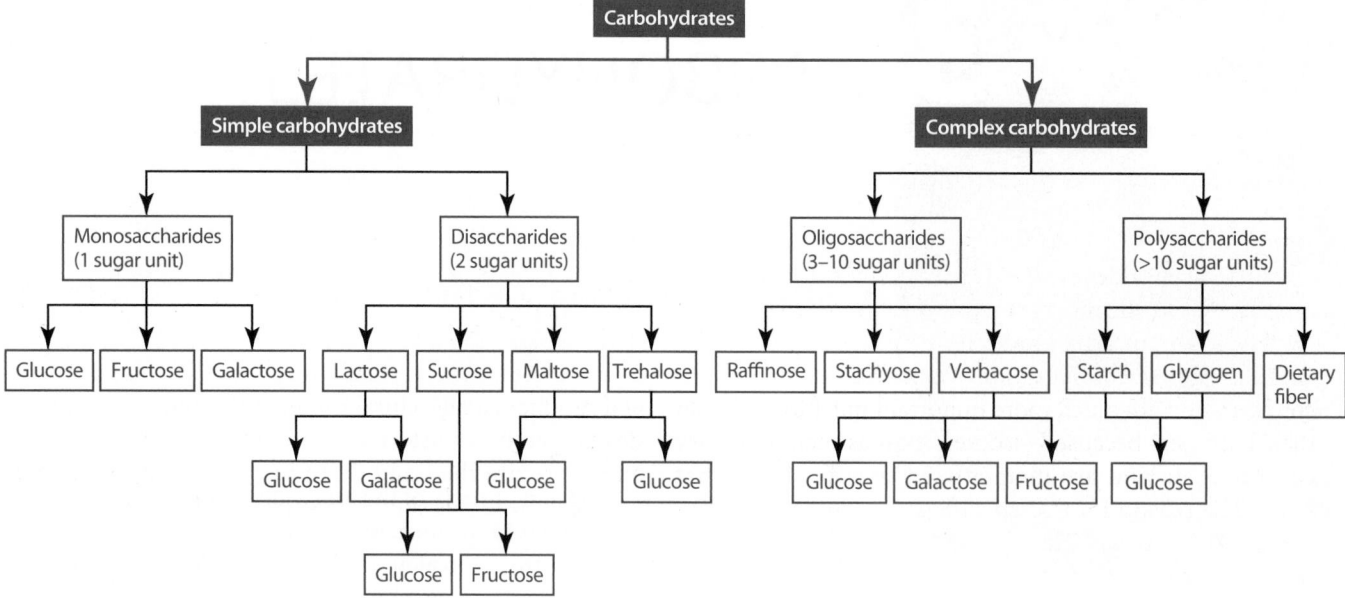

Figure 3.1 Classification of carbohydrates.
Source: Beerman/McGuire, Nutritional Sciences, 1/e. © Cengage Learning.

SIMPLE CARBOHYDRATES

Monosaccharides

As monosaccharides occur in nature or arise as intermediate products in digestion, they contain from three to seven carbon atoms and accordingly are termed trioses, tetroses, pentoses, hexoses, and heptoses. They cannot be further broken down with mild hydrolytic conditions, only with strong chemical oxidizing agents. In addition to hydroxyl groups, these compounds possess a functional carbonyl group, C=O, that can be either an aldehyde or a ketone. Hence, they are further designated as aldoses, sugars having an aldehyde group, and ketoses, sugars possessing a ketone group. These two classifications together with the number of carbon atoms describe a particular monosaccharide. For example, a five-carbon sugar having a ketone group is a ketopentose; a six-carbon aldehyde-possessing sugar is an aldohexose, and so forth.

Stereoisomerism: Chiral Carbons

A brief discussion of stereoisomerism—the occurrence of a molecule in different spatial configurations—as it relates to carbohydrates is provided here because most biological systems are stereospecific. (For a more extensive discussion refer to a general biochemistry text [1].)

Many organic substances, including carbohydrates, are optically active: If plane-polarized light is passed through a solution of the substances, the plane of light is rotated to the right (for dextrorotatory substances) or to the left (for levorotatory ones). The direction and extent of the rotation are characteristic of a particular compound and depend on the substance's concentration and temperature,

and the wavelength of the light. The right or left direction of light rotation is expressed as + (dextrorotatory) or − (levorotatory), and the number of angular degrees indicates the extent of rotation.

Optical activity is attributed to the presence of one or more asymmetrical or chiral carbon atoms in the molecule. **Chiral carbon** atoms have four different atoms or groups covalently attached to them. Aldoses with at least three carbon atoms and ketoses with at least four carbons have a chiral carbon atom. Because different groups are attached, it is not possible to move any two atoms or groups to other positions and rotate the new structure so that it can be superimposed on the original. Instead, when two of these molecules are side by side, repositioning groups in one creates a pair of molecules that are mirror images of each other. The molecules are said to be enantiomers, a special class within a broader family of compounds called **stereoisomers.** Diastereomers, another type of stereoisomers, are compounds having two or more chiral carbon atoms that have the same four groups attached but are not mirror images of each other.

If an asymmetrical substance rotates the plane of polarized light a certain number of degrees to the right, its enantiomer rotates the light the same number of degrees to the left. Enantiomers exist in D or L orientation, and if a compound is structurally D, its enantiomer is L. The D or L designation does not predict the direction of rotation of plane-polarized light, but rather is simply a structural analogy to the reference compound glyceraldehyde. Glyceraldehyde's D and L forms are, by convention, drawn as shown in Figure 3.2. Note that in the D configuration the —OH on the chiral carbon points to the right, and in the L configuration, to the left. Remember, these forms are not superimposable.

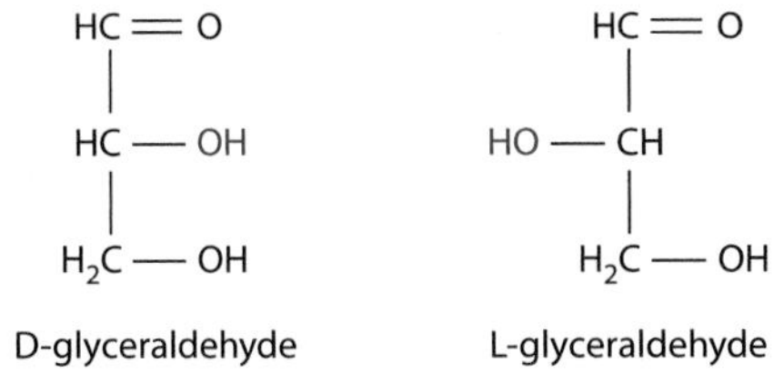

HC=O
|
HC—OH
|
H₂C—OH

D-glyceraldehyde

HC=O
|
HO—CH
|
H₂C—OH

L-glyceraldehyde

Figure 3.2 Structural formulas of the D and L configurations of glyceraldehyde.

Monosaccharides with more than three carbons have more than one chiral center. In such cases, the highest-numbered chiral carbon indicates whether the molecule is of the D or the L configuration. Monosaccharides of the D configuration are much more important nutritionally than their L isomers because D isomers exist as such in dietary carbohydrate and are metabolized specifically in that form. The reason for this specificity is that the enzymes involved in carbohydrate digestion and metabolism are stereospecific for D sugars, meaning that they react only with D sugars and are inactive toward L forms. The D and L forms of glucose and fructose are shown in Figure 3.3. Note that all of the —OH groups of the stereoisomers are flipped to the opposite side.

In Figure 3.3 the structures of glucose and fructose are shown as open-chain models, in which the carbonyl (aldehyde or ketone) functions are free. The monosaccharides generally do not exist in open-chain form, as explained later, but they are shown that way here to clarify the D-L concept and to illustrate the **anomeric carbon,** the carbon atom comprising the carbonyl function. Notice that the anomeric carbon is number 1 in the aldose (glucose)and number 2 in the ketose (fructose). This is due to the fact that the carbon bearing the most important functional group is given the lowest number possible.

Ring Structures

In solution, the monosaccharides do not exist in an open-chain form. They do not undergo reactions characteristic of true aldehydes and ketones. Instead, the molecules form a cyclic ring structure through a reaction between the carbonyl group and a hydroxyl group. If the cyclized sugar contains an aldehyde, it is called a hemiacetal; if the sugar contains a keto group, it is called a hemiketal. This formation of the cyclic structures forms an additional chiral carbon. Therefore, the participating groups within a monosaccharide are the aldehyde or ketone of the anomeric carbon atom and the alcohol group attached to the highest-numbered chiral carbon atom, as illustrated in Table 3.1 using the examples of D-glucose, D-galactose, and D-fructose. The formation of the hemiacetal or hemiketal produces a new chiral center at the anomeric carbon, designated by an asterisk in the structures in Table 3.1, and therefore the bond direction of the newly formed hydroxyl becomes significant. In the Fisher projections shown, the anomeric hydroxyls are arbitrarily positioned to the right, resulting in an alpha (α) configuration. If the anomeric hydroxyl were directed to the left, the structure would be in a beta (β) configuration. Cyclization to the hemiacetal or hemiketal can produce either the α- or the β-isomer. In aqueous solution, an equilibrium mixture of the α-, β-, and open isomers exists, with the concentration of the β form roughly twice that of the α form. In essence, the α-hemiacetal can change to the open structure and again form a ring with either the α or the β configuration.

Stereoisomerism among the monosaccharides, and also among other nutrients such as amino acids and lipids, has important metabolic implications because of the stereospecificity of certain metabolic enzymes. An interesting example of stereospecificity is the action of the digestive enzyme α-amylase, which hydrolyzes polyglucose molecules such as starches, in which the glucose units are connected through an α-linkage. Cellulose is also a polymer of glucose, but one in which the monomeric glucose residues are connected by β-linkages, and it is resistant to the α-amylase hydrolysis present in the human digestive system.

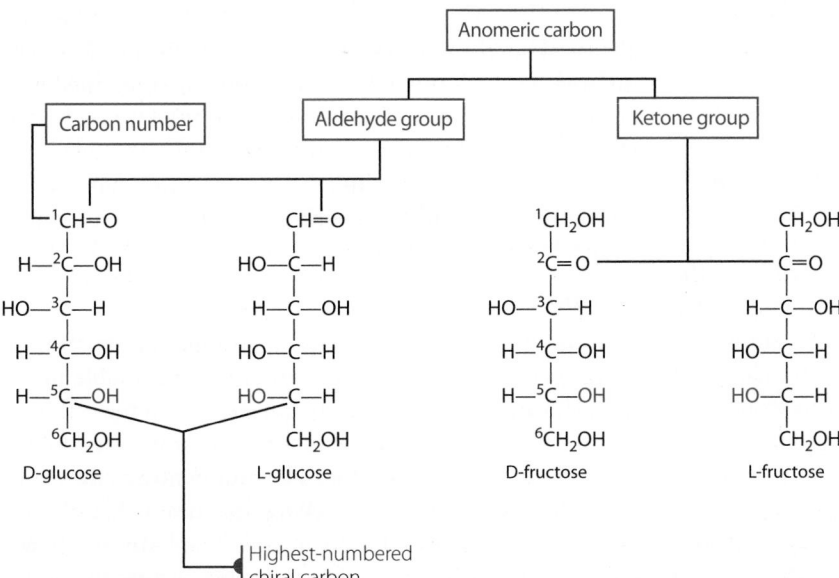

Figure 3.3 Structural (open-chain) models of the D and L forms of the monosaccharides glucose and fructose.

Table 3.1 Various Structural Representations among the Hexoses: Glucose, Galactose, and Fructose

Hexose	Fisher Projection	Cyclized Fisher Projection	Haworth	Simplified Haworth
α-D-glucose				
β-D-galactose				
β-D-fructose				

* Anomeric carbon.

Haworth Models

The structures of the cyclized monosaccharides are more conveniently and accurately represented by Haworth models. In such models the carbons and oxygen comprising the five- or six-membered ring are depicted as lying in a horizontal plane, with the hydroxyl groups pointing down or up from the plane. Those groups directed to the right in the open-chain structure point down in the Haworth model, and those directed to the left point up. Table 3.1 shows the structural relationship of simple projection and Haworth formulas for the major naturally occurring hexoses: glucose, galactose, and fructose. Remember that in solution the cyclic monosaccharides open and close to form an equilibrium between the α and the β forms. Regardless of how the cyclic structure is written, the molecule exists in both forms in solution unless the anomeric carbon has formed a chemical bond and is no longer able to open and close. The different ways of drawing the structures are presented here because all are used in the nutrition literature. Chemists often portray the structures to show the true bond angles. The structures can be shown in a boat configuration or a chair configuration. Additional information can be obtained from a biochemistry textbook [1].

Pentoses

Compared to the hexoses, pentose sugars furnish little dietary energy because relatively few are available in the diet. However, they are readily synthesized in the cell from hexose precursors and are incorporated into metabolically important compounds. The aldopentose ribose, for example, is a constituent of key nucleotides such as the adenosine phosphates—adenosine triphosphate (ATP), adenosine diphosphate (ADP), adenosine monophosphate

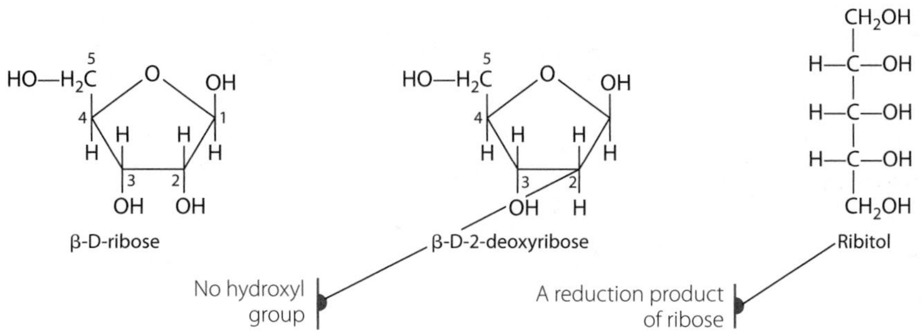

Figure 3.4 Structural formulas of the pentoses ribose and deoxyribose and of the alcohol ribitol.

(AMP), cyclic adenosine monophosphate (cAMP), and the nicotinamide adenine dinucleotides (NAD^+, $NADP^+$). Ribose and its deoxygenated form, deoxyribose, are part of the structures of ribonucleic acid (RNA) and deoxyribonucleic acid (DNA), respectively. Ribitol, a reduction product of ribose, is a constituent of the vitamin riboflavin and of the flavin coenzymes: flavin adenine dinucleotide (FAD) and flavin mononucleotide (FMN). The structural formulas of ribose, deoxyribose, and ribitol are depicted in Figure 3.4.

Amino and Acid Derivatives

Amino sugars, including glucosamine and galactosamine, occur in oligosaccharides and polysaccharides such as chitin and chrondroitin. The amino sugars have an amino group replacing the —OH on C2. Monosaccharides such as glucose can be enzymatically oxidized to glucuronic acid. Glucuronic acid is part of the glucuronic acid pathway (discussed later in this chapter) and is found in many glycoproteins, covered in Chapter 6.

Reducing Sugars

Monosaccharides that are cyclized into hemiacetals or hemiketals are sometimes called reducing sugars because they are capable of reducing other substances, such as the copper ion (from Cu^{2+} to Cu^+). This property is useful in identifying which end of a polysaccharide chain has the monosaccharide unit that can open and close. This role of reducing sugars is discussed in more detail in the section on polysaccharides.

High-Fructose Corn Syrup

A monosaccharide mixture of particular interest is what has been called high-fructose corn syrup (HFCS) or "corn sugar." HFCS is usually made up of 55% fructose and 45% glucose, though other mixtures are commercially available. Because of its use in sweetened beverages and other processed foods, the consumption of HFCS has increased dramatically during recent years. Because this increase in dietary fructose consumption has been concurrent with the increase in obesity and its complications within the population (see Chapter 8), concerns have been raised that a causal relationship between either HFCS or fructose consumption and obesity might exist. The Perspective at the end of this chapter will examine whether the epidemic of overweight and obesity is related specifically to increased fructose consumption.

Disaccharides

Disaccharides contain two monosaccharide units attached to one another through acetal bonds. Acetal bonds, also called glycosidic bonds because they occur in the special case of carbohydrate structures, are formed between a hydroxyl group of one monosaccharide unit and a hydroxyl group of a second monosaccharide, with the elimination of one molecule of water. The glycosidic bonds generally involve the hydroxyl group on the anomeric carbon of one member of the pair of monosaccharides and the hydroxyl group on carbon 4 or 6 of the second member. Furthermore, the glycosidic bond can be α or β in orientation, depending on whether the anomeric hydroxyl group was α or β before the glycosidic bond was formed and on the specificity of the enzymatic reaction catalyzing their formation. Specific glycosidic bonds therefore may be designated α(1-4), β(1-4), α(1-6), and so on. Disaccharides are major energy-supplying nutrients in the diet. The most common disaccharides in the diet are maltose, lactose, and sucrose (Figure 3.5).

Maltose

Maltose is formed primarily from the partial hydrolysis of starch and therefore is found in malt beverages such as beer and malt liquors. It consists of two glucose units linked through an α(1-4) glycosidic bond. The glucose unit on the right in Figure 3.5 is shown in the α form, although it also may exist in the β form.

Lactose

Lactose is found naturally only in milk and milk products. It is composed of galactose linked by a β(1-4) glycosidic bond to glucose. The glucose can exist in either the α or β form (Figure 3.5).

Sucrose

Sucrose (cane sugar, beet sugar) is the most widely distributed of the disaccharides and is the most commonly used natural sweetener. It is composed of glucose and fructose and is structurally unique in that its glycosidic bond involves the anomeric hydroxyl of both residues. The linkage is α with respect to the glucose residue and β with respect to the fructose residue (Figure 3.5). Because it has no free hemiacetal or hemiketal function, sucrose is not a reducing sugar.

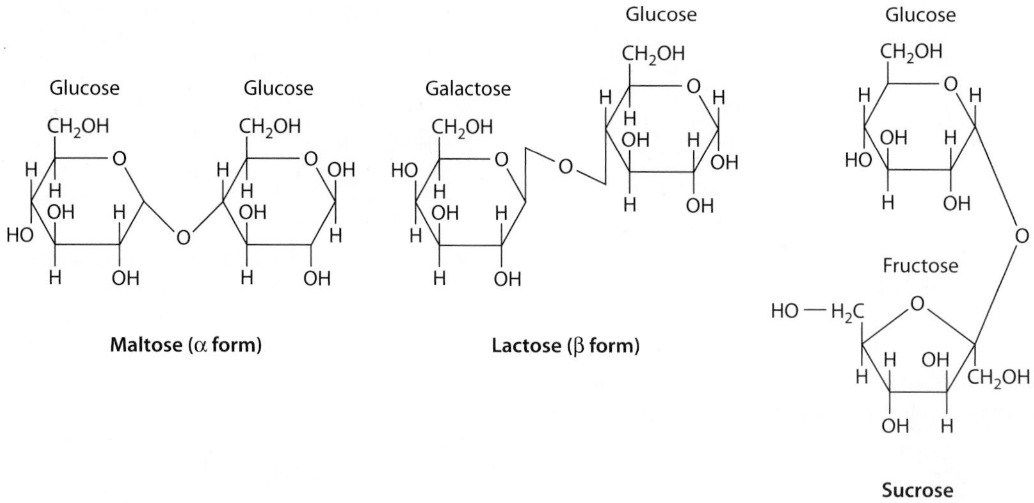

Figure 3.5 Common disaccharides.

Trehalose

Another disaccharide, trehalose, is found naturally in fungi (mushrooms) and in other foods of the plant kingdom. Trehalose is an $\alpha(1\text{-}1)$ linkage of two D-glucose molecules. It is a nonreducing sugar [2]. Since trehalose is digested slowly, provokes a low glycemic response, and possesses different physical and chemical properties from other sugars, it has become an ingredient in processed foods in Japan and other countries. It has been granted Generally Recognized as Safe (GRAS) status by the U.S. Food and Drug Administration (FDA) [2,3].

COMPLEX CARBOHYDRATES

Oligosaccharides

Raffinose (a trisaccharide), stachyose (a tetrasaccharide), and verbascose (a pentasaccharide) are made up of glucose, galactose, and fructose and are found in beans, peas, bran, and whole grains. Human digestive enzymes do not hydrolyze them, but the bacteria within the intestine can digest them. This is the basis for flatulence that occurs after eating these foods.

Polysaccharides

The glycosidic bonding of monosaccharide residues may be repeated many times to form high-molecular-weight polymers called polysaccharides. If the structure is composed of a single type of monomeric unit, it is called a homopolysaccharide. If two or more different types of monosaccharides make up its structure, it is called a heteropolysaccharide. Both types exist in nature; however, homopolysaccharides are of far greater importance in nutrition because of their abundance in many natural foods. The polyglucoses starch and glycogen, for example, are the major storage forms of carbohydrate in plant and animal tissues, respectively. Polyglucoses range in molecular weight from a few thousand to 500,000.

The reducing property of a saccharide is useful in describing polysaccharide structure by enabling one end of a linear polysaccharide to be distinguished from the other. In a polyglucose chain, for example, the glucose residue at one end of the chain has a hemiacetal group because its anomeric carbon atom is not involved in acetal bonding to another glucose residue. The residue at the other end of the chain is not in hemiacetal form because it is attached by acetal bonding to the next residue in the chain. A linear polyglucose molecule therefore has a reducing end (the hemiacetal end) and a nonreducing end (at which no hemiacetal exists). This notation is useful in designating at which end of a polysaccharide certain enzymatic reactions occur.

Starch

The most common digestible polysaccharide in plants is starch. Its two forms, amylose and amylopectin, are both polymers of D-glucose. The amylose molecule is a linear, unbranched chain in which the glucose residues are attached solely through $\alpha(1\text{-}4)$ glycosidic bonds. In water, amylose chains adopt a helical conformation, as shown in Figure 3.6a. Amylopectin, on the other hand, is a branched-chain polymer, with branch points occurring through $\alpha(1\text{-}6)$ bonds, as illustrated in Figure 3.6b. Both amylose and amylopectin occur in cereal grains, potatoes, legumes, and other vegetables. Amylose contributes about 15% to 20%, and amylopectin 80% to 85%, of the total starch content of these foods.

Glycogen

The major form of stored carbohydrate in animal tissues is glycogen, which is localized primarily in liver and skeletal muscle. Glycogen is even more highly branched than

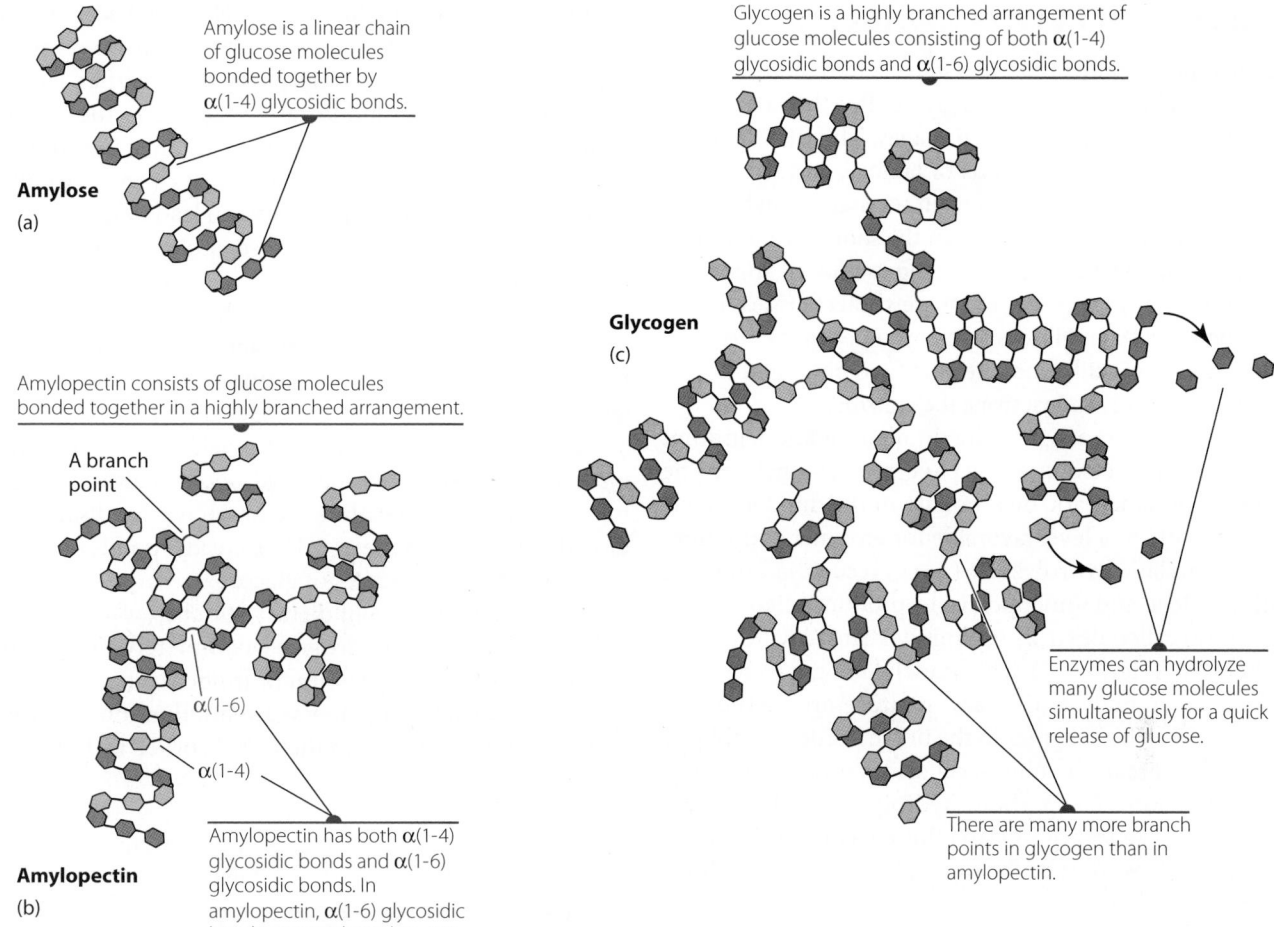

Amylose is a linear chain of glucose molecules bonded together by α(1-4) glycosidic bonds.

Amylose
(a)

Amylopectin consists of glucose molecules bonded together in a highly branched arrangement.

A branch point

α(1-6)

α(1-4)

Amylopectin
(b)

Amylopectin has both α(1-4) glycosidic bonds and α(1-6) glycosidic bonds. In amylopectin, α(1-6) glycosidic bonds occur at branch points.

Glycogen is a highly branched arrangement of glucose molecules consisting of both α(1-4) glycosidic bonds and α(1-6) glycosidic bonds.

Glycogen
(c)

Enzymes can hydrolyze many glucose molecules simultaneously for a quick release of glucose.

There are many more branch points in glycogen than in amylopectin.

Figure 3.6 Structure of starches and glycogen.
Source: Beerman/McGuire, Nutritional Sciences, 1/e. © Cengage Learning.

amylopectin (Figure 3.6c). The glucose residues within glycogen serve as a readily available source of glucose. When dictated by the body's energy demands, glucose residues are sequentially removed enzymatically from the nonreducing ends of the glycogen chains and enter energy-releasing pathways of metabolism. This process, called **glycogenolysis,** is discussed later in this chapter. The high degree of branching in glycogen and amylopectin offers a distinct metabolic advantage because it presents a large number of nonreducing ends from which glucose residues can be cleaved.

Cellulose

Cellulose is the major component of cell walls in plants and, like the starches, a homopolysaccharide of glucose. It differs from the starches in that the glycosidic bonds connecting the residues are β(1-4), rendering the molecule resistant to the digestive enzyme α-amylase, which is stereospecific to favor α(1-4) linkages. Because cellulose is not digestible by mammalian digestive enzymes, it is defined as a dietary fiber and is not considered an energy source. However, colonic bacteria can digest it and a

portion of the degradation products such as short-chain fatty acids may contribute a small amount to caloric intake. A more extensive discussion of fiber is presented in Chapters 2 and 4.

DIGESTION

Polysaccharides and disaccharides are the most important dietary carbohydrates nutritionally because free monosaccharides are not commonly present in the diet in significant quantities. However, some free glucose and fructose are present in honey, certain fruits, and the carbohydrates added to processed foods such as high-fructose corn syrup. Before dietary carbohydrates can be used by the body's cells they must first be absorbed from the gastrointestinal (GI) tract into the bloodstream, a process normally restricted to monosaccharides—the form of carbohydrates enterocytes can absorb. Poly-, tri-, and disaccharides therefore must be hydrolyzed. The hydrolytic enzymes involved are collectively called **glycosidases** or, alternatively, **carbohydrases.**

Digestion of Polysaccharides

The digestion of polysaccharides starts in the mouth. The key enzyme is salivary α-amylase, a glycosidase that specifically hydrolyzes α(1-4) glycosidic linkages. The β(1-4) bonds of cellulose, the β(1-4) bonds of lactose, and the α(1-6) linkages that form branch points in the starch amylopectin are resistant to this enzyme. Given the short period of time that food is in the mouth before being swallowed, this phase of digestion produces few mono-or disaccharides. However, the salivary amylase action continues in the stomach until the gastric acid penetrates the food bolus and lowers the pH sufficiently to inactivate the enzyme.

The starches move into the duodenum and jejunum, where they are acted upon by pancreatic α-amylase. The presence of pancreatic bicarbonate in the duodenum elevates the pH to a level favorable for enzymatic function. The α-amylase hydrolyzes α(1-4) glycosidic bonds in both amylose and amylopectin to produce oligosaccharides (also called dextrins or limit dextrins), maltose, and maltotriose (Figure 3.7). The branched oligosaccharides, trisaccharide maltotriose, and maltose are further digested by specific enzymes in the brush border. α-amylase can further break the oligosaccharides down to maltose and maltotriose. The partially hydrolyzed amylopectin is not fully digested by α-amylase; this enzyme's action stops several residues short of the α(1-6) bonds, leaving a limit dextrin. These limit dextrins are acted on by α-dextrinase (also called sucrase-isomaltase), which is attached to the brush border membrane. This enzyme contains two polypeptides with two active sites, one with specificity to α(1-4) linkages (sucrase) and the other with specificity to both α(1-4) and α(1-6) linkages (isomaltase). α-dextrinase is the only intestinal enzyme that will hydrolyze α(1-6) glycosidic bonds. Glucose is released from limit dextrins by the combined action of α-dextrinase and other brush border enzymes (Figure 3.7).

A portion of the starch of beans and certain vegetables and other resistant starches are not fully digested. This is partially due to the accessibility of the food to the enzyme and partially related to naturally occurring amylase inhibitors in some foods. α-amylase inhibitors are now being investigated as a potential means to impede digestion of dietary starch and combat the overweight and obesity problem [5].

Digestion of Disaccharides

Virtually no digestion of disaccharides or small oligosaccharides occurs in the mouth, stomach, or lumen of the small intestine. Digestion takes place almost entirely within the microvilli (the brush border) of the upper small intestine via disaccharidase activity, and the resulting monosaccharides immediately enter the enterocytes with the facilitation of specific transporters (discussed later) (Figures 2.10 and 2.11). Among the enzymes located on the enterocytes

are lactase, sucrase, maltase, and trehalase. Lactase catalyzes the cleavage of lactose to equimolar amounts of galactose and glucose. As was pointed out earlier, lactose has a β(1-4) linkage, and lactase is stereospecific for this β linkage. Lactase activity is high in infants, but in most mammals, including humans, it decreases a few years after weaning. This diminishing activity can lead to lactose malabsorption and intolerance. Lactose intolerance is particularly prevalent in African Americans, Jews, Arabs, Greeks, and some Asians. Many products that reduce the effects of lactose intolerance, including lactase that can be added to regular dairy products and lactose-free alternatives, are available.

Sucrase hydrolyzes sucrose to yield one glucose and one fructose residue. Maltase hydrolyzes maltose to yield two glucose units. Trehalase is a brush border disaccharidase that hydrolyzes the α(1-1) glycosidic bonds of trehalose to yield two molecules of glucose.

In summary, nearly all dietary starches and disaccharides ultimately are hydrolyzed completely by specific glycosidases to their constituent monosaccharide units. Monosaccharides, together with small amounts of remaining disaccharides, can then be absorbed by the intestinal mucosal cells.

ABSORPTION, TRANSPORT, AND DISTRIBUTION

The wall of the small intestine is composed of absorptive enterocytes and mucus-secreting goblet cells that line projections, called villi, that extend into the lumen. On the surface of the lumen side, the absorptive cells have hairlike projections called microvilli (the brush border). A square millimeter of cell surface is believed to have as many as 2×10^5 microvilli projections. The microstructure of the small intestinal wall is illustrated in Figures 2.10 and 2.11. The anatomic advantage of the villi-microvilli structure is that it presents an enormous surface area to the intestinal contents, thereby facilitating absorption. The absorptive capacity of the human intestine has been estimated to amount to about 5,400 g/day for glucose and 4,800 g/day for fructose—a capacity that would never be reached in a normal diet. Digestion and absorption of carbohydrates are so efficient that nearly all monosaccharides are usually absorbed by the end of the jejunum.

Absorption of Glucose and Galactose

Glucose, including that released in the brush border through the digestion of di- and trisaccharides, is absorbed into the intestinal mucosa cell by several pathways.

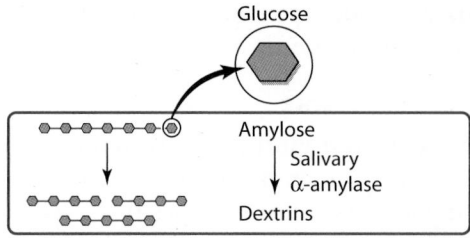

Glucose

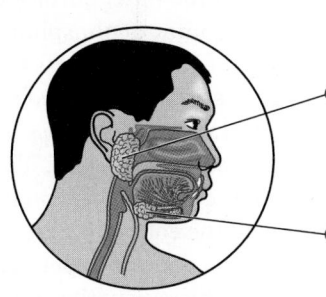

Amylose: Salivary glands release salivary α-amylase, which hydrolyzes α(1-4) glycosidic bonds in amylose, forming dextrins.

Amylopectin: Salivary glands release salivary α-amylase, which hydrolyzes α(1-4) glycosidic bonds in amylopectin, forming dextrins.

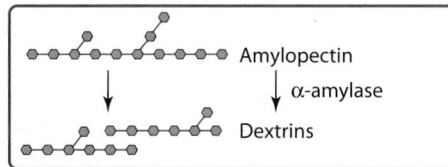

A. Digestion of amylose and amylopectin in the mouth

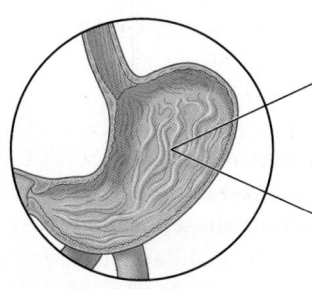

Amylose: Acidity of gastric juice destroys the enzymatic activity of α-amylase. The dextrins pass unchanged into the small intestine.

No further digestion

Amylopectin: Acidity of gastric juice destroys the enzymatic activity of salivary α-amylase. The dextrins pass unchanged into the small intestine.

No further digestion

B. There is no digestion of amylose and amylopectin in the stomach

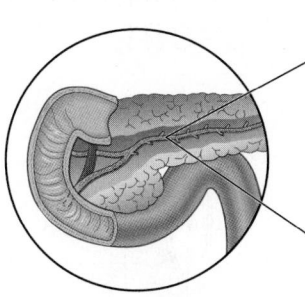

Amylose: The pancreas releases pancreatic α-amylase, which hydrolyzes α(1-4) glycosidic bonds, into the small intestine. Dextrins are broken down into maltose.

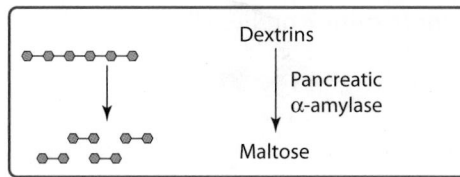

Amylopectin: The pancreas releases pancreatic α-amylase, which hydrolyzes α(1-4) glycosidic bonds to produce limit dextrins, maltotriose, isomaltose, and maltose. Hydrolysis stops 4 residues away from the α(1-6) bond.

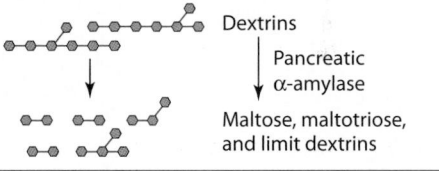

C. Digestion of amylose and amylopectin in the small intestine

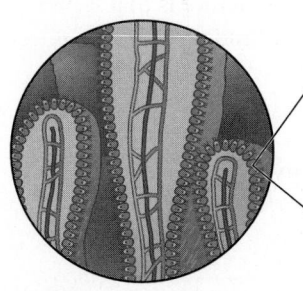

Amylose: Maltose is hydrolyzed by maltase, a brush border enzyme, forming free glucose.

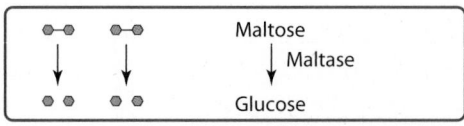

Amylopectin: Maltose, maltotriose, and limit dextrins are further hydrolyzed in the brush border by the enzyme maltase or sucrase-isomaltase (α-dextrinase) to glucose. α-dextrinase is the sole carbohydrase capable of hydrolysing α(1-6) glycosidic bonds.

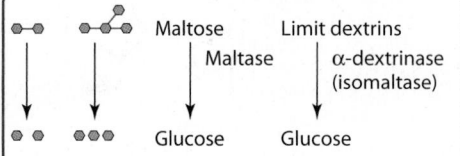

D. Digestion of amylose and amylopectin on the brush border of the small intestine

Figure 3.7 Digestion.
Source: Beerman/McGuire, Nutritional Sciences, 1/e. © Cengage Learning.

These include active transport and facilitated transport. Digestion has already been discussed.

Active Transport

The active transport mechanism for glucose and galactose absorption into enterocytes requires energy as ATP and the involvement of a specific receptor. The glucose-galactose receptor has been designated sodium-glucose transporter 1 (SGLT1) (Figure 3.8a). The SGLT1 simultaneously transports two substances (Na^+ and glucose or galactose) in the same direction and is thus a symporter. A mutation in the *SGLT1* gene is associated with glucose-galactose malabsorption. The transport protein of SGLT1 has two binding sites: One binds Na^+ and the other binds glucose. The glucose binding site is not available unless the transport protein has already bound a Na^+. The attachment of sodium to the carrier increases the transport protein's affinity for glucose. Sodium is moving down a concentration gradient because the intracellular concentration of Na^+ is low. When Na^+ is released inside the cell, the carrier's affinity for glucose is decreased, and the glucose is released into the cell. Na^+/K^+-ATPase then "pumps" the Na ions back out of the cell.

The SGLT1 is a Na^+/K^+-ATPase that is on the **apical** side (the intestinal lumen side) of the enterocyte and works by first combining with ATP in the presence of Na^+ on the inner surface of the cell membrane. The enzyme then is phosphorylated by the breakdown of ATP to adenosine diphosphate (ADP) and consequently is able to move three Na^+ out of the enterocyte. On the outer surface of the cell membrane, the ATPase becomes dephosphorylated by hydrolysis in the presence of K^+ and then is able to return two K^+ into the cell. The term *pump* is used because the Na and K ions are both transported across the membrane against their concentration gradients. This pump is responsible for most of the active transport in the body. This transport of glucose into the enterocyte is considered active in that the carriers needed are dependent upon the concentration gradients achieved by the action of Na^+/K^+-ATPase at the basolateral membrane. There is another Na^+/K^+-ATPase on the basolateral membrane (the portal vein side of the enterocyte) that maintains cation balance. The activity of the Na^+/K^+-ATPase is the major energy demand of the body at rest.

Facilitated Transport

All glucose absorption is not dependent upon SGLT1. At times of high glucose concentration in the intestinal mucosa, such as after a large carbohydrate meal, glucose is transported into the enterocyte by facilitated transporter type 2 (GLUT2). GLUT2 also transports glucose, galactose, and fructose out of the enterocyte and is located at the basolateral membrane. At times when the glucose concentration of the lumen of the intestine exceeds the blood

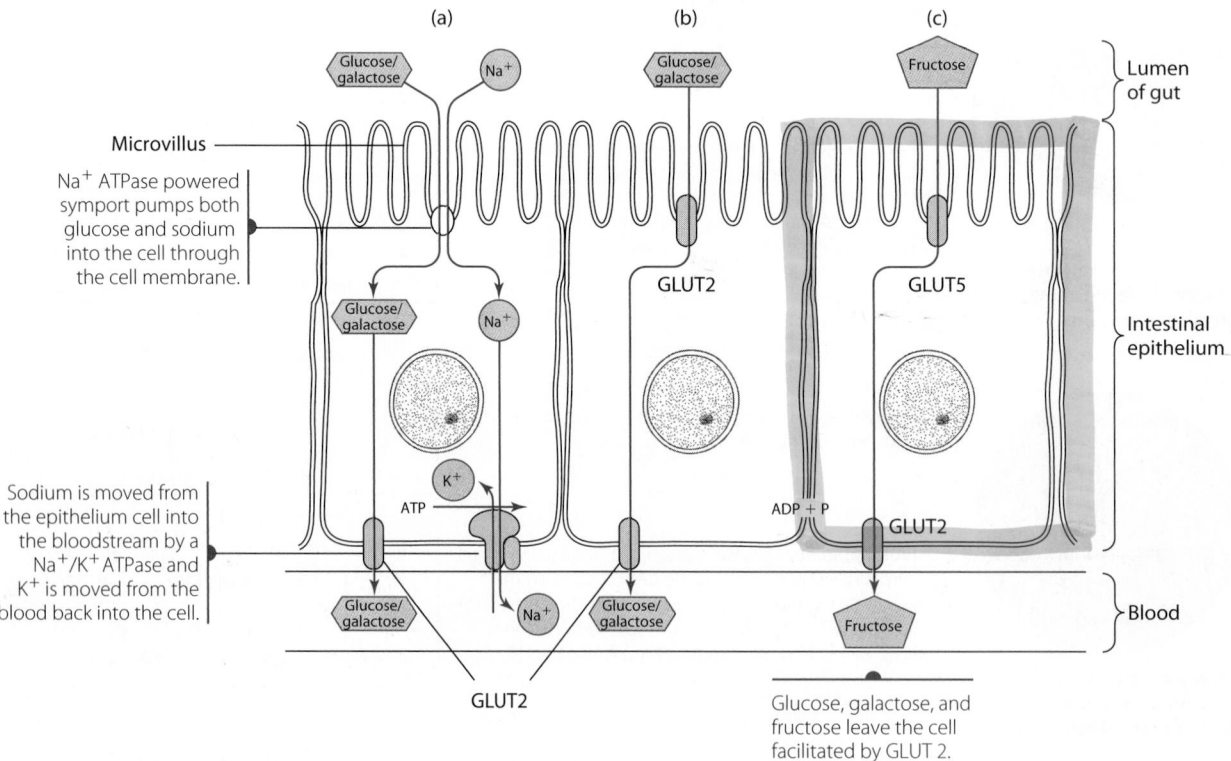

Figure 3.8 Transport of monosaccharides into enterocytes. (a) Active transport of glucose and galactose requiring ATP and Na^+. (b) Facilitated transport of glucose and galactose into the enterocyte by GLUT2 when the intestinal lumen glucose levels are high; glucose and galactose may also exit the cell with assistance from GLUT2. (c) Fructose entering the enterocyte via transport facilitated by GLUT5 and leaving the cell via transport facilitated by GLUT2.

concentration, intracellular GLUT2 is translocated to the apical membrane by the movement of the cytoskeleton and the contraction of myosin (as discussed in Chapter 1). GLUT2 has a high affinity for both glucose and fructose. After high-carbohydrate meals, more glucose (and fructose) is transported into the enterocyte by facilitated transport than by active transport using SGLT1.

The existence of GLUT2 in the apical membrane of human jejunal enterocytes has been demonstrated, with the amount present dependent upon the glucose concentration in the intestinal lumen. However, the control of GLUT2 translocation has been demonstrated only in experimental animals to date.

When insulin levels are high (with higher blood glucose levels) GLUT2 is translocated from the apical membrane back to intracellular vesicles. This has the effect of reducing intestinal glucose absorption when blood glucose levels are high. In insulin resistant individuals or those with type 2 diabetes the receptor is resistant to the effect of insulin, and the GLUT2 remains in the apical membrane. The result is that glucose continues to be absorbed at a higher rate [6,7]. There are other factors involved in the regulation of the amount of GLUT2 remaining in the membrane, such as sweetness receptors, high-fructose diets, high–saturated fat diets, and dietary artificial sweeteners. The regulation of GLUT2 in the apical membrane and all of the factors involved are not fully understood at this time.

Absorption of Fructose

[handwritten note: high concentration in the lumen? glucose enters the enterocyte ←]

...t into ...orter, ...r fructose [8]. ...ctive, ...of up-...lucose ...ent in ...previ-...ito the ...moves ...rocess ...t typi-...portal ...where ...es. Al-...though fructose is absorbed more slowly than glucose or galactose, which are actively absorbed, it is absorbed faster than sugar alcohols such as sorbitol and xylitol, which are absorbed purely by passive diffusion.

A large proportion of human subjects studied showed an inability to completely absorb doses of fructose in the range of 20 to 50 g [9]. Because fructose absorption is limited in nearly 60% of normal adults, intestinal distress, symptomatic of malabsorption, frequently appears following ingestion of 50 g or more of pure fructose [10]. This level of intake is readily achievable for individuals who consume 25 oz of a carbonated beverage sweetened with high-fructose corn syrup. The controversy surrounding the increase in high-fructose corn syrup in the food supply and its relation to health and obesity is discussed in the Perspective at the end of this chapter. It has been observed that the amount of fructose that can be consumed before malabsorption symptoms develop increases in the presence of high levels of glucose or sucrose; this may relate to the presence of GLUT2 in the apical membrane [10,11].

Facilitative Transport

Following transport of glucose, galactose, and fructose across the wall of the intestine, they enter the portal circulation, where they are carried directly to the liver. The liver is the major site of metabolism of galactose and fructose, which are readily taken up by the liver through specific hepatocyte receptors. The monosaccharides enter these liver cells by facilitated transport and subsequently are metabolized. Both fructose and galactose can be converted to glucose derivatives through pathways that are described later in this chapter. Once fructose and galactose are converted to glucose derivatives they have the same fate as glucose and can be stored as liver glycogen, returned to the bloodstream to maintain circulating glucose levels, or catabolized for energy according to the liver's energy demand. Little, if any, galactose and fructose are found in the peripheral blood, and these sugars are not directly subject to the strict hormonal regulation that is such an important part of glucose homeostasis. However, if their dietary intake is significantly higher than the normal percentage of total carbohydrate intake, they may be regulated indirectly as glucose because of their metabolic conversion to that sugar.

Glucose is nutritionally the most important monosaccharide because it is the exclusive constituent of starch and also occurs in each of three major disaccharides (Figure 3.1). Like fructose and galactose, glucose is extensively metabolized in the liver, but its removal by that organ is not as complete as in the case of fructose and galactose. The remainder of the glucose passes into the systemic blood supply and is then distributed among other tissues, such as muscle, kidney, brain, and adipose tissue. Glucose enters the cells in these organs by facilitated transport. In skeletal muscle and adipose tissue the process is insulin dependent, whereas in the liver, kidney, brain, and other tissues it is insulin independent. Because of the nutritional importance of glucose, the facilitated transport process by which it enters the cells of certain organs and tissues warrants a closer look. The following section explores the process in greater detail.

Glucose Transporters

Glucose is effectively used by a wide variety of cell types under normal conditions, and its concentration in the blood must be precisely controlled. Glucose plays a central role in metabolism and cellular homeostasis. Most cells in the body are dependent upon a continuous supply of glucose to supply energy in the form of ATP. The symptoms associated with diabetes mellitus are a graphic example of the consequences of a disturbance in glucose homeostasis.

The cellular uptake of glucose requires that it cross the plasma membrane of the cell. The highly polar glucose molecule cannot move across the cellular membrane by simple diffusion because it cannot pass through the nonpolar matrix of the lipid bilayer. For glucose to be used by cells, an efficient transport system for moving the molecule into and out of cells is essential. In certain absorptive cells, such as epithelial cells of the small intestine and renal tubule, glucose crosses the plasma membrane (actively) against a concentration gradient, pumped by an Na^+/K^+-ATPase symport system (SGLT1), as described previously. However, glucose is admitted to nearly all cells in the body by a carrier-mediated transport mechanism that does not require energy. A large number of transport proteins in the body facilitate the movement of specific substrates across cellular membranes into specific cells. The family of protein carriers involved in the transport of glucose is called glucose transporters, abbreviated GLUT.

GLUT Isoforms

A total of 14 individual glucose transport proteins have been identified, along with the genes that code for them [8]. The genome project has aided in this identification because, considered collectively, all transport proteins share a structure in common and have similar sequences in the genes that code for them. About 28% of the amino acid sequences are common within the family of transport

proteins. Each GLUT is an integral protein, penetrating and spanning the lipid bilayer of the plasma membrane. Twelve transmembrane α-helix segments are present in each of the transporters. Figure 3.9 shows a typical transporter, which is oriented so that hydrophilic regions of the protein chain protrude into the extracellular and cytoplasmic media, while the hydrophobic regions traverse the membrane, juxtaposed with the membrane's lipid matrix.

In its simplest form, a transporter protein:

- has a specific combining site for the molecule being transported
- undergoes a conformational change upon binding the molecule, allowing the molecule to be translocated to the other side of the membrane and released
- has the ability to reverse the conformational changes without the molecule being bound to the transporter so that the process can be repeated

This section will focus on the family of glucose transport proteins (GLUTs). Of the 14 GLUT isoforms that have been identified, only those that have been well studied and shown to have a major role in glucose metabolism are summarized in Table 3.2, though all 14 will be described briefly. All cells express at least one GLUT isoform on their plasma membrane. The different isoforms have distinct tissue distributions and biochemical properties, and they contribute to the precise disposal of glucose according to varying physiological conditions. Major characteristics of each of the GLUTs are: [8,12]

- GLUT1 was the first GLUT identified and the most intensely studied. As the most ubiquitously expressed GLUT, GLUT1 is responsible for the basic supply of glucose to erythrocytes, endothelial cells of the brain, and most fetal tissue. It supplies the glucose to the developing central nervous system during embryogenesis.

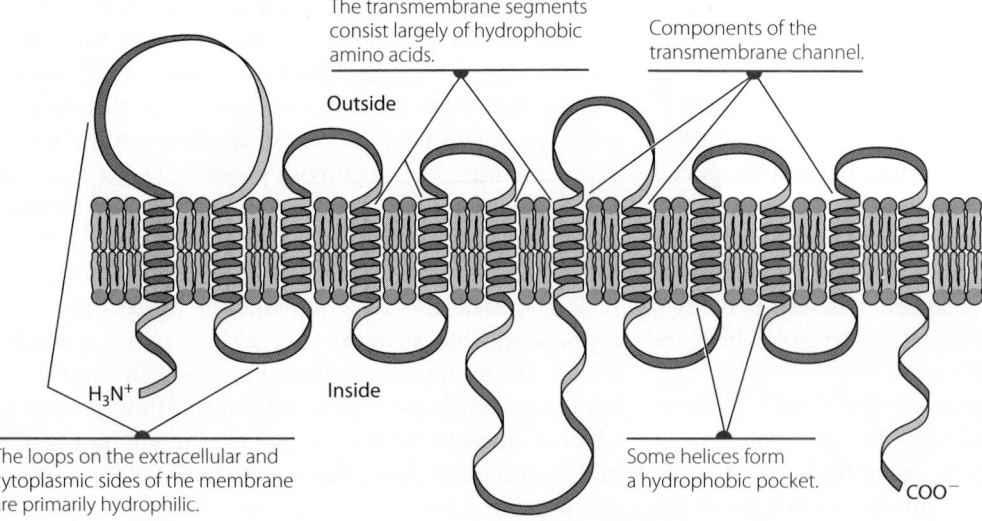

The transmembrane segments consist largely of hydrophobic amino acids.

Components of the transmembrane channel.

Outside

Inside

H_3N^+

The loops on the extracellular and cytoplasmic sides of the membrane are primarily hydrophilic.

Some helices form a hydrophobic pocket.

COO⁻

Figure 3.9 A model for the structural orientation of the glucose transporter.

Table 3.2 Glucose Transporters (GLUT)

Transporter Protein	Substrates	Major Sites of Expression
GLUT1	Glucose, galactose, mannose, glucosamine	Erythrocytes, central nervous system, blood-brain barrier, placenta, fetal tissues in general
GLUT2	Glucose, galactose, fructose, mannose, glucosamine	Liver, β-cells of pancreas, kidney, small intestine
GLUT3	Glucose, galactose, mannose, xylose, dehydroascorbic acid	Brain (neurons), spermatozoa, placenta, preimplantation embryos
GLUT4 (insulin dependent)	Glucose, glucosamine, dehydroascorbic acid	Muscle, heart, brown and white adipocytes
GLUT5	Fructose, but not glucose	Intestine, kidney, brain, skeletal muscle, adipose tissue

- GLUT2 is a low-affinity, high-capacity transporter with predominant expression in the β-cells of the pancreas, liver, small intestine, and kidney. As discussed previously, GLUT2 is involved in the transport of glucose and fructose from enterocytes into the portal blood, and when the concentration of glucose in the intestinal lumen is high, it transports glucose and fructose into the enterocyte. The rate of transport is highly dependent upon the blood glucose concentration. In the pancreas, GLUT2 appears to be the sensitive indicator of blood glucose levels and is involved in the release of insulin from the β-cells. High insulin levels cause GLUT2 to leave the plasma membrane of the enterocyte and return to storage vesicles.

- GLUT3 is a high-affinity glucose transporter with predominant expression in those tissues that are highly dependent upon glucose, such as the brain and neurons. It is also expressed in cells and tissues that have a high requirement for glucose such as spermatozoa, the placenta, and preimplantation embryos. Some data suggest that a possible disregulation of GLUT3 might lead to glucose deficits in the brain and thus to dyslexia in children.

- GLUT4 is the primary means by which insulin is responsible for the cellular uptake of glucose in muscle and adipose tissue. Other cells and tissues such as the liver, kidney, erythrocytes, and brain do not express GLUT4 and therefore are not dependent upon insulin for glucose uptake. One of the actions of insulin is to cause the translocation of GLUT4 from GLUT4 storage vesicles (GSV; discussed in the next section). A feature of type 2 diabetes, described in the Chapter 7 Perspective, is a resistance to insulin that prevents glucose uptake in muscle and adipose tissue.

- GLUT5 is specific for the transport of fructose and will not transport glucose. It is expressed primarily in the small intestine, but to a lesser degree in kidney, brain, skeletal muscle, and adipose tissue also.

- GLUT6 (which was formerly designated GLUT9) is expressed primarily in the brain, spleen, and peripheral leukocytes. It appears to transport hexoses only at higher concentrations.

- GLUT7 has been found in the small intestine and colon. It has a high affinity for glucose and fructose but does not bind galactose or xylose.

- GLUT8 (formerly GLUTXI) is expressed mainly in the testis with lower levels in the brain, adrenal gland, liver, spleen, brown adipose tissue, and lung. This GLUT has been studied mostly in animal models.

- GLUT9 is primarily detected in the liver and kidney, with lower levels found in the small intestine, placenta, lung, and leukocytes. The metabolic importance of GLUT9 is not fully understood. In addition to a high affinity for glucose and fructose, GLUT9's primary function appears to be the transport of uric acid.

- GLUT10 is present in the heart, lung, brain, liver, skeletal muscle, pancreas, placenta, and kidney. Its physiological role in humans is under investigation and is not fully understood at this time.

- GLUT11 has been cloned based on genomic information and is expressed in three isoforms. Its physiological role in humans has not been identified.

- GLUT12 has been identified in the skeletal muscle, heart, small intestine, and prostrate. The amount of GLUT12 found in the cellular membrane is increased by insulin (similar to GLUT4) in the normal individual, but not under conditions of obesity and type 2 diabetes that cause resistant insulin receptors. GLUT12 does not appear to be stored in storage vesicles and does not undergo cycling between storage vesicles and the membrane like GLUT4 does. The affinity of GLUT12 for glucose is unknown at this time, but it does transfer glucose, so there is some degree of affinity.

- GLUT13 is highly expressed in certain regions of brain and to a lower extent in adipose tissue and the kidney. This GLUT has no carbohydrate transport activity. It appears to transport H^+ and inositol. Its physiological role is not completely understood at this time.

- GLUT14 is similar (if not identical) to GLUT3 and possibly serves as a backup for that GLUT. It is expressed in the testis.

The current knowledge of GLUTs and their physiological actions has been acquired using molecular biology techniques. The genome project identified genes that had a high degree of similarity to the GLUTs, providing a reason and the tools to look for them in various tissues. The protein molecules were then cloned. Another technique that has been used, called the knockout mouse, blocks the expression of the specific gene under study. With this technique it is possible to determine what effect the absence of the GLUT has on the animal, and hence to learn more of its function.

Insulin

This section covers only the role of insulin in the cellular absorption of glucose. Blood glucose levels are maintained within a narrow range by a balance among glucose absorption from the intestine, production by the liver, and uptake and metabolism by the peripheral tissues. Insulin plays a central role in regulating the level of blood glucose during periods of feeding and fasting. In fact, this powerful anabolic hormone is involved in glucose, lipid, and amino acid/protein metabolism. Insulin's role in these activities will be discussed in the appropriate macronutrient chapters and summarized in Chapter 7.

The insulin-responsive transporter GLUT4 is synthesized on the ribosomes of the rough endoplasmic reticulum and then transferred to the Golgi apparatus, where it is packaged into GLUT4 storage vesicles (GSV). In the basal, unstimulated state of the adipocyte and skeletal muscle cells, GLUT4 resides in these structures [8,12,13]. When blood glucose levels are elevated, insulin is released by the β-cells of the pancreas. One role of insulin is inhibition of the synthesis of glucose (gluconeogenesis) by the liver (covered later in this chapter). Another role is to bind with specific insulin receptors on the cell membrane, which causes the GSV to translocate to the cell membrane (see Figure 3.10) [8,13]. Key to the ability of insulin to bind to the receptor site on the cell membranes of skeletal muscle, cardiac muscle, or adipose tissue cells are the activation of phosphatidylinositol-3-kinase (PI3-kinase) and the cascading reactions that follow. This activity is discussed more fully in Chapter 7. The net result of insulin's effects on the cell membrane is to cause translocation of GLUT4 to the cell membrane; this process can be simply described as follows:

❶ The biosynthesis of GLUT4 and its storage in GSVs are stimulated.

❷ The GSVs are transported to the cell membrane by elements of the cytoskeleton including the microtubules and actin.

❸ An interaction between GSVs and the plasma membrane occurs, mediated by a tethering complex, a step called tethering.

❹ The GVS docks with the plasma membrane in preparation for fusion.

❺ The lipid bilayers of the GSVs and plasma membrane fuse.

❻ Endocytosis—the GLUT4 becomes part of the plasma membrane and available for transporting glucose into the cell.

In the presence of insulin, GLUT4 continuously cycles through the endosomal system. In insulin resistant states or at low insulin levels, the GLUT4 stays in the GSV and its presence in the cell membrane is reduced. Interestingly, exercise causes similar translocation of GLUT4 from the GSVs to the cell membrane, though the mechanism of this translocation is poorly understood.

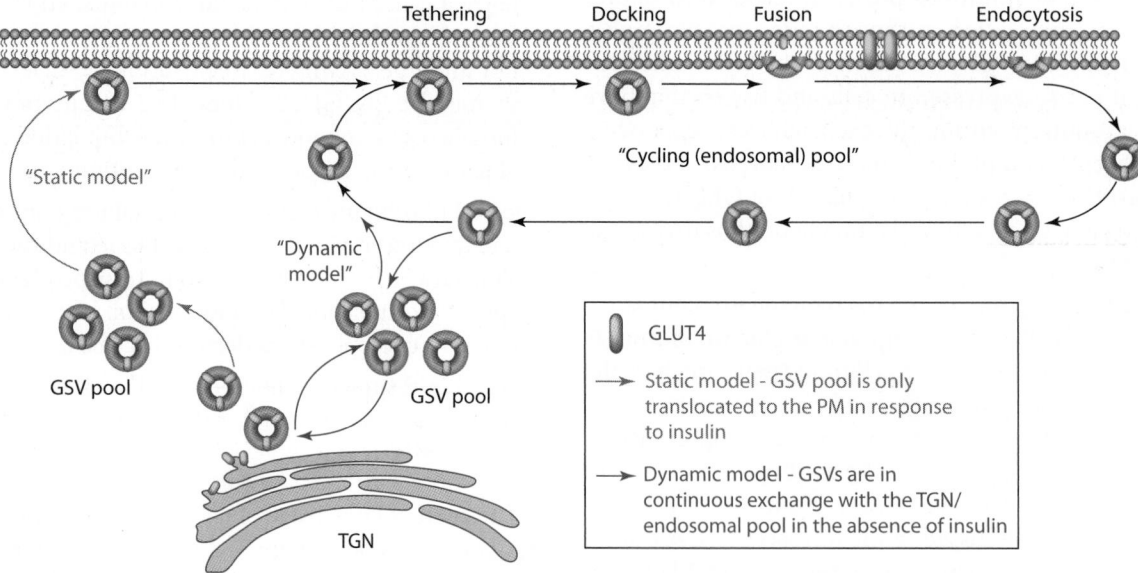

Figure 3.10 GLUT4 membrane trafficking pathways. GLUT4 is synthesized in the trans-Golgi network (TGN) and sorted to GLUT4 storage vesicles (GSVs). According to the static model, it remains in the GSV in the absence of insulin. With insulin action, GLUT4 gets translocated to the plasma membrane from the GSV. In the dynamic or cycling model, there is constant recycling of GLUT4 from the GSVs to the plasma membrane and back again. With insulin action, more of the GLUT4 remains in the plasma membrane.

Source: Adapted from Augstin R., Life, 2010;62:315–33, Figure 3B. Adapted by permission.

Glucose Entry into Interstitial Fluid

The endothelial tissue of which blood vessel walls are constructed is freely permeable to metabolites such as glucose. Some tissues, most notably the brain, possess an additional layer of epithelial tissue between the blood vessel and the cells of the brain. Unlike the endothelium, epithelial layers are not readily permeable to many substrates, and the passage of metabolites through them requires active transport or facilitative diffusion. For this reason, the epithelium is called the blood-tissue barrier of the body. Among the blood-tissue barriers studied—including those of the brain, cerebrospinal fluid, retina, testes, and placenta—GLUT1 appears to be the prime isoform for cross-barrier glucose transport [8], though other GLUTs appear to be involved (see Table 3.2).

Maintenance of Blood Glucose Levels

Maintenance of normal blood glucose concentration is an important homeostatic function and is a major function of the liver, skeletal muscle, and adipose tissue—which together represent the majority of the tissues in the body. Regulation is the net effect of the organs' metabolic processes that remove glucose from or return glucose to the blood. These pathways, which are examined in detail in the section "Integrated Metabolism in Tissues," are hormonally influenced, primarily by the antagonistic pancreatic hormones insulin and glucagon and to a lesser extent by the glucocorticoid hormones of the adrenal cortex. The rise in blood glucose following the ingestion of carbohydrate, for example, triggers the release of insulin while reducing the secretion of glucagon. Insulin is the only hormone that lowers blood glucose levels and is the primary anabolic hormone. Insulin stimulates the uptake of glucose, amino acids, and lipid, which leads to their conversion to storage forms in muscle and adipose tissue. The storage form for glucose, glycogen, is synthesized through the process called **glycogenesis**. Glucagon, the primary catabolic hormone, has the opposite effects of increasing the breakdown of liver glycogen (by a process called glycogenolysis) and lipid stored in adipose tissue and inhibiting the synthesis of proteins. Additional mechanisms to increase blood glucose levels include an increase in the secretion of glucocorticoid hormones, primarily cortisol. Glucocorticoids cause increased activity of hepatic gluconeogenesis, a process described in detail in a later section of this chapter.

GLYCEMIC RESPONSE TO CARBOHYDRATES

The rate at which glucose is absorbed from the intestinal tract appears to be an important parameter in controlling the homeostasis of blood glucose, insulin release, obesity, and possibly weight loss. The intense research of the last few years has led to the concepts of glycemic index (GI) and glycemic load (GL) [14,15], which are discussed in this section. Current research suggests roles for persistently elevated blood glucose, blood insulin levels, and obesity in the development of chronic diseases [16,17]. The role of these factors in the development of insulin resistance and type 2 diabetes is covered in Chapters 7 and 8. See also the Perspective on diabetes following Chapter 7.

Glycemic Index and Glycemic Load

The glycemic index is an alternative way to classify dietary carbohydrates by their impact on blood glucose levels caused by their ease of digestion and absorption. It has been suggested that the glycemic index (GI) and glycemic load (GL) offer a means to examine the relative risks of diets designed to prevent coronary heart disease (CHD) and obesity.

The effect that carbohydrate-containing foods have on blood glucose concentrations is called the glycemic response to the food. Some foods that are rapidly digested and absorbed (high-GI foods) cause a rapid rise in blood glucose levels that, because of the effect of insulin released in response, can subsequently lead to a rapid fall even below the fasting level. Other foods cause a slower and more extended rise with a lower peak level of glucose and insulin and a gradual fall (low-GI foods). The glycemic index concept was developed to provide a numerical value to represent the effect of a particular food on blood glucose levels. It provides a quantitative comparison between foods. The glycemic index is defined as the increase in blood glucose level above the baseline level (fasting level) during a 2-hour period following the consumption of a defined amount of carbohydrate (usually 50 g) compared with the same amount of carbohydrate in a reference food. A related quantitative measure, the glycemic load, considers both the quantity and the quality of the carbohydrate in a food. The glycemic load equals the glycemic index times the grams of carbohydrate in a typical portion of the food. A food's GI and GL can be quite different; for example, the carbohydrate in carrots has a high GI score, but the GL for carrots is low because a half-cup serving of carrots contains only 6.13 g of carbohydrate. The higher the GL, the greater the expected elevation in blood glucose and the insulinogenic effect of the food.

Some studies of GI values have used glucose as the reference food, while others used white bread. The reference food is assigned a score of 100. In practice, the glycemic index is measured by determining the elevation of blood glucose for 2 hours following ingestion and plotting the values against time. The area under the curve for the test food is divided by the area under the curve for the reference food, and the result is multiplied by 100 (Figure 3.11). If glucose is used as the reference food and assigned a glycemic index of 100, white bread has a GI of about 71. When white bread is used as the reference, some foods will have a glycemic index of greater than 100.

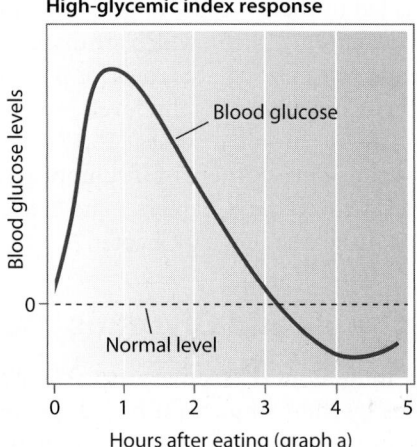

High-glycemic index response

Blood glucose levels

Blood glucose

Normal level

Hours after eating (graph a)

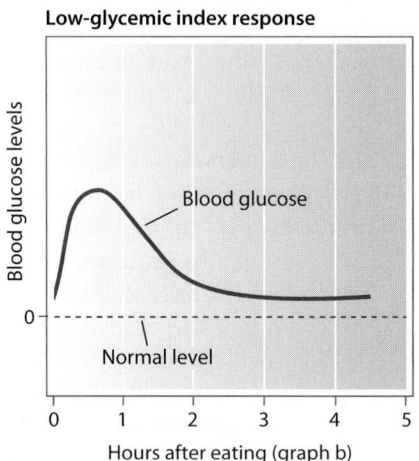

Low-glycemic index response

Blood glucose levels

Blood glucose

Normal level

Hours after eating (graph b)

Calculation of Glycemic Index

❶ The elevation in blood glucose level above the baseline following consumption of a high-glycemic index food or 50 g of glucose in a reference food (glucose or white bread). The glycemic index of the reference food is by definition equal to 100 (graph a).

❷ The elevation of blood glucose levels above the baseline following the intake of 50 g of glucose in a low-glycemic index food (graph b).

❸ The glycemic index is calculated by dividing the area under the curve for the test food by the area under the curve for the reference food and multiplying the result by 100.

Figure 3.11 Blood glucose changes following carbohydrate intake (glycemic index).
Source: Beerman/McGuire, Nutritional Sciences, 1/e. © Cengage Learning.

In some countries GI or GL is used or is being considered for use on food labels [18,19]. There are many potential criticisms of the use of GI and GL for labeling purposes, however, foremost the wide variation of GI values for apparently similar foods and between laboratories. Factors that may cause this variation include the amount of carbohydrate in the meal, composition of the

meal (particularly fiber, protein, and fat), previous meal composition, physical activity level of the subjects, choice of the reference food, and glucose tolerance of the subjects [18,19]. The variations observed could also reflect real differences among samples of the same food due to factors such as its food form, ripeness, location of growing, and variety. For example, the glycemic index for a baked russet potato is 76.5 and for an instant mashed potato is 87.7 (using glucose as the reference food) [20]. Even the temperature of the food can make a difference: A boiled red potato eaten hot (with the starch gelatinized) has a glycemic index of 89.4, but the same potato eaten cooler (with the starch back to a crystalline structure) has a glycemic index of 56.2 (Table 3.3).

Glycemic index and glycemic load have proven useful in evaluating the risk of developing chronic disease and obesity. Long-term consumption of a diet with a relatively high GL is associated with an increased risk of obesity, type 2 diabetes, and coronary heart disease [15–17,20,21]. The literature suggests that the longer and higher the elevation of blood glucose and insulin, the greater the risk of developing chronic diseases and obesity.

Many published tables provide the glycemic index for different foods. The most complete is an international table [22]. Selected examples from this publication have been reproduced in Table 3.3 along with the glycemic index of potatoes. Remember that the food products differ in different regions of the world. The glycemic indices listed in Table 3.3 are intended to be used to show trends, not to prepare diets.

INTEGRATED METABOLISM IN TISSUES

The metabolic fate of the monosaccharides depends to a great extent on the body's energy needs at the time. This section covers the individual pathways of carbohydrate metabolism. The following section addresses the ways metabolism is regulated, including allosteric mechanisms, substrate-level regulation, induction, post-translational modification, and translocation. Several terms used in carbohydrate metabolism sound and appear to be similar but are in fact quite different. The metabolic pathways of carbohydrate metabolism are listed below:

- **Glycogenesis:** The synthesis of glycogen
- **Glycogenolysis:** The breakdown of glycogen
- **Glycolysis:** The oxidation of glucose
- **Gluconeogenesis:** The production of glucose from noncarbohydrate intermediates
- **Pentose phosphate pathway (hexosemonophosphate shunt):** The production of five-carbon monosaccharides and nicotinamide adenine dinucleotide phosphate (NADPH)
- **Tricarboxylic acid (TCA) cycle:** The oxidation of pyruvate and acetyl-CoA to CO_2 and H_2O

Table 3.3 Glycemic Index of Common Foods with White Bread and Glucose Used as the Reference Food

Food Tested	Glycemic Index	
	White Bread = 100	Glucose = 100
White bread[1]	100	71
Baked russet potato[1]	107.7	76.5
Instant mashed potatoes[1]	123.5	87.7
Boiled red potato (hot)[1]	125.9	89.4
Boiled red potato (cold)[1]	79.2	56.2
Bran muffin[2]	85	60
Coca Cola[2]	90	63
Apple juice, unsweetened[2]	57	40
Tomato juice[2]	54	38
Bagel[2]	103	72
Whole-meal rye bread[2]	89	62
Rye-kernel bread[2] (pumpernickel)	58	41
Whole-wheat bread[2]	74	52
All-Bran cereal[2]	54	38
Cheerios[2]	106	74
Corn Flakes[2]	116	81
Raisin Bran[2]	87	61
Sweet corn[2]	86	60
Couscous[2]	81	61
Rice[2]	73	51
Brown rice[2]	72	50
Ice cream[2]	89	62
Soy milk[2]	63	44
Raw apple[2]	57	40
Banana[2]	73	51
Orange[2]	69	48
Raw pineapple[2]	94	66
Baked beans[2]	57	40
Dried beans[2]	52	36
Kidney beans[2]	33	23
Lentils[2]	40	28
Spaghetti, durum wheat (boiled)[2]	91	64
Spaghetti, whole meal (boiled)[2]	32	46
Sucrose[2]	83	58

[1]Source for data: Fernandes G, Velangi A, Wolever TM. Glycemic index of potatoes commonly consumed in North America. J Am Diet Assoc. 2005; 105:557–62.
[2]Source for data: Foster-Powell K, Holt SH, Brand-Miller JC. International table of glycemic and glycemic load: Values 2002. Am J Clin Nutr. 2002; 76:5–76.

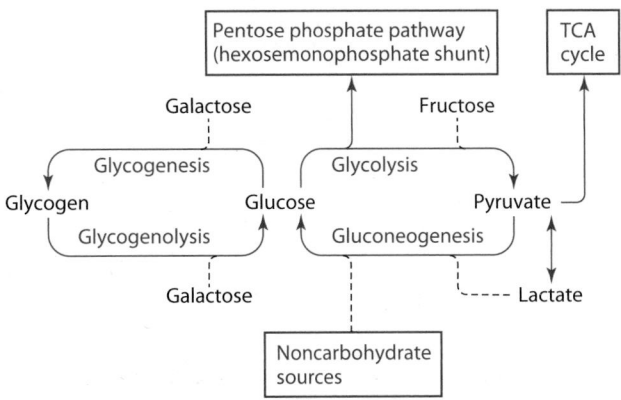

Figure 3.12 Integrated overview of carbohydrate metabolic pathways.

An integrated overview of these pathways is given in Figure 3.12. The metabolism of glycogen is covered first, followed by the energy-producing pathways (glycolysis and the TCA cycle). A detailed review of the pathways' intermediary metabolites and sites of regulation is provided in the sections that follow. The detailed pathways with the names of the chemicals and their structures are shown in the later figures. These are followed with a discussion of the individual reactions and additional comments that are particularly significant from a nutritional standpoint. Because of the central role of glucose in carbohydrate nutrition, its metabolic fate is featured here. The entry of fructose and galactose into the metabolic pathways is introduced later in the discussion.

Glycogenesis

The term *glycogenesis* refers to the pathway by which glucose ultimately is converted into its storage form glycogen—a process vital to ensuring a reserve of quick energy. This pathway is particularly important in hepatocytes because the liver is a major site of glycogen synthesis and storage. Glycogen accounts for as much as 7% of the weight of the liver. Liver glycogen can be broken down to glucose and reenter the bloodstream. Therefore, it plays an important role in maintaining blood glucose homeostasis. The other major site of glycogen storage is skeletal muscle. In human skeletal muscle, glycogen generally accounts for a little less than 1% of the weight of the tissue. Although the concentration of glycogen in the liver is greater, muscle stores account for most of the body's glycogen (~75%) because the muscle makes up a much greater portion of the body's weight than the liver does. The glycogen stores in muscle are an energy source within that muscle fiber and cannot directly contribute to blood glucose levels. (Muscle lacks the enzyme that converts the phosphorylated glucose back to free glucose.) We will discuss how metabolic products of glucose can return to the liver and be converted to glucose.

The initial part of the glycogenic pathway is illustrated in Figure 3.13. Glucose is first phosphorylated upon entering the cell, producing glucose-6-phosphate. In muscle cells, the enzyme catalyzing this phosphate transfer from ATP is hexokinase, a mixture of hexokinase isozymes type 1 and 2. The properties of this enzyme are shown

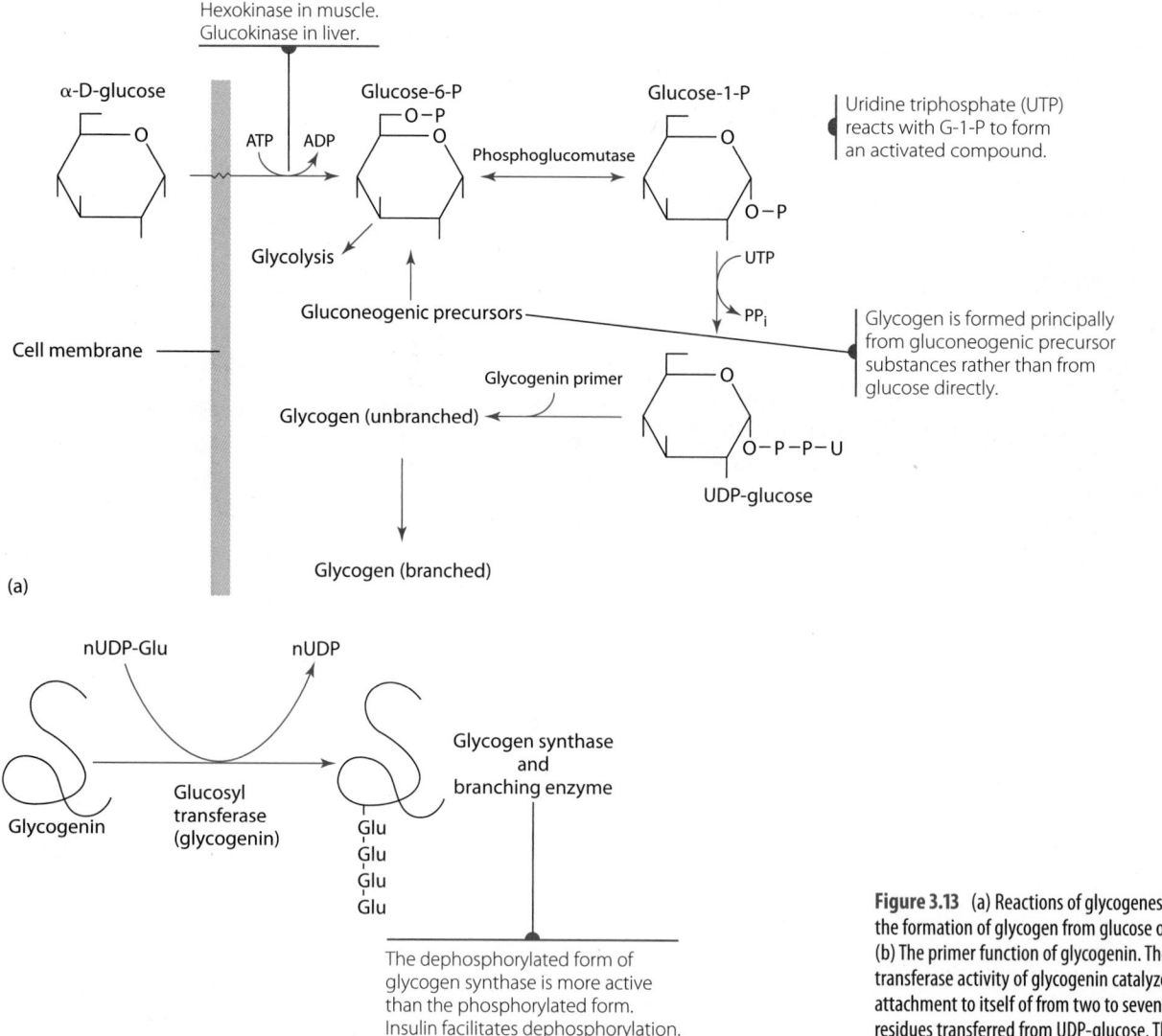

Figure 3.13 (a) Reactions of glycogenesis, by which the formation of glycogen from glucose occurs. (b) The primer function of glycogenin. The glucosyl transferase activity of glycogenin catalyzes the attachment to itself of from two to seven glucose residues transferred from UDP-glucose. The letter *n* represents an unspecified number of UDP-glucose molecules.

in Table 3.4. Muscle hexokinase is an allosteric enzyme that is negatively modulated by the product of the reaction, glucose-6-phosphate. This means that when the muscle cell has adequate glucose-6-P, additional glucose entering the cell is phosphorylated more slowly. Muscle hexokinase has a low K_m, which means it can function at maximum velocity when blood glucose levels are at normal (fasting) levels.

Glucose phosphorylation in the liver is catalyzed primarily by a hexokinase isozyme called glucokinase (sometimes called hexokinase 4). Although the reaction product, glucose-6-phosphate, is the same, interesting differences distinguish it from hexokinase 1 and 2 (Table 3.4). For example, muscle hexokinase is negatively modulated by glucose-6-phosphate, whereas liver glucokinase is not. This characteristic allows excess glucose entering the liver cell to be phosphorylated quickly and encourages glucose entry when blood glucose levels are elevated. Also, glucokinase has a much higher K_m than hexokinase, meaning that it can convert glucose to its phosphate form at a higher velocity should the blood concentration of glucose rise significantly (e.g., after a carbohydrate-rich meal).

Glycogen synthesis (glycogenesis) is initiated by the presence of glucose-6-phosphate. The phosphorylation

Table 3.4 Properties of Hexokinase and Hexokinase 4 (Glucokinase)

Hexokinase Types 1 and 2	Hexokinase Type 4 (Glucokinase)
Located in muscle	Located in liver and pancreas
Allosterically inhibited by glucose-6-P (its product)	Not inhibited by glucose-6-P
Low K_m; function at maximum velocity at fasting blood glucose concentrations	High K_m; functions at maximum velocity only when glucose levels are high (such as following a high-carbohydrate meal)
Not induced by insulin in normal individuals	Induced by insulin in normal individuals
Not induced by insulin in insulin resistant individuals	Not induced by insulin in insulin resistant individuals

of glucose as it enters the liver cell keeps the level of free glucose low, which enhances the entry of glucose into the liver cell due to the concentration gradient between the blood and the liver cell interior. Therefore, the liver has the capacity to reduce blood glucose concentration when it becomes high. Remember, the liver is not dependent upon insulin for glucose transport into the cell, but glucokinase is inducible by insulin. Insulin blood levels are increased by elevated blood glucose levels. Glucokinase activity is below normal in people with type 1 diabetes mellitus because they have low insulin levels, and the glucokinase is not induced. In type 2 diabetes the glucokinase is not induced by the insulin resistant membrane receptors. In either case, the low glucokinase activity contributes to the liver cell's inability to rapidly take up and metabolize glucose, which results even though GLUT2 of the liver is not regulated by insulin.

The next step in glycogenesis is the transfer of phosphate from the 6-carbon of the glucose to the 1-carbon in a reaction catalyzed by the enzyme phosphoglucomutase (Figure 3.13). Nucleoside triphosphates other than ATP sometimes function as activating substances in intermediary metabolism. In the next reaction of glycogenesis, energy derived from the hydrolysis of the α-β-phosphate anhydride bond of uridine triphosphate (UTP to UMP) allows the resulting uridine monophosphate to be coupled to the glucose-1-phosphate to form uridine diphosphate-glucose (UDP-glucose). Glucose is incorporated into glycogen as UDP-glucose. The reaction is catalyzed by glycogen synthase and requires some preformed glycogen as a primer, to which the incoming glucose units can be attached. The initial glycogen is formed by binding a glucose residue to a tyrosine residue of a protein called glycogenin. In this case, glycogenin acts as the primer. Additional glucose residues are attached by glycogen synthase to form chains of up to eight units. The role of glycogenin in glycogenesis has been reviewed [23]. In muscle the protein remains in the core of the glycogen molecule, but in the liver more glycogen molecules than glycogenin molecules are present, so the glycogen must break off of the protein. Glycogen synthase exists in an active (dephosphorylated) form and a less active (phosphorylated) form. Insulin facilitates glycogen synthesis by stimulating the dephosphorylation of glycogen synthase. The glycogen synthase reaction is the primary target of insulin's stimulatory effect on glycogenesis.

When six or seven glucose molecules are added to the glycogen chain, the branching enzyme transfers them to a C-6—OH group (Figure 3.14). Glycogen synthase cannot form the α(1-6) bonds of the branch points. This action is left to the amylo(1-4 → 1-6)-transglycosylase or branching enzyme, which transfers a seven-residue oligosaccharide segment from the end of the main glycogen chain to carbon number 6 hydroxyl groups. Branching within the glycogen molecule is important because it increases the molecule's solubility and compactness. Branching also

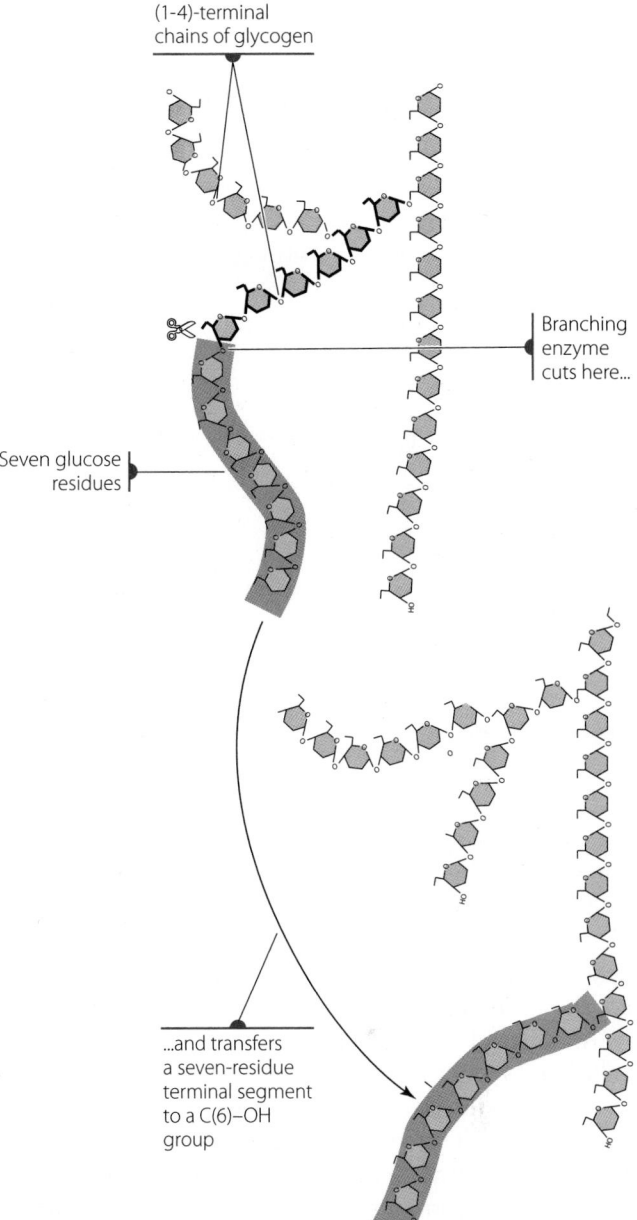

Figure 3.14 Formation of glycogen branches by the branching enzyme.

makes available many nonreducing ends of chains from which glucose residues can be cleaved rapidly and used for energy, in the process known as glycogenolysis and described in the following section. The overall pathway of glycogenesis, like most synthetic pathways, consumes energy because an ATP and a UTP are consumed for each molecule of glucose introduced.

Glycogenolysis

The potential energy of glycogen is contained within the glucose residues that make up its structure. In accordance with the body's energy demands, the residues can be systematically cleaved one at a time from the nonreducing

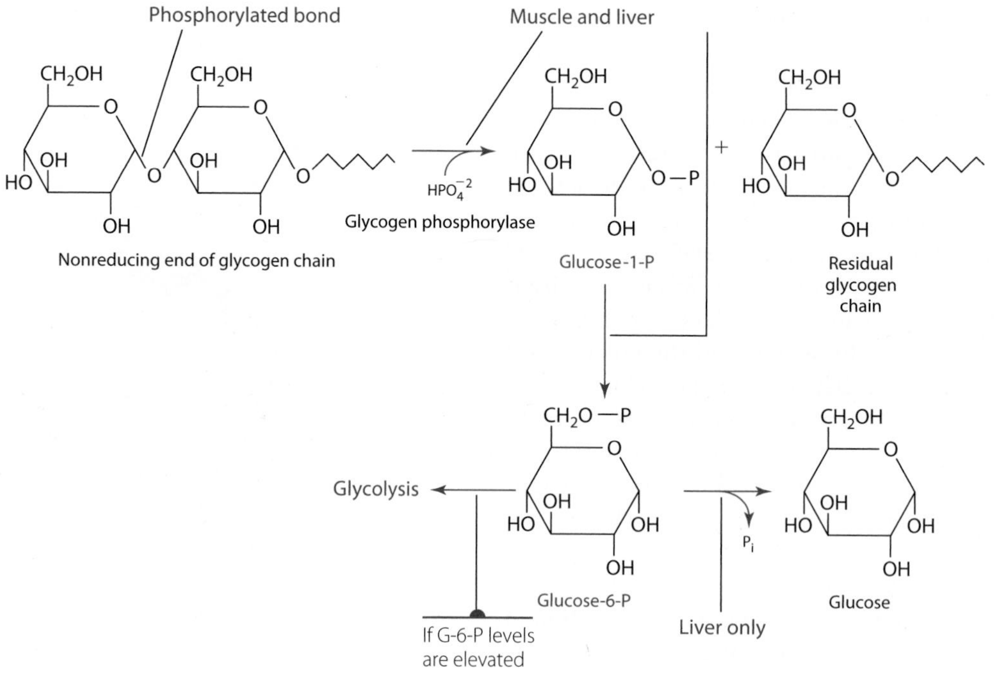

Figure 3.15 The reactions of glycogenolysis, by which glucose residues are sequentially removed from the nonreducing ends of glycogen segments.

ends of the glycogen branches and routed through energy-releasing pathways. The breakdown of glycogen into individual glucose units, in the form of glucose-1-phosphate, is called glycogenolysis and is catalyzed by the enzyme phosphorylase. The steps involved in glycogenolysis are shown in Figure 3.15.

Although glycogen phosphorylase cleaves $\alpha(1\text{-}4)$ glycosidic bonds, it cannot hydrolyze $\alpha(1\text{-}6)$ bonds. Phosphorylase acts repetitively along linear portions of the glycogen molecule until it reaches a point four glucose residues away from an $\alpha(1\text{-}6)$ branch point. Here the degradation process stops, resuming only after an enzyme called the debranching enzyme cleaves the $\alpha(1\text{-}6)$ bond at the branch point.

At times of heightened glycogenolytic activity, the formation of increased amounts of glucose-1-phosphate shifts the glucose phosphate isomerase reaction toward production of the 6-phosphate isomer. The glucose-6-phosphate can enter into the oxidative pathway for glucose (glycolysis) or become free glucose (in the liver or kidney). The conversion of glucose-6-phosphate to free glucose requires the action of glucose-6-phosphatase. This enzyme is not expressed in muscle cells or adipocytes. Therefore, free glucose can be formed only from liver or kidney glycogen and transported through the bloodstream to other tissues for oxidation.

Like its counterpart glycogenesis, glycogenolysis is highly regulated. Its catalyzing enzyme, phosphorylase, is regulated by both covalent and allosteric mechanisms. The regulation is different for the phosphorylation isozymes in muscle than in liver. The muscle and liver isozymes fulfill different physiological purposes: In muscle, the glucose is released from glycogen to provide glucose for energy within the cell, whereas in the liver the glucose is released to provide blood glucose. As phosphorylase is activated for glycogen phosphorylation, glycogen synthetase is inhibited.

Glycogenolysis Regulation

Covalent Regulation Covalent regulation of phosphorylase is enhanced by glucagon and the catecholamines, epinephrine and norepinephrine. These hormones cause a covalent modification of phosphorylase by converting it to an active form through the second messenger cAMP, which regulates the phosphorylation site of the enzymes involved, as discussed in Chapter 1. These hormones bind to a receptor on the cell membrane that causes adenyl cyclase to be activated to produce cAMP. The cAMP causes inactive phosphorylase kinase to become active by phosphorylating it. The active phosphorylase kinase plus ATP converts inactive (nonphosphorylated) phosphorylase b to active (phosphorylated) phosphorylase a. The phosphorylated phosphorylase is less sensitive to the allosteric activation discussed later in this chapter. Phosphorylase a can be converted back to the inactive form, phosphorylase b, by phosphoprotein phosphatase 1 (PP-1). A Nobel Prize was awarded for elucidating this pathway (Figure 3.16).

Allosteric Activation The allosteric activation of phosphorylase b is carried out by AMP to convert it to the

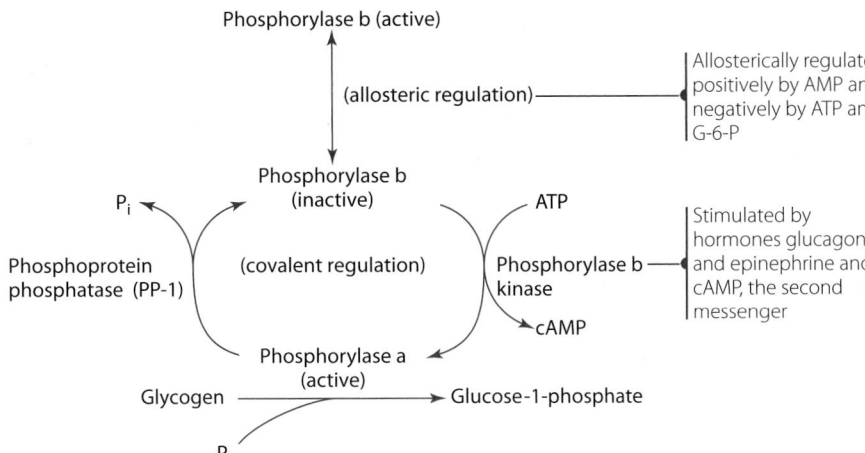

Figure 3.16 An overview of the regulation of glycogen phosphorylase. It is positively regulated covalently by cAMP and positively allosterically regulated by AMP. It is negatively regulated by ATP and glucose-6-P, which cause shifts in the equilibrium between the inactive and active ("b") forms.

active phosphorylase a. When energy levels are low, cellular ATP has been hydrolyzed to AMP, more energy is needed, and the phosphorylase a releases glucose-1-P. The AMP binds to an allosteric site on phosphorylase b, which increases the binding of the glycogen (see Figure 1.10). This allosteric site can also bind ATP, which is an allosteric inhibitor of the enzyme. Glucose-6-P and caffeine are also allosteric inhibitors of the enzyme.

Muscle Phosphorylase The muscle and liver phosphorylase are isozymes. The muscle enzyme releases glucose-1-P, which can be converted to glucose-6-P that enters into the glycolysis pathway to provide energy for the cell. Muscle phosphorylase is more sensitive to intracellular ligands such as AMP for activation. The muscle enzyme is inhibited by metabolites, ATP, glucose-6-P, and glucose. During times of stress the hormones epinephrine and norepinephrine stimulate cAMP synthesis and along with PP-1 covalently modify phosphorylase to the active form. Nervous stimulation and Ca^{+2} ions have the same effect.

Liver Phosphorylase Liver phosphorylase is less sensitive to intracellular ligands. It shows a weak increase in activity in the presence of AMP (10–20%) and is insensitive to inhibition by ATP or glucose-6-P. Liver phosphorylase is regulated by hormonal controls such as glucagon [24].

Glycolysis

Glycolysis is the pathway by which glucose is degraded into two 3-carbon units, pyruvate. From pyruvate, the metabolic course depends largely on the availability of reducing units in the cytosol, which is dependent upon the availability of oxygen within the cell. Glycolysis can function under either aerobic or anaerobic conditions. Under anaerobic conditions or in a situation without sufficient reducing equivalents due either to the lack of oxygen or

high cellular metabolism, pyruvate is converted to lactate. Under otherwise normal conditions, the conversion to lactate occurs mainly in times of strenuous exercise when the demand for oxygen by the working muscles exceeds that which is available. Lactate produced under anaerobic conditions can also diffuse from the muscle to the bloodstream and be carried to the liver for conversion to glucose. Under these anaerobic conditions, glycolysis releases a small amount of usable energy that can help sustain the muscles even in a state of oxygen debt. Providing this energy is the major function of the anaerobic pathway of glucose to lactate. Anaerobic glycolysis is the sole source of energy for erythrocytes because the red blood cell does not contain mitochondria. Both the brain and GI tract also produce much of their energy from glycolysis.

Under aerobic conditions, pyruvate can be transported into the mitochondria and participate in the TCA cycle, in which it becomes completely oxidized to CO_2 and H_2O. Complete oxidation is accompanied by the release of relatively large amounts of energy, much of which is salvaged as ATP by the mechanism of oxidative phosphorylation. The glycolytic enzymes function within the cytosol of the cell, but the enzymes catalyzing the TCA cycle reactions are located within the mitochondrion. Therefore, pyruvate must enter the mitochondrion for complete oxidation. Glycolysis followed by TCA cycle activity (aerobic catabolism of glucose) demands an ample supply of oxygen, a condition that generally is met in normal, resting mammalian cells. In a normal, aerobic situation, complete oxidation of pyruvate generally occurs, with only a small amount of lactate being formed. The primary importance of glycolysis in energy metabolism, therefore, is in providing the initial sequence of reactions (to pyruvate) necessary for the complete oxidation of glucose by the TCA cycle, which supplies relatively large quantities of ATP.

In cells that lack mitochondria, such as the erythrocyte, the pathway of glycolysis is the sole provider of ATP by the mechanism of substrate-level phosphorylation of ADP, discussed later in this chapter. Nearly all cell types conduct glycolysis, but most of the energy derived from carbohydrates originates in liver, muscle, and adipose tissue, which together constitute a major portion of total body mass. The pathway of glycolysis, under both aerobic and anaerobic conditions, is summarized in Figure 3.17. Also indicated in the figure is the mode of entry of glucose from glycogenolysis, dietary fructose, and dietary galactose into the pathway for metabolism. Following are comments on selected reactions (the numbers correspond to the numbers in Figure 3.17).

❶ The hexokinase/glucokinase reaction consumes 1 mol ATP/mol glucose. The properties of these enzymes were covered in Table 3.4. Glucokinase is present in the liver and pancreas. Hexokinase is located in muscle, adipose tissue, and the brain. As discussed earlier, the hexokinase in muscle has a low K_m, which means it can function at maximum velocity at normal blood glucose levels. When the muscle cell accumulates glucose-6-phosphate, the hexokinase is inhibited. Liver glucokinase, in contrast, has a high K_m, which means it requires a high concentration of glucose in blood to function at maximum velocity. The liver does not remove large quantities of glucose from blood unless blood glucose is elevated. Glucokinase in the liver is induced by insulin. Phosphorylating glucose serves to "prime" the glycolytic pathway, which energizes the molecule for subsequent reactions. Phosphorylated glucose cannot cross the cell membrane. Remember that glycogenolysis produces glucose-1-phosphate, which can be converted to glucose-6-phosphate without using an additional ATP.

❷ Glucose phosphoglucoisomerase (also called glucose phosphate isomerase) catalyzes movement of the carbonyl group from the first carbon (glucose) to the second carbon (fructose). This is an interconversion of isomers—glucose-6-P to fructose-6-P—and is reversible.

❸ The third reaction of glycolysis is the phosphorylation of fructose-6-phosphate to fructose-1,6-bisphosphate using an ATP. The term *bis* means that the two phosphates are on different carbons. (The prefix *di*, as in *dihydroxyacetone phosphate* in reaction 4, means that the two phosphates are attached to each other and to a single carbon atom.) The phosphofructokinase reaction is an important regulatory site. This step commits the cell to metabolize glucose rather than converting it to another sugar or storing it. Phosphofructokinase is modulated (by allosteric mechanisms) negatively by ATP and citrate (a product of the TCA cycle and an indication that energy needs are met). The inhibition by ATP is reversed by AMP, an indication that the cell needs more energy. There is a relationship among the levels of ATP, ADP, and AMP. They are interconverted by the reaction:

$$ADP + ADP \longleftrightarrow ATP + AMP$$

This reaction is catalyzed by adenylate kinase. When the reaction reaches equilibrium the quantity of ADP is about 10% of that of ATP, and AMP levels are less than 1% of those of ATP. Small changes in ATP are amplified in changes in AMP. The regulation of phosphofructokinase reactions is modulated by the relative amounts of ATP and AMP.

Phosphofructokinase is also regulated by fructose-2,6-bisphosphate, which is a potent allosteric activator that increases the affinity of the enzyme for its substrate, fructose-6-phosphate. Levels of fructose-2,6-bisphosphate are controlled by the enzyme phosphofructokinase-2. This enzyme is induced by glucagon and is different from the phosphofructokinase in the glycolytic pathway. Other activities of this enzyme will be discussed in the gluconeogenesis section of this chapter.

❹ Fructose bisphosphate aldolase cleaves hexose (fructose) bisphosphate into two triose phosphates, glyceraldehyde-3-phosphate (G-3-P), and dihydroxyacetone phosphate (DHAP).

❺ The isomers glyceraldehyde-3-phosphate and dihydroxyacetone phosphate are interconverted by the enzyme triosephosphate isomerase. In an isolated system, the equilibrium favors DHAP formation. In the cellular environment, however, it is shifted completely toward producing glyceraldehyde-3-phosphate because this metabolite is continuously removed from the equilibrium by the subsequent reaction catalyzed by glyceraldehyde-3-phosphate dehydrogenase.

❻ In this reaction, glyceraldehyde-3-phosphate is oxidized to a carboxylic acid, while inorganic phosphate is incorporated as a carboxylic phosphoric anhydride bond (a high-energy compound). The enzyme is glyceraldehyde-3-phosphate dehydrogenase, which uses NAD^+ as its hydrogen-accepting cosubstrate. Under aerobic conditions, the NADH formed is reoxidized to NAD^+ by O_2 through the electron transport chain in the mitochondria, as explained in the next section. The reason why O_2 is not necessary to sustain the reaction of converting glyceraldehyde-3-P to bis-P-glycerate is that under anaerobic conditions the NAD^+ consumed is restored by a subsequent reaction converting pyruvate to lactate (see reaction **⓫**).

❼ This reaction, catalyzed by phosphoglycerate kinase, exemplifies a substrate-level phosphorylation of ADP. A more detailed review of substrate-level phosphorylation, by which ATP is formed from ADP by the transfer of a phosphate from a high-energy donor molecule, is covered in the "Substrate-Level Phosphorylation" section. Two ATPs are synthesized because glucose (a hexose) makes two trioses. This reaction replaces the two ATPs used to prime glycolysis. Under conditions of high ATP (which means low ADP) the reaction can be reversed.

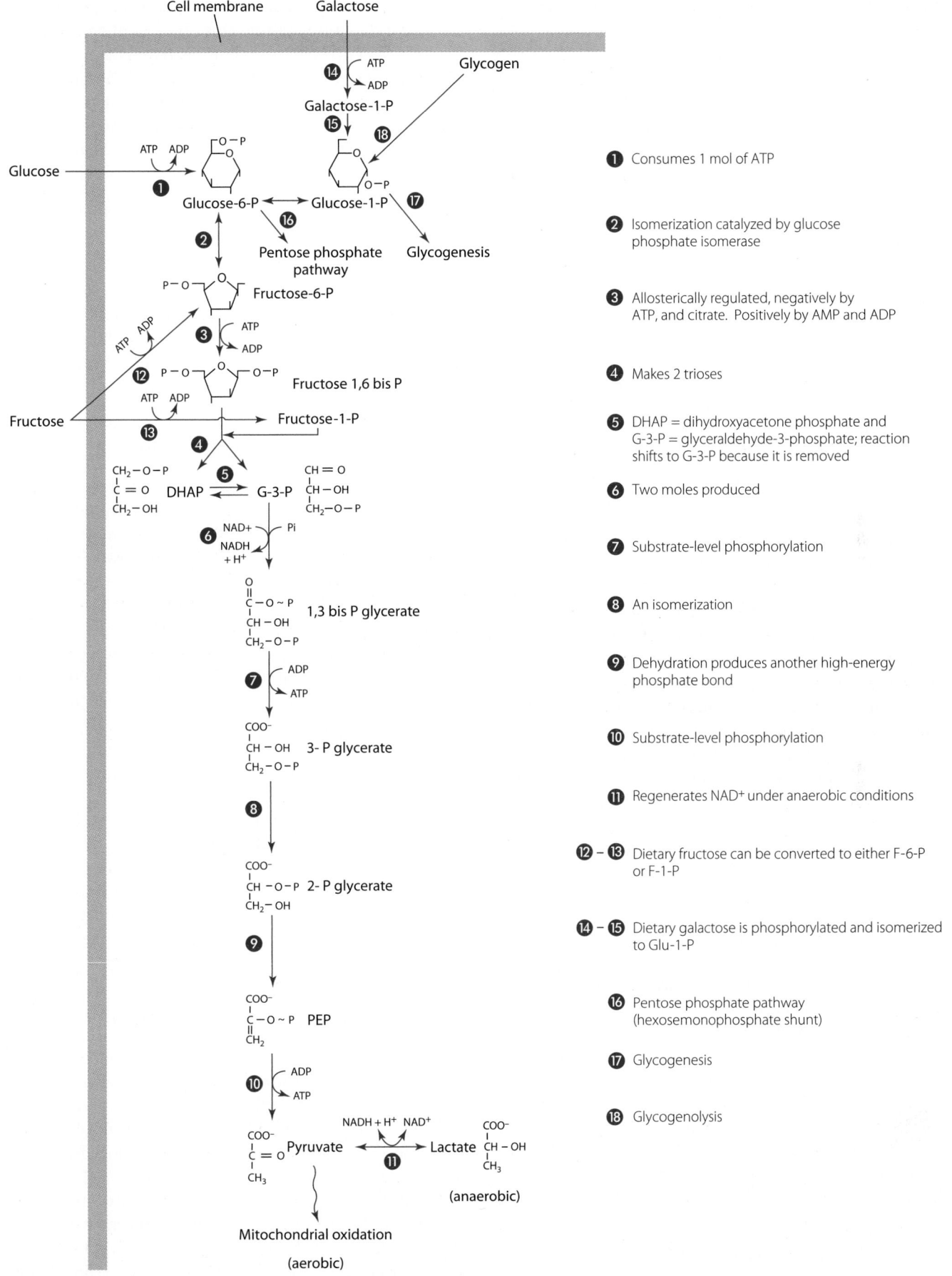

Figure 3.17 Glycolysis, indicating the mode of entry of glucose, fructose, glycogen, and galactose into glycolysis. Hydroxyl groups on ring structures are indicated by a line pointing above or below the ring.

8 Phosphoglycerate mutase catalyzes the transfer of the phosphate group from the number 3 carbon to the number 2 carbon of the glyceric acid.

9 Dehydration of 2-phosphoglycerate by the enzyme enolase introduces a double bond that imparts high energy to the phosphate bond.

10 Phosphoenolpyruvate (PEP) donates its phosphate group to ADP in a reaction catalyzed by pyruvate kinase to yield pyruvate. This is the second site of substrate-level phosphorylation of ADP in the glycolytic pathway to make two ATPs. Two ATPs were used to prime glycolysis, two were produced in reaction **7**, and two were produced in this reaction, for a net gain of two ATPs to this point. The hexose has now been split into two 3-carbon units. Phosphoenolpyruvate kinase is a highly regulated enzyme. It is activated allosterically by AMP and fructose-1,6-bisphosphate and inhibited by ATP, acetyl-CoA, and alanine. In the liver it is also regulated covalently by glucagon through the cAMP mechanism discussed earlier, which transfers a phosphoryl group from ATP. The phosphorylated enzyme is more sensitive to inhibition by ATP.

11 The lactate dehydrogenase reaction transfers two hydride ions from NADH and H$^+$ to pyruvate, reducing it to lactate. NAD$^+$ is formed in the reaction and can replace the NAD$^+$ consumed earlier under anaerobic conditions. This reaction is most active in situations of oxygen debt, as occurs in prolonged muscular activity. Under aerobic conditions, pyruvate enters the mitochondrion for complete oxidation via the tricarboxylic acid (TCA) cycle. A third important option available to pyruvate is its conversion to the amino acid alanine by amino transferase, a reaction by which pyruvate acquires an amino group from the amino acid glutamate (Chapter 6). The alternate pathways for pyruvate, together with the fact that pyruvate is also the product of the catabolism of various amino acids, makes pyruvate an important link between protein (amino acid) and carbohydrate metabolism.

12 and **13** These two reactions provide the means by which dietary fructose enters the glycolytic pathway. Fructose is an important factor in the average American diet, as nearly half the carbohydrate consumed is sucrose and high-fructose corn syrup, which is becoming more popular as a food sweetener (see the Perspective at the end of this chapter). In the liver, fructose is converted to fructose-1-phosphate by the enzyme fructokinase. The fructose-1-P is then converted into the two 3-carbon intermediates as in reaction **4**. In kidney and muscle, fructose is phosphorylated by hexokinase to form fructose-6-phosphate. This is a relatively unimportant reaction because the liver clears nearly all of the dietary fructose on the first pass. The hexokinase reaction is slow and occurs only in the presence of high levels of fructose.

14 and **15** Like glucose and fructose, galactose is first phosphorylated (by galactokinase) to form galactose-1-phosphate. The galactose-1-phosphate is converted to UDP-galactose, which is converted to UDP-glucose by subsequent reactions. The result of these reactions is the production of glucose-1-phosphate. The major dietary source of galactose is lactose, from which the galactose is released by lactase during absorption.

16 This is the point where glucose-6-phosphate enters into a pathway called the pentose phosphate pathway (hexosemonophosphate shunt), which is discussed later in this chapter.

17 and **18** This is the point of entry of glucose-1-phosphate into glycogenesis (the synthesis of glycogen) and of glucose-1-phosphate from glycogenolysis (the hydrolysis of glycogen) into glycolysis (glucose oxidative pathway).

The Tricarboxylic Acid Cycle

The tricarboxylic acid (TCA) cycle, also called the Krebs cycle or the citric acid cycle, is at the forefront of energy metabolism in the body. It can be thought of as the common and final catabolic pathway because products of carbohydrate, fat, and amino acids that enter the cycle can be completely oxidized to CO_2 and H_2O, with the accompanying release of energy. More than 90% of the energy released from food is estimated to occur as a result of TCA cycle oxidation. Not all the substances entering the cycle are totally oxidized, however. Some TCA cycle intermediates are used in the formation of glucose by the process of gluconeogenesis (discussed later), and some can be converted to certain amino acids by transamination (Chapter 6).

The TCA cycle is located within the mitochondrial matrix, either free or in the inner membrane. The energy output of the TCA cycle is attributed to mitochondrial electron transport, with oxidative phosphorylation being the source of ATP formation, as discussed later in this chapter. The oxidation reactions occurring in the cycle are actually dehydrogenations in which an enzyme catalyzes the removal of hydride ions to an acceptor cosubstrate such as NAD$^+$ or FAD. A hydride ion can be considered a proton coupled with two electrons. Because both the enzymes of the cycle and the enzymes and electron carriers of electron transport are compartmentalized within the mitochondria, the reduced cosubstrates, NADH and FADH$_2$, are readily reoxidized by O_2 through the electron transport chain, located in the mitochondrial inner membrane.

In addition to producing the reduced cosubstrates NADH and FADH$_2$, which furnish the energy when they are oxidized during electron transport, the TCA cycle produces most of the carbon dioxide through decarboxylation reactions. In terms of glucose metabolism, recall that two pyruvates are produced from one glucose molecule during cytoplasmic glycolysis. These pyruvates in turn are transported into the mitochondria, where decarboxylation leads to the formation of two acetyl-CoA units and two molecules of CO_2. The two carbons represented by the acetyl-CoA are incorporated into oxaloacetic acid to form citric acid and sequentially lost as two molecules of CO_2 through TCA cycle decarboxylations. Most of the CO_2 produced is exhaled through the lungs, although some is used in certain synthetic reactions called carboxylations.

TCA Pathway

The TCA cycle is shown in Figure 3.18. Acetyl-CoA couples with oxaloacetate to begin the pathway. Acetyl-CoA is formed from numerous sources, including the breakdown of fatty acids in the mitochondria, glycolysis in the cytosol, and certain amino acids. Pyruvate, the link between glycolysis and the TCA cycle, must enter the mitochondria to enter the TCA cycle. This is accomplished by complex reactions catalyzed by a multienzyme complex called the pyruvate dehydrogenase complex (PDC). This multienzyme system is made up of three enzymes: pyruvate dehydrogenase, dihydrolipoamide acetyltransferase, and dihydrolipoamide dehydrogenase. Several cofactors are required for the reaction, including coenzyme A (CoA), thiamin pyrophosphate, Mg^{2+}, NAD^+, FAD, and lipoic acid. Four vitamins, therefore, are necessary for the activity of the complex: pantothenic acid (a component of CoA), thiamin, niacin, and riboflavin. The role of these vitamins and others as precursors of coenzymes is discussed in Chapter 9. The net effect of the complex is decarboxylation (to produce CO_2) and dehydrogenation of pyruvate, with NAD^+ serving as the terminal hydrogen acceptor. The active sites of the three enzymes are packed closely together, which allows the passing of the product of one reaction to the next enzyme. This reaction yields energy because the reoxidation of the NADH produces ATP by oxidative phosphorylation. The reaction is regulated allosterically: negatively by ATP, acetyl-CoA, and NADH, and positively by NAD and ADP. The PDC is also regulated covalently. A Mg^{2+}-dependent enzyme, pyruvate dehydrogenase kinase, phosphorylates the complex when NADH and acetyl-CoA levels rise. Reactivation of the PDC occurs by the enzyme pyruvate dehydrogenase phosphatase, which removes the phosphate. Insulin and Ca^{+2} ions activate the kinase to activate the PDC.

The condensation of acetyl-CoA with oxaloacetate initiates the TCA cycle reactions. Following are comments on the individual reactions (Figure 3.18):

❶ The formation of citrate from oxaloacetate and acetyl-CoA is catalyzed by the enzyme citrate synthase. The reaction is regulated negatively by NADH and succinyl-CoA.

❷ The isomerization of citrate to isocitrate involves *cis* aconitate as an intermediate. The isomerization, catalyzed by aconitase, involves dehydration followed by sterically reversed hydration, resulting in the repositioning of the —OH group onto an adjacent carbon.

❸ Catalyzed by the enzyme isocitrate dehydrogenase, this is the first of four dehydrogenation reactions within the cycle. Energy is supplied from this reaction through the electron transport system by the reoxidation of the NADH. Note that the first loss of CO_2 in the cycle occurs at this site. The CO_2 arises from the spontaneous decarboxylation of an intermediate compound, oxalosuccinate (not shown). The reaction is positively modulated by ADP and negatively modulated by ATP and NADH.

❹ The decarboxylation and dehydrogenation of α-ketoglutarate is mechanistically identical to the pyruvate dehydrogenase complex reaction in its multienzyme-multicofactor requirement. In the reaction, called the α-ketoglutarate dehydrogenase reaction, NAD^+ serves as hydrogen acceptor, and a second carbon is lost as CO_2. The product of the reaction is succinyl-CoA. The pyruvate dehydrogenase, isocitrate dehydrogenase, and α-ketoglutarate dehydrogenase reactions account for the loss of the three carbons from pyruvate as CO_2.

❺ The NADH can pass through the electron transport system to make ATP via oxidative phosphorylation. Succinyl-CoA also contains a high-energy thioester bond that is hydrolyzed by the enzyme succinyl-CoA synthetase (also called succinyl thiokinase) and that releases sufficient energy to drive the phosphorylation of guanosine diphosphate (GDP) by inorganic phosphate. The resulting GTP can transfer its phosphate to ADP to make ATP in a reaction catalyzed by the enzyme nucleoside diphosphate kinase. This reaction is another example of ATP production through substrate-level phosphorylation. GTP can also serve as phosphate donor in certain phosphorylation reactions, for example, in reactions involved in gluconeogenesis or glycogenesis.

❻ The succinate dehydrogenase reaction uses FAD instead of NAD^+ as a hydrogen acceptor. The $FADH_2$ is reoxidized by electron transport by O_2 and produces ATP by oxidative phosphorylation. Succinate dehydrogenase is bound in the inner membrane of the mitochondria. Other TCA enzymes are found in the mitochondrial matrix.

❼ Fumarase incorporates the elements of H_2O across the double bond of fumarate to form malate.

❽ The conversion of malate to oxaloacetate completes the cycle. NAD^+ acts as hydrogen acceptor in this dehydrogenation reaction, which is catalyzed by malate dehydrogenase. This reaction is the fourth site of reduced cosubstrate formation (3-NADH and 1-$FADH_2$) and thus results in additional energy release in the cycle.

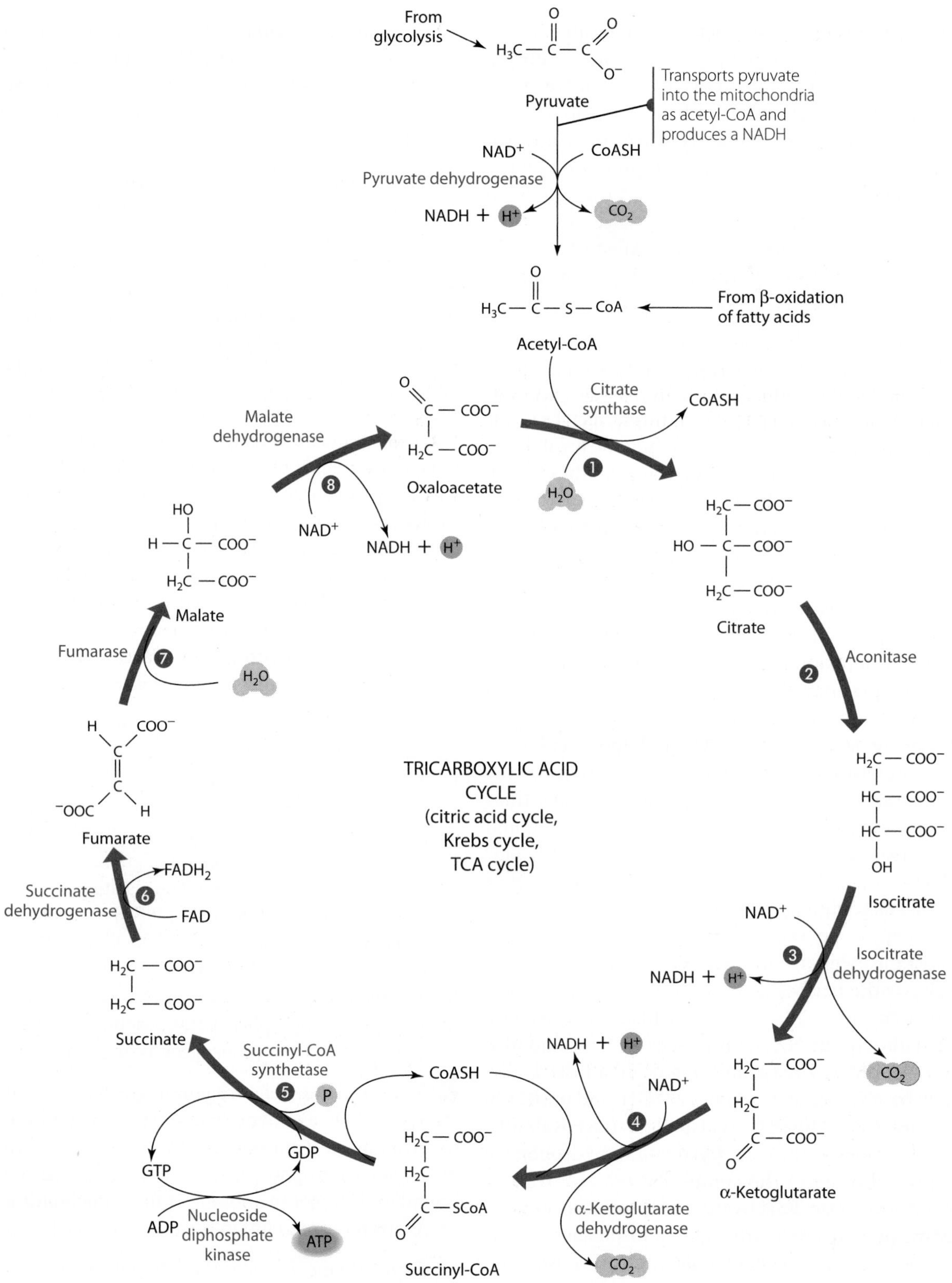

1. Acetyl-CoA adds 2 carbons to oxaloacetate to start the cycle.
2. Isomerization takes place by removing H_2O and then adding it back.
3. A CO_2 is lost and a NADH is produced.
4. Another CO_2 is lost and another NADH is produced.
5. A substrate-level phosphorylation.
6. FAD^+ is reduced to form $FADH_2$.
7. Add H_2O across the double bond.
8. Third NADH produced in the TCA cycle. One $FADH_2$ and one NADH produced in the conversion of pyruvate to acetyl-CoA.

Figure 3.18 The tricarboxylic acid (TCA) cycle.

ATPs Produced by Complete Glucose Oxidation

The complete oxidation of glucose to CO_2 and H_2O can be shown by this equation:

$$C_6H_{12}O_6 + 6\,O_2 \longrightarrow 6\,CO_2 + 6\,H_2O + \text{energy}$$

Complete oxidation is achieved by the combined reaction sequences of the glycolytic and TCA cycle pathways. The energy-conserving steps yield a net of two ATPs by substrate-level reactions in the glycolytic pathway and two ATPs (or one ATP and one GTP) by substrate-level reactions in the TCA cycle. In addition, there are three NADH and one [FAD] produced from each acetyl-CoA that goes through the TCA cycle. Two acetyl-CoAs are produced from each molecule of glucose, which releases two molecules of CO_2 and two NADH. In summary, one molecule of glucose produces:

- 6 molecules of CO_2 (released)
- 4 ATPs
- 10 NADH
- 2 [FAD]

The NADH and $FADH_2$ are in the matrix of the mitochondria and are oxidized by the electron transport chain and oxidative phosphorylation to ultimately produce ATP. By convention, it has been assumed in the past that 3 ATPS are formed by oxidative phosphorylation from NADH, and 2 ATPs are formed from $FADH_2$. As discussed later in this chapter, the actual number of ATPs formed from NADH is closer to 2.5; for $FADH_2$, it is 1.5. If the integers (3/2) are used for the number of ATPs produced from NADH/$FADH_2$, a total of 38 mol of ATP are formed. If we accept the 2.5/1.5 ratio, 32 mol of ATP are produced from each mol of glucose. Oxidative phosphorylation is only active under aerobic conditions. Under anaerobic conditions, only two ATPs are produced from each glucose at substrate level.

The actual number of ATPs formed aerobically from glucose varies. As will be discussed later, there are two different shuttle mechanisms to transport the electrons from NADH produced by the glycolytic pathway into the mitochondria. One mechanism, the glycerol-3-phosphate shuttle system, transfers the electrons to $FADH_2$ and therefore yields only 1.5 ATPs. The other shuttle system, the malate-aspartate shuttle, transfers the electrons to NADH inside the mitochondria and yields 2.5 ATPs.

Acetyl-CoA Oxidation and Tricarboxylic Acid Cycle Intermediates

A small but steady supply of four-carbon units is needed for the TCA cycle to oxidize all of the acetyl-CoA produced to CO_2 and H_2O. In the absence of four-carbon intermediates, ketoacidosis results. We will discuss this process briefly here and more extensively in Chapter 5. As we will discuss in Chapters 5 and 6, acetyl-CoA is

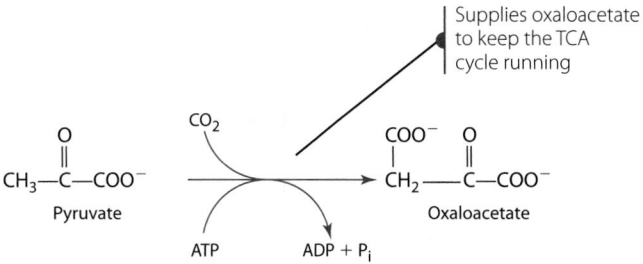

Figure 3.19 The reaction by which oxaloacetate is formed directly from pyruvate.

produced by fatty acid oxidation and amino acid catabolism, in addition to being derived from pyruvate as a result of glycolysis. An increase in acetyl-CoA leads to an imbalance between the amounts of acetyl-CoA and oxaloacetate, which condense one-to-one stoichiometrically in the citrate synthase reaction. To keep the TCA cycle functioning, oxaloacetate and/or other TCA cycle intermediates that can form oxaloacetate must be replenished in the cycle, and a mechanism for this does exist. Oxaloacetate, fumarate, succinyl-CoA, and α-ketoglutarate can all be formed from certain amino acids, but the single most important mechanism for ensuring an ample supply of oxaloacetate is the reaction that forms oxaloacetate (four carbons) directly from pyruvate (three carbons) by the addition of CO_2. This reaction, shown in Figure 3.19, is catalyzed by pyruvate carboxylase. The "uphill" incorporation of CO_2 is accomplished at the expense of ATP, and the reaction requires the participation of biotin (see Chapter 9). The conversion of pyruvate to oxaloacetate is called an **anaplerotic** (filling-up) process because of its role in restoring oxaloacetate to the cycle. Interestingly, pyruvate carboxylase is regulated positively by acetyl-CoA, thereby accelerating oxaloacetate formation in response to increasing levels of acetyl-CoA.

NADH in Anaerobic and Aerobic Glycolysis: The Shuttle Systems

Under anaerobic conditions, the NADH produced in the pathway of glycolysis (the glyceraldehyde-3-phosphate dehydrogenase reaction) cannot undergo reoxidation by mitochondrial electron transport because O_2 is the ultimate oxidizing agent in that system. Instead, NADH is used in the lactate dehydrogenase reduction of pyruvate to lactate, thereby becoming reoxidized to NAD^+ without involving oxygen. In this manner, NAD^+ is restored to sustain the glyceraldehyde-3-phosphate dehydrogenase reaction, allowing the production of lactate to continue in the absence of oxygen.

When glycolysis is operating aerobically, and the supply of oxygen is adequate to allow total oxidation of incoming glucose, lactate is not formed. Instead, pyruvate enters the mitochondrion and NAD^+ is reduced by the electron transport chain. NADH must be moved into the mitochondria, but it (or the electrons) cannot enter the mitochondrion directly. Instead, there are two separate shuttle systems that transfer reducing equivalents from NADH produced in the cytosol during glycolysis. These shuttle systems are specific to certain tissues. The glycerol-3-phosphate shuttle functions in the brain and skeletal muscle, whereas the more active malate-aspartate shuttle functions in the liver, kidney, and heart.

Glycerol-3-Phosphate Shuttle System Glycerophosphate produced by glycolysis is oxidized by two different glycerophosphate dehydrogenases, one in the cytoplasm and the other on the outer face of the inner mitochondrial membrane. The electrons in NADH are transferred to FAD^+, which results in production of only 1.5 ATPs per mole of cytosol-produced NADH. Therefore, if the glycerol-3-phosphate shuttle is in effect, only three ATPs are formed aerobically per mole of glucose by oxidative phosphorylation (Figure 3.20). This shuttle is not reversible.

Malate-Aspartate Shuttle System The most active shuttle compound, malate, is freely permeable to the inner mitochondrial membrane. Oxaloacetate from the cytosol is reduced by the NADH to form malate and NAD^+. The malate is oxidized by the enzyme malate dehydrogenase to oxaloacetic acid in the matrix of the mitochondria, producing NADH that enters the electron transport chain and generates about 2.5 ATPs per mole. The oxaloacetic acid undergoes transamination by aspartate amino transferase to form aspartate, which is freely permeable to the inner membrane and can move back out into the cytosol. The effect is that NADH moves into the mitochondria,

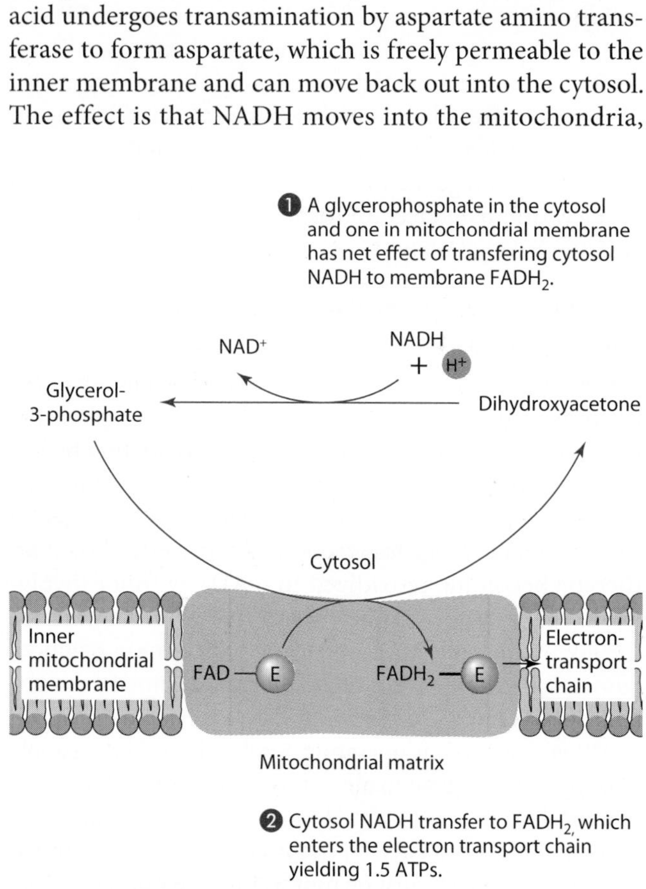

even though the inner mitochondrial membrane is impermeable to it (Figure 3.21). This shuttle is reversible.

Formation of ATP

Substrate-Level Phosphorylation

In discussing glycolysis and the TCA cycle it was shown that certain molecules were activated by phosphate group transfer from ATP and some compounds transferred their phosphate group to ADP to make ATP—that is, performed substrate-level phosphorylation. Phosphorylation itself is an endothermic reaction but is made possible by the highly exothermic hydrolysis of the terminal phosphate of ATP. Phosphorylation of ADP is accomplished by compounds having more energy than the amount needed ($\Delta G^0 = +7,300$ cal/mol or $+35.7$ kJ/mol) required for the reaction. Substrate-level phosphorylation is one mechanism to produce ATP from glycolysis and the TCA cycle.

Table 3.5 lists the standard free energy of hydrolysis of selected phosphate-containing compounds in both kcal and kJ. Phosphorylated molecules have a wide range of free energies of hydrolysis of their phosphate groups. Many of them release less energy than ATP, but some release more. Figure 1.16 gives the structures of phosphoenolpyruvate, 1,3-bisphosphoglycerate, and phosphocreatine, three compounds that have more free energy than ATP and are capable of phosphorylating ADP. The ΔG^0 of hydrolysis of the compounds, listed in Table 3.5, is called the phosphate group transfer potential and is a measure of the compounds' capacities to donate phosphate groups to other substances. The more negative the transfer potential, the more potent the phosphate-donating power. Therefore, a compound that releases more energy on hydrolysis of its phosphate can transfer that phosphate to an acceptor molecule having a relatively more positive transfer potential. For this transfer to occur in actuality, however, there must be a specific enzyme to catalyze the transfer. A phosphate group can be enzymatically transferred from ATP to glucose, a transfer that can be predicted from Table 3.5. It can also be predicted from Table 3.5 that compounds with a more negative phosphate group transfer potential than ATP can transfer phosphate to ADP, forming ATP.

❶ A glycerophosphate in the cytosol and one in mitochondrial membrane has net effect of transfering cytosol NADH to membrane FADH₂.

❷ Cytosol NADH transfer to FADH₂ which enters the electron transport chain yielding 1.5 ATPs.

Figure 3.20 Glycerol-3-phosphate shuttle.

Table 3.5 Free Energy of Hydrolysis (Phosphate Group Transfer Potential) of Some Phosphorylated Compounds

Compound	ΔG°(cal)	ΔG°(kJ)
Phosphoenolpyruvate	−14,800	−62.2
1,3-diphosphoglycerate	−11,800	−49.6
Phosphocreatine	−10,300	−43.3
ATP	−7,300	−35.7
Glucose-1-phosphate	−5,000	−21.0
Adenosine monophosphate (AMP)	−3,400	−9.2
Glucose-6-phosphate	−3,300	−13.9

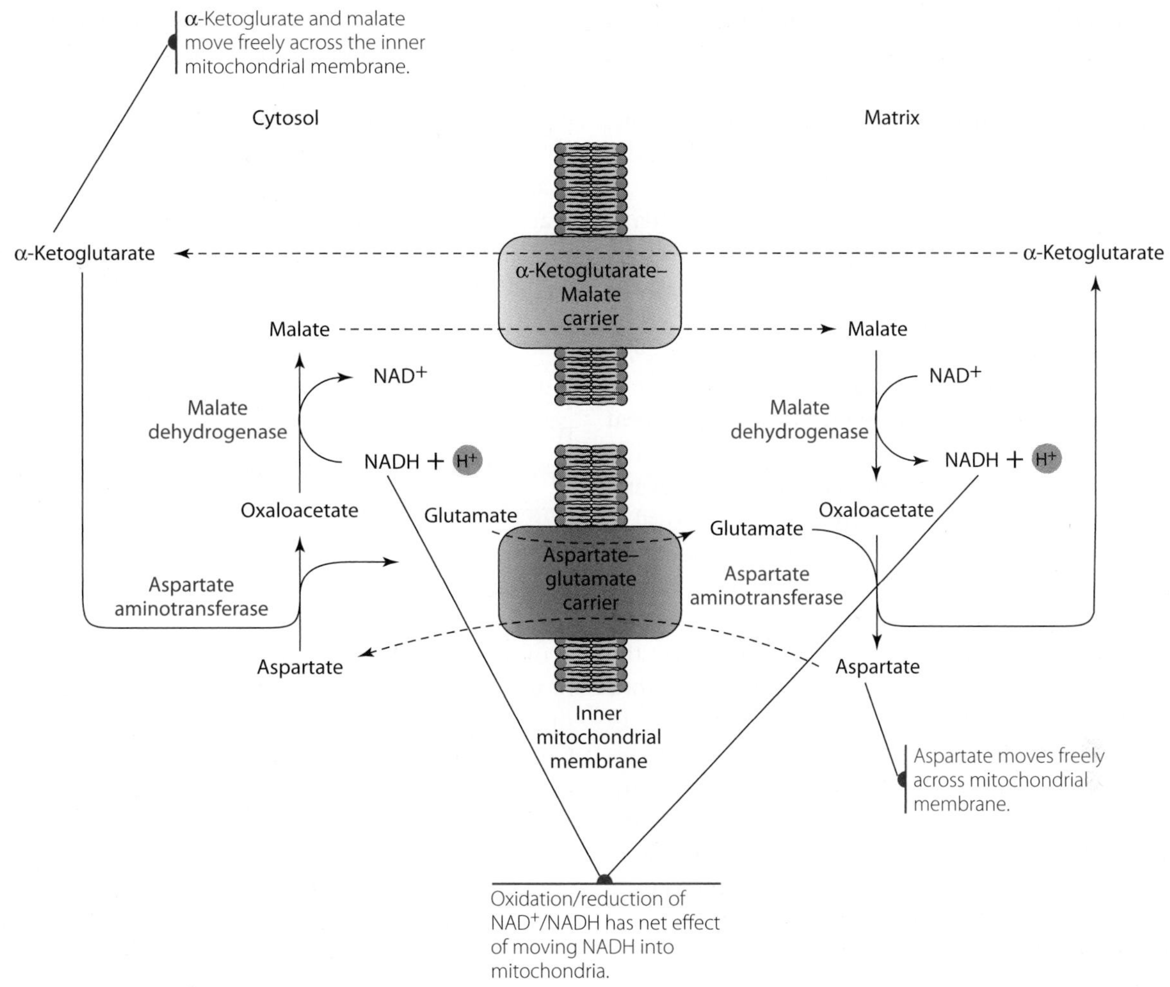

α-Ketoglurate and malate move freely across the inner mitochondrial membrane.

Cytosol

Matrix

α-Ketoglutarate ← - α-Ketoglutarate

α-Ketoglutarate–Malate carrier

Malate - → Malate

NAD⁺ → NAD^+

Malate dehydrogenase

Malate dehydrogenase

NADH + H⁺ → $NADH +$ H⁺

Oxaloacetate

Glutamate

Glutamate

Oxaloacetate

Aspartate–glutamate carrier

Aspartate aminotransferase

Aspartate aminotransferase

Aspartate

Aspartate

Inner mitochondrial membrane

Aspartate moves freely across mitochondrial membrane.

Oxidation/reduction of NAD⁺/NADH has net effect of moving NADH into mitochondria.

Figure 3.21 Malate-aspartate shuttle.

This kind of reaction does, in fact, occur in the hexokinase/glucokinase reactions. The phosphorylation of ADP by phosphocreatine, for example, represents an important mode for ATP formation in muscle, and the reaction exemplifies a substrate-level phosphorylation (Figure 3.22). The more important ATP-forming mechanisms from the standpoint of the amount produced are electron transport and oxidative phosphorylation, which are covered in the next section.

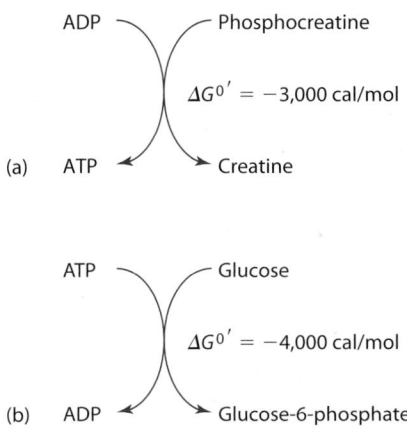

ADP ⟍ ⟋ Phosphocreatine

$\Delta G^{0\prime} = -3{,}000 \text{ cal/mol}$

(a) ATP ⟋ ⟍ Creatine

ATP ⟍ ⟋ Glucose

$\Delta G^{0\prime} = -4{,}000 \text{ cal/mol}$

(b) ADP ⟋ ⟍ Glucose-6-phosphate

Figure 3.22
(a) Example of high-energy phosphate bond being transferred from high-energy compound phosphocreatine to form ATP. (b) The transfer of the high-energy phosphate bond to a compound that becomes activated, allowing it to enter into the glycolytic pathway.

Biological Oxidation and the Electron Transport Chain

The major means by which ATP is formed from ADP is through the mechanism of oxidative phosphorylation. This process is discussed in detail here because ATP is the major supplier of energy from carbohydrates (and also lipids and amino acids). The energy required to form ATP is tapped from a pool of energy generated by the flow of electrons from substrate molecules undergoing oxidation and the translocation of protons (H^+) from the mitochondrial matrix to the space between the inner and outer membranes. The electrons from NADH or $FADH_2$ are then passed through a series of intermediate compounds and ultimately to molecular oxygen, which becomes reduced to H_2O in the process. The compounds participating in this sequential reduction-oxidation constitute the electron transport chain, also known as the respiratory chain because the electron transfer is linked to the uptake of O_2, which is made available to the tissues by respiration. (*Electron transport chain* is the more commonly used term.) The mitochondria contain the electron transport chain and are often called the power plants of the cell. The energy produced assumes the forms of chemical energy as ATP and heat to maintain body temperature. Therefore, the term *oxidative phosphorylation* is a descriptive blend of two simultaneous processes: electron transport and the oxidation of a metabolite by oxygen; and the phosphorylation of ADP to make ATP.

The processes of the cellular oxidation of nutrients, electron transport, and oxidative phosphorylation perform a unified function and should be thought of together. They are considered next in more detail. Oxidation of the energy nutrients from food (carbohydrates, protein, lipids, and alcohol) is what releases their inherent chemical energy and makes it available to the body either as heat or as ATP.

Cellular oxidation of a compound can occur by several different reactions: the addition of oxygen, the removal of electrons, and the removal of hydrogens plus electrons (hydride ions, atoms of H or ½ H_2, not protons or hydrogen ions). All these reactions are catalyzed by enzymes collectively termed oxidoreductases. Among these, the **dehydrogenases,** which remove hydrogens and electrons from nutrient metabolites, are particularly important in energy transformation. The hydrogens and electrons removed from metabolites by dehydrogenases generally produce NADH or [$FADH_2$], which are either in or shuttled into the mitochondria and move along the electron transport chain. Other oxidation reactions in which oxygen is incorporated into a compound or hydrogens are removed by enzymes other than dehydrogenases do not involve the electron transport chain. These reactions are catalyzed by a subgroup of oxidoreductase enzymes generally called oxidases and are not considered further in this section.

After oxidation of substrate molecules by a dehydrogenase enzyme, the hydride ions are transferred to a cosubstrate, such as the vitamin-derived nicotinamide adenine dinucleotide (NAD^+) or flavin mononucleotide (FMN). The structures of both the oxidized and reduced forms of these cosubstrates are shown in Figures 3.23 and 3.24. An example of the amount of energy released with oxidation of the fatty acid palmitate has already been discussed and is shown in Figure 1.13. The sequential arrangement of reactions in the electron transport chain is shown in Figure 3.25. Dashed lines outline the four complexes. Either NADH or [$FADH_2$] is the initial hydrogen acceptor for the electron transport chain. The hydrogens and electrons are then enzymatically transferred through the electron transport chain components and eventually to molecular oxygen, which becomes reduced to H_2O.

Anatomical Site for the Electron Transport Chain and Oxidative Phosphorylation

The structure of the mitochondrion is illustrated in Figures 1.6 and 1.7. Refer to Chapter 1 for a description of the outer membrane, which is permeable to most molecules smaller than 10 kilodaltons, and the inner membrane, which has very limited permeability. Remember that the enzymes of the TCA cycle, except for succinyl-CoA synthetase and those involved in fatty acid oxidation (discussed in Chapter 5), are located in the matrix of the mitochondria. The translocation of H^+ (protons) from within the matrix to the inner membrane space (the space between the cristae and outer membrane) provides much of the energy that drives the phosphorylation of ADP to make ATP. Note the respiratory stalks on the inner membrane (Figure 1.6), which also play an important role in the mechanism of oxidative phosphorylation. The electron transport chain starts with NADH or $FADH_2$, whether it is shuttled in from the cytosol, as discussed previously, or produced within the mitochondria.

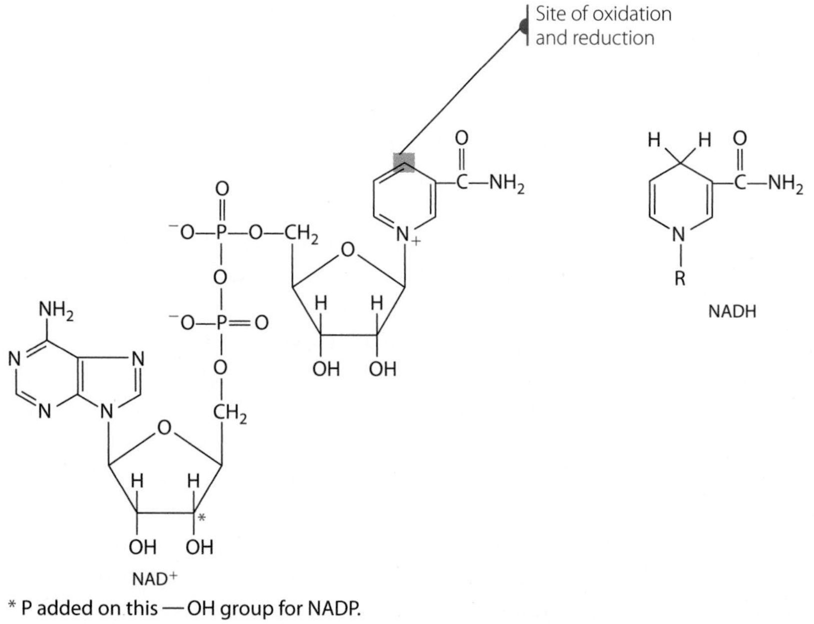

* P added on this —OH group for NADP.

Figure 3.23 Nicotinamide adenine dinucleotide (NAD^+) and its reduced form (NADH).

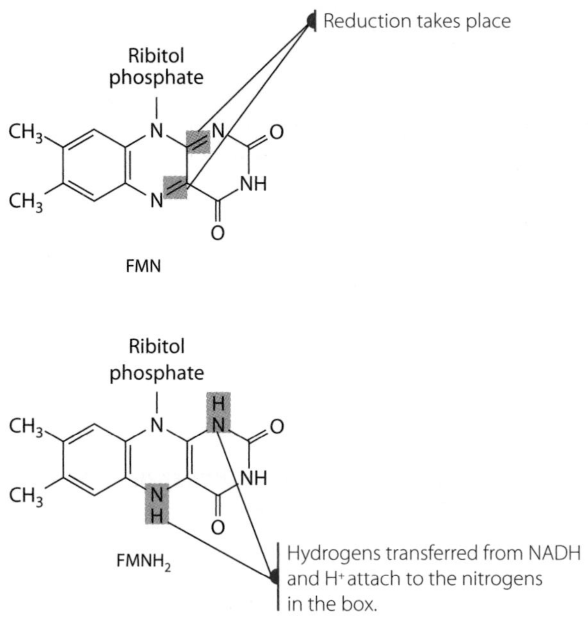

Ribitol
phosphate

Reduction takes place

FMN

Ribitol
phosphate

FMNH$_2$

Hydrogens transferred from NADH
and H$^+$ attach to the nitrogens
in the box.

Figure 3.24 Flavin mononucleotide (FMN) and its reduced form (FMNH$_2$).

Components of the Electron Transport Chain and Oxidative Phosphorylation

Glycolysis produces cytoplasmic NADH and FADH$_2$, and their shuttling into the mitochondria has already been discussed (Figures 3.20 and 3.21). Figure 3.26 presents a highly simplified overview of the electron transport chain. As indicated, the reactions actually take place in four distinct complexes of associated proteins and enzymes, which can be isolated and purified. Complex I,

NADH-coenzyme Q reductase, accepts electrons from NADH and is the link with glycolysis, the TCA cycle, and fatty acid oxidation. Complex II, succinate CoQ dehydrogenase, includes the membrane-bound succinate dehydrogenase that is part of the TCA cycle. Both Complex I and II produce CoQH$_2$. CoQH$_2$ is the substrate for Complex III, coenzyme Q–cytochrome c reductase. Complex IV is cytochrome oxidase. It is responsible for reducing molecular oxygen to form H$_2$O. The complexes work independently and are connected by mobile acceptors of electrons, coenzyme Q (CoQ) and cytochrome c. Each complex is discussed briefly here. For a more detailed explanation, consult a general biochemistry textbook [1].

Complex I: NADH–Coenzyme Q Oxidoreductase Complex I—also known as NADH dehydrogenase—transfers a pair of electrons from NADH to coenzyme Q. The structures of the oxidized and reduced forms of coenzyme Q are shown in Figure 3.27. Complex I is made of many polypeptide chains, a molecule of FMN, and several Fe-S clusters, along with additional iron molecules. The iron molecules bind with the sulfur-containing amino acid cysteine. The iron transfers one electron at a time, cycling between Fe^{+2} and Fe^{+3}. CoQ is a highly hydrophobic compound and it diffuses freely in the hydrophobic core of the inner membrane. The result of the multi-step reaction is the transfer of electrons and hydrogen from NADH to CoQ to form first CoQ hydroquinone and then CoQH$_2$ and actively transfer hydrogen ions from the matrix side of the inner mitochondrial membrane to the inner membrane space. The importance of the buildup of hydrogen ions in the inner membrane space is discussed in the following sections. The oxidation of NADH through the electron

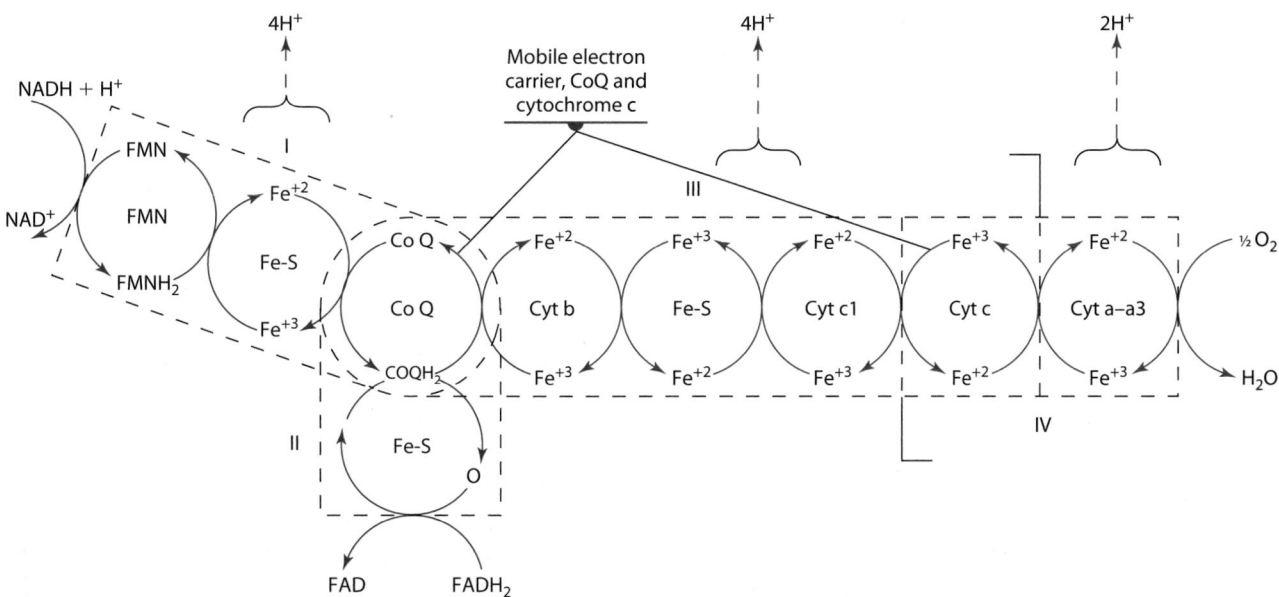

Figure 3.25 The sequential arrangement of the components of the electron transport chain, showing its division into four complexes, I, II, III, and IV. Coenzyme Q (ubiquinone) is shared by Complexes I, II, and III. Cyt c is shared by Complexes III and IV.

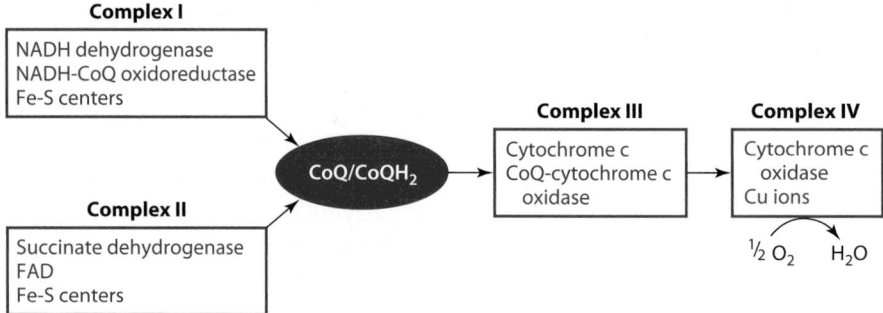

Figure 3.26 Schematic of electron transport modules connecting through coenzyme Q.

transport chain results in the synthesis of approximately 2.5 ATP molecules.

Complex II: Succinate Dehydrogenase Complex II is the succinate dehydrogenase enzyme, which is the only TCA cycle enzyme that is an integral part of the inner mitochondrial membrane. Beside the succinate dehydrogenase, complex II contains a FAD protein and Fe-S clusters (similar to those discussed previously). When succinate is converted to fumarate in the TCA cycle, FAD is reduced to $FADH_2$. The $FADH_2$ is oxidized with one electron transfer through the Fe-S centers to reduce coenzyme Q to coenzyme QH_2. Two protons are transferred to the inner mitochondrial space with the conversion of succinate to fumarate. The oxidation of $FADH_2$ through the electron transport chain results in the formation of approximately 1.5 molecules of ATP.

Complex III: Coenzyme Q–Cytochrome c Oxidoreductase Reduced coenzyme Q passes its electrons to cytochrome c in the third complex of the electron transport chain in a pathway known as the Q cycle. The complex contains three different cytochromes and Fe-S protein. The cytochromes contain heme molecules with an iron molecule

in the center. The iron in the center of the cytochromes is oxidized and reduced as electrons flow through. Electrons pass through the Q cycle in two phases. In the first phase a $CoQH_2$ passes one electron to form the semiquinone (one of the two hydroquinones oxidized), then another electron and hydrogen are transferred to the semiquinone to produce oxidized CoQ (quinone), releasing four protons to the inner membrane space. The electrons are then transferred to cytochrome c_1 (and associated cytochromes), and CoQ picks up two protons from the matrix, resulting in the reduction of a CoQ to $CoQH_2$. This means that two turns of the CoQ cycle result in the oxidation of $2CoQH_2$ to CoQ, the release of $4H^+$ in the inner membrane space, and the reduction of one CoQ to $CoQH_2$. Like coenzyme Q, cytochrome c is a mobile carrier. This characteristic means that cytochrome c is able to migrate along the membrane. Cytochrome c associates loosely with the inner mitochondrial membrane on the matrix side of the membrane. It can then pass its electrons on to cytochrome c oxidase in Complex IV, which is discussed next.

Complex IV: Cytochrome c Oxidase Complex IV is called cytochrome c oxidase. It accepts electrons from cytochrome c and catalyzes a four-electron reduction of oxygen to form water. This reaction is the final one in the oxidation of the energy-providing nutrients (carbohydrate, fat, protein, and alcohol) to produce usable chemical energy in the form of ATP. The structure of cytochrome c oxidase is known; it is made up of multiple subunits. Some of the subunits are encoded from nuclear DNA and some from mitochondrial DNA. These latter proteins contain the iron and copper. These metal ions cycle between their oxidized (Fe^{+3}, Cu^{+2}) and reduced (Fe^{+2}, Cu^{+1}) states. Cytochrome c oxidase also contains two cytochromes, cytochrome a and cytochrome a_3, which contain different heme moieties. Four protons are transported to the inner mitochondrial space.

Electron transport can carry on without phosphorylation, but the phosphorylation of ADP to form ATP (discussed in the next section) is dependent upon electron transport. A schematic of the inner mitochondrial membrane showing the four complexes of the electron

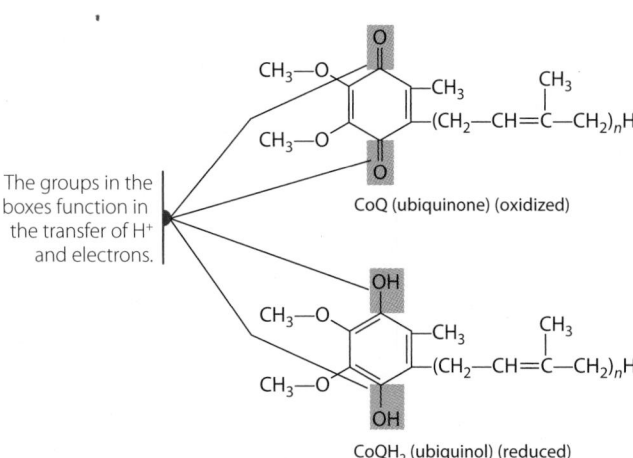

The groups in the boxes function in the transfer of H^+ and electrons.

CoQ (ubiquinone) (oxidized)

$CoQH_2$ (ubiquinol) (reduced)

Figure 3.27 Oxidized and reduced forms of coenzyme Q, or ubiquinone. The subscript n indicates the number of isoprenoid units in the side chain (most commonly 10). A one-electron transfer results in the formation of a semiquinone with only one of the quinone groups reduced.

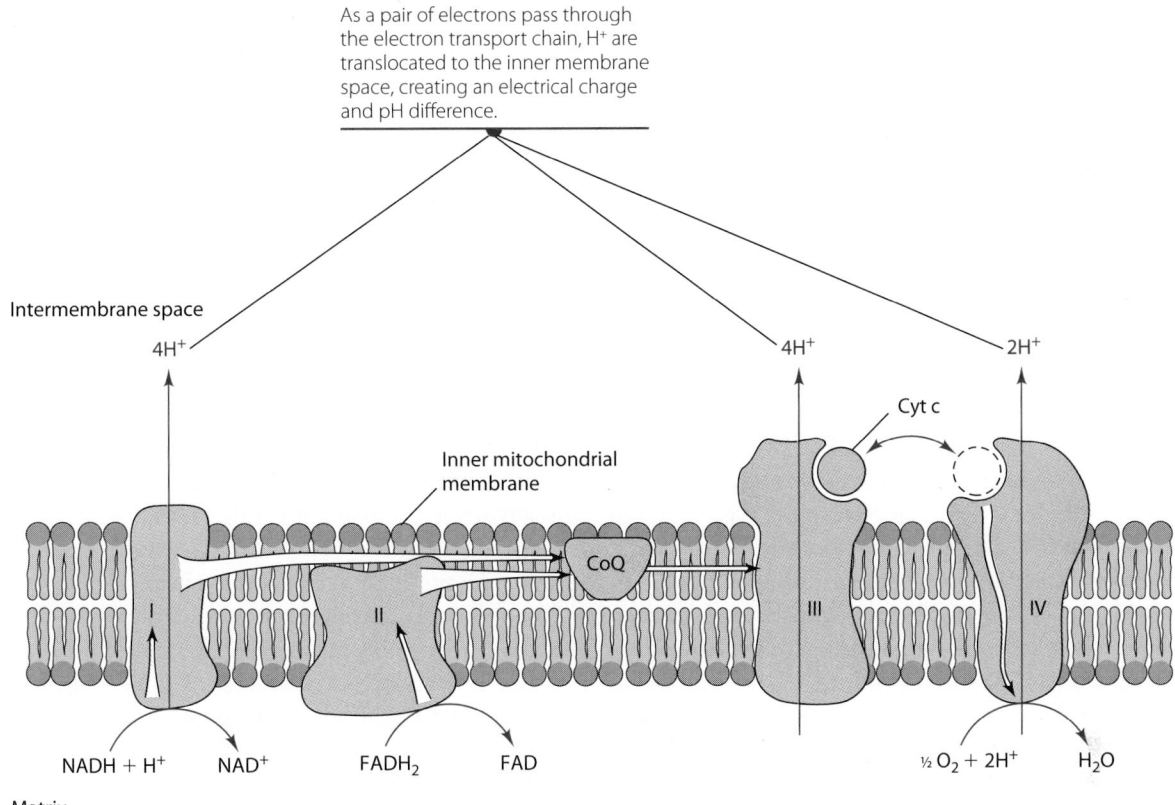

As a pair of electrons pass through the electron transport chain, H^+ are translocated to the inner membrane space, creating an electrical charge and pH difference.

Intermembrane space

$4H^+$

$4H^+$ $2H^+$

Cyt c

Inner mitochondrial membrane

CoQ

I   II   III   IV

NADH + H^+ NAD^+ $FADH_2$ FAD   ½ O_2 + $2H^+$ H_2O

Matrix

Figure 3.28 The spatial orientation of the complexes of the electron transport chain in the inner membrane of the mitochondrion.

transport chain is shown in Figure 3.28. The free energy change at various sites within the electron transport chain is shown in Table 3.6.

Phosphorylation of ADP to Form ATP

The intimate association of energy release with oxidation is exemplified by the oxidation of glucose to CO_2 plus water and energy discussed earlier in this chapter. Glycolysis occurs in the cytosol; the TCA cycle, electron transport, and oxidative phosphorylation occur in the mitochondria. It has already been established that the complete oxidation of 1 glucose yields either 30 or 32 ATPs. The complete biological oxidation of 1 mol of glucose yields approximately 700 kcal (or 2,937 kJ). The standard free energy for

the hydrolysis of ATP that has been used throughout this chapter is 7.3 kcal (30.5 kJ). However, standard conditions are at a concentration of 1 mol/L, whereas the concentration of ATP within the cell is closer to 1 to 5 mmol/L. The free energy of hydrolysis at this concentration is closer to 12 kcal (50 kJ). The free energies of other compounds with high phosphate transport potential like PEP, 1,3-bisphosphoglycerate, and phosphocreatine are also increased proportionally. It is more straightforward to use standard free energy in talking about these reactions. However, to determine the energy efficiency of the biological oxidation of glucose, the free energy of ATP under biological conditions must be considered. In living cells, 32 mol of ATP capture 384 kcal (32 × 12). The efficiency is therefore 384/700 × 100 or about 54% [1]. The remaining energy is released as heat. This is an efficient process as engines go.

The previous discussion on electron transport focused on the translocation of hydrogen ions from the matrix to the inner membrane space. This translocation is vital to the phosphorylation of ADP to form ATP. The translocation of hydrogen ions requires energy but in return creates a pool of potential energy. The generally accepted mechanism for the synthesis of ATP was first proposed by Peter Mitchell in 1961. He proposed that the energy stored in the difference in the concentration of H^+ between the matrix of the mitochondria and the inner mitochondrial space was the driving force for coupled ATP formation.

Table 3.6 Free Energy Changes at Various Sites within the Electron Transport Chain Showing Phosphorylation Sites

Reaction	$\Delta G^{\circ'}$ (cal/mol)	ADP Phosphorylation Site?
NAD+ ⟶ FMN	−922	No
FMN ⟶ CoQ	−15,682	Yes
CoQ ⟶ cyt b	−1,380	No
cyt b ⟶ cyt c1	−7,380	Yes
cyt c1 ⟶ cyt c	−922	No
cyt c ⟶ cyt a	−1,845	No
cyt a ⟶ ½O_2	−24,450	Yes

This proposal was called the chemiosmotic hypothesis. We will examine its main points to support our understanding of the coupling of phosphorylation with the electron transport chain. A recent review presents current research about proton translocation [25].

Translocation of H⁺ These energy relationships become important in understanding energy balance (discussed in Chapter 8). This area of research has been intense, and many components of the chemiosmotic hypothesis are supported by evidence. To determine if the pH gradient and electrical charge difference are sufficient to provide the energy for ATP synthesis, we must examine the number of H^+ translocated at each complex. Direct measurements have been difficult and not everyone agrees, but the consensus is that for every 2 electrons that pass through Complex I (NADH dehydrogenase) and Complex III, $4\ H^+$ are translocated by each complex for a total of 8. For Complex IV an additional $2\ H^+$ are translocated by each pair of electrons passing through the complex. No hydrogen ions are translocated in Complex II. This means that for every NADH oxidized to water, a total of 10 hydrogen ions are translocated from the matrix to the intermembrane space. The electrical charge across the inner membrane changes because of the positively charged hydrogen ions in the inner membrane space, a difference estimated to be approximately 0.18 volts. It is also assumed that the

pH difference between the mitochondrial matrix and the inner membrane is 1 unit. Using these assumptions, the free energy available is –94.49 kcal/mol (–23.3 kJ/mol). This is the potential free energy available to move protons back into the matrix of the mitochondria and at the same time couple phosphorylation of ADP to ATP with electron transport. Paul Boyer and John Walker shared the 1997 Nobel Prize for chemistry for their work on ATP synthase. A review of Paul Boyer's research on ATP synthase sums up several decades of work [26].

ATP Synthase Figure 3.29 illustrates electron transport and oxidative phosphorylation. The disparity in both the hydrogen ion concentration and electrical charge on either side of the inner membrane of the mitochondria has already been discussed. It is this proton gradient that provides the energy for ATP synthesis, which occurs with the aid of ATP synthase. ATP synthase is made up of two main components, F_0 and F_1, each with multiple subunits. F_0 is fixed in the membrane and F_1 sticks out of the membrane into the mitochondrial matrix (see Figure 1.6 to review the structure of mitochondria). Respiratory stalks extend from the cristae. If these stalks are removed, electron transport can proceed, but phosphorylation of ADP does not occur. Some of the subunits of F_1 are capable of rotating and have sites that bind ATP, ADP, and Pi. They also contain channels that allow proton movement through the membrane.

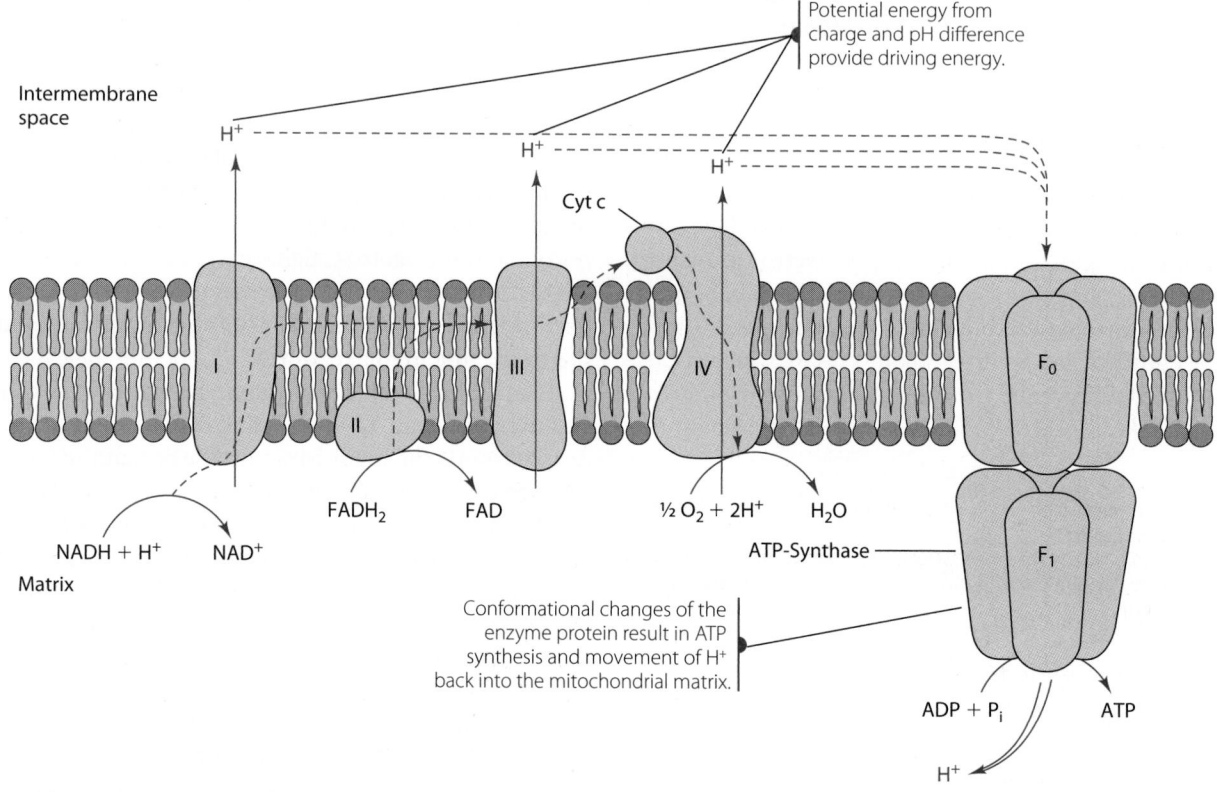

Figure 3.29 An illustration of oxidative phosphorylation coupled with ATP synthase. Energy from electron transport pumps protons into the intermembrane space from the matrix against a concentration gradient. The protons move back into the matrix through channels in the F_0F_1 ATP-synthase aggregate.

For each pair of electrons traversing complex IV, the rotating subunits of F_1 can complete 1 rotation and produce 3 ATPs. At the same time, protons from the intermembrane space are moved back into the matrix from the intermembrane space. The number of protons moved back depends upon the number of subunits in the rotating stalk (this can vary between 10 and 15). This results in from 3 to 5 protons per ATP formed moving back into the matrix. The return flow of protons furnishes the energy necessary for the synthesis of ATP from ADP and Pi. This has been an overview of the synthesis of ATP. The precise mechanism of phosphorylation is involved and requires the spatial movement of the subunits of ATP synthase [1].

ATP is synthesized in the mitochondrial space but must be moved to the cytoplasm to supply energy for the cell. There is an ATP-ADP translocase that shuttles ATP out of the mitochondria and ADP in. With the shuttle, the equivalent of one proton is moved from the cytosol to the mitochondrial matrix. Since the synthesis of one of ATP involves the movement of three protons from the cytosol to the matrix, with the translocase activity about four protons total are moved back into the matrix.

The previous discussion of the conversion of the chemical energy of carbohydrates to form ATP is an integral part of carbohydrate metabolism. The next sections cover other aspects of carbohydrate metabolism. Comprehensive reviews of electron transport, oxidative phosphorylation, and proton translocation are available to the interested reader [27–29].

The Pentose Phosphate Pathway (Hexosemonophosphate Shunt)

The pentose phosphate pathway (also called the hexosemonophosphate shunt) is one of the pathways that is available to glucose and is shown in Figure 3.30. It generates important intermediates not produced in other pathways. The pentose phosphate pathway has two important products:

- pentose phosphates, necessary for the synthesis of the nucleic acids found in DNA and RNA and for other nucleotides (Figure 3.4)
- the reduced cosubstrate NADPH, used for important metabolic functions, including the biosynthesis of fatty acids (Chapter 5), the maintenance of reducing substrates in red blood cells necessary to ensure the functional integrity of the cells, and drug metabolism in the liver

The cells of some tissues have a high demand for NADPH, particularly those that are active in the synthesis of fatty acids, such as cells of the mammary gland, adipose tissue, adrenal cortex, and liver. These tissues predictably engage the entire pentose phosphate pathway, recycling pentose phosphates back to glucose-6-phosphate to repeat the cycle and ensure an ample supply of NADPH.

The pathway reactions that include the dehydrogenase reactions and therefore the formation of NADPH from $NADP^+$ are called the oxidative reactions of the pathway. This segment of the pathway is illustrated on the left in Figure 3.30. The pentose phosphate pathway also synthesizes three-, four-, five-, six-, and seven-carbon sugars.

This pathway begins by oxidizing glucose-6-phosphate in two consecutive dehydrogenase reactions catalyzed by glucose-6-phosphate dehydrogenase (G-6-PD) and 6-phosphogluconate dehydrogenase (6-PGD). Both reactions require $NADP^+$ as cosubstrate, accounting for the formation of NADPH as a reduction product. The first reaction (G-6-PD) is irreversible and highly regulated. It is strongly inhibited by the cosubstrate NADPH and fatty acid CoAs. Pentose phosphate formation is achieved by the decarboxylation of 6-phosphogluconate to form the pentose phosphate, ribulose 5-phosphate, which in turn is isomerized to its aldose isomer, ribose 5-phosphate.

Pentose phosphates can subsequently be "recycled" back to hexose phosphates through the transketolase and transaldolase reactions illustrated in Figure 3.30. This recycling of pentose phosphates to hexose phosphates therefore does not produce pentoses, but it does ensure generous production of NADPH as the cycle repeats.

The re-formation of glucose-6-phosphate from the pentose phosphates, through reactions catalyzed by transketolase, transaldolase, and hexose phosphate isomerase, are called the nonoxidative reactions of the pathway and are shown on the right in Figure 3.30. Transketolase and transaldolase enzymes catalyze complex reactions in which three-, four-, five-, six-, and seven-carbon phosphate sugars are interconverted. These reactions are detailed in most comprehensive biochemistry texts [1].

The reversibility of the transketolase and transaldolase reactions allows hexose phosphates to be converted directly into pentose phosphates, bypassing the oxidative reactions. Therefore, cells that undergo a more rapid rate of replication and that consequently have a greater need for pentose phosphates for nucleic acid synthesis can produce these products in this manner.

The pathway's activity is low in skeletal muscle because of the limited demand for NADPH (fatty acid synthesis) in this tissue and also because of muscle's reliance on glucose and fatty acids for energy metabolism. Glucose-6-phosphate can be used for either glycolysis or for the pentose phosphate pathway. The choice is made based upon the cell's needs for energy (by assessing the ATP/ADP ratio) or for biosynthesis (by assessing the $NADP^+$/NADPH ratio). The level of NADPH is generally much higher than that of $NADP^+$.

Gluconeogenesis

D-glucose is an essential nutrient for most cells. The brain and other tissues of the central nervous system (CNS) and red blood cells are particularly dependent upon glucose as

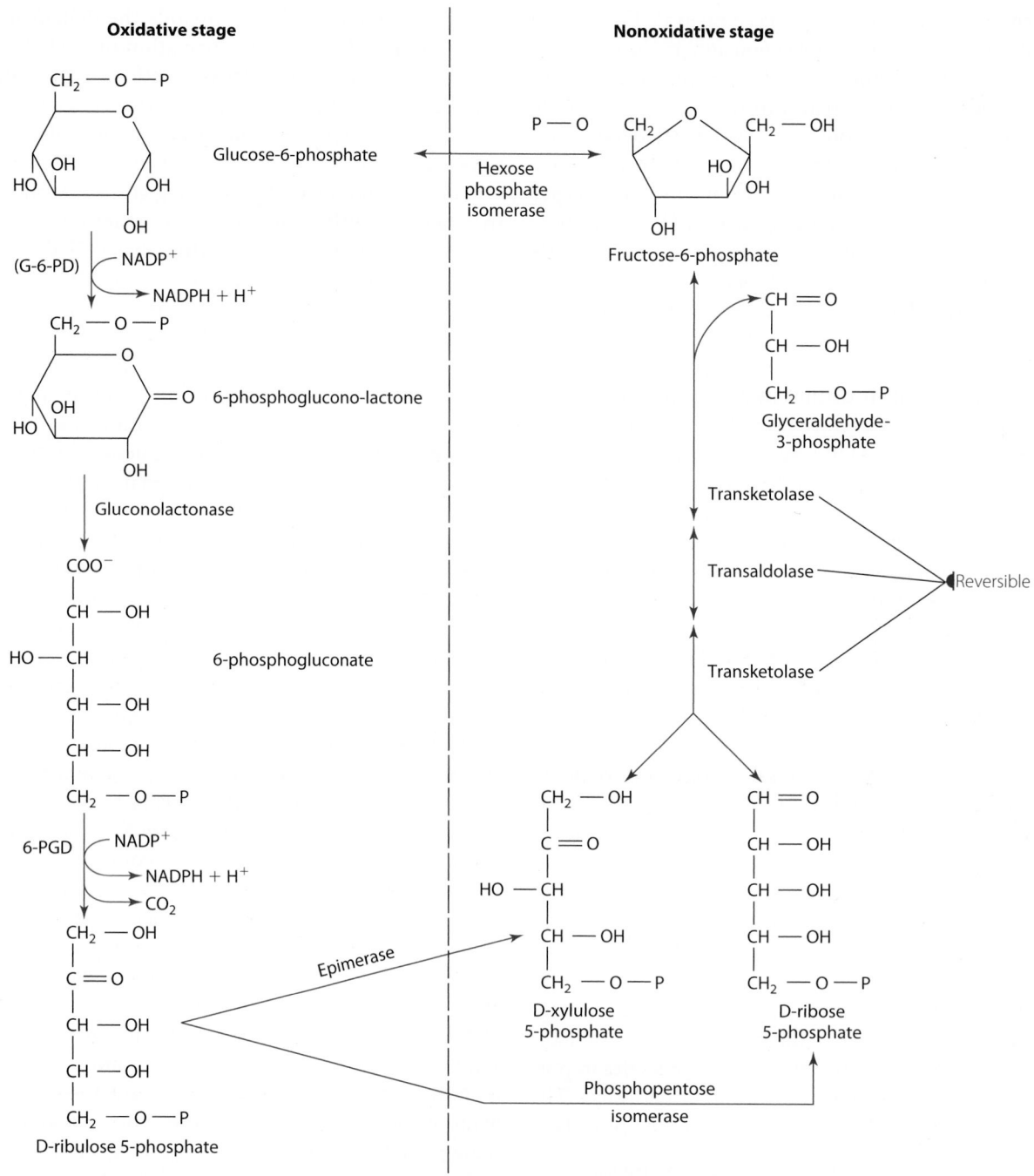

Figure 3.30 The pentose phosphate pathway (hexosemonophosphate shunt), showing the oxidative stage (left side of diagram) and the nonoxidative stage (right side of diagram). Abbreviations: G-6-PD, glucose-6-phosphate dehydrogenase; 6-PGD, 6-phosphogluconate dehydrogenase.

a nutrient. When dietary intake of carbohydrate is reduced and blood glucose concentration declines, hormones trigger accelerated glucose synthesis from noncarbohydrate sources. Lactate, pyruvate, glycerol (a catabolic product of triacylglycerols), and certain amino acids represent the important noncarbohydrate sources. The process of producing glucose from such compounds is termed **gluconeogenesis**. The liver is the major site of this activity, although under certain circumstances, such as prolonged starvation, the kidneys become increasingly important in

gluconeogenesis. The glucose formed by the liver and the kidney is mostly returned to the blood to maintain blood glucose levels. Note that intermediates of the TCA cycle can be converted to glucose, but fatty acids cannot. They are metabolized to acetyl-CoA (Chapter 5), which cannot be converted to glucose.

Gluconeogenesis essentially reverses the glycolytic pathway. It synthesizes glucose and consumes ATP and NAD^+ rather than producing ATP and NADH. Most of the cytoplasmic enzymes involved in glycolysis, which is

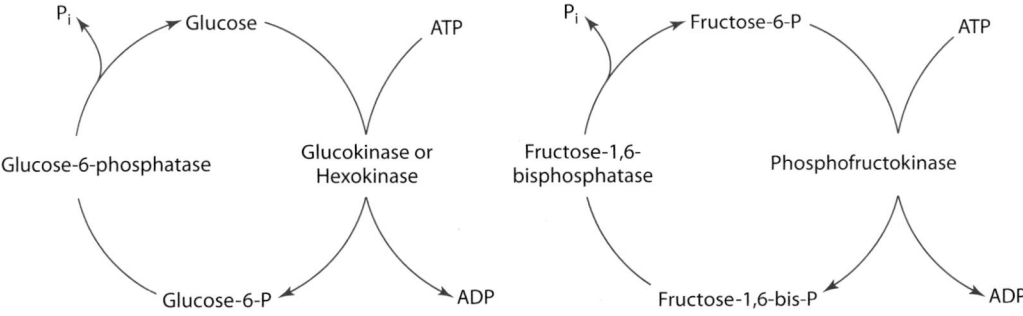

Figure 3.31 Glucokinase and phosphofructokinase reactions.

the conversion of glucose to pyruvate, catalyze their reactions reversibly and therefore provide the means for also converting pyruvate to glucose. When the cell is oxidizing glucose for energy, however, it does not need to make glucose from gluconeogenesis. Both the glycolytic pathway and gluconeogenesis must be regulated, and it is the nonreversible reactions that are regulated. Three reactions in the glycolytic sequence are highly exergonic, highly regulated, and *not* reversible: those catalyzed by the enzymes hexokinase (glucokinase), phosphofructokinase, and pyruvate kinase (sites 1, 3, and 10 in Figure 3.17). All of these reactions involve ATP and are unidirectional by virtue of the high, negative free energy change of the reactions. Therefore, the process of gluconeogenesis requires that these reactions be either bypassed or circumvented by other enzyme systems. The presence or absence of these enzymes determines whether a certain organ or tissue is capable of conducting gluconeogenesis. As shown in Figure 3.31, the glucokinase and phosphofructokinase reactions can be bypassed by specific phosphatases (glucose-6-phosphatase and fructose-1,6-bisphosphatase, respectively) that remove phosphate groups by hydrolysis.

The bypass of the pyruvate kinase reaction involves the formation of oxaloacetate as an intermediate. Mitochondrial pyruvate can be converted to oxaloacetate by pyruvate carboxylase, a reaction that was discussed earlier as an *anaplerotic* process. Oxaloacetate, in turn, can be decarboxylated and phosphorylated to phosphoenolpyruvate (PEP) by PEP carboxykinase, thereby completing the bypass of the pyruvate kinase reaction. The PEP carboxykinase reaction is a cytoplasmic reaction, however, and therefore oxaloacetate must leave the mitochondrion to be acted upon by the enzyme. The mitochondrial membrane, however, is impermeable to oxaloacetate, which therefore must first be converted to either malate (by malate dehydrogenase) or aspartate (by transamination with glutamate; see Chapter 6), both of which freely traverse the mitochondrial membrane. This mechanism is similar to the malate-aspartate shuttle previously discussed. In the cytosol, the malate or aspartate can be converted to oxaloacetate by malate dehydrogenase or aspartate aminotransferase (glutamate oxaloacetate transaminase), respectively.

The reactions of the pyruvate kinase bypass also allow the carbon skeletons of various amino acids to enter the gluconeogenic pathway, leading to a net synthesis of glucose. Such amino acids accordingly are called glucogenic. Glucogenic amino acids can be catabolized to pyruvate or to various TCA cycle intermediates or be anaerobically converted to glucose by leaving the mitochondrion in the form of malate or aspartate, as described. Reactions showing the entry of noncarbohydrate substances into the gluconeogenic system are shown in Figure 3.32, along with the bypass of the pyruvate kinase reaction.

Lactate Utilization

Effective gluconeogenesis accounts for the liver's ability to control the high levels of blood lactate that may accompany strenuous physical exertion. Muscle and adipose tissue, for example, lack the ability to form free glucose from noncarbohydrate precursors because they lack glucose-6-phosphatase. Thus, muscle and adipose lactate cannot serve as a precursor for free glucose within these tissues or contribute to the maintenance of blood glucose levels. Also, muscle cells convert lactate to glycogen but only slowly, especially in the presence of glucose (as when glucose enters muscle or adipose cells from the blood). How, then, is the high level of muscle lactate that can be encountered in situations of oxygen debt to be dealt with? Recovery is accomplished by the gluconeogenic capability of the liver. The lactate leaves the muscle cells and is transported through the general circulation to the liver, where it can be converted to glucose by the gluconeogenesis process just discussed. The glucose can then be returned to the muscle cells to reestablish homeostatic concentrations there. This circulatory transport of muscle-derived lactate to the liver and the return of glucose to the muscle is called the Cori cycle.

Efficient Glycogenesis

It has been previously discussed that the liver does not phosphorylate glucose at fasting levels. Liver glucose is, in fact, a poor precursor of liver glycogen except in the presence of gluconeogenic substances such as fructose, glycerol, or lactate. Glucose ingested during a meal is believed to take a somewhat roundabout path to glycogen. First it

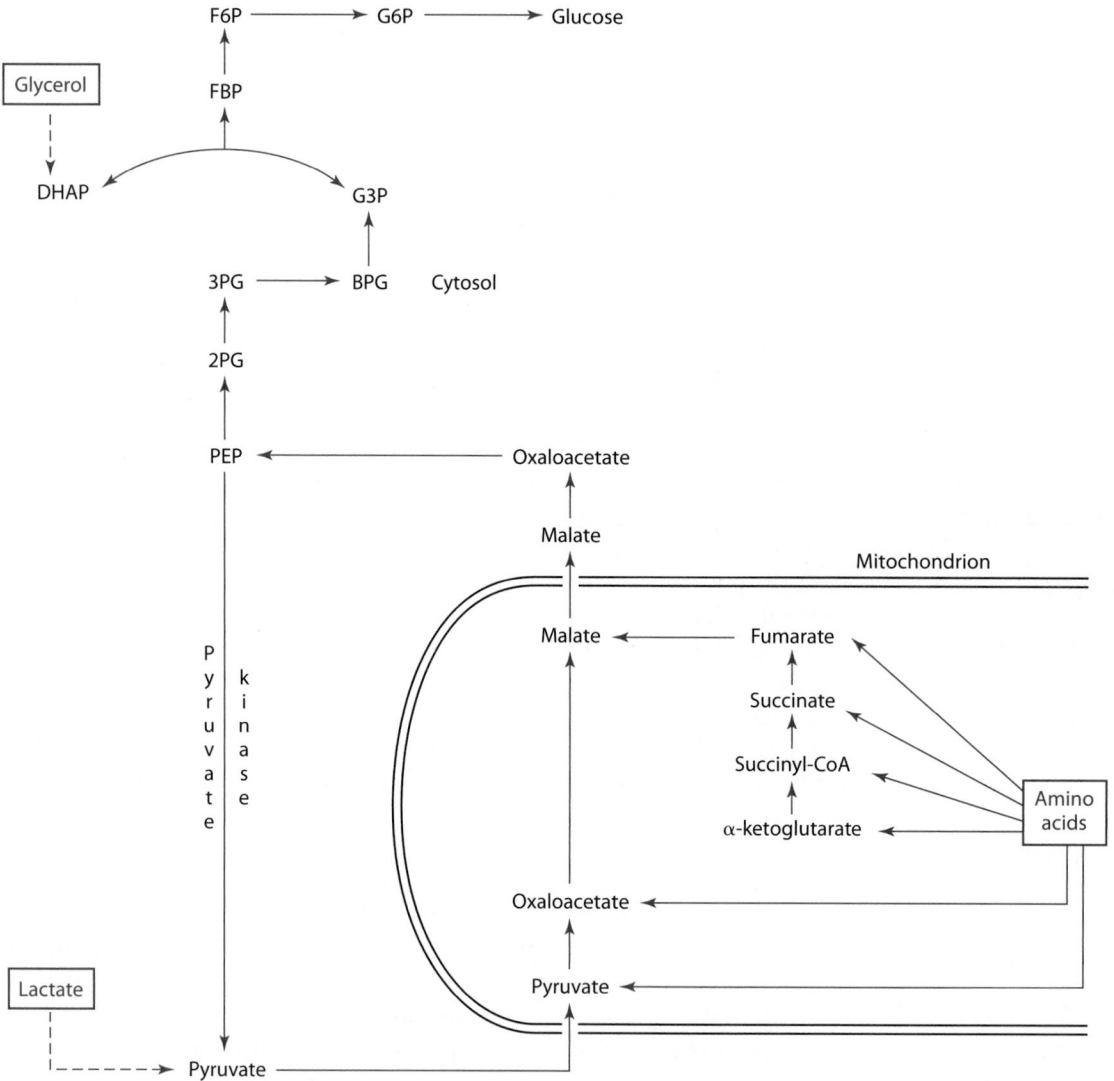

Figure 3.32 The reactions of gluconeogenesis, showing the bypass of the unidirectional pyruvate kinase reaction and the entry into the pathway of noncarbohydrate substances such as glycerol, lactate, and amino acids. Abbreviations: G6P, glucose-6-phosphate; F6P, fructose-6-phosphate; FBP, fructose-1,6-bisphosphate; DHAP, dihydroxyacetone phosphate; G3P, glyceraldehyde-3-phosphate; BPG, 1,3-bisphosphoglycerate; 3PG, 3-phosphoglycerate; 2PG, 2-phosphoglycerate; PEP, phosphoenolpyruvate.

is taken up by red blood cells and the brain and converted to lactate by glycolysis; then the lactate is taken up by the liver and converted to glucose-6-phosphate by gluconeogenesis (and ultimately to glycogen).

REGULATION OF METABOLISM

This section will focus on the general mechanisms used for regulation and then describe the regulation of glycolysis and gluconeogenesis as a more detailed example. The regulatory mechanisms for the other pathways are similar. The TCA cycle is the most prolific producer of ATP through oxidative phosphorylation and uses acetyl-CoA produced from glucose, fatty acids, and certain amino acids. The regulation of these pathways will be covered in the appropriate chapters.

The purpose of regulation of glycolysis and gluconeogenesis is to maintain homeostasis. The reactions of metabolism are altered to meet the nutritional and biochemical demands of the body. An excellent example of metabolic regulation is the reciprocal regulation of the glycolysis (catabolic) pathways and the gluconeogenic (anabolic) pathways. The glycolytic conversion of glucose to pyruvate liberates energy, whereas the reversal of the process from pyruvate to glucose (gluconeogenesis) consumes energy. The pyruvate kinase bypass in itself is energetically expensive, considering that 1 mol of ATP and 1 mol of GTP must be expended in converting intramitochondrial pyruvate to extramitochondrial PEP (Figure 3.32). It follows that among the factors that regulate the glycolysis/gluconeogenesis activity ratio is the body's need for energy. In a broad sense, regulation is achieved by four mechanisms:

- negative or positive modulation of allosteric enzymes by effector compounds

- hormonal activation by covalent modification or induction of specific enzymes
- directional shifts in reversible reactions by changes in reactant or product concentrations
- translocation of enzymes within the cell (covered in Chapter 1)

The concept of enzyme regulation was covered in Chapter 1, but a brief discussion of the principles is included here, with the regulation of carbohydrate metabolism in mind. This will be followed by a more detailed examination of the regulation of glycolysis and gluconeogenesis.

Allosteric Enzyme Modulation

Allosteric mechanisms can stimulate or suppress the enzymatic activity of a pathway. An allosteric, or regulatory, enzyme is said to be positively or negatively modulated. Modulators, which are usually compounds within the pathway, generally act by altering the conformational structure of the allosteric enzyme. Allosteric enzymes catalyze unidirectional, or nonreversible, reactions. The modulators of the enzymes of the unidirectional reactions must either stimulate or suppress a reaction in one direction only. General examples of allosteric modulators are presented in the following sections.

AMP, ADP, and ATP as Allosteric Modulators

An indication of the energy status of a cell and an important regulatory factor in energy metabolism is the ratio of the cellular concentrations of ADP (or AMP) to ATP. The usual breakdown product of ATP is ADP, but as ADP increases in concentration, some of it becomes enzymatically converted to AMP (to produce an ATP). Therefore, ADP and/or AMP accumulation can signify an excessive use of ATP and its depletion.

AMP, ADP, and ATP all act as modulators of certain allosteric enzymes, but the effect of AMP or ADP opposes that of ATP. For example, if ATP is abundant and ADP is scarce, additional energy is not needed. Energy-releasing (ATP-producing) pathways are negatively modulated, reducing the production of additional ATP. The reverse is also true; an increase in AMP (or ADP) concentration conversely signifies a depletion of ATP and the need to produce more of this energy source. In such a case, AMP or ADP can positively modulate allosteric enzymes of the energy-releasing pathways.

Two examples of positive modulation by AMP are its ability to cause a shift from the inactive form of phosphorylase b to an active form in glycogenolysis and the activation of phosphofructokinase in the glycolytic pathway discussed in the next paragraph. Increased levels of AMP are accompanied by an enhanced activity of either of these reactions that encourages glucose catabolism. The resulting shift in metabolic direction, as signaled by the AMP buildup, causes the release of energy as glucose is metabolized and helps restore depleted ATP stores.

Phosphofructokinase is modulated positively by AMP and ADP and negatively by ATP. As the store of ATP increases, slowing of the glycolytic pathway is called for. Phosphofructokinase is an extremely important rate-controlling allosteric enzyme and is modulated by a variety of substances. Its regulatory function has already been described in Chapter 1.

Other regulatory enzymes in carbohydrate metabolism that are modulated by ATP—all negatively—are pyruvate dehydrogenase complex, citrate synthase, and isocitrate dehydrogenase. Pyruvate dehydrogenase complex is positively modulated by AMP, and citrate synthase and isocitrate dehydrogenase are positively modulated by ADP.

Regulatory Effect of NADH/NAD$^+$ and NADPH/NADP$^+$

Another example of allosteric mechanisms is the ratio of NADH to NAD$^+$. NADH and NAD$^+$ can regulate their own formation through negative modulation. NADH is a product of glycolysis. Its buildup would indicate the pathway is not needed to produce additional ATP. If NAD$^+$ accumulates, the oxidative step in glycolysis would be favored. In the fasted state, the liver typically has a high NAD$^+$/NADH ratio (about 700, meaning that the level of NADH is low) and it produces more glucose than it needs through gluconeogenesis. However, muscle will be actively catabolizing glucose, and its NAD$^+$/NADH ratio will be lower and will favor lactate production. Dehydrogenase reactions, which involve the interconversion of the reduced and oxidized forms of the cosubstrate, are reversible. If metabolic conditions cause either NADH or NAD$^+$ to accumulate, the equilibrium is shifted to return the ratio to normal. Pyruvate dehydrogenase complex is positively modulated by NAD$^+$, whereas pyruvate kinase, citrate synthase, and α-ketoglutarate dehydrogenase are negatively modulated by NADH.

Whether the pentose phosphate pathway makes pentoses or NADPH is dependent upon the level of NADPH and NADP$^+$. Glucose-6-phosphate dehydrogenase is inhibited by high levels of NADPH and acetyl-CoA, which would indicate that demands for lipid biosynthesis are met. If the NADPH levels drop, the pathway can produce ribose. If the cell has more ribose than needed, the pathway follows the reaction on the right side of Figure 3.30 and makes more glucose and more NADPH.

Covalent Regulation

Covalent regulation is another mechanism of enzyme (resulting in pathway) regulation. This involves the binding of a group by a covalent bond and is one of the mechanisms by which hormones can exert their action. Examples include the covalent regulation of glycogen synthase and glycogen phosphorylase, enzymes discussed in the sections on glycogenesis and glycogenolysis, respectively. Phosphorylation inactivates glycogen synthase, whereas dephosphorylation activates it. In contrast, phosphorylation activates glycogen phosphorylase, and dephosphorylation inactivates it. These actions can be controlled by the actions of glucagon and epinephrine. Both hormones function by the phosphorylation of pathway enzymes through the second messenger cAMP.

Genetic Regulation

Another important example of enzyme regulation is through genetic control. The level of an enzyme can be either induced or suppressed. Such a change might arise through a prolonged shift in the dietary intake of certain nutrients. Induction stimulates transcription of new messenger RNA, programmed to produce the enzyme.

Specific hormones can influence (induce or suppress) the expression of a gene. One of the actions of certain hormones such as cortisol is to stimulate protein breakdown and decrease protein synthesis in skeletal muscle. In the liver, cortisol stimulates glycogen synthesis and gluconeogenesis by increasing the expression of several genes that encode for enzymes of the gluconeogenic pathway.

Directional Shifts in Reversible Reactions

Another control mechanism for pathways is based on enzyme kinetics, the concentration of the reactants and products in the cell. Most enzymes catalyze reactions reversibly, and the preferred direction in which a reversible reaction is proceeding at a particular moment is largely dependent upon the relative concentration of each reactant and product. An increasing concentration of one of the reactants drives or forces the reaction toward forming the other.

This concept is exemplified by the phosphoglucomutase reaction, which interconverts glucose-6-phosphate and glucose-1-phosphate and which functions in the pathways of glycogenesis and glycogenolysis (Figures 3.13 and 3.15). At times of heightened glycogenolytic activity (rapid breakdown of glycogen), glucose-1-phosphate concentration rises sharply, driving the reaction toward the formation of glucose-6-phosphate. With the body at rest, gluconeogenesis and glycogenesis are accelerated, increasing the concentration of glucose-6-phosphate. This increase in turn shifts the phosphoglucomutase reaction toward the formation of glucose-1-phosphate and ultimately glycogen.

Metabolic Control of Glycolysis and Gluconeogensis

Most enzymatic reactions are reversible, depending upon their free energy. Yet certainly in a given cell and generally in the cells of a particular organ the pathways are going in only one direction at a given time. The previous sections reviewed the different methods the body uses for controlling metabolic pathways. Glycolysis and gluconeogenesis provide examples of these control mechanisms in action. Figure 3.33 shows the reactions in both pathways that are under metabolic control by the mechanisms discussed, with the regulation of glycolysis on the left and that of gluconeogenesis on the right. The modulators that are activators are indicated by a plus sign, and those that are inhibitors by a minus sign.

The end result of gluconeogenesis is the formation of glucose, the molecule with which glycolysis begins. It is also true that the end product of glycolysis is pyruvate, and pyruvate is the first reactant of gluconeogenesis. As was pointed out earlier, however, gluconeogenesis is not simply the reversal of glycolysis. These two pathways are controlled reciprocally. Which of the two pathways is active at a given time depends upon the energy status of the cell. In glycolysis there are three regulated enzymes, all of which catalyze exergonic reactions: hexokinase (glucokinase), phosphofructokinase, and pyruvate kinase. These three reactions are replaced in the gluconeogenic pathway with those catalyzed by glucose-6-phosphatase; fructose-1,6-bisphosphatase; and pyruvate carboxylase-PEP-carboxykinase. The control of these reactions will be considered for each pathway. In gluconeogenesis, glucose-6-phosphatase is controlled by the level of substrate. Because the K_m for this enzyme is much higher than the level of glucose-6-P that is normally present, the reaction proceeds very slowly unless a high concentration of this substrate accumulates. A build-up of glucose-6-P is needed to activate the gluconeogenesis pathway.

The fate of pyruvate is strongly dependent upon acetyl-CoA levels. Acetyl-CoA inhibits the glycolytic enzyme pyruvate kinase allosterically and activates pyruvate carboxylase. This latter enzyme is found only in the mitochondria and is part of the gluconeogenic pathway that transfers mitochondrial pyruvate to PEP. If the TCA cycle is not active (adequate cellular ATP), the pyruvate is converted to glucose via gluconeogenesis.

Another control point for gluconeogenesis is the enzyme fructose-1,6-bisphosphatase, which is allosterically inhibited by AMP and activated by citrate. The effects of AMP and citrate on this enzyme are

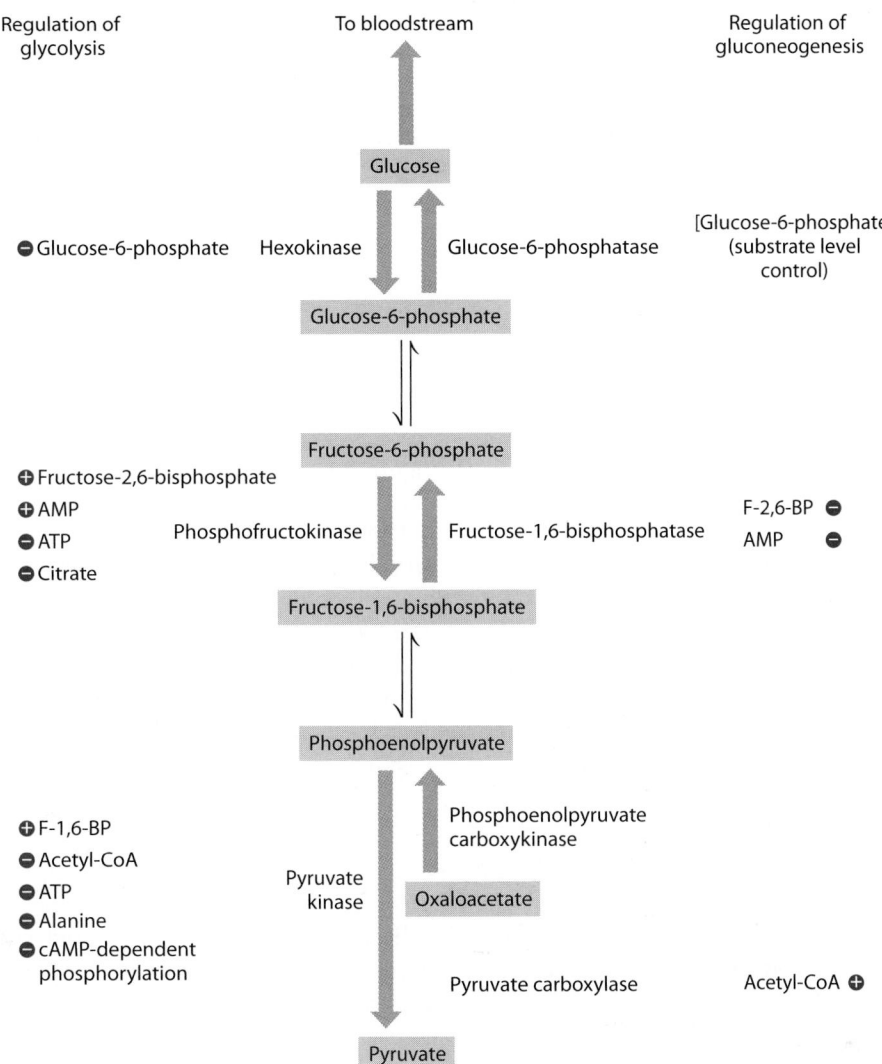

Figure 3.33 The principal regulatory mechanisms in glycolysis and gluconeogenesis. Non-reversible reactions of glycolysis and gluconeogenesis showing regulated steps. Inhibitors are indicated by minus signs and activators by plus signs.
Source: Garrett & Grisham, Biochemistry, 4th Edition. © Cengage Learning.

the opposite in glycolysis. When AMP levels are low (which means ATP is adequate) the gluconeogenesis pathway is active and glycolysis is reduced. Another allosteric regulator of fructose-1,6-bisphosphatase is fructose-2,6-bisphosphate. The levels of fructose-2,6-bisphosphate are controlled by the enzyme phosphofructokinase-2 (PFK-2). This enzyme is different than the phosphofructokinase of the glycolytic pathway. Fructose-6-phosphate (the substrate of phosphofructokinase of glycolysis) activates PFK-2, which would inhibit gluconeogenesis.

Another means of control for these two pathways is the level of enzymes. In glycolysis, glucokinase, phosphofructokinase, and pyruvate kinase are inducible enzymes, meaning that their concentrations can rise and fall in response to molecular signals such as a sustained change in the concentration of a certain metabolite. In the gluconeogenic pathway glucose-6-phosphatase, fructose bisphosphatase, PEP carboxykinase, and pyruvate carboxylase are inducible. The other enzymes of both pathways are constitutive (Chapter 1), meaning that their rate of synthesis is constant. Glucocorticoid hormones are known to stimulate gluconeogenesis by inducing the key gluconeogenic enzymes to form, and insulin may stimulate glycolysis by inducing increased synthesis of key glycolytic enzymes.

The interrelationship among pathways of carbohydrate metabolism is exemplified by the regulation of blood glucose concentration. The integration of the pathways, a topic of Chapter 7, is best understood after metabolism of

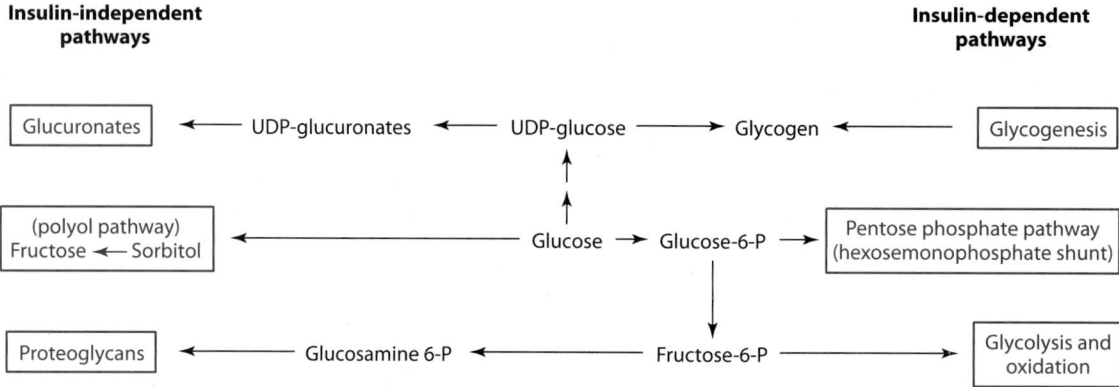

Figure 3.34 Insulin-independent and insulin-dependent pathways of glucose metabolism.

lipids and amino acids has been discussed (Chapters 5 and 6). Largely through the opposing effects of insulin and glucagon, the fasting serum glucose level normally is maintained within the approximate range of 80 to 100 mg/dL (4.5–5.5 mmol/L). Whenever blood glucose levels are excessive or sustained at high levels because insulin is insufficient, other insulin-independent pathways of carbohydrate metabolism for lowering blood glucose become increasingly active. Such insulin-independent pathways are indicated in Figure 3.34. The over activity of these pathways in certain tissues is believed to be partly responsible for the clinical manifestations of type 1 diabetes mellitus (see the Perspectives in Chapters 7 and 8).

SUMMARY

This chapter has dealt with a subject of vital importance in nutrition: the conversion of the energy contained within nutrient molecules into energy usable by the body. It examines an important food source of that energy, carbohydrates. The major sources of dietary carbohydrate are the starches and the disaccharides. In the course of digestion, these are hydrolyzed by specific glycosidases to their component monosaccharides, which are absorbed into the circulation from the intestine by active and facilitative transport. Glucose is transported into cells of various tissues, passing through the cells' outer membrane by facilitative transport by way of transporters. Different tissues use different GLUTs that are part of the family of glucose transporters. The GLUT4 that transports glucose into muscle and adipose tissue is stimulated by insulin. Insulin translocates the preformed GLUT4 from intracellular vesicles to the cell membrane. In the cells, monosaccharides first are phosphorylated at the expense of ATP and then can follow any of several integrated pathways of metabolism. Glucose is phosphorylated by hexokinase. In the muscle glucose is phosphorylated by hexokinase 1 and 2 and in the liver an isoenzyme of hexokinase called glucokinase is used. Fructose is phosphorylated mainly by fructokinase in the liver. Galactose is phosphorylated by galactokinase, also a liver enzyme.

During times of energy excess, cellular glucose and certain metabolites can be converted to glycogen, primarily in liver and skeletal muscle. Liver glycogen is mostly made from lactate, glycerol, or other TCA intermediates. When energy is needed it can be routed through the energy-releasing pathways of glycolysis and the tricarboxylic acid (TCA) cycle for ATP production. Glycolytic reactions convert glucose (or glucose residues from glycogen) to pyruvate. From pyruvate, either an aerobic course (complete oxidation in the TCA cycle) or an anaerobic course (to lactate) can be followed. Nearly all the energy formed by the oxidation of carbohydrates to CO_2 and H_2O is released via the TCA cycle, as reduced coenzymes are oxidized by mitochondrial electron transport. On complete oxidation, approximately 40% of this energy is retained in the high-energy phosphate bonds of ATP. The remaining energy supplies heat to the body.

Noncarbohydrate substances derived from the other major nutrients, glycerol from triacylglycerols (triglycerides) and certain amino acids, can be converted to glucose or glycogen by the pathways of gluconeogenesis. The basic carbon skeleton of fatty acids (metabolized to acetyl-CoA units) cannot be converted to a net synthesis of glucose, but some of the carbons from fatty acids find their way into the carbohydrate molecule. In gluconeogenesis, the reactions are basically the reversible reactions of glycolysis, shifted toward glucose synthesis in accordance with reduced energy demand by the body. Three kinase reactions occurring in glycolysis are not reversible, however, requiring the involvement of different enzymes and pathways to circumvent those reactions in the process of gluconeogenesis. Muscle glycogen provides a source of glucose for energy only for muscle fibers in which it is stored, because muscle lacks the enzyme glucose-6-phosphatase, which forms free glucose from glucose-6-phosphate. Glucose-6-phosphatase is active in the liver, however, which means that the liver can release free glucose from its glycogen stores into the circulation for maintaining blood glucose and for use by other tissues. The Cori cycle describes the liver's uptake and gluconeogenic conversion of muscle-produced lactate to glucose.

A metabolic pathway is regulated according to the body's need for energy or for maintaining homeostatic cellular concentrations of certain metabolites. Regulation is exerted mainly through hormones, through substrate concentrations (which can affect the velocity of enzyme reactions), and through allosteric enzymes that can be modulated negatively or positively by certain pathway products.

In Chapters 5 and 6, we will see that fatty acids and the carbon skeleton of various amino acids also are ultimately oxidized through the TCA cycle. The amino acids that do become TCA cycle intermediates, however, may not be completely oxidized to CO_2 and H_2O but instead may leave the cycle to be converted to glucose or glycogen (by gluconeogenesis) should dietary intake of carbohydrate be low. The glycerol portion of triacylglycerols enters the glycolytic pathway at the level of dihydroxyacetone phosphate, from which point it can be oxidized for energy or used to synthesize glucose or glycogen. The fatty acids of triacylglycerols enter the TCA cycle as acetyl-CoA, which is oxidized to CO_2 and H_2O but cannot contribute carbon for the net synthesis of glucose. This topic is considered further in Chapter 5.

These examples of the entrance of noncarbohydrate substances into the pathways discussed in this chapter are cited here to remind the reader that these pathways are not singularly committed to carbohydrate metabolism. Rather, they must be thought of as common ground for the interconversion and oxidation of fats and proteins as well as carbohydrate. Maintaining this broad perspective will be essential when we move on to Chapters 5 and 6, which examine the metabolism of lipids and proteins, respectively.

Much of the energy needs of the body are met by stored ATP. ATP can be generated by two distinct mechanisms:

1. the transfer of a phosphate group from compounds with a very–high-energy phosphate transfer potential to ADP, a process called substrate-level phosphorylation
2. oxidative phosphorylation, by which the energy derived from the translocation of H^+, which occurs during mitochondrial electron transport, is used to phosphorylate ADP to form ATP in the mitochondria

Oxidative phosphorylation is the major route for ATP production. Electron flow in the electron transport chain is from reduced cosubstrates to molecular oxygen. Molecular oxygen becomes the ultimate oxidizing agent and becomes H_2O in the process. The downhill flow of electrons and proton translocation generate sufficient energy to affect oxidative phosphorylation at multiple sites along the chain. The energy from this process that is not conserved as chemical energy (ATP) is given off as heat. About 60% of the energy assumes the form of heat.

Carbohydrate metabolism, including the energy-releasing, systematic oxidation of glucose to CO_2 and H_2O, exemplifies reactions of substrate-level and oxidative phosphorylation. Similar energy transfer happens with the lipid and amino acid pathways whenever a dehydration reaction occurs.

The pentose phosphate pathway generates important intermediates not produced in other pathways of the body, such as pentose phosphates for RNA and DNA synthesis and NADPH, which is used in the synthesis of fatty acids and in drug metabolism.

This chapter provides examples of the regulation of metabolism, an important topic in nutrition. This topic will be revisited several times in Chapters 7 and 8. Understanding the integration of metabolism and the control of energy balance is important. Much of the effects of exercise, disease, weight loss, and weight gain can be explained with these principles.

References Cited

1. Garrett RH, Grisham CM. Biochemistry. 4th ed. Belmont, CA: Thomson Brooks/Cole Publishers. 2010.
2. Richards AB, Krakowka S, Dexter LB, et al. Trehalose: a review of properties, history of use and human tolerance, and results of multiple safety studies. Food Chem Toxic. 2002; 40:871–98.
3. van Can JGP, Ijzerman TH, van Loon LJC, et al. Reduced glycaemic and insulinaemic responses following trehalose ingestion: implications for postprandial substrate use. Brit J Nutr. 2009; 102:1395–99.
4. Gray GM. Starch digestion and absorption in nonruminants. J Nutr. 1992; 122:172–77.
5. Obiro WC, Zhang T, Jiang B. The nutraceutical role of the Phaseolus vulgaris α-amylase inhibitor. Brit J Nutr. 2008; 100:1–12.
6. Kellett GL, Brot-Laroche E, Mace OJ, Leturque A. Sugar absorption in the intestine: the role of GLUT2. Annu Rev Nutr. 2008; 28:35–54.
7. Kellett GL, Brot-Laroche E. Apical GLUT2: a major pathway of intestinal sugar absorption. Diabetes. 2005; 54:3056–62.
8. Augustin R. The protein family of glucose transport facilitators: it is not only about glucose after all. Life. 2010; 62:315–33.
9. Riby J, Fujisawa T, Kretchmer N. Fructose absorption. Am J Clin Nutr. 1993; 58(suppl 5):S748–53.

10. Truswell AS, Seach JM, Thorburn AW. Incomplete absorption of pure fructose in healthy subjects and the facilitating effect of glucose. Am J Clin Nutr. 1988; 48:1424–30.

11. Jones HF, Butler RN, Brooks DA. Intestinal fructose transport and malabsorption in humans. Am J Physiol Gastrointest Liver Physiol. 2011; 300:G202–06.

12. Thorens B, Mueckler M. Glucose transporters in the 21st century. Am J Physiol Endocrinol Metab. 2010; 298:E141–45.

13. Larance M, Ramm G, James DE. The GLUT4 code. Mol Endocr. 2008; 22:226–33.

14. Ludwig DS. Glycemic load comes of age. J Nutr. 2003; 133:2695–96.

15. Esfahani A, Wong JMW, Mirrahimi AM, et al. Glycemic index: physiological significance. Am J Coll Nutr. 2009; 28:S439–45.

16. Brand-Miller J, McMillan-Price J, Steinbeck K, Caterson I. Dietary glycemic index: health implications. J Am Coll Nutr. 2009; 28:S446–49.

17. Jenkins DJA, Kendall CWC, Augustin LSA, et al. Glycemic index: overview of implications in health and disease. Am J Clin Nutr. 2002; 76:S266–73.

18. Aziz A. The glycemic index: methodological aspects related to the interpretation of health effects and to regulatory labeling. J AOAC Intnat. 2009; 92:879–87.

19. Venn BJ, Green TJ. Glycemic index and glycemic load: measurement issues and their effect on diet-disease relationships. Eu J Clin Nutr. 2007; 61:S122–31.

20. Fernandes G, Velangi A, Wolever TM. Glycemic index of potatoes commonly consumed in North America. J Am Diet Assoc. 2005; 105:557–62.

21. Liu S, Willett WC, Stampfer MJ, et al. A prospective study of dietary glycemic load, carbohydrate intake and risk of coronary heart disease in US women. Am J Clin Nutr. 2000; 71:1455–61.

22. Foster-Powell K, Holt SH, Brand-Miller JC. International table of glycemic index and glycemic load. Am J Clin Nutr. 2002; 76:5–56.

23. Smythe C, Cohen P. The discovery of glycogenin and the priming mechanism for glycogen biosynthesis. Eur J Biochem. 1991; 200:625–31.

24. Buchbinder JL, Bath BL, Fletterick RJ. Structural relationships among regulated and unregulated phosphorylases. Annu Rev Biophys Biomol Struct. 2001; 30:191–209.

25. Hosler J, Ferguson-Miller S, Mills D. Energy transduction: proton transfer through the respiratory complexes. Annu Rev Biochem. 2006; 75:165–87.

26. Boyer P. The ATP synthase-A splendid molecular machine. Annu Rev Biochem. 1997; 66:717–49.

27. Trumpower B, Gennis R. Energy transduction by cytochrome complexes in mitochondrial and bacterial respiration: the enzymology of coupling electron transfer reactions to transmembrane proton translocation. Annu Rev Biochem. 1994; 63:675–702.

28. Tyler D. ATP synthesis in mitochondria. In: The Mitochondrion in Health and Disease. New York: VCH Publishers, Inc. 1992 pp. 353–402.

29. Hatefi Y. The mitochondrial electron transport and oxidative phosphorylation system. Annu Rev Biochem. 1985; 54:1015–69.

Suggested Readings

McGarry JD, Kuwajima M, Newgard CB, Foster DW. From dietary glucose to liver glycogen: the full circle round. Ann Rev Nutr. 1987; 7:51–73.

The glucose paradox is emphasized, from the standpoint of its emergence, as are the attempts to resolve it.

Pilkis SJ, El-Maghrabi MR, Claus TH. Hormonal regulation of hepatic gluconeogenesis and glycolysis. Ann Rev Biochem. 1988; 57:755–83.

This is a brief, clearly presented summary of the effect of certain hormones on the important regulatory enzymes in these major pathways of carbohydrate metabolism.

Web Sites

www.nlm.nih.gov
National Library of Medicine
www.medscape.com/home
FromWebMD. Provides specialty information and education for physicians and other health professionals.
www.cdc.gov
Centers for Disease Control and Prevention
www.ama-assn.org
American Medical Association
http://vcell.ndsu.edu/animations/
A series of "Virtual Cell" animations demonstrating electron transport chain, ATP synthesis, insulin signaling, and other biological processes funded by the National Science Foundation. Other animations are applicable to other chapters and are a good resource.
www.hopkinsmedicine.org
A Web site from John Hopkins School of Medicine

HIGH-FRUCTOSE CORN SYRUP: JUST ANOTHER SWEETENER?

High-fructose corn syrup (HFCS) was introduced into the U.S. food supply during the early 1970s. Its per capita consumption continued to increase until the late 1990s. During this same time period and continuing into the current decade, the prevalence of obesity, particularly childhood obesity, expanded to near epidemic proportions. The obvious question was raised: Was this cause and effect? [1]. This Perspective examines the nature and uses of HFCS, the use of fructose as a sweetener, the potential metabolic consequences of the consumption of HFCS and fructose, and the changes in the intake of caloric sweeteners. Nutrition and health professionals, food scientists, and food industry representatives have not come to a consensus on the relation between HFCS and obesity independent of excess caloric consumption. This Perspective is not intended to resolve the issue but to present an overview of the evidence so that the interested reader can pursue the topic further and come to his or her own conclusions.

BACKGROUND ON HIGH-FRUCTOSE CORN SYRUP

HFCS is produced from starch derived from any of several commodities such as corn, rice, tapioca, wheat, potato, and cassava. In the United States most is produced from corn [2]. The starch is hydrolyzed and the glucose is partially converted to fructose enzymatically. HFCS is used in many foods beyond sweetened beverages, including sauces, salad dressings, desserts, dairy products, preserved fruit, and many more. This widespread use of HFCS makes it appear to be the major caloric sweetener in the food supply, but this is not the case. As shown in Figure 1, per capita consumption of HFCS rose between 1970 and 2008 (the latest data available), as sucrose consumption simultaneously declined [3]. The per capita use of both sweeteners leveled off about 1998, and the most recent data reported by the U.S. Department of Agriculture (USDA) suggest that the use of HFCS is trending down—as is total use of caloric sweeteners. If this turns out to be a continuing trend, it may be due to companies moving away from HFCS because of its negative press. The U.S. market share between sucrose and HFCS appears to be about equal. Worldwide, HFCS constitutes only about 8% of caloric sweeteners [4].

HFCS should not be confused with corn syrup (100% glucose) or crystalline fructose (100% fructose). Fructose is the sweetest monosaccharide and has a limited use as a specialty sweetener. HFCS is a mixture of fructose and glucose. The two most common mixtures are HFCS-55, which contains 55% fructose and 42% glucose, and HFCS-42, which contains 42% fructose and 53% glucose. Remember that sucrose contains 50% of each—one fructose and one glucose unit per sucrose molecule. Thus, though the name *high-fructose corn syrup* implies that it contains mostly fructose, it has a fructose to glucose ratio close to 50:50. In fact, all commercially used caloric sweeteners contain fructose in about the same proportions as HFCS. Other caloric sweeteners in use include honey (49% fructose, 43% glucose), molasses (50% fructose, 48% glucose), apple juice (59% fructose, 31% glucose), orange and grape juices (51% fructose, 49%glucose), and agave nectar (a mixture of ~50% fructose and glucose, depending on its plant source) [2].

Advantages of HFCS as a Sweetener

HFCS-55 has been formulated to be as sweet as sucrose. It also has other properties that increase its functionality in the food supply, including the capacity to retain moisture, enhance flavor, lower the food's freezing point, undergo fermentation, and create brown colors during baking [2,4]. In acidic products sucrose will hydrolyze to glucose and fructose and lose some of its sweetness, which is a problem for the beverage industry [4]. HFCS, in contrast, is already composed of monosaccharides and does not change with storage. HFCS also has a lower and more stable price than sucrose. HFCS is a liquid (syrup) and therefore more easily delivered (through pipes) than sucrose, a dry product that requires more labor-intensive handling.

HEALTH OUTCOMES RELATED TO CALORIC SWEETENERS

As stated previously, all caloric sweeteners contain both fructose and glucose at about the same level (50:50 fructose-glucose). A number of questions are being asked about the

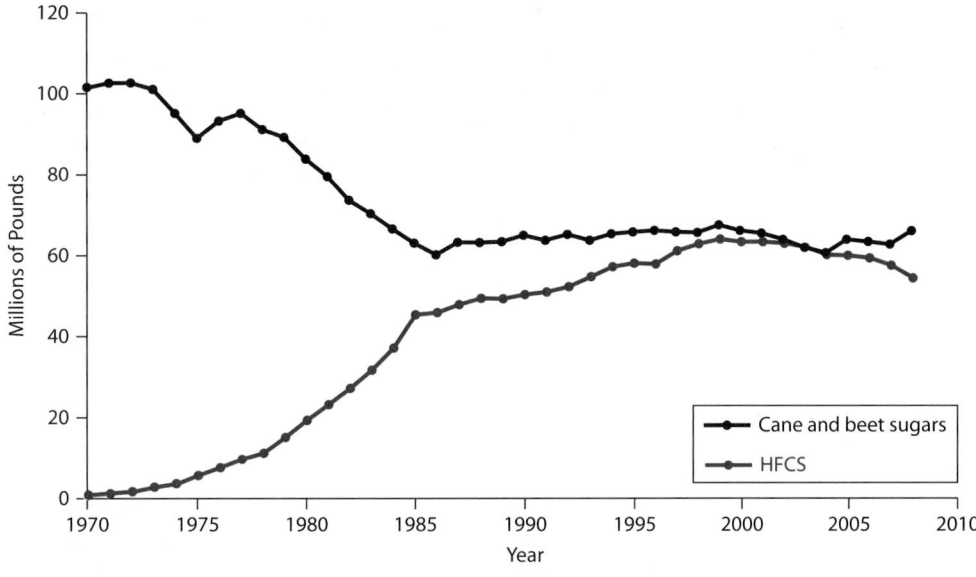

Figure 1 Per capita availability of cane and beet sugars and high-fructose corn syrup (HFCS).

health outcomes of caloric sweeteners in general—not just HFCS. Some of these questions are:

1. Do foods sweetened with caloric sweeteners encourage (or cause) an excess consumption of calories, which leads to obesity?

2. Is fructose consumption detrimental?

3. If fructose is detrimental, at what threshold of its contribution to the diet does it begin to cause a problem?

4. Considering the timing of the introduction of HFCS into the food supply and the concurrent rapid increase in the prevalence of overweight and obesity, is there something unique about HFCS that results in a cause and effect relationship between HFCS and obesity?

5. Is there a difference between any effects that HFCS might have on overweight or obese individuals as compared to normal-weight individuals?

These might sound like simple, straightforward questions that could be easily answered with well-designed, well-controlled animal and human experiments. However, this has not been the case, and there remains controversy about the proper design of such studies and interpretation of the results of research conducted to date. Though in reality the questions are intertwined, experiments must try to isolate the variables and provide answers one question at a time. The first three questions relate to all caloric sweeteners, including sucrose, honey, fruit juices, and HFCS. It is only questions 4 and 5 that relate to HFCS uniquely.

For decades, ongoing research with animal models has focused on sucrose, HFCS, or fructose by itself. This research on animals is well summarized in a recent review [5] and recaps the areas of concern for human consumption. Other recent reviews also summarize the evidence regarding health impacts of HFCS or fructose [6,7]. The abnormalities that have been demonstrated in animals to be caused by caloric sweeteners or fructose can be aggregated into the following areas [5]:

1. dyslipidemia, including serum levels of lipoproteins

2. lipid deposits in liver and skeletal muscle

3. impaired glucose homeostasis and insulin activity

4. high blood pressure

5. an increase in adipose tissue-related chronic disease risk factors

Some of these abnormalities, such as hypertension and increased chronic disease risk, are easily explained by the experimental conditions. Many of the studies fed diets providing greater than 30% of the calories as the caloric sweetener or fructose. These hypercaloric diets resulted in the animals becoming obese, and the observed pathological conditions are likely to be the result of the obesity. Animal models are useful in studying metabolic pathways and developing hypotheses for testing in humans, but they cannot take into account the unpredictable eating patterns of the free-living population.

Nonetheless, the results of this research with animal models and the correspondence of the introduction of HFCS into our food supply with the rapid increase in the prevalence of obesity have led to a controversy as to whether these same conditions are caused in people by consuming HFCS and/or fructose. Is the change in the prevalence of adult and childhood overweight and obesity between the early 1970s and 2008 [8,9] due to HFCS or fructose? The consumption of HFCS has stabilized or dropped in the last few years, while obesity rates have stayed about the same (high). Do the abnormalities observed in lab animals fed sweeteners develop similarly in humans who choose diets high in added sugars? Recent clinical trials have explored these questions.

Dyslipidemia and Deposition of Lipid in Liver and Skeletal Muscle

The metabolism of fructose is different than that of glucose and is discussed in the carbohydrate chapter (Chapter 3). In moderate doses, fructose is nearly completely removed from circulation by the liver and little appears in peripheral blood. However, with larger intakes (as might be obtained from large volumes of HFCS-sweetened carbonated beverages) there is a dose-related increase in fructose levels in peripheral blood [5].

Fructokinase (the enzyme that phosphorylates fructose to fructose-1-P) is expressed only in the liver, which limits the metabolism of fructose to that organ. The reaction it catalyzes is the first step in fructose metabolism to three-carbon moieties, which are mostly converted to glycogen or lactate. The metabolism of fructose to the three-carbon units produces available ATP, which promotes fatty acid synthesis. This, in turn, promotes the synthesis of triacylglycerols (TAG, or triglycerides), as discussed in Chapter 5. The liver exports much of these TAG as the lipoprotein VLDL, which is transferred to the serum [10]. Depending upon the rate of lipogenesis, all of the TAG synthesized may not be exported by the liver and some may be retained, resulting in fatty liver (not caused by alcohol). Thus, it seems logical that a high intake of fructose results in high blood TAG, increased lipogenesis, and fatty liver.

To test the lipogenic effect of simple sugars in humans, researchers administered 85 g of each of three caloric sweeteners—100% glucose, 50:50 glucose/fructose, and 25:75 glucose/fructose—as a bolus and then studied the levels of lipogenesis and insulin in their subjects over a 12-hour period [11]. They observed increased lipogenesis and a decreased insulin response with the 25:75 glucose/fructose mixture as compared to 100% glucose. Another study [12] examined the effect of consumption of either glucose- or fructose-sweetened beverages providing 25% of the subjects' energy for a 10-week period. For most of this period the subjects were on an ad libitum hypercaloric diet. The subjects of both groups gained weight, but only the fructose group gained visceral adipose (intra-abdominal fat) during the study period. Fasting TAG were elevated in the glucose group, but not the fructose group, whereas evidence of increased lipogenesis was found in the fructose group only. These results

are intriguing, but because the diets of both groups were hypercaloric, it remains questionable whether visceral fat deposition in the fructose group would still have increased had these subjects been in energy balance (no excess of calories).

Two long-term (4 to 6 weeks) studies were conducted examining the effects of fructose intake on plasma lipids [13,14]. In one study [13], fructose was provided at a level equivalent to the amount in a 2-L bottle of a sweetened beverage, given over the course of the day. The plasma TAG and glucose concentrations of subjects receiving the fructose were increased, but no lipid deposits in ectopic (nonadipose) tissue were observed. In the second study [14], fructose was fed to subjects at a level of 17% of energy needs, which is twice the average intake based upon a nationwide survey. One-third of the fructose was provided in natural foods (fruits and vegetables) and the remainder as a beverage. An increase of plasma TAG was observed in men but not women. Both studies provided energy based on needs (i.e., were not hypercaloric).

Weight Gain

Weight gain results when energy intake exceeds expenditure. There is no question that the U.S. population has increased its caloric intake by about 22% since about 1970 (3,200 kcal per capita per day in 1970 and 3,900 kcal per capita per day in 2006) [15]. Data on changes in daily energy expenditure are not as readily available, but most will agree that it has decreased over this same time period [5], which makes an even larger imbalance. Utilizing data from the USDA, the per capita calorie intake from different food groups over this same time period was examined; added sugars decreased by 1%, vegetables decreased by 1%, dairy decreased by 3%, and meat and eggs decreased by 3%. The food groups whose contribution to energy consumption increased were added fats (by 5%) and flour and cereal (by 3%) [reported in 3]. These data suggest that the increase in total per capita energy consumption was not due to added sugars.

Several studies have shown that children who consume more caloric, sweetened beverages are more likely to be overweight or obese [reported in 5]. That observation suggests a positive association between increased calorie intake and sweetened beverage consumption, but it does not prove that fructose causes weight gain. Significantly, the rate of obesity continued to increase after the consumption of HFCS peaked in 1999 and during successive years while HFCS use leveled off or dropped [3,9].

Mixed results have been obtained from intervention studies with HFCS or fructose. In studies that supplied an excess of calories, weight gain occurred in both the control group and the fructose group. In those studies where there was no increase in overall caloric consumption, subjects given fructose experienced no increase in body weight [13,14].

Impaired Glucose Homeostasis and Insulin Activity

Elevated levels of blood fructose do not elicit an insulin-release response from the pancreas (its cells lack GLUT5, the fructose transporter). Consuming fructose causes a small, if any, rise in plasma glucose levels, and therefore little or no release of insulin. This lack of an insulin response can impair insulin's actions within the liver but does not appear to affect the extrahepatic functions of insulin [16]. Because many of the studies tested hypercaloric diets, this is hard to assess. One of the studies discussed previously [13] that provided high-fructose diets at an energy level to maintain body weight (without increase for 4 weeks) found that insulin levels did not increase. There are other factors that control food intake that might be influenced by fructose, but the results of research into these factors are not definitive and will not be discussed in this Perspective. These hormonal controls of food intake and satiety are discussed in Chapter 8.

Conclusions

The information currently available cannot provide an unequivocal answer to the question of whether HFCS is just another caloric sweetener or if it is uniquely responsible for the increased prevalence of overweight and obesity. There has been an increase in energy intake among the U.S. population over the past several decades, and as a result, the prevalence of obesity has risen. In children, increased intake of caloric, sweetened beverages has contributed to the increase in energy intake and the resultant obesity.

Intervention studies with hypercaloric diets and high levels of fructose reported increased plasma TAG levels and increased lipid deposits in the visceral adipose tissue. In contrast, in other long-term intervention studies that fed diets that met calculated energy needs (were not hypercaloric), no weight gain or adipose deposition in ectopic tissue was observed, but there was an increase in plasma TAG and glucose levels. In one of the studies the plasma TAG was increased only in men and not in women.

There are still unanswered research questions [17]. Are there possible differential effects of dietary fructose and glucose on energy metabolism, or on the risk factors for chronic disease? If so, is there a dose response or threshold limit that triggers these differential effects? Does the potential risk of fructose relate to whether it is present as a disaccharide (purified or raw sucrose), a monosaccharide in a purified form, or a mixture of fructose and glucose, whether it is natural or manufactured? The effects of the fructose and HFCS are possibly dependent upon whether the individual is consuming just the energy to meet their needs or a hypercaloric diet. However, fructose might in some way facilitate the consuming of too many calories. Future scientific investigations may shed light on these and other mysteries as HFCS research continues.

References

1. Bray GA, Nielsen SJ, Popkin BM. Consumption of high-fructose corn syrup in beverages may play a role in the epidemic of obesity. Am J Clin Nutr. 2004; 79:537–43.
2. Moeller SM, Fryhofer SA, Osbahr III AJ, Robinowitz CB. The effects of high fructose corn syrup. Am Coll Nutr. 2009; 28:619–26.
3. U.S. Department of Agriculture, Economic Research Service. Caloric sweeteners availability: 1966–2008. http://www.ers.usda.gov/data/foodconsumption/nutrientavaildoc.htm. Accessed 6/13/2011.
4. White JS. Misconceptions about high-fructose corn syrup: is it uniquely responsible for obesity, reactive dicarbonyl compounds, and advanced glycation end products? J Nutr. 2009; 139:S1219–27.
5. Tappy L, Le KA. Metabolic effects of fructose and the worldwide increase in obesity. Physiol Rev. 2010; 90:23–46.
6. Gaby AR. Adverse effects of dietary fructose. Alternative Medicine Review. 2005; 10:294–306.
7. Ruxton CHS, Gardner EJ, McNutly HM. Is sugar consumption detrimental to health? a review of the evidence: 1995–1996. Crit Rev Food Sci Nutr. 2010; 50:1–19.
8. Flegal KM, Carroll MD, Ogden CL, Curtin LR. Prevalence and trends in obesity among US adults: 1999–2008. JAMA. 2010; 303:235–41.
9. Ogden CL, Carroll MD, Curtin LR, et al. Prevalence of high body mass index in US children and adolescents: 2007–2008. JAMA. 2010; 303:242–49.
10. Chong MF-F, Fielding BB, Frayn KN. Mechanisms for the acute effect of fructose on post prandial lipemia. Am J Clin Nutr. 2007; 85:1511–20.
11. Parks EJ, Skokan LE, Timlin MT, Dingfelder CS. Dietary sugars stimulate fatty acid synthesis in adults. J Nutr. 2008; 138:1039–46.
12. Stanhope KL, Schwarz JM, Keim NL, et al. Consuming fructose-sweetened, not glucose sweetened, beverages increases visceral adiposity and lipids and decreases insulin sensitivity in overweight/obese humans. J Clin Invest. 2009; 119:1322–34.
13. Le KA, Faeh D, Stettler R, et al. A 4-wk high-fructose diet alters lipid metabolism without affecting insulin sensitivity or ectopic lipids in healthy humans. Am J Clin Nutr. 2006; 84:1374–79.
14. Bantle JP, Raatz SK, Thomas W, Georgopoulos A. Effect of dietary fructose on plasma lipids in healthy subjects. Am J Clin Nutr. 2000; 72:1128–34.
15. U.S. Department of Agriculture, Economic Research Service: U.S. food supply: nutrients and other food components, per capita per day: 1909–2006. http://www.ers.usda.gov/data/foodconsumption/nutrientavaildoc.htm. Accessed 6/13/2011.
16. Dirlewanger M, Schneiter P, Jequier E, Tappy L. Effects of fructose on hepatic glucose metabolism in humans. Am J Physiol Endocrinol Metab. 2000; 279:E907–11.
17. Murphy SP. The state of the science on dietary sweeteners containing fructose: summary and issues to be resolved. J Nutr. 2009; 139:S1269–70.

4 FIBER

D IETARY FIBER WAS RECOGNIZED AGAIN as an important food component in the mid-1970s. Yet the concepts of fiber, originally called crude fiber or indigestible material, and its extraction from animal feed and forages were introduced in Germany during the 1850s. The crude fiber extraction method was used, even for human food, into the 1990s, despite the existence of better methodology and the inconsistent relationship between crude fiber and dietary fiber. Today, soluble and insoluble fibers may be extracted or, in some cases, manufactured in laboratories and added as an ingredient to create foods that contain what we now call *functional fiber*.

Results from extensive research devoted to dietary fiber during the last 30 or so years have demonstrated not only that fiber is important for gastrointestinal tract function but also that foods rich in fiber help prevent and manage a variety of diseases. The varied effects of fiber observed by researchers are related to the fact that dietary fiber consists of different components, each with its own distinctive characteristics. Examining these many components and their various distinctive characteristics emphasizes the fact that dietary fiber cannot be considered a single entity. This chapter addresses the definitions of dietary fiber and functional fiber; the relationship between plants and fiber; and the chemistry, intraplant functions, properties, and sources of fiber. It also reviews some relationships between fiber intake and disease as well as recommendations for fiber intake.

DEFINITIONS OF DIETARY FIBER AND FUNCTIONAL FIBER

With the publication of the 2002 Dietary Reference Intakes for Energy, Carbohydrate, Fiber, Fat, Protein, and Amino Acids by the National Academy of Sciences Food and Nutrition Board, uniform definitions for dietary fiber and functional fiber were established. **Dietary fiber** refers to nondigestible (by human digestive enzymes) carbohydrates and lignin that are intact and intrinsic in plants [1]. **Functional fiber** consists of nondigestible carbohydrates that have been isolated, extracted, or manufactured and have been shown to have beneficial physiological effects in humans [1]. The term *fiber* that appears on food labels reflects only dietary fiber. Table 4.1 lists dietary and functional fibers. Each fiber listed in Table 4.1 is discussed in this chapter in the "Chemistry and Characteristics of Dietary and Functional Fibers" section.

Table 4.1 Dietary and Functional Fibers

Dietary Fibers	Functional Fibers
Cellulose	Cellulose
Hemicellulose	Pectin
Pectin	Lignin[*]
Lignin	Gums
Gums	β-glucans
β-glucans	Fructans[*]
Fructans	Chitin and chitosan[*]
Resistant starches	Polydextrose and polyols[*]
	Psyllium
	Resistant dextrins[*]
	Resistant starches

[*]Data showing positive physiological effects in humans are needed.

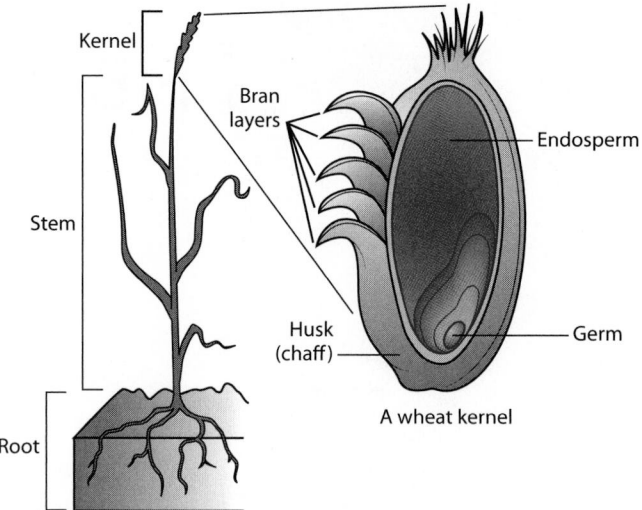

Figure 4.1 The partial anatomy of a wheat plant.

FIBER AND PLANTS

The plant cell wall consists of both a primary and a secondary wall and contains >95% of dietary fibers. The primary wall is a thin envelope that surrounds the contents of the growing cell. The secondary wall develops as the cell matures. The secondary wall of a mature plant contains many strands of cellulose arranged in an orderly fashion within a matrix of noncellulosic polysaccharides. The primary wall also contains cellulose, but in smaller amounts and less well organized. The hemicellulose content of plants varies but can make up 20% to 30% of the cell walls. Starch, the energy storage product of the cell, is found within the cell walls. Lignin deposits form in specialized cells whose function is to provide structural support to the plant. As the plant matures, lignin spreads through the intracellular spaces, penetrating the pectins. Pectins along with proteins are found in the middle lamella, which makes up the outer wall of the cell and functions as intercellular cement to unite the cell walls of adjacent cells. Lignin continues dispersing through intracellular spaces, but it also permeates the primary wall and then spreads into the developing secondary wall. As plant development continues further, suberin is deposited in the cell wall. Suberin is made up of a variety of substances, including phenolic compounds as well as long-chain alcohols and polymeric esters of fatty acids. Cutin, also made of polymeric esters of fatty acids, is a water-impermeable substance that is secreted onto the plant surface. Both suberin and cutin are enzyme and acid resistant. In addition to these substances, waxes (which consist of complex hydrophobic, hydrocarbon compounds) are found in many plants, coating the external surfaces.

Consuming plant foods provides fiber in the diet. The plant species, the part of the plant (leaf, root, stem), and the plant's maturity all influence the composition (cellulose, hemicellulose, pectin, lignin, etc.) of the fiber that is consumed. Figure 4.1 shows the anatomy of a wheat plant. Consuming a cereal such as wheat bran (which consists of the outer layers of cereal grains, as shown in Figure 4.1) provides primarily cellulose and hemicellulose along with lignin plus some β-glucans, raffinose, stachyose, and fructans. Eating fruits and vegetables provides almost equal quantities (~30%) of cellulose and pectin. This chapter reviews each of the dietary fibers, including their characteristics and functions, as well as foods rich in the particular fiber. Identifying the chemical characteristics and various intraplant functions and properties of these plant cell wall substances (or substances in contact with the wall) helps us to conceptualize how fiber components may affect physiological and metabolic functions in humans.

CHEMISTRY AND CHARACTERISTICS OF DIETARY AND FUNCTIONAL FIBERS

Cellulose

Cellulose is considered a dietary fiber as well as a functional fiber when added to foods. Chemical analysis shows cellulose (Figure 4.2a) to be a long, linear **polymer** (a high-molecular-weight substance made up of a chain of repeating units) of β (1-4)-linked glucose units. Cellulose is a main component of plant cell walls. Hydrogen bonding between sugar residues in adjacent, parallel-running cellulose chains imparts a microfibril three-dimensional structure to cellulose. Being a large, linear, neutrally charged molecule, cellulose is water insoluble, although it can be modified chemically (e.g., carboxymethyl cellulose, methylcellulose, and hydroxypropyl methylcellulose) to be more water soluble for use as a food additive. The extent to which cellulose is degraded by colonic bacteria varies, but generally it is poorly fermented. Some examples

(a) Cellulose

(b) Hemicellulose (major component sugars)

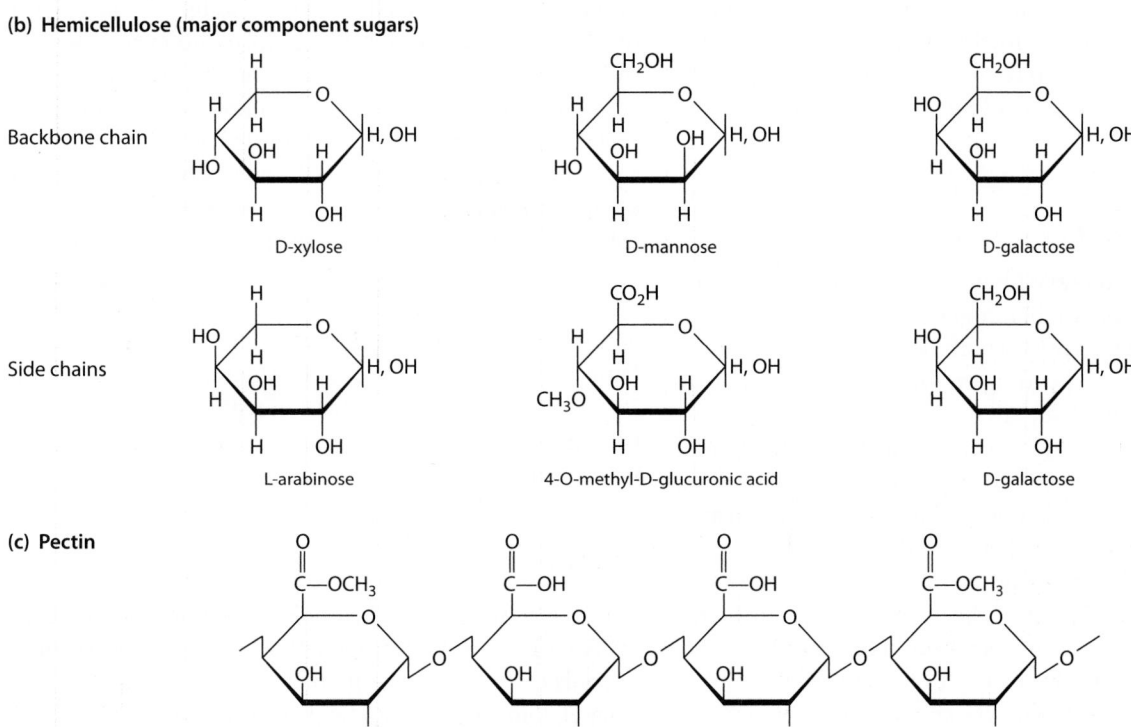

Backbone chain

D-xylose   D-mannose   D-galactose

Side chains

L-arabinose   4-O-methyl-D-glucuronic acid   D-galactose

(c) Pectin

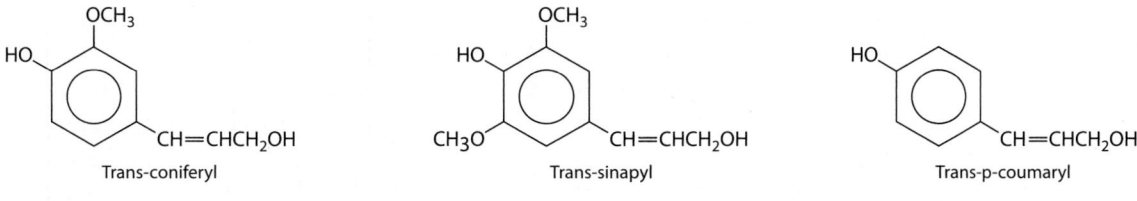

(d) Phenols in lignin

Trans-coniferyl   Trans-sinapyl   Trans-p-coumaryl

(e) Gum arabic

X: L-rhamnopyranose or
L-arabinofuranose
GALP: galactopyranose
GA: glucuronic acid

(f) β-glucan (from oats)

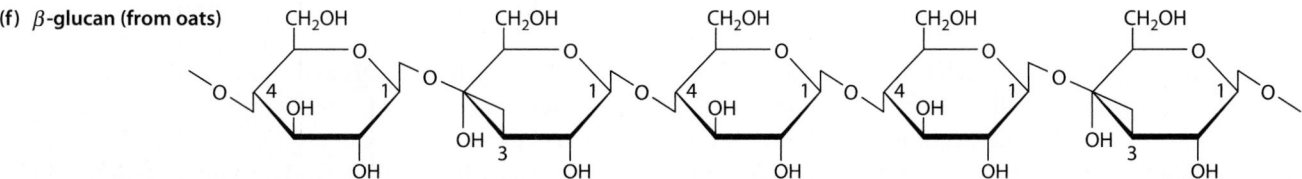

Figure 4.2 Chemical structures of dietary fibers and some functional fibers.

of foods high in cellulose relative to other fibers include bran, legumes, nuts, peas, root vegetables, vegetables of the cabbage family, the outer covering of seeds, and apples. Purified, powdered cellulose (usually isolated from wood) and modified cellulose are often added to foods, for example, as a thickening or texturing agent or to prevent caking or syneresis (leakage of liquid). Some examples of foods to which cellulose or a modified form of cellulose is added include breads, cake mixes, sauces, sandwich spreads, dips, frozen meat products (e.g., chicken nuggets), and fruit juice mixes.

Hemicellulose

Hemicellulose, a dietary fiber and a component of plant cell walls, consists of a heterogeneous group of polysaccharide substances that vary both between different plants and within a plant depending on location. Hemicelluloses contain a number of sugars in their backbone and side chains. The sugars, which form a basis for hemicellulose classification, include xylose, mannose, and galactose in the hemicellulose backbone and arabinose, glucuronic acid, and galactose in the hemicellulose side chains. The number of sugars in the side chains varies such that some hemicelluloses are relatively linear, whereas others are highly branched. Some of the sugars found in hemicelluloses are shown in Figure 4.2b. One example of a hemicellulose structure is β(1-4)-linked D-xylopyranose units with branches of 4-O-methyl D-glucopyranose uronic acids linked by α(1-2) bonds or with branches of L-arabinofuranosyl units linked by α(1-3) bonds. The sugars in the side chains confer important characteristics on the hemicellulose. For example, hemicelluloses that contain acids in their side chains are slightly charged and water soluble. Other hemicelluloses are water insoluble. Fermentability of the hemicelluloses by intestinal microflora (bacteria adapted to living in that specific environment) is also influenced by the sugars and their positions. For example, hexose and uronic acid components of hemicellulose are more accessible to bacterial enzymes than are the other hemicellulose sugars. Foods that are relatively high in hemicellulose include bran and whole grains as well as nuts, legumes, and some vegetables and fruits.

Pectins

Pectins are a family of polysaccharide compounds that in turn make up a larger family of pectic substances including pectins, pectic acids, and pectinic acids. Pectin is both a dietary fiber and a functional fiber. Galacturonic acid is a primary constituent of pectin and makes up its backbone structure. Pectin's backbone is usually an unbranched chain of α(1-4)-linked D-galacturonic acid units, as shown in Figure 4.2c. Many of the carboxyl groups of the uronic acid moieties exist as methyl esters. Other carbohydrates may be linked to the galacturonic acid chain. These additional sugars, sometimes found attached as side chains, include rhamnose, arabinose, xylose, fucose, and galactose; galactose may be present in a methylated form. Pectins form part of the primary cell wall of plants and part of the middle lamella. They are water soluble and gel-forming and have a high ion-binding potential. Because they are stable at low pH values, pectins perform well in acidic foods. In the body, pectins are almost completely metabolized (fermented) by colonic bacteria and are not a good fecal bulking agent. Rich sources of pectins include apples, strawberries, and citrus fruits. Legumes, nuts, and some vegetables also provide pectins. Commercially, pectins are usually extracted from citrus peel or apples and are added to many products. Pectin is added to jellies and jams to promote gelling. It is also added to fruit roll-ups, fruit juices, and icing or frosting, among other products. Pectin is added to some enteral nutrition formulas administered to tube-fed hospital patients to provide a source of fiber in their diets.

Lignin

Lignin is a highly branched polymer composed of phenol units with strong intramolecular bonding. The primary phenols that compose lignin include trans-coniferyl, trans-sinapyl, and trans-p-coumaryl, shown in Figure 4.2d. Lignin forms the structural components of plants and is thought to attach to other noncellulose polysaccharides such as heteroxylans found in plant cell walls. Lignin is insoluble in water, has hydrophobic binding capacity, and is generally poorly fermented by colonic bacteria. Some studies, however, report metabolism by gut flora to form the lignan enterolactone, a weak phytoestrogen [2]. Lignin is both a dietary fiber and a functional fiber. It is found especially in the stems and seeds of fruits and vegetables and in the bran layer of cereals. More specific examples of foods high in lignin include wheat, mature root vegetables such as carrots, flaxseed, and fruits with edible seeds such as strawberries.

Gums

Gums, also called *hydrocolloids,* represent a group of substances. Gums are secreted at the site of plant injury by specialized secretory cells and can be exuded from plants (i.e., forced out of plant tissues). Gums that originate as tree **exudates** include gum arabic, gum karaya, and gum ghatti; gum tragacanth is a shrub exudate. Gums are often highly branched and are composed of a variety of sugars and sugar derivatives. Galactose and glucuronic acid are prominent, as are uronic acids, arabinose, rhamnose, and mannose, among others. Gum arabic, shown in Figure 4.2e, contains a main galactose backbone joined by β(1-3) linkages and β(1-6) linkages along with side chains of galactose, arabinose, rhamnose, glucuronic acid, or methylglucuronic acid joined by β(1-6) linkages. The nonreducing ends terminate with a rhamnopyrosyl unit. Within the large intestine, gums are highly fermented by colonic bacteria. Of the tree exudates, gum arabic is most commonly used as a food additive to promote gelling, thickening, and stabilizing. The popularity of gum arabic is attributable to its physical properties, which include high water solubility, pH stability, and gelling characteristics. It is found in candies such as caramels, gumdrops, and toffees, as well as in other assorted products.

Guar gum and locust bean gum (also called carob gum) are made from the ground endosperm of guar seeds and locust bean seeds, respectively. These water-soluble gums consist mostly of galactomannans, the main component of the endosperm. Galactomannans contain a mannose backbone in 1-4 linkages and in a 2:1 or 4:1 ratio with galactose present in the side chains. Guar galactomannans have more branches than locust bean galactomannans. Both guar gum and locust bean gum are added as a thickening agent and water-binding agent (among other roles) to products such as bakery goods, sauces, dairy products, ice creams, dips, and salad dressings. Gums are also found naturally in foods such as oatmeal, barley, and legumes. Some gums (xanthan gum and gellan gum) can be synthesized by microorganisms. Gums are considered to be both dietary and functional fibers.

β-glucans

β-glucans are homopolymers of glucopyranose units (Figure 4.2f). This water-soluble, highly fermentable, dietary fiber is found in relatively high amounts in cereal brans, especially oats and barley, as well as in some mushrooms. Oat β-glucan consists of a chain of β-D-glucopyranosyl units joined mostly in β(1-4) linkages but also some β(1-3) linkages. β-glucans, extracted from cereals, are used commercially as a functional fiber because of their effectiveness in reducing serum cholesterol and postprandial (after-eating) blood glucose concentrations.

Fructans: Inulin, Oligofructose, and Fructooligosaccharides

Fructans, sometimes called *polyfructose,* including inulin, oligofructose, and fructooligosaccharides, are chemically composed primarily of fructose units in chains of varying length. Inulin consists of a fructose chain that contains from 2 to about 60 units, with β(2-1) linkages and a glucose molecule linked to the C-2 position of the terminal fructofuranose unit to create a nonreducing unit at the end of the molecule. Although human digestive enzymes are not able to hydrolyze the β(2-1) linkage, some bacteria, such as bifidobacteria, produce β-fructosidase, which can hydrolyze the β(2-1) linkage. Oligofructose is formed from the partial hydrolysis of inulin and typically contains between 2 and 8 fructose units; it may or may not contain an end glucose molecule. Fructooligosaccharides are similar to oligofructose, except that polymerization of fructooligosaccharides ranges from 2 to 4 units. Ingesting fructooligosaccharides and other fructans has been shown to promote the growth of bifidobacteria (i.e., fructans act as prebiotics) as discussed in more detail in the section on fermentable fibers as prebiotics and in the Perspective at the end of this chapter.

Fructans are found naturally in plants and are considered dietary fibers, but at present they are not reported in most food composition databases. The most common food sources of inulin and other fructans include chicory, asparagus, leeks, onions, garlic, Jerusalem artichokes, tomatoes, and bananas. Fresh artichoke, for example, contains about 5.8 g of fructooligosaccharides per 100 g, and minced dried onion flakes provide 4 g of fructooligosaccharides per 100 g [3]. Wheat, barley, and rye also contain some fructans. Fructans, when added to foods, are often synthesized from sucrose by adding fructose. The fibers also can be extracted and purified from plant sources for commercial use. Inulin is used to replace fat in fillings, dressings, and frozen desserts, to name a few examples. Oligofructose is added, for example, to cereals, yogurt, dairy products, and frozen desserts. With sufficient data showing positive physiological effects, fructans added to foods could be considered a functional fiber. Americans are thought to consume up to about 4 g of fructooligosaccharides each day from foods.

Resistant Starch

Resistant starch (RS) is starch that cannot be or is not easily enzymatically digested, and thus absorbed, by humans. There are four main types of resistant starch, numbered 1 to 4. The first type, designated RS_1, is starch found in cell walls that is inaccessible to amylase activity. Specifically, RS_1 resists digestion because it is located within a plant's cellulose wall, which cannot be penetrated or broken down (i.e., the enzyme amylase cannot physically reach the amylose). Food sources of RS_1 include whole or partially milled grains and seeds. Resistant starch designated RS_2 typically resists digestion because the starch is tightly packaged inside of granules within the plant cells. Remember, amylose's linear structure enables tight stacking of the amylose chains. This tight packaging is especially prevalent in high-amylose plant foods such as unripe (green) bananas, some legumes, raw potatoes, and some maize (which may contain up to 80% amylose).

Another type of resistant starch, designated RS_3, is called retrograde starch. The moist-heat cooking and cooling or extrusion of starchy foods typically generates RS_3. Foods rich in retrograde starch include cooked and cooled rice, pasta, potatoes, and high-amylose corn. In addition, the supplement wheat dextrin contains RS_3; it is made by extracting starch from cooked and cooled wheat flour. Similarly, chemical modifications of starch, such as the formation of starch esters, or cross-bonded starches, result in resistant starch called RS_4. Both RS_1 and RS_2 are considered dietary fibers, whereas RS_3 and RS_4 are considered functional fibers [1]. RS_3 and RS_4 may be partially fermented by colonic bacteria. Americans are thought to consume up to about 10 g of resistant starch daily. Consumption of up to 20 g of resistant starch has been recommended to obtain health benefits.

Chitin and Chitosan

Chitin is a straight-chain amino-polysaccharide polymer containing β(1-4)-linked glucose units. It is similar in structure to cellulose, but an N-acetyl amino group substitutes for the hydroxyl group at carbon 2 of the D-glucopyranose residue. Chitin can replace cellulose in the cell walls of some lower plants. It is also a component of the exoskeleton of insects and is found in the shells of crabs, shrimp, and lobsters. Chitin is insoluble in water.

Chitosan is a deacetylated form of chitin and thus is a polysaccharide made of glucosamine and N-acetyl glucosamine. Polymers of chitosan vary in their degree of acetylation. Like chitin, chitosan has a high molecular weight, is viscous, and is water insoluble. However, lower-molecular-weight chitosans, manufactured through hydrolysis, are less viscous and water soluble. As a positively charged molecule in gastric juice, chitosan has the ability to interact with or complex to dietary lipids, primarily unesterified cholesterol and phospholipids, which are negatively charged. Once formed, the chitosan-lipid complex is excreted in the feces. With additional data showing physiological benefits in humans, chitosan and chitin may be considered functional fibers [1].

Polydextrose and Polyols

Polydextrose is a polysaccharide consisting of glucose and sorbitol units that have been polymerized at high temperatures and under a partial vacuum. Polydextrose, available commercially, is added to foods as a bulking agent or as a sugar substitute. The polysaccharide is neither digested nor absorbed by the human gastrointestinal tract; however, it can be partially fermented by colonic bacteria and contributes to fecal bulk. Polyols such as polyglycitol and malitol are found in syrups. With sufficient data on physiological benefits, some polyols and polydextrose may be classified as functional fibers [1].

Psyllium

Psyllium, classified as a mucilage, is obtained from the husk of psyllium seeds (also called plantago or fleas seed). Products containing psyllium have high water-binding capacities and thus provide viscosity in solutions. Psyllium is soluble in water, has a structure similar to that of gums, and is considered a functional fiber. It is added, for example, to health products such as Metamucil for its laxative properties. Foods containing psyllium that bear a health claim are required to state on the label that the food should be eaten with at least a full glass of liquid and that choking may result if the product is not ingested with enough liquid [4]. In addition, the label should state that the food should not be eaten if a person has difficulty swallowing [4].

Resistant Dextrins

Resistant dextrins, also called *resistant maltodextrins,* are generated by treating cornstarch with heat and acid and then with the enzyme amylase. The resistant dextrins consist of glucose polymers containing α(1-4) and α(1-6) glucosidic bonds and α(1-2) and α(1-3) bonds. With sufficient data showing beneficial physiological effects, resistant dextrins may be considered functional fibers [1].

Table 4.2 lists food sources of different types of fibers. Cummings and Stephen [5] provide an excellent review of carbohydrate terminology and classification, including more information on the properties of various carbohydrates.

Table 4.2 Food Sources of Fiber

Type of Fiber	Examples of Food Sources
Cellulose	All plant foods, especially wheat bran, legumes, nuts, peas, root vegetables (such as carrots), vegetables of the cabbage family, celery, broccoli, coverings of seeds, and apples
Hemicellulose	Whole grains, especially bran, nuts, and legumes
Lignin	Whole grains, especially wheat bran, mature root vegetables (such as carrots), fruits with edible seeds (such as strawberries), and broccoli (especially the stalk)
Pectin	Citrus fruits, strawberries, apples, raspberries, legumes, nuts, some vegetables (such as carrots), and oat products
Gums	Oatmeal, barley, and legumes
β-glucans	Oat products, barley, and some mushrooms
Resistant starches	RS_1: partially milled grains and seeds; RS_2: unripe (green) bananas, legumes, raw potato, and high-amylose corn; RS_3: rice, pasta, cold cooked potatoes, and high-amylose corn
Fructans	Chicory, asparagus, onion, garlic, artichoke, tomatoes, bananas, rye, and barley
Chitosan, chitin	Shells of crab, shrimp, and lobster

SELECTED PROPERTIES AND PHYSIOLOGICAL AND METABOLIC EFFECTS OF FIBER

The physiological and metabolic effects of fiber vary based on the type ingested. Significant characteristics of dietary fiber that affect its physiological and metabolic roles include its solubility in water (as shown in Figure 4.3), its hydration or water-holding capacity and viscosity, its adsorptive attraction or ability to bind organic and inorganic molecules, and its degradability or fermentability by intestinal bacteria. The following sections review each of these characteristics and their effects on various physiological and metabolic processes. Figure 4.4 diagrams their relationships. However, as you study these characteristics and their effects on the body, remember that we eat foods with a mixture of dietary fiber, not foods with just cellulose, hemicellulose, pectins, gums, and so forth. Thus, the effects on the various body processes are not as straightforward as presented in this chapter and vary considerably based on the foods ingested.

Solubility in Water

Fiber is often classified as water soluble or water insoluble (Figure 4.3). Fibers that dissolve in hot water are soluble, and those that do not dissolve in hot water are insoluble. In general, water-soluble fibers include some hemicelluloses and pectins, gums, β-glucans, fructans (inulin, fructooligosaccharides), psyllium, and some resistant starches. Foods typically rich in soluble fiber include legumes, oats, barley, some fruits (berries, bananas, apples, pears), and some vegetables (carrots, broccoli, artichokes, onions). Cellulose, lignin, some hemicelluloses and pectins, some resistant starches, chitosan, and chitin are examples of dietary fibers classified as insoluble. Examples of foods rich in insoluble fiber include whole-grain products, wheat and corn bran, nuts, seeds, some vegetables, and some fruits. Generally, vegetables and most grain products contain more insoluble fibers than soluble fibers.

Solubility in water also may be used as a basis for broadly characterizing fibers. For example, soluble fibers generally delay gastric emptying, increase transit time (through slower movement) through the intestine, and decrease nutrient (e.g., glucose) absorption. In contrast, insoluble fibers decrease (speed up) intestinal transit time and increase fecal bulk. These actions (discussed in the following section) of the soluble and insoluble fibers in turn induce other physiological and metabolic effects.

Water-Holding/Hydration Capacity and Viscosity

Water-holding or hydration capacity of foods refers to the ability of fiber in food to bind water; think of fiber as a dry sponge that hydrates or soaks up water and digestive juices as it moves through the digestive tract. Many of the water-soluble fibers such as pectins, gums, and some hemicelluloses have a high water-holding capacity in comparison with fibers such as cellulose and lignin, which have a lower water-holding capacity. In addition, some water-soluble fibers such as pectin, β-glucans, psyllium, some gums like guar gum and some resistant starches form viscous (thick) solutions within the gastrointestinal tract (Figure 4.3). Soluble fibers may bind up to several times their weight in water, producing a viscous, slow-moving solution that often traps nutrients to slow down digestion and absorption within the digestive tract.

Water-holding capacity, however, does not depend just upon the fiber's solubility in water. The pH of the gastrointestinal tract, the size of the fiber particles, and the degree to which foods are processed also influence water-holding capacity and in turn its physiological effects. Coarsely ground bran, for example, has a higher hydration capacity than bran that is finely ground. Consequently, coarse bran with large particles holds water, increases fecal volume, and speeds up the rate of fecal passage through the colon.

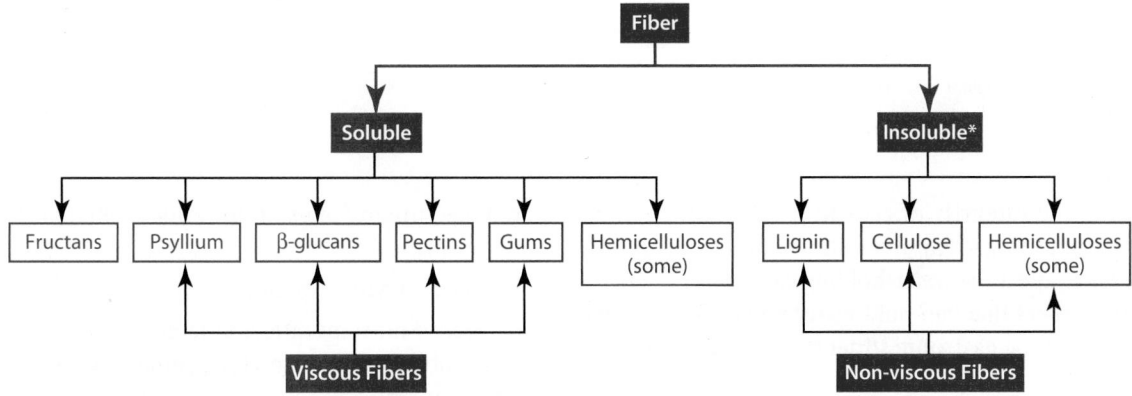

Figure 4.3 Fibers classified by solubility/insolubility in water and ability/inability to form viscous solutions.
*Other fibers that are considered less soluble or insoluble sometimes include some pectins, some resistant starches, chitosan, and chitin.

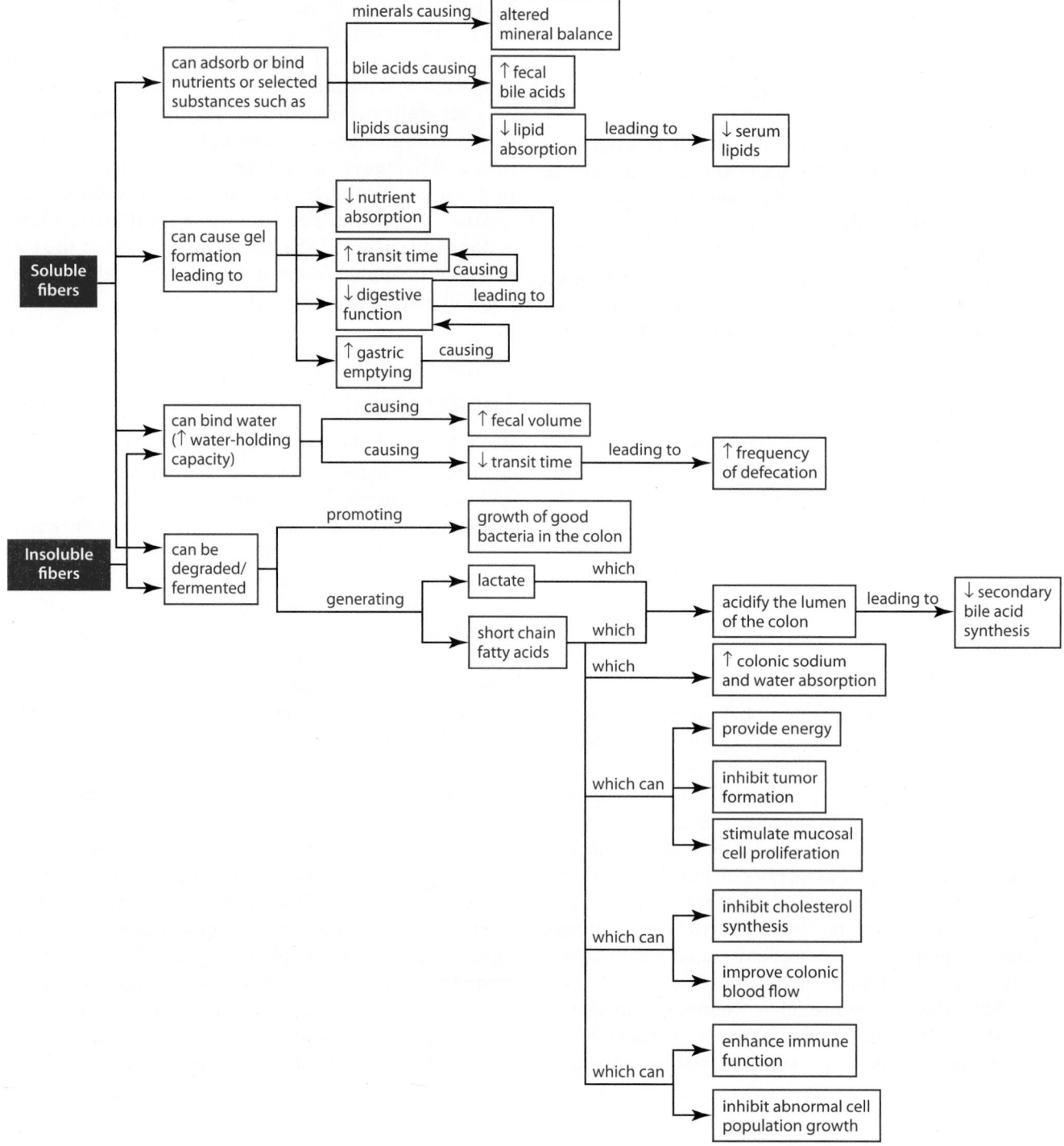

Figure 4.4 Gastrointestinal response to soluble and insoluble fibers.

Maintaining the integrity of cells in grains and legumes rather than subjecting them to traditional milling processes also appears to affect the water-holding capacity of fibers.

Ingesting fibers that can hold water and create viscous solutions within the gastrointestinal tract causes a number of effects:

- delayed (slowed) emptying of food from the stomach

- reduced mixing of gastrointestinal contents with digestive enzymes
- reduced enzyme function
- decreased nutrient diffusion rates (and thus delayed nutrient absorption), which attenuate the blood glucose response
- altered small intestine transit time

The following sections describe each of these effects.

Delayed (Slowed) Gastric Emptying

When fibers hydrate and form viscous gels within the stomach, the release of the chyme from the stomach (gastric emptying) into the duodenum (proximal small intestine) is delayed (slowed). Thus, nutrients remain in the stomach longer with these fibers than they would in the absence of the ingested fiber. This effect creates a feeling of postprandial (after-eating) satiety (fullness) and slows down the digestion process because carbohydrates and lipids that remain in the stomach undergo no digestion there and must move into the small intestine for further digestion to occur.

Reduced Mixing of Gastrointestinal Contents with Digestive Enzymes

The presence of fiber-rich viscous gels in the gastrointestinal tract provides a physical barrier that can impair the ability of the nutrients in the food to interact with the digestive enzymes. This interaction is critical for digestion to occur.

Reduced Enzyme Function

Viscous gel-forming fibers such as gums have been shown to interfere with the enzymatic hydrolysis of nutrients such as proteins and lipids within the gastrointestinal tract. Additionally, the viscous gel serves to trap nutrients and retard their ability to interact with digestive enzymes and to be absorbed into the intestinal cells. Whether fiber directly decreases the activity of the digestive enzymes and/or acts by reducing the rate of enzyme penetration into the food is unclear.

Decreased Nutrient Diffusion Rate—Attenuation of the Blood Glucose Response

Remember that for nutrients to be absorbed they must move from the lumen of the small intestine through a glycoprotein-rich (i.e., mucin-rich) water layer lying on top of the enterocytes and finally into the enterocyte. The fiber-associated decreased diffusion rate of nutrients through this water layer is thought to be caused by an increased thickness of the unstirred water layer due to the presence of the viscous fiber solution. In other words, the unstirred water layer becomes more viscous and resistant to nutrient movement, and without this movement nutrients cannot be absorbed into the enterocyte.

Another mechanism may also be responsible for decreased nutrient diffusion. Gums appear to slow glucose absorption by decreasing the convective movement of glucose within the intestinal lumen. Convective currents induced by peristaltic movements bring nutrients from the lumen to the enterocyte's cell membrane for absorption.

This decreased convective solute movement also may help explain why absorption of amino acids and fatty acids is decreased by viscous fiber. Ingesting viscous fibers such as gums, pectin, β-glucans, psyllium, and some resistant starch—and, to a variable extent, some chitosans, fructooligosaccharides, and polydextrose—has been shown to slow transit, delay glucose absorption, lower blood glucose concentrations, and affect the release of hormones (especially glucagon-like peptide 1 and insulin). Glucagon-like peptide 1 promotes tissue utilization of glucose, among other roles; increased release of glucagon-like peptide 1 associated with high-fiber diets may reduce insulin needs [6,7]. These traits are especially beneficial to someone with diabetes mellitus or prediabetes. In fact, specific food products for individuals with diabetes have been developed that are high in resistant starch (such as uncooked cornstarch) or contain other modified carbohydrates that resist digestive enzymes and are absorbed more slowly than other forms of carbohydrate. Consumption of such products permits the enjoyment of carbohydrate ingestion without excessive elevations in blood glucose concentrations and insulin needs and response.

A decreased nutrient diffusion rate may in turn result in nutrients "missing" their normal site of maximal absorption. For example, if a nutrient is normally absorbed in the proximal intestine but because of gel formation is "trapped" as part of the gel, then absorption cannot occur at this site. Should the nutrient be released from the gel, the release is most likely going to occur at a site distal to where the nutrient would normally have been absorbed. The extent to which nutrients are absorbed throughout the digestive tract varies with the individual nutrient.

Altered Small Intestine Transit Time

In general, soluble fibers typically delay (slow down or lengthen) small intestine transit time, whereas insoluble fibers speed up or shorten transit time within the small intestine. These changes in transit time, especially if it is shortened, may result in decreased nutrient absorption because the nutrients are in contact with enterocytes for too short a time.

Adsorption or Binding Ability

Some fiber components, especially lignin, gums, pectins, β-glucans, some hemicelluloses, and some modified forms of chitosans, have the ability to bind or adhere to (adsorb) substances such as enzymes and nutrients in the gastrointestinal tract. Maillard products also have this binding ability. Maillard products consist of enzyme resistant linkages between the amino group of amino acids, especially the amino acid lysine, and the carbonyl group of reducing sugars. Maillard products are formed during heat treatment, particularly in baking and frying foods, and typically cannot be digested by human digestive enzymes. Ingesting fibers with adsorption properties within the gastrointestinal tract may cause these physiological effects:

- diminished absorption of lipids
- increased fecal bile acid excretion
- lowered serum cholesterol concentrations (hypocholesterolemic properties)
- altered mineral, carotenoid, and phytochemical absorption

The mechanisms by which these effects occur vary considerably and are reviewed next.

Diminished Absorption of Lipids

Soluble fibers (especially pectin, gums, β-glucans, and some hemicelluloses) but also the insoluble fiber lignin and modified forms of chitosan may affect lipid absorption by adsorbing or interacting with fatty acids, cholesterol, and bile acids within the digestive tract. Fatty acids and cholesterol that are bound or complexed to fiber cannot form micelles and cannot be absorbed in this bound form; only free fatty acids, monoacylglycerols, and cholesterol can be incorporated into micelles, and it is the micelles that are needed for these end products of fat digestion to be transported through the unstirred water layers and into the enterocyte. Thus, fiber-bound lipids typically are not absorbed in the small intestine and pass into the large intestine, where they are excreted in the feces.

Increased Fecal Bile Acid Excretion

Adsorption of bile acids to fibers prevents the use of the bile acids for micelle formation. And, like fiber-bound fatty acids, bile acids bound to fiber cannot be reabsorbed and recirculated (enterohepatic recirculation). Fiber-bound bile acids typically enter the large intestine, where they are excreted in the feces.

Lowered Serum Cholesterol Concentrations (Hypocholesterolemic Properties)

The ability of some fibers to lower serum cholesterol concentrations is based on a couple of events. First, when the excretion of bile acids and cholesterol in the feces increases, less bile undergoes enterohepatic recirculation. A decrease in the bile acids returned to the liver and decreased cholesterol absorption lead to a decreased cholesterol content of liver cells. Decreased hepatic cholesterol promotes removal of low-density lipoprotein (LDL) cholesterol from the blood. The decrease in bile acids returned to the liver also necessitates the use of cholesterol for synthesis of new bile acids. The net effect is lower serum cholesterol concentrations. A second proposed mechanism for the hypocholesterolemic (lower blood cholesterol) effect of fiber is the shift in bile acid production away from cholic acid and toward chenodeoxycholic acid (the mechanism for the shift is not known). Chenodeoxycholic acid appears to inhibit 3-hydroxy 3-methylglutaryl (HMG)-CoA reductase, a regulatory enzyme necessary for cholesterol biosynthesis [8–10]. Decreased HMG-CoA reductase activity results in reduced hepatic cholesterol synthesis and theoretically lower blood cholesterol concentrations. A third hypothesis suggests that the production of propionic acid or other short-chain fatty acids (discussed in the section on fermentable fibers) through bacterial degradation of fiber lowers serum cholesterol concentrations, possibly through inhibitory effects on fatty acid and/or cholesterol synthesis. However, propionic acid fed to humans has had varying effects on serum cholesterol concentrations [8–10].

Ingestion of soluble fibers—especially psyllium, some gums (mainly guar gum), β-glucan, resistant dextrins, methylcellulose, and pectin—lowers serum cholesterol concentrations to varying degrees [6,8]. Variable effects on blood lipid concentrations also have been observed with ingestion of inulin, fructooligosaccharides, and chitosan supplements. The most well-studied cholesterol-lowering high-fiber foods/fibers are β-glucan from barley and oats, as well as psyllium; each of these has been studied sufficiently to have health claims (see the section titled "Health Claims and Food Labels"). Quantities of soluble fiber needed to lower serum lipid concentrations vary based on the fiber; effective LDL-cholesterol lowering quantities for pectin range from about 12 to 24 g, for guar gum about 9 to 30 g, for barley β-glucan and methylcellulose about 5 g, and for psyllium and oat β-glucan about 6 g [8]. To consume from foods the amount of soluble fiber necessary to lower serum lipids, one would need to ingest, for example, about 6 to 10 servings per day of soluble fiber–rich fruits and vegetables, or about 2 to 3 servings per day of legumes or oat- or barley-based cereals.

In addition to the ability of various fibers to lower serum cholesterol, other plant components, specifically phytostanols and sterols, also lower serum cholesterol by reducing the absorption of cholesterol into the enterocytes and/or by stimulating the transintestinal excretion of cholesterol. Daily consumption of plant sterols and stanols in amounts ranging from about 1.6 to 3 g/day has been shown to decrease total and LDL plasma cholesterol concentrations in people with normal and high blood lipid concentrations [11].

Altered Mineral, Carotenoid, and Phytochemical Absorption

Some fibers—especially those with uronic acid, such as hemicellulose, pectins, and gums—as well as fructose and galactose oligosaccharides can form cationic bridges with minerals within the gastrointestinal tract. Lignin, which has both carboxyl and hydroxyl groups, is also thought to affect mineral adsorption. The overall effect (positive or negative) that fiber has on mineral balance depends to some extent on its degree of fermentability or its accessibility to bacterial enzymes in the colon. Microbial proliferation from slowly fermentable fibers may result in increased binding of minerals within the new microbial cells and in the loss of minerals absorbed into the body. In contrast, the more rapidly fermentable fibers appear to have a favorable effect on mineral balance. The acidic environment generated by bacterial fermentation of some fibers is thought to increase mineral solubility, act with calcium to enhance activity of exchange system transporters, or both. Calcium, magnesium, zinc, and iron bound to these fiber components appear to be released as fermentation occurs and may be absorbed in the colon.

The absorption of carotenoids and some phytochemicals may be negatively affected by ingestion of fibers, especially pectin and guar gum. Reductions (33–74%) in the absorption of β-carotene, lycopene, lutein, and canthaxanthin have been demonstrated when pectin or guar gum is added to the diet.

Other bacterial actions, however, may improve phytochemical absorption. For example, polyphenols that are present in the diet as conjugated glycosides may be converted into unconjugated aglycones by bacterial action; the aglycones generated by the gut microbiota are often better absorbed than the initial conjugated form of the polyphenol found in the food. The beneficial effects of phytochemicals to health are discussed in the Perspective at the end of this chapter.

Degradability/Fermentability

Fiber reaches the colon undigested by human digestive enzymes. While both soluble and insoluble fibers can be degraded (fermented) to some extent, soluble fibers are usually fermented by colonic microflora to a greater degree than insoluble fibers. This section discusses first fermentable, then less- or nonfermentable fibers, and their effects on the body.

Fermentable Fibers

Intestinal bacteria utilizing their own enzymes digest the fiber/carbohydrates and other unabsorbed nutrients (such as some proteins or peptides) in a process called fermentation. Fermentation entails a variety of metabolic reactions and processes. Fermentation provides energy and other substances (such as nitrogen) for microbial growth as well as products (such as short-chain fatty acids) that may be used by the human host. Most fermentation occurs in the proximal (upper) colon—that is, by the cecum and in the ascending region of the colon. Fermentation of fiber diminishes as the undigested mass moves through the transverse and descending sections of the colon. The most fermentable of the fibers include fructans, galactooligosaccharides, pectin, gums, psyllium, β-glucans,

polydextrose, resistant dextrins, and RS_3. In addition to these fibers, some hemicelluloses are also fermentable, but their fermentation is much slower than that of the other fibers. Fibers that tend not be fermented include cellulose, carboxymethylcellulose, lignin, waxes, and RS_1.

Fermentable fibers provide many benefits to the body. For example, some fermentable fibers act as prebiotics. Fermentable fibers can also generate short-chain fatty acids for use by the body. Both of these roles are discussed hereafter.

Prebiotics In addition to being degraded by intestinal microflora, many fermentable fibers (but not all) have been shown to function as prebiotics. Prebiotics promote the colonic growth and/or activity of selected health-promoting species of bacteria. The fructans (inulin, oligofructose, and fructooligosaccharides), lactulose (a keto-analogue of lactose that consists of galactosyl β 1-4 fructose), transgalacto-oligosaccharides (a mixture of oligosaccharides derived from lactose), and galactose and soybean oligosaccharides have met the criteria as prebiotics. Galactose oligosaccharides and soybean oligosaccharides include raffinose, stachyose, and verbascose. Raffinose is a trisaccharide of fructose and glucose to which galactose is linked in an α(1–6) glycosidic linkage. Stachyose is similar to raffinose but has an additional galactose molecule, so it is a tetrasaccharide of fructose, glucose, and galactose to which another galactose is linked. Verbascose is an oligosaccharide containing fructose, glucose, and three galactose molecules. These sugars, shown in Figure 4.5, are found in a variety of peas and beans including soybeans, chickpeas, field peas, green peas, lentils, and mung, lima, snap, northern, and navy beans, among others. Galactose oligosaccharides are also found naturally in human milk.

Prebiotics typically stimulate the colonic growth and/or activity of lactobacilli and bifidobacteria, both health-promoting bacteria. The Perspective at the end of this chapter provides more information on the potential health benefits of prebiotics. See Chapter 2 for additional information on intestinal bacteria.

Short-Chain Fatty Acid Generation The principal metabolites of the fermentable fibers are lactic acid and short-chain fatty acids, formerly called volatile fatty acids because of their volatility in acidic aqueous solutions. The short-chain fatty acids include primarily acetic, butyric, and propionic acids. Other products of fiber fermentation are hydrogen, carbon dioxide, and methane gases that are excreted as flatus or expired by the lungs. Different fibers are fermented to different short-chain fatty acids in different amounts by different bacteria. For example, bacteroids that act on pectin generate acetic, propionic, and succinic acids, whereas eubacteria yield acetic, butyric, and lactic acids and bifidobacteria produce acetic and lactic acids from pectin fermentation. Typically, more acetic acid

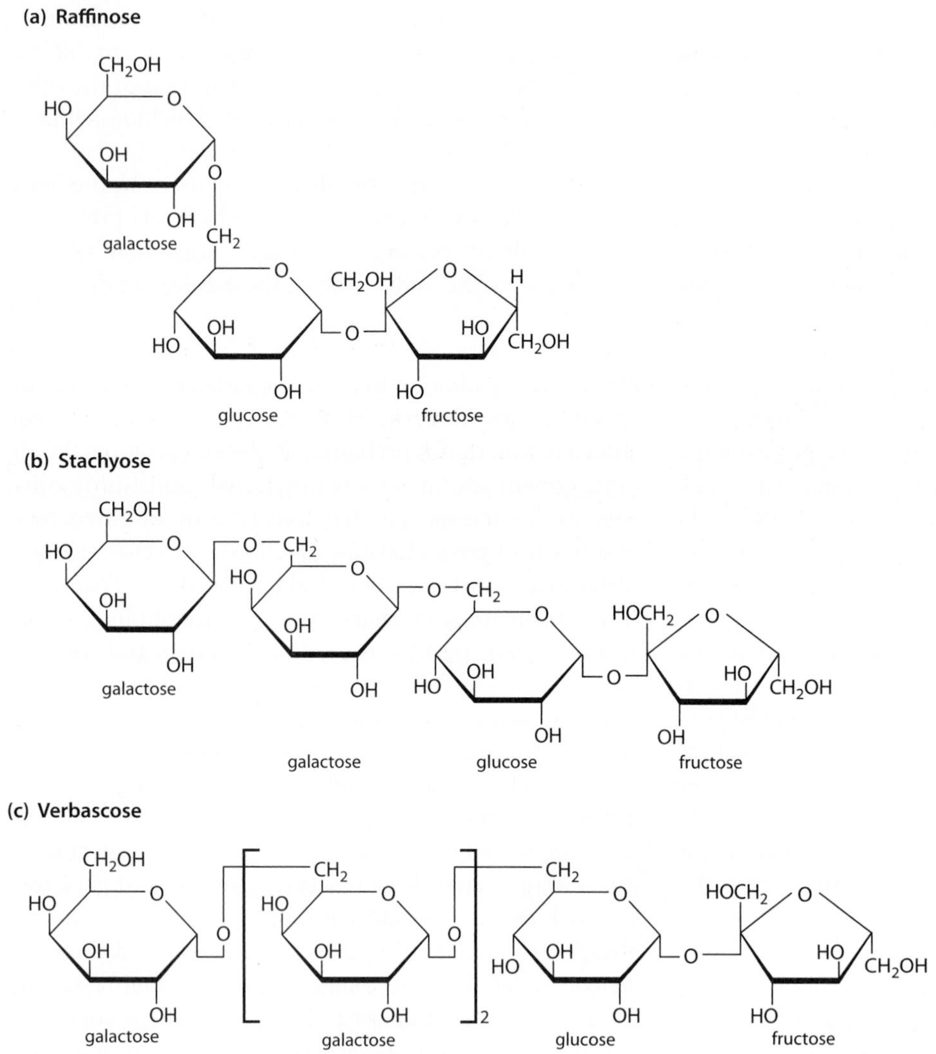

(a) Raffinose

(b) Stachyose

(c) Verbascose

Figure 4.5 Chemical structures of some galactose oligosaccharides that may promote the growth of healthy bacteria in the gastrointestinal tract.

is produced, followed in descending order by propionic acid, then butyric acid. All three of these acids have been shown to play important roles in the gastrointestinal tract, including:

- **Increased water and sodium absorption in the colon**: Short-chain fatty acids produced by fermentation are rapidly absorbed, and their absorption in turn stimulates water and sodium absorption into the mucosal cells of the colon.

- **Mucosal cell differentiation and proliferation**: Short-chain fatty acids generated from the degradation of dietary fiber in the colon stimulate the differentiation and proliferation of mucosal cells of the colon. The mechanism by which this process occurs is not yet understood.

- **Acidification of luminal environment and its effects**: The generation of short-chain fatty acids in the colon from bacterial fiber fermentation results in a decrease

in the pH of the colon's luminal environment. With the more acidic pH, free bile acids become less soluble. Furthermore, the activity of bacterial 7 α dehydroxylase diminishes (optimal pH ~6–6.5) and thus decreases the rate of conversion of primary bile acids to secondary (more cytotoxic) bile acids. With the lower pH, calcium, released with fiber degradation, binds bile and fatty acids. These latter two changes may be protective against colon cancer. In addition, the lower colonic pH favors the growth of beneficial lactobacilli and bifidobacteria and inhibits the growth of pH-sensitive pathogenic bacteria.

- **Provision of energy**: Short-chain fatty acids may be oxidized by the body for energy production; over 95% of the short-chain fatty acids are absorbed and utilized by the body. Short-chain fatty acids are thought to be absorbed into colonic cells by diffusion and/or anion exchange involving sodium and potassium. Butyric acid, and to some extent propionic acid, serves as a major energy source for colonic mucosal cells. In fact, butyric acid is thought to supply colonic cells with over two-thirds of their energy needs. Propionic acid not used by the colonic cells and acetic acid are transported from the colonic cells via the portal vein to the liver. In the liver, propionic acid is largely metabolized along with small amounts of acetic acid. Much of the propionic acid is converted to succinyl-CoA, which may be used by the liver for glucose or energy production. Most of the acetic acid passes through the liver and is used by other tissues, including skeletal and cardiac muscle and the kidneys and brain. Thus, fermentation of carbohydrates by colonic anaerobic bacteria makes available to the body some of the energy contained in undigested food. The exact amount of energy realized depends mostly upon the amount and type of dietary fiber that is ingested. It is estimated that the acids generated from the soluble fibers yield about 1.5 to 2.5 kcal/g; however, the slight decrease in the absorption of macronutrients may cancel out this small amount of energy generated from the short-chain fatty acids [12,13].

- **Inhibition of cholesterol synthesis:** The absorbed propionic acid generated by bacterial fiber fermentation has been shown to inhibit cholesterol synthesis in the liver [8–10]. This effect is thought to contribute in part to the cholesterol-lowering (hypocholesterolemic) effects observed with the ingestion of many soluble, fermentable fibers, as discussed under the subsection "Lowered Serum Cholesterol Concentrations (Hypocholesterolemic Properties)."

- **Improved colonic blood flow:** Short-chain fatty acids, especially propionic and acetic acids, generated by bacterial fiber fermentation improve blood flow in the colon and splanchnic (generally referring to organs in the abdominal cavity such as the liver, spleen, and intestines) region. These fatty acids are thought to directly affect smooth muscle as well as to interact with the enteric (intestinal) nervous system. This improved blood flow enhances both the delivery of nutrients to the colon and the transport of nutrients from the colon to the liver.

- **Enhanced immune function:** From Chapter 2 you may remember that over 50% of the body's lymphocytes as well as many other immune cells are found in the gastrointestinal tract. Short-chain fatty acids from bacterial fermentation are thought to stimulate the production of macrophages, T-helper lymphocytes, neutrophils, and antibodies to enhance immune system function. The acidic environment from the fatty acids also promotes both the growth of healthful bacteria and the production of mucin, which forms part of the physical barrier overlying intestinal cells. This increased mucin content provides a greater physical barrier and decreases the likelihood of pathogenic

bacterial colonization as well as bacterial translocation. Butyric acid appears to enhance cytokine production to augment immune system functions.

- **Trophic effects and prevention of abnormal cell populations:** The presence of butyric and propionic acids in the colon reduces mucosal atrophy. Moreover, these fatty acids, especially butyric acid, promote *in vitro* arrest of growth and differentiation as well as apoptosis in tumor cell lines. Thus, butyric and propionic acids appear to thwart the establishment of abnormal and potentially harmful cell populations.

Nonfermentable Fibers

Fiber components that are poorly or nonfermentable (principally cellulose and lignin, but also plant waxes and some resistant starches) or that are more slowly fermentable (such as some hemicelluloses) are also particularly valuable to colonic health. These fibers move through the gastrointestinal tract virtually unchanged and are excreted in the feces. While degradation of fermentable fibers provides energy for microbial growth, less fermentable or nonfermentable fibers play an important role in detoxification and in increasing fecal volume (bulk), as discussed next.

Detoxification Several attributes of colonic microbes facilitate detoxification. First, microbes can scavenge and sequester harmful substances such as nitrogenous wastes and toxins. For example, insoluble fibers may adsorb hydrophobic carcinogens to prevent their interaction with the colonic mucosa. Secondly, colonic bacteria or short-chain fatty acids from bacterial fermentation inhibit proliferation of tumor cells and delay tumor formation. Lastly, some bacteria, such as *Lactobacillus acidophilus*, may be able to inhibit the production of carcinogenic compounds.

Increased Fecal Volume (Bulk) In addition to its detoxifying role, fiber may promote increased fecal volume or bulk (i.e., stool mass). Fecal bulk consists of unfermented fiber, salts, water, and bacterial mass. In general, fecal bulk increases with increased bacterial proliferation. This increase occurs not only because of the mass of the bacteria but also because bacteria are about 80% water. Thus, with increased fecal bacteria present, mass increases, and so does the water-holding capacity of the feces.

In general, fecal bulk increases as fiber fermentability decreases. The rapidly fermentable fibers, such as pectins, gums, and β-glucans, appear to have little effect on fecal bulk but do provide degradation products to promote bacterial proliferation. Wheat bran is one of the most effective fiber laxatives because it can absorb three times its weight of water, thereby producing a bulky stool. Gastrointestinal responses to wheat bran as well as rice bran include increased fecal bulk, greater frequency of defecation, reduced (quicker) intestinal transit time, and decreased intraluminal pressure. Other fibers that have been shown to increase fecal bulk and decrease stool transit time to improve laxation include cellulose, psyllium, inulin, and oligosaccharides.

ROLES OF FIBER IN DISEASE PREVENTION AND MANAGEMENT

Diets rich in fiber are beneficial to varying degrees in the prevention and/or management of several health problems. In fact, a recent study examining fiber intake and total mortality and death found that dietary fiber intake was associated with a significantly lowered total risk of death in both men and women, and it lowered the risk of death from cardiovascular, infectious, and respiratory diseases by 24% to 56% in men and 34% to 59% in women [14]. Several systematic reviews and meta-analyses have been conducted to examine the relationships between intake of fiber and disease as well as between the intake of foods rich in fiber (most commonly whole grains or fruits and vegetables) and disease. The reviews and meta-analyses utilized a variety of studies (e.g., epidemiological studies, prospective cohort studies, and randomized controlled trials). Some of the results from such analyses are presented in the next four subsections.

Cardiovascular Disease

The ability of soluble fibers to lower serum cholesterol (i.e., exert a hypocholesterolemic effect), especially in those with high serum cholesterol concentrations, is beneficial since hypercholesterolemia is a risk factor for heart disease. However, it is not just the soluble fibers that are beneficial. While ingesting foods rich in insoluble fibers, such as corn, wheat, or rice bran, has been found to be less effective in lowering serum lipids, diets rich in whole grains (and thus also insoluble fibers) have been found to be generally protective against risk for heart disease [6,8,15,16]. High fiber intakes also have been associated both with lower blood pressure readings and with reductions in blood pressure among those with hypertension, a risk factor for heart disease [17–19]. The report of the Dietary Guidelines Advisory Committee states that there is a moderate body of evidence that dietary fiber from whole foods protects against cardiovascular disease [20]. Consistent evidence also has been reported for a moderate inverse relationship between intake of fruits and vegetables (primarily greater than five servings per day) and heart attack and stroke [20].

Diabetes Mellitus

The viscous gels formed with the ingestion of many of the soluble fibers also benefit those with diabetes mellitus [6,8,21]. Ingestion of diets rich in such fibers or of fiber supplements has been shown to improve glycemic control, largely through reduced rates of glucose absorption and insulin secretion, as well as improved insulin sensitivity. However, the Dietary Guidelines Advisory Committee [20] as well as others [6,22] consider the evidence for fiber's effectiveness limited. Evidence for a link between fruit and vegetable consumption and the development of type 2 diabetes is also considered limited and inconsistent [20].

Obesity and Weight Control

A generous fiber intake appears to have some benefits in terms of weight control. Fiber-rich foods tend to have a lower energy density and a higher volume, which can promote satiety. Moreover, high-fiber foods may reduce hunger (possibly through effects on satiety-inducing hormones such as glucagon-like peptide 1, ghrelin, and peptide YY) while simultaneously delaying gastric emptying and somewhat reducing nutrient utilization [6]. It has been generally concluded that it is of benefit to consume a high-fiber diet, a diet rich in whole grains, or fiber supplements for weight management. Additional studies also support reductions in body fat and waist circumference with high fiber intakes [23,24].

Gastrointestinal Disorders

An inadequate intake of fiber has been associated with several gastrointestinal conditions and disorders, including diverticular disease, constipation, and colon cancer. Diverticular disease has been frequently linked to diets low in fiber, and individuals with the condition are advised to consume diets rich in insoluble fiber [25,26]. Diverticula, protruding or bulging pouches of the wall of the colon, are thought to form when the colon's wall weakens. This weakening may result from years of constipation associated with low fecal bulk and straining to pass the hard fecal matter. (The straining increases the pressure inside the colon and weakens its walls.) When fecal matter becomes trapped in the diverticula, the pouches become inflamed (called diverticulitis) and the person experiences pain and sometimes fever, diarrhea, gastrointestinal bleeding, and infection. High-fiber (especially insoluble fiber) diets increase stool weight and fecal bulk to reduce straining and intra-colonic pressure; the increased fecal bulk also reduces the likelihood of fecal matter becoming trapped in the diverticula. Wheat bran, along with psyllium and cellulose, is especially effective at increasing fecal weight. However, whether a high-fiber diet reduces the likelihood of formation of new diverticula once the condition has developed is unclear [6].

The ability of insoluble fiber to increase stool weight and speed up (shorten) transit time may benefit those with constipation. Use of supplements or products such as Metamucil that are rich in psyllium is advocated for the treatment and prevention of constipation. Reviews of the literature, however, have not found sufficient evidence to formulate recommendations on fiber intakes needed for optimal gastrointestinal tract laxation function [6,20].

Risk of colon cancer may also be diminished by ingestion of fiber-rich diets (whole grains, fruits, and vegetables); however, evidence is limited [20,27–30]. Some of the many mechanisms of action that have been proposed for fiber's preventive role against colon cancer include:

- Fibers that adsorb primary bile acids to promote their fecal excretion exert a protective effect by decreasing their free concentration and availability for conversion to more harmful (carcinogenic) secondary bile acids.
- Fiber fermentation to short-chain fatty acids decreases the interluminal pH, which also decreases the conversion of primary bile acids (cholic acid and chenodeoxycholic acid) to secondary bile acids (such as deoxycholic acid and lithocholic acid), which have been shown to promote tumor generation.
- Fibers that increase fecal bulk decrease the intraluminal concentrations of procarcinogens and carcinogens and thereby reduce the likelihood of carcinogens interacting with colonic mucosal cells.
- Provision of a fermentable substrate to colonic bacteria alters bacteria species and numbers, which may inhibit proliferation or development of tumor cells or conversion of procarcinogens to carcinogens.
- A shortened fecal transit time decreases the time during which toxins can be synthesized and in which they are in contact with the colon.
- Fermentation of fiber may release fiber-bound calcium. The increased calcium in the colon may help eliminate the mitogenic advantage that cancer cells have over normal cells in a low-calcium environment.
- Butyric acid may slow the proliferation and differentiation of colon cancer cells.
- Insoluble fibers that resist degradation bind carcinogens, thereby minimizing the chances of interactions with colonic mucosal cells.

Unfortunately, not all studies have shown diminished risk of colon cancer with consumption of high-fiber diets. Further, intervention studies, such as the Polyp Prevention Trial, also have not found beneficial effects from ingestion of fiber-rich diets, as reviewed by Slavin [6] and others [20]. Enhanced development of colorectal cancers associated with high-fiber diets has been attributed to: (1) soluble fibers reducing the ability of insoluble fibers to adsorb hydrophobic carcinogens, and thus potentially allowing more carcinogens to enter the colon maintained in solution than adsorbed onto insoluble fibers; (2) the increased presence of carcinogens generated and deposited on the colonic mucosal surface following the degradation of soluble fibers; (3) soluble fibers crossing the intestinal epithelium and transporting with them carcinogens maintained in solution; and (4) soluble fibers reducing the reabsorption of primary bile salts and thereby increasing the chance for conversion to cytotoxic secondary bile acids [27–30].

Overall, little agreement exists among the numerous studies designed to determine the effects of fiber in the development, prevention, and/or treatment of colon cancer. While most of the evidence for the positive role of fiber in colon cancer prevention has come from epidemiological observations, variations in dietary factors (such as energy, protein, fat, vitamin D, calcium, and antioxidants) other than fiber intake have been noted in these studies and make interpretation of the findings difficult.

HEALTH CLAIMS AND FOOD LABELS

The Food and Drug Administration (FDA) has approved several health claims related to fiber. The claims typically focus on fruits, vegetables, and grain products. For example, for one claim, the food requirements include fruits, vegetables, or grain products that are low in fat and a good source of dietary fiber without fortification. An example of such a claim is "Low fat diets rich in fiber-containing grain products, fruits and vegetables may reduce the risk of some types of cancer, a disease associated with many factors" [4]. Another sample claim for fruits, vegetables, and grain products that are low in fat (saturated and total) and cholesterol and contain at least 0.6 g of soluble fiber per reference amount without fortification is "Diets low in saturated fat and cholesterol and rich in fruits and vegetables and grain products that contain some types of dietary fiber, particularly soluble fiber, may reduce the risk of heart disease, a disease associated with many factors" [4]. Another model claim—"Low fat diets rich in fruits and vegetables (foods that are low in fat and may contain dietary fiber, vitamin A, or vitamin C) may reduce the risk of some types of cancer, a disease associated with many factors"—has also been approved for fruits and vegetables that are a good source of vitamin A or C, or dietary fiber [4]. A fourth claim is associated with β-glucan from oat bran (containing at least 5.5% of β-glucan soluble fiber), rolled oats or oatmeal (containing at least 4% of β-glucan soluble fiber), whole oat flour (providing at least 4% of β-glucan soluble fiber), or psyllium husk with a purity of no less than 95%. An example related to this claim is

"Soluble fiber from foods such as [name of soluble fiber source and food product], as part of a diet low in saturated fat and cholesterol, may reduce the risk of heart disease. A serving of [name of food product] supplies [amount] grams of the [necessary daily dietary intake for the benefit] soluble fiber from [name of soluble fiber source] necessary per day to have this effect" [4]. The latter phrase (*as part of a diet low in saturated fat and cholesterol*) was included because the effects of soluble fiber on heart disease are thought to be less significant than the effects of a low–saturated fat diet.

The recommendation for fiber provided on the Nutrition Facts panel on foods is 25 g of dietary fiber for a 2,000-kcal diet. The dietary fiber content of foods is listed on the Nutrition Facts panel along with total carbohydrate, sugars, and other carbohydrate. Some food labels also provide a breakdown of the product's dietary fiber content into soluble and insoluble fibers. For example, the label on a box of raisin bran cereal might show that a serving (1 cup) provides 7 g of dietary fiber, with 6 g listed as insoluble and 1 g listed as soluble. Foods may be noted as an "excellent source of fiber" by the manufacturer if a serving of the food provides at least 20% of recommendations—that is, 0.20 × 25 g or 5 g of fiber. Foods may be considered a "good source of fiber" if they provide 10% of recommendations or 2.5 g of fiber/serving.

RECOMMENDED FIBER INTAKE

Recommendations for increasing the amount of fiber in the U.S. diet have come from several governmental and private organizations, each with a concern for improving the health of Americans [1,6,30–32]. The Dietary Guidelines suggest that Americans ingest 14 g of fiber per 1,000 kcal. In 2002, the National Academy of Sciences Food and Nutrition Board established Dietary Reference Intakes, specifically Adequate Intakes (AI), for fiber. Adequate Intakes of total fiber, representing the sum of dietary fiber and functional fiber, were established based upon amounts of fiber shown to protect against heart disease [1]. The recommendations for fiber intake for adults and children are shown in Table 4.3. Unfortunately, most Americans consume only about 15 g of fiber each day [1].

No Tolerable Upper Intake Level for dietary fiber or functional fiber has been established [1]. Tolerance to dietary fiber varies from person to person. The most common complaints with "over" consumption include abdominal discomfort, bloating, gas, and altered stool output. Ingestion of fiber in amounts greater than about 50 g may be considered excessive, at least in the United States.

Table 4.3 Recommended Fiber Intakes [1]

Population Group	Age (years)	Total Fiber (g)
Men	19 to 50	38
	≥ 51	31
Women	19 to 50	25
	≥ 51	21
Children	1 to 3	19
	4 to 8	25
Girls	9 to 18	26
Boys	9 to 13	31
	14 to 18	38

Dietary changes encouraged to accomplish an adequate fiber intake include the ingestion of:

- fiber-rich legumes
- at least 4½ cups of fruits and vegetables per day
- at least 3 ounces per day of whole grains

These recommendations are consistent with the U.S. Department of Agriculture's (USDA's) MyPlate [32].

Notice that recommendations that fiber intake be increased are interpreted in terms of dietary change rather than the addition to the diet of fiber supplements, which more than likely are devoid of other nutrients. It remains important to eat a variety of cereals, legumes, fruits, and vegetables so that variety in dietary fibers is maximized.

Table 4.4 shows the dietary fiber content of selected foods. A quick method for calculating typical dietary fiber intakes enables assessment in a clinical setting from a food history, 24-hour diet recall, or food record without using tables or computerized diet analysis programs. Because fiber-rich foods consist primarily of fruits, vegetables, grains, legumes, nuts, and seeds, the number of servings from each of these groups can be multiplied by the mean total fiber content of each food group [33]. For example, numbers of servings (size determined from the USDA data or food label) of fruits (not including juices) and vegetables are each multiplied by 1.5 g. The 1.5 g represents the average amount of dietary fiber per serving of fruit and per serving of vegetable. Numbers of servings of refined grains are multiplied by 1.0 g, and numbers of servings of whole grains are multiplied by 2.5 g. The totals from each of the four categories are summed and added to food-specific fiber values for legumes, nuts, seeds, and concentrated fiber sources; food-specific fiber values are obtained from databases [33]. The values calculated using this quick method are within 10% of the results obtained by looking up each individual food's fiber content [33].

Table 4.4 Dietary Fiber Content of Selected Foods* [34,35]

Food Group	Soluble Fiber (g / 100 g)	Insoluble Fiber (g / 100 g)	Total	Food Group	Soluble Fiber (g / 100 g)	Insoluble Fiber (g / 100 g)	Total
Fruits (raw)				Vegetables (cooked)			
Apple with skin	0.70	2.00	2.70	Asparagus			2.0
Banana	0.58	1.21	1.79	Broccoli	1.85	2.81	4.66
Grapes	0.24	0.36	0.60	Carrots	1.58	2.29	3.87
Mango	0.69	1.08	1.76	Cauliflower	0.70	3.50	4.20
Orange	1.37	0.99	2.35	Corn			2.0
Peach with skin	1.31	1.54	2.85	Lettuce (raw)			1.3
Pear with skin	0.92	2.25	3.16	Mushrooms			2.4
Pineapple	0.04	1.42	1.46	Potato baked			
Plum with skin	1.12	1.76	2.88	with skin	0.61	1.70	2.31
Strawberries	0.60	1.70	2.30	boiled, no skin	0.99	1.06	2.05
Watermelon	0.13	0.27	0.40	Grain and Grain Products			
Legumes/Beans (cooked)				Rice			
Black			8.7	white			0.3
Kidney	1.36	5.77	7.13	brown			1.8
Lima	1.02	4.21	5.23	Couscous			2.8
Navy			10.5	Bread			
Pinto	0.99	5.66	6.65	white			2.4
Nuts				whole grain			6.8
Almonds			12.3	Crackers (wheat)			10.6
Cashews			3.2	Cereals (cold)			
Pecans			9.6	All Bran			29.3
Peanuts			8.1	Raisin Bran			11.1
Walnuts			6.7	Corn Flakes			2.5
				Cheerios			10

*Soluble and insoluble fiber contents provided when available.

SUMMARY

Definitions have now been established for dietary and functional fibers. Dietary fibers are nondigestible carbohydrates and lignin that are intact and intrinsic in plants. Examples of dietary fibers include cellulose, hemicellulose, lignin, pectin, gums, β-glucans, fructans, and resistant starches. Functional fibers are nondigestible carbohydrates that have been isolated, extracted, or manufactured; they have been shown to have beneficial physiological effects in humans. Note that functional fibers, unlike dietary fibers, do not have to be intact or intrinsic only to plants. Functional fibers shown to have beneficial effects are cellulose, pectins, gums, β-glucans, psyllium, and resistant starches. Other fibers, including lignin, fructans, chitin, chitosan, polydextrose, polyols, and resistant dextrins, require additional studies.

The physiological effects of fiber in the gastrointestinal tract are as varied as the number of fiber components and are determined to a large extent by the types and amounts present. Some of the many characteristics of dietary and functional fibers shown to be beneficial include water-holding/hydration capacity and viscosity, adsorption or binding ability, and degradation/fermentability. To obtain fiber through the diet, food sources of fiber need to be varied and complementary. Assurance of a good intake of fiber requires consumption of a variety of high-fiber foods including whole-grain cereals and breads, legumes, fruits, and vegetables.

References Cited

1. Food and Nutrition Board. Dietary Reference Intakes for Energy, Carbohydrate, Fiber, Fat, Protein and Amino Acids. Washington DC: National Academy of Sciences, 2002.

2. Begum AN, Nicolle C, Mila I, et al. Dietary lignins are precursors of mammalian lignans in rats. J Nutr. 2004; 134:120–27.

3. Hogarth AJ, Hunter DE, Jacobs WA, et al. Ion chromatographic determination of three fructooligosaccharide oligomers in prepared and preserved foods. J Agric Food Chem. 2000; 48:5326–30.

4. FDA Food Guidance, Compliance and Regulatory Information. http://www.fda.gov/Food/GuidanceComplianceRegulatoryInformation/GuidanceDocuments/FoodLabelingNutrition/FoodLabelingGuide/ucm064919.htm

5. Cummings JH, Stephen AM. Carbohydrate terminology and classification. Eur J Clin Nutr. 2007; 61(suppl 1):S5–18.

6. Slavin JL. Position of the American Dietetic Association: health implications of dietary fiber. J Am Diet Assoc. 2008; 108:1716–31.

7. D'Alessio D. Glucagon-like peptide 1 (GLP-1) in diabetes and aging. J Anti-Aging Med. 2000; 3:329–33.

8. Anderson JW, Baird P, Davis RH, et al. Health benefits of dietary fiber. Nutr Rev. 2009; 67:188–205.

9. Lin Y, Vonk RJ, Stooff MJ, et al. Differences in propionate–induced inhibition of cholesterol and triacylglycerol synthesis between human and rat hepatocytes in primary culture. Brit J Nutr. 1995; 74:197–207.

10. Wright RS, Anderson JW, Bridges SR. Propionate inhibits hepatocyte lipid synthesis. Proc Soc Exp Biol Med. 1990; 195:26–29.

11. Moruisi K, Oosthuizen W, Opperman A. Phytosterols/stanols lower cholesterol concentrations in familial hypercholesterolemic subjects: a systematic review with meta-analysis. J Am Coll Nutr. 2006; 25:41–48.

12. Livesey G. Energy values of unavailable carbohydrate and diets: an inquiry and analysis. Am J Clin Nutr. 1990; 51:617–37.

13. Smith T, Brown JC, Livesey G. Energy balance and thermogenesis in rats consuming nonstarch polysaccharides of various fermentabilities. Am J Clin Nutr. 1998; 68:802–19.

14. Park Y, Subar AF, Hollenbeck A, Schatzkin A. Dietary fiber intake and mortality in the NIH-AARP diet and health study. Arch Intern Med. 2011; 171:1061–68.

15. Anderson JW. Whole grains protect against atherosclerotic cardiovascular disease. Proc Nutr Soc. 2003; 62:135–42.

16. Fardet A. New hypotheses for the health-protective mechanisms of whole-grain cereals: what is beyond fibre? Nutr Res Rev. 2010; 23:65–134.

17. Streppel MT, Arends LR, Veer P, et al. Dietary fiber and blood pressure: a meta-analysis of randomized placebo-controlled trials. Arch Intern Med. 2005; 165:150–56.

18. Whelton SP, Hyre AD, Pedersen B, et al. Effect of dietary fiber intake on blood pressure: a meta-analysis of randomized controlled clinical trials. J Hypertension. 2005; 23:475–81.

19. Flint AJ, Hu FB, Glynn RJ, et al. Whole grains and incident hypertension in men. Am J Clin Nutr. 2009; 90:493–98.

20. Report of the Dietary Guidelines Advisory Committee for the Dietary Guidelines for Americans 2010. http://www.cnpp.usda.gov/DGAs2010-DGACReport.htm. Accessed March 22, 2011.

21. Hopping BN, Erber E, Grandinetti A, et al. Dietary fiber, magnesium, and glycemic load after risk of type 2 diabetes in a multiethnic cohort in Hawaii. J Nutr. 2010; 140:68–74.

22. Franz MJ, Powers MA, Leontos C, et al. The evidence for medical nutrition therapy for type 1 and type 2 diabetes in adults. J Am Diet Assoc. 2010; 110:1852–89.

23. Du H, van der A DL, Boshuizen HC, et al. Dietary fiber and subsequent changes in body weight and waist circumference in European men and women. Am J Clin Nutr. 2010; 91:329–36.

24. Tucker LA, Thomas KS. Increasing total fiber intake reduces risk of weight and fat gains in women. J Nutr. 2009; 139:576–81.

25. Frieri G, Pimpo MT, Scarpignato C. Management of colonic diverticular disease. Digestion. 2006; 73(suppl 1):S58–66.

26. Eglash A, Lane CH, Schneider DM. Clinical inquiries: what is the most beneficial diet for patients with diverticulosis? J Fam Pract. 2006; 55:813–15.

27. Bingham SA, Day NE, Luben R, et al. Dietary fibre in food and protection against colorectal cancer in the European Prospective Investigation into Cancer and Nutrition (EPIC): an observational study. Lancet. 2003; 361:1496–1501.

28. Schatzkin A, Houw T, Park Y, et al. Dietary fiber and whole-grain consumption in relation to colorectal cancer in the NIH-AARP Diet and Health Study. Am J Clin Nutr. 2007; 85:1353–60.

29. Trock B, Lanza E, Greenwald P. Dietary fiber, vegetables, and colon cancer: critical review and meta-analyses of the epidemiologic evidence. J Natl Cancer Inst. 1990; 82:650–61.

30. Kushi LH, Byers T, Doyle C, et al. The American Cancer Society 2006 guidelines on nutrition and physical activity for cancer prevention: reducing the risk of cancer with healthy food choices and physical activity. Cancer J Clin. 2006; 56:254–81.

31. American Diabetes Association. Nutrition recommendations and interventions for diabetes. Diabetes Care. 2008; 31(suppl):S61–78.

32. U.S. Department of Agriculture MyPlate. U.S. Department of Agriculture. http://www.choosemyplate.gov/

33. Marlett JA, Cheung TF. Database and quick methods of assessing typical dietary fiber intakes using 228 commonly consumed foods. J Am Diet Assoc. 1997; 97:1139–48, 1151.

34. Li BW, Andrews KW, Pehrsson PR. Individual sugars, soluble and insoluble dietary fiber contents of 70 high consumption foods. J Food Comp & Anal. 2002; 15: 715–23.

35. U.S. Department of Agriculture Nutrient Data Laboratory. www.nal.usda.gov/fnic/foodcomp/search

PHYTOCHEMICALS AND HERBAL SUPPLEMENTS IN HEALTH AND DISEASE

Chapter 4 described some of the valuable properties of fiber that make it an important part of the diet. Yet, plant foods that are rich in fiber are also rich in thousands of phytochemicals. These Phytochemicals are themselves also a valuable dietary component. This Perspective reviews some of the active ingredients—that is, the phytochemicals—in herbs (as well as in many other plant foods) and provides an overview of some of the more common herbal supplements used to maintain health and treat disease.

Over the past decade the market for herbal supplements in the United States has exploded, bringing in several billion dollars per year in sales of the more than 500 herbs being marketed. The public's enthusiasm stems from a number of purported benefits of the use of various herbs (plants or particular parts of a plant such as the leaf, stem, root, bark, seed, flower, etc.). Some of the top-selling herbs in America include echinacea, ginseng, ginkgo biloba, garlic, saw palmetto, and milk thistle. The supposed benefits derived from the use of these herbs range from improved memory to relief from ailments such as depression or the common cold.

PHYTOCHEMICALS

Phytochemicals consist of a large group of nonnutrient compounds that are biologically active in the body. As implied by the name, phytochemicals are found in plants, including fruits, vegetables, legumes, grains, herbs, tea, and spices. Of the tens of thousands of phytochemicals, polyphenolic phytochemicals make up the largest group. Dietary intake of polyphenols is estimated at about 1 g/day in the United States.

The polyphenols, which include more than 8,000 compounds, can be divided into a variety of classes. One of the largest of these classes is the flavonoids, which includes several subclasses—flavonols, flavanols, flavones, flavanones, anthocyanidins, and isoflavones. Table 1 provides a list of the flavonoid subclasses along with food sources. In the flavonol subclass, the main flavonols include quercetin and kaempferol. These flavonols are widely found in foods, but the best sources of quercetin and kaempferol are onions, kale, leeks, broccoli, apples, blueberries, red wine, tea, and the herb ginkgo biloba. Flavanols, another subclass, are typically categorized based upon chemical structure. Monomer forms are called catechins, and condensed forms are called proanthocyanins or tannins. Tannins provide astringent properties to foods and beverages. Flavanol intake has been estimated at 20 to 60 mg/day in the United States [1]. Another category of flavonoids are flavones such as luteolin and apigenin; only

a few foods, parsley and some cereals, have been identified as rich sources of these flavones. The flavanones, another subgroup of the flavonoids, also consist of a just a few compounds: glycosides of naringenin in grapefruits, eriodictyol in lemons, and hesperetin in oranges. A glass of fruit juice such as orange juice is thought to provide about 40 to 140 mg of flavanone glycosides. Another flavonoid group is the anthocyanidins, the aglycone (unconjugated) form of anthocyanins. Anthocyanins are plant pigments found mostly in the skin of plants. Anthocyanins provide color (usually red, blue, or purple) to many fruits and vegetables. A 100 g serving of berries can provide up to 500 mg anthocyanins [1]. A final category of flavonoids listed in Table 1 is the isoflavones, which are found mostly in legumes, especially soybeans and their products. Isoflavones, along with lignans (found in seeds, whole grains, nuts, and some fruits and vegetables) and coumestans (found in broccoli and sprouts) are phytoestrogens. The two main plant isoflavones are genistein and daidzein.

The flavonoid group represents one class among the thousands of phytochemicals found in foods. Some additional phytochemicals are listed in Table 2, along with some of their food sources; these include phenolic acids, carotenoids (see also Chapter 10), terpenes, organosulphides, phytosterols, glucosinolates, and isothiocyanates, among others. Interest in the phenolic acid category has grown with the rise in coffee consumption in the United States and studies suggesting phenolic compounds exhibit bacteriostatic or antimicrobial activities (in other words, they are capable of inhibiting the growth of bacteria and microbial activities). Coffee is a rich source of phenolic acids that are typically categorized as either derivatives of hydroxybenzoic acid or hydroxycinnamic acid. Caffeic, ferulic, p-coumaric, and sinapic acids make up the main dietary hydroxycinnamic acids.

Caffeic and ferulic acids are thought to be more commonly consumed than the others, and estimated intake of the two acids is thought to be between 500 and 1,000 mg/day, especially among coffee drinkers [1]. Hydroxycinnamic acids also are found in other foods including vegetables, grains (outer layers), and fruits (especially blueberries, tomatoes, kiwis, plums, cherries, and apples). Examples of hydroxybenzoic acids include ellagic and gallic acids, which are found in especially high concentrations in red wine, tea, nuts, and berries.

Although Tables 1 and 2 provide examples of foods containing some phytochemicals, note that most plant foods contain multiple phytochemicals. Tomatoes, for example, may contain as many as 10,000 different phytochemicals. In addition, the phytochemicals' composition, digestibility, and absorbability can vary with the plant species, climate or environmental conditions in which the plant was grown, the plant's stage of ripeness, and the methods of storing and processing the plant, among other factors.

Most phytochemicals are found in foods in a variety of forms, and these forms influence the digestion and the absorption of the phytochemical. One common form of polyphenols in foods is as a glycoside conjugate. Some glycosides must be digested to aglycones (unconjugated forms) before being absorbed. Other phytochemicals are thought to be absorbed from the small intestine without extensive digestion. Further, many phytochemical glycosides are neither digested nor absorbed in the small intestine. The mechanisms for the absorption of most phytochemicals are thought to involve a carrier; however, the complete absorptive processes have not been elucidated. Some phytochemicals that are not absorbed in the small intestine have been shown to undergo degradation by colonic microflora. The bacteria hydrolyze the glycosides, generating aglycones that may undergo further

Table 1 Flavonoid Phytochemicals and Their Sources

Flavonoid Subclass	Phytochemicals	Sources
Flavonols	Quercetin, kaempferol, myricetin	Onions, tea, olives, kale, leaf lettuce, cranberries, tomatoes, apples, turnip greens, endive, ginkgo biloba
Flavanols	Catechins, epicatechins	Green tea, pears, wine, apples
Flavones	Apigenin, luteolin	Parsley, some cereals
Flavanones	Tangeritin, naringenin, hesperitin, hesperedin	Citrus fruits
Anthocyanidins	Cyanidin	Berries, cherries, plums, red wine
Isoflavones	Genistein, daidzein, equol	Legumes, especially soybeans, nuts, milk, cheese, flour, tofu, miso, soy sauce

Table 2 Phytochemicals and Their Sources

Phytochemical Class	Phytochemicals	Sources
Carotenoids	β-carotene, α-carotene, lutein, lycopene	Tomatoes, pumpkins, squash, carrots, watermelon, papayas, guavas
Terpenes	Limonene, carvone	Citrus fruits, cherries, ginkgo biloba
Organosulphides	Diallyl sulphide, allyl methyl sulphide, S-allylcysteine	Garlic, onions, leeks, cruciferous vegetables: broccoli, cabbage, Brussels sprouts, mustard, watercress
Phenolic acids	Hydroxycinnamic acids: caffeic, ferulic, chlorogenic, neochlorogenic curcumin	Blueberries, cherries, pears, apples, oranges, grapefruit, white potatoes, coffee beans, St. John's wort, echinacea
	Hydroxybenzoic acids: ellagic, gallic	Raspberries, strawberries, grape juice
Lignans	Secoisolariciresinol, mataresinol	Berries, flaxseed/oil, nuts, rye bran
Saponins	Panaxadiol, panaxatriol	Alfalfa sprouts, potatoes, tomatoes, ginseng
Phytosterols	β-sitosterol, campesterol, stigmasterol	Vegetable oils (soy, rapeseed, corn, sunflower)
Glucosinolates	Glucobrassicin, gluconapin, sinigrin, glucoiberin	Cruciferous vegetables (see above)
Isothiocyanates	Allylisothiocyanates, indoles	Cruciferous vegetables (see above)

metabolism to form various aromatic acids and may also affect the absorption of other phytochemicals.

Once absorbed, most polyphenolic metabolites are conjugated in the small intestine or liver. Conjugation usually involves methylation, sulfation, or glucuronidation. These conjugated metabolites are then transported in the blood bound to plasma proteins like albumin. The amount of the metabolites present in the plasma varies considerably with the type of polyphenolic phytochemical consumed, the food source, and the amount ingested, but little is known about the metabolism of all the different polyphenols in the body, and thus about what metabolites are present in the plasma after consumption of a specific polyphenol.

These differences in the metabolism of the thousands of phytochemicals in the body complicate the interpretation of research studies and the ability to make recommendations. Most studies have been done *in vitro*, in cultured cells, or in isolated tissues using specific glycosides or aglycone forms of the various phytochemicals. The forms of the polyphenolic phytochemicals used in the studies, however, have not been the same as the forms in which the polyphenolic phytochemicals are found in the body. Moreover, the amounts or concentrations of the phytochemical used in the studies have often been much higher than the amounts of the phytochemicals found naturally in the body.

Despite the problems with many of the studies, phytochemicals are strongly believed to play several important roles in the body. Flavonoids, for example, are found in cell membranes between the aqueous and lipid bilayers, where they exhibit antioxidant functions. Specifically, flavonoids can scavenge free radicals such as hydroxyl, peroxyl, alkyl peroxyl, and superoxide and can terminate chain reactions (see the Perspective in Chapter 10 for a discussion of free radicals and termination). Two characteristics determine whether a flavonoid is a good antioxidant: first, its ability to

donate a hydrogen atom from its phenolic hydroxyl group to the free radical (similar to vitamin E), and second, the ability of its phenolic ring to stabilize the unpaired electron. Antioxidant activity is also exhibited by polyphenols other than flavonoids and by lignans (found in a variety of plant foods), carotenoids (found in brightly colored fruits and vegetables), and resveratrol (found in grapes and peanuts). Because of these antioxidant functions, phytochemicals may potentially decrease the risk of cancer and of LDL cholesterol oxidation, which is associated with the development of atherosclerosis. The phytochemical-induced enhanced endothelial function and reduced platelet aggregation and adhesion may also diminish the risk of atherosclerosis and blood clot formation. Flavonoid consumption also has been suggested to lower the risk of developing diabetes mellitus.

In addition to antioxidant roles, some lignans and isoflavones exhibit antiestrogenic effects. Phytoestrogens such as the isoflavones are structurally similar to estrogen in that the phenol ring can bind to estrogen receptors on body cells. Soy products, rich in isoflavones, have been marketed for use by women during perimenopause to help alleviate some of the side effects of diminished natural estrogen in the body. In addition, the isoflavone genestein, along with lignans and some other flavonoids, has been shown to inhibit tumor formation and proliferation. Thus, teas (black and green) that are particularly rich in flavonoids are enjoying increased popularity. Glucosinolates and isothiocyanates, along with terpenes and some phenolic acids such as hydroxycinnamic acid, also appear to have some protective effects against cancer (tumor formation), and phytosterols and isoflavones exhibit cholesterol-lowering effects that may be protective against heart disease. In fact, soy products rich in isoflavones and margarines with added phytosterols are being marketed for use in the diets of people with hypercholesterolemia. Although much additional research is needed, studies strongly

suggest possible roles for phytochemicals in the prevention of cardiovascular disease, cancers, and osteoporosis.

Herbs are also rich sources of many phytochemicals. They have been used for decades, and sometimes centuries, in Asia and other parts of the world to prevent and treat a variety of health problems. The purported benefits of six commonly used herbs—echinacea, garlic, ginkgo biloba, ginseng, milk thistle, and St. John's wort—are discussed in the following sections.

ECHINACEA

Echinacea is derived from a native North American plant species characterized by spiny cone flowering heads, similar in appearance to the daisy. Three types of echinacea, *Echinacea angustifolia, E. pallida,* and *E. purpurea,* are available commercially. Several parts of the plant, including the roots, flowers (tops), or leaves either alone or in combination, are used in the preparation of dietary echinacea supplements. Liquid alcohol–based extracts of the roots (*E. angustifolia*) or the expressed juice of the aerial portion (*E. purpurea*) are commonly sold forms of the herb.

Several active ingredients are found in echinacea. Some of these are thought to include high-molecular-weight polysaccharides (such as heteroxylans, arabinogalactans, and rhamnogalactans), glycoproteins, flavonoids, alkamides (such as isoburylamide), alkenes, alkynes (such as polyacetylenes), and phenolic acids (caffeic and ferulic acid derivatives such as cichoric acid, echinacosides, and cynarin). One or more of these active ingredients are thought to stimulate components of the immune system. Examples of positive effects on the immune system include increased production of cytokines by macrophages, activation of T-cells, and increased phagocytic activity, among others. Because of these actions, the herb typically is recommended for treating colds, upper respiratory infections, or flulike symptoms. Its topical application also is recommended as an aid in the healing of superficial wounds as well as for psoriasis and eczema. Meta-analyses and reviews of studies examining the effectiveness of echinacea in treating colds and the flu have shown no benefit. A few trials studying the effectiveness of echinacea in treating upper respiratory infections suggest promising but inconclusive results.

Daily doses of the herb usually consist of 500 to 1,000 mg of ground herb or root in tablets or capsules or brewed as a tea, or 0.5 to 4 mL of liquid extracts or tinctures (depending on strength). Dosages are generally divided and ingested two to three times daily. A consecutive maximum limit of echinacea use of 6 to 8 weeks has been suggested, with use for 10 to 14 days thought to be sufficient, as the effectiveness of echinacea is thought to diminish over time. Major side effects from the use of echinacea have not been reported; however, allergic reactions may occur. Echinacea use by people with systemic or immune system dysfunction disorders is contraindicated.

GARLIC

Garlic (*Allium sativum*) is part of the *Liliaceae* family, belonging specifically to the genus *Allium.* Garlic is similar to onions (also members of the *Liliaceae* family), chives, and leeks;

all contain derivatives of the sulfur-containing amino acid cysteine, mainly S-allyl-L-cysteine sulfoxide, also known as *alliin*. Alliin (an odorless compound) may be converted to allicin (diallyldisulfide-S-oxide) in the presence of alliinase, which is exposed when garlic cells are destroyed by cutting or chewing, for example. Allicin degrades to diallyl disulfide, the main component in the odor of garlic, and to ajoene. Allicin-free components from garlic such as aged garlic extract also have been linked with health benefits.

These active components of garlic and garlic extracts (classified as organosulphides) have been shown in various studies to be antilipidemic, antithrombotic, antihypertensive, anticarcinogenic, antiglycemic, antioxidant, and immune enhancing. Meta-analyses of controlled clinical trials suggest (at present) small benefits of garlic primarily as a modest blood lipid–lowering agent (total and LDL cholesterol and triacylglycerols) and as an antithrombotic agent. Garlic has not been shown to decrease cancer risk.

Garlic is available naturally (in bulbs) or in more concentrated form as tablets or capsules. Typical daily dosages of garlic used in the studies ranged from about 600 to 900 mg of powdered garlic per day, or pills standardized to 0.6% to 1.3% allicin, equivalent to about 1.8 to 2.7 g or one-half to one clove of fresh garlic. Standardization, however, should not be based on allicin. In fact, commercial garlic preparations often do not contain garlic's active compounds. Garlic cloves, for example, contain about 0.8% alliin; however, little alliin may be retained in the making of garlic powder. Losses of allicin to varying degrees also occur. Side effects most commonly associated with garlic consumption include unpleasant body and breath odor, heartburn, flatulence, and other gastrointestinal tract problems. People taking aspirin or who are on anticoagulant therapies typically should avoid eating large amounts of garlic.

GINKGO BILOBA

Ginkgo biloba, from the *Ginkgoaceae* family, is a tall, long-living (as long as 1,000 years), deciduous tree with gray-colored bark. The tree is native to China and was introduced into North America in the 18th century. The fan-shaped leaves of ginkgo biloba are cultivated, formulated, and concentrated into an extract containing the active compounds. Pharmacologically active flavonoids found in the leaves include, for example, tannins and their glycosides. Some flavonoid glycosides and glucosides are quercetin and kaempferol 3-rhamnosides and 3-rutinosides. Terpenes, which are also active, consist of ginkgolides A, B, C, J, and M as well as bilobalides. Active ingredients in ginkgo biloba have been shown to induce peripheral vasodilation, reduce red blood cell aggregation and platelet activating factor, alter neurotransmitter receptors and levels, and exhibit antioxidant actions.

Ginkgo biloba is purported to improve arterial and venous blood flow, especially cerebral and peripheral vascular circulation, and to improve neurosensory function. Thus, the herb is often recommended for conditions in which poor circulation is a factor, such as intermittent claudication (pain, cramping, and fatigue in the leg muscles, which is usually a symptom of peripheral arterial occlusive disease), memory impairment, dementia, vertigo (dizziness), and tinnitus (ringing in the ears). Conclusions of meta-analyses and extensive reviews of studies examining the efficacy of ginkgo biloba are varied. For example, some, but not all, controlled clinical studies suggest that ginkgo extracts are more effective than a placebo in treating some cognitive disorders, some cerebral disorders, intermittent claudication, and vertigo; however, further clinical trials are needed. Generally, use of ginkgo biloba for cerebral insufficiency and memory impairment in the elderly and to treat intermittent claudication has produced promising results, but the data are not considered fully convincing. The herb has not been found to promote neurologic recovery after ischemic stroke or to improve memory.

Typical daily dosages of standardized ginkgo biloba extracts used in most clinical studies totaled about 120 mg (although higher dosages have been used). The ginkgo biloba dosages generally are divided and administered three times daily. Ginkgo biloba extracts typically are standardized to contain 22% to 27% flavonoids and 5% to 7% terpene lactones, of which 2.8% to 3.4% are ginkgolides and 2.6% to 3.6% are bilobalides. Benefits may not be observed for at least 6 weeks. Side effects that may be associated with the use of ginkgo biloba include headache, dizziness, palpitations, and mild gastrointestinal distress (nausea and abdominal pain). Contact with the whole plant may be associated with an allergic skin reaction. Interactions have been reported between ginkgo biloba and aspirin, and ginkgo biloba and warfarin (an anticoagulant).

GINSENG

Ginsengs are derived from several different species of the genus *Panax*. Both Asian (*P. ginseng*) and American (*P. quinquefolium*) ginsengs are derived from the genus *Panax*. However, these species should not be confused with Siberian or Russian ginsengs or with Brazilian and Indian ginsengs, which are derived from a different plant. Ginsengs are perennial shade plants native to Korea and China. Ginseng has been used as an herbal remedy in Asia for centuries. All parts of the plant contain pharmacologically active components; however, the root is the most often used portion of the herb. The active components of ginseng (roots) are a group of triterpenoid saponin glycosides collectively called ginsenosides. Two saponins in ginseng are panaxadiol and panaxatriol (panaxans).

Ginseng is purported to reduce fatigue and improve stamina and well-being, and thus to serve as an energy enhancer, or adaptogen. In other words, ginseng is said to increase the body's ability to resist or cope with stress and to help the body build vitality. In addition, it has been suggested that ginseng is anticarcinogenic and may function as an antioxidant. Although a few studies have demonstrated that ginseng modulates some central nervous system activities to enhance performance, improve mood, diminish fatigue, and improve reaction time, among other effects, results of numerous other studies and meta-analyses assessing the effects of ginseng on the body do not support the claims. In other words, the efficacy of ginseng has not been clearly established for any indication.

Recommended dosages of ginseng (as tablets) range from about 100 to 300 mg/day, to be taken in divided doses. Tinctures and fluid extracts also are available; extracts are usually standardized to contain 4% to 7% ginsenosides. Another form, ginseng root, is used in dosages of 0.6 to 2 g. For those using ginseng, daily use for a short duration is suggested. Problems with product quality are common; despite label reports, products often contain negligible to no ginseng. Side effects most often observed from the use of ginseng include headache, nausea, diarrhea, insomnia, and nervousness. Negative interactions have been reported between ginseng and warfarin (an anticoagulant), the monoamine oxidase inhibitor phenelzine, and alcohol. In addition, germanium, an ingredient in some ginseng preparations, has been reported to induce resistance to diuretics.

MILK THISTLE

Milk thistle (*Silybum marianum*), also called St. Mary's or Our Lady's thistle, is a tall (about 5 to 10 feet) herb with a milk sap and dark, shiny, prickly leaves with white veins. The herb is native to Europe (the Mediterranean area) but is also grown in California and the eastern part of the United States. Specific compounds found in the fruit in concentrations of about 1% to 4% include a variety of flavonolignans—silybin, isosilybin, dehydrosilybin, silydianin, and silychristin, among others—collectively called silymarin. The three main components are silybin, silydianin, and silychristin, with silybin being the most potent. Other active ingredients include apigenin, histamine, triamine, betaine, and others. Most commercial milk thistle products contain over a dozen of these flavonolignans along with other compounds.

Fruits or seeds of milk thistle have been used for centuries to treat a variety of problems, mostly those associated with the liver, such as cirrhosis and hepatitis. Milk thistle exhibits antioxidant properties and is thought to be cytoprotective. It is thought to help the liver's resistance to toxic insults, to promote regeneration of liver cells, and to prevent damage to liver cells. Improved immune function and antiinflammatory and antiproliferative activities also have been attributed to milk thistle. As an antioxidant, silybin combined with phosphatidylcholine as a phytosome is thought to preserve glutathione use in liver cells and has been shown in European studies to be hepatoprotective in doses up to about 360 mg. A 2-year Egyptian study reported no objective evidence of improvement in liver function in a group of people with hepatitis C ingesting silymarin; however, patients reported feeling better. The efficacy and effectiveness of milk thistle have not been established in the United States. While some small studies have suggested promising results in individuals with liver disease, results of other studies have not. Thus, conclusive evidence is lacking and further studies are needed to determine the value of milk thistle for preventing and treating liver diseases as well as various cancers.

Milk thistle is sold as capsules that usually provide about 140 mg silymarin. Standardized extracts of milk thistle provide 35 to 70 mg silymarin and are recommended three times daily to achieve beneficial effects. Milk thistle is not very soluble; typically, less than 50% is absorbed, unless it is made more water soluble as in the form of a phytosome. The herb appears to be fairly well tolerated; the only side effects reported include mild gastrointestinal distress and allergic reactions.

ST. JOHN'S WORT

St. John's wort (*Hypericum perforatum*) is a perennial herb that produces golden yellow flowers. The flowers are typically harvested, dried, and extracted using alcohol and water. Major ingredients include naphthodianthrones (such as hypericin and pseudohypericin), phloroglucinols (such as hyperforin and adhyperforin), various flavonoids and flavonols (such as hyperoside, quercitrin, isoquercitrin, rutin, kaempferol, and biapigenin, among others), proanthocyanidins, xanthones, and phenolic acids (including caffeic acid, chlorogenic acid, and ferulic acid). Hypericin and hyperforin are thought to be the main active ingredients. Extracts of St. John's wort (*wort* is an Old English word for "plant") are usually standardized to provide 0.3% hypericin.

St. John's wort has been shown to inhibit neurotransmitter metabolism (especially of norepinephrine, dopamine, and serotonin), modulate neurotransmitter receptor concentrations and sensitivity, and alter neurotransmitter reuptake in the central nervous system. Oral consumption of St. John's extracts is recommended to treat depression and anxiety. Oily hypericum preparations also are used topically to relieve inflammation and promote healing of, for example, first-degree burns, hemorrhoids, or minor wounds. Numerous studies and meta-analyses of studies have shown that use of St. John's wort is more effective than a placebo and similarly as effective as many antidepressant therapies in treating mild to moderate depressive disorders. Moreover, the herb is often safer with respect to the side effects typically associated with the use of some antidepressant drug regimens. However, St. John's wort has not been shown to be any more effective than a placebo in treating major depressive disorders.

Daily dosages of up to about 1,000 mg administered in divided doses are commonly recommended, with therapeutic regimens of 2–3 weeks needed before effects are expected. The herb is sold in tablets and capsules and in tea and tincture forms. Adverse effects associated with the use of St. John's wort may include headache, fatigue, gastrointestinal distress (nausea, abdominal pain), dizziness, confusion, restlessness, and photosensitivity. The photosensitivity occurs with high dosages or prolonged use and is manifested as dermatitis and mucous membrane inflammation with sunlight exposure. Interactions have been reported between St. John's wort and anticoagulants, oral contraceptive (birth control) agents, theophylline (used for asthma), cyclosporin (used to diminish risk of transplant rejection), digoxin (a heart contractility drug), and indinavir (an antiviral drug).

REGULATION OF HERBAL SUPPLEMENTS

The Dietary Supplement Health and Education Act of 1994 allows herbs and phytomedicinals to be sold as dietary supplements as long as health or therapeutic claims do not appear on the product label [2]. The act defines dietary supplements to include vitamins, minerals, herbal or botanical products, amino acids, metabolites, extracts, and other substances alone or in combination that are added to the diet [2]. Because herbal supplements need not comply with other laws, the consumer and retailer have no assurance that the herb in the supplement corresponds with the label description or that the correct part of the herb was used in the manufacturing process. In other words, quality assurance of herbs and phytomedicinals is generally lacking in the United States, and the reputation of the producer becomes extremely important. The act itself and reviews of the Dietary Supplement Health and Education Act of 1994 are available for additional or more specific information [2,3].

References Cited

1. Manach C, Scalbert A, Morand C, et al. Polyphenols: food sources and bioavailabity. Am J Clin Nutr. 2004; 79:727–47.
2. Dietary Supplement Health and Education Act, 103–417, 3.(a). 1994 bill/resolution.
3. FDA Dietary Supplements. http://www.fda.gov/Food/DietarySupplements/default.htm

Web Sites with Information on Phytochemicals and Herbs

www.herbalgram.org
www.nccam.nih.gov
www.naturaldatabase.com
www.nal.usda.gov/fnic/foodcomp/Data/isoflav/ isoflav.html
www.nal.usda.gov/fnic/foodcomp/Data/car98/car98.html
www.usp.org
www.fda.gov/Food/DietarySupplements/default.htm

Suggested Readings

ECHINACEA

Birt DF, Widrlechner MP, LaLone CA, et al. Echinacea in infection. Am J Clin Nutr. 2008; 87(suppl):S488–92.
Goel V, Lovlin R, Chang C, et al. A proprietary extract from the echinacea plant (*Echinacea purpurea*) enhances systemic immune response during a common cold. Phytotherapy Res. 2005; 19:689–94.
Linde K, Barrett B, Wolkart K, Bauer R, Melchart D. Echinacea for preventing and treating the common cold. Cochrane Database Syst Rev 2006; 1:CD000530.
Turner RB, Bauer R, Woelkart K, et al. An evaluation of Echinacea angustifolia in experimental rhinovirus infections. N Engl J Med. 2005; 353:314–18.
Weber W, Taylor J, Stoep A, et al. *Echinacea purpurea* for prevention of upper respiratory tract infections in children. J Alternative Complementary Med. 2005; 11:1021–26.

GARLIC

Gardner CD, Lawson LD, Block E. Effect of raw garlic vs commercial garlic supplements on plasma lipid concentrations in adults with moderate hypercholesterolemia: a randomized clinical trial. Arch Intern Med. 2007; 167:346–53.
Goncagul AE. Antimicrobial effect of garlic (Allium sativum). Anti-Infect Drug Disc. 2010; 5:91–93.
Jepson RG, Kleijnen J, Leng GC. Garlic for peripheral arterial occlusive disease. Cochrane Database Syst Rev. 2000; 2:CD000095.
Khoo YSK, Aziz Z. Garlic supplementation and serum cholesterol: a meta-analysis. J Clin Pharm Ther. 2009; 3 4:133–45.
Kim JY, Kwon O. Garlic intake and cancer risk: an analysis using the Food and Drug Administration's evidence-based review system for the scientific evaluation of health claims. Am J Clin Nutr. 2009; 89:257–64.
Reinhart KM, Talati R, White CM, Coleman CI. The impact of garlic on lipid parameters: a systematic review and meta-analysis. Nutr Res Rev. 2009; 22:39–48.
Simons S, Wollersheim H, Thien T. A systematic review on the influence of trial quality on the effect of garlic on blood pressure. Neth J Med. 2009; 67:212–19.

GINKGO BILOBA

Birks JG, Evans J. Ginkgo biloba for cognitive impairment and dementia. Cochrane Database Syst Rev. 2009; (1):CD003120.
Brown LA, Riby LM, Reay JL. Supplementing cognitive aging: a selective review of the effects of ginkgo biloba and a number of everyday nutritional substances. Exp Aging Res. 2010; 36:105–22.
Coley N, Andrieu S, Gardette V, et al. Dementia prevention: methodological explanations for inconsistent results. Epidemiol Rev. 2008; 30:35–66.
DeKosky ST, Williamson JD, Fitzpatrick AL, et al. Ginko biloba for prevention of dementia: a randomized controlled trial. JAMA. 2008; 300:2253–62.
Kaschel R. Ginkgo biloba: specificity of neuropsychological improvement, a selective review in search of differential effects. Hum Psychopharmacol. 2009; 24:345–70.
Nicolai SPA, Kruidenier LM, Bendermacher BLW, et al. Ginkgo biloba for intermittent claudication. Cochrane Database Syst Rev. 2009; (2):CD006888.
Weinmann S, Roll S, Schwarzbach C, et al. Effects of Ginkgo biloba in dementia: systematic review and meta-analysis. BMC Geriatrics. 2010; 10:14.

GINSENG

Geng J, Dong J, Ni H, et al. Ginseng for cognition. Cochrane Database Syst Rev. 2010;(12)CD007769.
Gorby HE, Brownawell AM, Falk MC. Do specific dietary constituents and supplements affect mental energy? Review of the evidence. Nutr Rev. 2010; 68:697–718.

Lu J, Yao Q, Chen C. Ginseng compounds: an update on their molecular mechanisms and medical applications. Curr Vasc Pharmacol. 2009; 7:293–302.

Qi L, Wang C, Yuan C. American ginseng: potential structure-function relationship in cancer chemoprevention. Biochem Pharmacol. 2010; 80:947–54.

MILK THISTLE

Abenavoli L, Capasso R, Milic N, Capasso F. Milk thistle in liver diseases: past, present, future. Phytother Res. 2010; 24:1423–32.

Deep G, Agarwal R. Antimetastatic efficacy of silibinin: molecular mechanisms and therapeutic potential against cancer. Cancer Metastasis Rev. 2010; 29:447–63.

Kidd PM. Bioavailability and activity of phytosome complexes from botanical polyphenols: the silymarin, curcumin, green tea, and grape seed extracts. Altern Med Rev. 2009; 14:226–46.

Vaid M, Katiyar SK. Molecular mechanisms of inhibition of photocarcinogenesis by silymarin, a phytochemical from milk thistle (Silybum marianum L. Gaertn.). Int J Oncol. 2010; 36:1053–60.

ST. JOHN'S WORT

Caccia S, Gobbi M. St. John's wort components and the brain: uptake, concentrations reached and the mechanisms underlying pharmacological effects. Curr Drug Metab. 2009; 10:1055–65.

Izzo AA, Ernst E. Interactions between herbal medicines and prescribed drugs: an updated systematic review. Drugs. 2009; 69:1777–98.

Linde K, Mulrow CD. St. John's wort for depression. Cochrane Database of Systematic Reviews. 2000; 2:CD000448.

Randlov C, Mehlsen J, Thomsen C, et al. The efficacy of St. John's wort in patients with minor depressive symptoms or dysthymia: a double-blind placebo-controlled study. Phytomedicine. 2006; 13:215–21.

Sarris J, Kavanagh DJ. Kava and St. John's Wort: current evidence for use in mood and anxiety disorders. J Altern Complement Med. 2009; 15:827–36.

Shelton RC. St John's wort (Hypericum perforatum) in major depression. J Clin Psychiatry. 2009; 70 (Suppl5):23–27.

ARE PREBIOTICS BENEFICIAL TO HEALTH?

From Chapter 4 you will remember that prebiotics are nondigestible food ingredients that serve as substrates to promote the colonic growth and/or activity of selected health-promoting species of bacteria. Three criteria must be satisfied for a food ingredient to be considered a prebiotic [1,2]. First, the ingredient must be able to resist both digestion (including gastric acidity and hydrolysis) by human enzymes and absorption. Second, the ingredient must serve as a substrate for fermentation by intestinal microorganisms belonging to the human microbiota. Third, the ingredient must selectively stimulate the growth and/or activity of health-promoting intestinal bacteria [1,2]. The main bacterial species associated with health and well-being in humans are those of the *Bifidobacterium* and *Lactobacillus* genera.

SOURCES OF PREBIOTICS

Food ingredients meeting the criteria for prebiotics include fructans (inulin, oligosaccharides, fructooligosaccharides), lactulose, soybean oligosaccharides, and galactooligosaccharides. The most common food sources of the fructans include chicory, asparagus, leeks, onions, garlic, Jerusalem artichokes, tomatoes, and bananas; however, inulin and oligofructose are sometimes added to foods such as fillings, dressings, cereals, yogurt, dairy products, and frozen desserts. Additionally, short-chain fructooligosaccharides (containing a maximum of five fructose units) are also sometimes added to meal replacement products and beverages intended for healthy individuals as well as to some enteral nutrition products intended for use in hospitalized patients receiving tube feedings. Galactose oligosaccharides are found in human milk and a variety of peas and beans including soybeans, chickpeas, field peas, green peas, lentils, and mung, lima, snap, northern, and navy beans, among others. Another ingredient under investigation as a prebiotic is resistant starch type 3, found naturally in cooked and cooled starchy products and sometimes added to breads and cereals. Prebiotics are considered Generally Recognized as Safe (GRAS) by the U.S. Food and Drug Administration.

BENEFITS OF PREBIOTICS

Some of the purported benefits of prebiotics ingestion are the same as those associated with fiber ingestion. The main benefits of prebiotics relate most directly to their stimulation of the growth and/or activity of healthful bacteria (primarily lactobacilli and bifidobacteria) in the colon as well as to the production of short-chain fatty acids (butyric, propionic, and acetic acids), which are generated with the fermentation of

the prebiotic by the bacteria in the colon. These effects, as well as other secondary actions, in turn impart additional health benefits (Figure 1), including stimulation of the immune system. For example, the short-chain fatty acids lower the pH of the colon to inhibit the growth of many pathogenic bacteria while also stimulating leukocytes and inducing cytokine and chemokine production. Gut-associated lymphoid tissue is also activated, and intestinal secretions of immunoglobulin A (IgA) and interferon are increased. Prebiotics are also associated with reduced production of inflammatory compounds. These immunostimulatory actions help protect the body.

The presence of increased concentrations of health-promoting bacteria also serves to inhibit the pathogenic bacteria's attachment to colonic cells, growth, and toxin production among species such as *Clostridium difficile*. Prebiotic use may also help to improve colonic integrity by enhancing mucosal morphology and thickening and increasing mucin production; these changes in turn improve the intestine's resistance to pathogenic bacterial colonization and bacterial translocation. The increase in fecal mass from the increased bacterial growth improves laxation. In addition, like many of the soluble fibers, some prebiotics may exhibit hypolipidemic

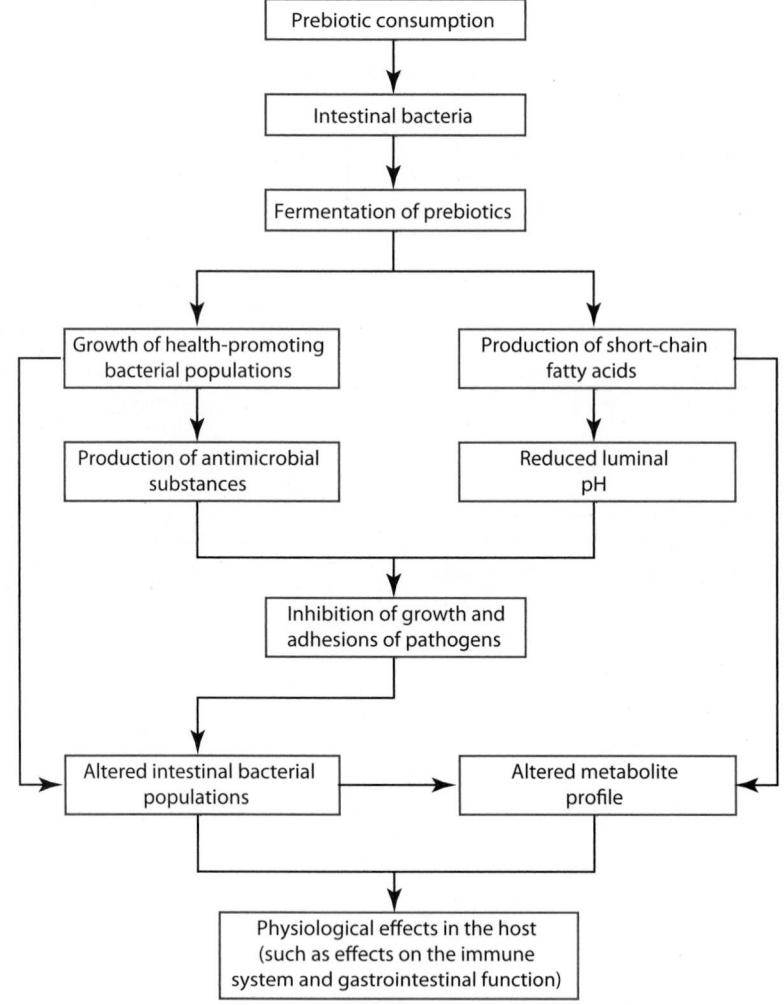

Figure 1 Selected mechanisms for some of the effects of prebiotic ingestion.
Sources: Adapted from D. Meyer, M. Stasse-Wolthuis. The bifidogenic effect of inulin and oligofructose and its consequences for gut health. European Journal of Clinical Nutrition (2007) 63, 1277−1289; A.P. Vos, L. M'Rabet, B. Stahl, G. Boehm, J. Garssen, Immune-modulatory effects and potential working mechanisms of orally applied nondigestible carbohydrates. Critical Reviews in Immunology, 27 (2): 97−140 (2007).

effects and attenuate the blood glucose response through either bacterial use of the nutrient (such as glucose) or inhibitory effects on its absorption. Prebiotics may also be able to bind to minerals as well as modulate the production of appetite-regulating neuropeptides and/or hormones; these actions in turn may improve mineral absorption and help with weight regulation, respectively. Thus, prebiotic use clearly has the potential to improve health.

Dosages of prebiotics needed to raise fecal counts of health-promoting bacteria in the colon range from about 2.5 to about 10 to 15 g daily and require about a week of administration to effect the increase [3-5]. Resistant starch intakes of 20 g daily and galactooligosaccharide intakes of up to 15 g/day have been recommended [6,7]. Because of differences in methodology, form and dose of substrate (prebiotic), duration, subjects, and types of measurements collected, comparisons of the efficacy of different prebiotics cannot be accurately made at this time [5,8]. Common side effects from prebiotic use are excessive gas, abdominal bloating, cramping, and osmotic diarrhea. These problems are more likely to occur when prebiotics are consumed in dosages of 40 to 50 g or more daily [4].

PREBIOTIC USE AND DISEASE PREVENTION AND/OR TREATMENT

The effectiveness of prebiotics in the prevention and/or treatment of a variety of health problems has been investigated; the evidence (discussed hereafter) may be divided into three main areas: gastrointestinal health, blood glucose control, and maintenance of a desirable blood lipid profile.

Gastrointestinal Health

Disorders for which the utility of prebiotics has been most studied include altered motility conditions such as diarrheal disorders and constipation and inflammatory intestinal conditions.

Diarrheal Disorders   Results of studies providing prebiotics to prevent or treat diarrhea—a common problem in people of all ages, from infants to the elderly—are inconclusive. Among infants ($n = 20$), a combination of oligofructose and galactooligosaccharides (1.8 g daily for 2 weeks) added to an infant formula (versus infant formula without prebiotics) has been shown to improve stool consistency and transit time [9]. However, a randomized controlled trial providing 0.55 g oligofructose per 15 g cereal versus no added oligofructose for 6 months in 282 infants did not alter the number of days the infants experienced diarrhea [10].

Reports of the effectiveness of prebiotics in those with antibiotic-associated diarrhea also have been mixed. In a study of 400 adults, 12 g fructooligosaccharides (versus a placebo) was not effective in preventing diarrhea in those taking broad-spectrum antibiotics [11]. However, in a randomized controlled trial, 12 g oligosaccharides (versus a placebo) for 30 days given along with antibiotics (metronidazole and vancomycin) reduced the incidence of relapse of diarrhea in 142 adults with diarrhea secondary to *Clostridium (C.) difficile* [12].

In addition to diarrheal problems among infants and those on antibiotics, travelers' diarrhea often affects individuals enjoying international travel. Less severe attacks of travelers' diarrhea were reported in 244 adults who received 10 g fructooligosaccharides versus placebo for 2 weeks prior to and during travel. However, the prevalence of diarrhea did not significantly differ between the two groups [7,13]. While the limited number of studies suggests some promising results, further research is needed regarding the efficacy of prebiotics in both the treatment and the prevention of diarrheal disorders.

Constipation   Constipation is another problem frequently experienced by individuals of all ages. Fructooligosaccharides and inulin use has been shown to improve intestinal motility through increases in microbial mass, increases in osmotic pressure in the colon, shortened transit time, and shortened time available for water absorption in the colon. The net effect of these changes is increased fecal weight and stool output and thus relief from constipation. Studies showing beneficial effects of prebiotics (versus placebo) in constipation relief have typically provided 15 g (up to about 40 g) fructooligosaccharides or inulin daily with significant increases in stool output in those receiving the prebiotics [5,7].

Inflammatory Bowel Diseases (Crohn's Disease and Ulcerative Colitis)   Both Crohn's disease and ulcerative colitis are inflammatory conditions affecting primarily the intestines and causing abdominal pain and diarrhea, among other symptoms. Reductions in mucosal inflammation as well as increased butyric acid concentrations were reported in 20 patients with ulcerative colitis (treated with a colectomy and the formation of an ileal-anal pouch and at risk for pouch inflammation) receiving 24 g inulin/day (versus placebo) for 3 weeks in a crossover design study [14]. Reductions in disease severity also were documented in 10 Crohn's disease patients receiving 15 g oligofructose/day for 3 weeks [15]. In contrast, disease activity scores did not significantly differ—though perceived gastrointestinal symptoms reported on a questionnaire were significantly reduced—among 15 patients with ulcerative colitis receiving mesalazine drug therapy and 12 g oligofructose plus inulin/day (versus a placebo) for 2 weeks [16]. Another randomized, placebo-controlled trial with over 100 patients with Crohn's disease found no benefit from the use of 15 g inulin-type fructans/day for 3 weeks on disease activity or number of patients entering remission [17]. At present, conclusions regarding the efficacy of prebiotic use in inflammatory bowel diseases cannot be drawn, and additional research is needed [18].

Irritable Bowel Syndrome   Irritable bowel syndrome is characterized by abdominal pain or discomfort that occurs in association with altered bowel habits over a period of at least 3 months. Several small studies providing prebiotics have been conducted in individuals with this condition, with mixed results. Patients with irritable bowel syndrome receiving 5 g fructooligosaccharides daily (versus those receiving a

placebo) for 6 weeks reported reductions in symptom scores [19]. Another 12-week study providing 3.5 to 7 g prebiotics daily versus a placebo to patients with irritable bowel syndrome showed improved stool consistency, reduced bloating, and improved anxiety scores [20]. In contrast, the use of 20 g fructooligosaccharides/day versus a placebo for 12 weeks in patients with irritable bowel syndrome did not significantly improve symptom scores [21]. Similarly, 4 weeks of oligofructose (6 g daily) use by 21 patients with irritable bowel syndrome did not improve symptom scores or transit time in a double-blind crossover trial [22]. Nonetheless, the positive results from some studies warrant further examination of the role of prebiotics in the management of irritable bowel syndrome [18,23].

Blood Glucose Control and Maintenance of a Desirable Blood Lipid Profile

Consumption of dietary fibers has been shown to attenuate the blood glucose response to a meal as well as to promote reductions in serum cholesterol concentrations, as discussed in Chapter 4. Prebiotics also have been tested in a limited number of studies to see if they can elicit similar changes. The results of most studies suggest that the use of fructooligosaccharides (given in doses of about 10.6 to 20 g daily for several weeks to 3 months) does not statistically improve blood glucose concentrations in those with hyperglycemia or euglycemia (normal blood glucose concentrations) [4]. At this time, because consistent benefits have not been observed with prebiotic administration, its use for blood glucose regulation in those with prediabetes or diabetes mellitus is not recommended. Reviews of multiple studies providing prebiotics (given in doses of about 7 to 20 g daily for about 3 to 10 weeks) to individuals with normal blood lipid concentrations also suggest little benefit from prebiotic supplementation [4,7]. In those with hyperlipidemia, while the results are mixed, the majority of the studies also suggest no benefits from prebiotic supplementation, but further research is needed [4,7,24].

In summary, prebiotic use enhances gastrointestinal tract and immune system functions. However, while the results from studies examining the effects of prebiotic use in treating and/or preventing health problems have been promising, they also have been primarily inconclusive. So, at present, to the question "Are prebiotics beneficial to health?" we must answer, Maybe.

References Cited

1. Gibson GR, Probert HM, van Loo J, et al. Dietary modulation of the human colonic microbiota: updating the concept of prebiotics. Nutr Res Rev. 2004; 17:259–75.

2. Gibson GR, Roberfroid MB. Dietary modulation of the human colonic microbiota: introducing the concept of prebiotics. J Nutr. 1995; 125:1401–12.

3. Bouhnik Y, Raskine L, Simoneau G, et al. The capacity of nondigestible carbohydrates to stimulate fecal

bifidobacteria in health humans: a double-blind, randomized placebo-controlled, parallel group, dose-response relation study. Am J Clin Nutr. 2004; 80:1658–64.

4. Kelly G. Inulin-type prebiotics: a review. Altern Med Rev. 2009; 14:36–55.

5. Meyer D, Stasse-Woltuis M. The bifidogenic effect of inulin and oligofructose and its consequences for gut health. Eur J Clin Nutr. 2009; 63:1277–89.

6. Douglas LC, Sanders ME. Probiotics and prebiotics in dietetics practice. J Am Diet Assoc. 2008; 108:510–21.

7. Macfarlane GT, Steed H, Macfarlane S. Bacterial metabolism and health-related effects of galacto-oligosaccharides and other prebiotics. J Appl Microbiol. 2008; 104:305–44.

8. Rycroft CE, Jones MR, Gibson GR, Rastall RA. A comparative in vitro evaluation of the fermentation properties of prebiotic oligosaccharides. J Applied Microbiol. 2001; 91:878–87.

9. Mihatsch WA, Hoegel J, Pohlandt F. Prebiotic oligosaccharides reduce stool viscosity and accelerate gastrointestinal transport in preterm infants. Acta Pediatr. 2006; 95:843–48.

10. Duggan C, Penny ME, Hibberd P. Oligofructose-supplemented infant cereal: 2 randomized, blinded, community-based trials in Peruvian infants. Am J Clin Nutr. 2003; 77:937–42.

11. Lewis S, Burmeister S, Cohen S, et al. Failure of dietary oligofructose to prevent antibiotic-associated diarrhea. Alimen Pharmacol Ther. 2005; 21:469–77.

12. Lewis S, Burmeister S, Cohen S, Brazier J. Effect of the prebiotic oligofructose on relapse of *Closteridium difficile*-associated diarrhea: a randomized control study. Clin Gastroenterol Hepatol. 2005; 3:442–48.

13. Cummings JH, Christie S, Cole TJ. A study of fructooligosaccharides in the prevention of travellers' diarrhoea. Alimen Pharmacol Ther. 2001; 15:1139–45.

14. Welters CF, Heineman E, Thunnissen FB. Effect of dietary inulin supplementation on inflammation of pouch mucosa in patients with an ileal pouch-anal anastomosis. Dis Colon Rectum. 2002; 45:621–27.

15. Lindsay JO, Whelan K, Stagg AJ. Clinical, microbiological, and immunological effects of fructooligosaccharide in patients with Crohn's disease. Gut. 2006; 55:348–55.

16. Casellas F, Borruel N, Torrejon A. Oral oligofructose enriched inulin supplementation in acute ulcerative colitis is well tolerated and associated with lowered faecal calprotection. Aliment Pharmacol Ther. 2007; 25:1061–67.

17. Benjamin JL, Hedin CRH, Koutsoumpas A. Randomized, double-blind, placebo-controlled trial of fructo-oligosaccharides in active Crohn's disease. Gut. 2011; 60:923–9.18.

18. Roberfroid M, Gibson GR, Hoyles L, et al. Prebiotic effects: metabolic and health benefits. Br J Nutr. 2010; 104(suppl 2):S1–63.

19. Paineau D, Payen F, Panserieu S. The effects of regular consumption of short-chain fructooligosaccharides on digestive comfort of subjects with minor functional bowel disorders. Br J Nutr. 2008; 99:311–18.

20. Silk DB, Davis A, Vulevic J. Clinical trial: the effects of a transgalactooligosaccharide prebiotic on faecal microbiota and symptoms in irritable bowel syndrome. Aliment Pharmacol Ther. 2009; 29:508–18.

21. Olesen M, Gudmand-Hoyer E. Efficacy, safety, and tolerability of fructooligosaccharides in the treatment of irritable bowel syndrome. Am J Clin Nutr. 2000; 72:1570–75.

22. Hunter JO, Tuffnell Q, Lee AJ. Controlled trial of oligofructose in the management of irritable bowel syndrome. J Nutr. 1999; 12(suppl):S1451–53.

23. Cabre E. Irritable bowel syndrome: can nutrient manipulation help? Curr Opin Clin Nutr Metab Care. 2010; 13:581–87.

24. Brighenti F. Dietary fructans and serum triacylglycerols: a meta analysis of randomized controlled trials. J Nutr. 2007; 137:S252–56.

Suggested Reading

Hempel S, Newberry S, Ruelaz A, et al. Safety of probiotics to reduce risk and prevent or treat disease. Available from www.ahrq.gov/clinic/tp/probiotictp.htm

Lomax AR, Calder PC. Prebiotics, immune function, infection and inflammation: a review of the evidence. Brit J Nutr. 2009; 101:633–58.

Roberfroid MB. Inulin-type fructans: Functional food ingredients. J Nutr. 2007; 137:S2493–2502.

Sabater-Molina M, Larque E, Torrella F, Zamora S. Dietary fructooligosaccharides and potential benefits on health. J Physiol Biochem. 2009; 65:315–28.

5 | LIPIDS

THE PROPERTY THAT SETS LIPIDS apart from other major nutrients is their solubility in organic solvents such as ether, chloroform, and acetone. If lipids are defined according to this property, which is generally the case, the range of their functions becomes broad: They serve not only as dietary sources of energy and constituents of cell and organelle membranes but also as the fat-soluble vitamins, corticosteroid hormones, and certain mediators of electron transport, such as coenzyme Q.

Among the many compounds classified as lipids, only a small number are important as dietary energy sources or as functional or structural constituents within the cell. The following classification is limited to those lipids germane to this section of the text, which deals with energy-releasing nutrients. Fat-soluble vitamins are discussed in Chapter 10.

1. Simple lipids
   a. Fatty acids
   b. Triacylglycerols, diacylglycerols, and monoacylglycerols
   c. Waxes (esters of fatty acids with higher alcohols)
      (1) Sterol esters (cholesterol–fatty acid esters)
      (2) Nonsterol esters (vitamin A esters, and so on)

2. Compound lipids
   a. Phospholipids
      (1) Phosphatidic acids (i.e., lecithin, cephalins)
      (2) Plasmalogens
      (3) Sphingomyelins
   b. Glycolipids (carbohydrate-containing)
   c. Lipoproteins (lipids in association with proteins)

3. Derived lipids (derivatives such as sterols and straight-chain alcohols obtained by hydrolysis of those lipids in groups 1 and 2 that still possess general properties of lipids)

4. Ethyl alcohol (though it is not a lipid per se, it does supply dietary energy, and its metabolism resembles lipid metabolism)

In the discussion of the structure and physiological function of lipids that follows, lipids have been grouped arbitrarily according to fatty acids, triacylglycerols (triglycerides), sterols and steroids, phospholipids, glycolipids, and ethyl alcohol. This grouping is more functional than structural.

STRUCTURE AND BIOLOGICAL IMPORTANCE

Fatty Acids

As a class, the fatty acids are the simplest of the lipids. They are composed of a straight hydrocarbon chain terminating with a carboxylic acid group. Therefore, fatty acids have a polar, hydrophilic end and a nonpolar, hydrophobic end that is insoluble in water (Figure 5.1). Fatty acids are components of the more complex lipids, discussed in later sections. They are of vital importance as an energy nutrient, furnishing most of the calories derived from dietary fat.

The lengths of the carbon chains of fatty acids found in foods and body tissues vary from 4 to about 24 carbon atoms. The fatty acids may be saturated (SFA), monounsaturated (MUFA, possessing 1 carbon-carbon double bond), or polyunsaturated (PUFA, having 2 or more carbon-carbon double bonds). PUFAs of nutritional interest may have as many as 6 double bonds. Where a carbon-carbon double bond exists,

there is an opportunity for either a *cis* or a *trans* geometric isomerism that significantly affects the molecular configuration of the molecule. The *cis* isomerism form results in the folding back and kinking of the molecule into a U-like orientation, whereas the *trans* form has the effect of extending the molecule into a linear shape similar to that of saturated fatty acids. The structures in Figure 5.1 illustrate saturation and unsaturation in an 18-carbon fatty acid and show how *cis* or *trans* isomerization affects the molecular configuration.

The more carbon-carbon double bonds occurring within a chain, the more pronounced is the bending effect. The degree of bending plays an important role in the structure and function of cell membranes. Most naturally occurring unsaturated fatty acids are of the *cis* configuration, although the *trans* form does appear in some natural fats and oils, and in dairy products and beef (*trans* fatty acids are produced by ruminant bacteria). Most *trans* fatty acids are derived from partially hydrogenated fats and oils.

Partial hydrogenation, a process commonly used in making margarine and frying oils, is designed to solidify

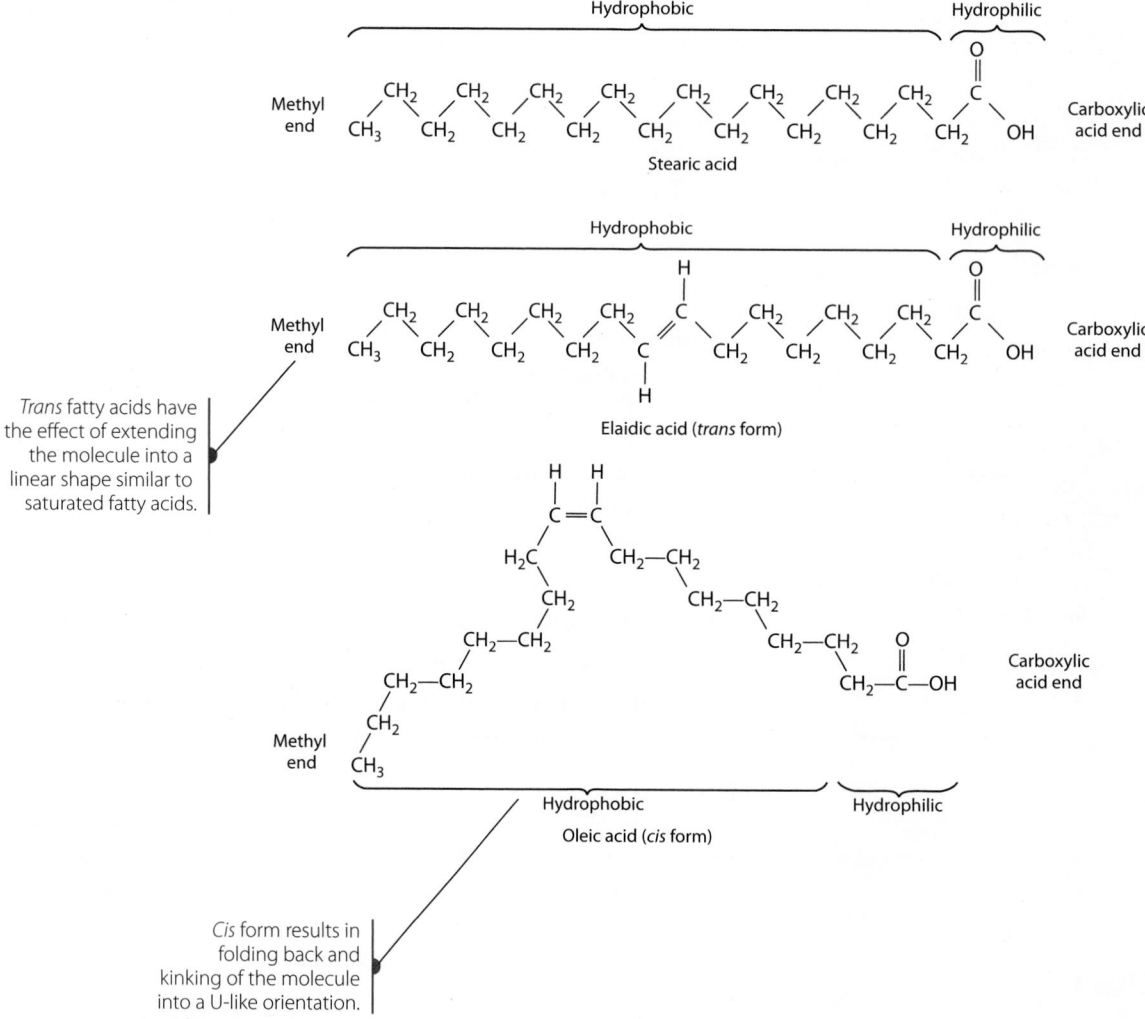

Trans fatty acids have the effect of extending the molecule into a linear shape similar to saturated fatty acids.

Cis form results in folding back and kinking of the molecule into a U-like orientation.

Figure 5.1 Structures of selected fatty acids.

vegetable oils at room temperature. Double bonds of *cis* orientation that are not reduced in the process undergo an electronic rearrangement to the *trans* form, which is energetically more stable. The availability of *trans* fatty acids in the typical U.S. diet has been estimated to be approximately 8.1 g/person/day, the major source being margarines and spreads [1]. More recent quantitative estimates are not available, but the requirement to list the amount of *trans* fatty acids on the food label should result in reduced consumption. Concerns have been raised about the possible adverse nutritional effects of dietary *trans* fatty acids, particularly their role in the etiology of cardiovascular disease (CVD). This topic is discussed in the section "Lipids, Lipoproteins, and Cardiovascular Disease Risk" in this chapter.

Fatty Acid Nomenclature

Two systems of notation have been developed to provide a shorthand way to indicate the chemical structure of a fatty acid. Both systems are used regularly and will be used interchangeably in the text for different purposes.

The delta (Δ) system of notation has been established to denote the chain length of the fatty acids and the number and position of any double bonds that may be present. For example, the notation 18:2 $\Delta^{9,12}$ describes linoleic acid. The first number, 18 in this case, represents the number of carbon atoms; the number following the colon refers to the total number of double bonds present; and the superscript numbers following the delta symbol designate the carbon atoms at which the double bonds begin. In this system, the numbering starts from the carboxyl end of the fatty acid.

A second commonly used system of notation locates the position of double bonds on carbon atoms counted from the methyl, or omega (ω), end of the carbon chain. For instance, the notation for linoleic acid would be 18:2 ω-6. Substitution of the omega symbol with the letter *n* has been popularized. Using this designation, the notation for linoleic acid would be expressed as 18:2 n-6. In this system, the total number of carbon atoms in the chain is given by the first number, the number of double bonds is given by the number following the colon, and the location

(carbon atom number) of the first double bond is given by the number following ω- or n-. This system of notation takes into account the fact that double bonds in a fatty acid are always positioned so that they are separated by three carbons. Thus, if you know the total number of double bonds and the location of the first relative to either the methyl or carboxylic end, you can determine the locations of the remaining double bonds.

Figure 5.2 demonstrates the designation of linoleic acid using each of the two systems: 18:2 $\Delta^{9,\,12}$ (delta); or 18:2 ω-6 or 18:2 n-6 (omega). The fatty acid α-linolenic acid, which contains three double bonds, is identified as 18:3 $\Delta^{9,\,12,\,15}$; or 18:3 ω-3 or 18:3 n-3.

Table 5.1 lists some naturally occurring fatty acids and their dietary sources. For unsaturated fatty acids, the table shows the Δ and ω system designations, and commonly used abbreviations. The list includes only those fatty acids with chain lengths of 14 or more carbon atoms because these fatty acids are most important both nutritionally and functionally. For example, palmitic acid (16:0), stearic acid (18:0), oleic acid (18:1), and linoleic acid (18:2) together account for >90% of the fatty acids in the average U.S. diet. However, shorter-chain fatty acids do occur in nature. Butyric acid (4:0) and lauric acid (12:0), for instance, are abundant in milk fat and coconut oil, respectively.

Most fatty acids have an even number of carbon atoms. The reason for this will be evident in the discussion of fatty acid synthesis. Odd-numbered-carbon fatty acids occur naturally to some extent in some food sources. For example, certain fish, such as menhaden, mullet, and tuna, as well as the bacterium *Euglena gracilis*, contain fairly high concentrations of odd-numbered-carbon fatty acids.

Essential Fatty Acids

If fat is entirely excluded from the diet of humans, a condition develops that is characterized by retarded growth, dermatitis, kidney lesions, and early death. Studies have shown that eating certain unsaturated fatty acids such as linoleic, α-linolenic, and arachidonic acids is effective in curing the conditions related to the lack of these fatty

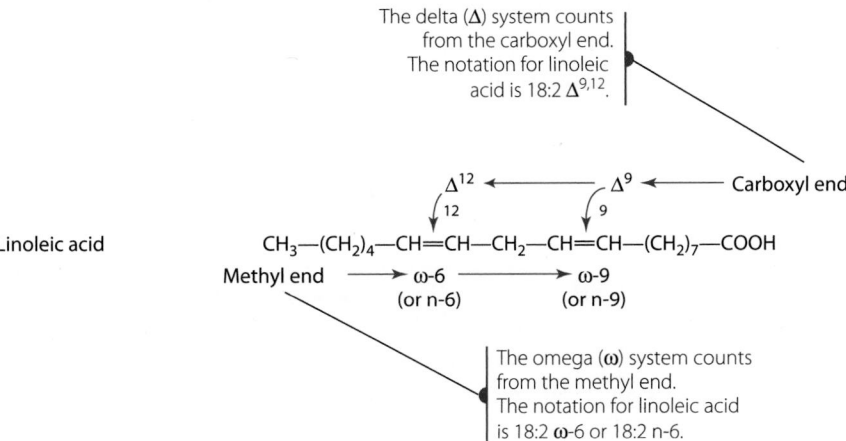

Linoleic acid

The delta (Δ) system counts from the carboxyl end. The notation for linoleic acid is 18:2 $\Delta^{9,12}$.

$$CH_3—(CH_2)_4—CH{=}CH—CH_2—CH{=}CH—(CH_2)_7—COOH$$

The omega (ω) system counts from the methyl end. The notation for linoleic acid is 18:2 ω-6 or 18:2 n-6.

Figure 5.2 The structure of linoleic acid, showing the two systems for nomenclature.

Table 5.1 Some Naturally Occurring Fatty Acids

Notation	Common Name	Formula	Source
Saturated Fatty Acids			
14:0	Myristic acid	$CH_3-(CH_2)_{12}-COOH$	Coconut and palm nut oils, most animal and plant fats
16:0	Palmitic acid	$CH_3-(CH_2)_{14}-COOH$	Animal and plant fats
18:0	Stearic acid	$CH_3-(CH_2)_{16}-COOH$	Animal fats, some plant fats
20:0	Arachidic acid	$CH_3-(CH_2)_{18}-COOH$	Peanut oil
24:0	Lignoceric acid	$CH_3-(CH_2)_{22}-COOH$	Most natural fats, peanut oil in small amounts
Unsaturated Fatty Acids			
16:1 Δ^9(n-7)	Palmitoleic acid	$CH_3-(CH_2)_5-CH=CH-(CH_2)_7-COOH$	Marine animal oils, small amount in plant and animal fats
18:1 Δ^9(n-9)	Oleic acid	$CH_3-(CH_2)_7-CH=CH-(CH_2)_7-COOH$	Plant and animal fats
18:2 $\Delta^{9,12}$(n-6)	Linoleic acid	$CH_3-(CH_2)_4-CH=CH-CH_2-CH=CH-(CH_2)_7-COOH$	Corn, safflower, soybean, cottonseed, sunflower seed, and peanut oils
18:3 $\Delta^{9,12,15}$(n-3)	α-linolenic acid	$CH_3-(CH_2-CH=CH)_3-(CH_2)_7-COOH$	Linseed, soybean, and other seed oils
20:4 $\Delta^{5,8,11,14}$(n-6)	Arachidonic acid	$CH_3-(CH_2)_3-(CH_2-CH=CH)_4-(CH_2)_3-COOH$	Small amounts in animal fats
20:5 $\Delta^{5,8,11,14,17}$(n-3)	Eicosapentaenoic acid	$CH_3-(CH_2-CH=CH)_5-(CH_2)_3-COOH$	Marine algae and fish that consume the algae
22:6 $\Delta^{4,7,10,13,16,19}$(n-3)	Docosahexaenoic acid	$CH_3-(CH_2-CH=CH)_6-(CH_2)_2-COOH$	Animal fats as phospholipid component, and marine algae and fish that consume the algae

acids. Two unsaturated fatty acids cannot be synthesized in animal cells but must be acquired in the diet from plant foods. The two essential fatty acids are linoleic acid (18:2 n-6) and α-linolenic acid (18:3 n-3). From linoleic acid, γ-linolenic (18:3 n-6) and arachidonic acids (20:4 n-6) can be formed in the body. An intermediate fatty acid in the pathway is eicosatrienoic acid. The pathway is

$$\text{linoleic acid (18:2 n-6)}$$
$$\downarrow$$
$$\gamma\text{-linolenic acid (18:3 n-6)}$$
$$\downarrow$$
$$\text{eicosatrienoic acid (20:3 n-6)}$$
$$\downarrow$$
$$\text{arachidonic acid (20:4 n-6)}$$

Linoleic and α-linolenic acids are essential because humans lack enzymes called Δ^{12} and Δ^{15} desaturases, which incorporate double bonds at these positions. These enzymes are found only in plants. Humans are incapable of forming double bonds beyond the Δ^9 carbon in the chain. If a $\Delta^{9,12}$ fatty acid is obtained from the diet, however, additional double bonds can be incorporated at Δ^6 (desaturation). Fatty acid chains can also be elongated by the enzymatic addition of two carbon atoms at the carboxylic acid end of the chain. These reactions are discussed further in the "Synthesis of Fatty Acids" section of this chapter.

n-3 Fatty Acids

Nutritional interest in the n-3 fatty acids has escalated enormously in recent years because of their reported hypolipidemic and antithrombotic effects. An n-3 fatty acid of particular interest is eicosapentaenoic acid (20:5 n-3; EPA) because it is a precursor of the physiologically important eicosanoids, discussed later in this chapter. Fish oils are particularly rich in n-3 fatty acids and therefore are the dietary supplement of choice in research designed to study their effects. Food sources and the tissue distribution of a few commonly occurring n-3 polyunsaturated fatty acids are given in Table 5.2.

Table 5.2 Dietary Sources and Tissue Distribution of the Major n-3 Polyunsaturated Fatty Acids

Major Members of Series	Tissue Distribution in Mammals	Dietary Sources
α-linolenic acid 18:3 n-3	Minor component of tissues	Some vegetable oils (soy, canola, linseed, rapeseed) and leafy vegetables
Eicosapentaenoic acid 20:5 n-3	Minor component of tissues	Fish and shellfish
Docosahexaenoic acid 22:6 n-3	Major component of membrane phospholipids in retinal photoreceptors, cerebral grey matter, testes, and sperm	Fish and shellfish

Triacylglycerols (Triglycerides)

Most stored body fat is in the form of triacylglycerols (TAG), which represent a highly concentrated form of energy. (*Triacylglycerols* is the currently accepted name that has replaced the older name *triglycerides* [TRIG or TG].) Triacylglycerols account for nearly 95% of dietary fat. Structurally, they are composed of a trihydroxyalcohol, glycerol, to which three fatty acids are attached by ester bonds, as shown in Figure 5.3; the formation of each of these ester bonds liberates a water molecule. The fatty acids may be all the same (a simple TAG) or different (a mixed TAG). The fatty acids in triacylglycerols can be all saturated, all monounsaturated, all polyunsaturated, or any combination of the three.

Carbons 1 and 3 of glycerol are not the same when viewed in a three-dimensional model. Also, when different fatty acids are attached to the first and third carbons of glycerol, the second carbon becomes asymmetric. (See Chapter 3 for a discussion of stereoisomerism.) Enzymes of the body are able to distinguish between the three carbons of glycerol and are generally quite specific. This specificity is important in digesting and synthesizing triacylglycerols, as will be discussed later in this chapter.

Acylglycerols may be composed of glycerol esterified to a single fatty acid (a monoacylglycerol, MAG) or to two fatty acids (a diacylglycerol, DAG), with the fatty acids attached to any of the three carbons of glycerol. Though present in the body only in small amounts, the mono- and diacylglycerols are important intermediates in some metabolic reactions and may be components of other lipid classes. They also may occur in processed foods, to which they can be added as emulsifying agents. A diacylglycerol oil is currently being marketed as a vegetable oil substitute; the manufacturer claims that using it in place of a TAG oil will result in less storage of body fat.

The specific glycerol hydroxyl group to which a certain fatty acid is attached is indicated by a numbering system for the three glycerol carbons, in much the same way as glyceraldehyde is numbered (Figure 3.2). This system is complicated somewhat by the fact that the central carbon of the glycerol is asymmetrical when different fatty acids are esterified at the two end carbon atoms and therefore may exist in either the D or the L form. A system of nomenclature called stereospecific numbering (*sn*) has been adopted in which the glycerol is presented as shown in Figure 5.3, with the C-2 hydroxyl group oriented to the left (L) and the carbons numbered 1 through 3 beginning at the top.

Triacylglycerols exist as fats (solid) or oils (liquid) at room temperature, depending on the nature of the component fatty acids. Triacylglycerols that contain a high proportion of relatively short-chain fatty acids or unsaturated fatty acids tend to be liquid (oils) at room temperature, whereas those made up of saturated fatty acids of longer chain length have a higher melting point and thus exist as solids. When used for energy, fatty acids are released in free (nonesterified or NEFA) form as free fatty acids (FFA) from the triacylglycerols in adipose tissue cells by the activity of lipases, and the FFAs are then transported by albumin to various tissues for oxidation.

Sterols and Steroids

This class of lipid is characterized by a four-ring core structure called the cyclopentanoperhydrophenanthrene, or steroid, nucleus. **Sterols** are monohydroxy alcohols of

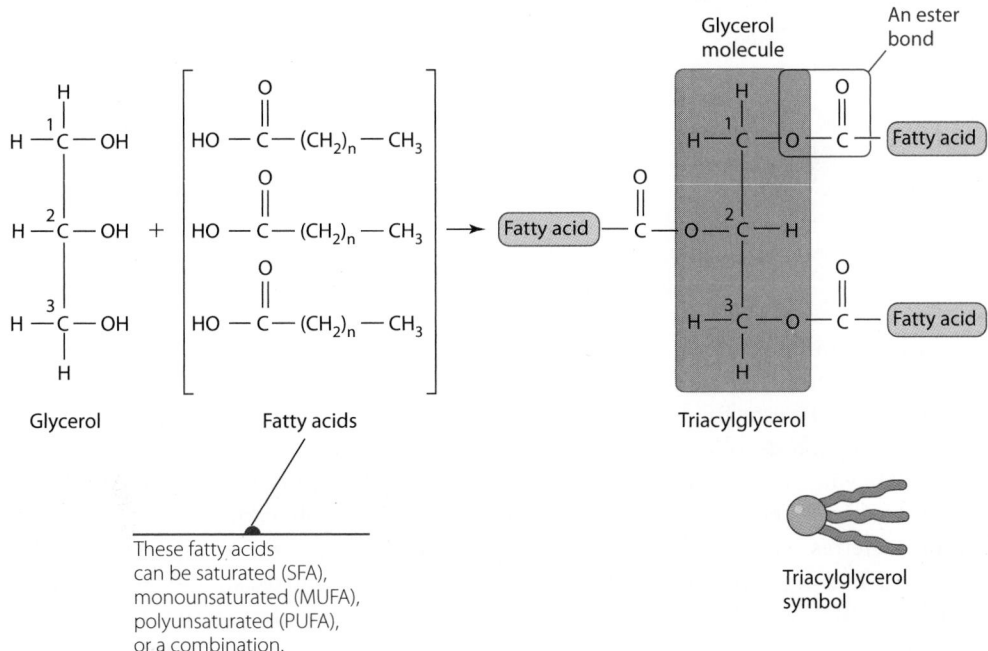

These fatty acids can be saturated (SFA), monounsaturated (MUFA), polyunsaturated (PUFA), or a combination.

Figure 5.3 Linkage of fatty acids to glycerol to form a triacylglycerol. Chain length of fatty acid is (n + 2).
Source: Beerman/McGuire, Nutritional Sciences, 1/e.
© Cengage Learning.

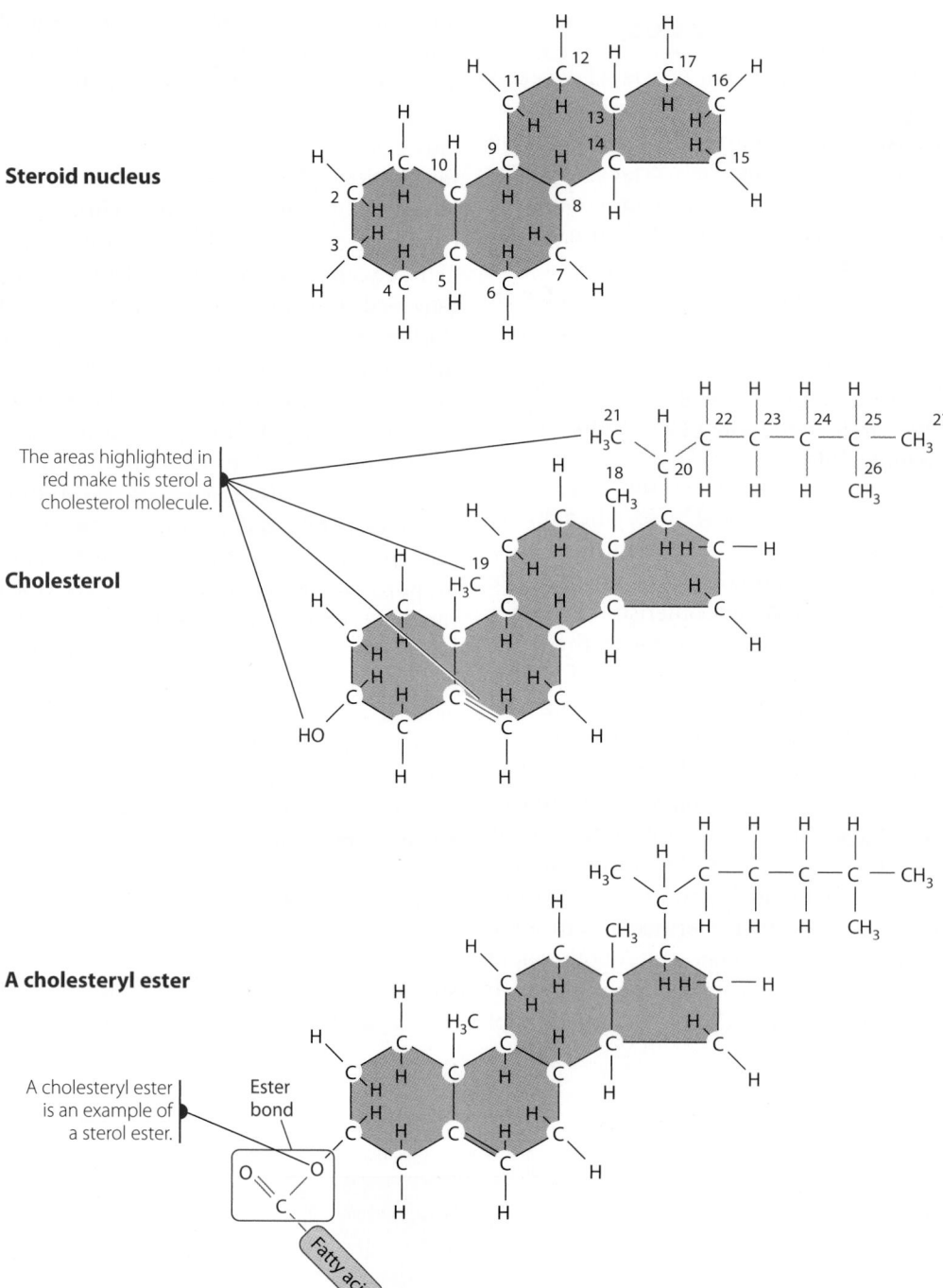

Figure 5.4 Structure of a sterol, cholesterol, and a cholesteryl ester.
Source: Beerman/McGuire, Nutritional Sciences, 1/e. © Cengage Learning.

steroidal structure. Cholesterol is the most common sterol in animals and is the precursor for other steroids. It can exist in free form, or the hydroxyl group can be esterified with a fatty acid. Many sterols other than cholesterol are found in plant tissues, and some interfere with cholesterol absorption. Most human enzyme systems are specific for cholesterol and do not react with plant sterols. The structure of cholesterol is shown in Figure 5.4, along with the numbering system for the carbons in the steroid nucleus and the side chain.

Meats, egg yolk, and dairy products, the common dietary sources of cholesterol, contain fairly large amounts. In the body, this sterol is an essential component of cell membranes, particularly the membranes of nerve tissue. Despite the bad press that cholesterol has garnered over the years because of its implication in cardiovascular disease, it serves as the precursor for many other important steroids in the body, including the bile acids; steroid sex hormones such as estrogens, androgens, and progesterone; the adrenocortical hormones; and vitamin D (cholecalciferol, the animal form). These steroids differ from one another in the arrangement of double bonds in the ring system, the presence of carbonyl or hydroxyl groups, and the nature of the side chain at C-17. All these structural modifications are mediated by enzymes that function as dehydrogenases, isomerases, hydroxylases, or desmolases. Desmolases remove or shorten the length of side chains on the steroid nucleus. The derivation of the various types of steroids from cholesterol is diagrammed in Figure 5.5. Although many physiologically active corticosteroid hormones, sex hormones, and bile acids exist, only representative compounds are shown. The biological importance and metabolic reactions of these compounds will be discussed later in this chapter. Sterols, together with phospholipids (considered next) comprise only about 5% of dietary lipids.

Phospholipids

As the name implies, **phospholipids** contain phosphate, as well as one or more fatty acid residues. Phospholipids are categorized into one of two groups called

glycerophosphatides and sphingophosphatides, depending upon whether their core structure is glycerol (glycerophosphatides) or the amino alcohol sphingosine (sphingolipids).

Glycerophosphatides

The building block of a glycerophosphatide is phosphatidic acid, formed by esterification of two fatty acids at C-1 and C-2 of glycerol and esterification of the C-3 hydroxyl with phosphoric acid (Figure 5.6). The fatty acid portion of the molecule is hydrophobic, while the phosphate and the polar head group are hydrophilic. In most cases, glycerophosphatides have a saturated fatty acid on position 1 and an unsaturated fatty acid on position 2. The structure in Figure 5.6 typifies a phosphatidate, a term that does not define a specific structure because different fatty acids may be involved. The conventional numbering of the glycerol carbon atoms is the same as that for triacylglycerols. From top to bottom, the numbering is *sn*-1, *sn*-2, and *sn*-3, provided the glycerol is written in the L configuration so that the C-2 fatty acid constituent is directed to the left, as

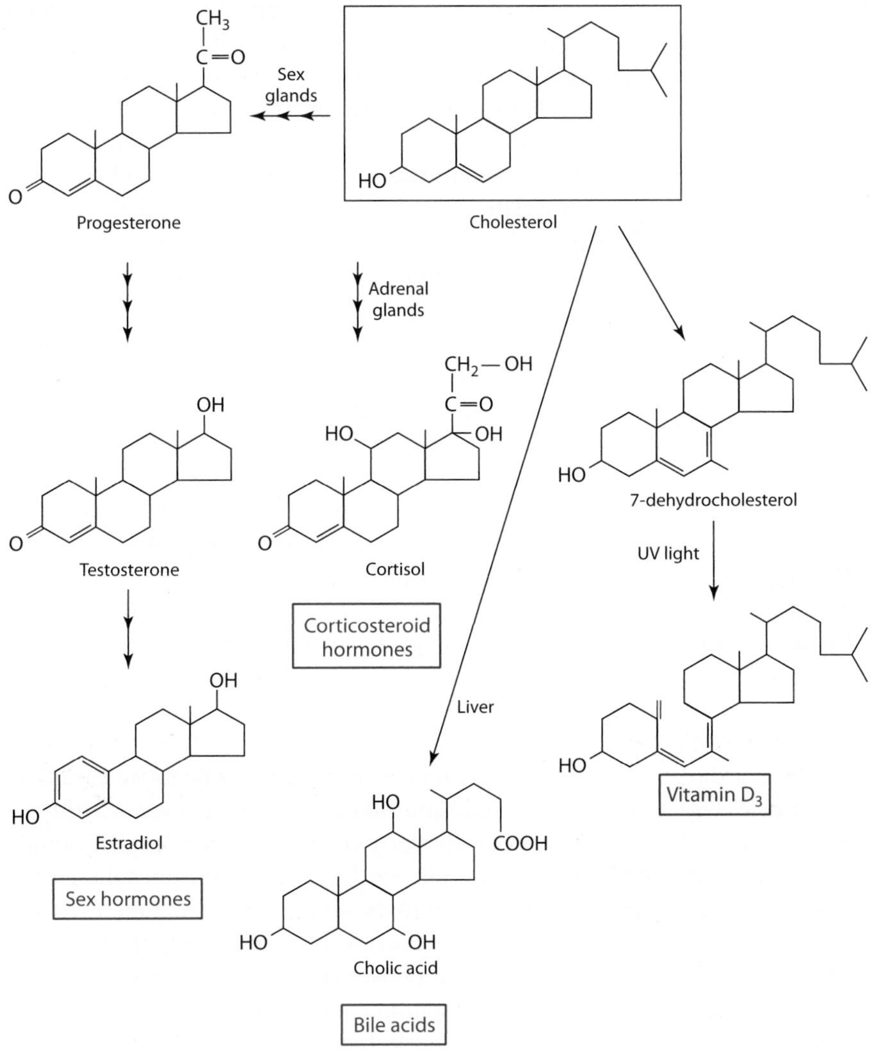

Figure 5.5 The formation of physiologically important steroids from cholesterol. Only representative compounds from each category of steroid are shown.

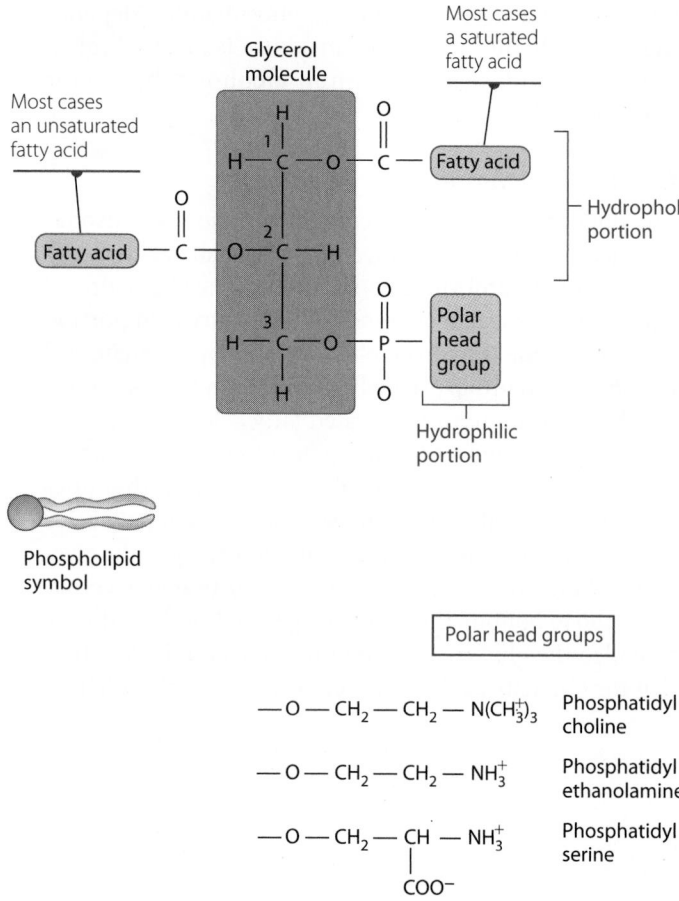

Phospholipid symbol

Figure 5.6 Typical structure of phospholipids.
Source: Beerman/McGuire, Nutritional Sciences, 1/e. © Cengage Learning.

shown in Figure 5.6. Phosphatidic acids form a number of derivatives with compounds such as choline, ethanolamine, serine, and inositol, each of which possesses an alcohol group through which a second esterification to the phosphate takes place (Figure 5.6). The compounds are named as the phosphatidyl derivatives of the alcohols, as indicated in the figure. A common phospholipid is phosphatidylcholine, which is better known by its common name, lecithin. The other phospholipids are formed by replacing the choline in the polar head group.

Diphosphatidylglycerol is another glycerophosphatide found in several tissues of the body. It is also called cardiolipin and was originally identified within heart muscle (Figure 5.7). Cardiolipin is located in the inner membrane of mitochondria and attaches cytochrome c to the membrane.

Biological Roles of Phospholipids

Phospholipids play several important roles in the body. Phospholipids are more polar than the triacylglycerols and sterols, and therefore tend to attract water molecules.

Because of this hydrophilic property, phospholipids are commonly expressed on the surface of blood-borne lipid particles, such as chylomicrons, thereby stabilizing the particles in the aqueous medium. Furthermore, glycerophosphatides are important components of cell and organelle membranes, where they serve as a conduit for the passage of water-soluble and fat-soluble materials across the membrane. In addition to lending structural support to the membrane, they serve as a source of physiologically active compounds. We will see later how arachidonate can be released on demand from membrane-bound phosphatidylcholine and phosphatidylinositol (another phospholipid) when it is needed for synthesis of **eicosanoids** (20-carbon fatty acids).

Phosphatidylinositol participates in several cell functions. For example, it plays a specific role in anchoring membrane proteins when the proteins are covalently attached to lipids. This function has been demonstrated by the fact that certain membrane proteins are released when cells are treated with a phosphatidylinositol-specific phospholipase C, which hydrolyzes the ester bond connecting the glycerol to the phosphate. Phosphatidylinositols anchor a wide variety of surface antigens and other surface enzymes in eukaryotic cells. In addition, certain hydrolytic products of phosphatidylinositol are active in intracellular signaling and act as second messengers in hormone function. An example of this role is the mechanism of action of insulin (discussed in Chapter 7). Phosphatidylinositol in the plasma membrane can be doubly phosphorylated by ATP, forming phosphatidylinositol-4, 5-bisphosphate. Stimulation of the cell by certain hormones, such as insulin, activates a specific phospholipase C, which produces inositol-1,4,5-trisphosphate and diacylglycerol from phosphatidylinositol-4,5-bisphosphate. Both of these products function as second messengers in cell signaling. Inositol-1,4,5-trisphosphate causes the release of Ca^{2+} held within membrane-bound compartments of the cell, triggering the activation of a variety of Ca^{2+}-dependent enzymes and hormonal responses [2]. Diacylglycerol binds to and activates an enzyme, protein kinase C, which transfers phosphate groups to several cytoplasmic proteins, thereby altering their enzymatic activities [3,4]. This dual-signal hypothesis of phosphatidylinositol hydrolysis is represented in Figure 5.8.

Sphingolipids

The 18-carbon amino alcohol sphingosine forms the backbone of the **sphingolipids.** Sphingosine (Figure 5.9) typically combines with a long-chain fatty acid through an amide linkage to form ceramide. Lipids formed from sphingosine are categorized into three subclasses: sphingomyelins, cerebrosides, and gangliosides. Of these, only the sphingomyelins are sphingophosphatides (Figure 5.10). The other two subclasses of sphingolipids contain no phosphate but instead possess a carbohydrate moiety. They are called

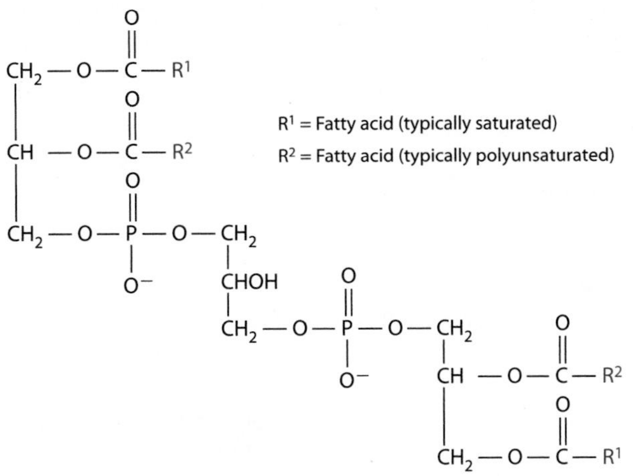

$$CH_2 - O - \overset{\overset{O}{\|}}{C} - R^1$$

$$CH - O - \overset{\overset{O}{\|}}{C} - R^2$$

R^1 = Fatty acid (typically saturated)

R^2 = Fatty acid (typically polyunsaturated)

$$CH_2 - O - \overset{}{\underset{O^-}{P}} - O - CH_2$$

CHOH

$$CH_2 - O - \overset{}{\underset{O^-}{P}} - O - CH_2$$

$$CH - O - \overset{\overset{O}{\|}}{C} - R^2$$

$$CH_2 - O - \overset{\overset{O}{\|}}{C} - R^1$$

Figure 5.7 Structure of diphosphatidylglycerol (cardiolipin).

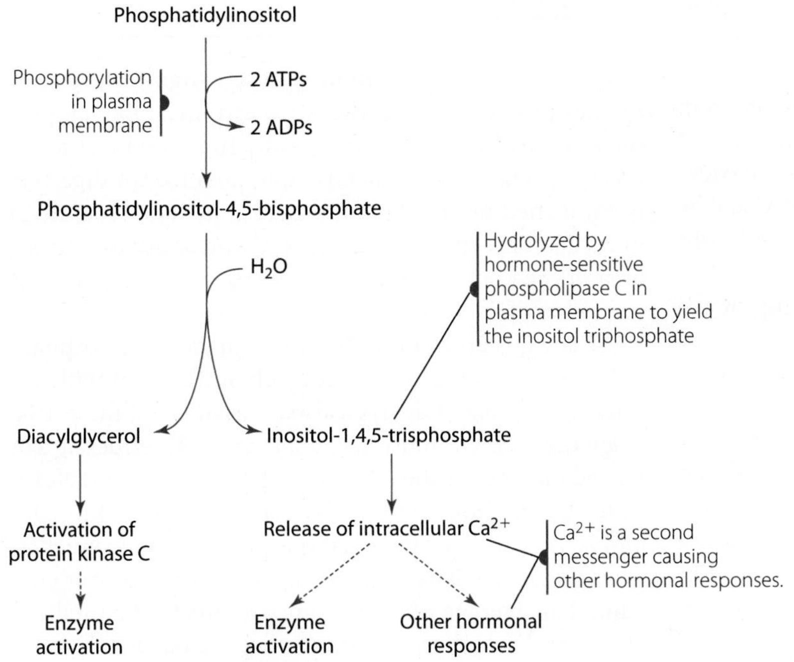

Phosphatidylinositol

Phosphorylation in plasma membrane — 2 ATPs
→ 2 ADPs

Phosphatidylinositol-4,5-bisphosphate

— H$_2$O

Hydrolyzed by hormone-sensitive phospholipase C in plasma membrane to yield the inositol triphosphate

Diacylglycerol   Inositol-1,4,5-trisphosphate

Activation of protein kinase C   Release of intracellular Ca^{2+} Ca^{2+} is a second messenger causing other hormonal responses.

Enzyme activation   Enzyme activation   Other hormonal responses

Figure 5.8 Phosphatidylinositol-4,5-bisphosphate, formed in the plasma membrane by phosphorylation of phosphatidylinositol.

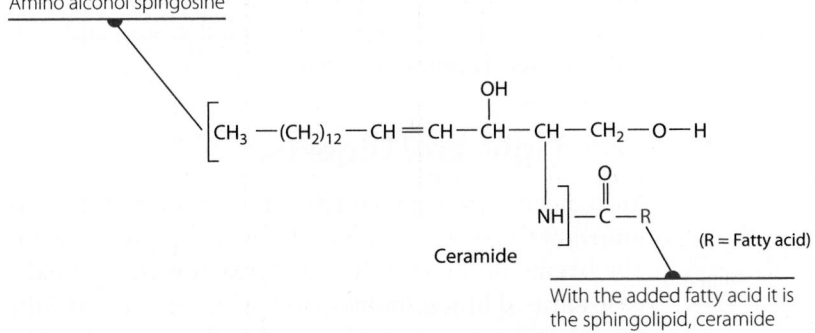

Amino alcohol spingosine

$$[CH_3 - (CH_2)_{12} - CH = CH - \overset{\overset{OH}{|}}{CH} - CH - CH_2 - O - H]$$

$$NH] - \overset{\overset{O}{\|}}{C} - R$$

(R = Fatty acid)

Ceramide

With the added fatty acid it is the sphingolipid, ceramide

Figure 5.9 Structure of the sphingolipidceramide.

glycolipids and are discussed in the next section. Sphingomyelins occur in plasma membranes of animal cells. They are particularly abundant in the myelin sheath of nerve tissues and thus important for nervous system function in higher animals. The sphingomyelins contain ceramide (a fatty acid residue attached in an amide linkage to the amino group of the sphingosine), which in turn is esterified to phosphorylcholine (Figure 5.10). Sphingomyelins can combine with either phosphorylcholine or phosphorylethanolamine.

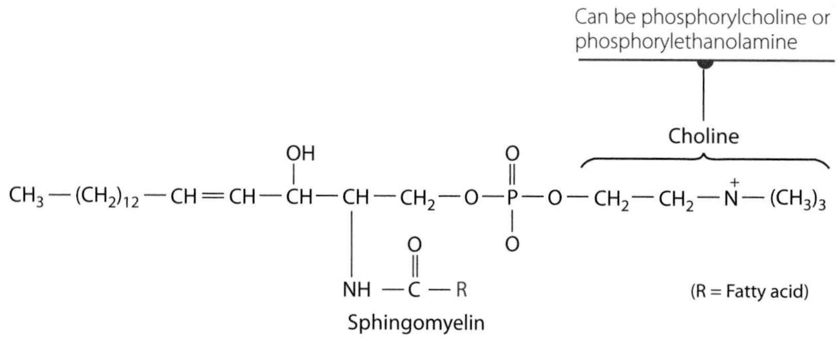

Can be phosphorylcholine or
phosphorylethanolamine

Choline

$$CH_3 - (CH_2)_{12} - CH = CH - \overset{\overset{\displaystyle OH}{|}}{CH} - CH - CH_2 - O - \overset{\overset{\displaystyle O}{\|}}{\underset{\underset{\displaystyle O}{|}}{P}} - O - CH_2 - CH_2 - \overset{+}{N} - (CH_3)_3$$

$$\underset{\underset{\displaystyle NH - \overset{\overset{\displaystyle O}{\|}}{C} - R}{}}{}$$

Sphingomyelin   (R = Fatty acid)

Figure 5.10 The structure of sphingomyelin.

Glycolipids

Glycolipids—so named because they have a carbohydrate component within their structure—can be subclassified into cerebrosides and gangliosides. Like the phospholipids, their physiological role is principally structural, and they contribute little as an energy source. Cerebrosides and gangliosides occur in the medullary sheaths of nerves and in brain tissue, particularly the white matter. As in the case of sphingomyelin, the sphingosine moiety provides the backbone for glycolipid structure. It is attached to a fatty acid by an amide bond, forming ceramide, as discussed previously. The glycolipids do not contain phosphate.

A cerebroside is characterized by the linking of ceramide to a monosaccharide unit such as glucose or galactose, producing either a glucocerebroside or a galactocerebroside (Figure 5.11).

Gangliosides resemble cerebrosides, except that the single monosaccharide unit of the cerebroside is replaced by an oligosaccharide containing various monosaccharide derivatives, such as N-acetyl neuraminic acid and N-acetyl galactosamine. Gangliosides are known to be involved in certain recognition events that occur at the cell surface.

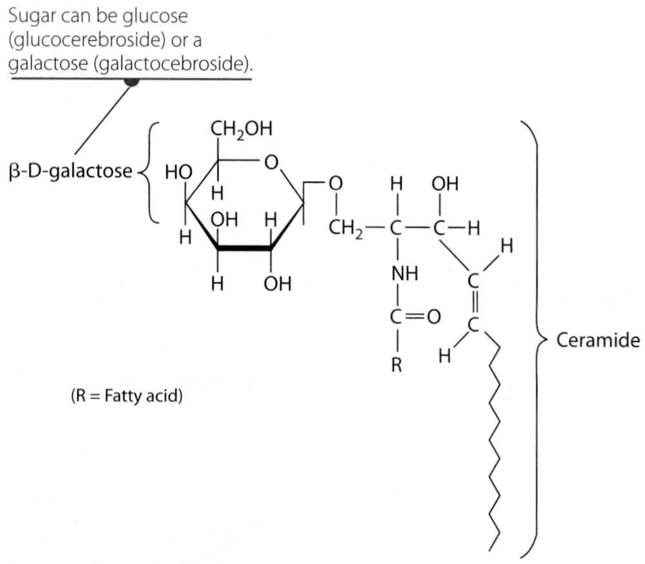

For example, they provide the carbohydrate determinants of the human blood groups A, B, and O.

DIGESTION

Because TAG are hydrophobic, their digestion poses a special problem in that digestive enzymes, like all proteins, are hydrophilic and normally function in an aqueous environment. The dietary lipid targeted for digestion is emulsified by an efficient process, mediated mainly by bile salts. This emulsification greatly increases the surface area of the dietary lipid, consequently increasing the accessibility of the fat to digestive enzymes.

Triacylglycerols, phospholipids (primarily phosphatidylcholine), and sterols (mainly cholesterol) provide the lipid component of the typical Western diet. Of these, triacylglycerols, commonly called fats or triglycerides, are by far the major contributor. The National Health and Nutrition Examination Survey (NHANES) conducted in 2007 and 2008 found that males 20 years and over consumed an average of 95 *g* daily and females 20 years and over consumed an average of 67 *g*. Compare this to the intake of cholesterol, which is 362 and 230 *mg* per day for the same groups, respectively [5]. Digestive enzymes involved in breaking down dietary lipids in the gastrointestinal tract are esterases that cleave the ester bonds within triacylglycerols (lipase), phospholipids (phospholipases), and cholesteryl esters (cholesterol esterase).

Triacylglycerol Digestion

Most dietary triacylglycerol digestion is completed in the lumen of the small intestine, although the process actually begins in the mouth and stomach with lingual lipase released by the serous gland, which lies beneath the tongue, and gastric lipase produced by the chief cells of the stomach. Basal secretion of these lipases apparently occurs continuously but can be stimulated by neural (sympathetic agonists), dietary (high fat), and mechanical (sucking and swallowing) factors. These lipases account for much of the limited digestion (10–30%) of TAG that occurs in the stomach. The lipase activity is made possible

Sugar can be glucose
(glucocerebroside) or a
galactose (galactocerebroside).

β-D-galactose

(R = Fatty acid)

Ceramide

Figure 5.11 A galactocerebroside.

by the enzymes' particularly high stability at the low pH of the gastric juices. Gastric lipase readily penetrates milk fat globules without substrate stabilization by bile salts, a feature that makes it particularly important for fat digestion in the suckling infant, whose pancreatic function may not be fully developed. Both lingual and gastric lipases act preferentially on triacylglycerols containing medium- and short-chain fatty acids. They preferentially hydrolyze fatty acids at the sn-3 position, releasing a fatty acid and 1,2-diacylglycerols as products. This specificity again is advantageous for the suckling infant because in milk, triacylglycerols' short- and medium-chain fatty acids are usually esterified at the sn-3 position [6]. Short- and medium-chain fatty acids are metabolized more directly than are long-chain fatty acids. Commercially available high-energy formulas for premature infants, which are rich in triacylglycerols containing short- and medium-chain fatty acids esterified at the sn-3 position, are designed to take advantage of the lipases' specificity. These products supply ample energy to the premature infant in a small volume [6–8].

For dietary TAG to be hydrolyzed by lingual and gastric lipases in the stomach, some degree of emulsification must occur to expose a sufficient surface area of the substrate. Muscle contractions of the stomach and the squirting of the fat through a partially opened pyloric sphincter produce shear forces sufficient for emulsification. Also, potential emulsifiers in the acid milieu of the stomach include complex polysaccharides, phospholipids, and peptic digests of dietary proteins. The presence of undigested lipid in the stomach delays the rate at which the stomach contents empty, presumably by way of hormones of the enterogastrone family such as secretin, which inhibits gastric motility. Dietary fats therefore have a "high satiety value."

Most TAG digestion occurs in the upper segment of the jejunum. The small intestine has the capacity to digest a large quantity of TAG: up to 600 g with 95% efficiency [9]. Significant hydrolysis and absorption, especially of the long-chain fatty acids, require less acidity, appropriate lipases, more effective emulsifying agents (bile salts), and specialized absorptive cells. These conditions are provided in the lumen of the upper small intestine. The partially hydrolyzed lipid emulsion leaves the stomach and enters the duodenum as fine lipid droplets. Effective emulsification takes place because as mechanical shearing continues, it is complemented by bile that is released from the gallbladder as a result of stimulation by the hormone cholecystokinin (CCK).

Refer to Chapter 2 for a discussion of the role of bile in digestion and the synthesis of bile from cholesterol. Figure 5.5 shows the oxidation of cholesterol to form cholic acid. The formation of conjugated bile salts from cholic acid is shown in Figure 5.12. Bicarbonate is released simultaneously with the release of pancreatic lipase, elevating the pH to a level suitable for pancreatic lipase activity. In combination with triacylglycerol breakdown products, bile

salts are excellent emulsifying agents. Their emulsifying effectiveness is due to their **amphipathic** properties; that is, they possess both hydrophilic and hydrophobic "ends." Such molecules tend to arrange themselves on the surface of small fat particles, with their hydrophobic ends turned inward and their hydrophilic regions turned outward toward the water phase. This chemical action, together with the help of peristaltic agitation, converts the fat into small droplets with a greatly increased surface area. The particles then can be readily acted upon by pancreatic lipase.

The action of pancreatic lipase on ingested triacylglycerols results in a complex mixture of diacylglycerols, monoacylglycerols, and free fatty acids. Its specificity is primarily toward sn-1-linked fatty acids and secondarily to sn-3 bonds. Therefore, the main path of this digestion progresses from TAG to 2,3-diacylglycerols to 2-monoacylglycerols. Only a small percentage of the triacylglycerols is hydrolyzed totally to free glycerol. The complete hydrolysis of triacylglycerols that does occur probably follows the isomerization of the 2-monoacylglycerol to 1-monoacylglycerol, which is then hydrolyzed, as shown in Table 5.3.

An inhibitor of gastric and pancreatic lipase, orlistat, has been developed to reduce the absorption of dietary triacylglycerols. It is marketed both as Xenical, a prescription-only product, and Alli, an over-the-counter product. The rationale for use is that when the hydrolysis of TAG is restricted, less dietary fat will be absorbed, resulting in decreased caloric intake. Xenical inhibits the absorption about 30% or by 200 kcal from fat per day.

The Role of Colipase

Pancreatic lipase activation is complex, requiring the participation of the protein colipase, calcium ions, and bile salts. Colipase is formed by the hydrolytic activation by trypsin of procolipase, also of pancreatic origin. It contains approximately 100 amino acid residues and possesses distinctly hydrophobic regions that are believed to act as lipid-binding sites. Colipase has been shown to associate strongly with pancreatic lipase and therefore may act as an anchor, or linking point, for attachment of the enzyme to the bile salt–stabilized micelles (described in the next section).

Cholesterol and Phospholipid Digestion

Cholesterol esters and phospholipids are hydrolyzed by a specific process described here. Esterified cholesterol undergoes hydrolysis to free cholesterol and a fatty acid in a reaction catalyzed by the enzyme cholesterol esterase.

The C-2 fatty acid of lecithin is hydrolytically removed by a specific esterase, phospholipase A$_2$, producing lysolecithin and a free fatty acid. The products of the partial digestion of dietary lipids, primarily 2-monoacylglycerols, lysolecithin, cholesterol, and fatty acids, combine with bile salts to

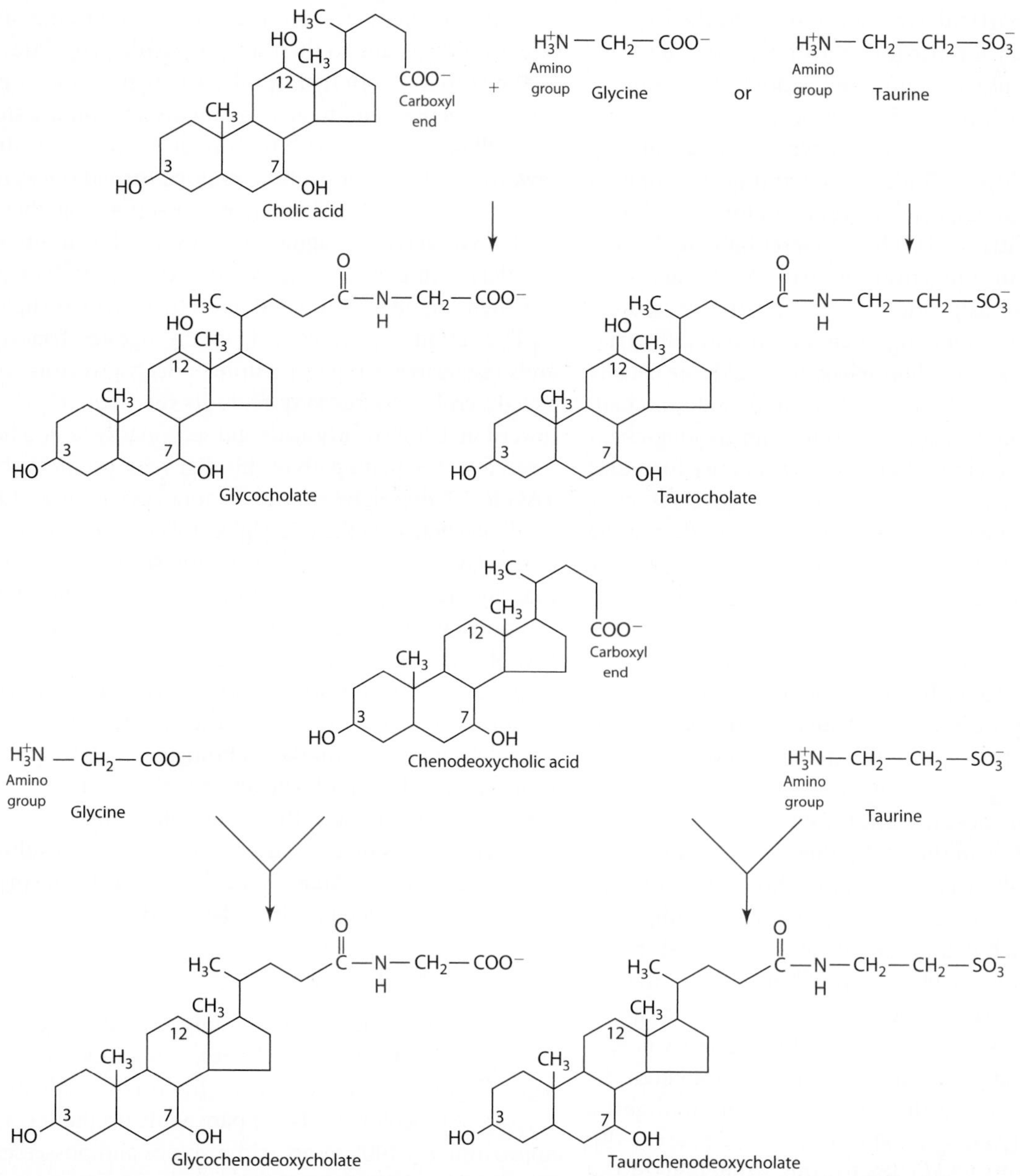

Figure 5.12 The formation of glycocholate, taurocholate, glycochenodeoxycholate, and taurochenodeoxycholate conjugated bile acids.

form negatively charged polymolecular aggregates called micelles. These aggregates have a much smaller diameter (~5 nm) than the unhydrolyzed precursor particles, allowing them access to the intramicrovillus spaces (50–100 nm) of the intestinal membrane. A summary of the digestion of lipids is shown in Table 5.3 and Figure 5.13.

ABSORPTION

Stabilized by the polar bile salts, the micellar particles are sufficiently water soluble to penetrate the unstirred water layer that bathes the enterocytes of the small intestine. Micelles are small enough to interact with the microvilli at the brush border, whereupon their lipid contents (which include FFA,

2-monoacylglycerols [2-MAG], 1-monoacylglycerols [1-MAG], cholesterol, cholesterol esters, and lysolecithin) move into the enterocytes.

Fatty Acid and Mono- and Diacylglycerol Absorption

The mechanism for moving fatty acids across the apical membrane is not fully understood. Two mechanisms have been suggested for the absorption of fatty acids (FA): a protein-independent diffusion model and a protein-dependent model, which uses fatty acid transport proteins (FATP). At least six different proteins have been suggested. Four of these FATP are produced in the

Table 5.3 Overview of Triacylglycerol Digestion

Location	Major events	Required enzyme or secretion	Details
Mouth	Triacylglycerol ↓ *Minor amount of digestion* → Triacylglycerols, diacylglycerols, and fatty acids	Lingual lipase produced in the salivary glands	**Diacylglycerol** Triacylglycerol $+ H_2O$ → Diacylglycerol + Fatty acid. Lingual lipase cleaves some fatty acids here.
Stomach	*Additional digestion* ↓ Triacylglycerol, diacylglycerol, and fatty acids	Gastric lipase produced in the stomach	**Diacylglycerol** Triacylglycerol $+ H_2O$ → Diacylglycerol + Fatty acid. Gastric lipase cleaves some fatty acids here.
Small intestine	*Phase I: Emulsification* ↓ Emulsified triacylglycerols, diacylglycerols, and fatty acid micelles ↓ *Phase II: Enzymatic digestion* ↓ Monoacylglycerols and fatty acids	Bile; no lipase / Pancreatic lipase produced in pancreas	**Monoacylglycerol** Triacylglycerol $+ H_2O$ → Monoacylglycerol + 2 Fatty acids. Pancreatic lipase cleaves some fatty acids here.

intestine and called FATP 1-4; the best characterized of these is FATP1. The predominant transport protein produced by the intestine is FATP4, which has been shown to have acyl-CoA transfer activity when identified in the endoplasmic reticulum (ER) of the enterocyte. FATP4 is not involved in moving the FA across the membrane; rather, a proposed mechanism for its function is the intracellular trapping of FA. Another FATP, FAT/CD36, has been shown to be involved in the absorption of FA into cells and also has a role in the FA absorption into enterocytes [9]. Neither the diffusion nor the carrier-protein mechanism requires energy for FA absorption into the enterocyte [10]. Although this process occurs in the distal duodenum and the jejunum, the bile salts are not absorbed at this point but instead are absorbed in the ileal segment of the small intestine. From there the bile salts are returned to the liver by way of the portal vein to be resecreted in the bile. This circuit is called enterohepatic circulation of the bile salts (see Chapter 2).

In the enterocyte the products of TAG digestion (FFA, MAG, and DAG) move to the endoplasmic reticulum (ER). After FFA, MAG, and DAG are absorbed into the enterocyte, specific binding proteins carry them to the ER. Here, acyltransferases transfer CoA-fatty acids onto the MAG and DAG to produce TAG. The assembly of TAG into chylomicrons is discussed later in this chapter. Note that triacylglycerols can also be synthesized from α-glycerophosphate in the enterocytes. This metabolite can be formed either from the phosphorylation of free glycerol or from reduction of dihydroxyacetone phosphate, an intermediate in the pathway of glycolysis (Figure 3.17).

Medium-chain fatty acids (those containing fewer than 10–12 carbon atoms) pass from the enterocyte directly into the portal blood, where they bind with albumin and are transported directly to the liver. As discussed later in this chapter, the long-chain fatty acids are added to MAG and DAG to form TAG that then are incorporated into

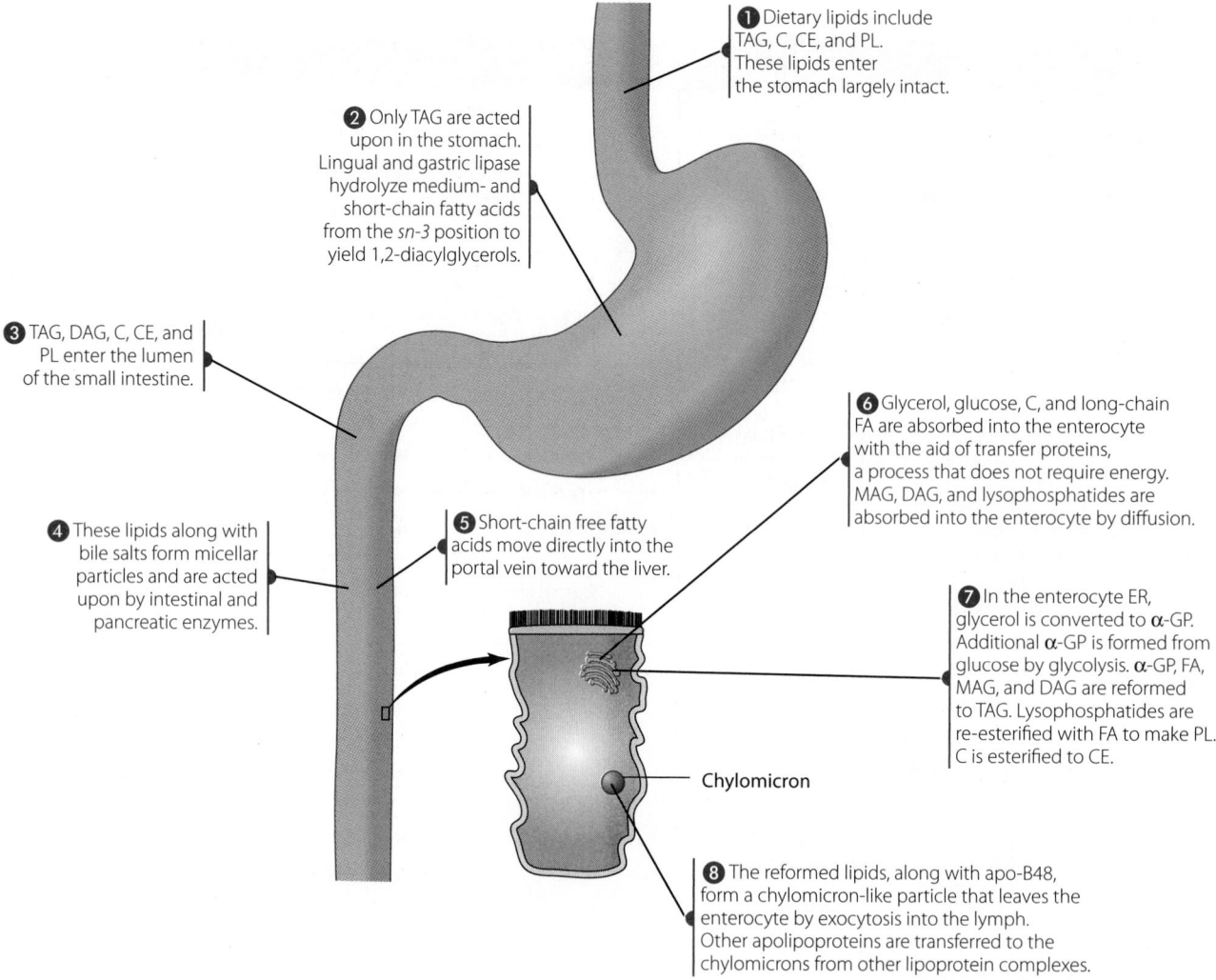

1 Dietary lipids include TAG, C, CE, and PL. These lipids enter the stomach largely intact.

2 Only TAG are acted upon in the stomach. Lingual and gastric lipase hydrolyze medium- and short-chain fatty acids from the *sn-3* position to yield 1,2-diacylglycerols.

3 TAG, DAG, C, CE, and PL enter the lumen of the small intestine.

4 These lipids along with bile salts form micellar particles and are acted upon by intestinal and pancreatic enzymes.

5 Short-chain free fatty acids move directly into the portal vein toward the liver.

6 Glycerol, glucose, C, and long-chain FA are absorbed into the enterocyte with the aid of transfer proteins, a process that does not require energy. MAG, DAG, and lysophosphatides are absorbed into the enterocyte by diffusion.

7 In the enterocyte ER, glycerol is converted to α-GP. Additional α-GP is formed from glucose by glycolysis. α-GP, FA, MAG, and DAG are reformed to TAG. Lysophosphatides are re-esterified with FA to make PL. C is esterified to CE.

Chylomicron

8 The reformed lipids, along with apo-B48, form a chylomicron-like particle that leaves the enterocyte by exocytosis into the lymph. Other apolipoproteins are transferred to the chylomicrons from other lipoprotein complexes.

Figure 5.13 Summary of digestion and absorption of dietary lipids.
Abbreviations: TAG = triacylglycerol, C = cholesterol, CE = cholesterol ester, PL = phospholipid, DAG = diacylglycerol, MAG = monoacylglycerol, FA = fatty acid, and α-GP = α-glycerolphosphate.

chylomicrons and enter the lymph. The different fates of the long- and short-chain fatty acids result from the specificity of the acyl-CoA synthetase enzyme for long-chain fatty acids only. Key features of intestinal absorption of TAG digestion products and resynthesis are depicted in Figure 5.13.

Cholesterol Absorption

As noted previously, U.S. males 20 years of age and over consume an average of 362 mg per day of cholesterol, while females over 20 years of age consume an average of 230 mg [5]. An additional 1 g (which is 1,000 mg!) is excreted by the liver into the intestine. Only about half of the intestinal cholesterol is absorbed; the remainder is excreted in the feces. Most of the cholesterol from the diet is the ester and must be hydrolyzed to free cholesterol to be absorbed. Cholesterol is found in the intestinal micelle, which must pass through the unstirred-water layer, which acts as a diffusion barrier at the lumen-enterocyte membrane interphase. Free cholesterol absorption is an energy-independent process and is facilitated by specific transporter proteins, such as the transmembrane protein Niemann-Pick C1 (NPC1L1) [11–13]. An inhibitor to this transporter, the drug ezetimibe, has been shown to bind with the enterocytes that express NPC1L1 and inhibits the absorption of cholesterol. Ezetimibe is a new drug and is prescribed to reduce cholesterol levels. Other transporters such as scavenger receptor class B type 1 are being investigated for their role in cholesterol absorption.

After the cholesterol is absorbed into the enterocyte and transported to the ER, it is esterified by two membrane-localized enzymes, acyl-CoA: cholesterol acyltransferase 1 and 2 (ACAT1 and ACAT2). These enzymes are highly specific for cholesterol and will not esterify plant sterols. Approximately 70% to 80% of cholesterol entering the lymphatic system is esterified. The reaction of cholesterol esters with apolipoproteins (protein components of lipoprotein complexes, designated "apo") and the formation of chylomicrons are discussed later in this chapter.

Chylomicron Formation

Lipids that are resynthesized in the ER of the enterocytes, along with fat-soluble vitamins, leave the enterocyte by exocytosis as chylomicrons or very-low-density lipoproteins (VLDLs). Chylomicrons are large TAG-rich spherical particles containing TAG, cholesteryl esters, phospholipids (PL), and vitamins A and E in the core and a monolayer of PL, free cholesterol, and protein on the surface. The protein added to the particle surface is a large hydrophobic apolipoprotein B-48 (apoB-48), which is an abridged version of the apolipoprotein (apoB-100, discussed later in this chapter) produced by the liver. It stabilizes the chylomicron in the aqueous environment of the circulation, which it will eventually enter. Other proteins associated with newly formed chylomicrons are apoA-1, apoA-4, and apoC. The apoB-48 protein is considered to be a constitutive protein (synthesized at a constant rate). Another protein that is required for the formation of the chylomicron is a fatty acid–binding protein (FABP), which is involved in the synthesis of TAG from MAG and DAG. The prechylomicron particles are pinched off the ER as lipid vesicles, which then fuse with the membrane of the Golgi apparatus. There, carbohydrate is attached to the protein coat, and the completed particles, now called chylomicrons, are transported to the cell membrane and moved into the lymphatic circulation by exocytosis. While chylomicrons are in circulation, additional lipoproteins (such as apoE) are transferred to them from other lipoprotein particles [10].

The enterocyte also produces a small amount of VLDL by a mechanism very similar to VLDL production in the hepatocyte. The VLDL lipoprotein produced by the hepatocyte contains a small amount of the apolipoproteins C and E. VLDL formation is discussed later in this chapter.

TRANSPORT AND STORAGE

Lipoprotein Complexes

Chylomicrons belong to a family of lipid-protein complexes (or particles) called **lipoproteins,** which get their name from the fact that they are made of lipids and proteins. Lipoproteins play an important role in transporting lipids, and serum lipoprotein patterns have been implicated as risk factors in chronic cardiovascular disease. The other lipoprotein complexes are very-low-density lipoproteins (VLDLs), intermediate-density lipoproteins (IDLs), low-density lipoproteins (LDLs), and high-density lipoproteins (HDLs).

Each of the lipoprotein complexes is associated with specific proteins called **apolipoproteins**. Apolipoproteins play an important role in the structural and functional relationships among the lipoproteins. Each of the lipoprotein complexes contains one or more types of apolipoproteins, but in general has only a single molecule of each type. This feature allows the blood levels of these apolipoproteins to be used to evaluate potential CVD risk. CVD risk will be discussed further in Chapter 7.

Chylomicrons transport dietary lipids. The other lipoproteins transport lipids produced endogenously, which are circulating lipids that do not arise directly from intestinal absorption but instead are processed through other tissues, such as the liver. Each lipoprotein complex has its own characteristic lipid and apolipoprotein composition, physical properties, and metabolic function. Initially, lipoproteins were separated from serum by electrophoresis and therefore were named based upon their movement in an electrical gradient. Later, they were separated by centrifugation and were named based upon their density. These names persist even though other methods are often used for their separation. Lipoproteins with higher concentrations of lipid have a lower density. Very-low-density lipoproteins (VLDLs or pre-β-lipoprotein) are mostly made in the liver; the primary function of these lipoproteins is to transport triacylglycerol made by the liver to other, nonhepatic tissues. VLDLs also contain cholesterol and cholesteryl esters. As TAG is removed from these lipoproteins, they undergo a brief stage as intermediate-density lipoproteins (IDLs). As further TAG is removed, IDLs become low-density lipoproteins (LDLs). (When LDLs were separated by electrophoresis, they were called β-lipoproteins.)

The role that all lipoproteins share is transporting lipids from tissue to tissue to supply the lipid needs of different cells. The arrangement of the lipid and protein components of a typical lipoprotein complex is represented in Figure 5.14. Note that more hydrophobic lipids (such as TAG and cholesteryl esters) are located in the core of the particle, whereas free cholesterol and the relatively more polar proteins and phospholipids are situated on the surface. This structure enhances their stability in an aqueous environment. As previously stated, lipoproteins differ according to the ratio of lipid to protein within the particle as well as in having different proportions of lipid types: triacylglycerols, cholesterol and cholesteryl esters, and phospholipids. Such compositional differences influence the density of the particle, which has become the physical characteristic used to differentiate and classify the various lipoproteins. In order of lowest (the most lipid) to highest density (the least lipid), the lipoprotein fractions are chylomicrons, VLDLs, IDLs, LDLs, and HDLs. The IDL complexes are short-lived in the bloodstream, however, and have little nutritional or physiological importance. Figure 5.15 shows the lipid and protein makeup of each of the lipoproteins.

Apolipoproteins

Apolipoproteins, the protein components of lipoprotein particles, tend to stabilize the lipoprotein complexes as they circulate in the aqueous environment of the blood, but they also have other important functions. They confer specificity on the lipoprotein complexes, allowing them to be

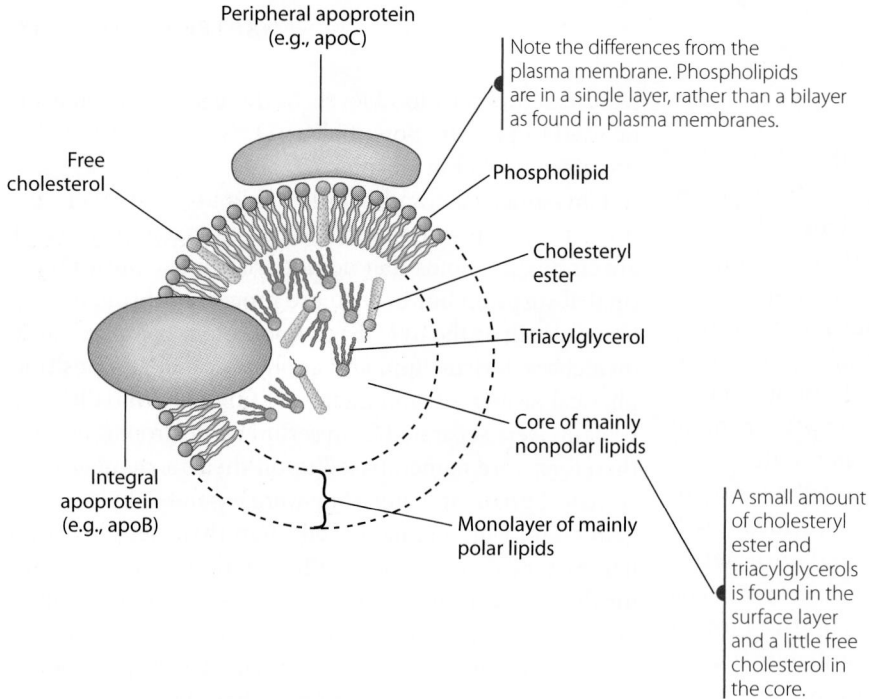

Peripheral apoprotein
(e.g., apoC)

Free
cholesterol

Integral
apoprotein
(e.g., apoB)

Phospholipid

Note the differences from the
plasma membrane. Phospholipids
are in a single layer, rather than a bilayer
as found in plasma membranes.

Cholesteryl
ester

Triacylglycerol

Core of mainly
nonpolar lipids

Monolayer of mainly
polar lipids

A small amount
of cholesteryl
ester and
triacylglycerols
is found in the
surface layer
and a little free
cholesterol in
the core.

Figure 5.14 Generalized structure of a plasma lipoprotein.

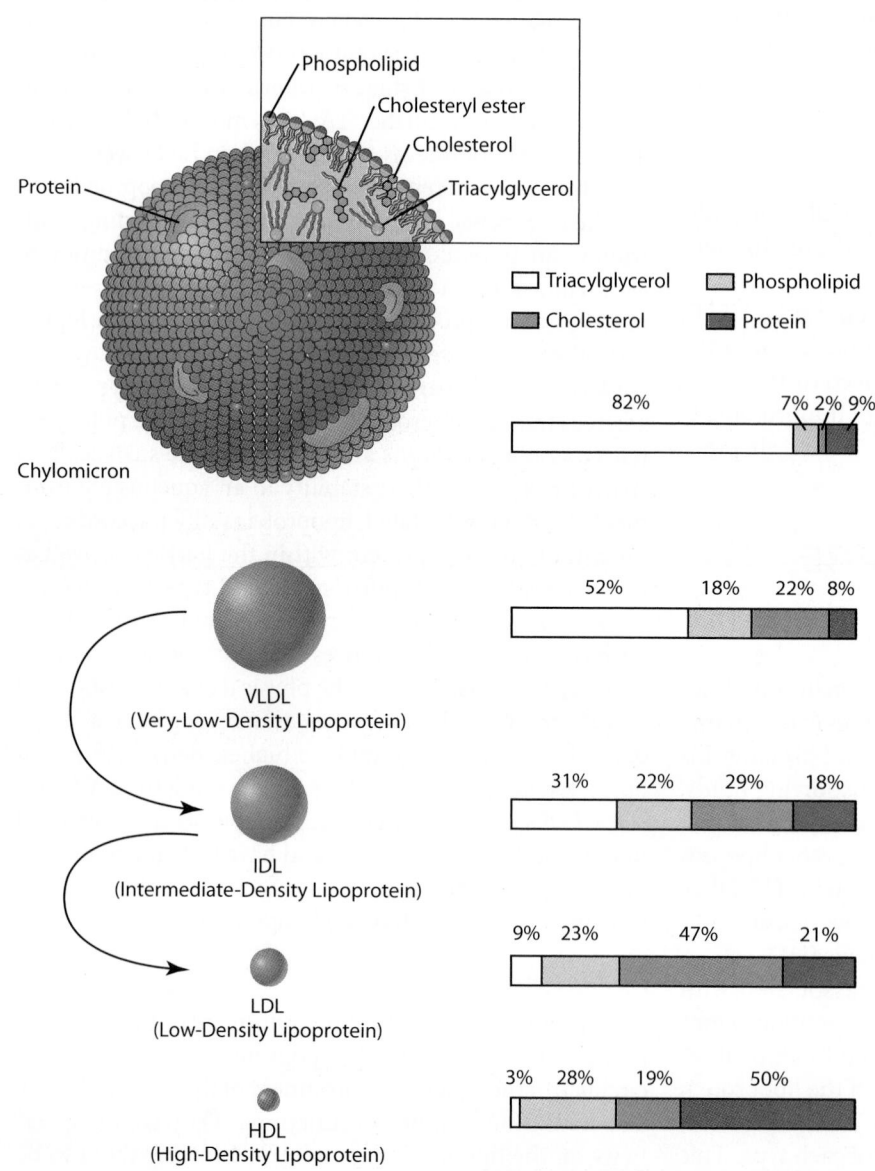

Phospholipid

Cholesteryl ester

Cholesterol

Triacylglycerol

Protein

□ Triacylglycerol   ░ Phospholipid

▓ Cholesterol   ■ Protein

Chylomicron

82%   7% 2% 9%

VLDL
(Very-Low-Density Lipoprotein)

52%   18%   22% 8%

IDL
(Intermediate-Density Lipoprotein)

31%   22%   29%   18%

LDL
(Low-Density Lipoprotein)

9%   23%   47%   21%

HDL
(High-Density Lipoprotein)

3%   28%   19%   50%

Figure 5.15 Lipid and protein of lipoprotein fractions.

Source: Beerman/McGuire, Nutritional Sciences, 1/e. © Cengage Learning.

recognized by specific receptors on cell surfaces. Apolipoproteins also stimulate certain enzymatic reactions, which in turn regulate the lipoproteins' metabolic functions.

A series of letters (A to E), with subclasses of each, are used to identify the various apolipoproteins. For convenience, they are usually abbreviated "apo" and followed by the identifying letter—that is, apoA-1, apoB-100, apoC-2, and so on. A partial listing of the apolipoproteins, together with their molecular weight, the lipoprotein complex with which they are associated, and their postulated physiological function, is found in Table 5.4. A brief overview of the lipoprotein particles' function is provided here. A more detailed description of their metabolism follows.

Chylomicrons

As discussed previously, re-formed lipid derived from dietary sources leaves the enterocytes largely in the form of chylomicrons, though small amounts of HDL and VLDL are produced by the enterocytes as well. Chylomicrons exit the enterocyte by exocytosis and first appear in the lymphatic vessels of the mesenteric region. They enter the bloodstream at a relatively slow rate, which prevents large-scale changes in the lipid content of peripheral blood. Entry of chylomicrons into the blood from the lymph can continue for up to 14 hours after consumption of a large meal rich in fat. The level of lipid in blood plasma usually peaks 30 minutes to 3 hours after a meal and returns to near normal within 5 to 6 hours. These times can vary, however, depending upon the stomach emptying time, which in turn depends upon the size and composition of the meal. The role of the chylomicron is to deliver dietary lipid mostly to tissues other than the liver, such as muscle and adipose tissue (80%). Much of the remaining lipid (20%) is delivered to the liver in the form of chylomicron remnants. Triacylglycerols, the most abundant lipid in the diet, are also the most abundant lipid in chylomicrons. As TAG is removed from chylomicrons, they undergo intravascular conversion to chylomicron remnants (structurally similar to VLDL).

Chylomicrons are transported by the blood throughout all tissues in the body, while undergoing intravascular hydrolysis at certain tissue sites. This hydrolysis occurs through the action of the enzyme lipoprotein lipase, which is associated with the endothelial cell surface of the small blood vessels and capillaries primarily in adipose tissue and muscle (but not in the liver). Its extracellular action on the circulating particles releases free fatty acids and diacylglycerols, which are quickly absorbed by the tissue cells. The large, triacylglycerol-laden chylomicrons account for the turbidity (milky appearance) of postprandial plasma. Because lipoprotein lipase is the enzyme that solubilizes these particles by its lipolytic action, it is sometimes referred to as clearing factor. The part of the chylomicron that is left following this lipolytic action is called a **chylomicron remnant**—a smaller particle, relatively lower in triacylglycerol, but richer in cholesterol and cholesteryl esters. These remnants are removed from the bloodstream by hepatocyte endocytosis following interaction of the remnant particles with specific receptors for apolipoprotein E or B/E on the cells [14,15].

Very-Low-Density Lipoprotein (VLDL) and Low-Density Lipoprotein (LDL)

Very-low-density lipoproteins are produced in the liver from endogenous triacylglycerol in much the same way as chylomicrons are produced in the enterocytes (Figure 5.16, in the next section). The lipid is synthesized in the smooth ER, transferred to the Golgi apparatus, and excreted from the cell along with the apolipoproteins B-100, apoC, and apoE by exocytosis. Circulating nascent VLDL is stripped of triacylglycerol by lipoprotein lipase at extrahepatic sites, in a manner similar to the removal of TAG from chylomicrons. As the TAG is removed from VLDL, a transient IDL particle is formed. The removal of TAG then

Table 5.4 Apolipoproteins of Human Plasma Lipoproteins

Apolipoprotein	Lipoprotein(s)	Molecular Mass (Da)	Additional Remarks
apoA-1	HDL, chylomicrons	28,000	Activator of lecithin: cholesterol acyltransferase (LCAT). Ligand for HDL receptor.
apoA-2	HDL, chylomicrons	17,000	Structure is two identical monomers joined by a disulfide bridge.
apoA-4	Secreted with chylomicrons but transfers to HDL	46,000	Associated with the formation of triacylglycerol- rich lipoproteins. Function unknown.
apoB-100	LDL, VLDL, IDL	550,000	Synthesized in liver. Ligand for LDL receptor.
apoB-48	Chylomicrons, chylomicron remnants	260,000	Synthesized in intestine.
apoC-1	VLDL, HDL, chylomicrons	7,600	Possible activator of LCAT.
apoC-2	VLDL, HDL, chylomicrons	8,916	Activator of extrahepatic lipoprotein lipase.
apoC-3	VLDL, HDL, chylomicrons	8,750	Several polymorphic forms depending upon content of sialic acids.
apoD	Subfraction of HDL	20,000	Function unknown.
apoE	VLDL, HDL, chylomicrons, chylomicron remnants	34,000	Present in excess in the b-VLDL. Ligand for chylomicron remnant receptor.

continues until a cholesterol-rich LDL particle remains. In this manner, chylomicrons and VLDLs are cleared from the plasma in a matter of minutes and a few hours, respectively, from the time they enter the bloodstream. As indicated in Table 5.4, the apolipoprotein apoC-2, an activator of lipoprotein lipase, is a component of both chylomicrons and VLDL—particles that are subject to lipoprotein lipase action. This is an example of the regulatory function of an apolipoprotein.

Within the muscle cell, the free fatty acids from VLDL and those derived from hydrolysis of the absorbed diacylglycerols are primarily oxidized for energy, with only limited amounts resynthesized for storage as triacylglycerols. Endurance-trained muscle, however, does contain TAG deposits. In adipose tissue, in contrast, the absorbed fatty acids are largely used to synthesize TAG, in keeping with that tissue's storage role.

Role of the Liver and Adipose Tissue in Lipid Metabolism

This section explains how the liver and adipose tissues are involved in lipid metabolism following a meal. Our normal eating pattern is to consume a meal, then fast for several hours before we eat again. During the day most of us are in a constant postprandial state. Our bodies have adapted to cope with the alternation between periods when extra nutrients flood the blood and those in which the levels of blood nutrients must be restored from tissue storage. A brief discussion of this process is provided in this section. A more in-depth description of fasting's effects on metabolism is presented in the Perspective following Chapter 6 and in Chapter 7, which covers interrelationships in the metabolism of energy-yielding nutrients.

Liver

The liver plays an important role in the body's use of lipids and lipoproteins. As discussed earlier, hepatic synthesis of the bile salts, indispensable for digesting and absorbing dietary lipids, is one of its functions. In addition, the liver is the key player in lipid transport because it is the site of synthesis of lipoproteins formed from endogenous lipids and apolipoproteins. The liver is capable of synthesizing new lipids from nonlipid precursors, such as glucose and amino acids. It can also take up and catabolize dietary lipids delivered to it in the form of chylomicron remnants and LDL, repackaging their lipids into HDL and VLDL forms. Remember that pathways of lipid, carbohydrate, and protein metabolism are integrated and cannot stand alone. Figure 5.16 summarizes exogenous lipid metabolism in the liver following a fatty meal.

In the postprandial (fed) state, glucose, amino acid, and medium-chain fatty acid concentrations rise in portal blood, which goes directly to the liver. There, the

glucose that was not taken up by other organs is taken up by the hepatocytes and phosphorylated for further metabolism. Glycogenesis occurs—utilizing three-carbon precursors (such as lactic acid), products of fructose metabolism, or freshly absorbed glucose—until the hepatic glycogen stores are repleted. Any excess glucose that is not needed for energy or glycogenesis can be converted to fatty acids. Remember from Chapter 3 that glucose is metabolized to triose phosphates and to pyruvate by glycolysis, and then to acetyl-CoA as it is transferred into the mitochondria. The acetyl-CoA can be transferred back to the cytosol (Chapter 3) and used to synthesize fatty acids. The glycerol needed for TAG is made from triose phosphates (such as glycerol-3-phosphate). Amino acids can also serve as precursors for lipid synthesis because they can be metabolically converted to acetyl-CoA and/or pyruvate. The synthesis of fatty acids, triacylglycerols, and glycerophosphatides is described in detail later in this chapter.

In addition to the newly synthesized lipid derived from nonlipid precursors, dietary lipid is also delivered to the liver in the form of chylomicron remnants and medium-chain fatty acids that were absorbed from the portal blood. The apolipoprotein E on the surface of the chylomicron remnants binds with specific receptors for apoE on the membranes of the vascular endothelial cells of the liver. The chylomicron remnant enters into the hepatocyte in the same manner as LDL (discussed later in this chapter). The lipid portion of the chylomicron remnant contains free fatty acids, monoacylglycerols, diacylglycerols, glycerol, cholesterol, and cholesterol esters.

Dietary free fatty acids of medium chain length delivered directly to the hepatic tissue can be used for energy or, following chain elongation, to resynthesize other lipid fractions. Cholesterol and cholesteryl esters from the chylomicron remnant may be used in several ways:

- converted to bile salts and secreted in the bile
- secreted into the bile as neutral sterol (such as cholesterol or cholesteryl ester)
- incorporated into VLDL or HDL and released into the blood

Newly synthesized TAG is combined with phospholipid, cholesterol, and proteins to form VLDLs and HDLs, which are released into the circulation. Because triacylglycerols can be formed from glucose, hepatic TAG production is accelerated when the diet is rich in carbohydrate. The additional triacylglycerols result in VLDL overproduction and may account for the occasional transient hypertriacylglycerolemia observed in healthy people when they consume diets rich in simple sugars (Figure 5.16).

The HDLs shown in Figure 5.16 are involved in reverse cholesterol transport and, when synthesized in the liver, are smaller than the VLDLs and contain less TAG. HDL

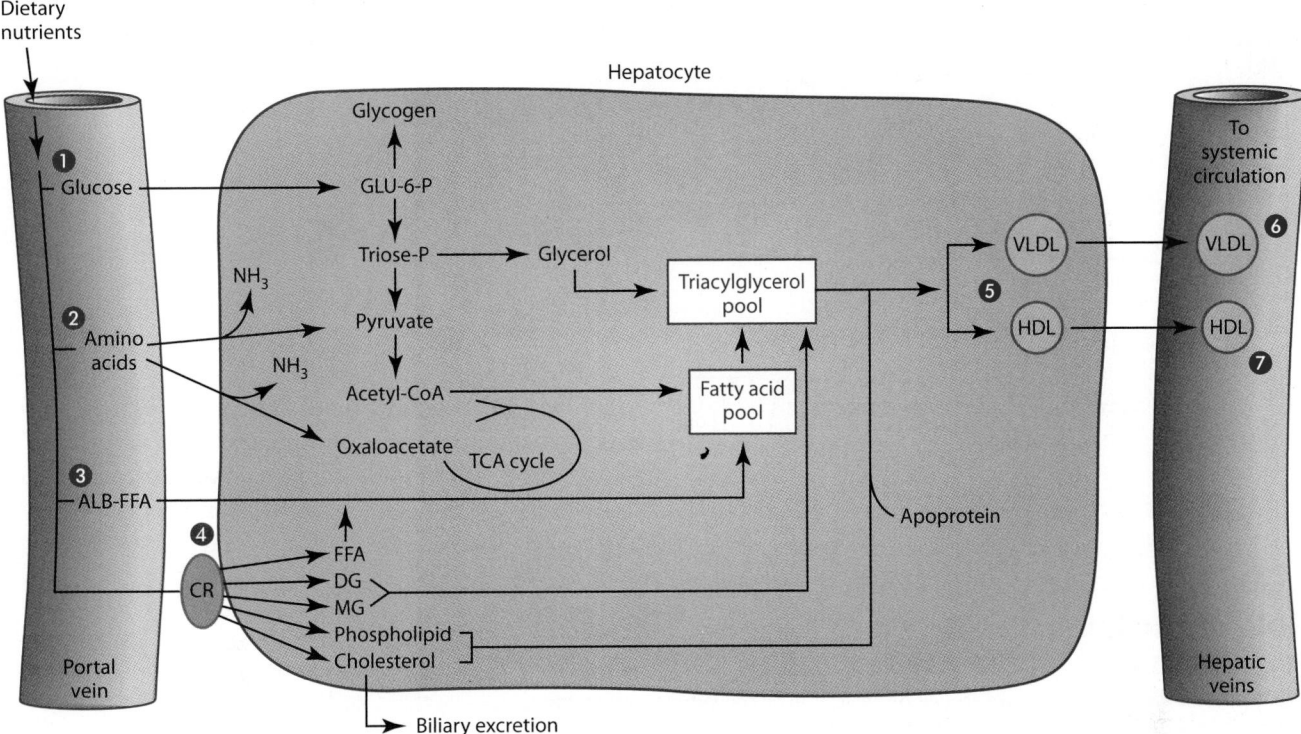

Dietary
nutrients

1 Dietary nutrients enter the liver through the portal vein. Glucose can be converted to glycogen or enter glycolysis.

2 Amino acids enter the amino acid pool and some are metabolized to produce pyruvate and oxaloacetate.

3 Short-chain FFA, bound to albumin, enter the fatty acid pool and are incorporated into TAG.

4 CR attach to apoA, E binding sites, enter the hepatocyte by endocytosis, and are taken up by a lysosome. FFA, MAG, DAG, and C are released. The lipids are reformed to TAG and CE and packaged.

5 TAG, C, and PL are packaged with apolipoproteins and enter the circulation as VLDLs or HDLs.

6 VLDLs deliver the meal's lipids to the non-hepatic tissue.

7 HDL is involved in reverse cholesterol transport.

Figure 5.16 Metabolism in the liver following a fatty meal.
Abbreviations: CR = chylomicron remnant, FFA = free fatty acid, MAG = monoacylglycerol, DAG = diacylglycerol, C = cholesterol, CE = cholesterol ester, TAG = triacylglycerol.

also possesses phospholipids and cholesterol in addition to TAG as its major lipid constituents. The role of HDL will be discussed later in this chapter.

Adipose Tissue

Adipose tissue shares with the liver an important role in metabolism of lipids as regards storage and maintenance of a constant supply. Unlike the liver, adipose tissue is not involved in the uptake of chylomicron remnants or the synthesis of endogenous lipoproteins. Adipose tissue is involved in absorbing TAG and cholesterol from chylomicrons through the action of lipoprotein lipase. Adipocytes are the major storage site for triacylglycerol, and a single large globule of fat constitutes over 85% of the volume of the adipose cell. TAG is in a continuous state of turnover in adipocytes; that is, constant lipolysis (hydrolysis) is countered by constant re-esterification to form TAG. These two processes are not simply forward and reverse directions of the same reactions but are different pathways involving different enzymes and substrates. Each of the processes is

regulated separately by nutritional, metabolic, and hormonal factors, the net effect of which determines the level of circulating fatty acids and the extent of adiposity.

A summary of lipid metabolism in an adipocyte is presented in Figure 5.17. In the fed state, metabolic pathways in adipocytes favor triacylglycerol synthesis. As in the liver, adipocyte fatty acids can be synthesized from glucose, a process strongly influenced by insulin. Insulin accelerates the entry of glucose into the adipose cells (the liver does not respond to this action of insulin). Insulin also increases the availability and uptake of fatty acids in adipocytes by stimulating hormone-sensitive lipoprotein lipase. The glycolytic breakdown of cellular glucose provides a source of glycerophosphate for re-esterification with the fatty acids to form triacylglycerols. Absorbed monoacylglycerols and diacylglycerols also furnish fatty acids for this resynthesis. Free glycerol is not used in the adipocyte, which does not contain the enzyme glycerol-3-phosphotase, and is returned to the blood. Plasma glycerol levels have thus been used as an indication of TAG

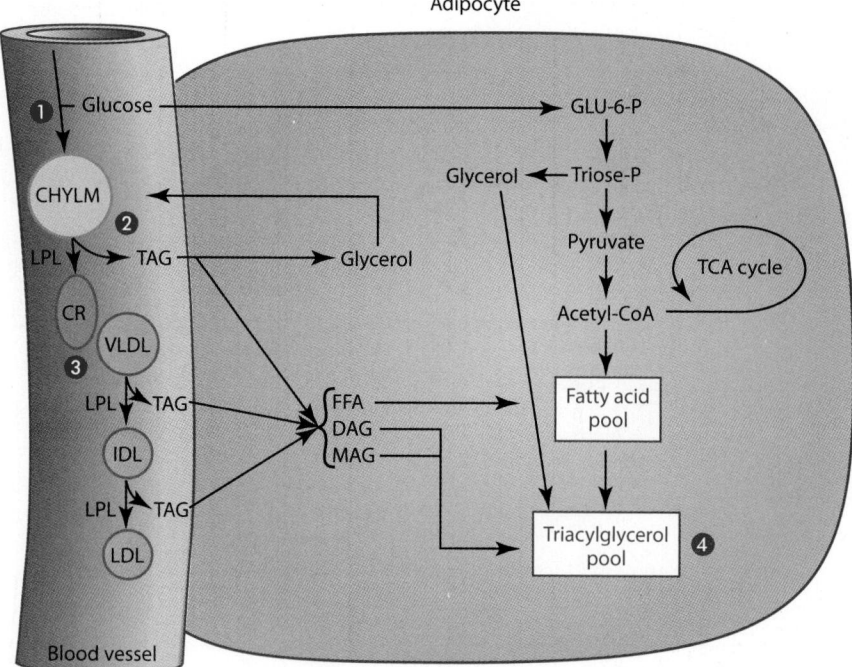

Adipocyte

❶ Glucose is metabolized to make acetyl-CoA, which can be converted to fatty acids.

❷ Lipoprotein lipase acts on TAG in chylomicrons (CHYLM) and free fatty acids (FFA), DAG, and glycero enter the adipocyte. Glycerol cannot be used and is excreted back into the bloodstream.

❸ Lipoprotein lipase acts on VLDL so TAG, FFA, diglycerides (DAG), monoglycerides (MAG), and cholesterol enter the cell.

❹ The pathways favor energy storage as TAG. Insulin stimulates lipogenesis by promoting entry of glucose into the cell and by inhibiting the lipase that hydrolyzes the stored TAG to FFA and glycerol.

Figure 5.17 Lipid metabolism in the adipose cell following a meal.
Abbreviations: CHYLM = chylomicron, DAG = diacylglycerol, MAG = monoacylglycerol, TAG = triacylglycerol, and FFA = free fatty acid.

turnover in adipose tissue. Insulin exerts its lipogenic action on adipose further by strongly inhibiting hormone-sensitive lipase, which hydrolyzes stored triacylglycerols, thus favoring TAG accumulation. Hormone-sensitive lipase is insulin sensitive, distinguishing it from the intravascular lipoprotein lipase that functions extracellularly.

Metabolism of Triacylglycerol during Fasting

To this point, this section has dealt with the role of the liver and adipose tissue in the fed state. In the fasting state, the metabolic scheme in these tissues shifts. For example, as blood glucose levels diminish, insulin concentration in blood falls, lowering the inhibition of the hormone-sensitive lipase, accelerating lipolytic activity in adipose tissue. The lipolytic activity produces free fatty acids and glycerol. Free fatty acids derived from adipose tissue circulate in the plasma in association with albumin and are taken up by the liver or muscle cells and oxidized for energy by way of acetyl-CoA formation. In the liver, some of the acetyl-CoA is diverted to produce ketone bodies, which can serve as important energy sources for muscle tissue and the brain during fasting and starvation. The liver continues synthesizing VLDLs and HDLs and releases them into circulation, though these processes are diminished in a fasting situation. Glucose (derived from liver glycogen) and free fatty acids (transported to the liver from adipose

tissue) become the major precursors for the synthesis of endogenous VLDL triacylglycerol [14]. As described previously, this lipoprotein then undergoes catabolism to IDL, transiently, and to LDL by lipoprotein lipase. Most of the plasma LDL is endogenous and is composed mostly of phospholipid and cholesterol, along with apolipoproteins (chiefly of the apoA series).

Metabolism of Lipoproteins

Chylomicrons and chylomicron remnants normally are not present in the blood serum during the fasting state. As described previously, chylomicrons are released from the intestinal endothelial cell (nascent chylomicron) and contain predominately TAG but also apolipoprotein B-48. The apoB-48 is a subset of the amino acid sequence of the apoB-100 produced by the liver. Other apolipoproteins such as apoB and E are transferred to chylomicrons during their circulation. The next section discusses the binding sites for lipid transport into the cells. The metabolic fate of chylomicrons is shown in Figure 5.18.

Low-Density Lipoprotein (LDL)

The fasting serum concentration of VLDL is low, compared with its concentration in postprandial serum, because of VLDL's rapid conversion to IDL and LDL. Therefore, the

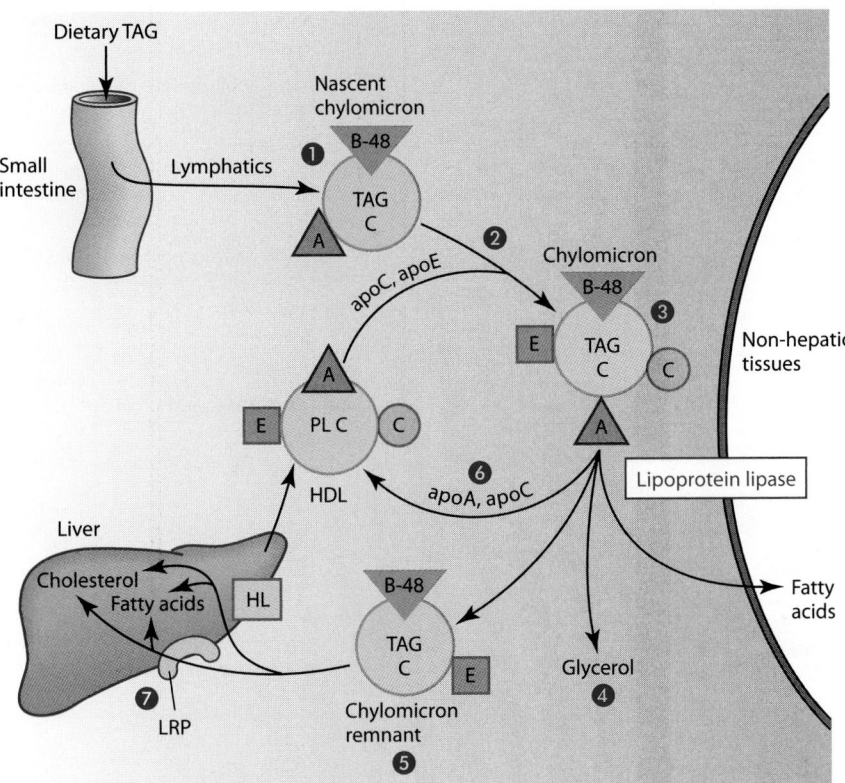

Figure 5.18 Fate of chylomicrons.

Abbreviations: TAG = triacylglycerol, PL = phospholipid, HL = hepatic lipase, LRP - LDL receptor protein, C = cholesterol and cholesterol esters.

Source: Modified from Harpers Illustrated Biochemistry, Figure 25-3, page 221, by R.K. Murray, D.K. Rodwell, and W. Victor, 27th edition (Lange Medical Books/McGraw Hill 2006).

major lipoproteins in fasting serum are LDL (derived from VLDL), HDL (synthesized mainly in the liver), and a very small amount of VLDL. As discussed earlier and summarized in Table 5.4, the apolipoproteins may regulate metabolic reactions within the lipoprotein particles and determine to a great extent how the particles interact with each other and with receptors on specific cells.

The LDL fraction is the major carrier of cholesterol, binding about 60% of the total serum cholesterol (Figure 5.15). Its function is to transport the cholesterol to tissues, where it may be used for membrane construction or for conversion into other metabolites, such as the steroid hormones. LDL interacts with LDL B-100 receptors on cells, an event that culminates in the removal of the lipoprotein from the circulation. LDL B-100 receptors are located on hepatocytes and on cells of nonhepatic tissue. The distribution of LDL among tissues may depend upon its rate of transcapillary transport as well as on the activity of the LDL receptors on cell surfaces. Once the LDL particle, complete with its lipid cargo, is bound to the receptor, both are internalized together by the cell. The particle's component parts are then degraded by lysosomal enzymes in the cell (Figure 5.19). The next section examines the LDL receptor in greater detail.

The LDL Receptor

The discovery of the LDL receptor in the late 1970s and early 1980s was an important biochemical event. This discovery is credited to Michael S. Brown, M.D., and Joseph L.

Goldstein, M.D., who received the 1985 Nobel Prize in Physiology and Medicine for it [16]. According to a recent review from these authors, the discovery stemmed from their search for the molecular basis for the clinical manifestation of hypercholesterolemia, and their research revealed the following facts about LDL and its connection to cholesterol metabolism [17].

LDL binds to normal fibroblasts (and other cells, particularly the hepatocytes and cells of the adrenal gland and ovarian corpus luteum) with high affinity and specificity. Membrane-bound LDL is internalized by endocytosis made possible by receptors on the cell membrane. These receptors are called LDL-apoB 100, E receptors and are the same receptors that remove chylomicron remnants from circulation. LDL receptors interact with lipoprotein particles that contain either apoB-100 or apoE, proteins carried on the surface of an LDL particle. The interaction between the receptors and these apolipoproteins is the key to the cell's internalization of the LDL. Figure 5.20 depicts the fate of the LDL particle following its binding to the membrane receptor. The membrane receptor with the LDL particle attached is taken into the cell by endocytosis. The LDL particle is taken up by a lysosome, and the receptor is released and returns to the surface of the cell. The receptor makes a round trip into and out of the cell about every 10 minutes during its 20-hour life span [16,17]. In the lysosome the protein and cholesteryl ester components are hydrolyzed by lysosomal enzymes into amino acids, FFA,

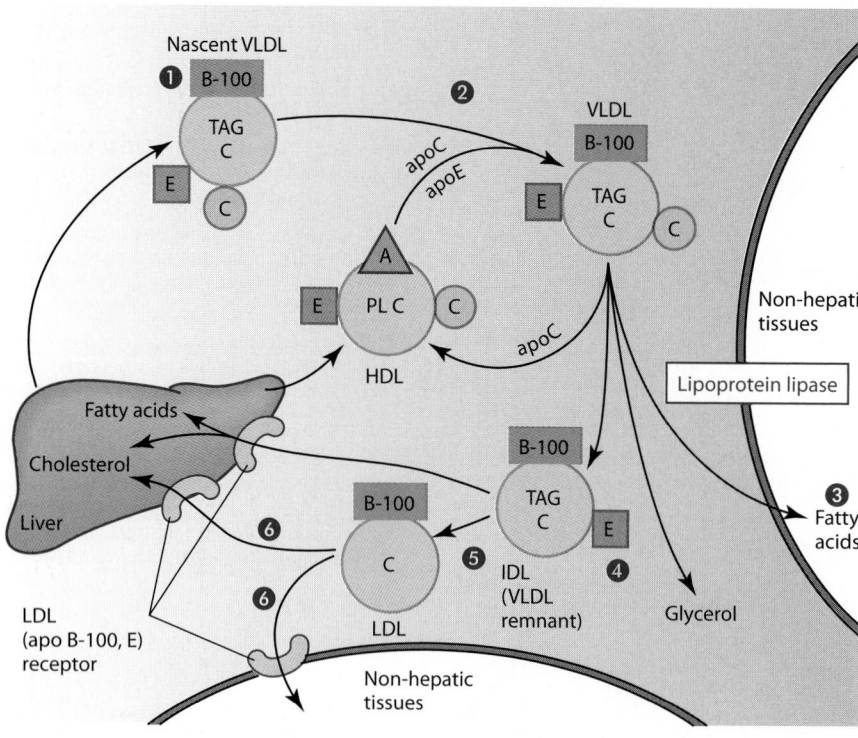

Figure 5.19 Fate of very-low-density lipoprotein (VLDL) and low-density lipoprotein (LDL).
Abbreviations: B-100, E = apolipoprotein B-100 and apolipoprotein E, TAG = triacylglycerol, C = cholesterol and cholesterol esters, and PL = phospholipid.
Source: Modified from Harpers Illustrated Biochemistry, Figure 25-4, page 222, by R.K. Murray, D.K. Rodwell, and W. Victor, 27th edition (Lange Medical Books/McGraw Hill 2006).

❶ Nascent VLDLs are made in the Golgi apparatus of the liver.

❷ Additional apolipoproteins C and E are transferred from HDL.

❸ The fatty acids from triacylglycerols (TAG) are hydrolyzed by lipoprotein lipase found in adipose, aorta, heart, spleen, etc. (non-hepatic tissue).

❹ As the TAG is removed from the VLDL, the particle becomes smaller and becomes an IDL.

❺ Further loss of TAG and it becomes a LDL.

❻ LDLs are taken up by B-100 receptors found in the liver and non-hepatic tissue.

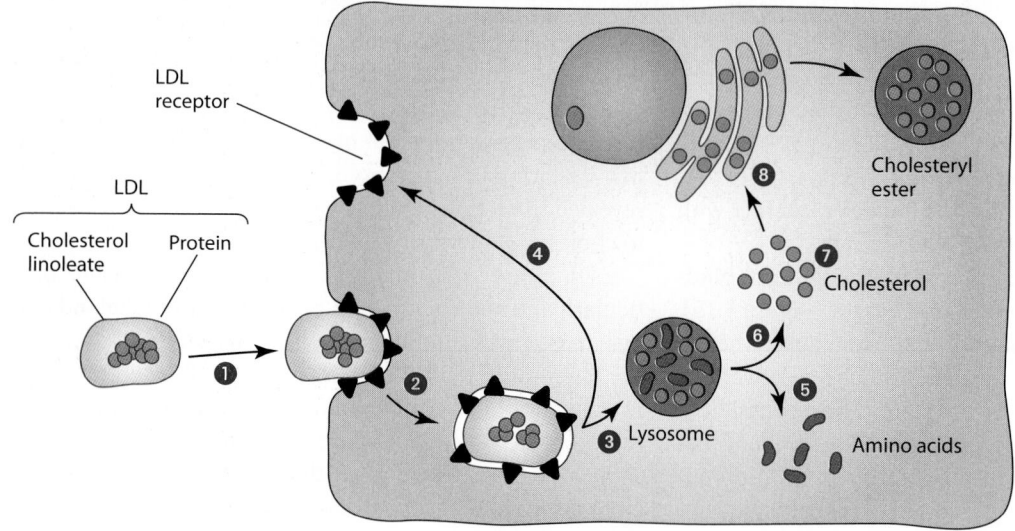

Figure 5.20 Sequential steps in endocytosis of LDL leading to synthesis of cholesteryl ester.
Source: M. Brown, J. Goldstein, 'Receptor mediated endocytosis: insights from the lipoprotein receptor system'. © 1986 The Noble Foundation. Used by courtesy of The Samuel Roberts Noble Foundation, Ardmore, OK.

❶ LDL particle with apoB and apoE attaches to the LDL receptor.

❷ Endocytosis of LDL particle and receptor.

❸ LDL particle fuses with lysosome.

❹ LDL receptor returns to the membrane surface.

❺ Proteins of LDL particle hydrolyzed to amino acids.

❻ Free cholesterol released from LDL particle.

❼ HMG-CoA reductase is involved in cholesterol synthesis. When excess cholesterol is present, HMG-CoA reductase and synthesis of LDL receptors are inhibited.

❽ Cholesterol transferred to Golgi, esterified with ACAT, and stored in the cell.

and free cholesterol. The resulting free cholesterol exerts the following regulatory functions:

- It modulates the activity of two microsomal enzymes, 3-hydroxy-3-methylglutaryl-CoA reductase (HMG-CoA reductase) and acyl-CoA: cholesteryl acyl transferase (ACAT).

- By lowering the concentration of receptor mRNA, it suppresses synthesis of LDL receptors, thereby preventing further entry of LDL into the cell.

Activity of the HMG-CoA reductase, the rate-limiting enzyme in cholesterol synthesis, is suppressed through decreased transcription of the reductase gene and the concomitant increased degradation of the enzyme. In contrast, ACAT is activated, promoting formation of cholesteryl esters that can be stored as droplets in the cytosol of the cell.

The number of receptors synthesized by cells varies according to cholesterol requirements. The LDL receptor has been found to be a transmembrane glycoprotein that, in the course of its synthesis, undergoes several carbohydrate-processing reactions. The carbohydrate moiety is important for proper functioning of the receptor, and its location on the molecule has been mapped. Maturation of the LDL receptor precursor proteins, like that of other proteins synthesized on the endoplasmic reticulum of the cell, occurs in the cell's Golgi apparatus. There the LDL receptors are targeted for their final destination (see Chapter 1). Incomplete or improper processing can prevent the receptor from reaching its proper destination on the plasma membrane.

The LDL receptor has been extensively studied since LDL-cholesterol is a known risk factor for cardiovascular disease. Genetic studies have identified naturally occurring mutations that result in abnormal LDL receptors that can cause hypercholesterolemia, termed familial hypercholesterolemia. This is just one of the causes of elevated LDL-cholesterol.

To summarize, the LDL fraction in normal lipid metabolism can be thought of as a depositor of cholesterol and other lipids in peripheral cells that possess the LDL receptor. Cells targeted by LDL include the cells of the vascular endothelium. It therefore follows that high concentration and activity of LDL have implications in the etiology of cardiovascular disease.

High-Density Lipoprotein (HDL)

Opposing LDL's cholesterol-depositing role is the HDL fraction of serum lipoproteins. Figure 5.21 provides a description of the metabolism of HDL. An important function of HDL is to remove unesterified cholesterol from cells and other lipoproteins, where it may have accumulated, and return it to the liver to be excreted in the bile—a task that has been called reverse cholesterol transport. Two key properties of HDL are necessary for this process to occur.

The first key property is HDL's ability to bind to receptors on both hepatic and extrahepatic cells. Receptors may be specific for HDL, but they also include the LDL receptor, to which HDL can bind through its apoE component. In other words, the LDL receptor recognizes both apoE and apoB-100. Consequently, it is called the apoB, E receptor. The implication is that HDL can compete with LDL at its receptor site [18].

The second key property of HDL is mediated through its apoA-1 component, which stimulates the activity of the enzyme lecithin: cholesterol acyltransferase (LCAT). This enzyme forms cholesteryl esters from free cholesterol by catalyzing the transfer of fatty acids (usually polyunsaturated) from the C-2 position of phosphatidylcholine to free cholesterol. The free cholesterol (recipient) substrate is derived from the plasma membrane of cells or

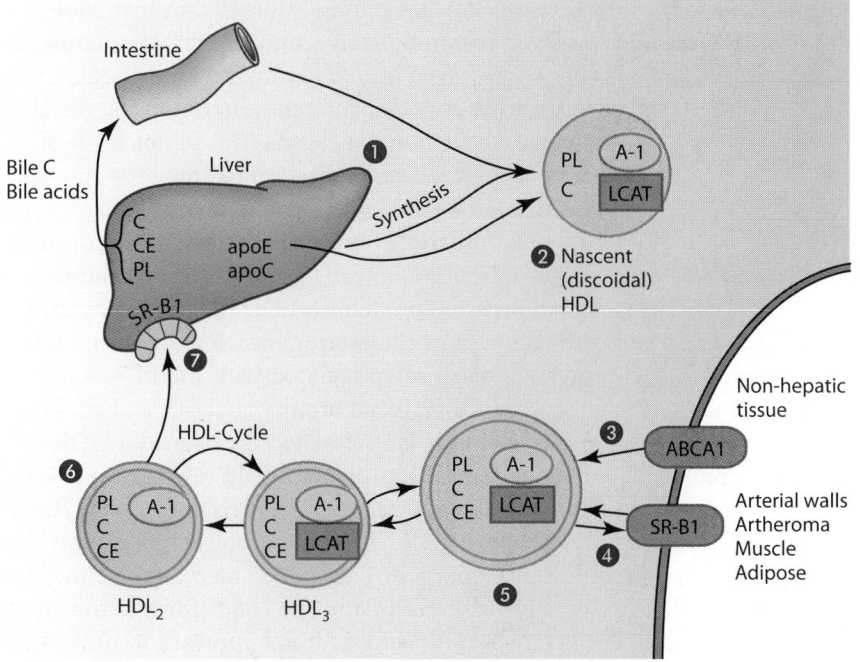

❶ HDL is synthesized primarily in the liver with a lesser amount from the intestine. apoE and apoC are synthesized in the liver and added to HDL.

❷ The nascent or discoidal HDL contains phospholipids (PL), cholesterol (C), and lecithin: cholesterol acyltransferase (LCAT).

❸ Receptors of the adenosine triphosphate (ATP)-binding cassette transporter family (ABCA1) transport cholesterol and PL to HDL unidirectionally.

❹ Receptors of the scavenger receptor family (SR-B1) transfer the lipids bidirectionally.

❺ As the HDL particle picks up PL and cholesterol esters (CE), a polar bilayer of PL is formed with a non-polar core of C and CE.

❻ The HDL spherical particle cycles in size and lipid content by transferring CE to the liver via the SR-B1 site; this is mediated by cholesterol ester transfer protein (CTEP). PL is transferred to the liver and lysolecithin is transferred to albumin.

❼ The life span of HDL is about 2 days and during this time it actively works at the reverse transport of cholesterol to the liver for excretion via bile.

Figure 5.21 Reverse cholesterol transport.
Source: Modified from Harpers Illustrated Biochemistry, Figure 25-5, page 223, by R.K. Murray, D.K. Rodwell, and W. Victor, 27th edition (Lange Medical Books/McGraw Hill 2006).

surfaces of other lipoproteins. Cholesteryl esters resulting from this reaction can then exchange readily among plasma lipoproteins, mediated by a transfer protein called cholesteryl ester transfer protein (CETP). LCAT, by taking up free cholesterol and producing its ester form, thus promotes the net transfer of cholesterol out of nonhepatic cells and other lipoproteins. Cholesteryl esters can then be transported directly to the liver in association with HDL or indirectly by LDL, following CETP transfer from HDL to LDL. Recall that either lipoprotein can bind to LDL (apoB, E) receptors.

After the cholesterol esters are deposited in the liver cells, they are hydrolyzed by cholesteryl esterase, and the free cholesterol is excreted in the bile as bile salt (Figure 5.12). This process is the major route by which cholesterol is excreted from the body. Reverse cholesterol transport benefits the cardiovascular system by reducing the amount of deposited cholesterol in the vascular endothelium, and thus the risk of fatty plaque formation and atherosclerosis. This delivery of cholesteryl esters to the liver (and the subsequent elimination of cholesterol) presumably explains the correlation of high HDL levels with reduced risk of CVD, a topic reviewed in the next section.

Additional functions of HDL have recently been suggested [19]. These include a role as an anti-inflammatory regulator through interactions with the vascular endothelium and circulating inflammatory cells. Some evidence supports the idea that HDL is an integral component of innate immunity. HDL has also been shown to have anti-apoptotic functions (Chapter 1) for a number of cell types, including vascular endothelial and smooth muscle cells, some leukocytes, pancreatic β cells, cardiomyocytes, and bone-forming cells. Further research will reveal its biological importance in these areas [19].

LIPIDS, LIPOPROTEINS, AND CARDIOVASCULAR DISEASE RISK

Atherosclerosis is a degenerative disease of the vascular endothelium. The principal players in the atherogenic process are cells of the immune system and lipid material, primarily cholesterol and cholesteryl esters. An early response to arterial endothelial cell injury is an increased adherence of monocytes and T lymphocytes to the area of the injury. **Cytokines,** protein products of the monocytes and lymphocytes, mediate the atherogenic process by chemotactically attracting phagocytic cells to the area. Additional exposure to a high level of circulating LDL and the deposition and oxidative modification of cholesteryl esters further promote the inflammatory process. The process is marked by the uptake of LDL by phagocytic cells that become engorged with lipid, called foam cells. Phagocytic

uptake is accelerated if the apoB component of the LDL is modified by oxidation. Lipid material, in the form of foam cells, may then infiltrate the endothelium. As lipid accumulates, the lumen of the blood vessel is progressively occluded. The deposited lipid, known to be derived from blood-borne lipids, is called fatty plaque. Atherosclerosis was once considered to be a disease caused by dyslipidemia, and the lipid theory of the pathophysiology of atherosclerosis has been well reviewed [20]. Now, however, atherosclerosis is considered to be a disease of both dyslipidemia and immunity. The Perspective at the end of this chapter discusses these more recently discovered immunological aspects of the disease [21].

Ever since plaque was found to be composed chiefly of lipids, an enormous research effort has been underway to investigate the possible link between dietary lipids and the development of atherosclerosis. The presumed existence of such a link has come to be known as the lipid hypothesis, which maintains that dietary lipid intake can alter blood lipid levels, which in turn initiate or exacerbate atherogenesis. The next section contains a brief account of the involvement of certain dietary lipids and fatty acids, and of genetically acquired apolipoproteins, in atherogenesis.

Cholesterol

At center stage in the lipid hypothesis controversy is cholesterol. The effects of dietary interventions designed to improve serum lipid profiles are often measured by the extent to which the interventions raise or lower serum cholesterol. This reasoning is justified in that cholesterol is a major component of atherogenic fatty plaque, and many studies have linked cardiovascular disease risk to chronically elevated serum cholesterol levels. Receiving the greatest attention, however, is not so much the change in total cholesterol concentration but how the cholesterol is distributed between its two major transport lipoproteins, LDL and HDL. Because cholesterol is commonly and conveniently quantified in clinical laboratories, assays can be used to establish LDL:HDL ratios by measuring the amount of cholesterol in each of the two fractions. Assayed cholesterol associated with the LDL fraction is designated LDL-C by laboratory analysts, and cholesterol transported in the HDL fraction is designated HDL-C.

Because maintaining relatively low serum levels of LDL and relatively high levels of HDL (a low LDL:HDL ratio) supports wellness, the concept of "good" and "bad" cholesterol emerged. The "good" form is the cholesterol associated with HDL, and the "bad" form is the cholesterol transported as LDL. It is important to understand, however, that cholesterol itself is not good or bad; rather, it serves as a proxy for the relative concentrations of LDL and HDL, ratios of which can indeed be good or bad. LDL:HDL ratios are, in fact, determined more reliably by measurements other than cholesterol content. For example, immunological methods for quantifying apoB (the major LDL apolipoprotein) and apoA-1 (the primary HDL apolipoprotein) are now widely used. Ratios of apoA to apoB then serve as an indicator of cardiovascular disease risk, with risk decreasing as the ratio decreases. Approximately one molecule of the apolipoprotein (apoB or apoA-1) is associated with each lipoprotein particle [22].

ApoB in the serum includes both apoB-48, made in the enterocyte, and apoB-100, made in the liver; the majority is apoB-100. This apolipoprotein is found in VLDLs, IDLs, and LDLs. The total moles of apoB present in the serum indicate the number of potentially atherogenic particles.

ApoA-1 is the major apolipoprotein in the HDL particles that are part of the reverse cholesterol system. HDL particles are antiatherogenic. They also have anti-inflammatory and antioxidant properties. A 2006 review provides more detailed information about the use of the apoB:apoA-1 ratio for assessing cardiovascular risk [23].

Associated with lower levels of LDL and higher levels of HDL is the level of total cholesterol, which is less often the focus of cardiovascular risk assessment. Among the reasons for cholesterol's "bad press" in connection with cardiovascular disease is the fact that cholesterol, and especially cholesteryl esters, are major components of fatty plaque. Contrary to widespread belief, changing the amount of cholesterol in the diet has only a minor influence on blood cholesterol concentration in most people. This is because compensatory mechanisms, such as HDL activity in scavenging excess cholesterol and the down-regulation of cholesterol synthesis by dietary cholesterol (discussed in the "Synthesis of Cholesterol" section later in this chapter), are engaged. Remember that dietary cholesterol is found in foods derived from animals, which are also a primary source of saturated fatty acids. It is well known, however, that certain individuals respond strongly, and others weakly, to dietary cholesterol (hyper- and hyporesponders). This phenomenon, which may have a genetic basis, is further complicated by the observation that considerable within-person variability exists independent of diet, a fact that clearly confounds the results of intersubject studies.

Several mechanisms may be considered when trying to account for differences in individual responses to dietary cholesterol, including differences in absorption or biosynthesis; formation of LDL and its receptor-mediated clearance; and rates of LDL removal and excretion. Evidence for hypo- and hyperresponders to changes in dietary cholesterol and other lipids has been accumulating for several decades. These studies have been summarized in a systematic review that includes the genetic variations [23]. It appears that the genes for apolipoproteins such as apoA, apoB, and apoE contribute to the heterogeneity in the lipid-related response to dietary intervention.

Saturated and Unsaturated Fatty Acids

Research examining the influence of various types of fatty acids on cardiovascular disease risk has focused on the effect that each kind has on the risk factors for coronary vascular disease (CVD) such as total serum cholesterol levels or LDL-C levels as biomarkers. The early literature dealing with the effect of dietary fats containing primarily saturated fatty acids (SFAs), monounsaturated fatty acids (MUFAs), polyunsaturated fatty acids (PUFAs), or *trans* fatty acids is extensive and uses these biomarkers as end points. These early research results generally led to the conclusion that SFAs are hypercholesterolemic, PUFAs are hypocholesterolemic, and MUFAs are neutral (neither increasing nor lowering serum cholesterol).

Scientific understanding of the role of dietary intake of lipids in cardiovascular disease risk has changed over time. Observational and intervention studies were initiated to determine the effects of lipid on biomarkers that are better predictors than LDL levels. Several of these studies have now been underway for 20 to 30 years or more, and this time span makes it possible to use disease end points (such as cardiovascular deaths or strokes) rather than risk factors. One large collaborative study examined data from 61 prospective studies from Western Europe and North America, Australia, Japan, and China. The meta-analysis included baseline measurements of total cholesterol and blood pressure for nearly 900,000 adults. During the 12 million person years of observations, there were 55,000 vascular deaths: 34,000 from ischemic heart disease (the blocking of a coronary artery); 12,000 from stroke; and 10,000 from other causes. The analysis revealed that the ratio of total cholesterol to HDL-C is a more informative predictor of ischemic heart disease mortality than is total cholesterol, HDL-C, or non–HDL-cholesterol. Non–HDL-cholesterol is obtained by subtracting HDL-C from total cholesterol and is mostly LDL-C [24]. This analysis confirmed that lowering cholesterol and blood pressure reduced cardiovascular deaths and was able to show that the nature of the reduction was age dependent. The analysis also showed that just a few years of statin therapy that reduced the LDL-C by about 50 mg/dL on average was able to reduce the incidence of ischemic heart disease and ischemic stroke by about a third. Statins are drugs used to inhibit HMG-CoA and block the synthesis of cholesterol. They are widely used to normalize blood cholesterol. Ischemic stroke is the brain damage caused by an area of the brain not having sufficient blood flow. This is in contrast to a hemorrhagic stroke, which results from a ruptured blood vessel. Elevated blood pressure is a risk factor for hemorrhagic stroke.

An expert panel at an invitation only symposium examined evidence for coronary heart disease (CHD) risk from epidemiologic, clinical, and mechanistic studies.

They found that not only was it important to reduce SFA intake, but it mattered what replaced SFAs in the diet. They concluded that when the energy from SFAs is reduced by 1% and the SFAs are replaced with PUFAs, the LDL-C is reduced and is likely to produce a 2% to 3% reduction in the incidence of CHD [25]. They also found no clear benefit of substituting carbohydrates for SFA, although there might be a benefit if the carbohydrate that was consumed had a low glycemic index. Likewise, another pooled analysis of 11 studies concluded that if energy from SFA is reduced by 5% and is replaced by an equivalent amount of PUFA, the risk of CHD is reduced. A 5% decrease in energy from SFA that is replaced with an equivalent amount of energy from carbohydrate, however, results in a slight increase in the correlation between carbohydrate and CHD risk [25–27]. These new studies also re-evaluate the statistical relation of MUFA to CHD and indicate that there does not appear to be one. MUFA has not been found to be protective. Epidemiologic and interventional studies suggest that although substituting MUFA-rich foods for SFA-rich foods in the diet can lower blood cholesterol concentrations, the substitution does not lower the extent of coronary artery atherosclerosis. Some evidence suggests that the source of the MUFA (from animals or plants) may influence the correlation between MUFA and CHD [27,28]. The collaborative study mentioned previously [24] states that even with the large number of subjects in their meta-analysis there is not sufficient data to demonstrate any correlation between MUFA and CHD.

The potential risk of CVD is actually more complicated than what is implied by considering the correlates to blood cholesterol or LDL-C. It involves a combination of genetics, dietary factors, level of obesity, exercise, and other lifestyle determinants. The ratio of total cholesterol to HDL-C has been found to be more predictive of cardiovascular deaths than the previously used risk factors, total cholesterol, or ratio of LDL-C to HDL-C. The cholesterolemic response to individual fatty acids, even those within a single fatty acid class, is heterogeneous. This heterogeneity is particularly noticeable among the long-chain saturated fatty acids. Strong evidence indicates that lauric (12:0), myristic (14:0), and palmitic (16:0) acids are all hypercholesterolemic, specifically raising LDL-C, with myristic acid (14:0) being the most potent in this respect. On the other hand, stearic acid (18:0), neutral in its effect, in fact is reputed to reduce levels of total cholesterol and LDL-C when compared to other long-chain saturated fatty acids. Therefore, stearic acid should not be grouped with shorter-chain SFAs with respect to LDL-C effects. Oleic acid (18:1) and linoleic acid (18:2 n-6) are more hypocholesterolemic than 12:0 and 16:0 fatty acids. Linoleate (18:2 n-6) is the more potent of the two, independently lowering total and LDL cholesterol [28].

Trans Fatty Acids

Double-bonded carbon atoms can exist in either a *cis* or a *trans* orientation, as shown in Figure 5.1. Though most natural fats and oils produced by plants or mammals contain only *cis* double bonds, some *trans* fatty acids are derived from the fats of ruminants, cows, sheep, and goats; others are made by food manufactures. For example, milk fat contains 4% to 8% *trans* fatty acids. Much larger amounts of *trans* fatty acids are industrially produced by partially hydrogenating natural fats and oils. *Trans* fatty acids are found in certain margarines and margarine-based products, shortenings, frying fats, and baked goods that use these products [29]. The hydrogenation of the fatty acids or TAG changes the melting point, giving the product a higher degree of hardness (so that it remains solid at room temperature) and plasticity (spreadability), which are desirable to both the consumer and the food manufacturer. Frying oils have also been hydrogenated to enhance their stability at frying temperatures. Higher frying temperatures reduce the uptake of the fat during cooking. During the dehydrogenation process, electronic shifts cause remaining, unhydrogenated *cis* double bonds to revert to a *trans* configuration that is energetically more stable. The most abundant *trans* fatty acids in the diet are elaidic acid (Figure 5.1) and its isomers, which are of an 18:1 structure, though 18:2 *trans* fatty acids are also found.

Food labeling regulations currently require products to specify the amount of *trans* fatty acids per serving. Food processors want to be able to label their products as having "zero *trans* fat." One means to accomplish this is to use a blend of natural oils containing a chain length and unsaturation level that provide the desired properties without any hydrogenation [30]. Note that labeling regulations permit a food containing less than 0.5 g of *trans* fat per serving to be labeled as providing zero. Consuming several foods labeled as containing zero *trans* fat can result in consuming more than the recommended level.

The reason for the concern about dietary *trans* fat is its association with increased levels of risk factors for cardiovascular and other chronic diseases. These include systemic inflammation, a decrease in HDL levels, and an increase in LDL levels. Some reports suggest that *trans* fat also increases adiposity and insulin resistance [31]. The American Heart Association and the Dietary Guidelines for Americans recommend that *trans* fatty acid intake be as low as possible (zero intake, though advisable, is not considered practical because of the small amount of natural *trans* fat in the food supply).

It has been reported that diets rich in *trans* fatty acids are as hypercholesterolemic as saturated fatty acids [32]. In fact, serum lipid profiles following feeding of a diet high in *trans* fatty acids may be even more unfavorable than those produced by saturated fatty acids because not only are total cholesterol and LDL cholesterol levels elevated, but the HDL cholesterol level is lowered. The study cited was criticized for using *trans* elaidic acids obtained by a process not typical of the hydrogenation of margarines and shortenings and also for including uncharacteristically large dietary amounts of the *trans* fatty acids in the study diet. However, reports from subsequent studies confirm that *trans* fat consumption elevates serum LDL-C while decreasing HDL-C and also raises total cholesterol:HDL-C ratios [33]. Another confirmatory investigation, conducted on a large group of healthy women over an 8-year period, matched *trans* fat intake with the incidence of nonfatal myocardial infarction or death from coronary heart disease [34]. Although the study indicated a positive correlation between *trans* fat intake and coronary heart disease, it did not escape criticism because the data were obtained by consumer questionnaires rather than by a randomized controlled study in which intake could be precisely monitored by researchers [35]. Furthermore, the *trans* fatty acids in the foods consumed by the subjects varied considerably, and a clear-cut dose-response relationship could not be demonstrated [36]. A more recent report from the Nurses' Health Study measured the amount of *trans* fatty acids in the erythrocytes of subjects at baseline and followed subjects for a 6-year period for nonfatal myocardial infarctions and coronary heart disease (CHD) deaths. Erythrocyte *trans* fatty acids were also measured in control subjects. This study used biomarkers for the *trans* fatty acids rather than food intake questionnaires to estimate the level of intake of *trans* fatty acids. The study showed a threefold increase in the risk of CHD between the bottom quartile of erythrocyte *trans* fatty acids and the top quartile [37].

Some reports exonerate *trans* fat of its alleged hypercholesterolemic properties. In a randomized crossover study involving hypercholesterolemic subjects, replacing butter with margarine in a low-fat diet actually lowered LDL-C and apolipoprotein B by 10%, while HDL-C and apolipoprotein A levels were unaffected [31,36]. Nonetheless, the adverse effects of dietary *trans* fatty acids on risk factors for chronic diseases include increased inflammation (increased levels of TNF [tumor necrosis factor], interleukin-6 [a prostaglandin], and C-reactive protein) and dyslipidemia (increased total serum cholesterol, LDL-C, apoB, triacylglycerols, and lipoprotein(a), and decreased HDL-C). There is also evidence for increased insulin resistance, and a potential for increase in weight gain and in visceral fat. A meta-analysis of large human studies indicates that each 2% increase in energy from *trans* fatty acids is associated with a 23% increase in CHD [31].

Lipoprotein(a)

Lipoprotein(a) (Lp(a)) is composed of a low-density lipoprotein (LDL) particle containing apoB and a covalently linked glycoprotein called apolipoprotein(a) (apo(a)). Apo(a) has a strong structural homology (similar amino acid sequence) with plasminogen. Plasminogen is the inactive precursor of the enzyme plasmin, which dissolves blood clots by its hydrolytic action on fibrin. Using a meta-analysis approach for analyzing human studies involving more than 11,000 subjects, it was reported that Lp(a) promotes increased risk for CHD. Apo(a) has several genetic isoforms that vary in size. The smaller–molecular-weight isoforms appear to be more pathogenic. The relative risk of CHD for the smaller Lp(a) isoforms is only about one-fourth as strong as the risk associated with elevated LDL levels [38].

Apolipoprotein E

There are three isoforms of apoE: apoE2, apoE3, and apoE4. As shown in Table 5.4, apoE is a structural component of HDL, VLDL, LDL, chylomicrons, and chylomicron remnants. The function of apoE that has been discussed is related to the LDL particle and the LDL receptor (Figure 5.20). One of the isoforms, apoE4, has been associated with multiple chronic diseases.

A single individual inherits one allele from each parent. About 25% of the Caucasian population has the apoE4 allele, and it has been known for many years that these individuals have an increased risk for CVD. Only part of this increased risk is considered to be due to the dysfunction in LDL and lipid metabolism. ApoE4 is thought to increase the risk of CVD at an earlier age [37]. ApoE has also been shown to increase oxidative stress and inflammation. ApoE is made by the liver, brain, and macrophages. Macrophage-derived apoE is abundant in atherosclerotic plaques, where it influences platelet aggregation, macrophage cholesterol efflux, expression of adhesion molecules, and inhibition of smooth muscle proliferation and migration [40]. See the Perspective at the end of this chapter for more about the role of inflammation in atherosclerosis.

There are also several neurological consequences of apoE4. For example, it has been shown to be a risk factor in early onset of Alzheimer's disease, poorer outcomes following traumatic brain injury, and postoperative cognitive dysfunction. The mechanism for its association with these diseases is not fully understood, but it is thought to be related to the increased oxidative stress and pro-inflammatory properties of apoE4 compared to the other isoforms of apoE. It is interesting that CVD risk is greater in smokers with apoE4 than nonsmokers. Some of the association of apoE4 with diseases is still controversial and must await additional research for confirmation [41].

INTEGRATED METABOLISM IN TISSUES

Catabolism of Triacylglycerols and Fatty Acids

The complete hydrolysis of triacylglycerols yields glycerol and three fatty acids. In the body, this hydrolysis occurs largely through the activity of lipoprotein lipase of the vascular endothelium in nonhepatic tissue and through an intracellular lipase that is active both in the liver and (particularly) in adipose tissue. The intracellular lipase is activated by hormones such as epinephrine, glucagon, and adrenocorticotropic hormone (ACTH). The hormone attaches to a receptor on the cell membrane and by the way of the second messenger cyclic andenosine monophosphate (cAMP) and adenylcyclase, the triacylglycerol lipase is phosphorylated to the active form. The lipase hydrolyzes one fatty acid at a time, leaving three fatty acids and glycerol. Glycerol cannot be metabolized by adipose tissue. The glycerol portion can be used for energy by the liver and by certain other tissues that have the enzyme glycerokinase, through which glycerol is converted to glycerol phosphate. Glycerol phosphate can enter the glycolytic pathway at the level of dihydroxyacetone phosphate, from which point either energy oxidation or gluconeogenesis can occur (review Figure 3.17).

Fatty acids are a rich source of energy; on an equal-weight basis they surpass carbohydrates in this property. This occurs because fatty acids exist in a more reduced state than that of carbohydrate and therefore undergo a greater extent of oxidation en route to CO_2 and H_2O. Many tissues are capable of oxidizing fatty acids by way of a mechanism called β-oxidation, described later in this chapter. When the fatty acid enters the cell, it is first activated by coenzyme A to acyl-CoA, in an energy-requiring reaction catalyzed by cytoplasmic fatty acyl-CoA synthetase (Figure 5.22). The reaction consumes two high-energy phosphate bonds to yield AMP. This is equivalent to using two ATPs. The pyrophosphate that is produced is quickly hydrolyzed, which ensures that the reaction is irreversible.

Mitochondrial Transfer of Acyl-CoA

The oxidation of FA occurs primarily within the mitochondrion and produces energy through oxidative phosphorylation (Chapter 3). Peroxisomal β-oxidation of FA also occurs but is not a major source of energy. Peroxisomes are involved in shortening long-chain acyl-CoAs and detoxifying other lipids. Short-chain fatty acids can pass directly into the mitochondrial matrix and form acyl-CoA derivatives in the matrix. Long-chain fatty acids and their CoA derivatives are incapable of crossing the inner mitochondrial membrane (but can cross the permeable outer membrane), so a membrane transport system is necessary. The carrier molecule for this system is carnitine (see Chapter 9), which can be synthesized in humans from lysine and methionine, and is found in high concentration in muscle. The activated fatty acid (acyl-CoA) is joined covalently to carnitine at the cytoplasmic side of the outer mitochondrial membrane by the transferase enzyme carnitine acyltransferase I (CAT I). Carnitine: acylcarnitine transferase moves the acylcarnitine across the inner membrane; then a second transferase, carnitine acyltransferase II (CAT II), located on the inner face of the inner membrane, releases the acyl carnitine to form acyl-CoA and carnitine (Figure 5.23).

β-Oxidation of Fatty Acids

The oxidation of the activated fatty acid in the mitochondrion occurs through a cyclic degradative pathway by which two-carbon units in the form of acetyl-CoA are cleaved one acetyl-CoA at a time from the carboxyl end. The reactions of β-oxidation—specifically, of the saturated FA palmitate—are summarized in Figure 5.24. The activated palmitoyl-CoA is acted upon by the enzyme acyl-CoA dehydrogenase to produce a double bond between the α- and β-carbons. There are four such dehydrogenases, each specific to a range of chain lengths. The enzymes specific for longer chain lengths are bound to the inner membrane and those for shorter chain lengths are free in the matrix. The unsaturated acyl-CoA adds the elements of water in a stereospecific way across the double bond to form a β-hydroxyacyl-CoA with the aid of the enzyme enoyl-CoA hydratase, sometimes called crotonase. The β-hydroxy group is then oxidized to a ketone

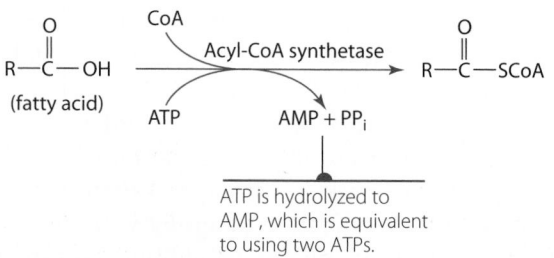

Figure 5.22 Activation of fatty acid by coenzyme A.

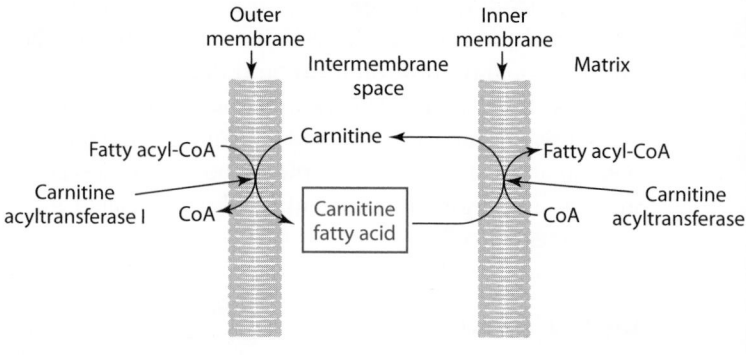

Figure 5.23 Membrane transport system for transporting fatty acyl-CoA across the inner mitochondrial membrane.

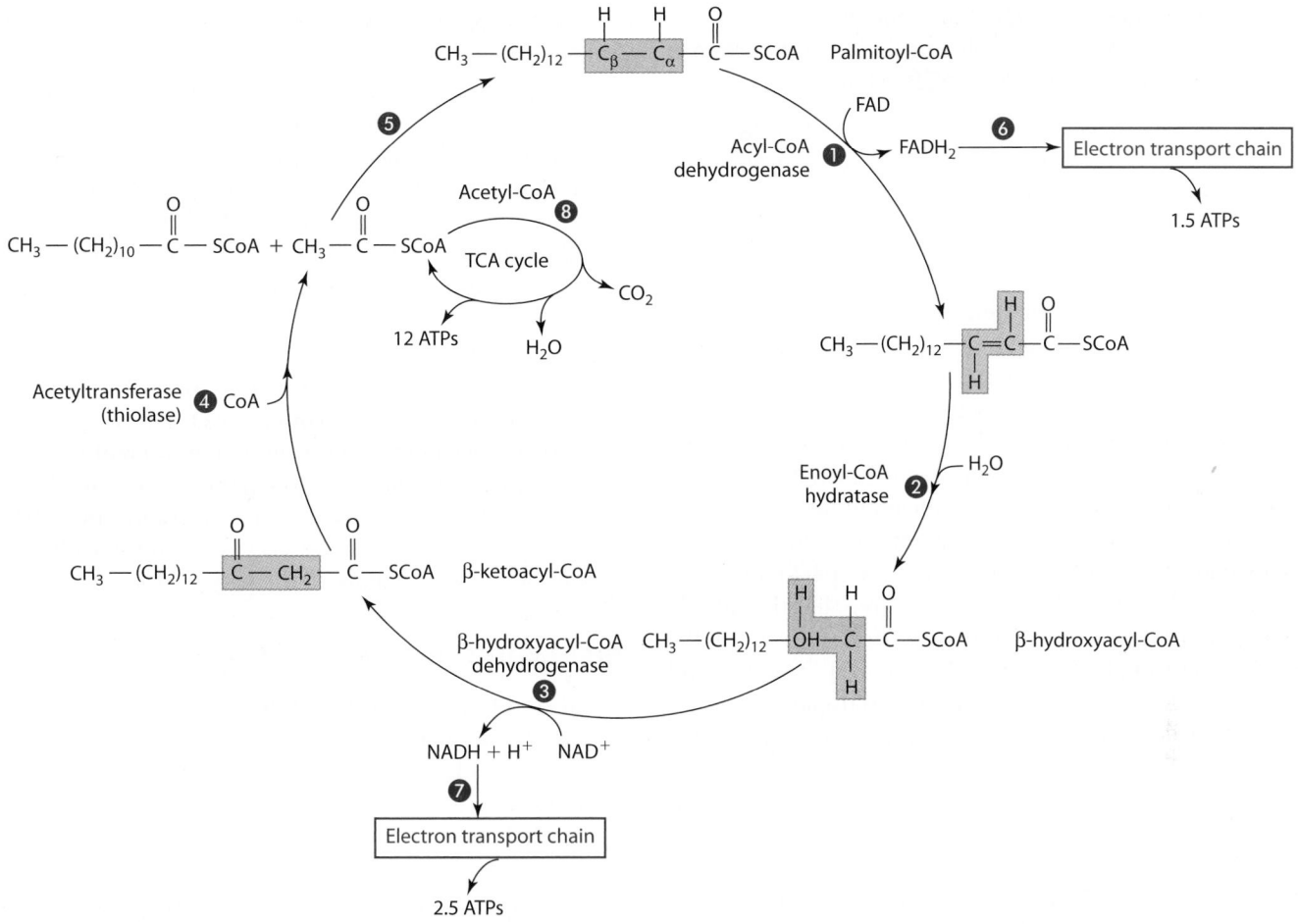

Figure 5.24 The mitochondrial β-oxidation of an activated fatty acid using palmitate as an example.

① The formation of a double bond between the α– and β–carbons is catalyzed by acyl-CoA dehydrogenase. There are four such dehydrogenases, each specific to a range of chain lengths.

② The unsaturated acyl-CoA adds the elements of water in a stereospecific way. The reaction is catalyzed by enoyl-CoA hydratase, sometimes called crotonase.

③ The β–hydroxy group is oxidized to the ketone by the NAD⁺—requiring enzyme β-hydroxyacyl-CoA dehydrogenase.

④ The β–ketoacyl-CoA is cleaved by acyl transferase (also called thiolase), resulting in the insertion of CoA and the cleavage at the β–carbon. The products of this reaction are acetyl-CoA and a saturated CoA-activated fatty acid having two fewer carbons than the original fatty acid.

⑤ This entire sequence of reactions is repeated, with two carbons being removed with each cycle.

⑥ A $FADH_2$ is oxidized by the electron transport system and produces 1.5 ATPs.

⑦ A NADH is produced and is oxidized by the electron transport system to produce about 2.5 ATPs.

⑧ Each acetyl-CoA is further oxidized by the TCA cycle to produce 10 ATPs.

by the NAD^+-requiring enzyme β-hydroxyacyl-CoA dehydrogenase, producing a NADH that can enter the electron transport chain to produce about 2.5 ATPs. The β-ketoacyl-CoA is cleaved by acyl transferase (thiolase), resulting in the insertion of another CoA and cleavage at the β-carbon. The products of this reaction are acetyl-CoA and a saturated CoA-activated fatty acid that has two fewer carbons than the original fatty acid. The acetyl-CoA enters the TCA cycle for further oxidation and the activated fatty acid with two fewer carbons continues the β-oxidation cycle, losing two carbons with each turn. For additional detail on these reactions, consult a biochemistry textbook such as [40].

Energy Considerations in Fatty Acid Oxidation

The complete β-oxidation of one palmitic acid—including oxidation of the $FADH_2$ and NADH produced during β-oxidation and of each of the acetyl-CoAs through the TCA cycle—yields about 106 molecules of ATP. The activation of a fatty acid requires 2 high-energy bonds per molecule of fatty acid oxidized. Each cleavage of a saturated carbon-carbon bond yields 4 ATPs, 1.5 by oxidation of $FADH_2$ and 2.5 by oxidation of NADH by oxidative phosphorylation. The acetyl-CoAs are oxidized to CO_2 and water in the TCA cycle, and for each acetyl-CoA oxidized, 10 ATPs (or their equivalent) are produced (see Chapter 3). Using the example of palmitate (16 carbons), we can summarize the yield of ATP as follows:

7 carbon-carbon cleavages	$7 \times 4 = 28$
8 acetyl-CoAs oxidized	$8 \times 10 = \underline{80}$
Total ATPs produced	108
2 ATPs for activation	-2
Net ATPs	106

As nearly one-half of dietary and body fatty acids are unsaturated, they provide a considerable portion of lipid-derived energy. They are catabolized by β-oxidation in the mitochondrion in nearly the same way as their saturated counterparts, except that one fewer fatty acyl-CoA dehydrogenase reaction is required for each double bond present. This is because the double bond introduced into the saturated fatty acid by the reaction occurs naturally in unsaturated fatty acids. However, the specificity of the enoyl-CoA hydratase reaction requires that the double bond be between the second and third carbon for the hydration to take place, and the "natural" double bond may not occupy the Δ^2 position. For example, after three cycles of β-carbon oxidation, the position of the double bond in what was originally a Δ^9 monounsaturated fatty acid will occupy a Δ^3 position. Figure 5.25 shows 18:1 Δ^9 undergoing three cycles of β-oxidation. At the end of the third cycle, the fatty acid is a Δ^3 fatty acid. The presence of a specific enoyl-CoA-isomerase then shifts the double

bond from a *cis* Δ^3 to *trans* Δ^2, allowing the hydrase and subsequent reactions to proceed. The oxidation of an unsaturated fatty acid results in somewhat less energy production than oxidation of a saturated fatty acid of the same chain length because for each double bond present 1 $FADH_2$-producing fatty acyl-CoA dehydrogenase reaction is bypassed, resulting in 1.5 fewer ATPs.

Although most fatty acids metabolized are composed of an even number of carbon atoms, small amounts of fatty acids having an odd number of carbon atoms are also used for energy. β-oxidation occurs as described, with the liberation of acetyl-CoA until a residual propionyl-CoA remains. The subsequent oxidation of propionyl-CoA requires reactions that use the vitamins biotin and B_{12} in a coenzymatic role (Figure 5.26). Because the succinyl-CoA formed in the course of these reactions can be converted into glucose, the odd-numbered carbon fatty acids are uniquely glucogenic among all the fatty acids.

Formation of Ketone Bodies

In addition to its direct oxidation through the TCA cycle, acetyl-CoA may follow other catabolic routes in the liver, one of which is the pathway by which the so-called **ketone bodies** (acetoacetate, β-hydroxybutyrate, and acetone) are formed, a process called **ketogenesis**. Acetoacetate and β-hydroxybutyrate are not oxidized further in the liver but instead are transported by the blood to

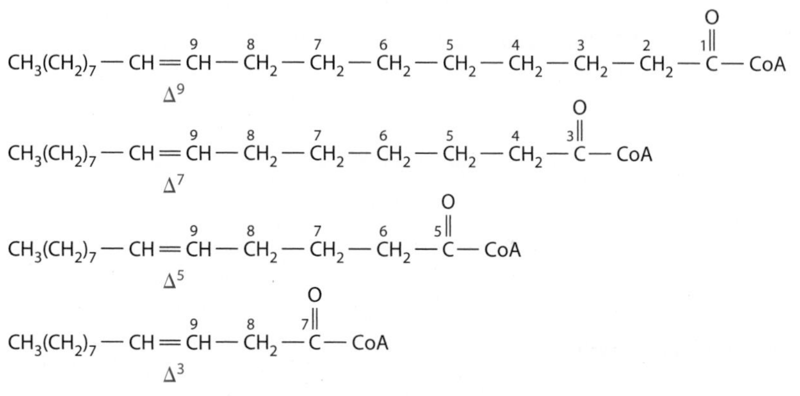

Figure 5.25 Sequential β-oxidation of oleic acid, showing the location of the double bond using the Δ nomenclature system. Numbers above the carbons represent the original carbon numbers of oleic acid.

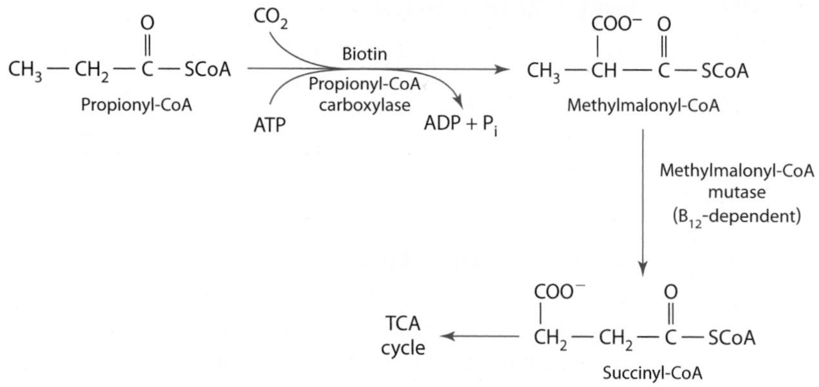

Figure 5.26 Oxidation of propionyl-CoA.

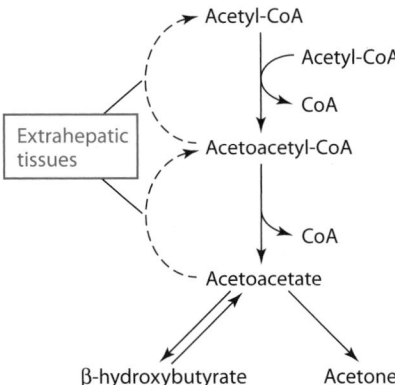

Figure 5.27 Steps in ketone body formation.

peripheral tissues, where they can be converted back to acetyl-CoA and oxidized through the TCA cycle. The steps in ketone body formation, which occurs only in the mitochondria, are shown in Figure 5.27. The reversibility of the β-hydroxybutyrate dehydrogenase reaction, together with enzymes present in extrahepatic tissues that convert acetoacetate to acetyl-CoA (shown by broken arrows in Figure 5.27), reveals how the ketone bodies can serve as a source of fuel in these tissues. Ketone body formation is actually an "overflow" pathway for acetyl-CoA use, providing another way for the liver to distribute fuel to peripheral cells.

Normally, the concentration of the ketone bodies in the blood is very low, but it may reach very high levels in situations of accelerated fatty acid oxidation combined with low carbohydrate intake or impaired carbohydrate use. Such a situation would occur in uncontrolled diabetes mellitus, in starvation, or with consumption of a very-low-carbohydrate diet. Recall from Chapter 3 that for the TCA cycle to function, the supply of four-carbon units must be adequate. These intermediates are formed mainly from pyruvate (formed during glycolysis). When the supply of carbohydrate is inadequate, there is insufficient glucose for glycolysis to occur at a normal rate and less pyruvate is produced. Thus the pool of oxaloacetate (made from pyruvate), with which the acetyl-CoA normally combines for oxidation in the TCA cycle, is reduced. As carbohydrate use diminishes, oxidation of fatty acids accelerates to provide energy through the production of TCA cycle substrates (acetyl-CoA). This shift to fat catabolism, coupled with reduced oxaloacetate availability, results in an accumulation of acetyl-CoA. As would be expected, a sharp increase in ketone body formation follows, resulting in the condition known as ketosis. Ketosis can be dangerous because it can disturb the body's acid-base balance (two of the ketone bodies are, in fact, organic acids). However, the liver's ability to deliver ketone bodies to peripheral tissues such as the brain and muscle is an important mechanism for providing fuel in periods of starvation. In short, it is the lesser of two evils.

Catabolism of Cholesterol

Unlike the triacylglycerols and fatty acids, cholesterol is not an energy-producing nutrient. Its four-ring core structure remains intact in the course of its catabolism and is eliminated as such through the biliary system, as described earlier in this chapter. Cholesterol, primarily in the form of its ester, is delivered to the liver chiefly in the form of chylomicron remnants, as well as in the form of LDL-C and HDL-C. The cholesterol that is destined for excretion either is hydrolyzed by esterases to the free form, which is secreted directly into the bile canaliculi, or it is first converted into bile acids before entering the bile. It is estimated that neutral sterol, most of which is cholesterol, represents about 55%, and bile acids and their salts about 45%, of total sterol excreted.

The key metabolic changes in the cholesterol-to-bile acid transformation are:

- reduction in the length of the hydrocarbon side chain at C-17
- addition of a carboxylic acid group on the shortened chain
- addition of hydroxyl groups to the ring system of the molecule

The effect of these reactions is to enhance the water solubility of the sterol, facilitating its excretion in the bile. Cholic acid, whose structure is shown in Figure 5.12, has hydroxyl groups at C-7 and C-12 in addition to the C-3 hydroxyl of the native cholesterol. The other major bile acids differ from cholic acid only in the number of hydroxyls attached to the ring system. For example, chenodeoxycholic acid has hydroxyls at C-3 and C-7, deoxycholic acid at C-3 and C-12, and lithocholic acid at C-3 only. Other bile acids are formed through the conjugation of these compounds with glycine or taurine, which attaches through the carboxyl group of the steroid. These reactions are shown in Figure 5.12.

Recall that the enterohepatic circulation can return absorbed bile salts to the liver. Bile salts returning to the liver from the intestine repress the formation of an enzyme that catalyzes the rate-limiting step in the conversion of cholesterol into bile acids. If the bile salts are prevented from returning to the liver, the activity of this enzyme increases, stimulating the conversion of cholesterol to bile acids and leading to their excretion. The removal of bile salts is exploited therapeutically in treating hypercholesterolemia by using unabsorbable, cationic resins that bind bile salts in the intestinal lumen and prevent them from returning to the liver.

Synthesis of Fatty Acids

Aside from linoleic acid and α-linolenic acid, which are essential and must be acquired from the diet, the body is capable of synthesizing fatty acids from simple precursors. The

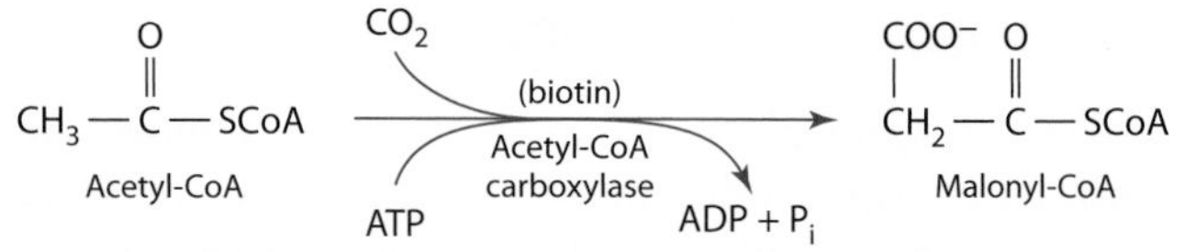

Figure 5.28 Formation of malonyl-CoA from acetyl-CoA and CO$_2$ (carboxylation reaction).

basic process involves the sequential assembly of a "starter" molecule of acetyl-CoA with units of malonyl-CoA, the CoA derivative of malonic acid. Ultimately, however, all the carbons of a fatty acid are contributed by acetyl-CoA because malonyl-CoA is formed from acetyl-CoA and CO$_2$. This reaction occurs in the cytosol. It is catalyzed by acetyl-CoA carboxylase, a complex enzyme containing biotin as its prosthetic group. The role of biotin in **carboxylation** reactions (such as this one), which involve the incorporation of a carboxyl group into a compound, is discussed in Chapter 9. ATP furnishes the energy to attach the new carboxyl group to acetyl-CoA (Figure 5.28).

Nearly all acetyl-CoA production occurs in the mitochondria. It is formed there from pyruvate oxidation, from the oxidation of fatty acids, and from the degradation of the carbon skeletons of some amino acids (see Chapter 6). Some acetyl-CoA is formed in the cytosol from amino acid catabolism. The synthesis of fatty acids is localized in the cytosol, but acetyl-CoA produced within the mitochondrial matrix is unable to exit through the mitochondrial membrane. Instead, the major mechanism for the transfer of acetyl-CoA to the cytosol is its reaction with oxaloacetate to form citrate, which can pass through the inner membrane. In the cytosol, citrate lyase converts the citrate back to oxaloacetate and acetyl-CoA. This reaction, shown here, is essentially the reversal of the citrate synthetase reaction of the TCA cycle, except that it requires expenditure of ATP.

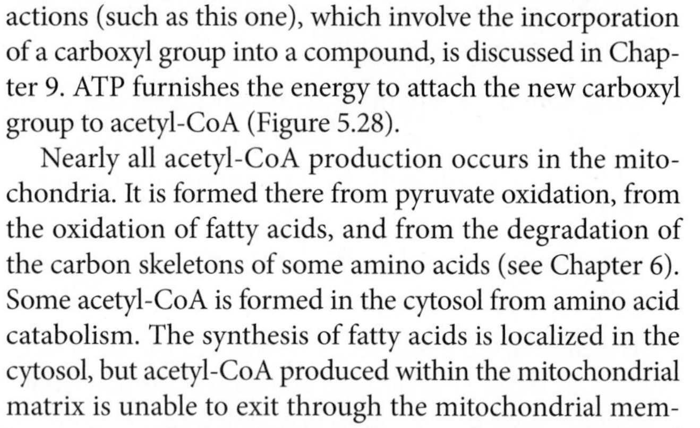

The enzymes involved in fatty acid synthesis are arranged in a complex called the fatty acid synthase system, which is found in the cytosol. Key components of this complex are the acyl carrier protein (ACP) and the condensing enzyme

(CE), both of which possess free —SH groups to which the acetyl-CoA and malonyl-CoA building blocks attach. ACP is structurally similar to CoA (Figure 9.18). Both possess a 4′-phosphopantetheine component (pantothenic acid coupled through β-alanine to thioethanolamine) and phosphate. The thioethanolamine contributes the free —SH group to the complex. The free —SH of the condensing enzyme is contributed by the amino acid cysteine.

Before the actual steps in the elongation of the fatty acid chain can begin, the two sulfhydryl groups must be "loaded" correctly with malonyl and acetyl groups. Acetyl-CoA is transferred to ACP, with the loss of CoA, to form acetyl-ACP. The acetyl group is then transferred again to the —SH of the condensing enzyme, leaving available the ACP—SH, to which malonyl-CoA attaches, again with the loss of CoA. This loading of the complex can be represented as in Figure 5.29. The extension of the fatty acid chain then proceeds through the following sequential steps, which also are shown schematically in Figure 5.30 along with the enzymes and cofactors catalyzing their actions. The enzymes catalyzing these reactions are also part of the fatty acid synthase complex along with ACP and CE.

The first step is the coupling of the carbonyl carbon of the acetyl group to the C-2 of malonyl-ACP with the elimination of the malonyl carboxyl group as CO$_2$. The β-ketone is then reduced, with NADPH serving as hydrogen donor. (The NADPH is generated by the pentose phosphate pathway in the cytosol, as discussed in Chapter 3.) This alcohol is dehydrated, yielding a double bond. The double bond is reduced to butyryl-ACP, again with NADPH acting as reducing agent. The butyryl group is transferred to the CE, exposing the ACP sulfhydryl site, which accepts a second molecule of malonyl-CoA. A second condensation reaction takes place, coupling the butyryl group on the CE to C-2 of the malonyl-ACP. The six-carbon chain is then reduced and transferred to CE in a repetition of steps 2 through 5. A third molecule of malonyl-CoA attaches at ACP—SH, and so forth. The completed fatty acid chain is hydrolyzed from the ACP without transfer to the CE. The normal product of the fatty acid synthase system is palmitate, 16:0. It can in turn be lengthened by fatty acid elongation systems to stearic acid, 18:0, and even longer saturated fatty acids. Elongation occurs by the addition of two-carbon units at the carboxylic acid end of the chain. Furthermore, by **desaturation** reactions, palmitate and stearate can be converted to their corresponding Δ^9 monounsaturated fatty acids,

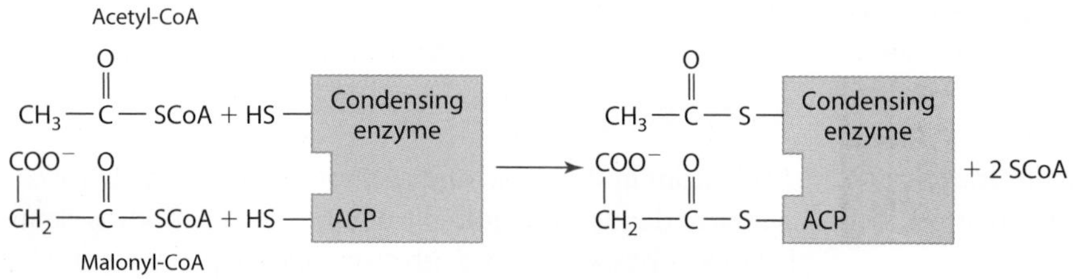

Figure 5.29 "Loading" of sulfhydryl groups into the fatty acid synthase system.

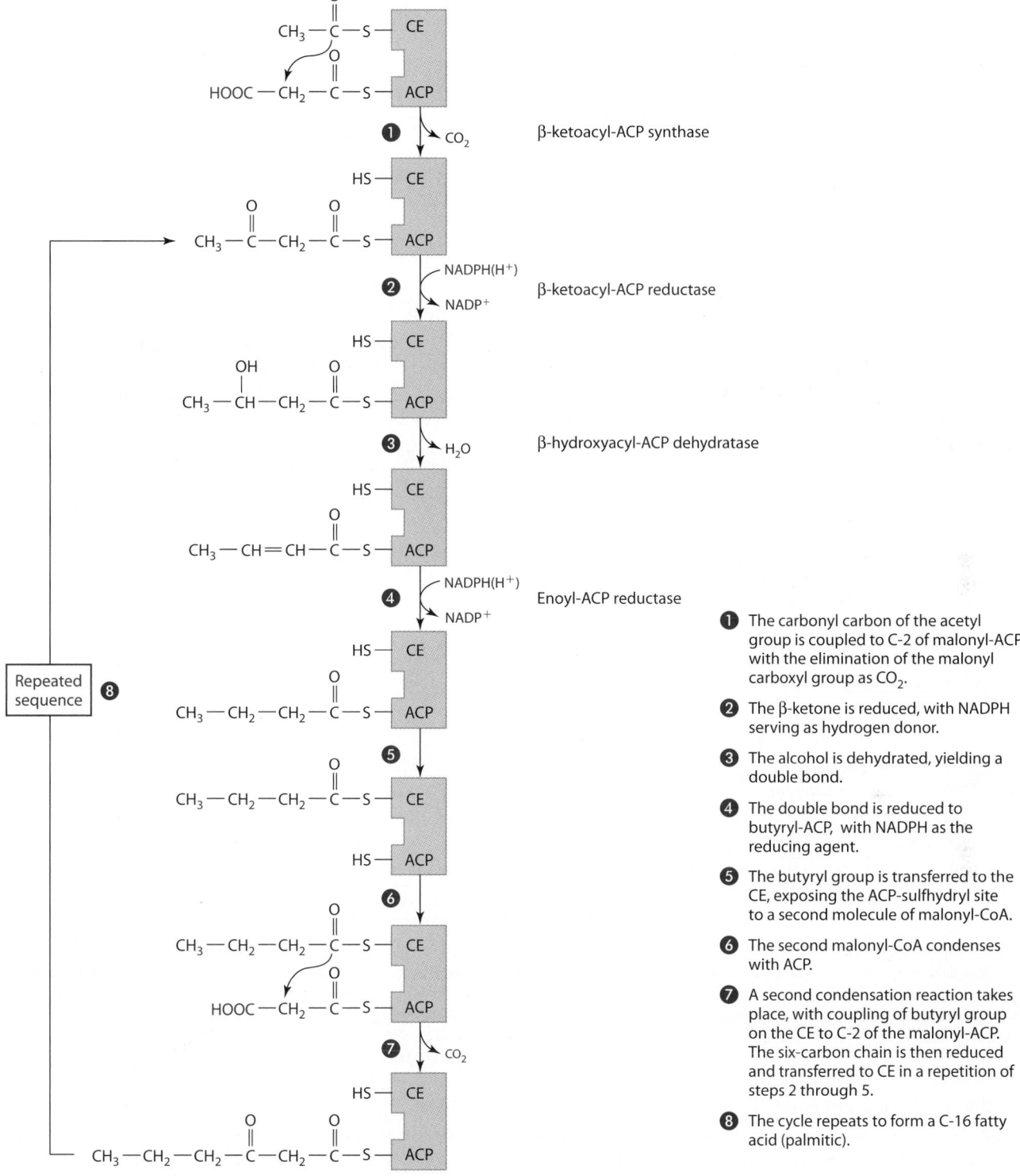

Figure 5.30 The steps in the synthesis of fatty acid. CE (condensing enzyme) and ACP (acyl carrier protein) are members of a complex of enzymes referred to as the fatty acid synthase system.

1. The carbonyl carbon of the acetyl group is coupled to C-2 of malonyl-ACP with the elimination of the malonyl carboxyl group as CO_2.

2. The β-ketone is reduced, with NADPH serving as hydrogen donor.

3. The alcohol is dehydrated, yielding a double bond.

4. The double bond is reduced to butyryl-ACP, with NADPH as the reducing agent.

5. The butyryl group is transferred to the CE, exposing the ACP-sulfhydryl site to a second molecule of malonyl-CoA.

6. The second malonyl-CoA condenses with ACP.

7. A second condensation reaction takes place, with coupling of butyryl group on the CE to C-2 of the malonyl-ACP. The six-carbon chain is then reduced and transferred to CE in a repetition of steps 2 through 5.

8. The cycle repeats to form a C-16 fatty acid (palmitic).

palmitoleic acid (16:1) and oleic acid (18:1), respectively. Fatty acid desaturation reactions are catalyzed by enzymes referred to as mixed-function oxidases, so called because two different substrates are oxidized: the fatty acid (by removal of hydrogen atoms to form the new double bond) and NADPH. Oxygen is the terminal hydrogen and electron acceptor to form H_2O.

Essential Fatty Acids

Recall that human cells cannot introduce additional double bonds beyond the Δ^9 site because they lack enzymes called Δ^{12} and Δ^{15} desaturases. That is why linoleic acid (18:2 $\Delta^{9,12}$; LA, n-6) and α-linolenic acid (18:3 $\Delta^{9,12,15}$; ALA, n-3) are essential fatty acids. These fatty acids can be acquired from plant sources because plant cells do

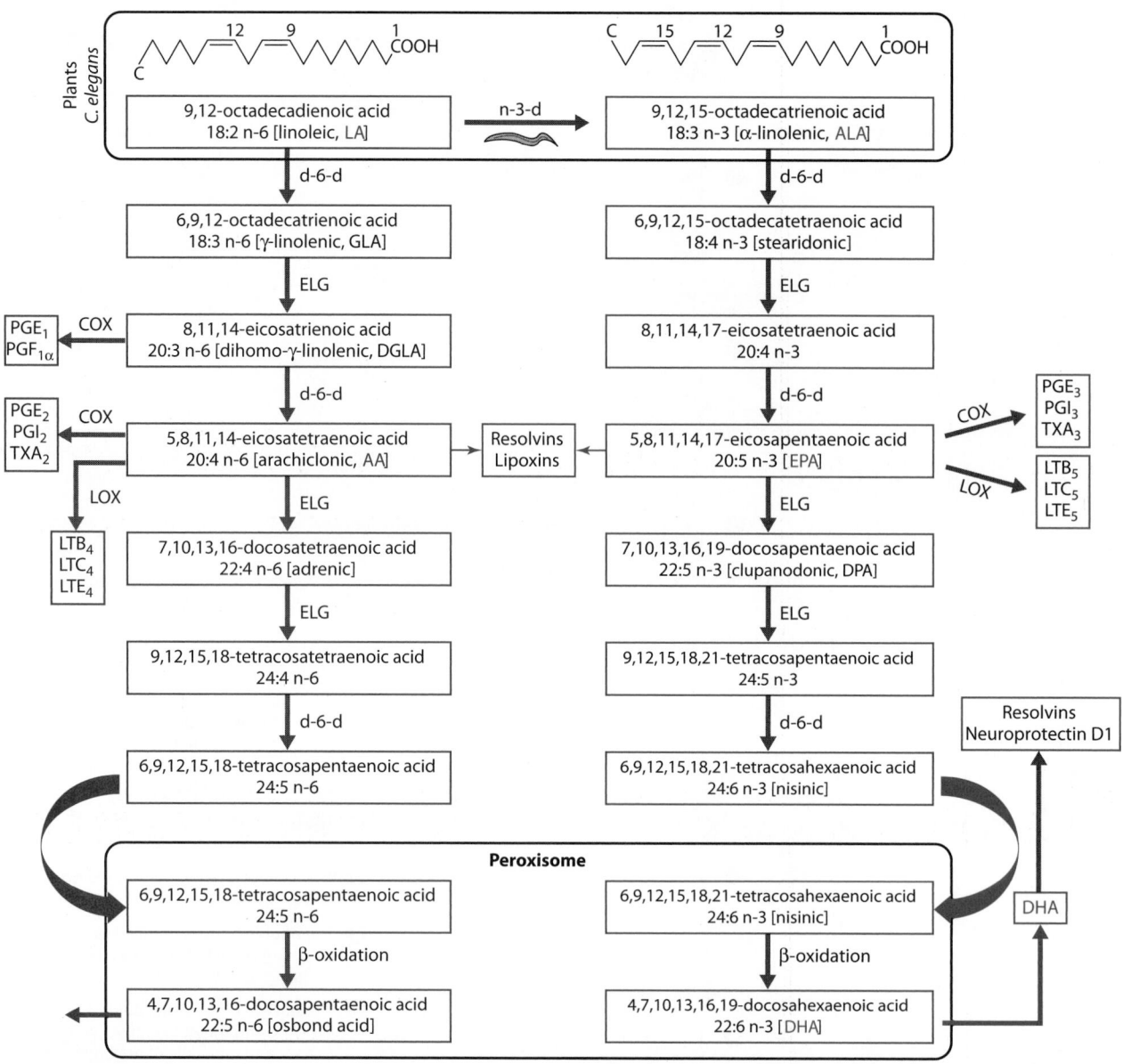

Figure 5.31 PUFA biosynthesis. The IUPAC names (all-*cis*) and the common names (in square brackets) with abbreviations are reported. ELG indicates elongase, while d-6-d and d-5-d indicate delta desaturases. In plants, an n-3 desaturase (n-3-d) converts LA to ALA. Mammals convert LA and ALA to long-chain fatty acids using a series of desaturation and elongation reactions in the ER. However, the synthesis of DHA from 24:6 n-3 and osbond acid (22:5 n-6) from 24:5 n-6 requires the synthesis of 24:6 n-3 and 24:5 n-6 in the ER, and their passage into the peroxisome, where they undergo one cycle of beta-oxidation to produce DHA and osbond acid, which move back to the ER (red arrows). Formation of resolvins and protectins from DHA is also shown.

Source: Russo, G.L., Dietary n−6 and n−3 polyunsaturated fatty acids: From biochemistry to clinical implication in cardiovascular prevention. Biochemical Pharmacology, 77; 2009:937-946. Reprinted by permission.

have the desaturase enzymes. The Western diet favors linoleic acid (n-6) and once it is acquired, longer, more highly unsaturated fatty acids can be formed from it by a combination of elongation and desaturation reactions. ALA (n-3) follows a similar pattern and, in parallel reactions, enzymes function to make similar compounds that are biologically active. Figure 5.31 outlines the biosynthesis of various PUFAs from LA and ALA, listing their chemical and common names. The biologically active compounds derived from these PUFAs are also shown, along with the enzymes involved. These compounds include eicosanoids—**prostaglandins**, prostacyclins, **thromboxanes**, and **leukotrienes**—produced from both LA (n-6) and ALA (n-3). Resolvins and neuroproctectins

come from DHA [41]. The steps in their syntheses and their activity are discussed later in this chapter.

The essential fatty acids enter the smooth ER for further metabolism. LA undergoes a desaturation by the enzyme delta-6-desaturase (d-6-d) to form γ-linolenic acid (18:3 n-6). The next step is an elongation catalyzed by the enzyme elongase (ELG) to form dihomo-γ-linolenic acid (20:3 n-6). Arachidonic acid (AA; 20:4 n-6) is then formed by a second desaturation. ALA (n-3) undergoes comparable reactions to form eicosapentaenoic acid (EPA; 20:5 n-3). Since the n-6 and n-3 fatty acids follow the same pathway with the same enzymes, they compete, and an excess of one family causes a significant change in the conversion of the other family [42]. The eicosanoids (both n-6 and n-3) are esterified with the glycerol backbone to form phospholipids or triacylglycerols and transferred to membranes. AA is predominant in membranes, so n-6 biosynthesis predominates. AA and EPA go through further elongation and desaturations in the smooth ER to form tetracosapentoenoic acid (24:5 n-6) and tetracosahexaenoic acid (24:6 n-3). These fatty acids are transferred to the peroxisome, where they undergo β-oxidation to form docososapentanoic acid (22:5 n-6) and docosahexaenoic acid (DHA; 22:6 n-3). The next section discusses the eicosanoids of physiological importance.

Eicosanoids: Fatty Acid Derivatives of Physiological Significance

AA-, ALA-, EPA-, and DHA-containing phospholipids or TAG are incorporated into any of the cell's membranes or the neutral lipid. The higher the degree of unsaturation among the fatty acids within a membrane, the greater the fluidity of that membrane. The membrane's fluidity is an important determinant for the hormone-receptor binding sites. For example, it has been hypothesized that insulin resistance might be associated with the development of cells with a rigid membrane, which limits the expression of insulin receptors and reduces their number [43].

When eicosanoids are synthesized the polyunsaturated fatty acid precursors are mobilized from the phospholipids or TAG by phospholipase A2. Further reactions can then produce the biologically active eicosanoids, as shown in Figure 5.31. Note that AA (n-6) produces the eicosanoids in what is called the 2 and 4 series, while EPA produces eicosanoids in the 1 and 3 series. Cyclo-oxygenases and lipoxygenases convert AA to the prostaglandin-2-, thromboxane-2-, and leukotriene-4-series; various hydroperoxy- and hydroxyl-eicosatetraenoic acid (HPETE and HETE) derivatives; and lipoxinA_4. EPA is metabolized to the eicosanoids of the prostaglandin-3-, leukotriene-5-, and thromboxane-3-series. DHA can be metabolized to other active compounds such as resolvins, docosatrienes, and neuroprotectins.

Opposing Effects of n-6 and n-3 Fatty Acid–Derived Eicosanoids

Table 5.5 highlights the effects of individual messengers derived from AA (n-6), EPA, and DHA (n-3). Note that most of the AA-derived messengers are pro-inflammatory or show other disease-propagating effects, whereas n-3 derivatives oppose these effects. Mediators of the n-6 prostaglandin family are pro-arrhythmic, while the messengers derived from EPA and DHA (n-3) are anti-arrhythmic,

Table 5.5 n-3 and n-6 Fatty Acid-Derived Messengers and Their Physiological Effects

Messenger Classes	Arachidonic Acid (n-6)–Derived Messengers	Physiological Effects	EPA- and DHA (n-3)-Derived Messengers	Physiological Effects
Prostaglandins	PGD_2		PGD_3	
	PGE_2	Pro-arrhythmic	PGE_3	Anti-arrhythmic
	PGF_2		PGF_3	
	PGI_2	Pro-arrhythmic	PGI_3	Anti-arrhythmic
Thromboxanes	TXA_2	Platelet activator	TXA_3	Platelet inhibitor
	TXB_2	Vasoconstriction	TXB_3	Vasodilation
Leukotrienes	LTA_4		LTA_5	
	LTB_4	Pro-inflammatory	LTB_5	Anti-inflammatory
	LTC_4		LTC_5	
	LTC_4		LTD_5	
	LTD_4		LTE_5	
Epoxyeclosatrienoic derivitives	5,6-EET			
	8,9-EET			
	11,12-EET	Pro-inflammatory		
	14,15-EET			
Hydroxyleicosatetraenoic derivatives	5-HETE			
	12-HETE			
	15-HETE			
Lipoxins	LXA_4			
Resolvins			RVE1	Anti-inflammatory
			RVD	Anti-inflammatory
Neuroprotectin			NPD1	Anti-inflammatory

Source: Based on data from Heird W., Lapillonne A., The role of essential fatty acids in development. Annu Rev Nutr. 2005;25:549–71.

anti-inflammatory, or vasodilators. Thromboxanes (TXB_2) produced from AA (n-6) activate platelets (which promote blood clots) and cause vasoconstriction (which raises blood pressure); in opposition, the thromboxane TXB_3 (n-3) inhibits platelets and causes vasodilation. Similarly, whereas leukotriene (LTB_4 n-6) from AA is pro-inflammatory and leads to the production of inflammatory cytokines, the corresponding leukotriene (LTB_5 n-3) from EPA and DHA is anti-inflammatory and actually blocks the biosynthesis of the inflammatory leukotriene derived from AA. Other anti-inflammatory derivatives of EPA include resolvins (RV1 or RVD) and nuclear receptors (NF).

These effects may help explain why individuals consuming larger quantities of the n-3 fatty acids are less susceptible to sudden cardiac deaths due to arrhythmias. Epidemiological data suggest that significant reductions in sudden death from cardiovascular episodes (likely from arrhythmias) result from consumption of more fish, and similar results have been seen with supplementation with fish oils (EPA and DHA) or with ALA [42]. The cardioprotective effects of n-3 have long been recognized and are the basis of the recommendation for the increased consumption of fish, particularly deep-water fish such as herring, salmon, and tuna [42]. Populations that consume more fish such as the Greenland Inuits and Japanese have lower incidences of fatal myocardial infarction, atherosclerosis, and other ischemic pathologies. In experimental trials, benefits have been shown most consistently among subjects that consume one or more meals featuring fish per week rather than fish oil supplements. n-3 fatty acids seem to particularly benefit the nervous system, where DHA is concentrated and appears to function in photoreceptors and synaptic membranes. DHA thus plays roles in vision, neuroprotection, successful aging, and memory in addition to its anti-inflammatory and inflammation-resolving properties as compared to n-6 PUFAs. A recent review covers the **signal-lipidomics** of DHA [43]; this broad research area encompasses cellular and molecular signaling pathways regulated by DHA, its bioactive derivatives, and its receptor-mediated actions.

Essential Fatty Acids in Development

Both n-6 and n-3 essential fatty acids are found in both adults and infants, and are metabolized by the same series of desaturases and elongases to longer-chain polyunsaturated fatty acids as described previously. Deficiency symptoms for the n-6 series that have been identified in adults include poor growth and scaly skin lesions. Deficiency symptoms for the n-3 series include neurological and visual abnormalities. Human infants have been observed to have similar neurological abnormalities when maintained on a regimen that was lacking in 18:3 n-3. Human milk contains more of the essential fatty acids (though the level varies) than most infant formulas do, as well as the elongated derivatives EPA and DHA. There is evidence that n-3 essential fatty acids are necessary for neural tissue and retinal

photoreceptor membranes. Both term and preterm infants can convert n-3 essential fatty acids to the long-chain polyunsaturated fatty acids, but whether they can convert them at an adequate rate to meet their needs is unclear. n-3 essential fatty acid deficiency appears to be more common among preterm infants than term infants. Infant formulas containing 22:6 n-3 and 20:4 n-6 are now available [44].

Impact of Diet on Fatty Acid Synthesis

The rate of fatty acid synthesis can be influenced by diet. Diets high in simple carbohydrates and low in fats induce a set of lipogenic enzymes in the liver. This induction is exerted through the process of transcription, leading to elevated levels of the mRNA for the enzymes. The transcriptional response is triggered by an increase in glucose metabolism, and the triggering substance, though not positively identified, is thought to be glucose-6-phosphate [45]. Other studies have confirmed that a very low-fat, high-sugar diet causes an increase in fatty acid synthesis and in palmitic acid–rich, linoleic acid–poor VLDL triacylglycerols. Furthermore, the effect may be reduced if starch is substituted for the sugar, possibly owing to the slower absorption of starch-derived glucose and a lower postprandial insulin response [46].

Synthesis of Triacylglycerols

The biosyntheses of triacylglycerols and glycerophosphatides share common precursors and are considered together in this section. The precursors are CoA-activated fatty acids and glycerol-3-phosphate, the latter produced either from the reduction of dihydroxyacetone phosphate or from the phosphorylation of glycerol. These and subsequent reactions of the pathways are shown in Figure 5.32, which depicts two pathways for lecithin synthesis from diacylglycerol. The de novo pathway of lecithin synthesis is the major route. However, the importance of the salvage pathway increases when a deficiency of the essential amino acid methionine exists.

Synthesis of Cholesterol

Nearly all tissues in the body are capable of synthesizing cholesterol from acetyl-CoA. The liver accounts for about 20% of endogenous cholesterol synthesis. Among the extrahepatic tissues, which are responsible for the remaining 80% of cholesterol synthesis, the intestine is probably the most active. The cholesterol production rate, which includes both absorbed cholesterol and endogenously synthesized cholesterol, approximates 1 g/day. Compare this with the recommended dietary intake limit of about 300 mg/day. The average cholesterol intake is considered to be about 300 mg/day, only about half of which is absorbed. Endogenous synthesis therefore accounts for more than two-thirds of the daily total.

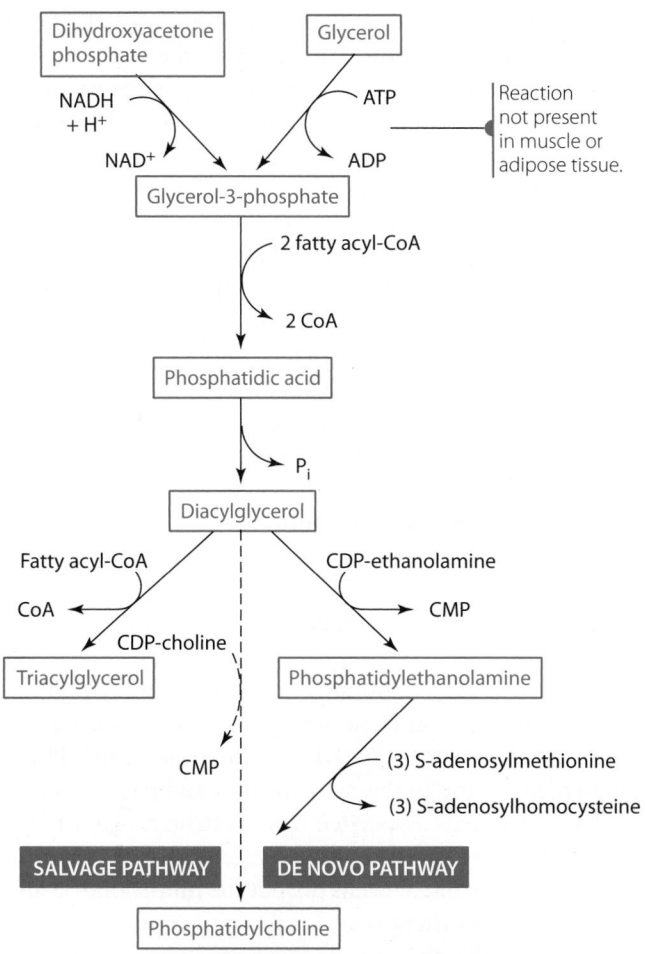

Figure 5.32 A schematic summary of the synthesis of triacylglycerols and lecithin showing that precursors are shared. In lecithin formation, three moles of activated methionine (S-adenosylmethionine) introduce three methyl groups in the de novo pathway, and choline is introduced as CDP (cytidine diphosphate)-choline in the so-called salvage pathway.

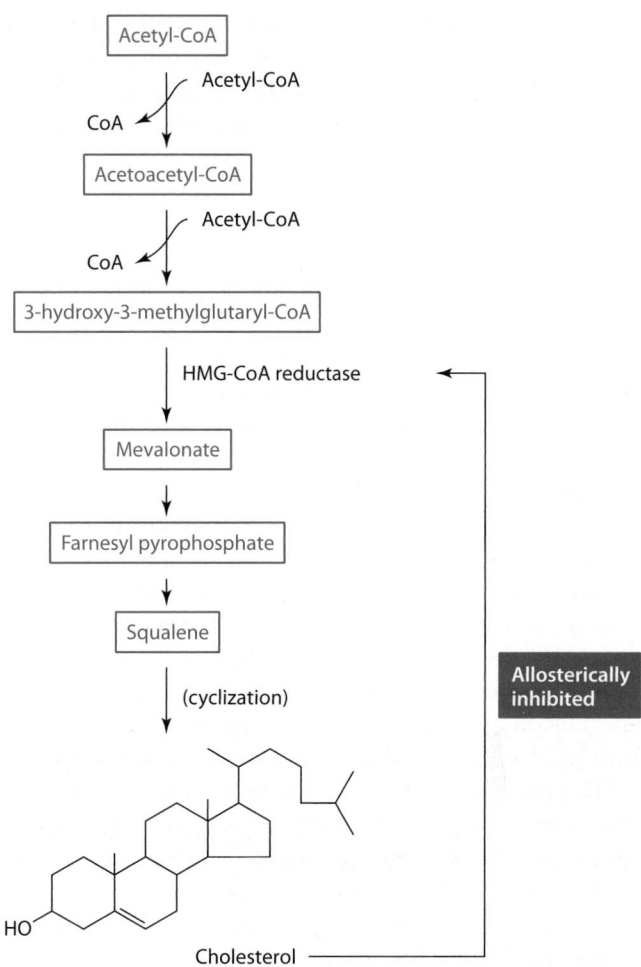

Figure 5.33 An overview of the pathway of cholesterol biosynthesis in the hepatocyte indicating the negative regulatory effect of cholesterol on the HMG-CoA reductase reaction.

At least 26 steps are known to be involved in the formation of cholesterol from acetyl-CoA. The individual steps are not provided here, but the synthesis of cholesterol can be thought of as occurring in three stages:

❶ a cytoplasmic sequence by which 3-hydroxy-3-methylglutaryl-CoA (HMG-CoA) is formed from 3 mol of acetyl-CoA

❷ the conversion of HMG-CoA to squalene, including the important rate-limiting step of cholesterol synthesis, in which HMG-CoA is reduced to mevalonic acid by HMG-CoA reductase

❸ the formation of cholesterol from squalene

As total body cholesterol increases, the rate of synthesis tends to decrease. This is known to be caused by a negative feedback regulation of the HMG-CoA reductase reaction. This suppression of cholesterol synthesis by dietary cholesterol seems to be unique to the liver and is not much evident in other tissues. The effect of feedback control of biosynthesis depends to a great extent upon the amount of cholesterol absorbed. The suppression is not sufficient to prevent an increase in the total body pool of cholesterol when dietary intake is high. A family of drugs called statins are HMG-CoA inhibitors and are widely used to block endogenous cholesterol synthesis. A brief scheme of hepatic cholesterol genesis and its regulation is shown in Figure 5.33.

REGULATION OF LIPID METABOLISM

The regulation of fatty acid oxidation is closely linked to carbohydrate status. Fatty acids formed in the cytosol of hepatocytes can either be converted into triacylglycerols and phospholipids or be transported via carnitine into the mitochondrion for oxidation. The enzyme carnitine acyl transferase I, which catalyzes the transfer of fatty acyl groups to carnitine (Figure 5.23), is specifically inhibited by malonyl-CoA. Recall that malonyl-CoA is the first intermediate in the synthesis of fatty acids. Therefore, it is logical that an increase in the concentration of malonyl-CoA would promote fatty acid synthesis while inhibiting fatty acid oxidation. Malonyl-CoA concentration increases whenever a person is well supplied with carbohydrate. Excess glucose that cannot be oxidized through the glycolytic pathway or stored as glycogen is converted to triacylglycerols for storage, using the available malonyl-CoA. Therefore, glucose-rich cells do not actively oxidize fatty acids for energy. Instead, a switch to lipogenesis is stimulated, accomplished in part by inhibition of the entry of fatty acids into the mitochondrion.

Blood glucose levels can affect lipolysis and fatty acid oxidation by other mechanisms as well. Hyperglycemia triggers the release of insulin, which promotes glucose transport into the adipose cell and therefore promotes lipogenesis. Insulin also exerts a pronounced antilipolytic effect. Hypoglycemia, on the other hand, results in a reduced intracellular supply of glucose, thereby suppressing lipogenesis. Furthermore, the low level of insulin accompanying the hypoglycemic state would favor lipolysis, with a flow of free fatty acids into the bloodstream. Low glucose levels also stimulate fatty acid oxidation in the manner described in the "Formation of Ketone Bodies" section of this chapter. In this case, accelerated oxidation of fatty acids follows the reduction in TCA cycle activity, which in turn results from inadequate oxaloacetate availability.

The key enzyme for the mobilization of fatty acids is hormone-sensitive triacylglycerol lipase, found in adipose tissue cells. Lipolysis is stimulated by hormones such as epinephrine and norepinephrine, adrenocorticotropic hormone (ACTH), thyroid-stimulating hormone (TSH), glucagon, growth hormone, and thyroxine. Insulin, as mentioned earlier, antagonizes the effects of these hormones by inhibiting the lipase activity.

An important allosteric enzyme involved in the regulation of fatty acid biosynthesis is acetyl-CoA carboxylase, which forms malonyl-CoA from acetyl-CoA (Figure 5.28). This enzyme, which functions in the cytosol, is positively stimulated by citrate, but in its absence is barely active. Recall that citrate is part of the shuttle for moving acetyl-CoA from the mitochondria (a major site of production) to the cytosol, where fatty acids are synthesized. Citrate is continuously produced in the mitochondrion as a TCA cycle intermediate, but its concentration in the cytosol is normally low. When mitochondrial citrate concentration increases, it can escape to the cytosol because the mitochondrial membrane is permeable to citrate. In the cytosol it acts as a positive allosteric signal to acetyl-CoA carboxylase, thereby increasing the rate of formation of malonyl-CoA, which results in lipogenesis. The result of citrate accumulation is that excess acetyl-CoA is diverted to fatty acid synthesis and away from TCA cycle activity.

Acetyl-CoA carboxylase can be modulated negatively by palmitoyl-CoA, which is the end product of fatty acid synthesis. This situation would most likely arise when free fatty acid concentrations increase as a result of insufficient glycerophosphate, with which fatty acids must combine to form triacylglycerols. Deficient glycerophosphate levels would likely stem from inadequate carbohydrate

availability. In such a situation, regulation would logically favor fatty acid oxidation rather than synthesis.

Serum cholesterol levels are of great interest to researchers because of their correlation to the risk of CVD. The regulation of cholesterol homeostasis is associated with its effect on LDL receptor concentration and on the activity of regulatory enzymes such as acyl-CoA: cholesterol acyltransferase (ACAT) and hydroxymethylglutaryl-CoA (HMG-CoA) reductase. Cholesterol's feedback suppression of HMG-CoA reductase has been discussed and is shown in Figure 5.33. The combination of increasing ACAT activity (the conversion of free cholesterol to cholesteryl esters) and decreasing numbers of LDL receptors reduces the accumulation of cholesterol in vascular endothelial and smooth muscle cells. Figure 5.20 illustrates these mechanisms of control.

BROWN FAT THERMOGENESIS

Brown adipose tissue obtains its name from its high degree of vascularity and the abundant mitochondria present in its adipocytes. Recall that the mitochondria are pigmented, owing to the cytochromes and perhaps other oxidative pigments associated with electron transport. Not only do brown fat cells contain larger numbers of mitochondria than white fat cells do, but the mitochondria also are structurally different and contain uncoupling protein 1 to promote **thermogenesis** (heat production) at the expense of producing ATP. Brown fat also is derived from a different embryological origin than white fat [47].

Brown fat mitochondria have special H^+ pores in their inner membranes, formed by integral uncoupling protein 1 (UCP 1). UCP 1 is a translocator of protons, which allows the external H^+ pumped out of the mitochondrial matrix by electron transport to flow back into the matrix and thus become unavailable to drive F_0F_1 ATP synthase, the site of phosphorylation. Remember that it is the H^+ gradient that causes the conformational changes that result in the phosphorylation of ADP to produce ATP. Figure 5.34 illustrates how the proposed mechanism of brown fat thermogenesis relates to the chemiosmotic theory of oxidative phosphorylation. Membrane pores of brown fat mitochondria allow the cycling of protons, which lowers the proton concentration in the inner membrane space and results in heat generation rather than ATP production. This cycling appears to be regulated by the 32,000-dalton UCP 1.

Two types of external stimuli trigger thermogenesis: (1) ingestion of food and (2) prolonged exposure to cold temperature. Both of these events stimulate the tissue via sympathetic innervation via the hormone norepinephrine. The sympathetic signal has a stimulatory and hypertrophic effect on brown adipose tissue. This effect enhances expression of the UCP 1 in the inner membrane of the mitochondrion and accelerates synthesis of

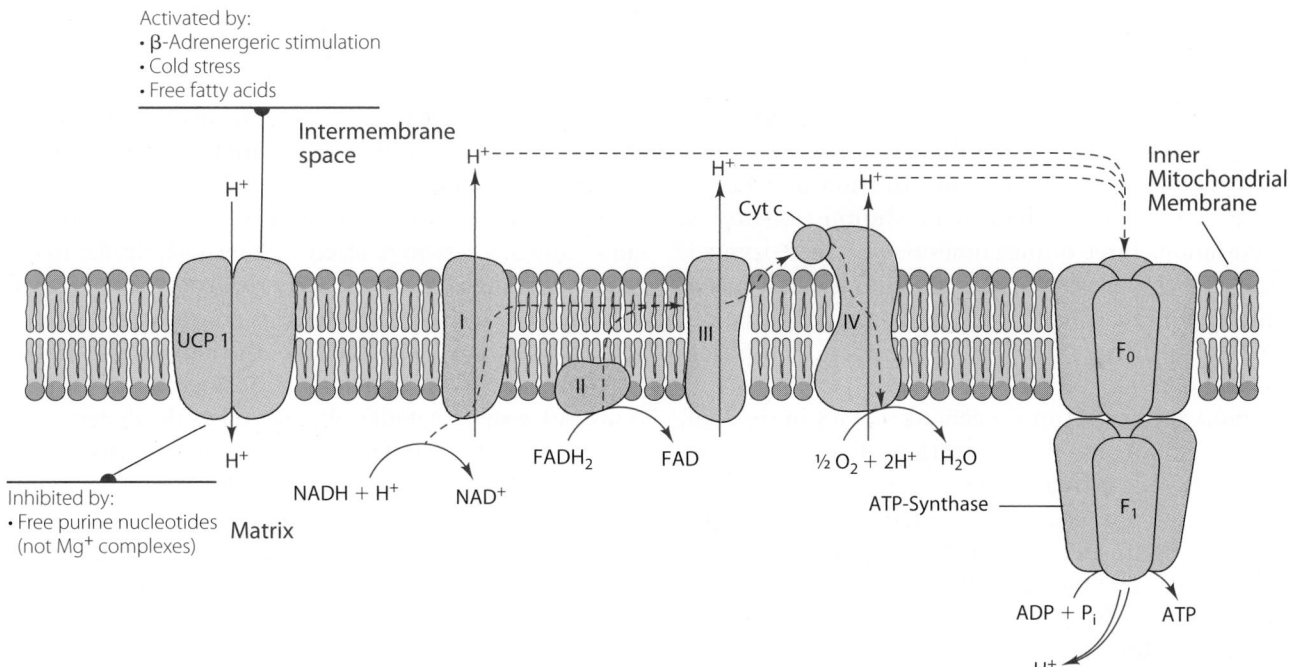

Figure 5.34 A Schematic of the inner membrane of a mitochondrion from brown adipose tissue showing uncoupling protein 1 (UCP 1), the components of the electron transport chain, and ATP synthase. H^+ are translocated to the intermembrane space by electron transport and flow back into the mitochondrial matrix by ATP synthase and UCP 1 when it is activated. UCP 1 is activated by β-adrenergic stimulation, cold stress, and free fatty acids. It is inhibited by free purine nucleotides (not complexed with Mg^+) such as ADP, ATP, GDP, and GTP.

lipoprotein lipase and glucose transporters to make more fatty acids and glucose available [47] to meet the higher metabolic demand. Theoretically, then, weight reduction should accompany a higher activity of brown fat, and, indeed, a possible link between obesity and deficient brown fat cell function has been researched [47]. Obese individuals seem to have less brown fat than nonobese individuals. Better understanding of the brown adipose tissue's activity may increase the potential for enhancing energy expenditure by increasing its quantity or activity through new drugs.

ETHYL ALCOHOL: METABOLISM AND BIOCHEMICAL IMPACT

Ethyl alcohol (ethanol) is neither a carbohydrate nor a lipid. Though empirically ethanol's structure (CH_3—CH_2—OH) most closely resembles a carbohydrate, its metabolism most closely resembles fatty acid catabolism. We have chosen to review it in this chapter for several reasons. First, it is a common dietary component, being consumed in the form of alcoholic beverages such as beer, wines, and distilled spirits. Second, the pathways that oxidize ethyl alcohol also oxidize (or detoxify) other exogenous substances in the body. Although ethanol is not a "natural" nutrient, it does have caloric value (its calories are "empty," that is, devoid of beneficial nutrients). Each gram of ethanol yields 7 kcal, and ethanol may account for up to 10% of the total energy intake of moderate consumers and up to 50% for alcoholics. Because of its widespread consumption and relatively high caloric potency, it commands attention in a nutrition textbook.

Ethanol is readily absorbed through the entire gastrointestinal tract. It is transported unaltered in the bloodstream and then oxidatively degraded in tissues, primarily the liver, first to acetaldehyde and then to acetate. In tissues other than the liver, as well as in the liver itself, the acetate subsequently is converted to acetyl-CoA and oxidized via the TCA cycle. At least three enzyme systems are capable of ethanol oxidation:

- alcohol dehydrogenase (ADH)
- the microsomal ethanol oxidizing system (MEOS; also known as the cytochrome P-450 system)
- catalase, in the presence of hydrogen peroxide

Of these, the catalase-H_2O_2 system is the least active, probably accounting for <2% of in vivo ethanol oxidation. Therefore, we will not discuss the catalase system further. Nearly all ingested ethanol is oxidized by hepatic (and, to some extent, gastric) alcohol dehydrogenase and hepatic microsomal cytochrome P-450 systems.

The Alcohol Dehydrogenase (ADH) Pathway

ADH is a soluble enzyme functioning in the cytosol of hepatocytes. It is an ordinary NAD^+-requiring dehydrogenase and is known to be able to oxidize ethanol to acetaldehyde. The NADH formed by the reaction can be oxidized by mitochondrial electron transport by way of the NADH shuttle systems (see Chapter 3), thereby giving rise to ATP formation by oxidative phosphorylation. The K_m of alcohol dehydrogenase for ethanol is approximately 1 millimolar, or about 5 mg/dL. (K_m is reviewed in Chapter 1, in the section dealing with enzymes.) This means that at this cellular concentration of ethanol, ADH is functioning at half its maximum velocity. At concentrations three or four times the K_m, the enzyme is saturated with the ethanol substrate and is catalyzing at its maximum rate. Concentrations of ethanol in the cell more than four times the K_m level cannot be completely oxidized by ADH.

Because ethanol is an exogenous dietary ingredient, there is no "normal" concentration of ethanol in the cells or the bloodstream. The so-called toxic level of blood ethanol, however, is considered to be in the range of 50 to 80 mg/dL and is defined by its pharmacological actions. The high lipid solubility of ethanol allows it to passively enter cells with ease. If its cellular concentration reaches a level even one-third or one-fourth of that of the blood at toxic levels, ADH becomes saturated by the substrate and will be functioning at its maximum velocity. The excess, or "spillover," ethanol then must be metabolized by alternate systems, the most important of which is the microsomal ethanol oxidizing system (MEOS), described next. The depletion of NAD$^+$ brought about by the high level of activity of ADH can also force the shift to the microsomal system, which does not require NAD$^+$ for its oxidative reactions. The depletion of NAD$^+$ alters the NAD$^+$: NADH ratio and impairs NAD$^+$-requiring reactions such as the TCA cycle, gluconeogenesis, and fatty acid oxidation. The buildup of acetyl-CoA encourages fatty acid synthesis in the liver and with time can lead to TAG accumulation in this organ [40].

Alcohol dehydrogenase is also active in gastric mucosal cells. Interestingly, there appears to be a significant gender difference in the level of its activity in these cells. Young (premenopausal) females develop higher blood alcohol levels than male counterparts with equal consumption and consequently display a lower tolerance for alcohol and are at greater risk of toxic effects in the liver. The lower level of alcohol dehydrogenase activity in the female gastric mucosa is believed to account for this observation [48,49].

The Microsomal Ethanol Oxidizing System (MEOS)

Despite its name, the microsomal ethanol oxidizing system (MEOS) is able to oxidize a wide variety of compounds in addition to ethanol, including fatty acids, aromatic hydrocarbons, steroids, and barbiturate drugs. The oxidation occurs through a system of electron transport, similar to the mitochondrial electron transport system described in detail in Chapter 3. Because the MEOS is microsomal (isolated ER) and associated with the smooth endoplasmic reticulum, it is sometimes referred to as the microsomal electron transport system. Another distinction of the system is its requirement for a special cytochrome called cytochrome P-450, which acts as an intermediate electron carrier. Cytochrome P-450 is not a single compound but rather exists as a family of structurally related cytochromes, the members of which share the property of absorbing light that has a wavelength of 450 nm.

Ethanol oxidation by the MEOS involves several linked oxidation reactions of NADPH, FAD, FMN, and cytochrome P-450 that result in the simultaneous oxidation of reduced cytochrome P-450 and oxidation of ethanol to acetaldehyde by molecular oxygen. Because two substrates are oxidized concurrently, the enzymes involved in the oxidations are commonly called mixed-function oxidases. Both oxygen atoms are reduced to H_2O, and therefore two H_2O molecules are formed in the reactions. Microsomal electron transport of the MEOS is shown in Figure 5.35. Acting as carriers of electrons from NADPH to oxygen are FAD, FMN, and a cytochrome P-450 system.

An important feature of the MEOS is that certain of its enzymes, including the cytochrome P-450 units, are inducible by ethanol—particularly at higher concentrations of ethanol. With increased synthesis of these substances, the hepatocytes can metabolize ethanol much more effectively, thereby establishing a state of metabolic tolerance. Compared with a normal (nondrinking or light-drinking) subject, an individual in a state of metabolic tolerance to ethanol can ingest larger quantities of the substance before showing the effects of intoxication. When enzyme induction occurs, however, it can also accelerate the metabolism of other substances metabolized by the microsomal system. In other words, tolerance to ethanol induced by heavy drinking can render a person tolerant to other substances as well.

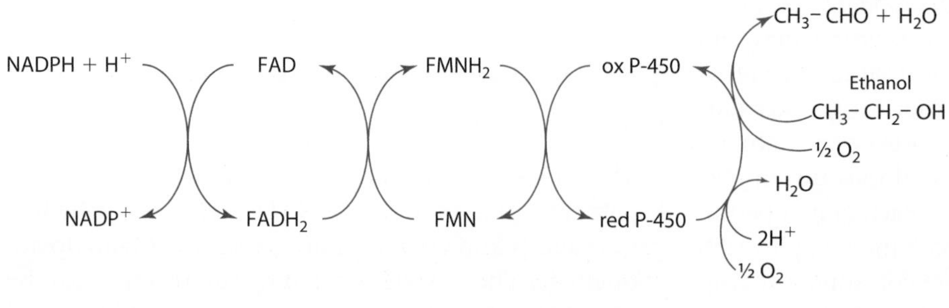

Figure 5.35 The microsomal ethanol oxidizing system (MEOS). Both ethanol and NADPH are oxidized by molecular oxygen in this electron transfer scheme. Because two substrates are oxidized, enzymes involved in the oxidation are referred to as mixed-function oxidases.

Alcoholism: Biochemical and Metabolic Alterations

Excessive consumption of ethanol can lead to alcoholism, defined by the National Council on Alcoholism as consumption that is capable of producing pathological changes. Alcoholism is a serious socioeconomic and health problem, exemplified by the fact that in the United States alcohol is the third leading preventable cause of death [50]. The well-known consequences of alcoholism—fatty liver, hepatic disease (cirrhosis), lactic acidosis, and metabolic tolerance—can be explained by the manner in which ethanol is metabolized. Basically, the consequences of excessive alcohol intake are explainable by metabolic effects of (1) acetaldehyde toxicity, (2) elevated NADH: NAD^+ ratio, (3) metabolic competition, and (4) induced metabolic tolerance.

Acetaldehyde Toxicity

Both the ADH and MEOS routes of ethanol oxidation produce acetaldehyde, which is believed to exert direct adverse effects on metabolic systems. For example, acetaldehyde is able to attach covalently to proteins, forming protein adducts. Should the adduct involve an enzyme, the activity of that enzyme could be impaired. Acetaldehyde has also been shown to impede the formation of microtubules in liver cells and to cause the development of perivenular fibrosis, either of which is believed to initiate the events leading to cirrhosis. These and other possible adverse effects of acetaldehyde are reviewed by Lieber [51].

Alcoholic cirrhosis was once thought to be caused by malnutrition because the drinker satisfied his or her caloric needs with the empty calories of alcohol at the expense of a nutritionally balanced diet. In view of the effect of high levels of acetaldehyde on hepatocyte structure and function, however, chronic overindulgence is now known to cause cirrhosis even when nutritional deficiency is absent and the alcohol is co-ingested with an enriched diet.

High NADH:NAD^+ Ratio

The oxidation of ethanol increases the concentration of NADH at the expense of NAD^+, thereby elevating the NADH:NAD^+ ratio. This occurs because both ADH and acetaldehyde dehydrogenase use NAD^+ as a cosubstrate. NADH is an important regulator of certain dehydrogenase reactions. The rise in concentration of NADH represents an overproduction of reducing equivalents, which in turn acts as a signal for a metabolic shift toward reduction—namely, hydrogenation. Such a shift can account for the fatty liver (through the anabolic activity producing fatty acids) and lactic acidemia (high blood-lactate levels resulting from increased reduction of pyruvate to lactic acid) that often accompany alcoholism. For example, lactic acidemia can be attributed in part to the direct effect of NADH in shifting the lactate dehydrogenase (LDH) reaction toward the

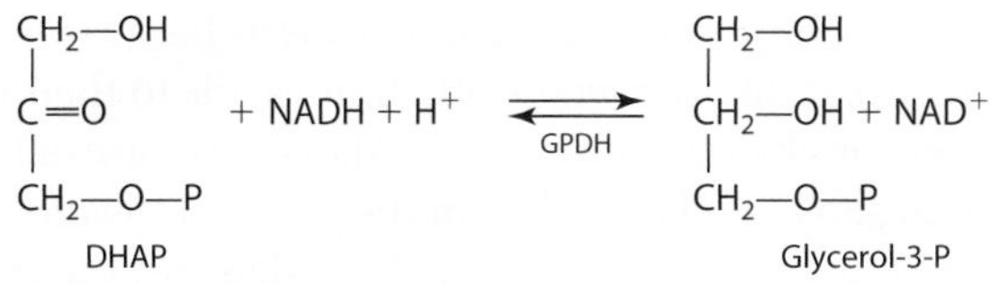

Figure 5.36 The reduction of dihydroxyacetone phosphate (DHAP) to glycerol-3-P, producing NAD^+ from NADH.

formation of lactate. The reaction, which follows, is driven to the right by the high concentration of NADH:

$$\text{Pyruvate} + \text{NADH} + \text{H}^+ \xrightarrow{\text{LDH}} \text{Lactate} + \text{NAD}^+$$

Lipids accumulate in most tissues in which ethanol is metabolized, resulting in fatty liver, fatty myocardium, fatty renal tubules, and so on. The mechanism appears to involve both increased lipid synthesis and decreased lipid removal and can be explained in part by the increased NADH:NAD^+ ratio. As NADH accumulates, it slows dehydrogenase reactions of the TCA cycle, such as the isocitrate dehydrogenase and α-ketoglutarate dehydrogenase reactions, thereby slowing the overall activity of the cycle. This results in an accumulation of citrate, which positively regulates acetyl-CoA carboxylase. Acetyl-CoA carboxylase, which converts acetyl-CoA into malonyl-CoA by the attachment of a carboxyl group, is the key regulatory enzyme for the synthesis of fatty acids from acetyl-CoA. The high NADH:NAD^+ ratio therefore directs metabolism away from TCA cycle oxidation and toward fatty acid synthesis.

Also contributing to the lipogenic effect of alcoholism is the effect of NADH on the glycerophosphate dehydrogenase (GPDH) reaction. This reaction, shown in Figure 5.36, favors the reduction of dihydroxyacetone phosphate (DHAP) to glycerol-3-phosphate if NADH concentration is high. Glycerol-3-phosphate provides the glycerol component in the synthesis of triacylglycerols. Therefore, a high NADH:NAD^+ ratio stimulates the synthesis of both the fatty acids and the glycerol components of triacylglycerols, contributing to the cellular fat accumulation that develops in alcoholism.

A rise in NADH concentration also affects the glutamate dehydrogenase (GluDH) reaction (Figure 5.37), resulting in impaired gluconeogenesis. The GluDH reaction

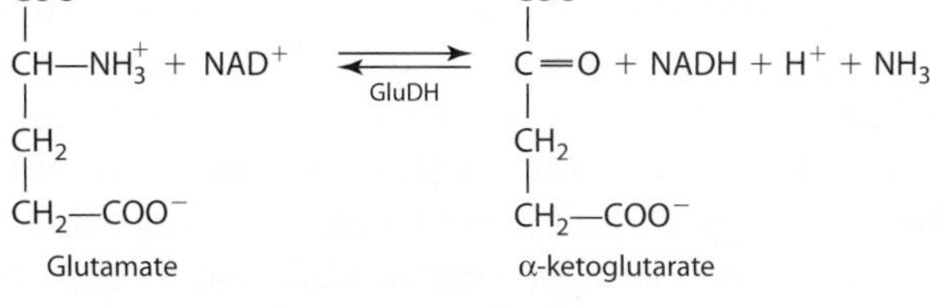

Figure 5.37 The reversible reaction of glutamate and NAD + forming α-ketoglutarate, NADH, and ammonia, catalyzed by glutamate dehydrogenase (GluDH).

is extremely important in gluconeogenesis because of the role it plays in the conversion of amino acids to their carbon skeletons by transamination and in the release of their amino groups as NH_3. A shift in the reaction toward glutamate because of the elevated NADH depletes the availability of α-ketoglutarate, which is the major acceptor of amino groups in the transamination of amino acids.

Substrate Competition

A well-established nutritional problem associated with excessive alcohol metabolism is a deficiency of vitamin A. Two aspects of ethanol interference with normal metabolism probably can account for this problem. One is the effect of ethanol on retinol dehydrogenase, the cytoplasmic enzyme that converts retinol to retinal. Retinal is required for the synthesis of photo pigments used in vision. Retinol dehydrogenase is thought to be identical to ADH, and therefore ethanol competitively inhibits the hepatic conversion of retinol to retinal. In addition to this substrate competition effect, ethanol may interfere with retinol metabolism through induced metabolic tolerance.

Induced Metabolic Tolerance

As explained earlier, ethanol can induce enzymes of the MEOS, causing an increased rate of metabolism of substrates oxidized by this system. Retinol, like ethanol, spills over into the MEOS when ADH is saturated and NAD^+ stores are low because of heavy ingestion of ethanol. Ethanol induction of retinol-metabolizing enzymes then can occur. The specific component of the MEOS known to be induced by heavy consumption of ethanol has been designated cytochrome P-4502E1 (CYP2E1). Although induction accelerates the hepatic oxidation of retinol, the oxidation product is not retinal but other polar, inert products of oxidation. The hepatic depletion of retinol can therefore be attributed to its accelerated metabolism, which is secondary to ethanol induction of a metabolizing enzyme. In effect, the alcoholic subject becomes tolerant to vitamin A, necessitating a higher dietary intake of the vitamin to maintain normal hepatocyte concentrations.

Alcohol in Moderation: The Brighter Side

Alcohol is a nutritional "Jekyll and Hyde," and which face it flaunts is clearly a function of the extent to which it is consumed. We focused earlier on the effects of alcohol at high intake levels and the negative impact of alcoholism on metabolism and nutrition. Epidemiological data from worldwide studies consistently demonstrate there is an inverse association between moderate alcohol or wine intake and coronary heart disease. Positive effects of alcohol or wine intake on oxidative stress, insulin insensitivity, diabetes mellitus, and inflammation have been shown [52].

Ethanol is known to elevate the level of high-density lipoprotein (HDL) in serum and to lower the amount of serum lipoprotein (a) [53]. Both effects favor a decrease in cardiovascular disease risk. In addition to the epidemiological data, prospective studies have shown that alcohol intake correlates with serum HDL-C levels to explain 50% to 70% of the inverse association of alcohol with risk of CHD [54]. The suggested mechanism is HDL's ability to protect against the deposition of arterial fatty plaque (atherogenesis), whereas high levels of lipoprotein(a) appear to promote it. The effects of these and other lipoproteins on atherogenesis were discussed earlier in this chapter. Dementia shares several risk factors with cardiovascular disease. A U-shaped relationship of alcohol intake with risk of dementia has been reported, indicating a beneficial effect of moderate consumption.

Among the three classes of alcoholic beverages—wine, beer, and distilled spirits—the strongest correlations are with the amount of ethanol consumed and not the individual types of beverages. The common belief is that distilled spirits and beer have about equal benefits and wine has somewhat more, but scientific data that substantiates that belief has not been reported. Wine does have strong antioxidant properties, particularly red wine. Most of the antioxidant chemicals in grapes are found in the skin and seeds. The skin is included in the production of red wine. The polyphenols and a variety of other antioxidants that can reduce reactive oxygen species (ROS) are present. ROS contribute to the oxidative stress that causes inflammation and contributes to coronary vascular disease [55].

SUMMARY

The hydrophobic character of lipids makes them unique among the major nutrients, requiring special handling in the body's aqueous milieu. Ingested fat must be finely dispersed in the intestinal lumen to present a sufficiently large surface area for enzymatic digestion to occur. In the bloodstream, reassembled lipid must be associated with proteins to ensure its solubility in that environment while undergoing transport. The major sites for

the formation of lipoproteins are the intestine, which produces them from diet-derived lipids, and the liver, which forms lipoproteins from endogenous lipids. Central to the processes of fat transport and storage is adipose tissue, which accumulates fat as triacylglycerol when the intake of energy-producing nutrients is greater than the body's caloric needs. When energy demands so dictate, fatty acids are released from storage and transported to other tissues for oxidation. The mobilization follows the adipocyte's response to specific hormonal signals that stimulate the activity of the intracellular lipase.

Fatty acids are a rich source of energy. Their mitochondrial oxidation furnishes large amounts of acetyl-CoA for TCA cycle catabolism, and in situations of low carbohydrate intake or use, as occurs in starvation or diabetes, the rate of fatty acid oxidation increases significantly with concomitant acetyl-CoA accumulation. This causes an increase in the level of ketone bodies, organic acids that can be deleterious through their disturbance of acid-base balance but that also are beneficial as sources of fuel to tissues such as the muscle and brain in periods of starvation.

Although the lipids are thought of first and foremost as energy sources, some can be identified with intriguing hormone-like functions ranging from blood pressure alteration and platelet aggregation to enhancement of immunological surveillance. These potent bioactive substances are the prostaglandins, thromboxanes, and leukotrienes, all of which are derived from the fatty acids arachidonic acid (n-6), eicosatetraenoic acid (n-3), and docosahexaenoic acid (n-3).

Dietary lipid has been implicated in atherogenesis, the process leading to development of the degenerative cardiovascular disease called atherosclerosis. Major considerations in preventing and controlling this disease have been the concentration of cholesterol in the blood serum and the relative hypocholesterolemic or hypercholesterolemic effect of certain diets. Saturated fatty acids having medium-length chains, along with unsaturated *trans* fatty acids, are alleged to be hypercholesterolemic, whereas polyunsaturated *cis* fatty acids tend to lower serum cholesterol.

Fats can be synthesized by cytosolic enzyme systems when energy production by carbohydrate is adequate. The synthesis begins with simple precursors such as acetyl-CoA and can be triggered by hormonal signals or by elevated levels of citrate, which acts as a regulatory substance. Blood glucose concentration also acts as a sensitive regulator of lipogenesis, which is stimulated when a hyperglycemic state exists.

Ethanol is catabolized ultimately to acetyl-CoA, furnishing energy through its TCA cycle oxidation. The nutritional complexities of alcohol abuse were discussed.

References Cited

1. Hunter JE. Dietary *trans* fatty acids: review of recent human studies and food industry responses. Lipids. 2006; 41:967–92.
2. Berridge M. Inositol triphosphate and calcium signalling. Nature. 1993; 361:315–25.
3. Berridge MJ. Inositol triphosphate and diacylglycerol: two intersecting second messengers. Ann Rev Biochem. 1987; 56:159–93.
4. Zorzano A, Palacin M, Guma A. Mechanisms regulating glut4 transporter expression and glucose transport in skeletal muscle. ActaPhysiol Scand. 2005; 183:43–58.
5. U.S. Department of Agriculture, Agriculture Research Service. 2010 Nutrient intakes from food: mean amounts consumed per individual, by gender and age. In: *What we eat in America*, NHANES 2007–2008. www.ars.usda.gov/ba/bhnrc/fsrg. Accessed September 9, 2011.
6. Lindquist S, Hernell O. Lipid digestion and absorption in early life. Curr Opin Clin Nutr Metab Care. 2010; 13:314–20.
7. Mu H, Porsgaard T. The metabolism of structured triacylglycerols. Progress in Lipid Research. 2005; 44:430–48.
8. Black DD. Development and physiological regulation of intestinal lipid absorption.I. Development of intestinal lipid absorption: cellular events in chylomicron assembly and secretion. Am J Physiol Gastrinest Liver Physiol. 2007; 293:G519–24.
9. Mansbach CM II, Gorelick F. Development and physiological regulation of intestinal lipid absorption. II. Dietary lipid absorption, complex lipid synthesis, and the intracellular packaging and secretion of chylomicrons. Am J Physiol Gastrointest Liver Physiol. 2007; 293:G645–50.
10. Iqbal J, Hussain MM. Intestinal lipid absorption. Am J Physiol Endocrinol Metab. 2009; 296:E1183–94.
11. Jia L, Betters JL, Yu L. Niemann-Pick C1-Like 1 (NPC1L1) protein in intestinal and hepatic cholesterol transport. Ann Rev Physiol. 2011; 73:239–59.
12. Brown MJ, Yu L. Protein mediators of sterol transport across intestinal brush border membrane. Sub-Cellular Biochem. 2010; 51:337–80.
13. Wang DQ-H. Regulation of intestinal cholesterol absorption. Annu Rev Physiol. 2007; 69:221–48.
14. Redgrave TG. Chylomicron metabolism. Biochem Soc Transactions. 2004; 32:79–82.
15. Griffin BA, Fielding BA. Postprandial lipid handling. Curr Opin Clin Nutr Metab Care. 2001; 4:93–98.
16. Brown MS, Goldstein JL. A receptor-mediated pathway for cholesterol homeostasis. Science. 1986; 232:34–47.
17. Goldstein JL, Brown MS. The LDL receptor. Aterioscler Thromb Vasc Biol. 2009; 29:431–38.
18. van der Velde A. Reverse cholesterol transport: from classical view to new insights. World J Gastroenterol. 2010; 16:5908–15.
19. Gordon SM, Hofmann S, Askew DS, Davidson WS. High density lipoprotein: not just about lipid transport anymore. Trends Endocrin Metab. 2011; 22:9–15.
20. Ross R. The pathogenesis of atherosclerosis: a prospective for the 90s. Nature. 1993; 362:801–09.
21. Libby P, Ridker PM, Hansson GK. Progress and challenges in translating the biology of atherosclerosis. Nature. 2011; 473:317–25.
22. Walldius G, Junger I. The apoB/apoA-1 ratio: a strong, new risk factor for cardiovascular disease and a target for lipid-lowering therapy: a review of the evidence. J Int Med. 2006; 259:493–519.
23. Prospective Studies Collaboration. Blood cholesterol and vascular mortality by age, sex and blood pressure: a meta-analysis of individual data from 61 prospective studies with 55,000 vascular deaths. Lancet. 2007; 370:1829–39.
24. Astrup A, Dyerberg J, Elwood P, et al. The role of reducing intakes of saturated fat in the prevention of cardiovascular disease: where does the evidence stand in 2010? Am J. ClinNutr. 2011; 93:684–88.
25. Micha R, Mozaffarind D. Saturated fat and cardiometabolic risk factors, coronary heart disease, stroke, and diabetes: a fresh look at the evidence. Lipids. 2010; 45:893–905.
26. Jakabsen MU, O'Reilly EJ, Heitnann BL, et al. Major types of dietary fat and risk of coronary heart disease: a pooled analysis of 11 cohort studies. Am J ClinNutr. 2009; 89:1425–32.
27. Degirolamo C, Rudel LL. Dietary monounsaturated fatty acids appear not to provide cardioprotection. Curr Atheroscler Rep. 2010; 12: 391–96.

28. Kris-Etherton P, Yu S. Individual fatty acid effects on plasma lipids and lipoproteins: human studies. Am J Clin Nutr. 1997; 65 (suppl):S1628–44.

29. Remig R, Franklin B, Margolis S, Kostas G. *Trans* fats in America: a review of their use, consumption, health implications and regulation. J Am Diet Asoc. 2010; 110:585–92.

30. Teegala SM, Willett WC, Muzaffarian D. Consumption and health effects of *trans* fatty acids: a review. J of AOAC Intnat. 2009; 92:1250–57.

31. Mensink RP, Katan MB. Effect of dietary *trans* fatty acids on high density and low density lipoprotein cholesterol levels in healthy subjects. N Engl J Med. 1990; 323:439–45.

32. Willett WC, Stampfer MJ, Manson JE, et al. Intake of *trans* acids and risk of coronary heart disease among women. Lancet. 1993; 341:581–85.

33. Shapiro S. Do *trans* fatty acids increase the risk of coronary artery disease? a critique of the epidemiologic evidence. Am J Clin Nutr. 1997; 66(suppl):S1011–17.

34. Kris-Etherton P, Dietschy J. Design criteria for studies examining individual fatty acid effects on cardiovascular disease risk factors: human and animal studies. Am J Clin Nutr. 1997; 65(suppl):S1590–96.

35. Sun Q, Ma J, Campos H, et al. A prospective study of *trans* fatty acids in erythrocytes and risk of coronary heart disease. Circulation. 2007; 115:1858–65.

36. Chisholm A, Mann J, Sutherland W, et al. Effect on lipoprotein profile of replacing butter with margarine in a low fat diet: randomized crossover study with hypercholesterolaemic subjects. BMJ. 1996; 312:931–38.

37. Erqou S, Thompson A, Angelantonio ED, et al. Apolipoprotein (a) isoforms and the risk of vascular disease. J Am Cardio. 2010; 55:2160–67.

38. Kolovou GD, Anagnostopoulou KK. Apolipoprotein E polymorphism, age and coronary heart disease. Age Res Rev. 2007; 6:94–108.

39. Jofre-Monseny L, Minihane AM, Rimbach G. Impact of ApoE genotype on oxidative stress, inflammation and disease risk. Mol Nutr Food Res. 2008; 52:131–45.

40. Garrett RH, Grisham CM. Biochemistry. 4th ed. Belmont CA: Thomson Brooks/Cole Publishers. 2010.

41. Russo GL. Dietary n-6 and n-3 polyunsaturated fatty acids: from biochemistry to clinical implication in cardiovascular prevention. Biochem Pharmacol. 2009; 77:937–46.

42. Schmitz G, Ecker J. The opposing effects of n–3 and n–6 fatty acids. Prog Lipid Res. 2008; 47:147–55.

43. Bazan NG, Molina MF, Gordon WC. Docosahexaenoic acid signalolipidomics in nutrition: significance in aging, neuroinflammation, macular degeneration, Alzheimer's, and other neurodegenerative diseases. Annu Rev Nutr. 2011; 31:321–51.

44. Heird W, Lapillonne A. The role of essential fatty acids in development. Annu Rev Nutr. 2005; 25:549–71.

45. Towle H, Kaytor E, Shih H. Regulation of the expression of lipogenic enzyme genes by carbohydrate. Annu Rev Nutr. 1997; 17:405–33.

46. Hudgins L, Seidman C, Diakun J, Hirsch J. Human fatty acid synthesis is reduced after the substitution of dietary starch for sugar. Am J Clin Nutr. 1998; 67:631–39.

47. Ravussin E, Galgani J. The implication of brown adipose tissue for humans. Annu Rev Nutr. 2011; 31:33–47.

48. Frezza M, di Padova C, Pozzato G, et al. High blood alcohol levels in women: the role of decreased alcohol dehydrogenase activity and first pass metabolism. N Engl J Med. 1990; 322:95–99.

49. Thomasson R. Gender differences in alcohol metabolism: physiological responses to ethanol. Recent Dev Alcohol. 1995; 12:163–79.

50. Mokdad AH, Marks JS, Stroup, DF, Gerberding JL. Actual causes of death in the United States: 2000. J Am Med Assoc. 2004; 291:1238–46.

51. Lieber CS. The discovery of the microsomal ethanol oxidizing system and its physiologic and pathologic role. Drug Metab Rev. 2004; 36:511–29.

52. Ferreira MP, Willoughby D.Alcohol consumption: the good, the bad, and the indifferent. Appl Physiol Metab. 2008; 33:12–20.

53. Valimaki M, Laitnen K, Ylikahri R, et al. The effect of moderate alcohol intake on serum apolipoprotein A-1-containing lipoproteins and lipoprotein (a). Metabolism. 1991; 40:1168–72.

54. Collins MA, Neafsey EJ, Mukamal KJ, et al. Alcohol in moderation, cardioprotection and neuroprotection: epidemiological considerations and mechanistic studies. Clin Exp Res. 2009; 33:206–19.

55. Walzem RL. Wine and health: state of proofs and research needs. Inflammo pharmacology. 2008; 16:265–71.

Suggested Readings

Brown MS, Goldstein JL. A receptor-mediated pathway for cholesterol homeostasis. Science. 1986; 232:34–47.

Goldstein JL, Brown MS. The LDL receptor. Artioscler Thromb Vasc Biol. 2009; 29:431–38.

These are excellent step-by-step reviews of the research resulting in the delineation of the LDL receptor, its mechanisms of cholesterol homeostasis, and the therapeutic implications of these mechanisms. The second article updates the information on LDL receptors with more recent findings.

Budowski P. Ω-3 fatty acids in health and disease. In: Bourne GH, ed. World Review of Nutrition and Dietetics. 1988; 57:214–74.

The structural aspects, sources, and antithrombotic actions of the Ω-3 fatty acids are thoroughly reviewed, along with the eicosanoids and their multiplicity of physiological functions.

Web Sites

www.nal.usda.gov
   This takes you to the National Agriculture Library and from there you can link to the U.S. Government Food and Nutrition Information Center.
www.heart.org
   American Heart Association
www.eatright.org
   American Dietetic Association

THE ROLE OF LIPOPROTEINS AND IMMUNITY IN ATHEROGENESIS

Cardiovascular disease (CVD) is currently the leading cause of morbidity and mortality in the western countries. Within the next 15 years it is expected to become the leading cause of death in the world [1] as a result of the rapid increase in the prevalence of coronary artery disease (CAD) in developing countries and Eastern Europe coupled with the rising incidence of obesity and diabetes in the Western countries [2]. Atherosclerosis is a chronic inflammatory disease as well as a disorder of lipid metabolism. Chapter 5 covered the role played by disorders in lipid and lipoprotein metabolism in the development of CVD. A major component of the development of CVD is the process of atherogenesis, the formation of atheromatous plaque in the inner lining of the arteries. There are still many aspects of atherogenesis we do not fully understand, but considerable insight has been gained beyond the classical view of a couple of decades ago. The classical view postulated an ever-increasing plaque with a concomitant decrease in size of the lumen, much like the accumulation of rust in a water pipe, caused by alterations in lipid metabolism [3]. It is now recognized that plaque development is caused by the combination of inflammation and dyslipidemia. Under normal circumstances, the components of blood—red cells, white cells, and platelets—flow past the inner lining without adhering to it. Fatty streaks are prevalent but asymptomatic in young people; they may at some point cause symptoms or just disappear. So what happens to start the process that causes a plaque to form, and what triggers a plaque to produce thrombosis (a clot)? Just how is inflammation involved? This Perspective explores the current understanding of atherosclerosis.

Inflammation is just one part of the body's innate immune response to tissue damage or a foreign object. Inflammation is a nonspecific response to injury in which phagocytic cells, neutrophils and macrophages, play an important role. The inflammation response is similar regardless of the cause of the damage. Typically, when there is an injury the local macrophages release cytokines, which are chemicals released by leukocytes that function as mediators for the inflammation response [4].

Larger arteries are considered to be elastic—they contain the protein elastin—and do not restrict flow to any great extent. The medium- to small-size arteries, often called arterioles, make up most of the arterial bed that restricts blood flow and increases blood pressure. Of these, smaller coronary arteries are a special example. Unlike peripheral arteries, coronary arteries fill when the heart is in diastole (relaxed) and empty during systole (contracted). If a coronary artery contains an

atherosclerotic plaque and develops a clot, an infarct occurs and can cause death of the cardiac muscle [5]. These smaller arteries do not contain the elastin protein but do contain more smooth muscle. Their walls are made up of three layers: the inner layer or tunica intima, the middle layer or tunica media, and the outer layer or adventia. This outer layer contains connective tissue, nerve endings, mast cells, fibroblasts, and micro-vessels. The innermost layer, the intima, includes a monolayer of endothelial cells that are in contact with the blood plus a small layer of smooth muscle cells under the endothelial cells. The middle layer also contains smooth muscle cells along with a variety of other cell types.

When these arteries are subjected to any of several negative stimuli associated with risk factors for CVD such as hypertension, dyslipidemia, or pro-inflammatory mediators, the endothelial cells produce proteins on their outer matrix that act as an adhering factor. The platelets, the first blood component to interact with the endothelial cells, further change the cell surface, allowing leukocytes (white blood cells) to begin to attach to the endothelial cells. The first cells to attach are the macrophages, which release cytokines, which in turn call in additional leukocytes. The most common type of leukocyte, and the most numerous among the leukocytes adhering to the endothelial cells, is the monocyte. The monocytes are directed into the intima by pro-inflammatory effectors such as cytokines or tumor-necrosis factor (TNF). The monocytes differentiate into macrophages and take up the lipid-rich LDL particles containing cholesterol and cholesterol esters by endocytosis. When they have engulfed sufficient fatty particles they are called foam cells because of their microscopic appearance. The cytokines and TNF attract additional monocytes into the intima and media. Other leukocytes such as T-cells and mast cells also accumulate in the media. As the atheroma progress, additional smooth muscle cells from the media are attracted into the intima and then proliferate in response to platelet-derived growth factors. The smooth muscle cells produce the extracellular proteins collagen and elastin, forming a fibrous cap that covers the plaque [5].

The plaque can enlarge and thus narrow the lumen of the artery so that it begins to impede the blood flow; it may or may not progress to clot formation. The balance between inflammation and anti-inflammatory activity controls the progression of the atherosclerosis [2]. The thrombus (clot) is most likely to form when the fibrous cap is physically disrupted, which can be caused by several mechanisms [5]. The immune cells that have been attracted to the plaque,

including activated macrophages, T-cells, and mast cells, produce a variety of molecules that can destabilize the plaque. These include inflammatory cytokines, activated oxygen species, proteases, coagulation factors, and vasoactive molecules [2]. Some of the smooth muscle cells and macrophages die, leaving lipid droplets and crystals of cholesterol that enhance the plaque's lipid core. The polyunsaturated fatty acids and cholesterol can be oxidized by the reactive oxygen species, producing epoxy fatty acids or oxysterols. The macrophages also produce pro-coagulant factors that make the lipid core more thrombogenic.

Known risk factors for CVD can initiate the pathogenic pathway. For instance, hypertension can increase arterial wall tension, leading to a disturbed repair process and aneurysm formation. Also, angiotensin (Chapter 12) is a major pressor hormone that alters the endothelial membrane and can be the first factor to initiate the leukocyte adherence. Cigarette smoking and diabetes likewise alter endothelial function, which increases the risk for atheroma, but the mechanism is unknown. Once the process begins with leukocyte adherence the cascade of events described previously follows, and plaque development is the result. However, if LDL levels are reduced, the plaque formation is retarded.

Recent research demonstrates that inflammation plays a key role in atherogenesis within small- to mid-size arteries, including coronary arteries. Immune cells and pro-inflammatory effectors are prominent in the early formation of the atherogenic plaque. The atherogenic plaque would not be such a problem if it were not for its tendency to rupture and the subsequent clot formation. The known CVD risk factors also alter the expression of certain pro-inflammatory genes. Certain areas in the genome are associated with myocardial infarction [2].

HDL plays an important role in modifying plaque formation and development. HDL particles are involved in reverse cholesterol transport, as described in the previous chapter. HDL particles also have anti-inflammatory actions. The cholesteryl ester transfer protein (CTEP) facilitates the exchange of cholesterol esters in HDL for triacylglycerol in the LDL particles, which removes some of the oxidized lipid. The anti-inflammatory properties of HDL reverse some of the inflammation that drives the deposition of new lipid.

In summary, CVD was once thought to be due primarily to dyslipidemia, but it is now known that inflammation plays a major role in its development. Following damage in the intima of the smaller arteries caused by one of the CVD risk factors (oxidized cholesterol, free radicals, high blood pressure, etc.) local macrophages are called in, and they release cytokines. The cytokines release a series of chemicals that increase the ability of protein to attach to the intima cell wall and summon additional leukocytes. The monocytes differentiate into macrophages and begin to engulf LDL particles, which contain cholesterol and cholesterol esters. As the atheromatous plaque develops, a fibrous cap is formed. The plaque can grow or stay stable. The stability of the plaque is often dependent upon the fibrous cap staying intact. If it is disrupted, a thrombosis is likely to form, which can cause a closure of that artery or a blockage downstream. If an artery is blocked, the surrounding muscle does not receive sufficient oxygen and may die. With this increased understanding of the role of inflammation in atherosclerosis, the prevention and treatment of CVD—one of the leading causes of death—can go beyond managing dyslipidemia to focus on reducing inflammation as well.

References Cited

1. Shibata N, Glass CK. Macrophages, oxysterols and atherosclerosis. Circ J. 2010; 74:2045–51.

2. Hansson GK. Inflammation, atherosclerosis, and coronary artery disease. New Engl J Med. 2005; 352:1685–95.

3. Libby P. Inflammation and cardiovascular disease mechanisms. Am J Clin Nutr. 2006; 83:S456–60.

4. Sherwood L. Human Physiology: From Cells to Systems. 7th ed. Belmont, CA: Brooks/Cole.2010.

5. Libby P, Ridker PM, Hansson GK. Progress and challenges in translating the biology of atherosclerosis. Nature. 2011; 473:317–25.

6 PROTEIN

THE IMPORTANCE OF PROTEIN IN NUTRITION and health cannot be over-emphasized. It is quite appropriate that the Greek word chosen as a name for this nutrient is *proteos*, meaning "primary" or "taking first place." Proteins are found throughout the body, with over 40% of body protein found in skeletal muscle, over 25% found in body organs, and the rest found mostly in the skin and blood. Proteins are essential nutritionally because of their constituent amino acids, which the body must have to synthesize its own variety of proteins and nitrogen-containing molecules that make life possible. Each body protein is unique in the characteristics and sequence pattern of the amino acids that comprise its structure. This chapter focuses first on classifications of amino acids. Next, sources and digestion of protein to provide amino acids to the body are reviewed, along with how the amino acids are subsequently absorbed and metabolized in cells. The body's use of amino acids to make proteins and nitrogen-containing nonprotein compounds as well as the functional roles of these proteins and compounds in the body are also presented. Lastly, changes in the body's protein (lean) mass with aging are covered, as are recommended intakes of protein, protein quality, assessment of protein and amino acid needs, and protein deficiency.

AMINO ACID CLASSIFICATION

Amino acids may be classified in a variety of ways, including by structure, net charge, polarity, and essentiality. This section addresses each of these four classifications.

Structure

Structurally, all amino acids have a central carbon (C), at least one amino group ($-NH_2$), at least one carboxy (acid) group ($-COOH$), and a side chain (R group) that makes each amino acid unique. The generic amino acid may be represented as follows:

$$H_2N-CH-COOH$$
$$|$$
$$R$$

However, depending upon the pH of the environment, the amino and carboxy groups can accept or donate H^+, and thus the amino group may be represented as $^+NH_3$ and the carboxy group as COO^-. The distinctive characteristics of the side chains of the amino acids that make up a polypeptide bestow on a protein its structure and influence its functional role in the body. These same distinctive characteristics determine whether certain amino acids can be synthesized in the body or must be ingested. Furthermore, these characteristics program the various amino acids for their specific metabolic pathways in the body.

The differences among the side chains of the amino acids commonly found in body proteins are shown in Table 6.1. This division of amino acids based upon structural similarities is one approach used to classify amino acids; dividing amino acids based upon the presence or absence of a net charge is another.

Table 6.1 Structural Classification of Amino Acids

1. With aliphatic/nonpolar side chains
Glycine (Gly)   Alanine (Ala)   Valine (Val)

Leucine (Leu)   Isoleucine (Ile)

2. With side chains containing hydroxylic (OH) groups*
Serine (Ser)   Threonine (Thr)

3. With side chains containing sulfur atoms
Cysteine (Cys)   Methionine (Met)

4. With side chains containing acidic groups or their amides
Aspartic acid (Asp)   Glutamic acid (Glu)

Asparagine (Asn)   Glutamine (Gln)

5. With side chains containing basic groups
Arginine (Arg)   Lysine (Lys)   Histidine (His)

6. With side chains containing aromatic ring
Phenylalanine (Phe)   Tyrosine (Tyr)   Tryptophan (Trp)

*Although tyrosine contains a hydroxyl group, it is classified as an amino acid containing an aromatic ring (see Group 6).

Table 6.1 (*Continued*)

7. *Imino acids*
Proline (Pro)

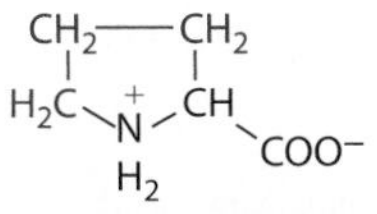

8. *Amino acids formed posttranslationally*
Cystine (Cys-S-S-Cys)

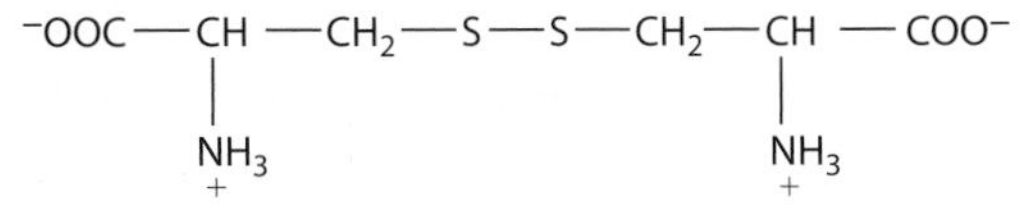

Hydroxylysine (Hyl)

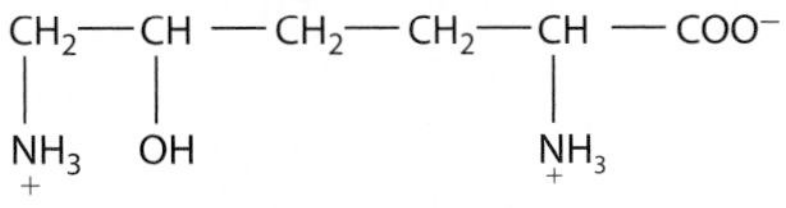

Hydroxyproline (Hyp)

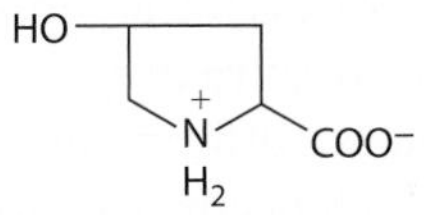

3-methylhistidine (3-meHis)

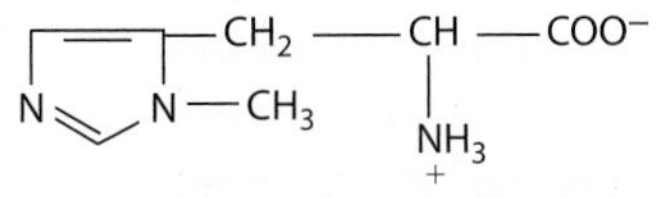

Net Electrical Charge

Table 6.1 shows the structures of amino acids as they exist in an aqueous solution at the physiological pH, approximately 6 to 8, of the human body. Amino acids in an aqueous solution are ionized. The term *zwitterion,* or dipolar ion, is applied to amino acids with no carboxy or amino groups in their side chain to generate an additional charge to the molecule. Zwitterions have no net electrical charge because their side chains are not charged, and the one positive and one negative charge from the amino and carboxy groups, respectively, in their base structure cancel each other out. Amino acids with no net charge, also called neutral amino acids (and listed in Table 6.2A), do not migrate substantially if placed in an electric field.

$$H_3N^+—CH—COO^-$$
$$|$$
$$R$$

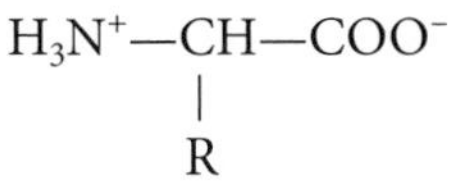

Two groups of amino acids (Table 6.2B) exhibit a net charge. Because of the presence of an additional carboxy group in the side chain, the dicarboxylic (also called acidic) amino acids aspartic acid and glutamic acid exhibit a net negative charge at pH 7; these forms of the amino acids are called aspartate and glutamate. Dicarboxylic amino acids or proteins with a high content of dicarboxylic amino acids migrate toward the anode if placed in an electric field. In contrast, because of the presence of an additional amino group in the side chain, the basic (also called dibasic) amino acids (lysine, arginine, histidine) exhibit a net positive charge at pH 7. These amino acids or proteins rich in them will migrate toward the cathode if placed in an electrical field.

Polarity

The tendency of an amino acid to interact with water at physiological pH—that is, its polarity—represents another means of classifying amino acids. Polarity depends upon the side chain or R group of the amino acid. Amino acids are classified as polar or nonpolar, although they can have varying levels of polarity. Polar charged amino acids include both the dicarboxylic (aspartic acid and glutamic acid) and basic (lysine, arginine, histidine) amino acids, as shown in the second column of Table 6.2C. Polar charged amino acids interact with aqueous environments, can form salt bridges, and can interact with electrolytes and minerals such as potassium, chloride, and phosphate.

Table 6.2A Neutral Amino Acids

Alanine	Glycine	Phenylalanine	Trytophan
Asparagine	Isoleucine	Proline	Tyrosine
Cysteine	Leucine	Serine	Valine
Glutamine	Methionine	Threonine	

Table 6.2B Amino Acids Exhibiting a Net Charge

Negatively Charged Amino Acids	Positively Charged Amino Acids
Aspartic acid	Arginine
Glutamic acid	Histidine
	Lysine

Table 6.2C Polar and Nonpolar Amino Acids

Polar Neutral Amino Acids	Polar Charged Amino Acids	Nonpolar Neutral Amino Acids	Relatively Nonpolar Amino Acids
Asparagine	Arginine	Alanine	Phenylalanine
Cysteine	Lysine	Glycine	Tryptophan
Glutamine	Histidine	Isoleucine	Tyrosine
Serine	Glutamate	Leucine	
Threonine	Aspartate	Methionine	
		Proline	
		Valine	

The neutral amino acids interact with water to different degrees and can be divided into polar, nonpolar, and relatively nonpolar categories, as listed in the first, third, and last columns of Table 6.2C. The side chains of polar neutral amino acids (first column of Table 6.2C) contain functional groups—such as the hydroxyl group for serine and threonine, the sulfur atom for cysteine, and the amide group for asparagine and glutamine—that can interact through hydrogen bonds with water (the aqueous environment of cells). Polar amino acids are generally found on the surfaces of proteins. If not found on the surface, they are oriented inward and function at a protein's (such as an enzyme's) binding site.

In contrast, the amino acids listed in the third column of Table 6.2C contain side chains that do not interact with water and are categorized as nonpolar or hydrophobic (water fearing). As Table 6.2C reveals, the aromatic amino acids are considered relatively nonpolar. Tyrosine, for example, because of its hydroxyl group on the phenyl ring, can to a limited extent form hydrogen bonds with water—hence the term *relatively nonpolar*. Because they do not interact with water, the nonpolar (and often the relatively nonpolar) amino acids are typically found compacted (e.g., attracted by van der Waal forces) and oriented toward or within the central region or core portion of proteins.

Essentiality

While amino acids can be classified based upon structure or properties such as net charge and polarity, in 1957 Rose [1] categorized the amino acids found in proteins as nutritionally essential (indispensable) or nutritionally nonessential (dispensable). In the context of nutrition, the term *essential* or *indispensable* means that the body cannot make the nutrient (in this case the amino acid), and that it must be supplied by diet. Back in the 1950s, only eight amino acids—leucine, isoleucine, valine, lysine, tryptophan, threonine, methionine, and phenylalanine—were considered essential for adult humans. Histidine was later added as an essential amino acid. Table 6.2D lists the essential amino acids.

Identifying amino acids strictly as nonessential/dispensable or essential/indispensable is an inflexible classification, however, that allows no gradations, even in decidedly different or changing physiological circumstances. Therefore, a third category has been added: conditionally or acquired indispensable amino acids.

Table 6.2D Essential/Indispensable Amino Acids

Phenylalanine	Methionine	Isoleucine
Valine	Tryptophan	Leucine
Threonine	Histidine	Lysine

Table 6.2E Conditionally Indispensable Amino Acids and Their Precursors

Amino Acid	Precursor(s)
Tyrosine	Phenylalanine
Cysteine	Methionine, serine
Proline	Glutamate
Arginine	Glutamine or glutamate, aspartate
Glutamine	Glutamate, ammonia

A dispensable amino acid may become indispensable if an organ fails to function properly. For example, neonates born prematurely often have immature organ function and are unable to synthesize some nonessential amino acids, such as cysteine and proline. Immature liver function or liver disease (cirrhosis) impairs both phenylalanine and methionine metabolism, which occur primarily in the liver. Consequently, the amino acids tyrosine and cysteine, normally synthesized via phenylalanine and methionine catabolism, respectively, become indispensable until normal organ function is established. Inborn errors of amino acid metabolism, which result from genetic disorders in which key enzymes in amino acid metabolism lack sufficient enzymatic activity, represent another situation in which dispensable amino acids become indispensable. People with classic phenylketonuria (PKU) exhibit little to no activity for phenylalanine hydroxylase, the enzyme that converts phenylalanine to tyrosine. Without adequate hydroxylase activity, tyrosine is not synthesized in the body and must be provided completely by diet; in other words, tyrosine is indispensable for those with PKU. Some examples of conditionally indispensable amino acids are listed in Table 6.2E, along with their usual amino acid precursors.

SOURCES OF AMINO ACIDS

Amino acids are derived from protein. Both dietary (exogenous) and endogenous proteins provide the body with amino acids for use. Dietary (exogenous) sources of protein include:

- animal products such as meat, poultry, fish, eggs, and dairy products (with the exception of butter, sour cream, and cream cheese)
- plant products such as grains, grain products, legumes, and vegetables

Following ingestion, exogenous proteins serve as sources of the essential amino acids, nonessential amino acids, and the additional nitrogen needed to synthesize more nonessential amino acids and nitrogen-containing compounds in the body. The differences between animal and plant proteins are discussed in the section on protein quality at the end of this chapter.

Endogenous proteins presented to the digestive tract represent another source of amino acids and nitrogen. Endogenous proteins include:

- desquamated mucosal cells, which generate about 50 g of protein per day

- digestive enzymes and glycoproteins, which generate about 17 g of protein each day [2]

The digestive enzymes and glycoproteins are derived from digestive secretions of the salivary glands, stomach, intestine, liver, and pancreas. The intestinal cells contain a variety of proteins (such as apoproteins, structural proteins, cytosolic enzymes) that when sloughed into the gastrointestinal tract are degraded. Most of these endogenous proteins, which may total about 70 g or more per day, are digested and provide amino acids that are available for absorption. Digestion of protein and absorption of amino acids are crucial for optimal protein nutriture.

DIGESTION

Macronutrient digestion in general terms is covered in Chapter 2. Chapter 2 also covers in a more comprehensive manner the regulation of many of the digestive secretions. This section covers only protein digestion within the gastrointestinal tract organs (Figure 6.1 and Table 6.3), with an emphasis on the major enzymes responsible for protein digestion. As no appreciable digestion of protein occurs in the mouth or esophagus, this discussion focuses first on the stomach.

Stomach

The digestion of protein begins in the stomach with the action of hydrochloric acid (HCl), which is found in gastric juice. The hydrochloric acid content of the gastric juice results in a gastric pH of about 1 to 2 and enables denaturation (disruption) of the quaternary, tertiary, and secondary structures of protein (shown later in Figures 6.17–6.19). Denaturants such as hydrochloric acid break apart hydrogen and electrostatic bonds to unfold or uncoil the protein; however, peptide bonds are not affected by the hydrochloric acid. Hydrochloric acid does, however, begin pepsin activation from pepsinogen, which is secreted by gastric chief cells. Pepsin, once formed, is catalytic against pepsinogen as well as other proteins.

$$\text{Pepsinogen} \xrightarrow{\text{HCl or pepsin}} \text{Pepsin}$$

Pepsin functions as an endopeptidase (meaning that it hydrolyzes interior peptide bonds within proteins or

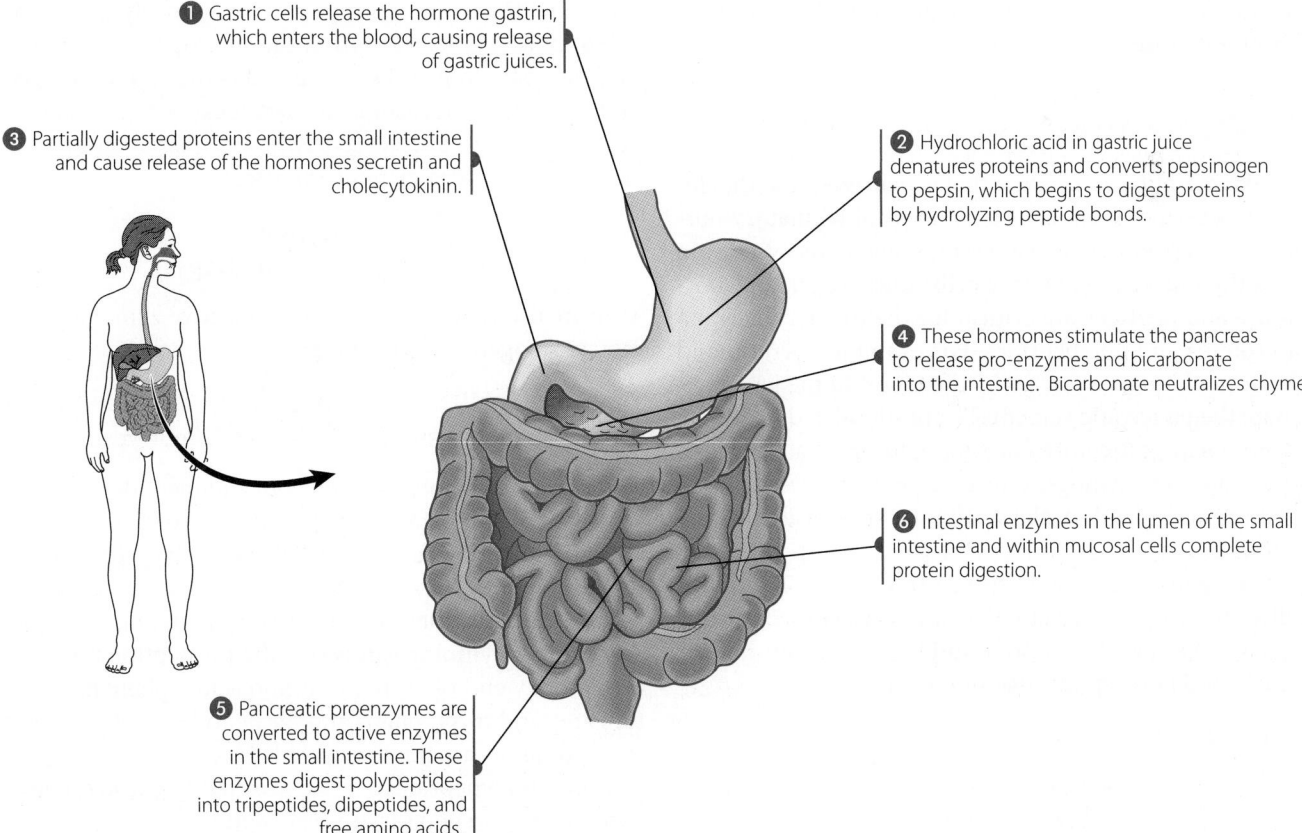

❶ Gastric cells release the hormone gastrin, which enters the blood, causing release of gastric juices.

❸ Partially digested proteins enter the small intestine and cause release of the hormones secretin and cholecytokinin.

❷ Hydrochloric acid in gastric juice denatures proteins and converts pepsinogen to pepsin, which begins to digest proteins by hydrolyzing peptide bonds.

❹ These hormones stimulate the pancreas to release pro-enzymes and bicarbonate into the intestine. Bicarbonate neutralizes chyme.

❻ Intestinal enzymes in the lumen of the small intestine and within mucosal cells complete protein digestion.

❺ Pancreatic proenzymes are converted to active enzymes in the small intestine. These enzymes digest polypeptides into tripeptides, dipeptides, and free amino acids.

Figure 6.1 An overview of protein digestion.
Source: Derived from Beerman/McGuire, Nutritional Sciences, 1/e. © Cengage Learning.

Table 6.3 Some Enzymes Responsible for the Digestion of Protein

Zymogen	Enzyme or Activator	Enzyme	Site of Activity	Substrate (peptide bonds adjacent to)	End product(s)
Pepsinogen	HCl or pepsin $\longrightarrow$	Pepsin	Stomach	Most amino acids, including aromatic, dicarboxylic, leu, met	Peptides
Trypsinogen	Enteropeptidase or Trypsin $\longrightarrow$	Trypsin	Intestine	Basic amino acids	Smaller peptides, some free amino acids
Chymotrypsinogen	Trypsin $\longrightarrow$	Chymotrypsin	Intestine	Aromatic amino acids, met, asn, his	Smaller peptides, some free amino acids
Procarboxypeptidases	Trypsin $\longrightarrow$	Carboxypeptidase	Intestine		
		A		C-terminal neutral amino acids	Free amino acids
		B		C-terminal basic amino acids	Free amino acids
		Aminopeptidases	Intestine	N-terminal amino acids	Free amino acids

polypeptides) at a pH < ~3.5. Specifically, pepsin attacks peptide bonds adjacent to the carboxy end of a relatively wide variety of amino acids (i.e., pepsin has low specificity), including leucine; methionine; the aromatic amino acids (phenylalanine, tyrosine, and tryptophan); and the dicarboxylic amino acids (glutamate and aspartate).

The end products of gastric protein digestion include primarily large polypeptides, along with some oligopeptides (short chains of amino acids peptide bonded to each other) and free amino acids. These end products are emptied in an acidic chyme through the pyloric sphincter into the duodenum (the proximal or upper part of the small intestine) for further digestion.

Small Intestine

The chyme-nutrient mixture that is delivered into the duodenum further stimulates the release of regulatory hormones and peptides such as secretin and cholecystokinin from the mucosal endocrine cells; these regulatory hormones and peptides are critical for the further digestion of proteins and polypeptides. For example, secretin and cholecystokinin are carried by the blood to the pancreas, where the pancreatic acinar cells are stimulated to secrete alkaline pancreatic juice containing bicarbonate, electrolytes, water, and zymogens. In addition to pancreatic juice, the Brunner's glands of the small intestine release mucus-rich secretions.

Zymogens (initially discussed in Chapter 2 and also called proenzymes because they are inactive) secreted by the pancreas into the intestine and further responsible for protein and polypeptide digestion include:

- trypsinogen
- chymotrypsinogen
- procarboxypeptidases A and B

Within the small intestine, these inactive zymogens must be chemically altered to be converted into their respective active enzymes capable of protein hydrolysis. The activation of trypsinogen by enteropeptidase is important since the formation of trypsin facilitates activation of other zymogens. Yet, while trypsinogen activation is important in the intestine, extensive damage would occur should trypsinogen become active within the pancreas. To prevent this, the pancreas produces a compound called trypsin inhibitor.

$$\text{Trypsinogen} \xrightarrow{\text{Enteropeptidase}} \text{Trypsin}$$

Enteropeptidase (an endopeptidase formerly known as enterokinase) is secreted from the enterocyte in response to cholecystokinin and secretin and converts trypsinogen to trypsin. Once trypsin is formed, it can act (like enteropeptidase but to a lesser extent) on trypsinogen to yield active proteolytic enzymes (proteases).

$$\text{Trypsinogen} \xrightarrow{\text{Trypsin}} \text{Trypsin}$$

Trypsin also serves to activate the inactive zymogen chymotrypsinogen as shown here:

$$\text{Chymotrypsinogen} \xrightarrow{\text{Trypsin}} \text{Chymotrypsin}$$

Trypsin and chymotrypsin are both endopeptidases. Trypsin is specific for peptide bonds at the carboxy end of basic amino acids (lysine and arginine). Excess trypsin also acts by negative feedback to inhibit trypsinogen synthesis by pancreatic cells, thereby regulating pancreatic zymogen secretion. Chymotrypsin is specific for peptide bonds at the carboxy end of aromatic amino acids (phenylalanine, tyrosine, and tryptophan) and for peptide bonds adjacent to methionine, asparagine, and histidine.

Procarboxypeptidases are converted to carboxypeptidases by trypsin and serve as exopeptidases.

$$\text{Procarboxypeptidases} \xrightarrow{\text{Trypsin}} \text{Carboxypeptidases}$$

These exopeptidases attack peptide bonds at the carboxy (C)-terminal end of polypeptides to release free amino acids. Carboxypeptidases are zinc dependent, specifically requiring zinc at the enzyme's active site. Carboxypeptidase A hydrolyzes peptides with C-terminal aromatic or aliphatic (nonpolar) neutral amino acids. Carboxypeptidase B cleaves basic amino acids from the C-terminal end to generate free basic amino acids as end products.

Several peptidases are produced by enterocytes, including those in the ileum, enabling peptide digestion and amino acid absorption to occur in the distal small intestine. Some of these intestinal peptidases include the following:

- aminopeptidases, which vary in specificity, cleave amino acids from the amino/(N)-terminal end of oligopeptides
- dipeptidylaminopeptidases, some of which are magnesium dependent, hydrolyze dipeptides
- tripeptidases, which are specific for selected amino acids, hydrolyze tripeptides to yield a dipeptide and a free amino acid

Not all tripeptides, however, undergo additional digestion to produce free amino acids at the brush border of enterocytes. Triglycine and proline-containing peptides tend to be absorbed intact and hydrolyzed within the enterocyte. The digestive process is influenced to some extent by the free amino acid end products, which can sometimes inhibit the activity of brush border peptidases (a process called end product inhibition) to diminish digestion.

Protein digestion yields two main end products: peptides (principally dipeptides and tripeptides) and free amino acids. To be used by the body, these end products must next be absorbed.

ABSORPTION

Absorption is the process by which the end products of digestion are transported from the lumen of the gastrointestinal tract, most often the intestine, into the body. To get into the blood for transport to tissues, amino acids must cross two intestinal membranes, the brush border (also called apical) membrane and the basolateral (also called serosal) membrane. This section of the chapter addresses transporters found in cell membranes that carry amino acids into and out of cells.

Intestinal Brush Border Membrane Absorption

Amino Acid Transport

Amino acid absorption occurs along the entire small intestine, but most amino acids are absorbed in the duodenum and upper jejunum. The absorption of amino acids into enterocytes requires carriers; however, paracellular absorption—that is, absorption via passage through the tight junctions of enterocytes or by transcellular endocytosis—can occur in occasional situations in which large volumes of hypotonic fluids containing some amino acids have been ingested. Transport systems for amino acids have been traditionally designated using a lettering system, with a further distinction that uppercase letters be used for sodium dependence and lowercase letters for sodium independence; however, not all systems (e.g., the L, which is sodium independent) follow this rule. Moreover, with most of the systems now cloned, amino acid transporters are being reclassified and characterized in further detail. Table 6.4 lists some of the transport systems responsible for carrying amino acids across the brush border membrane into the intestinal cell and some examples of amino acids that are carried by each of these transport systems. The older nomenclature has been retained in this text because it facilitates associations between the transporter names and the amino acids carried by the transporters.

The transporters vary in mechanism of action. Some transporters, such as the y^+, t, asc, $b^{o,+}$, and x_c^-, are passive and function as exchangers or uniporters. Other carriers are active and are driven by one or more transmembrane ion gradients. For example, with the X_{AG}^- transporter (antiporter), glutamate, H^+, and three Na^+ enter the cell in exchange for one K^+, and with the N system, glutamine and Na^+ enter the cell in exchange for H^+.

Most amino acids are thought to be transported across the enterocyte brush border membrane by sodium-dependent transporters, as shown in Figure 6.2. With this mechanism, first sodium binds to the carrier. This binding of sodium appears to increase the carrier's affinity for

Table 6.4 Some Systems Transporting Amino Acids across the Intestinal Cell Brush Border Membrane

Amino Acid Transport Systems	Sodium Required	Examples of Substrates Carried
L	No	Leucine, other neutral amino acids
B	Yes	Phenylalanine, tyrosine, tryptophan, isoleucine, leucine, valine
IMINO	Yes	Proline, glycine
y^+	No	Basic amino acids
X_{AG}^-	Yes	Aspartate, glutamate
$B^{o,+}$	Yes	Most neutral and basic amino acids
$b^{o,+}$	No	Most neutral and basic amino acids
y^{+L}	No/Yes	Basic and neutral amino acids
ASC	Yes	Alanine, serine, cysteine
t	No	Tryptophan, phenylalanine, tyrosine
asc	No	Similar to ASC
N	Yes	Glutamine, asparagine, histidine
ag	No	Aspartate, glutamate

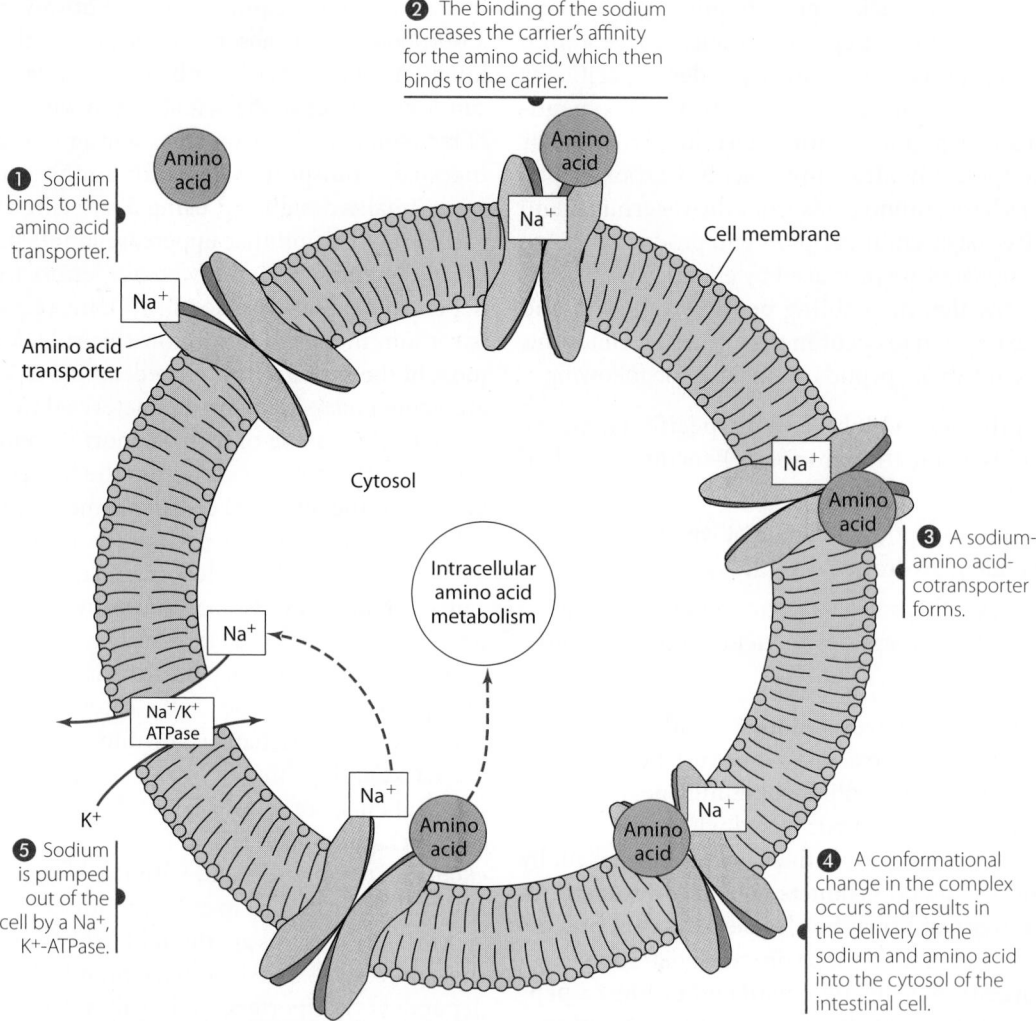

❷ The binding of the sodium increases the carrier's affinity for the amino acid, which then binds to the carrier.

❶ Sodium binds to the amino acid transporter.

Amino acid

Amino acid

Na⁺

Cell membrane

Na⁺

Amino acid transporter

Cytosol

Na⁺

Amino acid

❸ A sodium–amino acid–cotransporter forms.

Intracellular amino acid metabolism

Na⁺

Na⁺/K⁺ ATPase

Na⁺

K⁺

❺ Sodium is pumped out of the cell by a Na⁺, K⁺-ATPase.

Na⁺

Amino acid

Amino acid

Na⁺

❹ A conformational change in the complex occurs and results in the delivery of the sodium and amino acid into the cytosol of the intestinal cell.

Figure 6.2 Sodium (Na⁺) dependent transport of an amino acid into a cell.

the amino acid, which then binds to the carrier. However, for the transport of some amino acids, these first two steps may be reversed; that is, the binding of the amino acid may precede the binding of the sodium. Once the sodium–amino acid–transporter complex forms, a conformational change in the complex results in the delivery of the sodium and amino acid into the cytosol (cytoplasm) of the enterocyte. The sodium is subsequently pumped out of the cell by a Na⁺/K⁺-ATPase.

The affinity (K_m) of a carrier for an amino acid is influenced both by the hydrocarbon mass of the amino acid's side chain and by the net electrical charge of the amino acid. As the hydrocarbon mass of the side chain increases, affinity increases [3]. Thus, the branched-chain amino acids typically are absorbed faster than smaller amino acids. Neutral amino acids also tend to be absorbed at higher rates than basic or acidic amino acids. Essential (indispensable) amino acids are absorbed faster than nonessential (dispensable) amino acids, with methionine, leucine, isoleucine, and valine being the most rapidly absorbed [3]. The most slowly absorbed amino acids are the two acidic

amino acids, glutamate and aspartate, both of which are nonessential [3]. Changes in de novo synthesis of specific amino acid carriers help to ensure adequate capacity.

However, ingesting large quantities of one amino acid or a particular group of amino acids that use the same carrier system may create, depending upon the amount ingested, competition among the amino acids for absorption. The result may be that the amino acid present in highest concentration is absorbed but also may impair the absorption of the other, less concentrated amino acids carried by that same system. Thus, amino acid supplements may result in impaired or imbalanced amino acid absorption. Moreover, absorption of peptides (discussed in the next section) is more rapid than absorption of an equivalent mixture of free amino acids. Also, nitrogen assimilation following ingestion of protein-containing foods is superior to that following ingestion of free amino acids. In other words, free amino acids have no absorptive advantage. Moreover, the supplements are usually expensive, do not typically taste very good, and may cause gastrointestinal distress.

Peptide Transport

Peptide (primarily dipeptide and tripeptide) transport across the brush border membrane of the enterocyte is accomplished by a transport system different from those that transport amino acids. One transport system designated PEPT1 appears to transport all di- and tripeptides. This transport of peptides across the brush border membrane using PEPT1 is associated with the comovement of protons (H^+) and thus depolarization of the brush border membrane. An area of low pH lying adjacent to the brush border surface of the enterocyte provides the driving force for the H^+ gradient. Thus, as shown in Figure 6.3, as the dipeptide or tripeptide is transported into the enterocyte, an H^+ ion also enters the enterocyte. The transport of the H^+ into the enterocyte results in an intracellular acidification. The H^+ ions are pumped back out into the lumen in exchange for Na^+ ions. An Na^+/K^+-ATPase allows for Na^+ extrusion at the basolateral membrane to maintain the gradient.

Although peptides, like amino acids, compete with one another for transporters, peptide transport appears to occur more rapidly than amino acid transport and is thought to represent the primary means by which most amino acids enter the intestinal cell. In other words, the majority of amino acids are absorbed as peptides. Peptides, once within the enterocytes, are generally hydrolyzed by cytosolic peptidases to generate free intracellular amino acids. Intact peptides, however, can be found occasionally in circulation, and this is thought to result from entry of peptides into the body via paracellular (also called intercellular) routes. With illnesses, especially those affecting the intestines (such as inflammatory bowel diseases or celiac disease), the gastrointestinal tract can become more

permeable, thus increasing the likelihood of peptides appearing intact in the blood.

Peptides found in the blood are thought to be hydrolyzed by peptidases or proteases in the plasma, at the cell membrane (especially in the liver, kidneys, and muscle), or, following transport into tissues, intracellularly in the cytosol or in various organelles. Peptide transport into renal tubular cells is influenced by the net charge of the amino acid at the amino (N-) and the carboxy (C-) terminal. Peptides containing either basic or acidic amino acids at either the N- or C- terminal have lower affinity for transport than peptides with neutral side chains at these positions.

The ability to administer peptides directly into the blood as in parenteral nutrition is of nutritional significance since some amino acids (e.g., tyrosine, cysteine, and glutamine) are insoluble or unstable in their free form. Administration of the peptide form, since it can be used by tissues, thus allows nutrients to be provided in situations in which traditional free amino acid parenteral mixtures are ineffective.

Intestinal Basolateral Membrane Transport

For amino acids to enter the blood and be used by other body tissues, the amino acids must be transported across the basolateral (also called serosal) membrane of the enterocyte and into interstitial fluid, where they enter the blood through capillaries of the villi for transport into the portal vein leading to the liver and other tissues. The carriers found in the enterocyte's basolateral membrane are generally the same as those found in the membranes of nonepithelial cells of the body. Most basolateral membrane transporters for amino acids (listed in Table 6.5) are sodium independent.

The significance of the amino acid transporters becomes extremely apparent when people are born without the ability to make a properly working transporter due to a genetic defect. Lysinuric protein intolerance, for example,

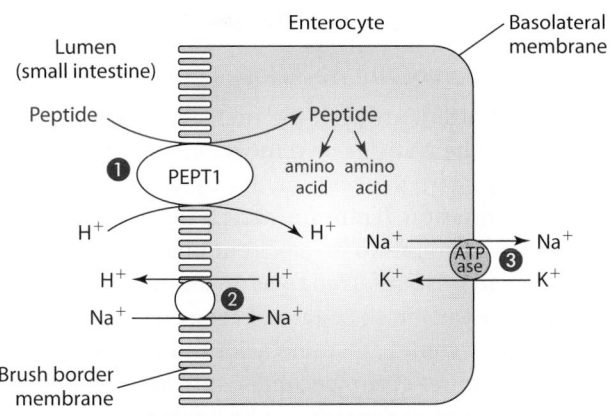

❶ Peptides are transported into the intestinal cell along with H^+.

❷ The H^+ are pumped back into the intestinal lumen in exchange for Na^+.

❸ A Na^+, K^+ ATPase pumps Na^+ out of the cell in exchange for K^+ across the basolateral membrane.

Figure 6.3 Peptide transport. Peptides are transported across the brush border membrane of the intestinal epithelial mucosal cell.

Table 6.5 Some Systems Transporting Amino Acids across the Intestinal Cell Basolateral Membrane

Amino Acid Transport System	Sodium Required	Examples of Substrates Carried
L	No	Leucine, other neutral amino acids
y^+	No	Basic amino acids
$b^{0,+}$	No	Neutral and basic amino acids
t	No	Phenylalanine, tyrosine, tryptophan
X^-_{AG}	Yes	Aspartate and glutamate
A	Yes	Alanine, other short-chain, polar, neutral amino acids
ASC	Yes	Alanine, cysteine, serine, other three- and four-carbon amino acids
asc	No	Same substrates as ASC
GLY	Yes	Glycine

results from defects in the basic amino acid transporters in the intestine, liver, and kidneys. The defects cause poor absorption of lysine, arginine, and ornithine into the body and thus low plasma concentrations and availability of these amino acids for protein synthesis and for urea cycle activity. Symptoms of the disorder include hyperammonemia, growth retardation, muscle weakness, hepatomegaly, and hypotonia, among other problems. Nutrition support involves a protein-restricted diet to help minimize the hyperammonemia and supplements of citrulline to help improve arginine and ornithine production in the body. Likewise, the critical role of transporters is illustrated by the condition called Hartnup disease, an autosomal recessive genetic disorder that affects absorption of tryptophan and other neutral amino acids (likely the B transport system) into intestinal and kidney cells. People with Hartnup disease malabsorb tryptophan, among other amino acids, and often develop a niacin deficiency if not treated with large doses of niacin (recall that tryptophan is a precursor of niacin).

Amino Acid Absorption into Extraintestinal Tissues

After amino acids are transported out of the enterocyte, they enter portal blood and are transported to the liver. Uptake of the amino acids into liver cells (hepatocytes), as well as cells of the kidney and other organs, occurs by some carrier systems similar to those found in the intestinal cell membranes. The sodium-dependent N system is especially prominent in the periportal cells of the liver and functions as an antiporter to take up sodium and glutamine in exchange for H^+. The process occurs in reverse in the perivenous hepatic cells; glutamine is released in exchange for H^+. Hormones and cytokines, such as interleukin-1 and tumor necrosis factor α, influence amino acid transport. System A in hepatocytes, for example, is induced by glucagon and provides amino acid substrates for gluconeogenesis. System GLY is sodium dependent and specific for glycine; two sodium ions are transported for each glycine. The γ-glutamyl cycle is thought to be involved in amino acid transport through membranes of renal tubular cells, erythrocytes, and perhaps neurons. In the γ-glutamyl cycle, glutathione acts as a carrier of neutral amino acids into cells. The cycle is depicted in detail in Figure 6.4. Briefly, glutathione reacts with γ-glutamyl transpeptidase located in cell membranes, forming a γ-glutamyl enzyme complex, which binds a neutral amino acid at the cell surface and transports it into the cytosol for use.

AMINO ACID METABOLISM

The liver is the primary site for the uptake of most amino acids following ingestion of a protein-containing meal. The liver is thought to monitor the absorbed amino acids and to adjust the rate of their metabolism (including catabolism or breakdown of amino acids, and anabolism or use of amino acids for synthesis) according to the needs of the body. In this section of the chapter, an overview of amino acid catabolism will be presented first. The specific catabolism of individual amino acids along with some other uses of individual amino acids will be reviewed next. A later section discusses the anabolic uses of some amino acids for the synthesis of proteins and nitrogen-containing nonprotein compounds.

Amino Acid Catabolism Overview

Liver cells have a high capacity for the uptake and catabolism of amino acids. Catabolism of amino acids occurs to varying degrees in different tissues both during fasting periods and immediately after eating (the postprandial period). In fact, after a meal, the liver takes up about 50% to 65% of amino acids from portal blood. The liver is the main site for the catabolism of the indispensable amino acids, with the exception of the branched-chain amino acids, which tend to be utilized to a greater extent by muscle and other organs such as the heart. Within the liver, the periportal hepatocytes catabolize most amino acids with the exception of glutamate and aspartate, which are metabolized to a greater extent by perivenous hepatocytes. The liver derives up to 50% of its energy (ATP) from amino acid oxidation; the energy generated may in turn be used for gluconeogenesis or urea synthesis, among other needs, depending upon the body's state of nutriture. This section on amino acid catabolism focuses on the reactions that occur as amino acids are broken down in cells, including first the transamination and/or deamination of amino acids and then the disposal of ammonia. It next discusses the uses of the carbon skeleton of amino acids as well as some other uses of amino acids.

Transamination of Amino Acids

Frequently (but not always), the first step in amino acid catabolism is the transfer or removal of an amino acid's amino group. The process occurs by transamination and/or deamination. Transamination reactions involve the transfer of an amino group from one amino acid to an α-keto acid (also referred to as an amino acid carbon skeleton). The carbon skeleton/α-keto acid that gains the amino group becomes an amino acid, and the amino acid that loses its amino group becomes an α-keto acid. A generic transamination reaction can be written as:

$$\text{amino acid}_1 + \text{α-keto acid}_2 \longrightarrow \text{α-keto acid}_1 + \text{amino acid}_2$$

These reactions are important for the synthesis of many of the body's dispensable amino acids.

Transamination reactions are catalyzed by enzymes called aminotransferases/transaminases. These enzymes typically require vitamin B_6 in its coenzyme form, pyridoxal phosphate (PLP). Some examples of aminotransferases

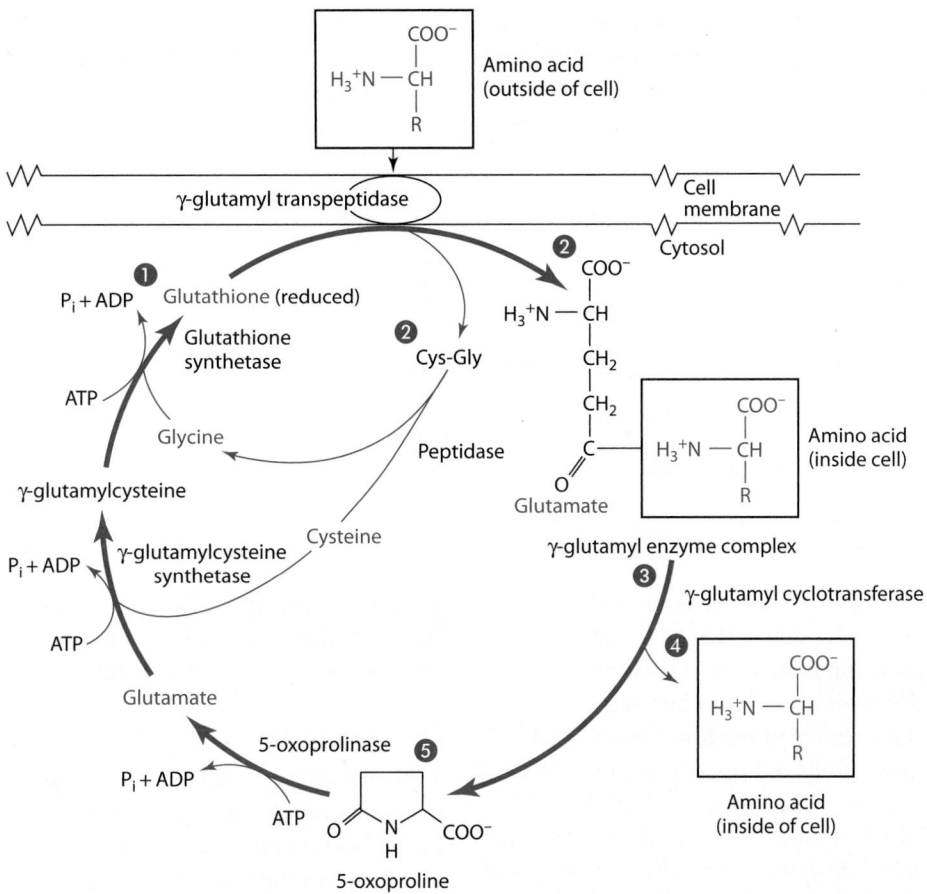

❶ Glutathione reacts with γ-glutamyl transpeptidase to form a γ-glutamyl enzyme complex.

❷ The glutamate portion of glutathione remains attached to the enzyme complex while cysteinyl-glycine (Cys-Gly) is released and an amino acid binds to the glutamate enzyme complex. The cysteinyl-glycine is eventually cleaved into its constituent amino acids by a cytosolic peptidase.

❸ γ-glutamyl cyclotransferase cleaves the peptide bond between the amino acid and the γ-carbon of the glutamate enzyme complex.

❹ The free amino acid can be used within the cell.

❺ 5-oxoproline generated from step 3 is used to reform glutamate and via several steps glutathione (step 1).

Figure 6.4 The γ-glutamyl cycle for transport of amino acids.

include tyrosine aminotransferase, branched-chain aminotransferases, alanine aminotransferase (ALT; formerly called glutamate pyruvate transaminase and abbreviated GPT), and aspartate aminotransferase (AST; formerly called glutamate oxaloacetate transaminase and abbreviated GOT). These last two aminotransferases (ALT and AST) are among the body's most active and involve three key amino acids and α-keto acids—alanine and its α-keto acid pyruvate, glutamate and its α-keto acid α-ketoglutarate, and aspartate and its α-keto acid oxaloacetate—as shown and described in Figure 6.5. Specifically, ALT transfers amino groups from alanine to an α-keto acid (e.g., α-ketoglutarate), forming pyruvate and another amino acid (e.g., glutamate), respectively. Similarly, AST transfers amino groups from aspartate to an α-keto acid (e.g., α-ketoglutarate), yielding oxaloacetate and another amino acid (e.g., glutamate), respectively. These reactions are reversible, and because glutamate and α-ketoglutarate readily transfer and/or accept amino groups, these compounds play central roles in amino acid metabolism.

Aminotransferases are found in varying concentrations in different tissues. For example, AST is found in higher concentrations in the heart than in the liver, muscle, and other tissues. In contrast, ALT is found in higher concentrations in the liver than in the heart but is also found in moderate amounts in the kidneys and small amounts in other tissues. Normal serum concentrations of these enzymes are low; however, with injury or disease to an organ, serum enzyme concentrations rise and can serve as an indicator of organ damage. For example, with liver damage, higher than normal blood concentrations of AST and ALT as well as other enzymes normally found in the liver such as alkaline phosphatase and lactate dehydrogenase are observed. With heart damage (as may occur with a heart attack), enzymes that are normally found in the heart, such as AST, "leak" out into the blood and serve as indicators of heart cell damage.

Interestingly, α-keto acids are sometimes used nutritionally. In kidney failure, nitrogenous compounds that

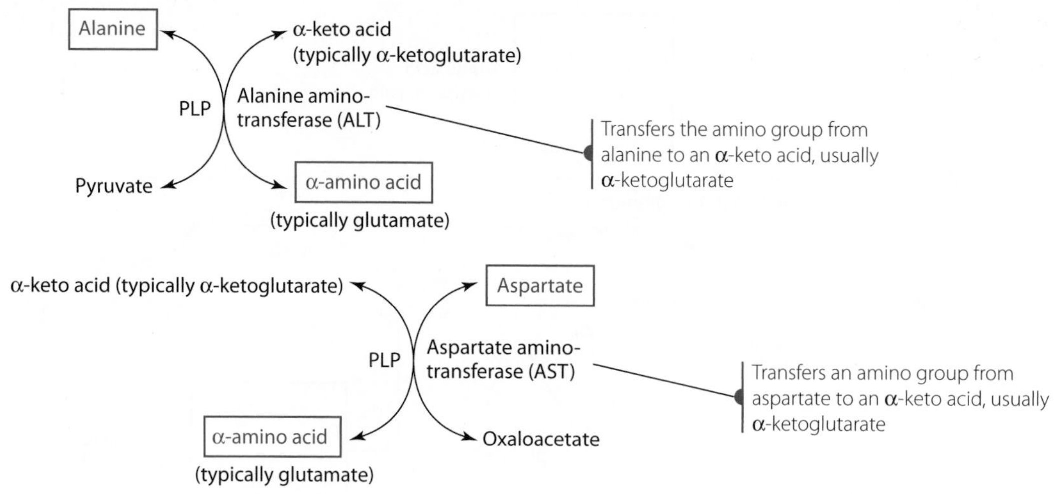

Figure 6.5 Transamination reactions.

are normally excreted in the urine accumulate in the blood. The provision of α-keto acids of some of the essential amino acids to someone with kidney failure allows some of the body's excess nitrogen to be used to aminate the α-keto acids. This results in the lowering of blood nitrogen concentrations while also providing the individual with essential nutrients. Three amino acids (lysine, histidine, and threonine), however, cannot undergo transamination to any appreciable extent; thus, these amino acids cannot be given effectively as α-keto acids.

Deamination of Amino Acids

In contrast to transamination reactions, deamination reactions involve only the removal of an amino group from an amino acid, with no transfer of the amino group to another compound. Some amino acids that are more commonly deaminated include glutamate, histidine, serine, glycine, and threonine; however, many of these same amino acids also can be transaminated. The enzymes carrying out the deamination reactions are generally lyases, dehydratases, or dehydrogenases and produce an α-keto acid and ammonia or an ammonium ion. Figure 6.6 shows the deamination of the amino acid threonine by threonine dehydratase (which deaminates and dehydrates threonine) to form α-ketobutyrate and ammonia. At the body's physiological

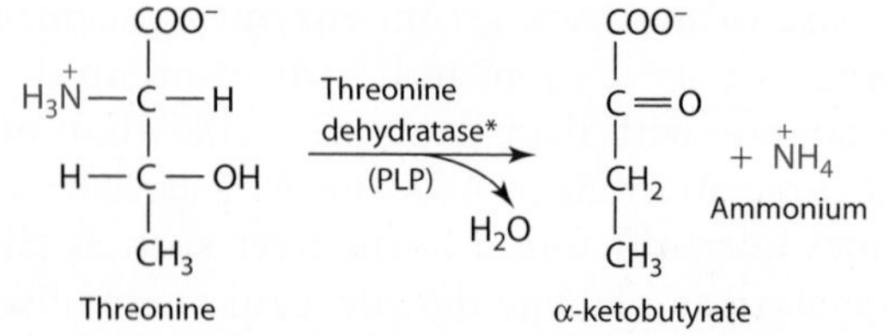

*The enzyme is called *dehydratase* rather than *deaminase* because the reaction proceeds by loss of elements of water. In the deamination, the amino group from the amino acid is removed. Vitamin B_6 as PLP is required by the enzyme.

Figure 6.6 The deamination of the amino acid threonine. In the deamination, the amino group from the amino acid is removed.

pH, ammonia is typically converted to the ammonium ion; however, the reaction is reversible. The next section addresses the disposal of ammonia by the body.

Disposal of Ammonia

The ammonia or ammonium ions generated by deamination reactions are not the only source of ammonia found in the body. Major sources of ammonia and/or ammonium ions in the body include:

- formation in the body from chemical reactions such as deamination
- generation by the deamidation of the amide groups from glutamine and asparagine
- ingestion and absorption from foods (e.g. cheeses, processed meats)
- generation by the bacterial lysis of urea and amino acids in the gastrointestinal tract and subsequent absorption through the enterocyte into the body

Typically three enzymes—glutamate dehydrogenase, glutamine synthetase, and carbamoyl phosphate synthetase I (as part of the urea cycle)—assist in the removal of the ammonia/ammonium ions from body cells. These enzymes are found in high concentrations in the liver but are also found in other organs.

Glutamate and Glutamine Synthesis Glutamate dehydrogenase readily uses an ammonia or ammonium ion ($^+NH_4$) and α-ketoglutarate to make the amino acid glutamate, as shown here:

$$^+NH_4 + \text{α-ketoglutarate} + \text{NADPH} \longleftrightarrow \text{Glutamate} + \text{NADP}^+ + H_2O$$

The glutamate generated in this reversible reaction can then release the ammonia or ammonium ion for the synthesis of either urea or a dispensable amino acid.

Glutamine synthetase can also use ammonia or an ammonium ion for the amidation of glutamate's gamma carboxy group to form glutamine in an ATP-dependent reaction that also requires magnesium or manganese as follows:

$$^+NH_4 + \text{Glutamate} + \text{ATP} \longrightarrow \text{Glutamine} + \text{ADP} + P_i$$

Glutamine's functions, including its role in ammonia transport, are discussed further in this chapter in the "Interorgan Flow of Amino Acids and Organ-Specific Metabolism" section.

While the liver's perivenous cells and other body tissues readily synthesize glutamate and glutamine from ammonia or ammonium ions, the periportal hepatocytes are active in ureagenesis using (from portal blood) ammonia that was ingested in foods or obtained from bacterial synthesis in the intestine. These same periportal cells are responsible for almost all amino acid catabolism, so ammonia and ammonium ions generated during amino acid degradative reactions also can be immediately taken up for urea synthesis.

The Urea Cycle The urea cycle, discovered by Sir Hans Krebs, functions in the liver and is extremely important for the removal of ammonia and ammonium ions from the body. Figure 6.7 reviews key compounds of the urea cycle and shows its relationship with amino acids and the tricarboxylic acid (TCA), also known as the Krebs, cycle. The five reactions of the urea cycle are broken down in the following list of reactions:

- Ammonia (NH_3) (or an ammonium ion) combines with CO_2 (or HCO_3^-) to form carbamoyl phosphate

in a reaction catalyzed by mitochondrial carbamoyl phosphate synthetase I (CPSI) and using 2 mol of ATP and Mg^{2+}. N-acetyl-glutamate (NAG), made in the liver and intestine, is required as an allosteric activator to allow ATP binding.

- Carbamoyl phosphate reacts with ornithine in the mitochondria, using the enzyme ornithine transcarbamoylase (OTC), to form citrulline. Citrulline in turn inhibits OTC activity.

- Aspartate reacts with citrulline once it has been transported into the cytosol. This step, catalyzed by argininosuccinate synthetase, is the rate-limiting step of the cycle. ATP (two high-energy bonds) and Mg^{2+} are required for the reaction, and argininosuccinate is formed. Argininosuccinate, arginine, and AMP + PP_i inhibit the enzyme.

- Argininosuccinate is cleaved by argininosuccinase in the cytosol to form fumarate and arginine. Both fumarate and arginine inhibit argininosuccinase activity. Argininosuccinase is found in a variety of tissues throughout the body, especially the liver and kidneys. High concentrations of arginine increase the synthesis of N-acetylglutamate (NAG), which is needed in the reaction for the synthesis of carbamoyl phosphate in the mitochondria.

- Urea is formed and ornithine is re-formed from the cleavage of arginine by arginase, a manganese-requiring hepatic enzyme. Arginase activity is inhibited by both ornithine and lysine, and may become rate limiting under conditions that limit manganese availability or that alter its affinity for manganese [4].

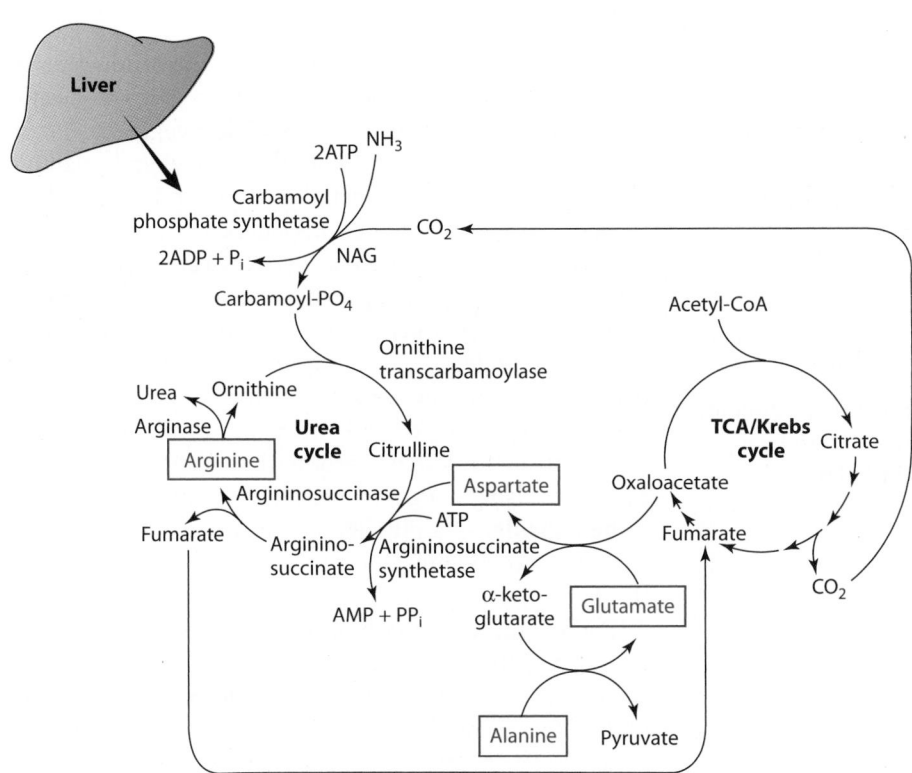

Figure 6.7 Interrelationships of amino acids and the urea and TCA/Krebs cycles in the liver. The individual reactions in the urea cycle are discussed in the text.

Overall, the urea cycle uses four high-energy bonds. The urea molecule derives one nitrogen from ammonia, a second nitrogen from aspartate, and its carbon from CO_2/HCO_3^-. Once formed, urea typically travels in the blood to the kidneys for excretion in the urine; however, up to about 25% of urea may be secreted from the blood into the intestinal lumen, where it may be degraded by bacteria to yield ammonia.

Activities of urea cycle enzymes fluctuate with diet and hormone concentrations. For example, with low-protein diets or acidosis, urea synthesis diminishes and urinary urea nitrogen excretion decreases significantly. Thus, substrate availability results in short-term changes in the rate of ureagenesis. In the healthy individual with a normal protein intake, blood urea nitrogen (BUN) concentrations range from about 8 to 20 mg/dL, and urinary urea nitrogen represents about 80% of total urinary nitrogen. Glucocorticoids and glucagon, which promote amino acid degradation, typically increase mRNA for the urea cycle enzymes.

Several defects (genetic mutations) have been identified in urea cycle enzymes. Urea cycle enzyme defects typically result in high levels of blood ammonia (hyperammonemia) and necessitate a protein-restricted diet. Urea synthesis is also diminished and blood ammonia concentrations increased in those with advanced liver disease. The elevated blood ammonia concentrations observed in liver disease are thought to contribute to hepatic encephalopathy, characterized by brain dysfunction (coma). Medical treatment for encephalopathy involves decreasing blood ammonia concentrations. Drugs such as lactulose are given to acidify the gastrointestinal tract contents and promote the diffusion of the ammonia out of the blood and into the gastrointestinal tract. Further, antibiotics are prescribed that promote the destruction of intestinal tract bacteria that generate ammonia.

Metabolism of the Carbon Skeleton/α-Keto Acid: An Overview

As outlined in Figure 6.8, once an amino group has been removed from an amino acid, the remaining part is called a carbon skeleton or α-keto acid.

$$\text{Amino acid} \longrightarrow \text{NH}_2 + \text{carbon skeleton/} \atop \text{α-keto acid}$$

Carbon skeletons of amino acids can be further metabolized with the potential for multiple uses in the cell, depending upon the original amino acid from which they were derived. An amino acid's carbon skeleton, for example, can be used to produce:

- energy
- glucose
- ketone bodies
- cholesterol
- fatty acids

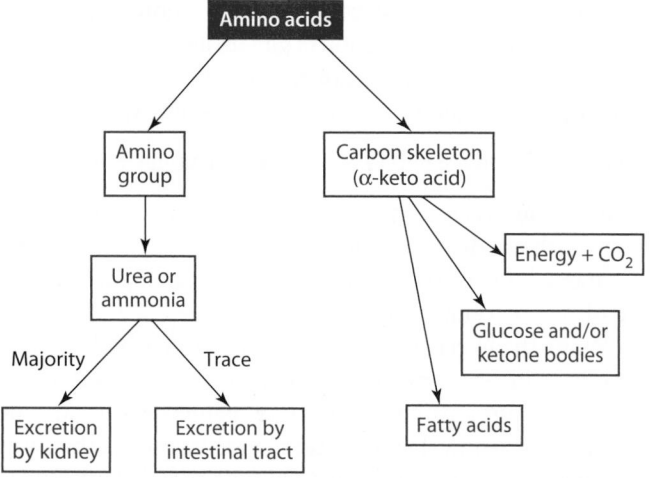

Figure 6.8 Possible fates of amino acids upon catabolism.

Whereas all amino acids can be completely oxidized to generate energy, not all amino acids can be used, for example, for the synthesis of glucose. Furthermore, the fate of the amino acid's carbon skeleton depends upon the body's physiological and nutritional state.

Energy Generation The complete oxidation of amino acids generates energy, CO_2/HCO_3^-, and ammonia/ ammonium ions. Amino acids are used for energy in the body when diets are inadequate in energy (measured in kilocalories, abbreviated *kcal*). The oxidation of selected amino acids is presented in later subsections addressing hepatic catabolism and uses of amino acids.

Glucose and Ketone Body Production The production of glucose from a noncarbohydrate source such as amino acids is known as gluconeogenesis. Gluconeogenesis occurs primarily in the liver but also in the kidneys and small intestine; it is discussed in detail in Chapter 3. The carbon skeletons of several amino acids can be used to synthesize glucose. For example, oxaloacetate (the carbon skeleton of aspartate) and pyruvate (the carbon skeleton of alanine) may be used to produce glucose in body cells. In addition, the carbon skeleton of asparagine can be converted into oxaloacetate, and the carbon skeletons of glycine, serine, cysteine, tryptophan, and threonine can be converted into pyruvate for glucose production. Valine and methionine are also glucogenic, yielding succinyl-CoA. Thus, to be considered a glucogenic amino acid, catabolism of the amino acid must yield pyruvate or intermediates of the TCA cycle.

For an amino acid to be considered ketogenic, the catabolism of the amino acid must generate acetyl-CoA or acetoacetate, which are used for the formation of ketone bodies. Some amino acids are both glucogenic and ketogenic. Phenylalanine and tyrosine, for example, can be degraded to form fumarate (an intermediate of the TCA cycle), which can be used to form glucose, but also acetoacetate, which can be used to synthesize ketone bodies. Isoleucine is partially glucogenic, generating succinyl-CoA, but also ketogenic, yielding acetyl-CoA as well upon its catabolism. Threonine is partially glucogenic, yielding succinyl-CoA or pyruvate depending upon its pathway of degradation, and partially ketogenic when degraded by another pathway to acetyl-CoA. Tryptophan is also considered partially ketogenic and partially glucogenic. Tryptophan yields acetyl-CoA as well as pyruvate upon catabolism. Leucine and lysine are the only totally ketogenic amino acids and upon catabolism generate acetyl-CoA. Figure 6.9 shows the general fates of amino acid carbon skeletons with respect to key intermediates of metabolism.

The conversion of amino acids to glucose is accelerated by a high blood glucagon to insulin ratio and by high blood cortisol concentrations. Glucagon concentrations are generally elevated in the blood when blood glucose concentrations are low, as may occur in between meals or with a fast causing depletion of liver glycogen stores. Blood glucagon (and in some cases cortisol along with epinephrine) is also elevated in the presence of infection or trauma/injury and in certain disease states such as untreated diabetes mellitus and liver disease, to name a few.

Cholesterol Production The oxidation of several amino acids, including isoleucine, leucine, lysine, tryptophan, and threonine, yields acetyl-CoA, which can be metabolized to produce cholesterol (Figure 6.9). Leucine, however, is also the only amino acid whose catabolism directly generates β-hydroxy β-methylglutaryl-CoA, an intermediate (shown later in Figure 6.36) in cholesterol synthesis. Moreover, leucine oxidation produces another metabolite, β-hydroxy β-methylbutyrate (HMB), which appears to promote de novo cholesterol synthesis in muscle, enabling cell growth and function. This topic is further discussed in the "Skeletal Muscle" section and more specifically in the "Isoleucine, Leucine, and Valine Catabolism" section. Cholesterol synthesis is discussed in detail in Chapter 5.

Fatty Acid Production In times of excess energy and protein intakes coupled with adequate carbohydrate intake, the carbon skeleton of amino acids may be used to synthesize fatty acids. Leucine, for example, is used to synthesize fatty acids in adipose tissue. Leucine's catabolism is shown later in Figure 6.36. Fatty acid synthesis is discussed in Chapter 5.

Hepatic Catabolism and Uses of Aromatic Amino Acids

The details of the metabolism of selected amino acids and the formation of TCA cycle and non–TCA cycle intermediates are discussed in following sections. The catabolism

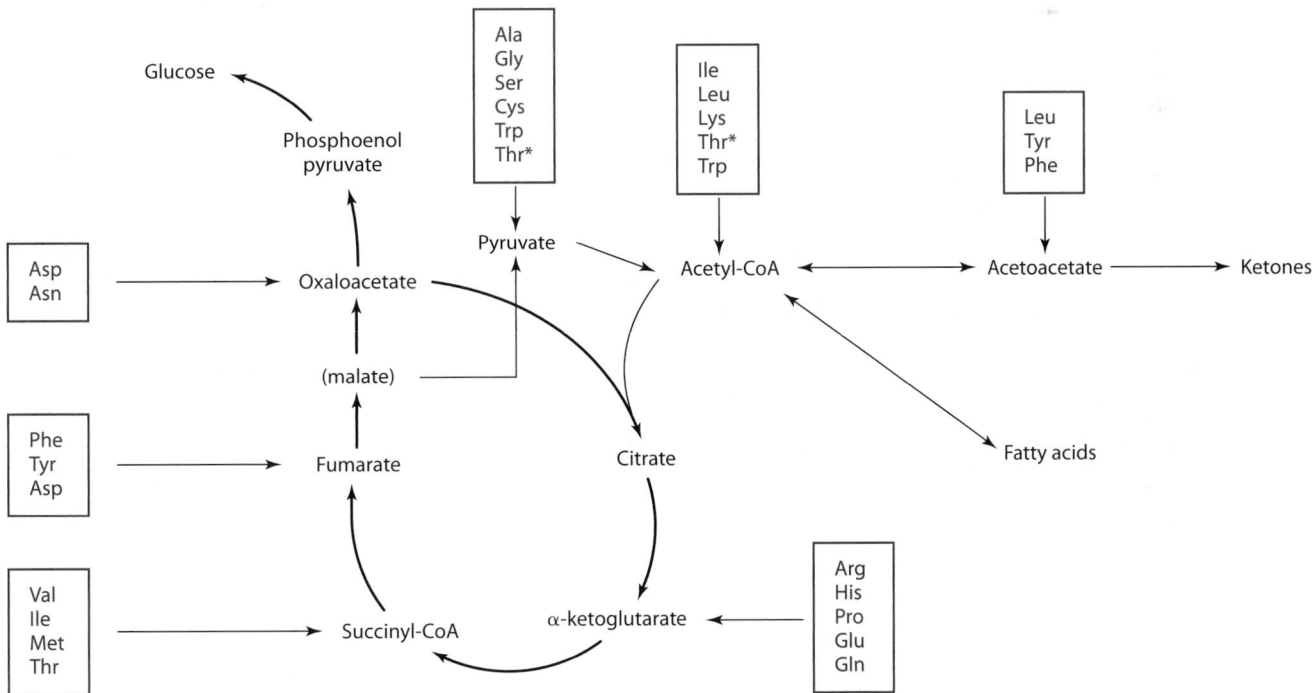

*Physiological contribution unclear

Figure 6.9 The fate of amino acid carbon skeletons. Ketogenic: Lys and Leu; partially ketogenic and glucogenic: Phe, Ile, Thr, Trp, Tyr; glucogenic: Ala, Gly, Cys, Ser, Asp, Asn, Glu, Gln, Arg, Met, Val, His, Pro.

of the amino acids is categorized primarily according to their structural classification, although also by net charge for the basic amino acids. The aromatic amino acids are discussed first, followed by the sulfur-containing amino acids, the branched-chain amino acids, the basic amino acids, and lastly other selected amino acids.

Amino acid catabolism occurs in most body tissues, although the liver plays a primary role for some amino acids (such as the aromatic and sulfur-containing amino acids) more than for others. For example, in advanced liver disease, the inability of the liver to take up and catabolize certain amino acids is evidenced by the increased plasma concentrations of both the aromatic amino acids—phenylalanine, tyrosine, and tryptophan—and the sulfur-containing amino acids methionine and cysteine.

Phenylalanine and Tyrosine

As shown in Figures 6.9 and 6.10, phenylalanine and tyrosine are partially glucogenic because they are degraded to fumarate. In addition, phenylalanine and tyrosine are catabolized to acetoacetate and thus are partially ketogenic.

- The first step in the degradation of phenylalanine (Figure 6.10) is specific to the liver and the kidneys. Phenylalanine is converted to tyrosine by the enzyme phenylalanine hydroxylase, also called a monooxygenase. This enzyme is iron dependent, and vitamin C and tetrahydrobiopterin are required for the reaction. Enzyme activity is regulated by phosphorylation/dephosphorylation with glucagon promoting phosphorylation and enzyme activity. Insulin has the opposite effect.

- Tyrosine degradation (Figure 6.10) begins with transamination by a vitamin B_6–dependent tyrosine aminotransferase to yield p-hydroxyphenylpyruvate. Higher tyrosine concentrations as well as high cortisol levels promote increases in tyrosine aminotransferase activity. The compound p-hydroxyphenylpyruvate, once formed, is then decarboxylated by a dioxygenase to

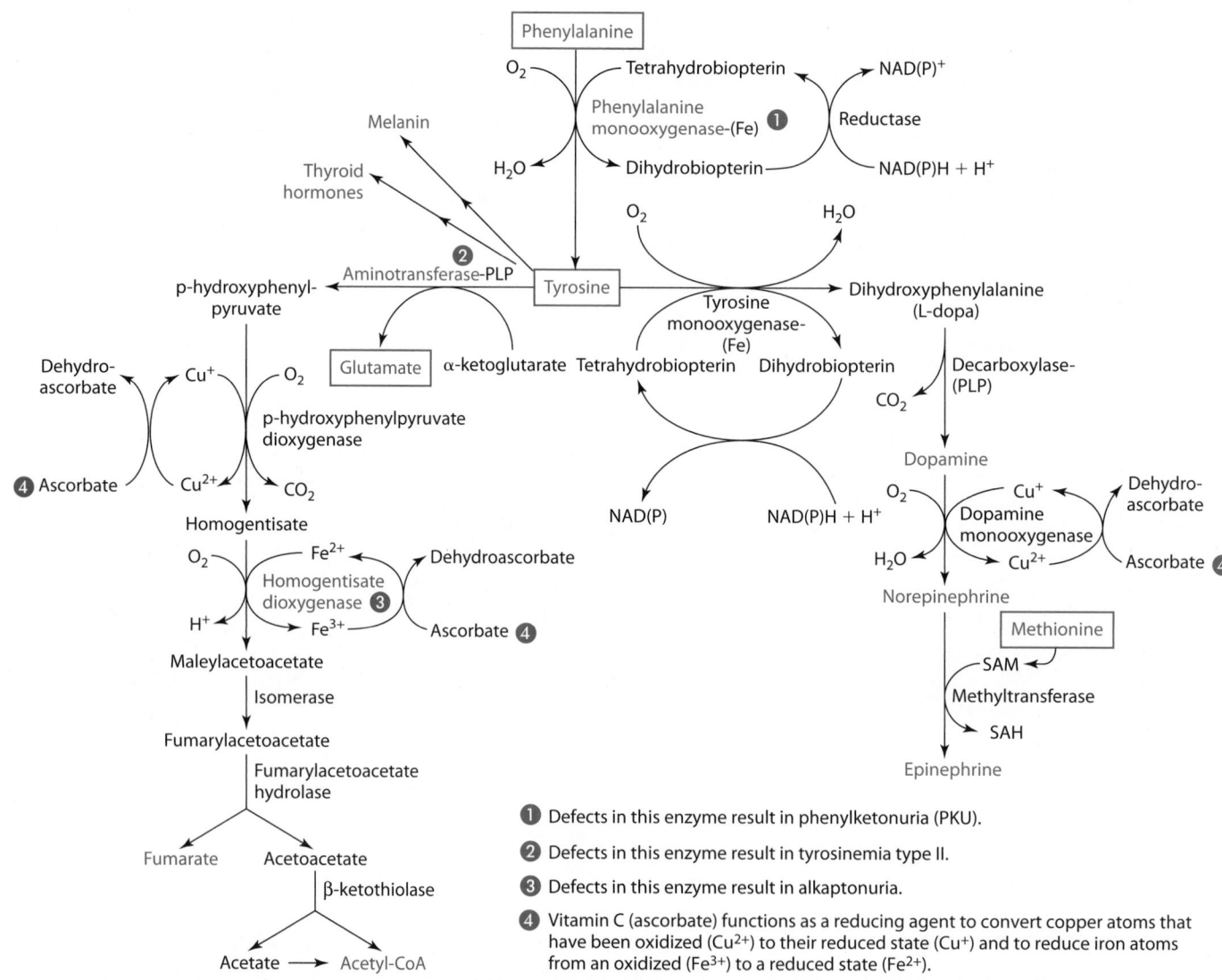

Figure 6.10 Phenylalanine and tyrosine metabolism.

generate homogentisate. Homogentisate dioxidase converts homogentisate to maleylacetoacetate, which is then isomerized to fumarylacetoacetate. A hydrolase converts fumarylacetoacetate into fumarate (a TCA cycle intermediate) and acetoacetate, which may be further metabolized to acetyl-CoA for energy or ketone body production.

Tyrosine also can be used to synthesize other compounds in other cells of the body. Some of these uses are mentioned hereafter and shown in Figure 6.10 as well as later in Figure 6.16.

- In neurons and the adrenal medulla, for example, tyrosine is used for the synthesis of neurotransmitters and hormones, respectively. The initial reaction involves tyrosine hydroxylase (also called monooxygenase), an iron-dependent enzyme that hydroxylates tyrosine to generate 3,4-dihydroxyphenylalanine (L-dopa). Subsequent reactions utilizing L-dopa yield the catecholamines (dopamine, norepinephrine, and epinephrine). The catecholamines function as neurotransmitters in the nervous system; however, in circulation they (especially epinephrine) function as hormones and have major effects on nutrient metabolism.

- In melanocytes in the skin, eye, and hair cells, tyrosine is converted through multiple reactions into melanin. The reactions occur within melanosomes, membrane-bound organelles found in the melanocytes. Melanin is a pigment that gives color to skin, eyes, and hair.

- In the thyroid gland, tyrosine is taken up and used with iodine to synthesize thyroid hormones. These reactions are discussed in detail in the section on iodine in Chapter 13.

Disorders of Phenylalanine and Tyrosine Metabolism Several inborn errors of phenylalanine and tyrosine metabolism have been identified and are shown in Figure 6.10. The autosomal recessive genetic disorder phenylketonuria (PKU) occurs when the activity of phenylalanine hydroxylase, which converts phenylalanine to tyrosine, is defective. It is one of the most prevalent disorders of amino acid metabolism, with an incidence of about 1 in 10,000 in the United States. This enzymatic defect results in a buildup of phenylalanine and phenylalanine metabolites (phenyllactate, phenylpyruvate, and phenylacetate) in the blood and other body fluids. In addition, because phenylalanine's conversion to tyrosine is impaired, blood tyrosine concentrations diminish. If untreated, PKU causes neurologic problems such as seizures and hyperactivity, among other problems. The disorder is treated with a phenylalanine-restricted diet, which means that ingestion of protein-containing foods is extremely limited, and tyrosine must be added to the diet because it cannot be made in the body. In addition, labels on products that contain aspartame (brand name Equal) must have a warning indicating that the product contains phenylalanine and thus its use must be restricted by those with PKU.

Impaired activity of the enzyme tyrosine aminotransferase, which converts tyrosine to p-hydroxyphenylpyruvate, results in another inborn error of metabolism called tyrosinemia type II. Tyrosinemia type II has a worldwide incidence of about 1 in 250,000. This form of tyrosinemia is characterized by high plasma tyrosine concentrations, skin and eye lesions, and impaired mental development. People with the disorder must consume a diet restricted in both phenylalanine and tyrosine.

Another genetic disorder involving tyrosine degradation is alkaptonuria, which results from defective homogentisate dioxygenase activity. The condition is not common worldwide (affecting 1 in 250,000 to 1 million); however, in Slovakia it affects about 1 in 19,000. Homogentisate dioxygenase normally converts homogentisic acid to maleylacetoacetate. Alkaptonuria is characterized by high concentrations of homogentisic acid in body tissues and fluids. The homogentisic acid oxidizes and turns a dark color, thus making the urine appear black when exposed to air. People with this disorder often experience joint problems (such as arthritis) as the homogentisic acid accumulates in connective tissues. Dietary treatment is not usually prescribed.

Tryptophan

Another aromatic amino acid metabolized principally by the liver is tryptophan. Its metabolism is shown in Figure 6.11. Tryptophan is partially glucogenic, because it is catabolized to form pyruvate; it is also partially ketogenic, forming acetyl-CoA as shown in Figure 6.9.

- The first step in tryptophan catabolism yields N-formylkynurenine. The enzyme tryptophan dioxygenase, which catalyzes this first reaction, is a heme-iron–containing enzyme. The enzyme is induced by glucagon as well as cortisol.

- Further catabolism of N-formylkynurenine yields formate and kynurenine. Kynurenine may be metabolized to 3-hydroxykynurenine by a monooxygenase. The 3-hydroxykynurenine may be converted to 3-hydroxyanthranilate and alanine by kynureninase, a vitamin B_6 (PLP)–dependent enzyme. Alanine formed from tryptophan degradation can be transaminated to form pyruvate, hence the glucogenic nature of tryptophan.

- Further catabolism of 3-hydroxyanthranilate results in the formation of 2-amino 3-carboxymuconic 6-semialdehyde. This compound is further metabolized to produce many additional compounds, including picolinate (a possible binding ligand for minerals), and 2-aminomuconic 6-semialdehyde, which is further metabolized in several reactions to acetyl-CoA (a ketogenic intermediate).

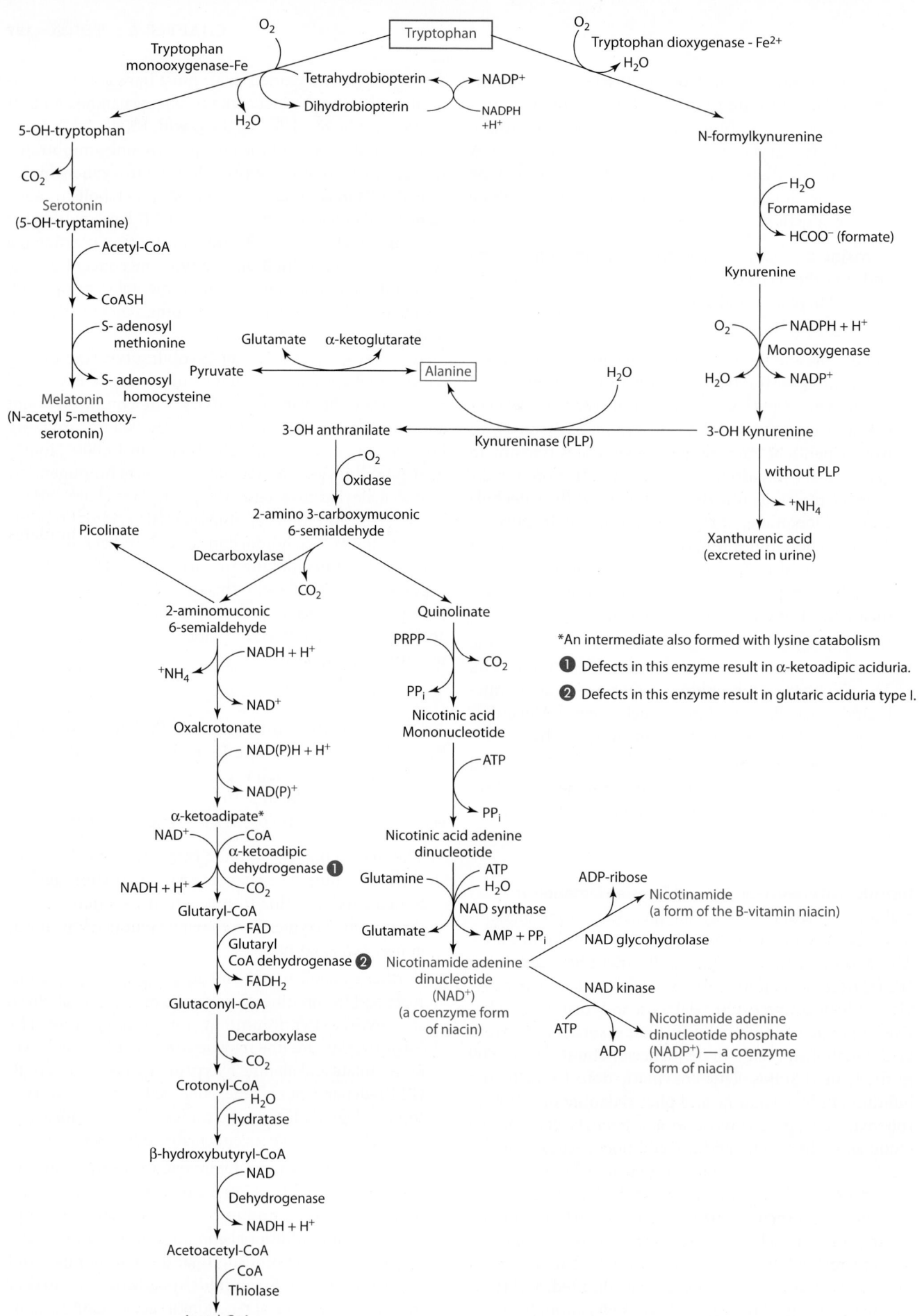

Figure 6.11 Tryptophan metabolism.

Tryptophan also has other fates in the body, as shown in Figure 6.11 and later in Figure 6.16. For example:

- The metabolism of tryptophan through N-formylkynurenine generates the B-vitamin niacin as nicotinamide as well as its coenzyme form nicotinamide adenine dinucleotide (NAD) phosphate (NADP). Thus, deficient protein intake limits niacin synthesis in the body.

- In addition, tryptophan is used for the synthesis of serotonin (5-hydroxytryptamine) and melatonin (N-acetyl 5-methoxyserotonin). Melatonin is made primarily in the pineal gland, which lies in the center of the brain. Melatonin synthesis and release correspond with darkness; the hormone is thought to be involved mainly with the regulation of circadian rhythms and sleep. Supplement use has been helpful for some people with jet lag. Serotonin functions throughout the body but especially in the gastrointestinal tract. It promotes vasoconstriction and smooth muscle contraction. It also functions as a neurotransmitter; see the "Brain and Accessory Tissues" section later in this chapter.

Disorders of Tryptophan Metabolism As part of tryptophan's degradative pathway in which 2-aminomuconic 6-semialdehyde is converted in multiple reactions to acetyl-CoA, defective activities of two enzymes have been documented. One genetic disorder, α-ketoadipic aciduria, results from the defective activity of α-ketoadipic dehydrogenase, which converts α-ketoadipate to glutaryl-CoA. With this disorder, lysine, tryptophan, α-aminoadipate, α-ketoadipate, and α-hydroxyadipate build up in the blood and other body fluids. Infants with this disorder become hypotonic, acidotic, and experience seizures and a number of motor and developmental problems. Nutrition support requires a lysine- and tryptophan-restricted diet because this set of reactions is common in both tryptophan and lysine degradation. A second disorder related to this pathway also may occur. Glutaric aciduria (or acidemia) type 1, an autosomal recessive condition, results from the defective activity of the riboflavin-dependent enzyme glutaryl-CoA dehydrogenase, which converts glutaryl-CoA to glutaconyl-CoA. As with α-ketoadipic aciduria, the enzyme glutaryl-CoA dehydrogenase is critical to the catabolism of tryptophan (Figure 6.11) as well as lysine (shown later in Figure 6.13). In glutaric aciduria type 1, glutaryl-CoA builds up and is converted to glutaric acid, which also accumulates in body fluids. Over time, affected infants develop acidosis, ataxia, seizures, and macrocephaly, among other problems. Treatment requires a diet restricted in both lysine and tryptophan (because both produce glutaryl-CoA). For some individuals, riboflavin supplements have been shown to enhance glutaryl-CoA dehydrogenase activity.

Hepatic Catabolism and Uses of Sulfur (S)-Containing Amino Acids

The catabolism of methionine, an S-containing essential amino acid, occurs to a large extent in the liver and generates another S-containing nonessential amino acid, cysteine.

Methionine

Oxidation of methionine yields succinyl-CoA, and thus it is a glucogenic amino acid (Figure 6.9). Some of methionine's uses in the body are shown later in Figure 6.16. Methionine metabolism, shown in Figure 6.12, is briefly described here.

- The first step in methionine catabolism is the conversion of methionine to S-adenosyl methionine (SAM) by methionine adenosyl transferase (present in high concentrations in the liver) in an ATP-requiring reaction. SAM has many functions in the body. SAM promotes further methionine catabolism; it stimulates cystathionine synthase, which converts homocysteine to cystathionine. SAM also inhibits methylene tetrahydrofolate (THF) reductase activity, which forms the 5-methyl THF (also called N5-methyl THF) needed to regenerate methionine from homocysteine. Thus, SAM (when present in higher concentrations) facilitates the degradation of methionine and not its resynthesis. SAM also has other functions. SAM serves as the principal methyl donor in the body and, as such, is required for the synthesis of carnitine, creatine, epinephrine, and melatonin. It is also needed for the metabolism of arsenic. Furthermore, the methyl groups from SAM are used to methylate DNA, and thus affect gene expression. In addition, SAM may be decarboxylated to form S-adenosyl methylthiopropylamine, an intermediate in the synthesis of the polyamines—putrescine, spermidine, and spermine. Polyamines are important in cell division and growth.

- The removal or donation of the methyl group from SAM yields the compound S-adenosyl homocysteine (SAH). SAH can be converted to homocysteine by the enzyme S-adenosyl homocysteine hydrolase. Homocysteine, once formed, can be converted back to methionine either in a betaine-dependent reaction or in a vitamin B_{12} (as methylcobalamin)– and folate (as 5-methyl THF)–dependent reaction. Betaine, obtained from diet or generated in the liver from choline oxidation, provides a methyl group that is transferred to homocysteine by the hepatic enzyme betaine homocysteine methyltransferase. With the loss of the methyl group, betaine becomes dimethylglycine. Dimethylglycine can be further demethylated to generate glycine. In the vitamin B_{12}– and folate-dependent remethylation reaction (Figure 6.12), methylcobalamin

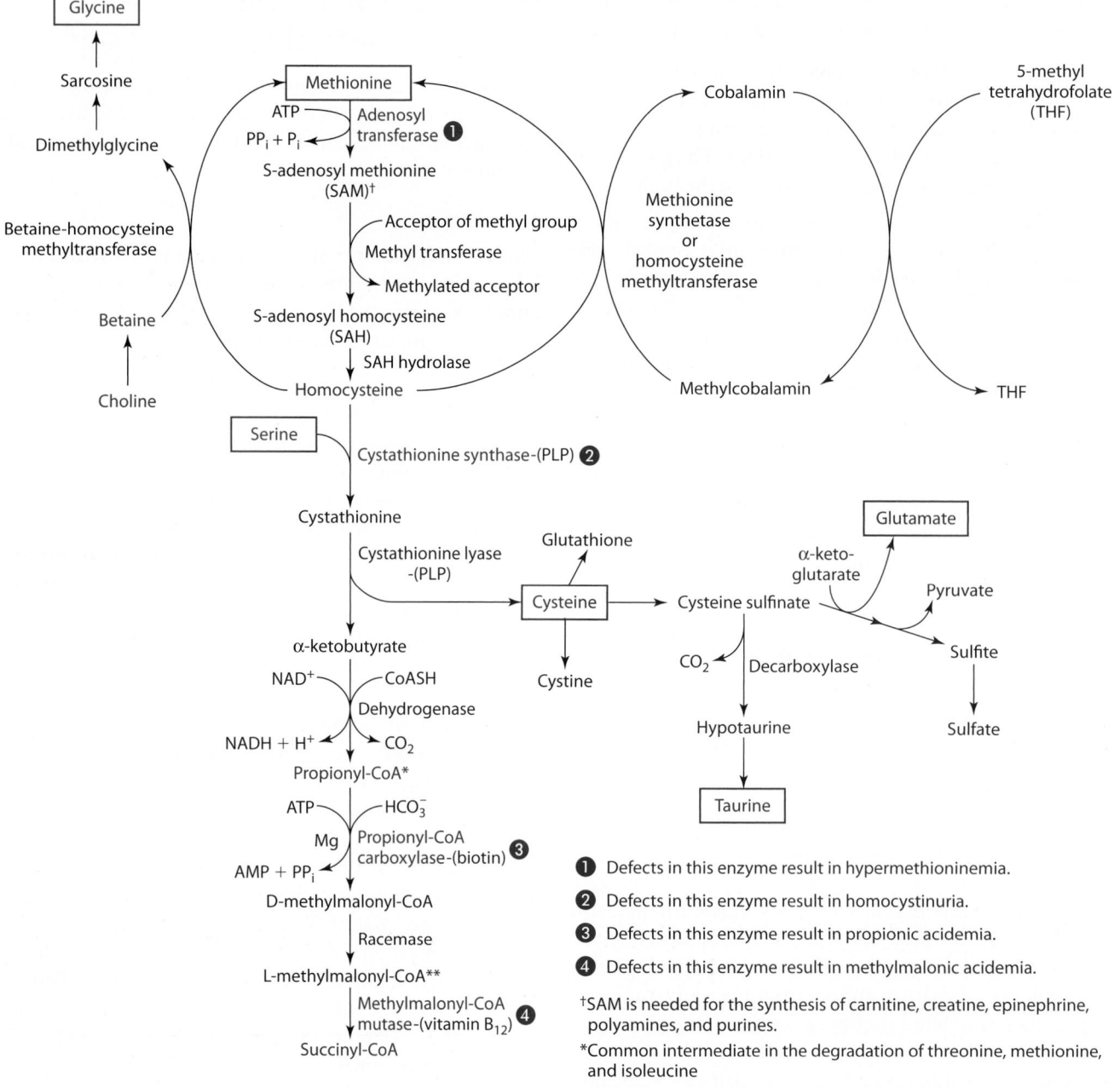

Figure 6.12 Methionine and cysteine metabolism.

directly provides the methyl group to remethylate homocysteine to form methionine. Methylcobalamin receives the methyl group from 5-methyl THF. Elevated plasma homocysteine concentrations have been shown to interfere with collagen cross-linking in bone and may increase fracture risk. High plasma homocysteine concentrations also have been found to be a risk factor for heart disease and may develop if folate, vitamin B_{12}, and/or vitamin B_6 status is poor. A discussion of the importance of adequate folate, vitamin B_{12}, and vitamin B_6 nutriture and heart disease is found in Chapter 9 in the sections on folate and vitamin B_{12}.

- To be further metabolized in the body, homocysteine must react with the amino acid serine, forming cystathionine through the action of cystathionine (β) synthase. The presence of vitamin B_6 in its coenzyme form (PLP) is necessary for this reaction to occur, hence the need for adequate vitamin B_6 status to prevent elevated blood homocysteine concentrations.

- Further catabolism of cystathione requires additional coenzymes. Cystathionine is cleaved by cystathionine β lyase, another vitamin B_6–dependent enzyme, to form the dispensable amino acid cysteine. Also generated in the reaction is α-ketobutyrate, which is further decarboxylated to propionyl-CoA. The conversion of homocysteine to cysteine by cystathionine synthase and cystathionine lyase is sometimes called the transulfuration pathway. These reactions occur in the liver, but also in the kidneys, intestine, and pancreas.

- Propionyl-CoA (made from α-ketobutyrate) is next converted to D-methylmalonyl-CoA by the biotin-dependent enzyme propionyl-CoA carboxylase. D-methylmalonyl-CoA is then converted to L-methyl-malonyl-CoA by a racemase. Then L-methyl-malonyl-CoA is converted by methylmalonyl-CoA mutase, a vitamin B_{12}–dependent enzyme, to the TCA cycle intermediate succinyl-CoA. These reactions are shown in Figure 6.12.

Disorders of Methionine Metabolism Defects in methionine adenosyl transferase, the enzyme that converts methionine to S-adenosyl methionine (SAM), result in the genetic disorder hypermethioninemia. This condition is characterized by high blood concentrations of methionine and thus treatment necessitates a diet restricted in methionine but containing increased cysteine.

Defects in cystathionine β synthase, which converts homocysteine to cystathionine, result in the genetic disorder homocystinuria. The condition affects about 1 in 200,000 to 300,000 people worldwide, but about 1 in 65,000 in Ireland. People with this condition exhibit high blood homocysteine and methionine concentrations, and low blood cysteine concentrations. The high plasma homocysteine concentrations can promote blood clot (thrombi) formation. Other selected manifestations include skeletal problems, osteoporosis, ocular changes, and mental retardation. Treatment requires a diet low in methionine (and thus low intakes of normal protein-containing foods), added cysteine, and in some cases supplements of betaine and folate.

The genetic disorder propionic acidemia (with an incidence of about 1 in 35,000 to 70,000 but as many as 1 in 1,000 in Greenland and 1 in 2,000 to 3,000 in Saudi Arabia) results from defects in the activity of propionyl-CoA carboxylase, a biotin-dependent enzyme. Another disorder caused by genetic errors in the same pathway is methylmalonic acidemia, which results from impaired methylmalonyl-CoA mutase activity. Methylmalonic acidemia affects about 1 in 48,000. Propionic acidemia is characterized by the accumulation of propionic acid in body fluids, and in methylmalonic acidemia both propionic and methylmalonic acids (as well as other compounds such as methylcitrate, 3-hydroxy propionate, and tiglic acid) accumulate in body fluids. Infants exhibit excessive vomiting, ketoacidosis, hypertonia, failure to thrive, and respiratory difficulties, among other problems. Because propionyl-CoA and thus methylmalonyl-CoA are generated from not only methionine, as shown in Figure 6.12, but also from the degradation of both threonine (shown later in Figure 6.15) and isoleucine, and because the degradation of valine produces methylmalonyl-CoA (see later Figure 6.36), the diets of people with either of these conditions require restriction of multiple amino acids. In addition, odd-chain fatty acids and polyunsaturated fatty acids (in excessive amounts) generate propionyl-CoA and thus must be restricted. In some cases, biotin supplements have been shown to improve the activity of propionyl-CoA carboxylase, but a restricted diet is still typically needed. Similarly, vitamin B_{12} supplements can sometimes improve methylmalonyl-CoA mutase activity in some people with methylmalonic acidemia (recall that methylmalonyl-CoA mutase is vitamin B_{12} dependent).

Cysteine

- Cysteine is a nonessential amino acid. Hepatic concentrations of free cysteine appear to be tightly controlled. Cysteine is used like other amino acids for protein synthesis. It is also used to synthesize glutathione. Cysteine is also converted by cysteine dioxygenase to cysteine sulfinate, which is used to produce the amino acid taurine (Figure 6.12).

- Taurine, a β-amino sulfonic acid, is made in the liver but concentrated in muscle and the central nervous system; it is also found in smaller amounts in the heart, liver, and kidneys, among other tissues. Although taurine is not involved in protein synthesis, it is important in the retina, where it is thought to exhibit antioxidant properties and help maintain the structure and function of the photoreceptor cells. Taurine is thought to maintain membrane stability by scavenging peroxidative (e.g., oxychloride) products. Taurine also functions in the liver and intestine as a bile salt, taurocholate, and in the central nervous system as an inhibitory neurotransmitter.

- Cysteine degradation (Figure 6.12) yields pyruvate and sulfite. Sulfite is converted by sulfite oxidase (an iron- and molybdenum-dependent enzyme) to sulfate, which can be excreted in the urine or used to synthesize sulfolipids and sulfoproteins.

Hepatic Catabolism and Uses of Branched-Chain Amino Acids

The liver plays only a minor role in the initial catabolism of the three branched-chain amino acids, isoleucine, leucine, and valine. Transaminase activity needed to remove the amino groups is minimal in the liver, although hepatic transferases increase in response to glucocorticoid (cortisol) release, as may occur with infection or trauma, or prolonged fasting. Thus, under normal circumstances, the branched-chain amino acids typically remain in circulation and are taken up and transaminated primarily by the skeletal muscle, but also by the heart, kidneys, diaphragm, and adipose tissue, if needed. Alpha-keto acids of the branched-chain amino acids, generated from branched-chain amino acid transamination, may be used within the tissues or released into circulation. The liver, among other organs, can further catabolize these α-keto acids. Additional information on branched-chain amino acid metabolism is found under "Skeletal Muscle" in the "Interorgan 'Flow' of Amino Acids and Organ-Specific Metabolism" section of this chapter.

Hepatic Catabolism and Uses of Basic Amino Acids

Lysine

The catabolism of lysine, a totally ketogenic amino acid, generates acetyl-CoA, as shown in Figures 6.13 and 6.9. Lysine and tryptophan degradation share a common intermediate, α-ketoadipate, and thus share some common reactions. Lysine has another important use in the body. After being methylated using SAM (made from methionine), lysine is used in the synthesis of carnitine, which is needed for fatty acid oxidation. This use of lysine is shown later in Figure 6.23.

Disorders of Lysine Metabolism Defects in lysine degradation by glutaryl-CoA dehydrogenase and α-ketoadipate dehydrogenase result in glutaric aciduria type 1 and α-ketoadipic aciduria, respectively, as discussed in the "Disorders of Tryptophan Metabolism" section and shown in Figure 6.11.

Arginine

Arginine is metabolized mostly in the liver and kidneys but also in the intestine. It is a glucogenic amino acid, as its catabolism generates the TCA cycle intermediate

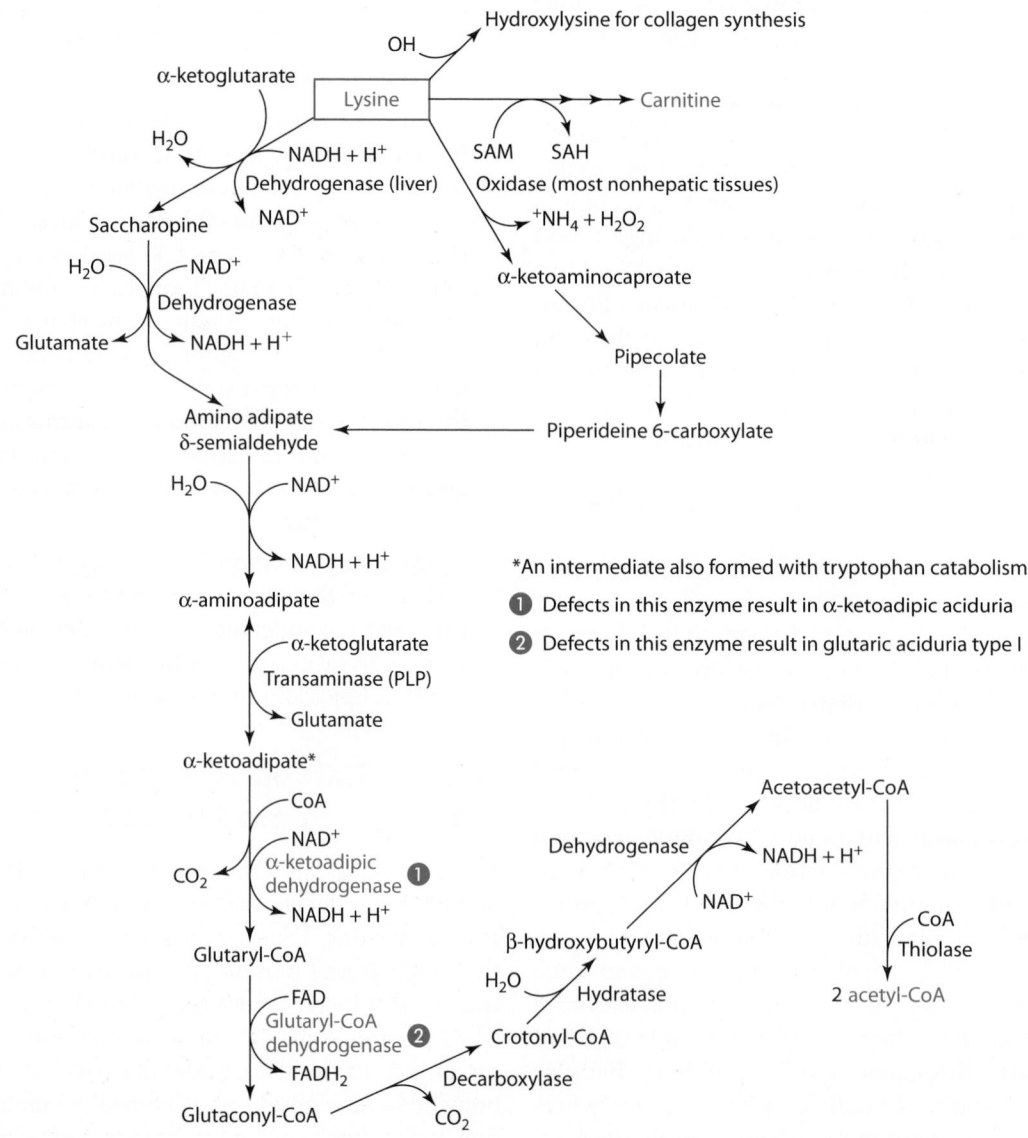

Figure 6.13 Lysine metabolism.

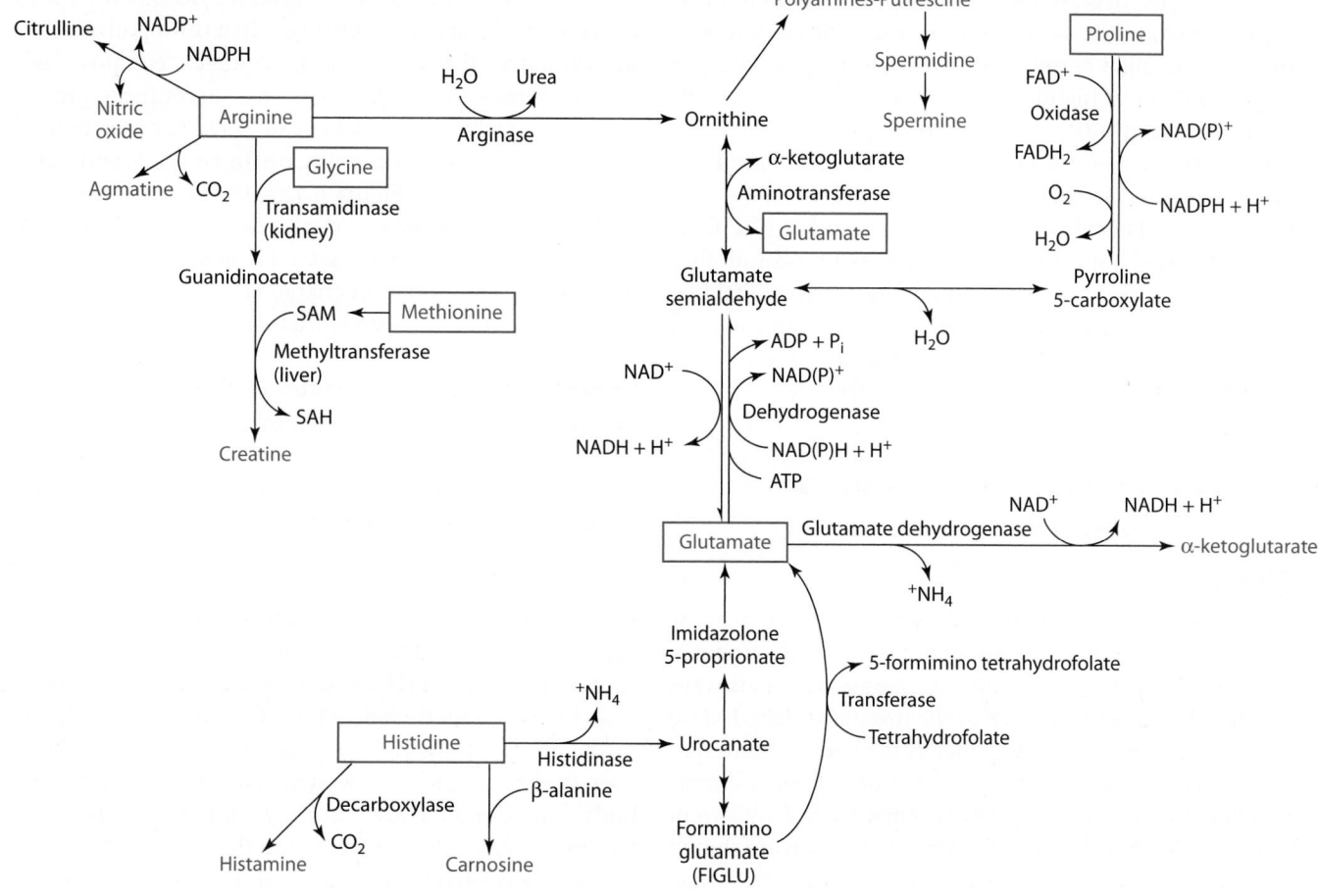

Figure 6.14 Arginine, proline, histidine, and glutamate metabolism.

α-ketoglutarate (Figure 6.9). Arginine, however, also has several other uses in the body, as shown in Figure 6.14 and later in Figure 6.16. In the liver, it is primarily degraded as part of the urea cycle to form urea and ornithine. Ornithine may be decarboxylated to form polyamines (putrescine, spermine, and spermidine), or it may be transaminated by ornithine aminotransferase to form, through a series of reactions, the amino acid proline. Polyamines are thought to function in cell signaling, growth, and proliferation. In the kidneys, arginine is used with glycine to produce guanidinoacetate; guanidinoacetate is then released into the blood and travels to the liver, where it is converted into creatine. Agmatine made in the brain and central nervous system, among other organs, from the decarboxylation of arginine is involved in neuromodulary functions. In endothelial cells, cerebellar neurons, neutrophils, and splanchnic tissues, arginine is used via nitric oxide synthase for nitric oxide production. Nitric oxide is involved in a variety of physiological processes including regulation of blood pressure (relaxation of vascular smooth muscle) and intestinal motility, inhibition of platelet aggregation, and macrophage function. Nitric oxide also can combine with glutathione to form glutathionylated nitric oxide, a compound that in turn is known to stimulate the

glutathionylation of proteins. This posttranslational modification is thought to affect the function and stability of many cellular proteins.

Histidine

Histidine degradation is also shown in Figure 6.14. It is a gluconeogenic amino acid yielding α-ketoglutarate (Figure 6.9). Histidine also has several other uses in the body, as depicted later in Figure 6.16. It may combine with β-alanine to generate carnosine. Carnosine is discussed in more detail in the section of this chapter on nitrogen-containing nonprotein compounds. In addition, through a vitamin B$_6$–dependent decarboxylation reaction, the amine histamine also can be formed from histidine. Histamine functions in the brain as a neurotransmitter. In the gastrointestinal tract, it has many roles including the stimulation of gastric secretions such as hydrochloric acid. In mast cells (found throughout the body in locations such as within the nose and mouth, blood vessels, and internal body surfaces) and in white blood cells (especially basophils), histamine exhibits immunologic roles. It stimulates constriction of bronchial smooth muscle and causes dilation or increased permeability of capillaries to facilitate white blood cell infiltration and phagocytosis of foreign antigens. This increased permeability may result in flushing (redness) of the skin and in the escaping of fluid into tissues, causing a runny nose and watery eyes. Another interesting fate of histidine in the body relates to its post-translational modification in some proteins. Specifically, histidine, in some body proteins like actin in muscle, becomes methylated and when the protein is broken down, the methylated histidine, called 3-methylhistidine (see Table 6.1), is released but cannot be reused to synthesize another protein. Because it cannot be reused, the 3-methylhistidine is excreted in the urine and is often used as an index of muscle catabolism. This topic is also discussed in the "Skeletal Muscle" section later in this chapter.

Hepatic Catabolism and Uses of Other Selected Amino Acids

Threonine

Threonine can be metabolized by three different pathways and consequently is both glucogenic and ketogenic (Figure 6.9). One of the more commonly used pathways of degradation is through cytosolic threonine dehydratase to generate α-ketobutyrate, which is further catabolized to propionyl-CoA, then to D-methylmalonyl-CoA, L-methylmalonyl-CoA, and ultimately succinyl-CoA, as shown in Figure 6.15. These latter steps in the catabolism are shared with methionine and isoleucine, and in part with valine. Alternately, threonine may be degraded by mitochondrial threonine dehydrogenase to form aminoacetone, which is converted to methylglyoxal and then pyruvate.

This pathway is thought to be used if cytosolic threonine concentrations are relatively high. In a third pathway, the mitochondrial threonine cleavage complex (composed of a dehydrogenase and a ligase) converts threonine to glycine and acetylaldehyde; acetylaldehyde is further metabolized to acetate and then to acetyl-CoA in an ATP- and CoA-dependent reaction (Figure 6.15). Threonine is found in fairly high concentrations relative to other amino acids in the glycoproteins of mucus. Consequently, in situations of intestinal inflammation characterized by excess mucus production, threonine needs are thought to be elevated.

Disorders of Threonine Metabolism Defects in two steps of threonine metabolism from propionyl-CoA to succinyl-CoA can lead to propionic acidemia and methylmalonic academia, as shown in Figure 6.15 and previously discussed in the "Disorders of Methionine Metabolism" section.

Glycine and Serine

Glycine and serine are produced from one another in a reversible reaction that requires folate in its coenzyme forms tetrahydrofolate (THF) and 5,10 methylene THF (also called N5 N10 methylene THF). Glycine is converted to serine mainly in the kidneys (Figure 6.15). Glycine, however, is also needed for the synthesis of other important body compounds (shown in Figure 6.16), including glutathione, creatine, porphyrins, and the bile salt glycocholate. Serine is used for the synthesis of ethanolamine and choline for phospholipids. See also the discussion on the kidney in the "Interorgan 'Flow' of Amino Acids and Organ-Specific Metabolism" section later in this chapter.

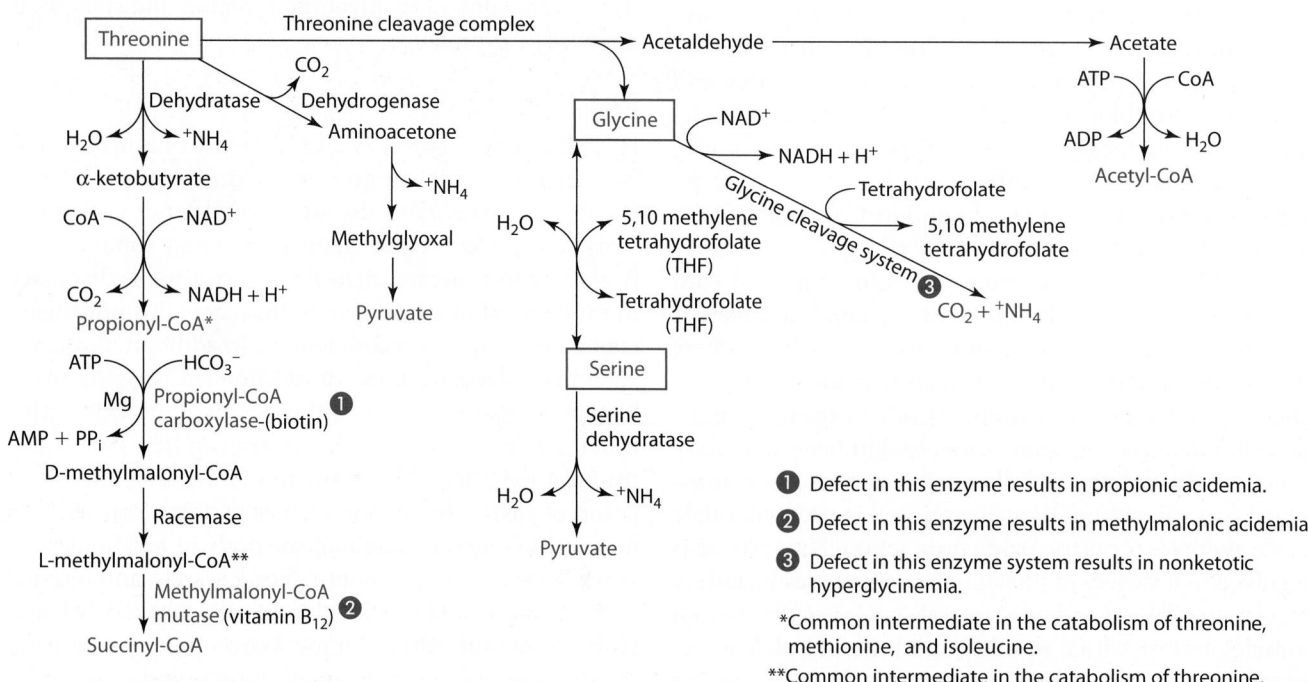

Figure 6.15 Threonine, glycine, and serine metabolism.

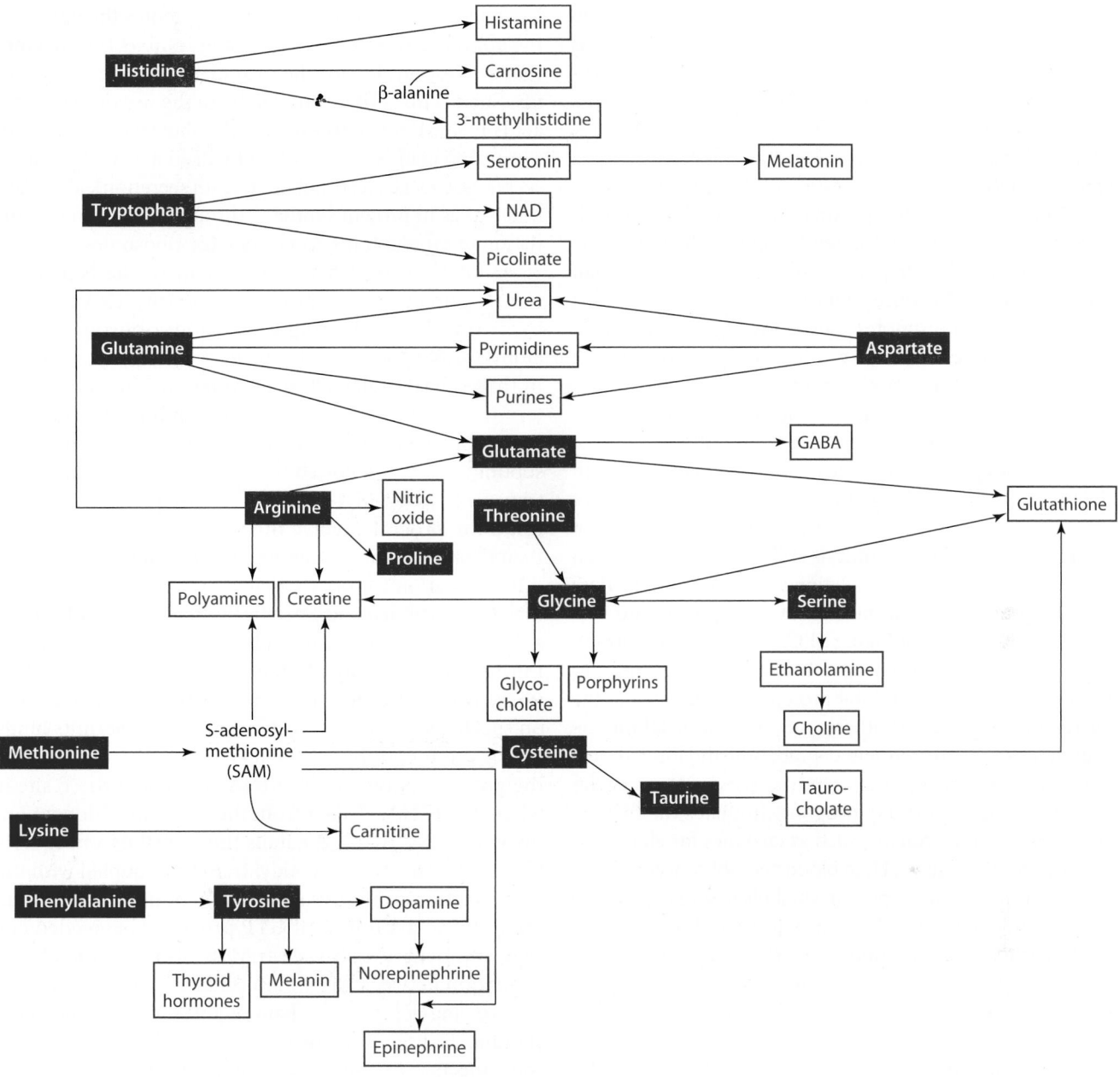

Figure 6.16 A summary of the uses of selected amino acids for the synthesis of nitrogen-containing compounds and selected biogenic amines, hormones, and neuromodulators.

Disorders of Glycine Metabolism Impaired catabolism of glycine, caused by an autosomal recessive defect in the mitochondrial glycine cleavage system, results in nonketotic hyperglycinemia. This enzyme complex normally converts glycine into ammonia and carbon dioxide and requires folate as tetrahydrofolate (Figure 6.15). Defects in four different genes that code for the complex have been reported. Infants with the condition exhibit seizures, neurologic deterioration, flaccidity, and lethargy, among other problems. Blood and other body fluids contain increased glycine concentrations. A low-protein diet is necessary for people with nonketotic hyperglycinemia.

Figure 6.16 provides a summary of many of the compounds generated from individual amino acids. The next section of the chapter further elaborates on anabolic uses of amino acids in the body.

PROTEIN SYNTHESIS

Anabolism, including protein synthesis, increases in tissues following the ingestion of food. Food, of course, provides the amino acids necessary to build body proteins. However, the form and nature of the dietary protein may influence amino acid utilization within the body. For example, amino acids released following ingestion and digestion of "fast proteins," which include whey protein, soy protein, amino acid mixtures, and protein hydrolysates (e.g., partially hydrolyzed protein), appear to be utilized differently in the body when compared with amino acids released following ingestion and digestion of "slow proteins" such as casein. Fast protein ingestion causes plasma amino acids to rise more quickly and to higher concentrations, but also to fall more quickly, than ingestion of equal amounts of slow proteins. Ingestion of slow proteins results in lower and prolonged plasma amino acid concentrations and better nitrogen (protein) retention than ingestion of fast proteins. The hyperamino-acidemia (higher than normal amino acid concentrations in the blood) after fast protein ingestion promotes transiently higher amino acid deamination rates and urea production than slow protein ingestion. In addition, amino acids from fast proteins appear to be used more for splanchnic protein synthesis versus peripheral or skeletal muscle protein synthesis.

Hormones play a major role in amino acid utilization in the body. During prolonged periods in which food is not eaten (termed postabsorptive), such as during the overnight hours or a fast, protein synthesis still occurs but at a much lower rate, and protein degradation predominates. The degradative processes are stimulated by epinephrine and cortisol release and by the higher glucagon to insulin ratio in the blood. This higher glucagon to insulin ratio diminishes both insulin's ability to inhibit protein degradation and the overall rate of protein synthesis. Yet, while skeletal muscle experiences the most protein degradation and limited protein synthesis during postabsorptive periods, the glucagon to insulin ratio favoring glucagon stimulates the hepatic synthesis of some proteins, such as enzymes for gluconeogenesis and ureagenesis. High blood cortisol concentrations further promote muscle protein catabolism and hepatic use of the amino acids for gluconeogenesis and ureagenesis. Blood cortisol concentrations typically increase with infection and injury/trauma but also with depletion of hepatic glycogen stores, as occurs during an extended fast.

In contrast to the general catabolic nature of glucagon, epinephrine, and cortisol, other hormones in the body, such as growth hormone and insulin, are anabolic. Insulin, for example, which is secreted in response to a rise in blood glucose and to a rise in some blood amino acid concentrations (as occurs with food consumption), generally increases protein synthesis and decreases protein degradation. This effect occurs to a greater extent if both carbohydrate- and protein-containing foods are coingested versus ingestion of either carbohydrate or protein alone. To promote protein synthesis, insulin, for example, affects (generally stimulates) the transcellular movement of amino acid transporters to the cell membrane for use and increases the overall activity of amino acid transporters, including systems A, ASC, and N in the liver, muscle, and other tissues. Insulin also antagonizes the activation of some enzymes responsible for amino acid oxidation (degradation); the phosphorylation and thus activation of phenylalanine hydroxylase (which degrades phenylalanine), for instance, is inhibited by insulin. Thus, insulin promotes the uptake of the amino acids into the tissues and inhibits the enzymes that are responsible for the degradation of the amino acids. Such actions of insulin facilitate the use of the amino acids for protein synthesis. Insulin, however, along with the amino acid leucine (which by itself acts as an insulin secretogogue, i.e., it stimulates insulin secretion), also plays other roles in protein synthesis through effects on the initiation of protein translation along the ribosomes.

As described in Chapter 1, protein synthesis involves transcription of a gene into messenger (m) RNA followed by its translation. During translation, ribosomes move along mRNA to synthesize proteins; the process occurs in three phases referred to as initiation, elongation, and termination. Initiation involves the binding of eukaryotic initiation factors (eIF)-1A and eIF-3 to the 40S ribosomal subunit, which is followed by the delivery of the initiation transfer (t)RNA, Met-tRNAi^{MET}. Subsequent steps in the initiation process involve the formation of the 48S and then the 80S initiation complexes of the ribosome. Several other initiation factors participate in these steps, as does the amino acid leucine. Specifically, leucine stimulates the assembly of eIF-4F, a three-subunit complex that binds to mRNA caps and poly (A) tails needed for the initiation. Phase two, elongation, follows initiation and also occurs on specific sites of the ribosome: the A site permits binding of the incoming aminoacyl-tRNA, the P site is for the growing polypeptidyl-tRNA chain, and the E site is where the tRNAs detach from the ribosome. Elongation, involving sites A and P, entails the arrival of aminoacyl-tRNAs and successive peptidyl transfers, coupled with the translocation of the ribosome one codon further along the mRNA. Hydrolysis of GTP provides the needed energy and occurs with each translocation. Peptide bond formation between the amino acids as they are added to the growing polypeptide chain requires the 50S ribosomal subunit. Termination, the last step, occurs when the ribosome meets with a stop codon in the mRNA.

Multiple factors influence translation. Thus, each cellular protein exhibits a specific and characteristic rate of synthesis. Translation is affected by the amount and stability of mRNA, the ribosome number (amount of ribosomal RNA, or rRNA), the activity of the ribosomes (rapidity of translation, or peptide formation), the presence of amino acids in the appropriate concentrations to attach to the tRNA, and the hormonal environment, which in turn can be influenced by nutrients. Some amino acids may even regulate the expression of some genes through interactions with amino acid–responsive elements in the gene's promoter region. Amino acids, for example, can promote changes in cell volume and protein synthesis through intracellular signaling pathways. Leucine and a leucine metabolite, β-hydroxy-β-methylbutyrate (HMB), for instance, promote protein synthesis through increased phosphorylation of mammalian target of rapamycin (mTOR).

mTOR, a large protein kinase, mediates the effects of insulin on protein synthesis through different multiprotein complexes but also exerts effects on protein synthesis that are independent of insulin. Chapter 1 provides additional information on transcription and translation, as well as DNA and RNA.

PROTEIN STRUCTURE AND ORGANIZATION

Proteins begin to fold and take "shape" as they are synthesized by the ribosomes. The shape or structure and organization of proteins are designated as primary, secondary, tertiary, and quaternary, although not all proteins have this fourth level (see Figures 6.17–6.20). The primary structure of a protein represents the amino acid sequence of the protein. The secondary structure is the coiling, folding, and/or bending of the protein. Various interactions between and among amino acids within the proteins contribute to the overall levels of organization. For example, hydrogen bonds contribute to the secondary structures of proteins. Hydrogen (H) bonds are weak electrical attractions that can occur between hydrogen atoms and negatively charged atoms such as oxygen or nitrogen. Electrostatic attractions, also called ionic attractions or salt bonds, occur between oppositely charged (acidic and basic) side chains of amino acids, such as lysine ($+1$) and glutamate (-1), to impact the

secondary structure. In addition, hydrophobic interactions occur between the side chains of nonpolar amino acids. The interactions can generate particular structures, such as the α-helix and β-pleated sheet; the presence of these structures provides important attributes, including added stability, strength, and rigidity, to proteins. The α-helix and β-pleated sheet are particularly abundant in proteins with structural roles, such as collagen, elastin, and keratin.

The overall or total three-dimensional configuration of the protein is referred to as the tertiary structure. For example, the tertiary structures of globular proteins, which are named for their spherical shape, generally contain multiple α-helices and β-pleated sheets. Myoglobin, calmodulin, and many enzymes and serum proteins are globular proteins. The quaternary structure results from two or more polypeptide chains interacting. Some of the same interactions contributing to the secondary structure also contribute to these additional levels of organization and include the clustering of hydrophobic amino acids toward the center of the protein and the electrostatic attraction of oppositely charged amino acids. In addition to the weak noncovalent hydrogen, electrostatic, and hydrophobic bonding, strong covalent bonding (involving electron sharing) may occur. One of the more commonly formed covalent bonds occurs between cysteine residues where the —SH groups are oxidized to form disulfide bridges (—S—S—), as shown in Figure 6.19b. Together, the interactions among the amino acid side chains determine the

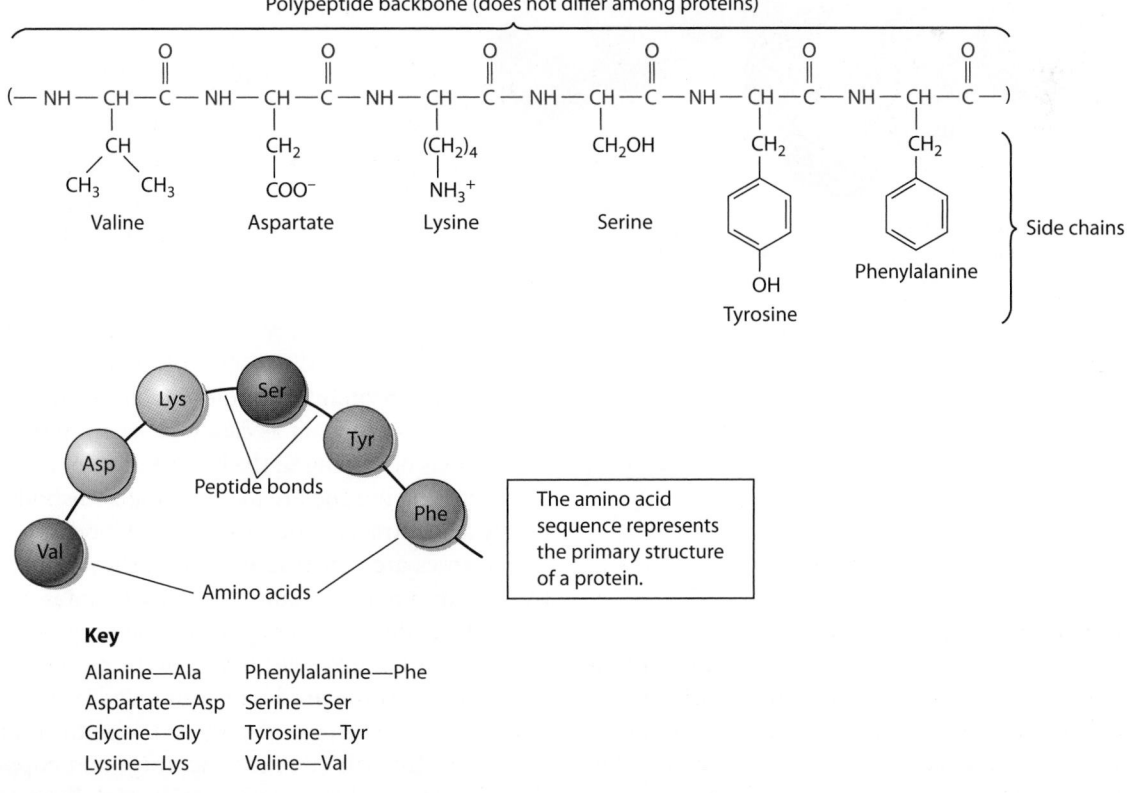

Figure 6.17 The primary structure of a protein.
Source: Derived from Beerman/McGuire, Nutritional Sciences, 1/e. © Cengage Learning.

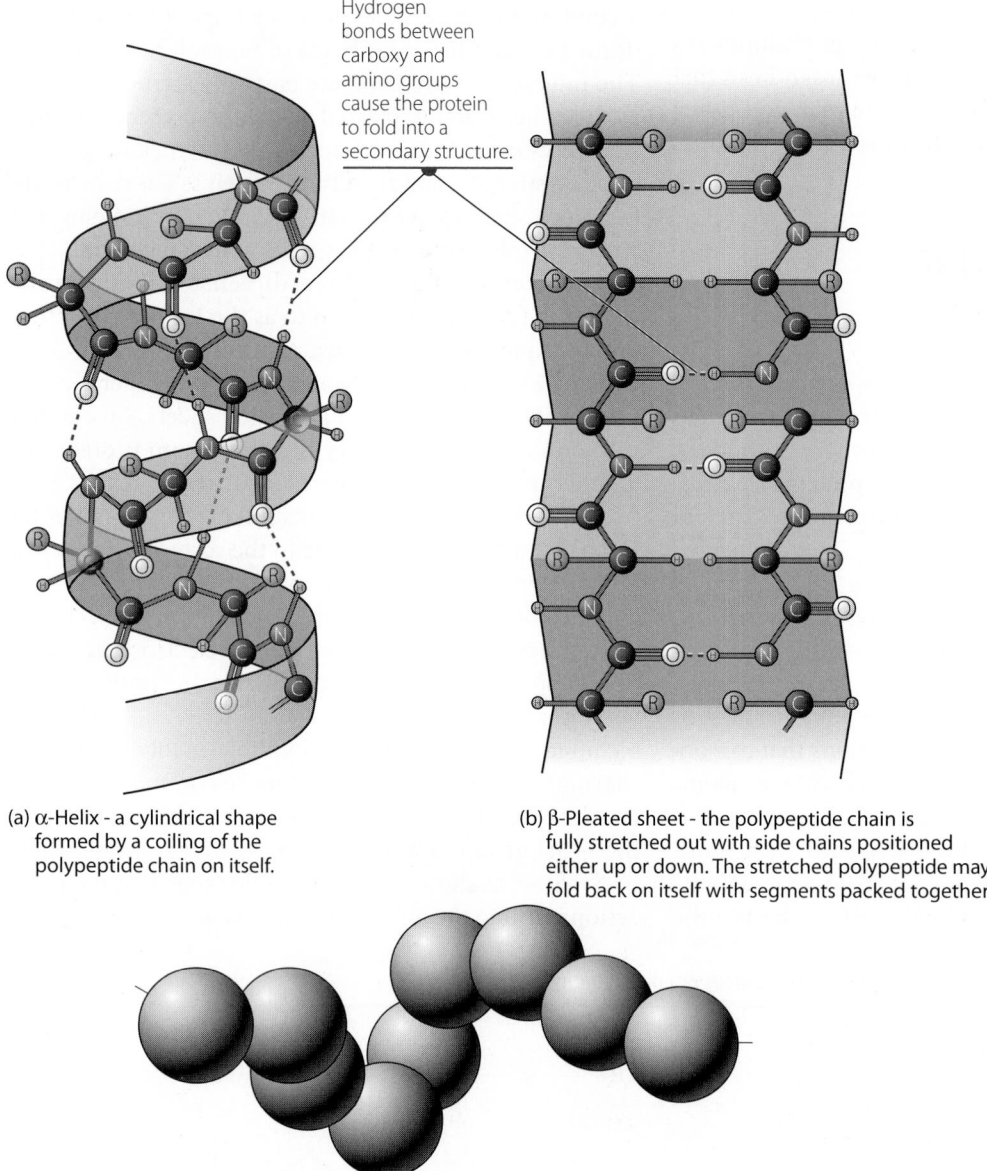

Hydrogen bonds between carboxy and amino groups cause the protein to fold into a secondary structure.

(a) α-Helix - a cylindrical shape formed by a coiling of the polypeptide chain on itself.

(b) β-Pleated sheet - the polypeptide chain is fully stretched out with side chains positioned either up or down. The stretched polypeptide may fold back on itself with segments packed together.

(c) Random coil - an unstable structure formed due to the presence of certain amino acids whose side chains interfere with one another.

Figure 6.18 Secondary structure of proteins.
Source: Derived from Beerman/McGuire, Nutritional Sciences, 1/e. © Cengage Learning.

protein's overall shape and, therefore, influence the protein's function in the body.

FUNCTIONAL ROLES OF PROTEINS AND NITROGEN-CONTAINING NONPROTEIN COMPOUNDS

The molecular architecture and activity of living cells depend largely on proteins, which make up over half of the solid content of cells and which show great variability in size, shape, and physical properties. Their physiological roles also are quite variable, and because of this variability, categorizing proteins according to their functions can be helpful in the study of human metabolism.

Catalysts

Enzymes are protein molecules (generally designated by the suffix *-ase*) that act as catalysts: They change the rate of reactions occurring in the body. Enzymes are necessary for sustaining life and are found in the body both intracellularly and extracellularly (e.g., in the blood).

Enzymes are constructed so that they combine selectively with other molecules (called substrates) in the cell. The active site on the enzyme (a small region usually in a crevice of the enzyme) is where the enzyme and substrate bind and the product is generated. Some enzymes, however, require a cofactor or coenzyme to carry out the reaction. Minerals such as zinc, iron, and copper function as cofactors for some enzymes. *Metalloprotein* is the name typically used for proteins to which minerals are

(a)

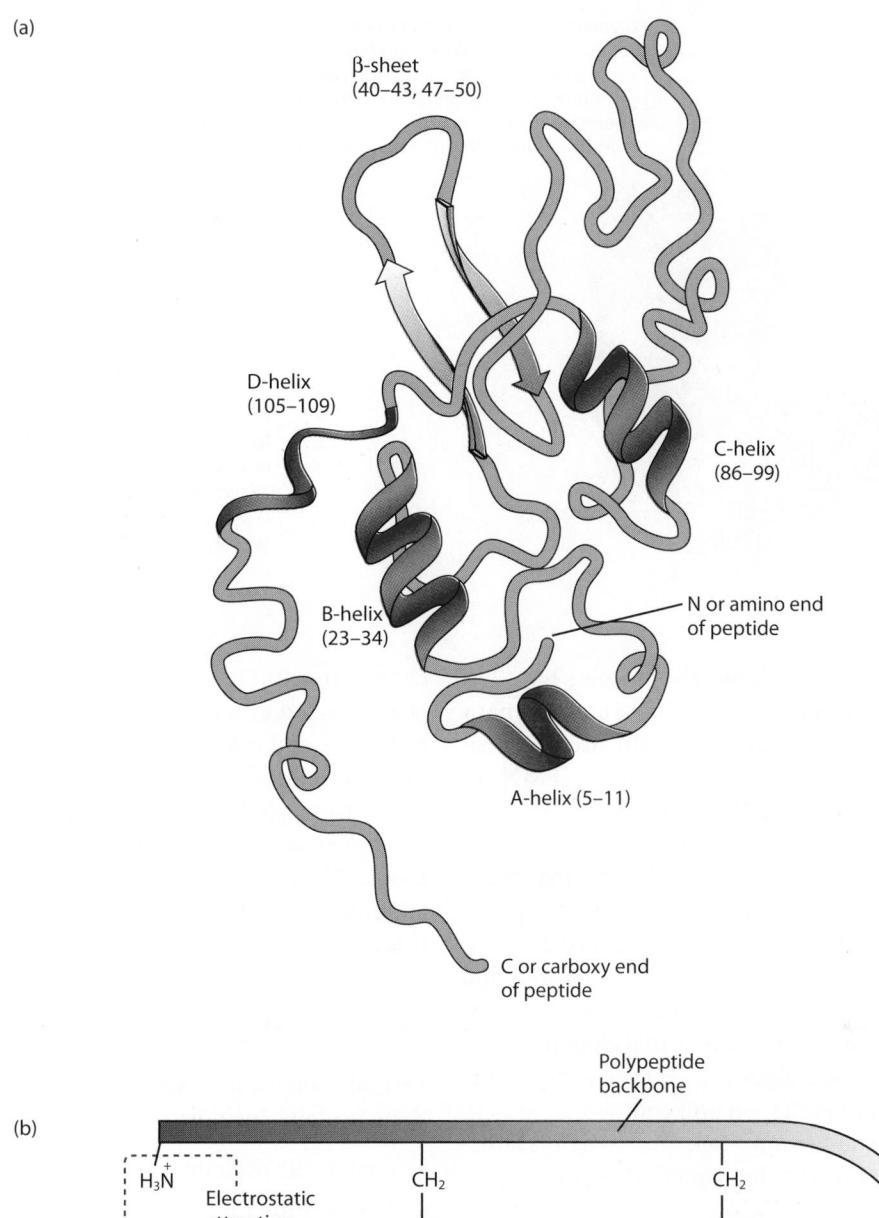

(b)

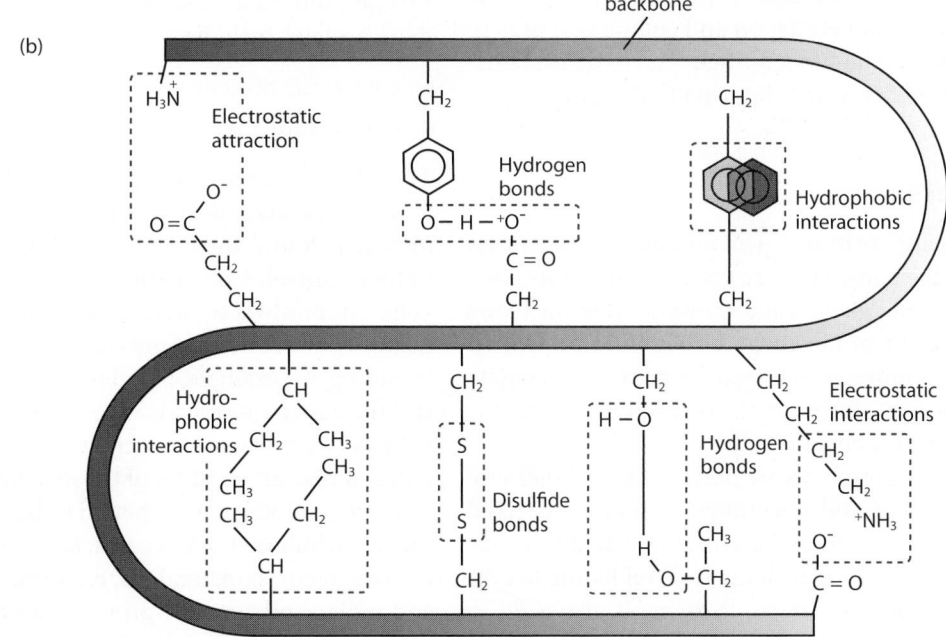

Figure 6.19 (a) The tertiary structure of the protein α-lactalbumin. (b) Examples of interactions found in tertiary structures.

Source: Adapted from D.B. Marks, A.D. Marks, and C.M. Smith, Basic Medical Biochemistry. Copyright © 1996 by Lippincott, Williams & Wilkins. Reprinted by permission.

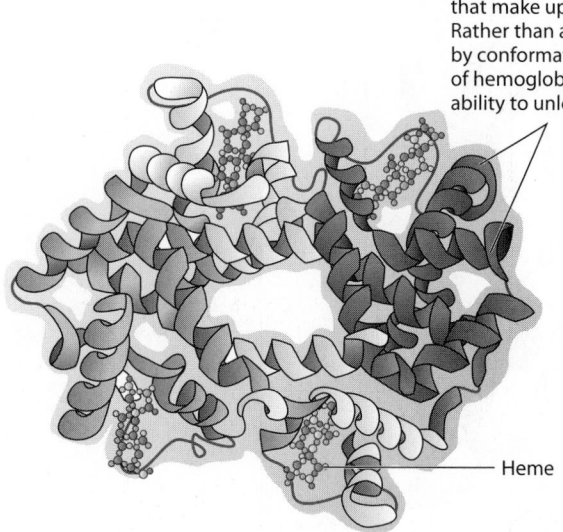

Polypeptide chains - Each of the 4 polypeptide chains that make up hemoglobin can bind one oxygen atom. Rather than acting independently, the subunits cooperate by conformational changes so as to enhance the affinity of hemoglobin for oxygen in the lungs and to increase its ability to unload oxygen to peripheral tissues.

Heme

Figure 6.20 Quaternary structure of the hemoglobin protein. Quaternary proteins are characterized by interactions between 2 or more (usually 2 or 4) polypeptide chains. The aggregated form is called an oligomer. The polypeptide chains (called subunits) making up the oligomer are held together by hydrogen bonds and electrostatic salt bridges.
Source: Derived from Beerman/McGuire, Nutritional Sciences, 1/e. © Cengage Learning.

complexed. Some, but not all, metalloproteins have enzymatic activity. B vitamins serve as coenzymes for many enzymes. *Flavoprotein* is the term generally used for protein enzymes bound to flavin mononucleotide (FMN) or flavin adenine nucleotide (FAD), coenzyme forms of the B vitamin riboflavin. Most human physiological processes require enzymes to promote chemical changes that could not otherwise occur. Some examples of different types of enzymes include dehydrogenases, which remove or transfer hydrogens; kinases, which add phosphate groups; and isomerases, which transfer atoms within a molecule. Some examples of physiological processes that depend upon enzyme function include digestion, energy production, blood coagulation, and excitation and contraction of neuromuscular tissue. The section titled "Catalytic Proteins" in Chapter 1 provides further information on enzymes.

Messengers

Some proteins are hormones. **Hormones** act as chemical messengers in the body. They are synthesized and secreted by endocrine tissue (glands) and transported in the blood to target tissues or organs, where they bind to protein receptors on membranes. Hormones generally regulate metabolic processes, for example, by promoting enzyme synthesis or affecting enzyme activity.

Whereas some hormones are derived from cholesterol and classified as steroid hormones, others are derived from one or more amino acids. The amino acid tyrosine, for example, is used along with the mineral iodine to synthesize the thyroid hormones. Tyrosine is also used to synthesize the catecholamines, including dopamine, norepinephrine, and epinephrine. The hormone melatonin is derived in the brain from the amino acid tryptophan. Other hormones are made up of one or more polypeptide chains. Insulin, for example, consists of two polypeptide chains linked by a disulfide bridge. Glucagon, parathyroid hormone, and calcitonin each consist of a single polypeptide chain. Many other peptide hormones, such as adrenocorticotropic hormone (ACTH), somatotropin (growth hormone), and vasopressin (also known as antidiuretic hormone, ADH), have important roles in human metabolism and nutrition. These hormones are discussed throughout this chapter and the book.

Structural Elements

Several proteins have structural roles in the body. Some of these proteins include:

- contractile proteins
- fibrous proteins

The two main contractile proteins, actin and myosin, are found in cardiac, skeletal, and smooth muscles. Skeletal muscle is found throughout the body and is under voluntary control. Contraction is calcium induced and involves not only actin and myosin, but also troponin and tropomyosin. Smooth muscle is found in many tissues including, for example, blood vessels, the lungs, the uterus, and the gastrointestinal tract. Smooth muscle is under involuntary control and contracts in response to calcium-induced phosphorylation of the structural protein myosin.

Fibrous proteins, which tend to be somewhat linear in shape, include collagen, elastin, and keratin and are found in bone, teeth, skin, tendons, cartilage, blood vessels, hair, and nails. Collagen is a group of well-studied proteins. Each type of collagen is made of three polypeptide (tropocollagen) chains that are cross-linked for strength. These chains, rather than forming specific secondary structures (α-helices or β-pleated sheets, discussed in the protein structure section), form a helical arrangement. The amino acid composition of the chains is rich in the amino acids glycine and proline. In addition, collagen contains two hydroxylated amino acids—hydroxylysine and hydroxyproline—that are not found in other proteins. Collagen polypeptides are also attached to carbohydrate chains and thus are considered to be glycoproteins. Other structural proteins, such as elastin, are associated with proteoglycans. Both glycoproteins and proteoglycans are conjugated proteins and are discussed further in the "Other Roles" section.

Buffers

Proteins, because of their constituent amino acids, can serve as buffers in the body and thus help to regulate acid-base balance. A **buffer** is a compound that ameliorates a change in pH that would otherwise occur in response to the addition of alkali or acid to a solution. The pH of the blood and other body tissues must be maintained within an appropriate range. Blood pH ranges from about 7.35 to 7.45, whereas cellular pH levels are often more acidic. For example, the pH of red blood cells is about 7.2, and that of muscle cells is about 6.9. The H^+ concentration within cells is buffered by both the phosphate system and the amino acids in proteins. The protein hemoglobin, for example, functions as a buffer in red blood cells. In the plasma and extracellular fluid, proteins and the bicarbonate system serve as buffers. The buffering ability of proteins can be illustrated by the reaction $H^+ +$ protein $\longleftrightarrow$ Hprotein and is shown in Figure 6.21.

Fluid Balancers

In addition to acid-base balance, proteins influence fluid balance through their presence in the blood and in cells. More specifically, proteins help attract and keep water inside a particular area and contribute to osmotic pressure. Diminished blood/plasma concentrations of proteins, such as albumin (the most abundant of the proteins in the blood), result in a decrease in plasma osmotic pressure. When protein concentrations in the blood are less dense than normal, fluid "leaks" out of the blood and into interstitial spaces and causes swelling (edema). Restoring adequate concentrations of protein in the blood (e.g., by infusing albumin intravenously) promotes diffusion of water from the interstitial space back into the blood.

Immunoprotectors

Immunoprotection is provided to the body in part by a group of proteins called **immunoproteins,** also called immunoglobulins (Ig) or antibodies (Ab). These immunoproteins, of which there are five major classes (IgG, IgA, IgM, IgE, and IgD), are Y-shaped proteins made of four polypeptide chains (two small chains called light [L] chains and two large chains called heavy [H] chains). The immunoglobulins are produced by plasma cells derived from B-lymphocytes, a type of white blood cell. Immunoglobulins function by binding to antigens—which typically consist of foreign substances, such as bacteria or viruses that have entered the body—and inactivating them. By complexing with antigens, immunoglobulins create immunoprotein-antigen complexes that can be recognized and destroyed through reactions with either complement proteins or cytokines. The complement proteins (approximately 20) are produced primarily in the liver and circulate in the blood and extracellular fluid. Cytokines are produced by white blood cells such as T-helper (CD4) cells and macrophages. In addition, white blood cells such as macrophages and neutrophils also destroy foreign antigens through the process of phagocytosis.

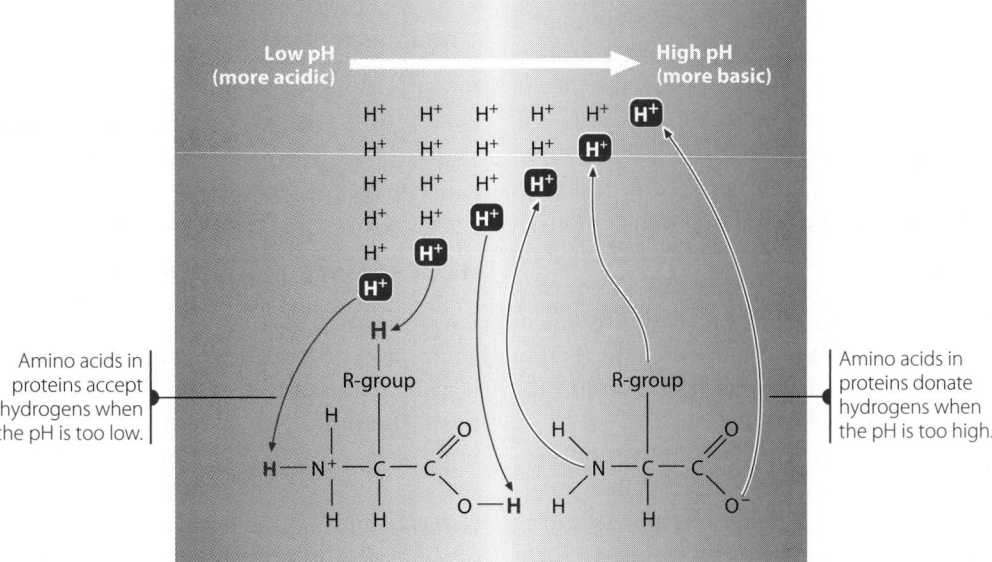

Figure 6.21 The role of the amino acid in pH balance.
Source: Derived from Beerman/McGuire, Nutritional Sciences, 1/e. © Cengage Learning.

Transporters

Transport proteins are a diverse group of proteins that combine with other substances (especially vitamins and minerals, but also other nutrients) to provide a means of carrying those substances within the blood, into cells, out of cells, or within cells. Transport proteins in cell membranes, for example, carry and thus regulate the flow of nutrients into and out of cells. Several types of transporters exist in cell membranes. Some transporters (called uniporters) carry only one substance across cell membranes; other transporters (called symporters) carry more than one substance. For example, many amino acid transporters in the intestinal cell's brush border membrane function as uniporters or symporters. Antiporters, another type of cell membrane protein transporter, function by exchanging one substance for another. For example, the Na^+, K^+-ATPase pump transports three sodium ions out of the cell in exchange for two potassium ions, which enter the cell. Proteins in cell membranes can also carry substances other than amino acids. For example, the protein Ctr transports copper into intestinal cells. The protein hemoglobin, found in red blood cells, transports oxygen and carbon dioxide.

The concentration of total protein in human plasma typically ranges up to about 7.5 g/dL. Of the hundreds of proteins in the blood, several serve as transporters. Lipoproteins, for example, transport cholesterol and triacylglycerol in the blood; the proteins in the lipoproteins are actually a group of about 10 different apoproteins that both enable lipid transport and direct the lipoproteins to cells for use.

A few transport proteins of clinical significance include albumin, transthyretin, and retinol-binding protein. Albumin, the most abundant of the plasma proteins, transports nutrients such as tryptophan, fatty acids, and vitamin B_6; some minerals including zinc, calcium, and small amounts of copper; and some drugs. The protein is synthesized by the liver and released into the blood; changes in osmotic pressure and osmolality affect its rate of synthesis. A healthy person makes about 9 to 12 g of albumin per day [5]. Albumin is often used to assess an individual's protein status, specifically visceral (internal organ) protein status. Because of albumin's relatively long half-life (~14–18 days), however, it is not as good or as sensitive an indicator of visceral protein status as some of the other plasma proteins. The half-life is the time it takes for 50% of the amount of a protein such as albumin (or nonprotein compound) to be degraded.

Two other proteins synthesized by the liver and released into plasma are transthyretin (also called prealbumin) and retinol-binding protein. Retinol-binding protein, as its name implies, transports retinol (a form of vitamin A) but also thyroid hormone. Transthyretin and retinol-binding protein, like albumin, are also used as biochemical indicators of visceral protein status. Because transthyretin and retinol-binding protein have relatively shorter half-lives (~2 days and 12 hours, respectively) than albumin, they are more sensitive indicators of changes in visceral protein status. The concentrations of albumin, prealbumin, and retinol-binding protein diminish in the blood over varying time periods (depending on their half-life) in people, for example, who have ingested inadequate dietary protein. Typically, plasma concentrations of albumin < 3.5 g/dL, prealbumin (transthyretin) < 18 mg/dL, and retinol-binding protein < 2.1 mg/dL suggest inadequate visceral protein status. Such people need a diet high in energy (kcal) and protein to promote improvements (assuming the liver is healthy) in status.

Some transport proteins found in the blood are classified according to size and charge using the procedure protein electrophoresis. Globulins, a heterogeneous group of proteins with diverse transport functions, are identified using this method. Most globulins are synthesized in the liver, with the exception of the gamma globulins (antibodies), which are made mostly by plasma cells (mature B-lymphocytes). The four classes of globulins are listed here, along with some examples of proteins comprising each class and their transport roles:

- α1-globulins: glycoproteins, high-density lipoproteins (for lipid transport)
- α2-globulins: glycoproteins, haptoglobin (for free hemoglobin transport), ceruloplasmin (for copper transport and oxidase activity), prothrombin (for blood coagulation), and very-low-density lipoproteins (for lipid transport)
- β-globulins: transferrin (for iron and other mineral transport) and low-density lipoproteins (for lipid transport)
- γ-globulins: immunoglobulins or antibodies (for immunoprotection)

Some hospital laboratories report serum albumin concentrations relative to globulin concentrations. Normally, albumin concentrations slightly exceed globulin concentrations.

Acute Phase Responders

Another role of a specific group of proteins, called acute phase or positive acute phase reactant proteins, is as responders in times of acute (sudden), critical illness. These proteins are made in the liver as part of the body's response to infection (sepsis), injury, or inflammation. Some examples of these acute phase proteins are C-reactive protein, fibronectin, orosomucoid (also called α1-acid glycoprotein), haptoglobin, serum amyloid A, α2-macroglobulin, ceruloplasmin, and metallothionein. Collectively, these proteins perform a variety of functions that protect the body, such as stimulating the immune system, promoting wound healing, and chelating and removing free iron from circulation to prevent its use by bacteria for growth. C-reactive protein is used clinically to evaluate inflammation in patients. The concentration of this protein rises dramatically within a few hours of inflammation such as that caused by an infection. Diminishing concentrations of C-reactive protein suggest the possibility of a less catabolic state. The Perspective at the end of this chapter provides a more detailed discussion of some additional functions of these acute phase proteins and the body's response to metabolic stress.

Other Roles

Proteins carry out many additional roles in the body. For example, in cell membranes, proteins function in cell adhesion, and some further serve to transmit signals into and out of the cell. The protein opsin is important for vision (as discussed under the section on vitamin A in Chapter 10). Proteins also serve as receptors on cell membranes. Proteins can function in storage roles. For example, some minerals like copper, iron, and zinc are stored in body tissues bound to proteins; these proteins are often called metalloproteins.

For some proteins, exact roles have yet to be clearly defined. The body generates a group of proteins called stress or heat shock proteins (abbreviated *hsp*). These proteins are categorized by molecular weight (e.g., hsp 60, hsp 70, hsp 90) and are synthesized in response to stress, including heat stress and oxidative stress. Exercise and other physical activity in warm environments, among other conditions, promotes the synthesis of these proteins. The amino acid glutamine appears to enhance the expression of some heat shock proteins during critical illness (oxidative stress). More specifically, glutamine is thought to be necessary for the activation of specific transcription factors required for heat shock protein synthesis. While heat shock proteins are essential to cellular survival, their exact functions remain unclear. Hsp 70 induction, for example, appears to improve cell survival in the presence of cytotoxins and to reduce organ dysfunction. Some heat shock proteins are thought to facilitate protein folding (i.e., the formation of the secondary and tertiary protein structures) as the proteins are synthesized. Another hypothesized role of the heat shock proteins is the repair of denatured or injured proteins.

Many proteins in the body are conjugated proteins—that is, proteins that are joined to nonprotein components. Glycoproteins, one type of conjugated protein, represent a huge group of proteins with multiple functions. **Glycoproteins** consist of a protein covalently bound to a carbohydrate component. The carbohydrate in glycoproteins generally includes short chains of glucose, galactose, mannose, fucose, N-acetylglucosamine, N-acetylgalactosamine, and acetylneuraminic (sialic) acid at the terminal end of the oligosaccharide chain. The carbohydrate portion of the glycoprotein can make up as much as 85% of the glycoprotein's weight. The carbohydrate component is bound typically through an N-glycosidic linkage with asparagine's amide group in its side chain or through an O-glycosidic linkage with the hydroxy group in serine's or threonine's side chain. Glycoproteins are found in the blood, on the outer surface of plasma membranes, and in association with the extracellular matrix (which surrounds and supports some body cells). In the extracellular matrix of bone, for example, glycoproteins play structural roles. Mucus, which is found in body secretions, is rich in glycoproteins. Mucus both lubricates and protects epithelial cells in the body. Some of the body's hormones (such as thyrotropin) and blood proteins (such as transthyretin and immunoglobulins) are glycoproteins.

Another group of conjugated proteins is the proteoglycans, which are found in every tissue of the body. Most proteoglycans are associated with the extracellular matrix but also with other structural matrix components, where they form cross-links to enhance strength and resilience and to modulate adhesion and communication between cells and between the extracellular matrix and cells. **Proteoglycans** are macromolecules consisting of a core protein covalently conjugated, typically by O-glycosidic or N-glycosylamine linkages, to one or more glycosaminoglycans. Glycosaminoglycans consist of long chains of repeating disaccharides, comprise up to 95% of the weight of the proteoglycan, and are the main site of the proteoglycan that interacts with cell surface proteins or extracellular matrix proteins. Examples of glycosaminoglycans include hyaluronic acid (found in high concentrations in cartilage), chondroitin sulfate (found in high concentrations in bone and cartilage), keratan sulfate and dermatan sulfate (found in the cornea of the eye), and heparan sulfate (found in high concentrations in plasma cell membranes).

Nitrogen-Containing Nonprotein Compounds

In addition to their use in the synthesis of body proteins, amino acids are used to synthesize nitrogen-containing compounds that are not proteins but nonetheless play important roles in the body. The purpose of the next section of this chapter is to address the roles of some nutritionally significant nitrogen-containing nonprotein compounds (Table 6.6). Not included in this review, however, are a number of biogenic amines, neurotransmitters, and neuropeptides that are synthesized from amino acids in many glands, tissues, and organs throughout the body. A discussion of these compounds is found in this chapter in the "Brain and Accessory Tissues" section. Some of the compounds also are mentioned in sections that discuss the metabolism of amino acids.

Table 6.6 Sources of Nitrogen for Some Nitrogen-Containing Nonprotein Compounds

Nitrogen-Containing Nonprotein Compound	Constituent Amino Acids
Glutathione	Cysteine, glycine, glutamate
Carnitine	Lysine, methionine
Creatine	Arginine, glycine, methionine
Carnosine	Histidine, β-alanine
Choline	Serine

Glutathione

Glutathione (Figure 6.22) is a tripeptide synthesized from three amino acids—glycine, cysteine, and glutamate—in most body cells. Its synthesis occurs in two steps, both ATP dependent. First, the γ carboxy group of glutamate is attached to the amino group of cysteine by γ glutamyl cysteine synthetase to form a peptidic γ linkage. In the second step, glutathione synthetase creates a peptide bond between the amino group of glycine and the carboxy group of cysteine to produce glutathione. The availability of cysteine appears to be the major factor influencing glutathione synthesis, although synthesis can be affected by administration of any of the precursor substrates or via activity of glutathione peroxidase and reductase, which catalyze other glutathione-dependent reactions.

Glutathione is referred to as a thiol because it contains a sulfhydryl (-SH) group in its reduced form (designated GSH). Glutathione can also be found in cells in its oxidized form (designated GSSG) and attached to proteins (up to about 15%). Normally, the ratio of GSH to GSSG in cells is >10 to 1; the GSH to GSSG ratio represents an indicator of the cell's redox state. In fact, the ratio of GSH to GSSG is thought to be the most important regulator of the cellular redox potential.

Glutathione is found in the cytosol of most cells of the body, but small amounts also are found within cell organelles and in the plasma. Glutathione has several functions in the body. It is a major antioxidant with the ability to scavenge free radicals (O_2^- and $OH^•$), thereby protecting critical cell components and SH-containing proteins against oxidation. With the enzyme glutathione peroxidase, glutathione protects cells by reacting with hydrogen

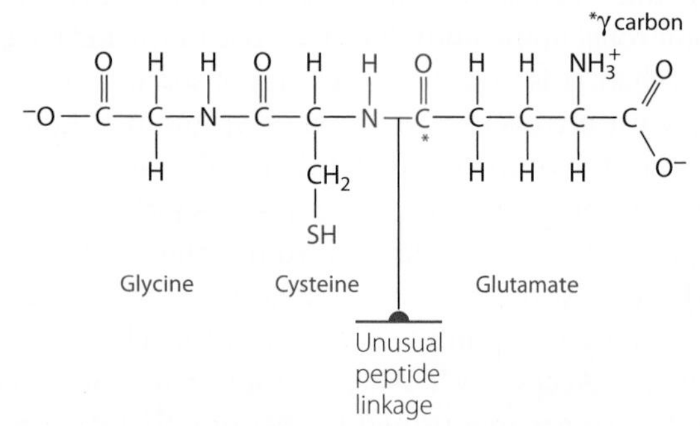

peroxides (H_2O_2) and lipid hydroperoxides (LOOHs) before they can cause damage. Glutathione also transports amino acids as part of the γ-glutamyl cycle (Figure 6.4) in some tissues. It participates in the synthesis of leukotriene (LT) C4, which mediates the body's response to inflammation. Glutathione is also involved in the conversion of prostaglandin H2 to prostaglandins D2 and E2 by endoperoxide isomerase. Glutathione can conjugate with nitric oxide to form S-nitrosoglutathione.

Glutathione synthesis is sensitive to protein intake and pathological conditions. Hepatic, intestinal, and systemic GSH concentrations decline with poor protein intake as well as during inflammation and disease; this decline negatively impacts the body, necessitating strategies to enhance or at least maintain GSH concentrations. Glutathione is discussed further in the section on selenium in Chapter 13.

Carnitine

Carnitine, another nitrogen-containing compound, is made (Figure 6.23) from the amino acid lysine that has been methylated; the methyl groups are derived from S-adenosyl methionine (SAM), which is made in the body from the oxidation of the amino acid methionine. Following lysine methylation, trimethyllysine undergoes hydroxylation at the 3 position to form 3-OH trimethyllysine. Hydroxytrimethyllysine is further metabolized to generate γ-butyrobetaine and subsequently carnitine. Iron, vitamin B_6 (as pyridoxal phosphate, PLP), vitamin C, and niacin participate in the synthesis of carnitine. In addition to being synthesized in the liver and kidneys, carnitine is found in foods, especially meats such as beef and pork. In these foods, carnitine may be free or bound (as acylcarnitine) to long- or short-chain fatty acid esters. Carnitine from food or supplements is absorbed in the proximal small intestine by sodium-dependent active transport and passive diffusion; diffusion typically predominates with ingestion of supplements providing 0.5 to 6 g [6]. Approximately 54% to 87% of carnitine intake is absorbed. Intestinal absorption of carnitine is thought to be saturated with intakes of about 2 g [7]. Muscle represents the primary carnitine pool, although no carnitine is made there. Intramuscular concentrations of carnitine are generally 50 times greater than usual plasma concentrations. Carnitine homeostasis is maintained principally by the kidney, with >90% of filtered carnitine and acylcarnitine being reabsorbed.

Carnitine, found in most body tissues, is needed for the transport of fatty acids, especially long-chain fatty acids, across the inner mitochondrial membrane for oxidation. The inner mitochondrial membrane is impermeable to long-chain (10) fatty acyl-coenzyme (Co) As. This role of carnitine is discussed in more detail in Chapter 5. Carnitine is also needed for ketone catabolism for energy. Carnitine also forms acylcarnitines from short-chain acyl-CoAs. These acylcarnitines may serve to buffer the free CoA pool.

Figure 6.22 The structure of glutathione in its reduced form (GSH).

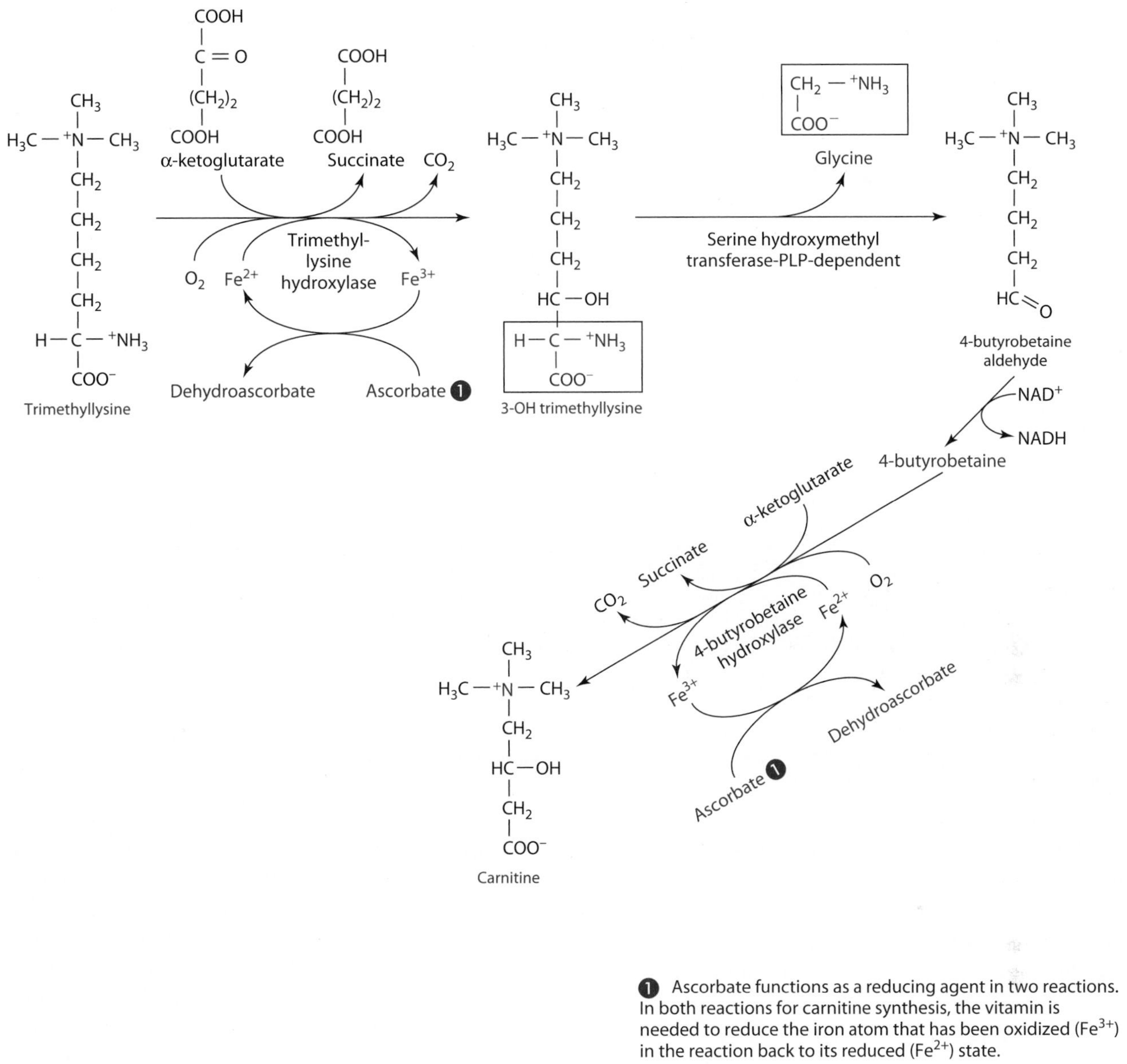

Figure 6.23 Carnitine synthesis.

Carnitine deficiency, though rare, results in impaired energy metabolism. Advertisements marketing carnitine supplements to help burn fat or supply energy are making false claims. Furthermore, although repeated use of carnitine supplements has been shown to increase plasma and muscle carnitine, studies have not uniformly shown improved physical performance [6]. Other studies, however, have shown beneficial effects of carnitine supplementation in people with a variety of cardiac problems and diabetes.

Creatine

Creatine (Figure 6.24), a key component of the energy compound creatine phosphate, also called phosphocreatine, can be obtained from foods (primarily meat and fish) or synthesized from three amino acids in the body.

The first step in the synthesis of creatine occurs in the kidneys, where arginine and glycine react to form guanidinoacetate by the action of L-arginine:glycine amidinotransferase. In this reaction, the guanidinium (also called the amidino) group of arginine is transferred to the amino group of glycine; the remainder of the arginine molecule is released as ornithine. The next step in the synthesis of creatine is the methylation of guanidinoacetate by guanidinoacetate methyltransferase. This step occurs in the liver using SAM (S-adenosyl methionine) as a methyl donor.

Once synthesized, creatine is released into the blood for transport to tissues. About 95% of body creatine is in muscle, with the remaining 5% in organs such as the kidneys and brain. In tissues, creatine is found both in free form as creatine and in its phosphorylated form. The

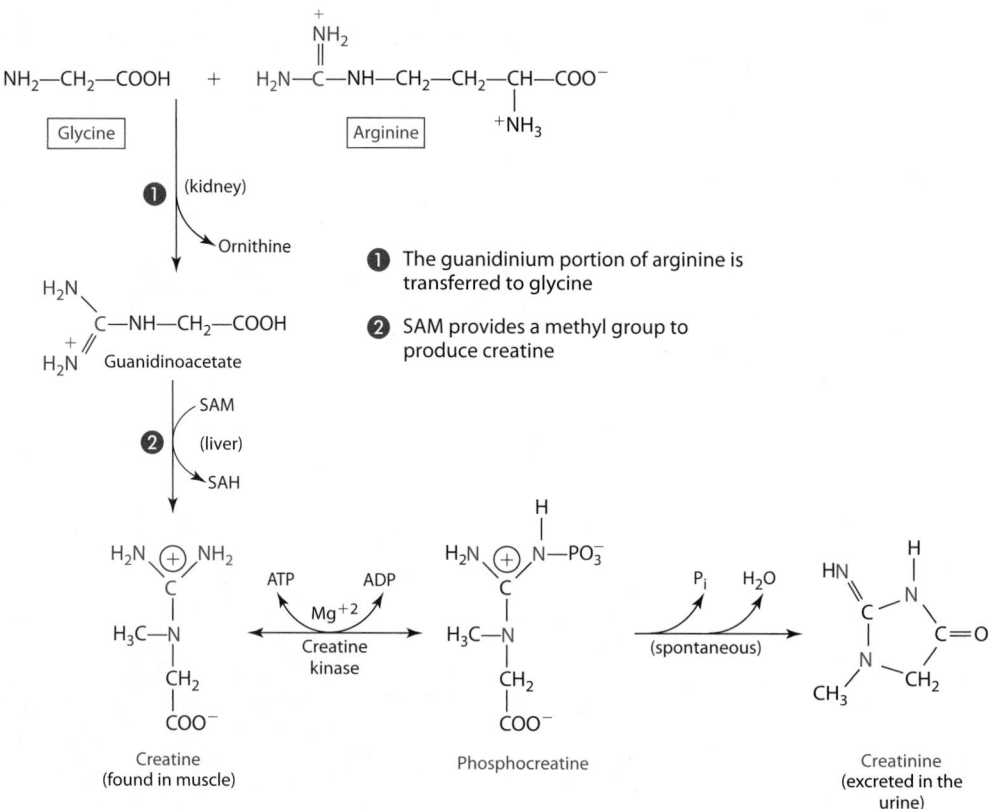

Figure 6.24 The synthesis of creatine from glycine and arginine in the kidney and liver. The conversion of creatine to phosphocreatine in the muscle and its spontaneous cyclization to creatinine.

phosphorylation of creatine to form phosphocreatine is shown here:

$$\text{Creatine} \xrightarrow[\text{ATP} \quad \text{ADP}]{\text{Creatine kinase—Mg}^{2+}} \text{Phosphocreatine}$$

Phosphocreatine functions as a "storehouse for high-energy phosphate." In fact, over half of the creatine in muscle at rest is in the form of phosphocreatine. Phosphocreatine replenishes ATP in a muscle that is rapidly contracting. Remember, muscle contraction requires energy. This energy is obtained with the hydrolysis of ATP. However, the ATP in muscle can suffice for only a fraction of a second. Phosphocreatine, stored in the muscle and possessing a higher phosphate group transfer potential than ATP, can transfer a phosphoryl group to ADP, thereby forming ATP or assisting in ATP regeneration, providing energy for muscular activity. Creatine kinase, also called creatine phosphokinase (abbreviated CK or CPK), catalyzes the phosphate transfer in active muscle, as shown here:

$$\text{Phosphocreatine} \xrightarrow[\text{ADP} \quad \text{ATP}]{\text{Creatine kinase—Mg}^{2+}} \text{Creatine}$$

Creatine kinase is made up of different subunits in different tissues. For example, in the heart, creatine kinase is made up of two subunits designated M and B. (The brain and muscle also have creatine kinase, but in these tissues the enzyme is made up of the BB and MM subunits, respectively.) Damage to the heart, as with a heart attack, causes the enzyme to "leak" out of the heart and reach elevated concentrations in the blood. Thus, an elevation in CK-MB in the blood along with other indicators is used to diagnose a heart attack. Similarly, damage to skeletal muscle, as may occur with trauma, results in elevations of CK-MM in the blood.

The availability of phosphocreatine and its use by muscle are thought to delay the breakdown of muscle glycogen stores, which upon further catabolism also can be used by muscle for energy. Creatine and creatine phosphate do not remain indefinitely in muscle; rather, both slowly but spontaneously cyclize (as shown in Figure 6.24) because of nonreversible, nonenzymatic dehydration. This cyclization of creatine and phosphocreatine forms creatinine. Once formed, creatinine leaves the muscle, passes across the glomerulus of the kidneys, and is excreted like other nitrogenous waste products (e.g., urea, ammonia, uric acid) in the urine. Creatinine clearance is sometimes used as a means of estimating kidney function. The urinary excretion of creatinine is used as an indicator of existing muscle mass, as discussed later in the section under "Skeletal Muscle"

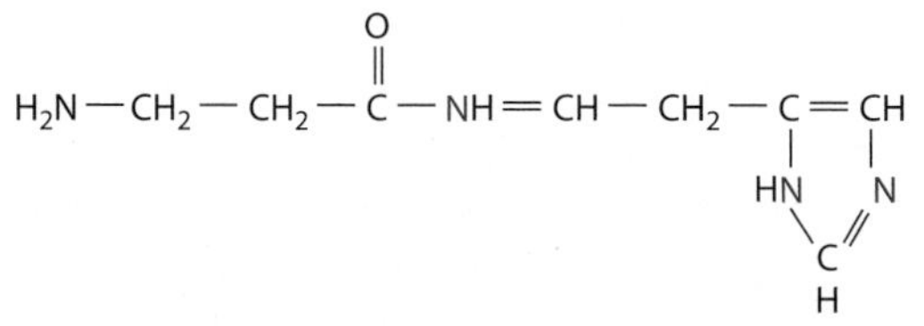

H₂N — CH₂ — CH₂ — C(=O) — NH = CH — CH₂ — C = CH with imidazole ring (HN, N, C, H)

Figure 6.25 Carnosine.

titled "Indicators of Muscle Mass and Muscle/Protein Catabolism." Not all creatinine, however, gets excreted in the urine. Small amounts may be secreted into the gut and, like urea, metabolized by bacteria in the intestine.

Because creatine plays such a vital role in energy production in muscle, it is a popular supplement. Creatine supplements have been shown to increase (~20–50%) muscle creatine concentrations and the amount of short-duration, high-intensity exercise (such as sprints and power-type activities separated by intervals of recovery) that can be performed [8–10]. Typical loading dosages were 5 g of creatine monohydrate taken four times daily for a total of 20 g/day for 4 to 6 days, followed by ongoing ingestion of creatine in doses of 2 to 5 g daily. Side effects associated with long-term use of creatine are unknown.

Carnosine

Carnosine (also called β-alanyl histidine; Figure 6.25) is made in the body from the amino acid histidine and β-alanine in an energy-dependent reaction catalyzed by carnosine synthetase. In the body, carnosine is synthesized and found largely in the cytosol of skeletal and cardiac muscle, but is also found in the brain, kidneys, and stomach. Related compounds include a methylated form of carnosine known as anserine (β-alanyl methylhistidine) and homocarnosine (γ-aminobutyryl histidine), among others. Carnosine also is available in foods, primarily meats, and may be digested into histidine and β-alanine in the intestine or possibly absorbed intact by peptide transporters. While not all of the functions of carnosine have been identified, some studies have shown that carnosine acts as both a buffer and an antioxidant within cells; it may also reduce calcium needs for muscle contractility. β-alanine supplementation increases muscle carnosine concentrations; however, the identification of side effects and benefits of such supplementation requires additional research [11,12].

Choline

Choline (Figure 6.26) is made in the body from methylation of the amino acid serine using S-adenosyl methionine (SAM). Choline is also found free in foods in small

CH₃ — ⁺N(CH₃)(CH₃) — CH₂ — CH₂OH

Figure 6.26 Choline.

amounts but is more commonly found in foods as part of the phospholipid lecithin (phosphatidyl choline). Foods rich in lecithin include eggs, liver and other organ meats, muscle meats, shrimp, cod, salmon, wheat germ, and legumes such as soybeans and peanuts. Lecithin is also added to many foods as an emulsifier.

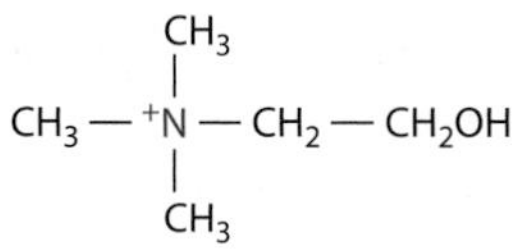

In the body, choline has several functions, including roles as a methyl donor, in the formation of platelet aggregating factor, and in the secretion of very-low-density lipoproteins from the liver. It is also needed to synthesize spingomyelin, phosphatidyl choline, and the neurotransmitter acetylcholine.

To be converted to acetylcholine, free choline crosses the blood-brain barrier and enters cerebral cells from the plasma through a specific choline transport system. Within the presynaptic terminal of the neuron, acetylcholine is formed by the action of choline acetyltransferase as follows:

Choline + acetyl-CoA ⟶ Acetylcholine + CoA

The acetyl-CoA needed for the reaction is thought to arise from glucose metabolism by neural glycolysis and the action of the pyruvate dehydrogenase complex. Concentrations of choline in cholinergic neurons typically are below the K_m of choline acetyltransferase; thus, the enzyme normally is not saturated. Choline also can be recycled—that is, acetylcholinesterase can hydrolyze acetylcholine following synaptic transmission, and phospholipases can liberate choline from lecithin and spingomyelin as needed.

Choline is oxidized in the liver and kidneys. In the liver, choline oxidation generates betaine, which functions as a methyl donor to regenerate methionine from homocysteine. Further metabolism of betaine (also called trimethylglycine) generates dimethyl glycine (also called sarcosine), which may be catabolized to glycine, methylene tetrahydrofolate (a coenzyme form of folate), carbon dioxide, and an ammonium ion. These reactions are shown in the section of Chapter 9 on folate (specifically, the amino acid metabolism of serine and glycine).

Experimental diets devoid of choline can result in decreases in plasma choline and phosphatidylcholine concentrations as well as alterations in some liver enzymes. Animals devoid of dietary choline develop a fatty liver accompanied by some hepatic necrosis. Low intakes of both choline and betaine have been associated with inflammation. The Food and Nutrition Board has suggested that an Adequate Intake is 425 mg and 550 mg of choline daily for adult females and males, respectively [13]. Such intakes are easily obtained through dietary consumption of animal products and foods containing fats. A Tolerable Upper Intake Level of 3.5 g of choline daily also has been set [13]. The **Tolerable Upper Intake Level** represents the highest level of daily intake that is likely to pose no risks of adverse health effects to most people in the general population [13].

Purine and Pyrimidine Bases

Nitrogenous bases, along with a five-carbon sugar and phosphoric acid, are needed for the synthesis of two nucleic acids, deoxyribonucleic acid (DNA) and ribonucleic acid (RNA), in the body. It is amino acids that provide the source for the nitrogen in these bases. The nitrogenous bases can be divided into two categories: pyrimidines and purines. The pyrimidines are six-membered rings containing nitrogen atoms in positions 1 and 3. The pyrimidine bases include uracil, cytosine, and thymidine. Deoxycytidine and thymidine (also called deoxythymidine) are found in DNA. Cytidine and uridine are present in RNA. The purines are made up of two fused rings with nitrogen atoms in positions 1, 3, 7, and 9. The purine bases include adenine and guanine and are found in DNA as deoxyadenosine and deoxyguanosine and in RNA as adenosine and guanosine. A brief review of purine and pyrimidine synthesis and degradation follows.

The synthesis of the nitrogen-containing bases used to make nucleic acids and nucleotides occurs for the most part de novo in the liver. The individual steps in pyrimidine synthesis are shown in Figure 6.27. First, synthesis of the pyrimidines uracil, cytosine, and thymine (or in nucleotide form UTP, CTP, and TTP, respectively) is initiated by the formation of carbamoyl phosphate from the amino acid glutamine, CO_2, and ATP. The enzyme carbamoyl phosphate synthetase II catalyzes this reaction in the cytosol and is distinct from carbamoyl phosphate synthetase I, which is needed in the initial step of urea synthesis and is found in the mitochondria. Second, carbamoyl phosphate reacts with the amino acid aspartate to form N-carbamoyl aspartate. Aspartate transcarbamoylase catalyzes the reaction, which is the committed step in pyrimidine biosynthesis. Following several additional reactions, detailed in Figure 6.27, uridine monophosphate (UMP) is synthesized. Defects in the activity of either OMP decarboxylase used to make UMP (reaction 6, Figure 6.27) or orotate phosphoribosyl transferase (reaction 5, Figure 6.27) cause the genetic disorder orotic aciduria. This condition is characterized by megaloblastic anemia, leukopenia, retarded growth, and the excretion of large amounts of orotic acid in the urine.

The interconversions among the pyrimidine nucleoside triphosphates are shown in Figure 6.28 and discussed next. Once uridine monophosphate (UMP) is formed, it may react with other nucleoside di- and triphosphates.

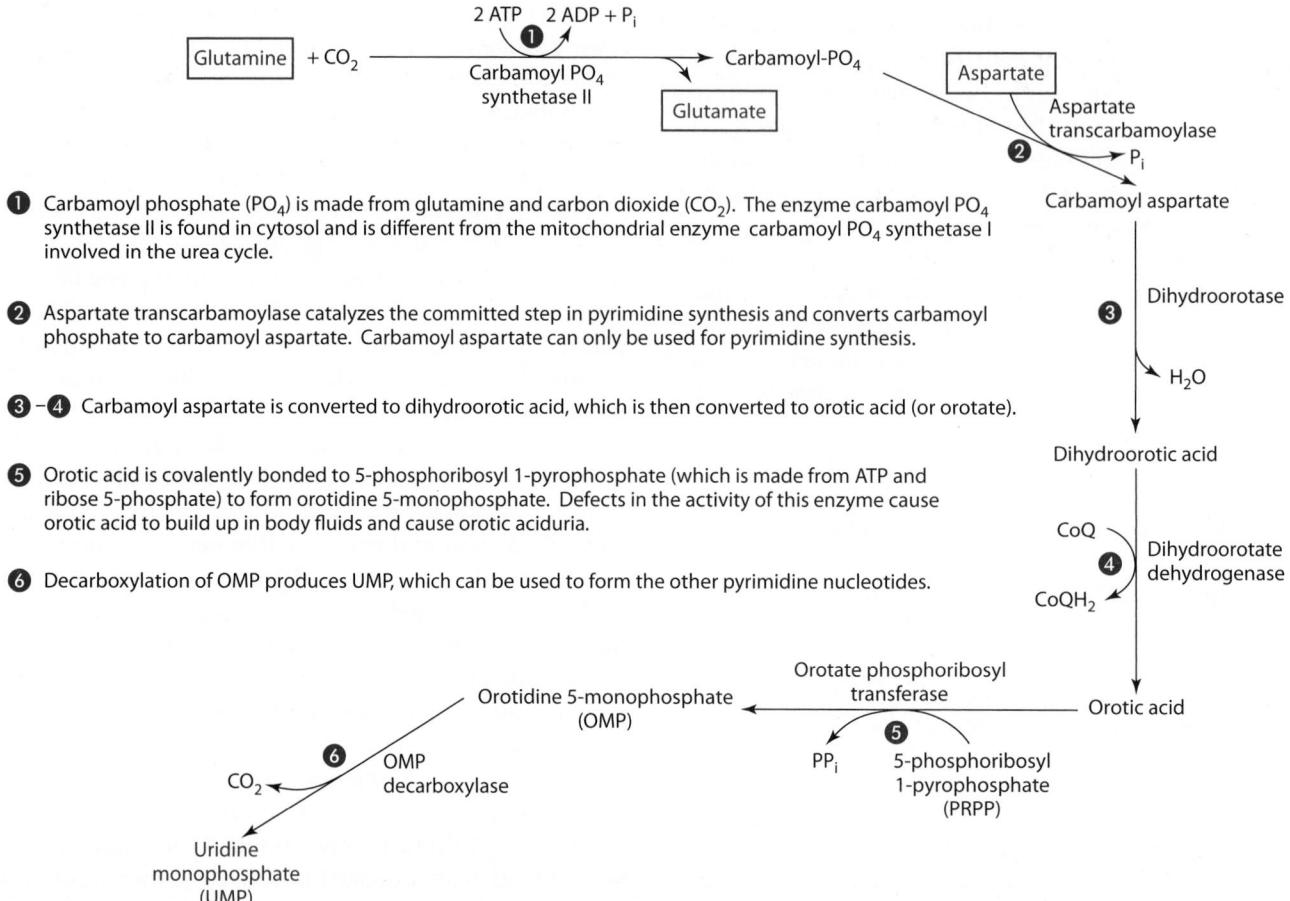

❶ Carbamoyl phosphate (PO_4) is made from glutamine and carbon dioxide (CO_2). The enzyme carbamoyl PO_4 synthetase II is found in cytosol and is different from the mitochondrial enzyme carbamoyl PO_4 synthetase I involved in the urea cycle.

❷ Aspartate transcarbamoylase catalyzes the committed step in pyrimidine synthesis and converts carbamoyl phosphate to carbamoyl aspartate. Carbamoyl aspartate can only be used for pyrimidine synthesis.

❸–❹ Carbamoyl aspartate is converted to dihydroorotic acid, which is then converted to orotic acid (or orotate).

❺ Orotic acid is covalently bonded to 5-phosphoribosyl 1-pyrophosphate (which is made from ATP and ribose 5-phosphate) to form orotidine 5-monophosphate. Defects in the activity of this enzyme cause orotic acid to build up in body fluids and cause orotic aciduria.

❻ Decarboxylation of OMP produces UMP, which can be used to form the other pyrimidine nucleotides.

Figure 6.27 The initial reactions of pyrimidine synthesis.

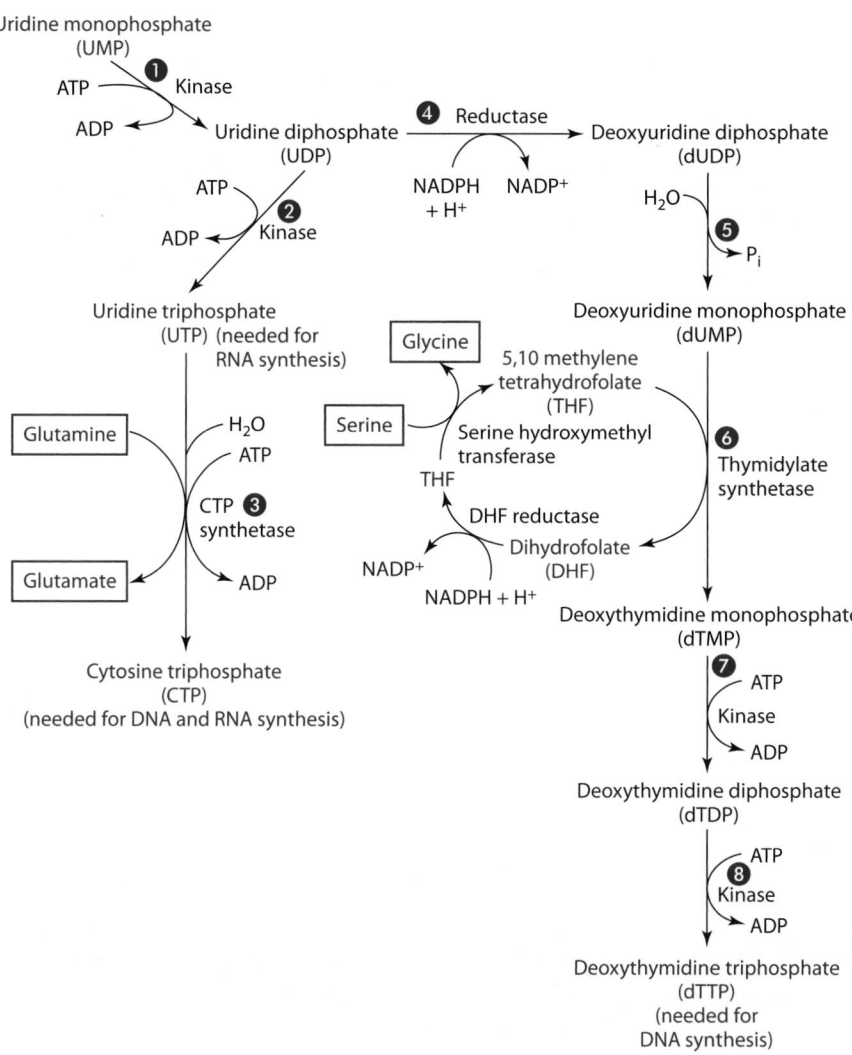

The following are the numbered steps shown in the figure:

❶ UMP reacts with ATP to generate uridine diphosphate (UDP).

❷ UDP is then converted to uridine triphosphate (UTP).

❸ UTP is used with the amino acid glutamine (Gln) to make cytosine triphosphate (CTP).

❹ UDP can be reduced using NADPH + H⁺ in a reaction that also involves riboflavin and thioredoxin to form deoxyuridine diphosphate (dUDP).

❺ dUDP can be converted to deoxyuridine monophosphate (dUMP).

❻ dUMP can be converted to deoxythymidine monophosphate (also referred to as thymidine monophosphate and abbreviated dTMP or TMP, respectively) by the enzyme thymidylate synthetase. Folate as 5,10 methylene tetrahydrofolate (THF) provides a one-carbon unit to convert dUMP to dTMP. The dihydrofolate (DHF) that is formed must be converted back to THF for the cycle to continue. This reaction is catalyzed by DHF reductase, which is the target for the anti-cancer drug methotrexate.

❼ dTMP can be phosphorylated using ATP to form deoxythymidine diphosphate (dTDP).

❽ dTDP can be phosphorylated using ATP to form deoxythymidine triphosphate (dTTP), which is needed for DNA synthesis.

Figure 6.28 The formation of the pyrimidine nucleoside triphosphates UTP, CTP, and TTP for DNA and RNA synthesis.

UMP can be converted to uridine diphosphate (UDP) utilizing ATP. UDP can be converted to uridine triphosphate (UTP) also using ATP, and UTP can be converted to cytosine triphosphate (CTP) using ATP and an amino group from glutamine. Alternately, UDP can be reduced to deoxy(d)UDP by ribonucleotide reductase; this reaction requires riboflavin as $FADH_2$ and the protein thioredoxin. DeoxyUDP can then be converted to dUMP. The formation of deoxythymidine (also called thymidine) monophosphate (dTMP or TMP) from dUMP is catalyzed by thymidylate synthetase; the reaction requires the coenzyme form of folate 5,10 methylene tetrahydrofolate and forms dihydrofolate (DHF). Dihydrofolate reductase is needed to convert DHF to tetrahydrofolate, which is then converted to 5,10 methylene tetrahydrofolate and thus allows for dTMP synthesis. DeoxyTMP can be phosphorylated to form deoxythymidine diphosphate (dTDP) and then phosphorylated again to produce deoxythymidine triphosphate (dTTP or abbreviated TTP). Thus, through these reactions CTP, (d)TTP, and UTP have been generated and can be used for the synthesis of DNA and RNA. The pyrimidine ring structure and its sources of carbon and nitrogen atoms along with the structures of the pyrimidine bases are shown in Figure 6.29. CTP is also used in phospholipid synthesis, and UTP is used to form activated intermediates in the metabolism of various sugars. Drugs used to treat cancer often target key enzymes needed for the synthesis of purines or pyrimidines, which are needed by both healthy and cancer cells to grow and multiply. The drug methotrexate, for example, inhibits dihydrofolate reductase activity and thereby decreases dTMP (and thus TTP) formation. Rapidly dividing cells such as cancer cells are more susceptible to the effects of these drugs.

The purine bases adenine and guanine (Figure 6.29) are synthesized de novo as nucleoside monophosphates by sequential addition of carbons and nitrogens to ribose-5-phosphate that has originated from the hexose monophosphate shunt. As shown in Figure 6.30, in the initial reaction, ribose 5-phosphate reacts with ATP to form

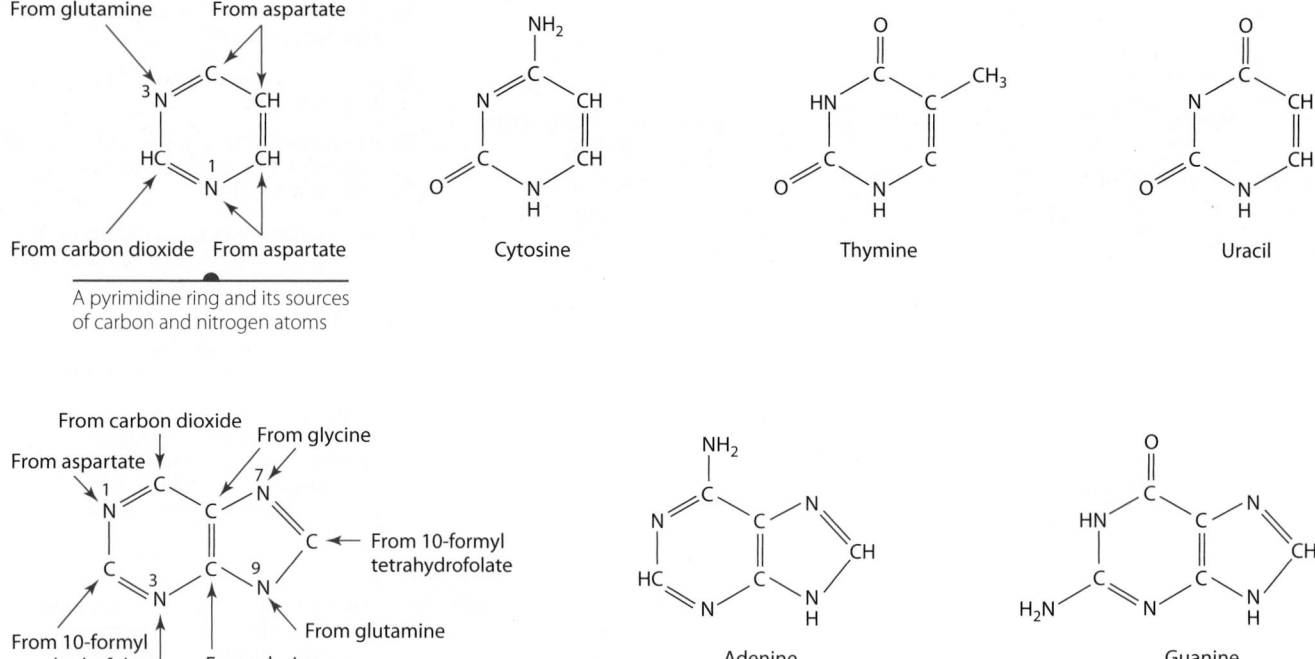

Figure 6.29 The pyrimidine and purine ring structures and the pyrimidine and purine bases. Cytosine, adenine, and guanine are found in both DNA and RNA. Thymine is found in DNA and uracil only in RNA.

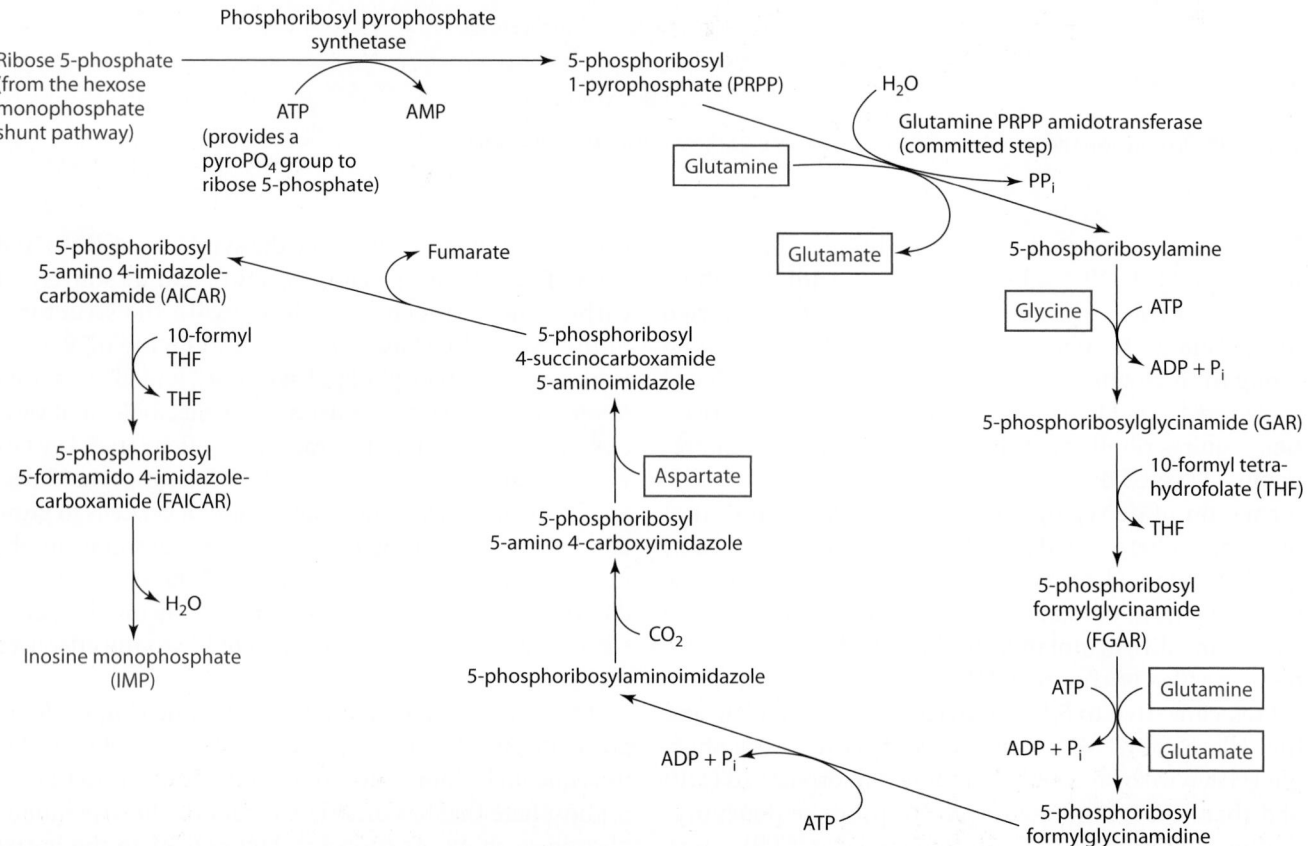

Figure 6.30 Synthesis of inosine monophosphate (IMP), which is used to synthesize other purine nucleotides.

5-phosphoribosyl 1-pyrophosphate (PRPP). Glutamine then donates a nitrogen to form 5-phosphoribosylamine. This step represents the committed step in purine nucleotide synthesis. Next in a series of reactions, nitrogen and carbon atoms from glycine are added, formylation occurs by tetrahydrofolate, another nitrogen atom is donated by the amide group of glutamine, and ring closure occurs. Another set of reactions involving the addition of carbons from carbon dioxide and from 10-formyl THF (from folate) and a nitrogen from aspartate occurs. The net result of all of these reactions is the formation of a purine ring. The ring (Figure 6.29) is thus derived from components of several amino acids, including glutamine, glycine, and aspartate, as well as from folate and CO_2.

The formation of purine nucleoside triphosphates for DNA and RNA synthesis is shown in Figure 6.31. Inosine monophosphate (IMP) is used to synthesize adenosine monophosphate (AMP) and guanosine monophosphate (GMP). AMP and GMP are phosphorylated to ADP and GDP, respectively, by ATP. The deoxyribotides are formed at the diphosphate level by converting ribose to deoxyribose, thereby producing dADP and dGDP. ADP can be phosphorylated to ATP by oxidative phosphorylation; the remaining nucleotides are phosphorylated to their triphosphate form by ATP.

Purine nucleotides also can be synthesized by the salvage pathway, which requires much less energy than de novo synthesis. In the salvage pathway, the purine base adenine reacts with 5-phosphoribosyl 1-pyrophosphate (PRPP) to form AMP + PP_i in a reaction catalyzed by adenine phosphoribosyl transferase. The purine guanine also can react with PRPP to form GMP + PP_i. Hypoxanthine can react with PRPP to form IMP + PP_i. These last two reactions are catalyzed by hypoxanthine-guanine phosphoribosyl transferase. Defects in this enzyme cause the disorder Lesch-Nylan syndrome, a genetic X-linked condition characterized most notably by self-mutilation, such as the biting off of one's fingers, and premature death. Other symptoms include mental retardation and the accumulation of hypoxanthine, phosphoribosyl pyrophosphate, and uric acid in body fluids.

Degradation of pyrimidines involves the sequential hydrolysis of the nucleoside triphosphates to mononucleotides, nucleosides, and, finally, free bases. This process can be accomplished in most cells by lysosomal enzymes. During catabolism of pyrimidines, the ring is opened with the production of CO_2 and ammonia from the carbamoyl portion of the molecule. The ammonia can be converted into urea and excreted. Malonyl-CoA and methylmalonyl-CoA, produced from the remainder of the ring, follow

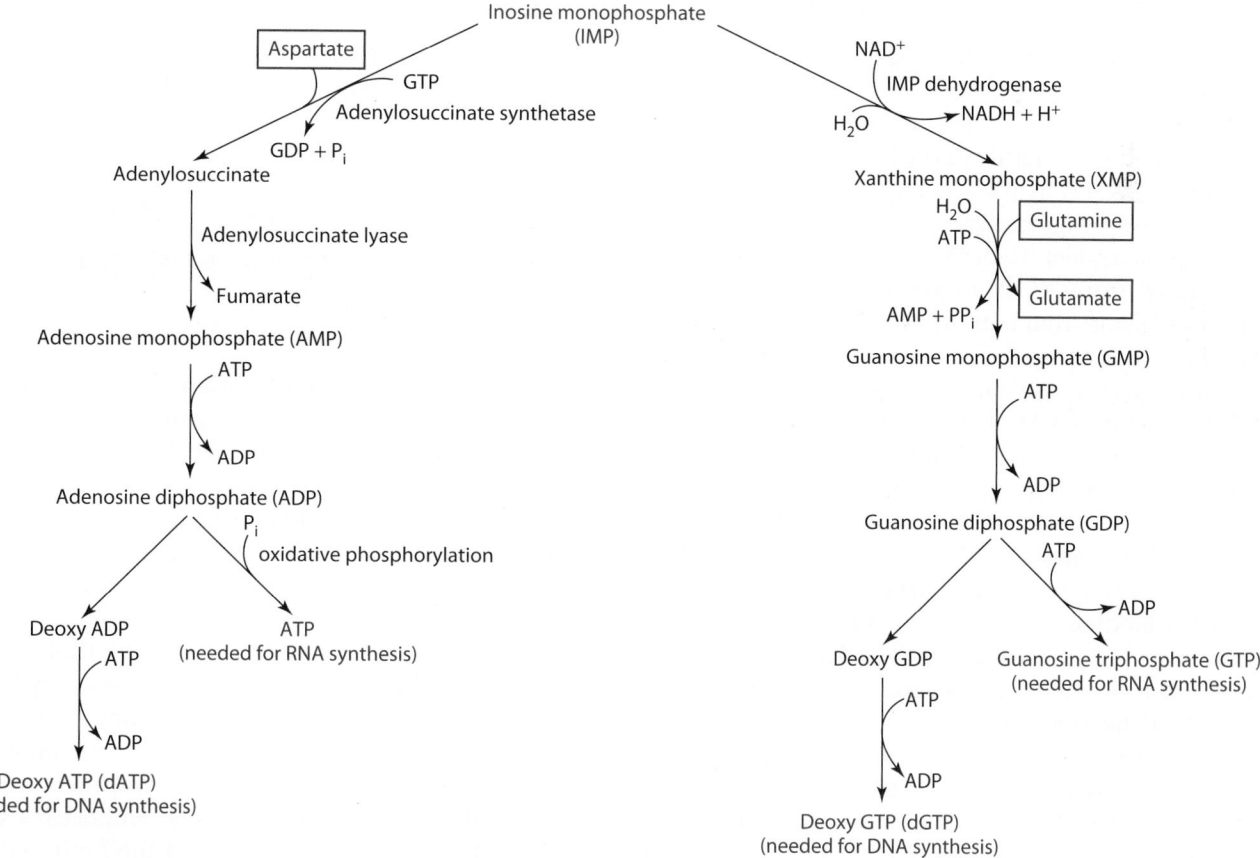

Figure 6.31 The formation of purines and nucleoside triphosphates needed for DNA and RNA synthesis.

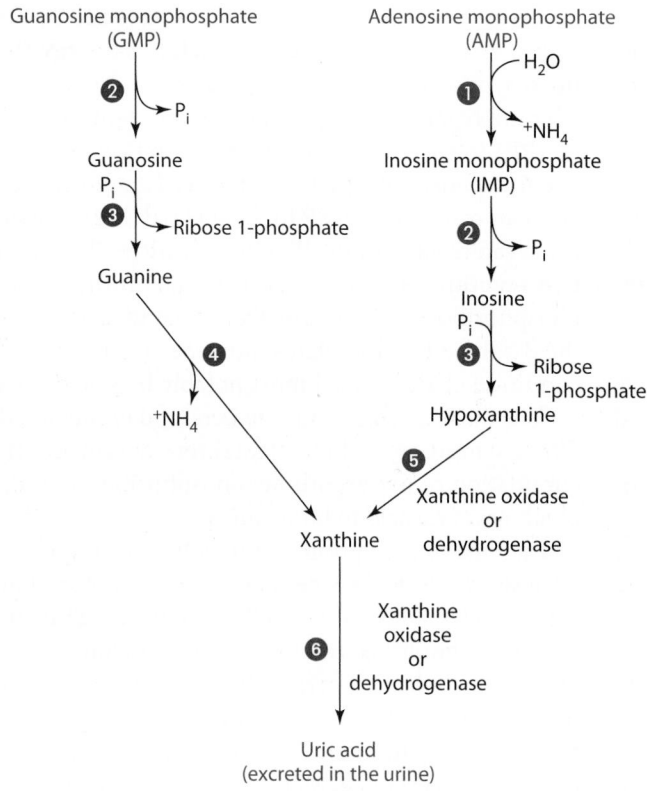

Guanosine monophosphate (GMP)

Adenosine monophosphate (AMP)

❶ AMP is deaminated to produce IMP

❷ IMP and GMP are dephosphorylated, generating inosine and guanosine, respectively

❸ A ribose is removed from the inosine and guanosine to form hypoxanthine and guanine, respectively

❹ Guanine is deaminated to form xanthine

❺ Hypoxanthine is converted to xanthine

❻ Xanthine is converted to uric acid, which is excreted in the urine

Figure 6.32 The degradation of the purines AMP and GMP generates uric acid.

their normal metabolic pathways, thus requiring no special excretion route.

Purines (GMP and AMP) are progressively oxidized for degradation primarily in the liver, yielding xanthine, which is converted to uric acid for excretion (Figure 6.32). Xanthine dehydrogenase and oxidase, both molybdenum- and iron-dependent flavoenzymes, convert hypoxanthine (generated from AMP) to xanthine and also convert xanthine (made from both AMP and GMP) to uric acid. Xanthine oxidase uses molecular oxygen and generates hydrogen peroxide, while xanthine dehydrogenase uses NAD^+ and forms $NADH + H^+$. The uric acid that is produced is normally excreted in the urine, although up to 200 mg also may be secreted into the digestive tract. In the disorder gout and in renal failure, uric acid accumulates in the body, causing painful joints among other problems. Allopurinol is one of several drugs used to treat gout; it works by binding to the enzyme xanthine oxidase to prevent its interaction with xanthine and hypoxanthine and thus diminish uric acid production. The oxidase (rather than the dehydrogenase) form of the enzyme predominates in several body tissues under conditions of oxygen deprivation (as with a heart attack). A problem in this situation is that when oxygen delivery relieves this deprivation, hydrogen peroxide and free radical production both increase and may further damage the injured tissues.

Research involving introduction of enzymes and antioxidant nutrients to help minimize tissue damage with reoxygenation is ongoing.

INTERORGAN "FLOW" OF AMINO ACIDS AND ORGAN-SPECIFIC METABOLISM

While tissues and organs use amino acids to synthesize proteins and some nitrogen-containing compounds, the metabolism of the amino acids varies to some extent among the different organs. In many instances, the products generated from amino acid metabolism in one organ may be needed by another organ, creating a dependence between organs. This interdependence begins with the intestinal cells, which are the first cells of the body to receive dietary amino acids. The first part of this section will cover amino acid metabolism by intestinal cells, followed by a discussion of amino acids in the plasma and then the specific roles that glutamine and alanine play among body tissues. Lastly, specific uses of amino acids by other selected tissues and organs such as skeletal muscle, the kidneys, and the brain will be presented.

Intestinal Cell Amino Acid Metabolism

Intestinal cells use amino acids for energy production as well as for the synthesis of proteins and nitrogen-containing compounds. Some of the uses of amino acids in enterocytes include:

- structural proteins
- nucleotides
- apoproteins necessary for lipoprotein (chylomicron) formation
- new digestive enzymes
- hormones
- nitrogen-containing compounds

In addition, amino acids may be totally or partially metabolized within intestinal cells. It is estimated that the intestine (which represents about 3–6% of the body weight) uses 30% to 40% and splanchnic tissues use up to 50% of some of the essential amino acids absorbed from the diet [14]. Moreover, the intestines are thought to use up to about 90% of glutamate absorbed from the diet [14]. The next five subsections discuss the metabolism of glutamine, glutamate, aspartate, arginine, and methionine in intestinal cells. Figure 6.33 provides a partial overview of intestinal cell amino acid metabolism.

Intestinal Glutamine Metabolism

Glutamine serves several roles in intestinal cells. It is degraded extensively by intestinal cells as a primary source of energy. It also has been shown to have trophic (growth)

effects, stimulating gastrointestinal mucosa cell proliferation. Consequently, glutamine helps to prevent both atrophy of gut mucosa and bacterial translocation. In addition, glutamine has been shown to enhance the synthesis of heat shock proteins. It is also needed in large quantities along with threonine for the synthesis of mucins found in gastrointestinal tract mucus secretions. These roles of glutamine in the gastrointestinal tract have prompted several companies to enrich enteral and parenteral (intravenous) nutrition products with glutamine. When glutamine is provided through tube feedings, over 50% of glutamine is extracted by the splanchnic (visceral) bed. It is estimated that the human gastrointestinal tract uses up to 10 g of glutamine per day, and that the cells of the immune system use over 10 g per day. In addition to dietary glutamine, much of the body's glutamine that is produced by the skeletal muscles (and to lesser extents by the lungs, brain, heart, and adipose tissue) is released and taken up, mostly by the intestinal cells.

Glutamine not used for energy production within the intestine also may be partially catabolized to generate ammonia and glutamate. The ammonia enters the portal blood for uptake by the liver or may be used within the intestinal cell for carbamoyl phosphate synthesis. The glutamate thus formed is discussed next.

Intestinal Glutamate Metabolism

In the intestinal cell, glutamate arises directly from diet or from glutamine metabolism. It is often transaminated with pyruvate to form α-ketoglutarate and alanine (Figure 6.33); the alanine typically enters portal blood for transport to the liver. Glutamate not used for alanine

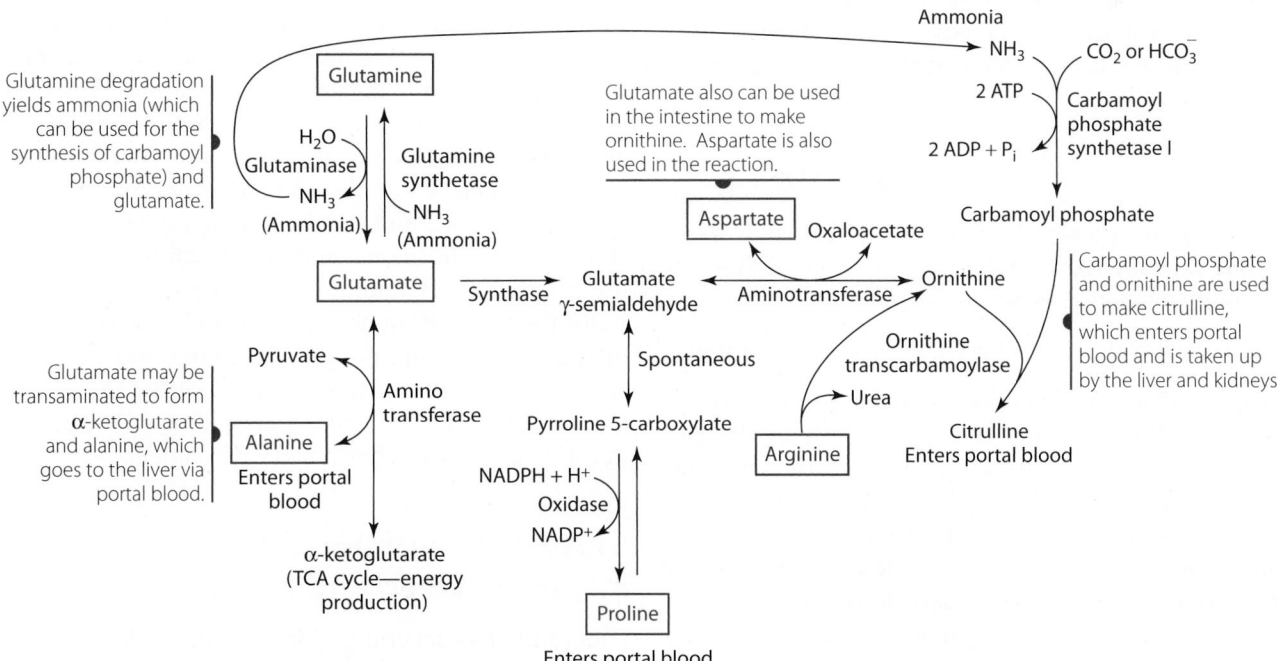

Figure 6.33 A partial overview of amino acid metabolism in the intestinal cell.

synthesis is often used with glycine and cysteine to make glutathione, or it may be used to synthesize proline, as shown here:

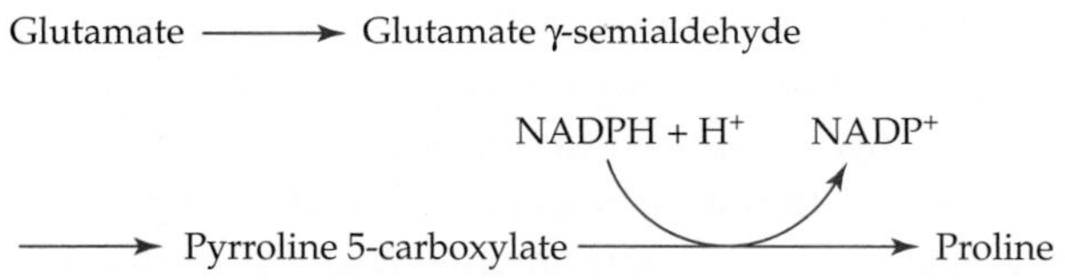

Glutamate $\longrightarrow$ Glutamate γ-semialdehyde

$$\text{NADPH} + \text{H}^+ \quad \text{NADP}^+$$

$\longrightarrow$ Pyrroline 5-carboxylate $\longrightarrow$ Proline

The majority of proline synthesis is thought to occur through intestinal cell glutamate metabolism. Proline is then released into portal blood for delivery to the liver. Lastly, glutamate may be used along with aspartate to synthesize ornithine, which in turn may be released into portal blood or can be used to make citrulline (Figure 6.33). Thus, very little glutamate leaves the intestinal cell as glutamate and enters portal blood.

Intestinal Aspartate Metabolism

In addition to metabolism of glutamine and glutamate, metabolism of aspartate from the diet generally occurs within intestinal cells. Aspartate most often undergoes transamination to generate oxaloacetate; aspartate's amino group in turn is used to synthesize ornithine. Very little aspartate (like glutamate) leaves the intestinal cells as aspartate and is found in portal blood.

Intestinal Arginine Metabolism

Arginine is also used by intestinal cells. Up to 40% of dietary arginine is oxidized in enterocytes, yielding citrulline and urea [15]. Carbamoyl phosphate is synthesized in intestinal cells by the action of carbamoyl phosphate synthetase I using ammonia (NH_3), carbon dioxide (CO_2) or bicarbonate (HCO_3^-), and ATP, as shown in Figure 6.33 and here:

$$\text{NH}_3 + \text{HCO}_3^- + 2\text{ATP} \longrightarrow \text{Carbamoyl} \atop \text{phosphate} + 2\text{ADP} + \text{P}_i$$

The carbamoyl phosphate in turn is used along with ornithine to synthesize citrulline in a reaction catalyzed by ornithine transcarbamoylase, as follows:

$$\text{Carbamoyl phosphate} + \text{Ornithine} \longrightarrow \text{Citrulline}$$

Citrulline that is made in the enterocytes is released into blood and then typically taken up, mostly by the kidneys, which use it for arginine synthesis; the liver may also take up the citrulline as needed for the urea cycle. Because of the role of the intestine in citrulline synthesis and the need for citrulline in arginine synthesis, arginine production can be impaired in individuals with intestinal injury. In such a situation, arginine becomes a conditionally essential amino acid and either arginine or citrulline must be supplemented in the diet.

Intestinal Methionine (and Cysteine) Metabolism

Methionine also is metabolized by intestinal cells. Studies suggest that up to 52% of methionine intake is metabolized in the gut [4]. Cysteine, generated from methionine or obtained directly from diet, is used in the intestinal cells to make glutathione. Alternately, cysteine is metabolized primarily (70–90%) to taurine, and to a lesser extent (10–30%) to pyruvate and sulfite [4]. These reactions can be reviewed in Figure 6.12.

Amino Acids in the Plasma

After ingestion of a protein-containing meal, amino acid concentrations typically rise in the plasma for several hours, then return to basal concentrations. In basal situations or between meals, plasma amino acid concentrations are relatively stable and are species-specific; however, absolute concentrations of specific amino acids in the plasma vary from person to person.

Amino acids circulating in the plasma and found within cells arise from digestion and absorption of dietary (exogenous) protein as well as from the breakdown of existing body (endogenous) tissues. These endogenous amino acids intermingle with exogenous amino acids to form a "pool" totaling about 150 g. The pool includes amino acids in the plasma as well as amino acids in the cytosol of body cells. Reuse of endogenous amino acids is thought to represent the primary source of amino acids for protein synthesis. Despite differences in protein intake and rates of degradation of tissue proteins, the pattern of the amino acids in the amino acid pool appears to remain relatively constant, although the pattern is quite different from that found in body proteins.

The total amount of the essential amino acids found in the pool is less than that of the nonessential amino acids. The essential amino acids found in greatest concentrations are lysine and threonine. Of the nonessential amino acids, those found in greatest concentrations are alanine, glutamate, aspartate, and glutamine. In fact, up to 80 g of glutamine can be found in the body's amino acid pool.

Amino acids within the pool, regardless of source, are taken up by tissues and metabolized in response to various stimuli such as hormones and physiological state. Tissues, for example, extract amino acids for energy production or for the synthesis of nonessential amino acids, protein, nitrogen-containing nonprotein compounds, biogenic amines, neurotransmitters, neuropeptides, hormones, glucose, fatty acids, or ketones, depending on the person's nutritional status and hormonal environment.

Glutamine and the Muscle, Intestine, Liver, and Kidneys

Glutamine has several major roles in the body, one of which is in ammonia transport. Whereas ammonia arising in the liver from amino acid reactions is typically shuttled into the urea cycle, this is not true in other tissues. In extrahepatic tissues, especially the muscle but also the lungs, heart, brain, and adipose, glutamine synthetase catalyzes the utilization of ammonia or ammonium ions with glutamate in an ATP-dependent reaction to form glutamine. It is estimated that the body produces 40 to 80 g glutamine per day. Ammonia is typically generated in these cells by amino acid deamination and deamidation. In muscle it also forms from AMP deamination; AMP is generated in the muscle with ATP degradation as occurs rapidly with exercise. Glutamate is formed in muscle and other cells from the transamination of the branched-chain amino acids with α-ketoglutarate to form branched-chain α-keto acids and glutamate, respectively. As shown in Figure 6.34, ammonia generated from AMP deamination combines with the glutamate to produce glutamine.

The glutamine that is formed in the muscle is released into the blood and transported for use by other tissues. Whereas the cells of the gastrointestinal tract as well as the immune system (lymphocytes, monocytes, and macrophages) rely on glutamine catabolism for energy production, glutamine in the liver and kidneys is utilized differently. In the absorptive state (or during periods of alkalosis), liver glutaminase activity increases, yielding ammonia for the urea cycle. In an acidotic state, the use of glutamine for the urea cycle diminishes, and the liver releases glutamine into the blood for transport to and uptake by the kidneys for use in acid-base balance. In the renal tubular cells, glutamine is catabolized by glutaminase to yield ammonia and glutamate. The glutamate may be further catabolized by glutamate dehydrogenase to yield α-ketoglutarate plus another ammonia. Ammonia reacts with H^+ to form an ammonium ion in the lumen of the kidney tubule; the ammonium ion is then excreted in the urine. Renal glutaminase activity and ammonia excretion increase with acidosis and decrease with alkalosis.

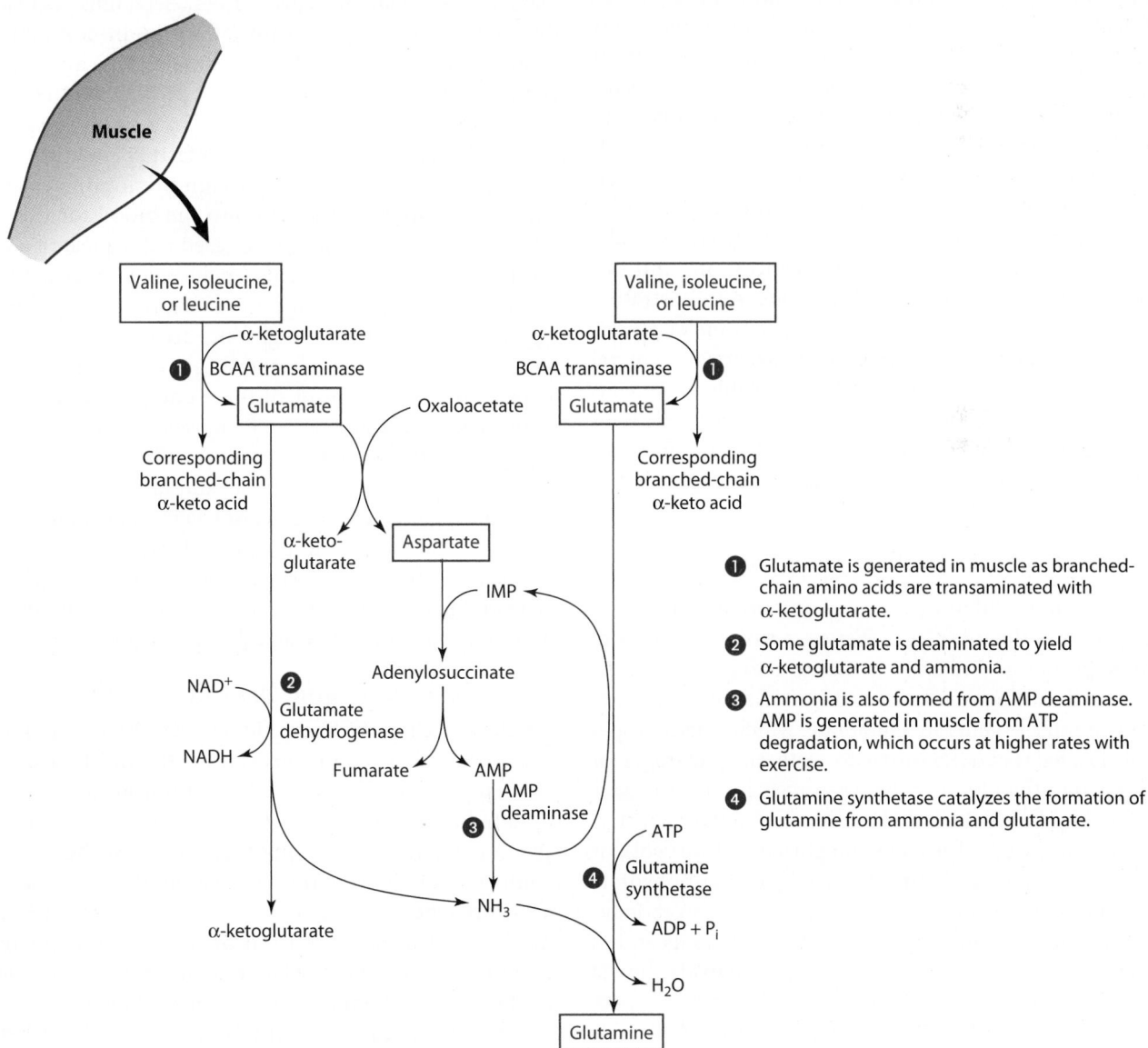

Figure 6.34 Some pathyways of glutamine generation in muscle.

Glutamine use by cells increases dramatically with hypercatabolic conditions such as infection and trauma. In these conditions muscle glutamine release increases but cannot meet other cellular demands. Thus, glutamine stores can become depleted and several cell functions may become impaired. Remember, glutamine is involved in several important body functions that are especially critical with illness/injury. To briefly review, glutamine is used extensively by immune system cells. Glutamine promotes proliferation of these cells and glutamine metabolites are used directly by these cells, for example, for purine and pyrimidine synthesis. Purines and pyrimidines are required in large quantities by activated lymphocytes and macrophages. Expression of cell surface activation markers and production of cytokines such as interferon and tumor necrosis factor alpha by lymphocytes and lymphokine-activated killer cell activity also depend on glutamine. Further, phagocytes require adequate glutamine availability. Glutamine also promotes the synthesis of heat shock/stress proteins, which help protect body cells. Glutamine prevents atrophy of the intestine, protects against intestinal bacterial translocation, and serves as the major substrate for energy production for intestinal cells. Finally, glutamine, along with alanine, uptake into cells promotes increases in cell volume with possible associated regulatory roles in intermediary metabolism. Glutamine supplementation, about 20 to 25 g/day, typically normalizes plasma glutamine concentrations and improves outcomes in critically ill patients. Administration of glutamine as a dipeptide (alanyl-glutamine or glycyl-glutamine) is needed in either an intravenous or enteral solution because the amino acid is not stable in aqueous solutions used in feeding. Dipeptidases on the surface epithelium of blood vessels are thought to hydrolyze the dipeptide so that the glutamine is available for use.

Alanine and the Liver and Muscle

In addition to glutamine, the amino acid alanine is also important in the intertissue (between tissues) transfer of amino groups generated from amino acid catabolism. As discussed in the previous section, transamination reactions in muscle generate glutamate, which is used, especially in a fed state/after eating, to synthesize glutamine for release into the blood. In between meals, with excessive glucose need, with increased use as with illness (characterized by increased release of epinephrine and cortisol), or in situations such as fasting marked by low carbohydrate (liver glycogen) stores and a glucagon to insulin ratio favoring glucagon, glutamate typically transfers its amino group to pyruvate, generated from glucose oxidation via glycolysis, to form α-ketoglutarate and alanine, respectively. Once made, the alanine is released from the muscle into the blood for travel to the liver. Within the liver, alanine undergoes transamination back to pyruvate, which is

then used to remake glucose. The glutamate that is generated with transamination can undergo deamination to provide ammonia for urea synthesis. These reactions are known as the glucose-alanine or alanine-glucose cycle and are shown in Figure 6.35. The glucose that is generated from the alanine is subsequently released into the blood, where it is available to be taken up and used by muscle. Muscle cells use the glucose through glycolysis and generate pyruvate. The formed pyruvate is again available for transamination to re-form alanine. This alanine-glucose cycle serves to transport nitrogen to the liver for conversion to urea while also allowing needed substrates to be regenerated.

Skeletal Muscle

About 40% of the body's protein is found in muscle, and skeletal muscle mass represents about 43% of the body's mass. Uptake of amino acids by the skeletal muscles readily occurs following ingestion of a protein-containing meal. During this time, skeletal muscles typically experience a net protein synthesis (i.e., protein synthesis is greater than protein degradation). In a postabsorptive state such as between meals or in a fasting situation, the reverse is true. Protein degradation predominates and amino acids may be released into the blood for use by other tissues. While alanine is released in the greatest concentration, other amino acids (including phenylalanine, methionine, lysine, arginine, histidine, tyrosine, proline, tryptophan, threonine, and glycine) are released in lesser quantities. However, further studies investigating the effects of meals containing all three energy nutrients on amino acid uptake and output by muscle are needed.

Like other tissues, muscles preferentially catabolize some amino acids more than others; six amino acids (aspartate, asparagine, glutamate, leucine, isoleucine, and valine) appear to be catabolized to greater extents in the skeletal muscle than other tissues. The catabolism of the branched-chain amino acids (isoleucine, leucine, valine) is discussed in the following subsection and shown in Figure 6.36.

Isoleucine, Leucine, and Valine Catabolism

Muscle, as well as the heart, kidneys, diaphragm, adipose tissue, and other organs (except, for the most part, the liver), possesses branched-chain aminotransferases, located in both the cytosol and mitochondria and responsible for the transamination of all three branched-chain amino acids. Following transamination, the α-keto acids of the branched-chain amino acids either remain within muscle for further oxidation or may be transported (bound to albumin) in the blood to other tissues (including the liver) for reamination or further catabolism.

After transamination, the branched-chain α-keto acids are decarboxylated in an irreversible reaction by the branched-chain α-keto acid dehydrogenase (BCKAD)

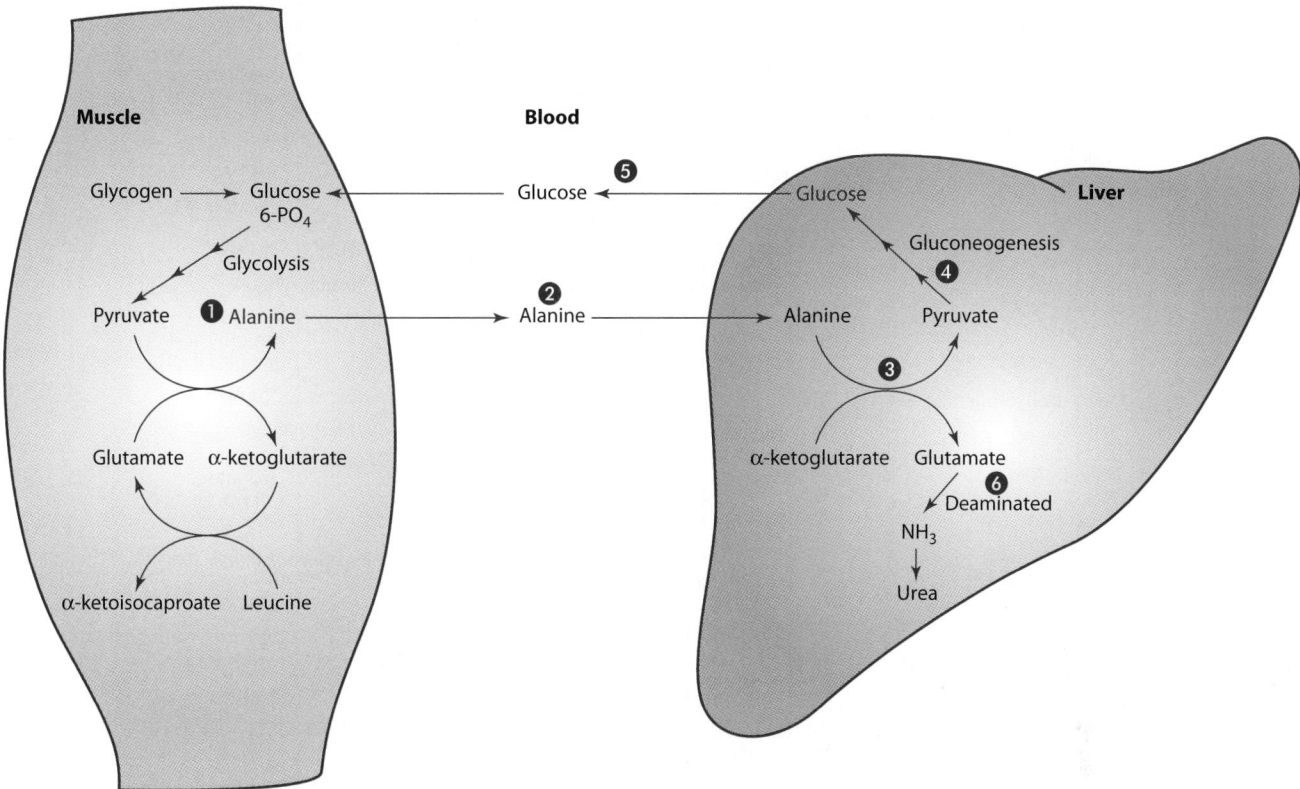

① Alanine is formed in muscle cells from transamination with glutamate (generated from leucine transamination) and from pyruvate (generated from glucose oxidation via glycolysis).

② Alanine travels in the blood to the liver.

③ In the liver, alanine is transaminated with α-ketoglutarate to form pyruvate.

④ Pyruvate can be converted back to glucose in a series of reactions.

⑤ The glucose is released from the liver into the blood for uptake by tissues such as muscle, which use glucose for energy.

⑥ The glutamate formed in the liver can be deaminated to release ammonia; the ammonia is used in the liver for urea production.

Figure 6.35 The alanine–glucose cycle: alanine generation in muscle, glucose generation in the liver.

complex. BCKAD is a large multienzyme complex made up of three subunits: E1α, E1β, and E2. This enzyme complex is found in the mitochondria of many tissues, including liver, muscle, heart, kidneys, intestine, and brain. It is highly regulated through phosphorylation (inactivation) and dephosphorylation (activation) mechanisms involving kinase and phosphatase proteins that act on the E1α subunit and through end product inhibition. This enzyme operates in a fashion similar to the pyruvate dehydrogenase complex (see Chapter 3) in that it requires thiamin in its coenzyme form TDP/TPP, niacin as NADH, and Mg^{2+} and CoA(SH) from pantothenic acid. A genetic defect diminishing BCKAD complex activity results in maple syrup urine disease (MSUD). MSUD necessitates a diet restricted in leucine, isoleucine, and valine intakes. The condition affects about 1 in 225,000 individuals worldwide, but in the Mennonite population in the United States it impacts about 1 in 150.

The details of the oxidation of the three branched-chain amino acids are shown in Figure 6.36. As with other amino acids, the complete oxidation of branched-chain amino acids yields products that are glucogenic and/or ketogenic. Valine oxidation yields succinyl-CoA. Thus, valine is considered glucogenic. The end products of isoleucine catabolism are succinyl-CoA and acetyl-CoA, which are glucogenic and ketogenic, respectively. The complete oxidation of leucine results in acetyl-CoA and acetoacetate formation; acetoacetate may be further metabolized to form acetyl-CoA (Figure 6.36). Leucine is thus totally ketogenic.

Other common intermediates are formed during branched-chain amino acid oxidation. Isoleucine, for example, generates propionyl-CoA, which is a common intermediate in the degradative pathways of methionine and threonine. Valine catabolism generates methylmalonyl-CoA, a common intermediate in the degradative pathways of methionine, threonine, and isoleucine. Defective propionyl-CoA carboxylase and methylmalonyl-CoA mutase activities (resulting in propionic acidemia and methylmalonic acidemia, respectively) thus necessitate restricted

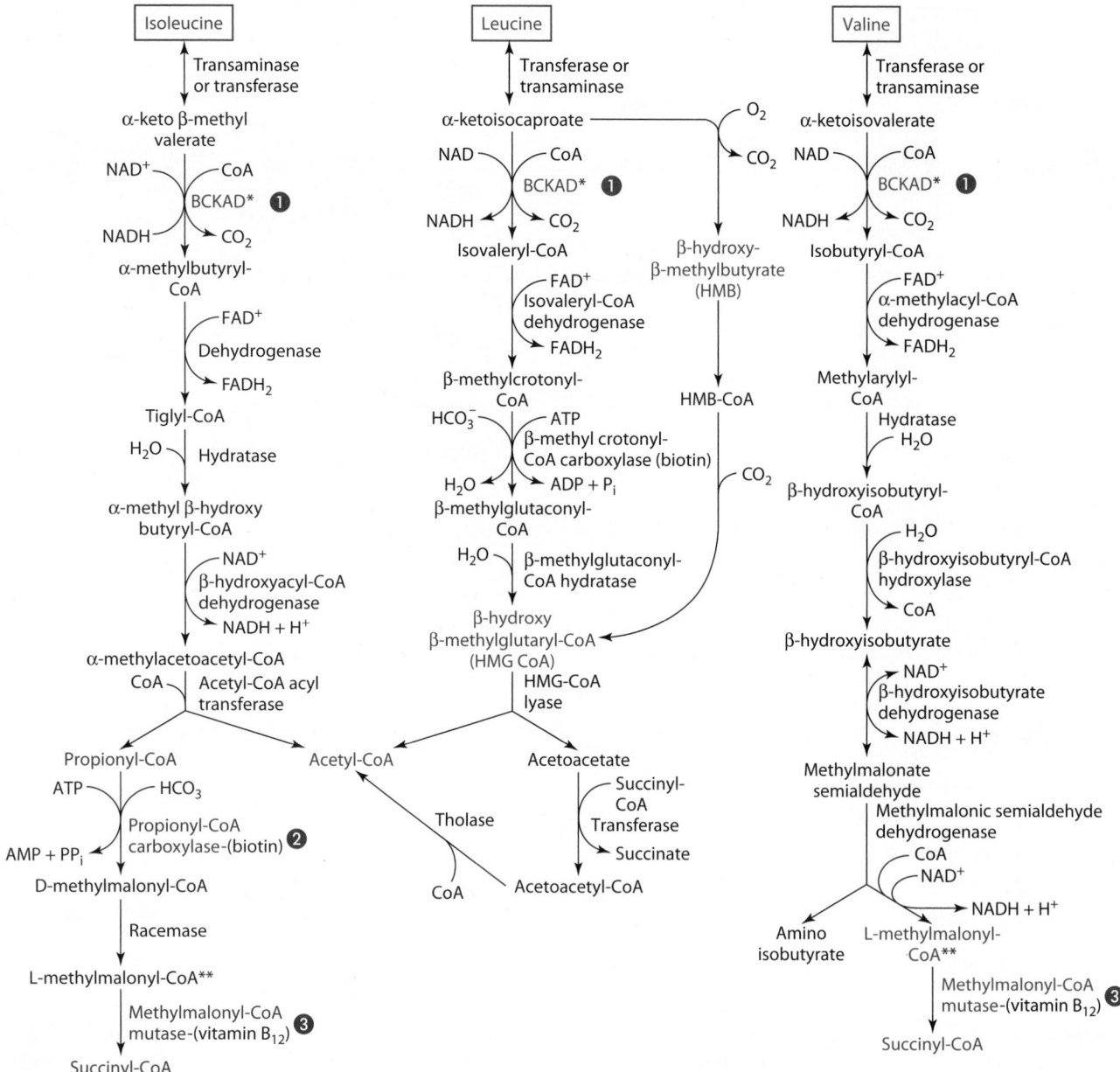

*Branched-chain α-keto acid dehydrogenase (BCKAD), requiring thiamin as TDP/TPP, niacin as NADH, and Mg^{2+} and CoA from pantothenate

**Common intermediate in the catabolism of methionine, threonine, isoleucine, and valine

❶ Defect in this enzyme complex causes maple syrup urine disease.

❷ Defect in this enzyme results in propionic acidemia.

❸ Defect in this enzyme results in methylmalonic acidemia.

Figure 6.36 Branched-chain amino acid metabolism.

dietary intakes of valine and isoleucine, as well as the previously discussed threonine and methionine. (See the "Disorders of Methionine Metabolism" section.)

Leucine's metabolism also generates β-hydroxy β-methylbutyrate (HMB) (Figure 6.36). HMB is important for the production of β-hydroxy β-methylglutaryl (HMG)-CoA, a precursor for de novo cholesterol synthesis in the muscle. It appears that with some illnesses and with muscle damage, HMG-CoA concentrations may be

inadequate to support cholesterol synthesis. Supplementation with HMB, usually as calcium HMB monohydrate (about 3 g per day given in divided doses), provides cells with a source of HMG-CoA to maintain cholesterol synthesis and thus cell function. In addition, HMB appears to attenuate both muscle proteolysis and depression of muscle protein synthesis to improve lean muscle mass. Atrophy of muscle with muscle damage or secondary to conditions such as cancer, sepsis, and acquired immune deficiency syndrome (AIDS) among others is due primarily to the activity of the ubiquitin-proteasome pathway (see the "Catabolism of Tissue Proteins" section); HMB appears to inhibit this pathway as well as to stimulate protein synthesis through mTOR. HMB's effects have been demonstrated in healthy individuals as well as in those with conditions typically associated with muscle loss such as cancer and AIDS.

Defects in some enzymes responsible for leucine degradation have been documented and are noted in Figure 6.36. Defects in isovaleryl-CoA dehydrogenase result in isovaleric acidemia. Although fairly rare, it is one of the more prevalent disorders of leucine metabolism, affecting about 1 in 250,000 worldwide but about 1 in 62,000 in Germany. Defects in β-methyl crotonyl-CoA carboxylase cause β-methyl crotonylglycinuria. Impaired activity of β-methylglutaconyl-CoA hydratase causes β-methylglutaconic aciduria and altered activity of β-hydroxyl β-methylglutaryl (HMG)-CoA lyase causes β-hydroxyl β-methylglutaric aciduria. Each of these disorders results in the production and accumulation of numerous acids and other compounds in body fluids, causing acidosis, dehydration, neurological problems, seizures, coma, and mental retardation, among other problems. A leucine-restricted diet is typically prescribed for these conditions. In some cases, to prevent toxic compounds from accumulating, supplements of carnitine and glycine may be needed. Fat restriction is also needed for those with HMG-CoA lyase deficiency.

Leucine is one of the few amino acids that is completely oxidized in the muscle for energy. Leucine is oxidized in a manner similar to fatty acids, and its oxidation results in the production of 1 mol of acetyl-CoA and 1 mol of acetoacetate. Complete oxidation of leucine generates more ATP molecules on a molar basis than complete oxidation of glucose. Leucine appears to be preferentially oxidized during fasting situations. During fasting, leucine concentrations rise in the blood and muscle, and the capacity of the muscle to degrade leucine increases concurrently. This supplies the muscle with the equivalent of 3 mol of acetyl-CoA per molecule of leucine oxidized; the acetyl-CoA produces energy for the muscle while simultaneously inhibiting the oxidation of pyruvate, which is derived from glucose oxidation via glycolysis. Pyruvate is then transaminated to alanine and transported via the blood to the liver (see the previous section "Alanine and the Liver and Muscle").

Indicators of Muscle Mass and Muscle/Protein Catabolism

While proteolysis of muscle generates amino acids that are released into the plasma for circulation to and use by other tissues, changes in plasma amino acid concentrations do not reflect changes in muscle mass. Instead, two previously mentioned compounds, creatinine and 3-methylhistidine,

are used as indicators of existing muscle mass and muscle degradation, respectively. Urinary creatinine excretion is used to assess muscle mass because creatinine is the degradation product of creatine, which constitutes a fairly standard proportion of muscle (approximately 0.3–0.5% of muscle mass by weight). Urinary creatinine excretion reflects about 1.7% of the total creatine pool per day and is expressed per 24 hours, as a coefficient based upon weight or height; however, because of variation in muscle creatine content, urinary creatinine is not always an accurate indicator of muscle mass.

The urinary excretion of 3-methylhistidine is used an indicator of muscle catabolism (degradation). As mentioned under the section on histidine in "Hepatic Catabolism and Uses of Basic Amino Acids," the amino acid histidine is found in high concentrations as 3-methylhistidine in the muscle protein actin. Because 3-methylhistidine cannot be reused for protein synthesis following protein degradation and is excreted in the urine, its urinary excretion can be measured and serves as an indicator of muscle breakdown. A drawback to its use, though, is that actin is not found only in muscle but appears to occur in other body tissues, including the intestine and platelets, which have high turnover rates. Thus, urinary 3-methylhistidine excretion also may represent an index of protein breakdown for many nonmuscle tissues in the body.

Kidneys

The kidneys preferentially take up and metabolize a number of amino acids and nitrogen-containing compounds (see Figure 6.37). The kidneys' roles include:

- glutamine catabolism for acid-base balance
- glycine catabolism for acid-base balance
- serine synthesis from glycine
- arginine and glycine use to form guanidinoacetate for creatine synthesis
- glutathione catabolism
- arginine synthesis from citrulline
- tyrosine synthesis from phenylalanine
- histidine generation from carnosine degradation

In fact, the kidneys are considered to be the major site in the body for arginine, histidine, serine, and perhaps tyrosine production [16].

Glutamine uptake by the kidneys has been estimated at 7 to 10 g per day [16] but increases dramatically during periods of acidosis, while glutamine uptake by the intestine, liver, and other organs is diminished. Especially in acidotic conditions, glutamine and then glutamate are deamidated in the kidneys, resulting in the two ammonias. In the kidney's tubular lumen, the ammonias combine with H^+ ions and form ammonium ions, which are

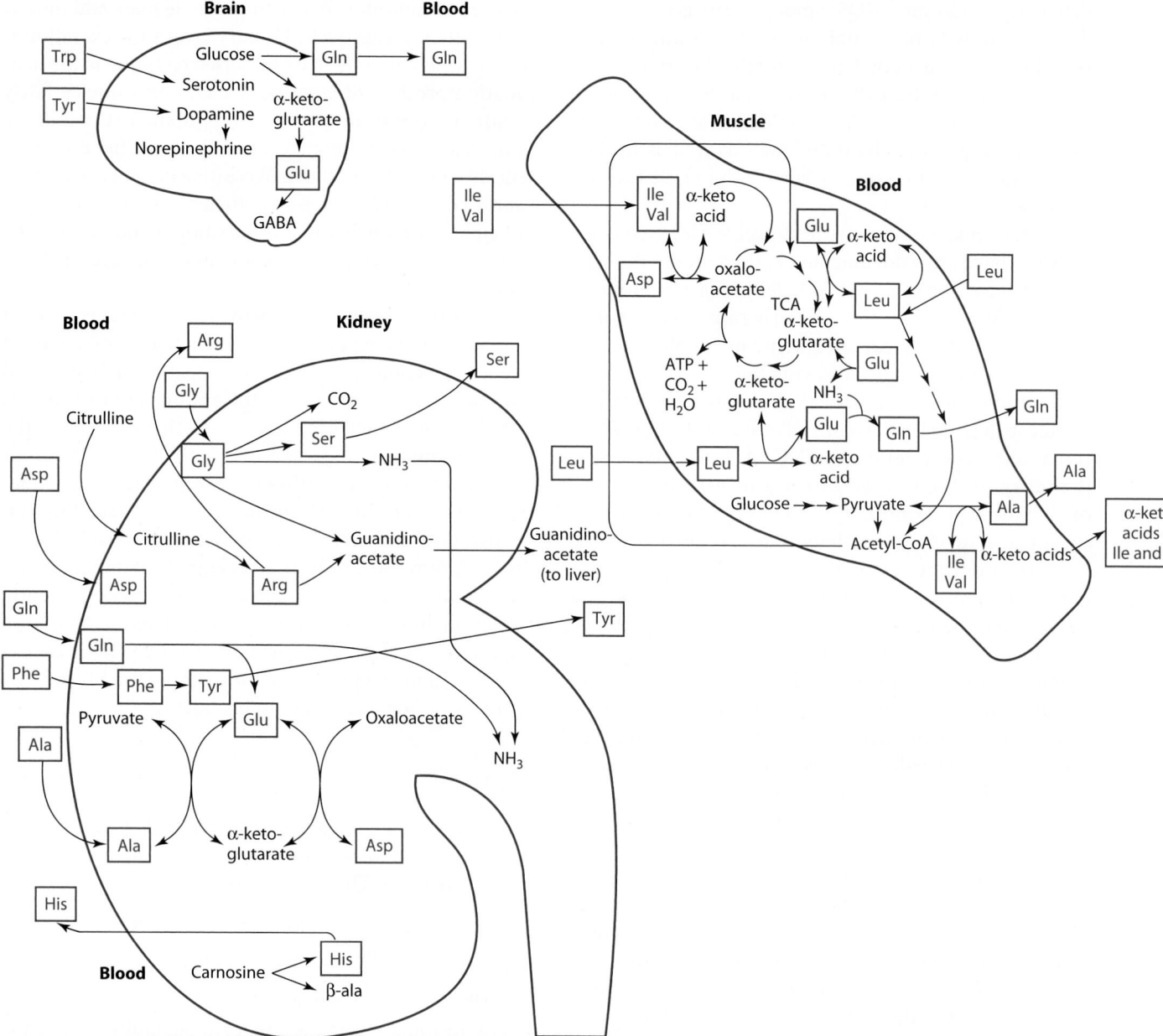

Figure 6.37 Amino acid metabolism in selected organs.

excreted in the urine. H$^+$ ions enter the tubular lumen in exchange for Na$^+$. In the lumen, the H$^+$ ions may also react with bicarbonate (HCO$_3^-$) to form water and carbon dioxide and with dibasic phosphate (HPO$_4^{2-}$) to form monobasic phosphate (H$_2$PO$_4^-$). Glycine utilization by the kidneys under acidotic conditions is similar to glutamine utilization; glycine is degraded, forming ammonia and carbon dioxide. The ammonia then enters into the tubular lumen, where it reacts with H$^+$ ions, forming ammonium ions that are excreted in the urine. The loss of the H$^+$ from the body serves to increase pH from an acidotic state toward a normal value of about 7.35 to 7.45.

Under healthy (nonacidotic) conditions, glycine is used by the kidneys (proximal tubule) for the synthesis of the amino acid serine. The kidneys also use glycine along with arginine for the synthesis of guanidinoacetate; this compound then travels to the liver, where it is used to generate creatine. The kidneys are thought to take up about 1.5 g of glycine per day [16]. Glycine, however, is also generated from glutathione catabolism in the proximal tubules of the kidneys.

Most arginine that is made in the body for tissue use is made in the kidneys from citrulline that was generated in the intestines and has been extracted from the blood; remember, the arginine made in the liver is immediately degraded to form urea and is thus not available to body tissues. It is estimated that the kidneys extract about 1.5 g of citrulline per day from the blood and release about 2 to 4 g of arginine daily [16].

Phenylalanine catabolism to tyrosine in the kidneys also has been demonstrated. It is estimated that the kidneys take up about 0.5 to 1 g of phenylalanine from the blood each day and releases about 1 g of tyrosine [16]. In addition to phenylalanine degradation, carnosine is oxidized by the kidneys, releasing histidine for use by other body tissues.

The kidneys also can generate glucose for the body. The kidneys, like the liver and to some extent like the small intestine, have the enzymes necessary for gluconeogenesis. See Chapter 3 for a detailed description of these reactions.

The role of the kidneys in nitrogen metabolism cannot be overemphasized. The organ is responsible for ridding the body of nitrogenous wastes that accumulate in the blood plasma. Kidney glomeruli act as filters of blood plasma, and all the constituents in plasma, with the exception of plasma proteins, move into the filtrate. Essential nutrients such as sodium, amino acids, and glucose are actively reabsorbed as the filtrate moves through the tubules. Many other substances are not actively reabsorbed and must either move along an electrical gradient or move osmotically with water to enter the tubular cells. The amount of these substances that enters the tubular cells, then, depends upon how much water moves into the cells and how permeable the cells are to the specific substances. The cell membranes are relatively impermeable to urea and uric acid, and are particularly impermeable to creatinine, little/none of which is typically reabsorbed.

Nitrogenous wastes found in the urine are listed in Table 6.7. About 80% of nitrogen is lost in the urine as urea under normal conditions. In acidotic conditions, urinary urea nitrogen losses decrease and urinary excretion of ammonium ions rises. In addition to urea and ammonia, usual nitrogenous wastes found in the urine include creatinine and uric acid, with lesser or trace amounts of creatine (<100 mg/day), protein (<100 mg/day), amino acids (<700 mg/day), and hippuric acid (<100 mg/day). Hippuric acid results from the conjugation of the amino acid glycine and benzoic acid, which is generated mostly in the liver from the catabolism of aromatic compounds. Because the benzoic acid is not water soluble, it must be conjugated for excretion. Trace amounts of other nitrogen-containing compounds such as porphobilinogen and metabolites of tryptophan also may be present in the urine. In addition to urinary nitrogen losses, nitrogen may be lost in the feces and sweat, and with the loss of hair and skin cells. These losses are referred to as insensible nitrogen losses.

Brain and Accessory Tissues

The brain has a high capacity for the active transport of amino acids. In fact, the brain has transport systems for neutral, basic, and acidic amino acids. The transporters for some of the amino acids are almost fully saturated at normal plasma concentrations; this is especially true of the transporters for the large neutral amino acids like the branched-chain and the aromatic amino acids, which can compete with each other for the common carriers. The effects of this competition become especially apparent in conditions in which the blood concentrations of any of the branched-chain or aromatic amino acids become elevated. For example, in untreated PKU, elevations in blood phenylalanine result in increased uptake of this amino acid by the brain. In untreated MSUD, elevations in blood leucine, isoleucine, and valine result in the increased uptake of these amino acids (at the expense of the aromatic amino acids) into the brain. Moreover, in liver disease, the concentrations of the aromatic amino acids exceed those of the branched-chain amino acids and cause increased uptake of the aromatic amino acids by the brain. The elevations of amino acids in the brain alter brain function, causing a variety of neurologic problems such as impaired brain development and altered behavior and mental function, among other manifestations.

While it is clear that conditions like liver disease and inborn errors of amino acid metabolism can alter the brain's uptake of selected amino acids and cause neurological and behavioral changes, such effects have not been demonstrated consistently in healthy individuals who attempt to alter behavior by altering dietary intakes of nutrients. For example, ingestion of carbohydrate (without ingestion of protein) has been shown to increase the brain's uptake of tryptophan and raise serotonin concentrations but does not always result in the expected behavioral effects (such as feeling calm and relaxed) of elevated serotonin. In other words, varying nutrient intakes, including carbohydrate and protein, by eating selected foods is thought to have little effect on the brain's serotonergic function.

Neurotransmitters and Biogenic Amines

Neurotransmitters are compounds generated in the body that transmit signals from a neuron to a target cell across a synapse. Neurotransmitters are stored or packaged in the nerve axon terminal as vesicles or granules until stimuli arrive to effect their release into the synaptic cleft and allow for their binding to receptors on the post-synaptic side of the synapse. Neurotransmitter action on the cell

Table 6.7 Nitrogen-Containing Waste Products Excreted in the Urine

Compound	Approximate Amount Excreted/Day	
	g/day	mmol/N
Urea	5–20	162–650
Creatinine	0.6–1.8	16–50
Uric acid	0.2–1.0	4–20
Ammonia	0.4–1.5	22–83

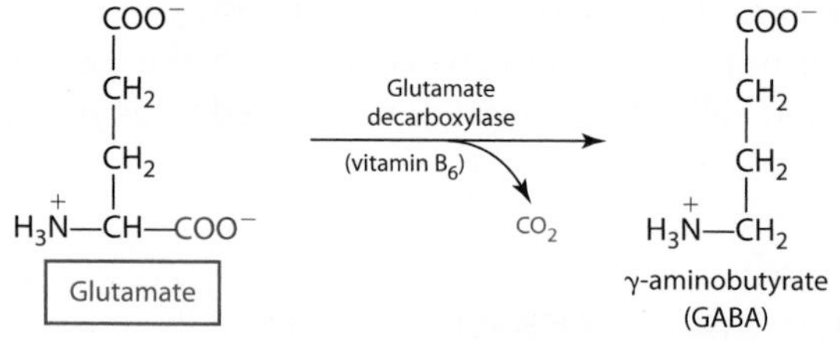

Figure 6.38 GABA synthesis from the amino acid glutamate.

membranes typically elicits an action or electrical potential. Several amino acids act directly as neurotransmitters in the body, including:

- Glycine, which acts primarily in the spinal cord as an inhibitory neurotransmitter.
- Taurine, which is thought to function as an inhibitory neurotransmitter.
- Aspartate, which is derived chiefly from glutamate through aspartate aminotransferase activity common in neural tissue, and is thought to act as an excitatory neurotransmitter in the central nervous system.
- Glutamate, which acts primarily in the brain and spinal cord as an excitatory neurotransmitter. Glutamate also can be decarboxylated in a vitamin B_6-(PLP)–dependent reaction to synthesize the neurotransmitter γ-amino butyric acid (GABA) (Figures 6.37 and 6.38). GABA functions in the brain as an inhibitory neurotransmitter.

Amino acids that are excitatory work by stimulating receptors on postsynaptic membranes; this stimulation in turn propagates the nerve impulse. In contrast, amino acids that are inhibitory retard the postsynaptic neuron from propagating nerve impulses.

Many amino acids are catabolized within the brain and nervous system to generate biogenic amines. These biogenic amines also may function as neurotransmitters.

Some of these amino acids and the amines they produce include:

- Tryptophan, which is used to synthesize serotonin (Figures 6.37 and 6.39). Serotonin functions as an excitatory neurotransmitter (biogenic amine) in the central nervous system and in circulation as a potent vasoconstrictor and stimulator of smooth muscle contraction. Serotonin affects sleep, mood, and appetite, as well as memory and learning (e.g., cognitive functions).
- Tyrosine, which is used in sympathetic neurons to make catechol derivatives, collectively called catecholamines (dopamine, norepinephrine, and epinephrine; Figures 6.37 and 6.40). In the brain and neurons, the catecholamines function as neurotransmitters. Dopamine affects a variety of behaviors as well as coordination of movement. Norepinephrine plays roles in alertness and sleep. Epinephrine is found in low concentrations in the brain; however, in circulation, it functions as a hormone with major (primarily catabolic) effects on nutrient metabolism.
- Histidine, which is decarboxylated to generate histamine (shown previously in Figure 6.14). The neurotransmitter histamine mediates attention and alertness, among other possible roles.

Once neurotransmitters and biogenic amines have exerted their actions, the fastest mechanism for their inactivation is uptake by adjacent cells or synaptic terminals. Enzymes responsible for catecholamines and serotonin degradation include monoamine oxidase and aldehyde dehydrogenase; catechol-O-methyltransferase (which is found in the liver, kidneys, and smooth muscle but not the neurons) also can methylate the catecholamines to effect their slower degradation after transport via the blood. The well-known interaction between medications known as monoamine oxidase inhibitors and foods high in amines such as tyramine is discussed in the Chapter 13 Perspective on nutrient-drug interactions.

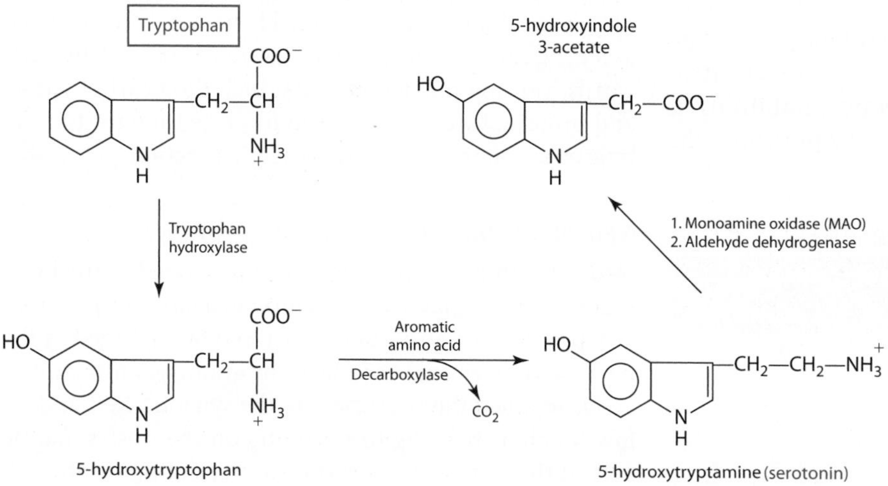

Figure 6.39 Serotonin synthesis (from tryptophan) and degradation.

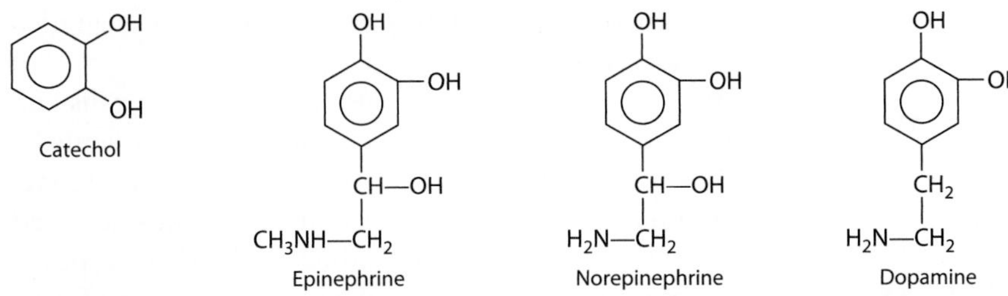

Figure 6.40 The structures of the catecholamines. The synthesis of these compounds is shown in Figure 6.10.

Other neurotransmitters are degraded by other pathways; histamine, for example, is catabolized by diamine oxidase.

Neuropeptides

Neuropeptides (also referred to as neuroactive peptides) are small proteinlike compounds that are similar to neurotransmitters but have more diverse effects. They are derived from amino acids but are not necessarily biogenic amines. The central nervous system abounds in neuropeptides; in fact, many of the same peptides that were discussed in Chapter 2 in association with the intestinal tract are also found associated with the central nervous system.

Neuropeptides perform a variety of functions. Some peptides act as hormone-releasing factors; ACTH, for instance, is involved with cortisol release. Some, such as somatotropin or growth hormone, have endocrine effects. Others, such as the enkephalins, have modulatory actions on transmitter functions, mood, or behavior. The enkephalins and endorphins, though similar to natural opiates, possess a wide range of functions, including affecting pain sensation, blood pressure, body temperature, body movement, hormone secretion, feeding, and modulation of learning ability. Some additional examples of neuropeptides include alpha melanocyte-stimulating hormone, neuropeptide Y, agouti-related peptide, ghrelin, and neurotensin, to name a few.

The neurosecretory cells of the hypothalamus are foremost in the secretion of the neuropeptides. Those that have hormone action move out of the axons of the nerve cells into the pituitary, from which they are secreted. This linkage between the nervous system and the pituitary is of great significance in the overall control of metabolism because the pituitary gland is primary in coordinating the various endocrine glands scattered throughout the body.

Neuropeptides are expressed and released by neurons. Because the nucleus and ribosomes in neurons are found in the cell body and dendrites, the neuropeptides, once made, must travel to the end of the axon to be stored in vesicles for future release. The neuropeptides are typically stored as inactive precursor polypeptides, which must be cleaved to generate an active neuropeptide, as shown here:

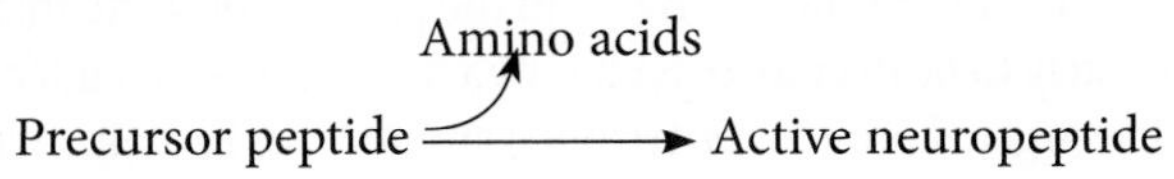

Amino acids

Precursor peptide ⟶ Active neuropeptide

Following synthesis of the active neuropeptide, it is released by exocytosis to perform its function at the membrane. After performing its function, the neuropeptide is hydrolyzed to its constituent amino acids.

Other Metabolic Roles of Amino Acids

While amino acids play important roles as neuropeptides, biogenic amines, and neurotransmitters in the brain and nervous system, they also serve other important functions. Glutamate is of significance as a means of ridding the brain of ammonia. Little glutamate is transported into the brain from the blood; rather, glucose that has been transported into the brain is metabolized to α-ketoglutarate, which can be converted to glutamate through reductive amination. Whenever excessive ammonia is present in the brain, glutamine is formed through the action of glutamine synthetase, which is highly active in neural tissues. A glutamate-glutamine cycle in the brain is thought to function as follows. Neurons take up glutamine and convert it to glutamate using glutaminase. The glutamate is released into the synapse (extracellular fluid) and then is taken up by astrocytes. Astrocytes convert the glutamate back to glutamine. The glutamine is then released. It can be reused by the neuron, but it is also freely diffusible and can move easily into the blood or cerebrospinal fluid, thereby allowing the removal of 2 mol of toxic ammonia from the brain. Any condition that causes an unusual elevation of blood ammonia (such as hepatic encephalopathy associated with advanced liver disease) can interfere with normal brain function, and treatment usually employs several strategies to reduce the blood ammonia concentration.

Leucine, as well as the other branched-chain amino acids, also provides the brain with nitrogen (amino groups). Astrocytes are thought to initially take up leucine and, using aminotransferases, remove its amino group for synthesis of glutamate and glutamine. Leucine's α-keto acid (α-ketoisocaproate), which is synthesized when the amino group is removed, is then taken up by neurons and reaminated to leucine using glutamate. Leucine and the other branched-chain amino acids are thought to provide 30% to 50% of the amino groups used by the brain for glutamate synthesis [17].

CATABOLISM OF TISSUE PROTEINS

Protein synthesis and protein degradation (i.e., protein turnover) are under independent controls but together account for about 10% to 25% of resting energy expenditure [18]. Rates of synthesis can be high, as with protein accretion during growth. Alternately, protein degradation can predominate, as during illness. Rates of protein turnover also vary among the body tissues, as is evidenced in the more rapid turnover of visceral protein as compared with skeletal muscle. Yet, because of its mass, muscle accounts for about 25% to 35% of all protein turnover in the body.

Degradation of proteins occurs primarily by the action of proteases, which are compartmentalized in the cytosol in lysosomes or proteasomes. The contributions of the lysosomes and proteasomes in proteolysis vary depending upon the tissue and the physiological status. Nonetheless, the constant degradation of proteins is of prime importance because it ensures a flux of amino acids through the cytosol that can be used for cellular growth and/or maintenance. This section of the chapter provides information on two main systems responsible for protein degradation within cells.

Lysosomal Degradation

Lysosomes are cell organelles (about 0.2–0.5 μm in diameter) that act like a cellular garbage digestive system to degrade proteins, nucleic acids, lipids, and carbohydrates, among other compounds. Lysosomes are found in all mammalian cells with the exception of red blood cells but in varying numbers. For example, skeletal muscles contain few lysosomes, whereas hepatocytes are particularly rich in lysosomes.

Lysosomes acquire proteins (and other substances) for degradation from extracellular sites, from the cell membrane, and from intracellular sites. Endocytosis is responsible for the internalization of most extracellular proteins as well as integral membrane proteins. The endocytosed proteins are sequestered in endosomes, which then fuse with lysosomes. The lysosomes contain a variety of digestive enzymes, including protein-digesting endopeptidases and exopeptidases known as cathepsins. Examples of cathepsins (designated by letters), which vary in specificity, include B, H, and L (cysteine proteases) and cathepsin D (an aspartate protease). These lysosomal enzymes, however, are active only at an acidic pH, which is achieved by a proton pump in the lysosomal membrane. This pump actively transports protons (H^+) from the cytosol into the lysosome to lower the lysosomal pH. Once activated, the proteases and other enzymes digest cellular proteins and components. No energy is needed for lysosomal digestion. The amino acids released from lysosomal proteolysis can be reused by the cell for protein synthesis or degraded based upon cellular needs.

Autophagy ("self-eating") also occurs within cells and involves the degradation of cytosolic cell constituents by the lysosomal pathway. There are three main types: macroautophagy, microautophagy, and chaperone-mediated autophagy. The most well-studied of the three types is macroautophagy, which involves sequestration of portions of the cytosol into vesicles called autophagosomes and subsequent fusion of the autophagosomes with lysosomes. Following acidification of the fused autophagosome-lysosome environment by proton pumps, proteins are digested by the lysosomal proteases. Autophagy is thought to be responsible for the degradation of longer-lived intracellular proteins as well as cellular organelles and macromolecules. Autophagy is induced under some pathological conditions and under conditions of nutrient deprivation. For example, autophagy in liver cells is enhanced by glucagon and suppressed by insulin and amino acids. The high glucagon:insulin ratio is consistent with conditions in which cells are nutritionally (amino acid) deprived. In liver cells, cellular uptake and accumulation of three amino acids—leucine, phenylalanine, and tyrosine—and increases in cell volume associated with the sodium-dependent cellular uptake of alanine, glutamine, and proline inhibit autophagy. The exact mechanisms by which this inhibition occurs are not known.

Proteasomal Degradation

In addition to lysosome-mediated cellular protein degradation, proteasomes (protease systems or complexes) also degrade proteins. Proteasomes are large, oligomeric structures with a central cavity for degradation. They are found in both the cytosol and nucleus of cells in two forms: 20S and 26S. The 20S proteasome consists of several subunits, of which three are responsible for protein degradation, specifically cleaving peptide bonds on the carboxy sides of acidic, basic, and hydrophobic amino acids. The 20S proteasome can be found bound by a 19S regulatory complex or cap to form a 26S proteasome, the form responsible for energy- and ubiquitination-dependent roles.

Ubiquitination is an ATP-dependent process by which proteins that are to be degraded are ligated to **ubiquitin**, a 76-amino acid polypeptide (Figure 6.41). The attachment of ubiquitin in effect marks the protein for degradation; however, before the ubiquitin can be linked to a protein, it must first be activated. Ubiquitin is activated by the enzyme E1. E1 is a subunit of the ubiquitin enzyme system, which hydrolyzes ATP to form a thiol ester with the carboxy end of ubiquitin. This activated ubiquitin is transferred to another enzyme protein, E2. Next, the carboxy end of ubiquitin is ligated by E3 to the protein substrate that is ultimately to be degraded. E3 has two distinct sites that interact with a targeted protein's N-terminal amino acid. Proteins with

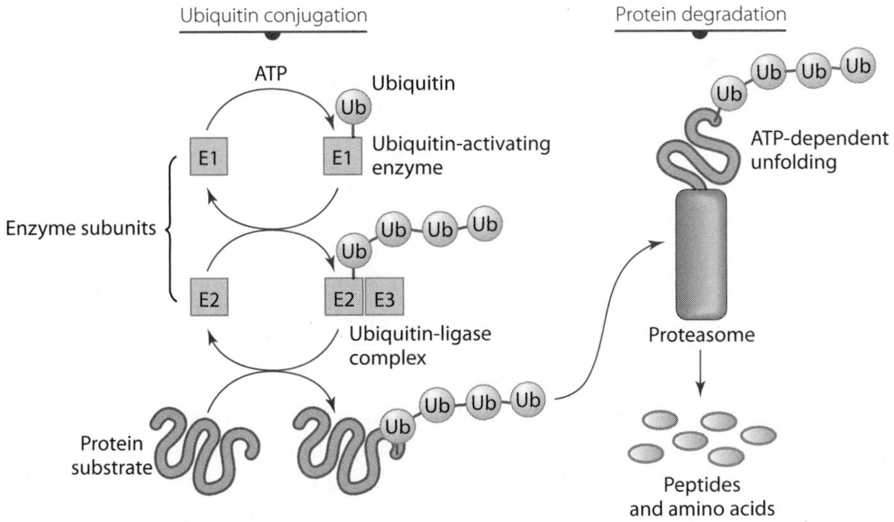

Figure 6.41 Proteasomal degradation of a protein.
Source: Adapted from 'The ubiquitin-proteasome proteolysis pathway: potential for target of disease intervention' by Breen, H.B. and Espat, N.J., 'Journal of Parenteral and Enteral Nutrition' 2004; 28:272–277. Copyright © 2004 by Sage Publications. Reprinted by permission of SAGE Publications.

N-terminal basic or large hydrophobic amino acids such as lysine, arginine, histidine, leucine, isoleucine, asparagine, glutamine, tryptophan, phenylalanine, and tyrosine are typically susceptible to degradation by the proteasomal system. One or more (typically five) ubiquitin proteins bind to a protein substrate; at least four ubiquitin proteins appear to be needed to ensure recognition and degradation by the 26S proteasome. ATP is required to unfold the tertiary and secondary structures of the proteins. Once ubiquitins are ligated to the protein to be degraded and the protein structure permits, proteases present as part of the proteasome degrade the ubiquitinated proteins in a series of reactions. Following proteolysis, ubiquitin is released for reuse, and the amino acids from the degraded protein can be reused.

The proteasomal system accounts for the majority of proteolysis in skeletal muscle. However, in muscle and perhaps other tissues (including neurons and the brain), another group of proteases, called calpains, also may initially participate. Calpains are calcium-activated proteases and are designated as 1, micro- or μ-calpain, and 2, milli- or m-calpain, with the nomenclature indicative of the different levels of calcium needed for activation. In muscle the calpain proteases appear to work in sequence with the proteasomal system, whereby the calpain proteases initiate the degradation of damaged/oxidized myofibrillar proteins. The released myofilaments are then ligated to ubiquitin for further degradation. The calpains also appear to play a role in protein synthesis by reducing the initiation of translation through inhibition of mTOR (which normally stimulates protein translation).

Proteasomal degradation is thought to be responsible for the degradation of abnormal, damaged, denatured, or mislocated proteins and of regulatory proteins that typically have short half-lives (often less than 30 minutes). Some peptides generated from proteasomal digestion of abnormal, mutant, or foreign proteins have been shown to bind to components of the body's immune system for antigen presentation; this process helps the body to further mount an immune response, enabling swift destruction of bacteria and viruses that have entered the body. Proteasomal degradation also has been shown to increase during starvation as well as in pathological conditions such as sepsis, cancer, and trauma. Cytokines are thought to be involved (in part) with its activation. A metabolite of leucine, β-hydroxy β-methylbutyrate (HMB), however, appears to be able to attenuate protein degradation by the proteasomal pathway, possibly by phosphorylating (inactivating) kinases that are involved in the expression of the proteasome. Regulation of this system is not completely understood.

CHANGES IN BODY MASS WITH AGE

The reference figures shown in Table 6.8, first developed in the 1970s, provide information on body composition, including muscle mass, based upon average physical dimensions from measurements of thousands of people who participated in various surveys [19]. These figures are a frame of reference with which to examine gender differences in body composition; they are not representative of an "ideal" body composition. As seen in Table 6.8, the reference man weighs 29.26 lb (13.3 kg) more and is 4 inches (~10 cm) taller than the reference woman (nonpregnant). Muscle accounts for 44.7% and body fat 15% (with 3% essential fat) of body weight in the male, whereas muscle is only 36.0% and body fat is 27% (12% essential fat) of body weight in the female. Essential fat is fat associated with bone marrow, the central nervous system, viscera (internal organs), and cell membranes, and in females, essential fat also includes fat in mammary glands and the pelvic region.

Table 6.8 Body Composition of Reference Man and Woman

Reference Man	Reference Woman
Age: 20–24 yr	Age: 20–24 yr
Height: 68.5 in (174 cm)	Height: 64.5 in (164 cm)
Weight: 154 lb (70 kg)	Weight: 125 lb (56.8 kg)
Total fat: 23.1 lb (10.5 kg) (15.0% body weight)	Total fat: 33.8 lb (15.4 kg) (27.0% body weight)
Storage fat: 18.5 lb (8.4 kg) (12.0% body weight)	Storage fat: 18.8 lb (8.5 kg) (15.0% body weight)
Essential fat: 4.6 lb (2.1 kg) (3.0% body weight)	Essential fat: 15.0 lb (6.8 kg) (12.0% body weight)
Muscle: 69 lb (31.4 kg) (44.7% body weight)	Muscle: 45 lb (20.5 kg) (36.0% body weight)
Bone: 23 lb (10.4 kg) (14.9% body weight)	Bone: 15 lb (6.8 kg) (12.0% body weight)
Remainder: 38.9 lb (17.7 kg) (25.3% body weight)	Remainder: 31.2 lb (14.2 kg) (25.0% body weight)

Sources: Adapted from Behnke A.R., Wilmore J.H., Evaluation and Regulation of Body Build and Composition. Englewood Cliffs, NJ: Prentice Hall, 1974; and Katch F.I., McArdle W.D., Introduction to nutrition, exercise, and health, 4th ed., Philadelphia: Lea & Febige, 1993, p. 235.

The difference in body composition is influenced not only by gender but also by other factors, including age, race, heredity, and stature. The influence of gender on body composition appears to exist from birth but becomes dramatically evident at puberty and continues throughout life. In both sexes, serum testosterone levels rise during adolescence; however, the increase is much greater in boys, whose testosterone values approach 10 times those of girls. As a result of this higher testosterone production and a growth spurt of longer duration, boys gain considerably more lean body mass than girls. Increased estrogen and progesterone concentrations and a shorter growth spurt duration contribute to greater gains in fat mass in females versus males during adolescence. The female achieves maximum lean body mass by about age 18 years, whereas the male continues accretion of lean body mass until about age 20 years. Such differences in lean body mass are largely responsible for the gender difference in nutrient requirements.

After 25 years of age, weight gain usually results from body fat accretion. As an example, healthy young (about age 25 years) men may average 20% body fat, while 55-year-old healthy men more likely average 30% body fat, and those who are 75 years old average 35% body fat. More marked increases occur in females than in males. In addition to the fat gains, lean body mass decreases (due primarily to a decrease in protein synthesis and body cell mass) with aging. Adults may gain about 1 lb of fat and lose about ½ lb of muscle (while often maintaining about the same or only a slight increase in body weight) between ages 30 and 60 years. The decline in muscle mass occurs predominantly after age 50 years at a rate of about 1% to 2% per year. Skeletal muscle loss may be (in part) due to decreased physical activity and altered protein metabolism;

the latter is thought to result from diminished anabolic hormone concentrations. A further effect of the decreased muscle mass with aging is a decrease in total body water, which is greater in females than in males. More specifically, extracellular fluid volume remains virtually unchanged, whereas interstitial fluid decreases, while plasma volume increases. Atrophy of organs as well as loss of bone mass also occurs with aging. The loss of bone mass is discussed in the Perspective at the end of Chapter 11.

Sarcopenia (*sarx* referring to "flesh" in Greek and *penia* meaning "loss" or "low") is an age-associated condition in which there is a loss of muscle and consequently decreased strength along with decreased metabolic rate. Specifically, skeletal mucle fiber numbers are diminished and the cross-sectional area of the remaining muscle fibers is reduced. Impaired muscle function results in increased risk of falls, diminished performance/physical disability, and frailty. Causes of sarcopenia are not completely understood but are thought to be multifactorial. Age-related loss of alpha motor neuron input to muscle is thought to be one major cause of the condition; this innervation is vital to muscle mass maintenance and strength. Age-associated oxidative damage in muscle also contributes, as it results in atrophy and loss of muscle fibers and muscle function. Moreover, with aging, the oxidized proteins generated in muscle may not be completely removed; this accumulation of "oxidized debris" diminishes muscle function and strength. Another cause of sarcopenia is likely the diminished concentrations of estrogen and testosterone, which normally have anabolic effects on muscle; the diminished hormone concentrations result in increased production of inflammatory cytokines (interleukins [IL] 1 and 6, tumor necrosis factor α, for example), which cause further catabolic effects. Altered insulin and growth hormone concentrations, which influence protein synthesis and degradation, also play roles in sarcopenia, as do the reduced protein intake and physical inactivity that can occur with aging. While prevention of sarcopenia may not be possible, the effects can be at least reduced by consumption of adequate protein (at least the Recommended Dietary Allowance [RDA]) and energy in combination with routine (about two to three times per week) resistance (strength) training.

PROTEIN QUALITY AND PROTEIN AND AMINO ACID NEEDS

Dietary protein is required by humans because it contributes to the body's supplies of indispensable amino acids and the nitrogen needed for the synthesis of the dispensable amino acids. The quality of a protein depends to some extent upon its digestibility but primarily on its indispensable amino acid composition—both the specific amounts and the proportions of these amino acids. Protein-containing foods can be divided into two categories:

- high-quality or complete proteins
- low-quality or incomplete proteins

A **complete protein** contains all the indispensable amino acids in the approximate amounts needed by humans. Sources of complete proteins are mostly foods of animal origin such as milk, yogurt, cheese, eggs, meat, fish, and poultry. The exceptions are gelatin, which is of animal origin but lacks the indispensable amino acid tryptophan, and soy protein, which is of plant origin but is a complete protein. **Incomplete proteins**, or low-quality proteins, are derived from plant foods such as legumes, vegetables, cereals, and grain products. Most plant foods tend to have too little of one or more particular indispensable amino acids. The term *limiting amino acid* is used to describe the indispensable amino acid that is present in the lowest quantity in the food. Listed in Table 6.9 are examples of incomplete protein–containing foods and their limiting amino acid(s). Unless carefully planned, a diet containing only low-quality proteins may result in inadequate availability of selected amino acids and may inhibit the body's ability to synthesize its own body proteins. The body cannot make a protein if an amino acid is missing.

To ensure that the body receives all the indispensable amino acids, certain proteins can be ingested together or combined so that their amino acid patterns become complementary. This practice or strategy is called mutual supplementation. For example, legumes, with their high content of lysine but low content of sulfur-containing amino acids, complement the grains, which are more than adequate in methionine and cysteine but limited in lysine. The lacto-ovo vegetarian should have no problem with protein adequacy because when milk and eggs are combined—even in small amounts—with plant foods, the indispensable amino acids are supplied in adequate amounts. One exception is the combination of milk with legumes. Although milk contains more methionine and cysteine per gram of protein than do the legumes, it still fails to meet the standard of the ideal pattern for the sulfur-containing amino acids.

The digestibility of proteins is also important for amino acid use. The digestibility of a protein is a measure of the amounts of amino acids that are absorbed following ingestion of the given protein. Animal proteins have been found to be about 90% to 99% digestible, whereas plant proteins are about 70% to 90% digestible. Meat and cheese, for example, have a digestibility of 95%, and eggs are 97%

Table 6.9 Examples of Incomplete Protein–Containing Foods

Food Source of Incomplete Protein	Limiting Amino Acid(s)
Wheat, rice, corn, other grains and grain products	Lysine, threonine (sometimes), and tryptophan (sometimes)
Legumes	Methionine

digestible. Cooked split peas are about 70% digestible, and tofu is about 90% digestible. Both the digestibility of a protein and its amino acid content affect protein quality.

Evaluation of Protein Quality

Several methods are available to determine the protein quality of foods. A few of these methods are discussed in this section.

Protein Digestibility Corrected Amino Acid Score

The protein digestibility corrected amino acid score (PD-CAAS) is a commonly used indicator of protein quality. In fact, foods intended for individuals over 1 year of age or with health claims must use the protein digestibility corrected amino acid score method to provide information on the product's food label. This method involves comparing the amount of the limiting amino acid for a test protein to the amount of the same amino acid in 1 g of a reference protein (usually egg or milk). The value is then multiplied by the test protein's digestibility, as shown in the following formula.

$$\text{PDCAAS (\%)} = \frac{\text{Amount (mg) of limiting amino acid in 1 g test protein}}{\text{Amount (mg) of same amino acid in 1 g reference protein}} \times \frac{\text{True}}{\text{digestibility (\%)}}$$

Examples of foods with a PDCAAS of 100 include milk protein (casein), egg white, ground beef, and tuna, along with some other animal products. Soybean protein has a PDCAAS of 94, and the values for various lentils, peas, and legumes range from <50 to about 70.

An alternate approach to this method involves a comparison of the amino acid composition of a test protein with a reference *pattern* (as opposed to reference protein). The reference pattern that has been selected for use for all people (except infants) is the amino acid requirements of preschool children age 1 to 3 years. The requirements of preschool children, which include needs for growth and development, are higher for each amino acid than are those of adults (who are not undergoing growth and development) and thus are considered to meet or exceed the needs of older people. This overall approach permits evaluation of the protein's ability to meet the nitrogen and indispensable amino acid requirements of people.

The scoring pattern, expressed as (mg amino acid)/(g protein), is calculated by dividing the requirements of individual indispensable amino acids (in mg) for children by the protein requirements (in g). The scoring pattern for foods intended for children age 1 year or older and for older age groups is shown in Table 6.10, along with the recommended amino acid scoring pattern for infant formulas

Table 6.10 Amino Acid Scoring/Reference Patterns and Whole-Egg Pattern [20]

Amino Acid	Infants (mg/g protein)	Children and Adults (mg/g protein)	Whole Egg (mg/g protein)
Histidine	23	18	22
Isoleucine	57	25	54
Leucine	101	55	86
Lysine	69	51	70
Methionine + cysteine	38	25	57
Phenylalanine + tyrosine	87	47	93
Threonine	47	27	47
Tryptophan	18	7	17
Valine	56	32	66

and foods, which is based upon the amino acid composition of human milk [20]. Table 6.10 also shows the whole-egg pattern.

Protein Efficiency Ratio

The protein efficiency ratio (PER) represents body weight gained on a test protein divided by the grams of protein consumed. This method of assessing protein quality is used by food manufacturers for infant formulas and baby foods and is reported on the product's food label. To calculate the PER of proteins, young growing animals are typically placed on a standard diet with about 10% (by weight) of the diet as test protein. Weight gain is measured for a specific time period and compared to the amount of the protein consumed. The PER for the protein is then calculated using the following formula:

$$PER = \frac{\text{Gain in body weight (g)}}{\text{Grams of protein consumed}}$$

To illustrate, the PER for casein (a protein found in milk) is 2.5; thus, rats gain 2.5 g of weight for every 1 g of casein consumed. However, a food with a PER of 5 does not have double the protein quality of casein, with a PER of 2.5. Furthermore, although the PER allows determination of which proteins promote weight gain (per g of protein ingested) in growing animals, no distinction is made regarding the composition (fat or muscle/organ) of the weight gain.

In addition to protein digestibility corrected amino acid score and protein efficiency ratio, which are used for nutrition labeling purposes, other methods—chemical or amino acid score, biological value, and net protein utilization—may be used to determine protein quality. A discussion of these methods follows.

Chemical or Amino Acid Score

The chemical score (also called the amino acid score) involves determination of the amino acid composition of a test protein. This procedure is done in a chemical laboratory using either an amino acid analyzer or high-performance liquid chromatography techniques. Only the indispensable amino acid content of the test protein is determined. The value is then compared with that of the reference protein, for example, the amino acid pattern of egg protein (considered to have a score of 100). The amino acid/ chemical score of a food protein can be calculated as follows:

$$\text{Score of test protein} = \frac{\begin{array}{c}\text{Indispensable amino acid}\\\text{in food protein (mg/g protein)}\end{array}}{\begin{array}{c}\text{Content of same amino acid in}\\\text{reference protein (mg/g protein)}\end{array}}$$

The amino acid with the lowest score on a percentage basis in relation to the reference protein (egg) becomes the first limiting amino acid, the one with the next lowest score is the second limiting amino acid, and so on. For example, if after testing all amino acids, lysine were found to be present in the lowest amount relative to the reference protein (e.g., 85%), the test protein's chemical score would be 85. The amino acid present in the lowest amount is the limiting amino acid and determines the amino acid or chemical score for the protein. Table 6.10 gives the amino acid pattern in whole egg. Comparison of the quality of different food proteins against the standard of whole-egg protein can be valuable but probably is not nearly as important to adequate protein nutriture as comparison with reference patterns for the various population groups.

Biological Value

The biological value (BV) of proteins is another method used to assess protein quality. BV is a measure of how much nitrogen is retained in the body for maintenance and growth rather than absorbed. BV is most often determined in experimental animals, but it can be determined in humans. Subjects are fed a nitrogen-free diet for a period of about 7 to 10 days and then fed a diet containing the test protein in an amount equal to their protein requirement for a similar time period. Nitrogen that is excreted in the feces and in the urine during the period when subjects consumed the nitrogen-free diet is analyzed and compared to amounts excreted when the subjects consumed the test protein. In other words, the change in urinary and fecal nitrogen excretion between the two diets is calculated. The BV of the test protein is determined through the use of the following equation:

$$\text{BV of test protein} = \frac{I - (F - F_0) - (U - U_0)}{I - (F - F_0)} \times 100$$

$$= \frac{\text{Nitrogen retained}}{\text{Nitrogen absorbed}} \times 100$$

where I is intake of nitrogen, F is fecal nitrogen while subjects are consuming a test protein, F_0 is endogenous fecal nitrogen when subjects are maintained on a nitrogen-free diet, U is urinary nitrogen while subjects are consuming a test protein, and U_0 is endogenous urinary nitrogen when subjects are maintained on a nitrogen-free diet.

Foods with a high BV are those that provide the amino acids in amounts consistent with body amino acid needs. The body retains much of the absorbed nitrogen if the protein is of high BV. Eggs, for example, have a BV of 100, meaning that 100% of the nitrogen absorbed from egg protein is retained. Although the BV provides useful information, the equation fails to account for losses of nitrogen through insensible routes such as the hair and nails. This criticism is true of any method involving nitrogen balance studies. A further consideration is that proteins exhibit a higher BV when fed at levels below the amount necessary for nitrogen equilibrium, and retention decreases as protein intake approaches or exceeds adequacy.

Net Protein Utilization

Another measure of protein quality, similar to nitrogen balance studies, is net protein utilization (NPU). NPU measures retention of food nitrogen consumed rather than retention of food nitrogen absorbed. NPU is calculated from the following equation:

$$\text{NPU of test protein} = \frac{I - (F - F_0) - (U - U_0)}{I} \times 100$$

$$= \frac{\text{Nitrogen retained}}{\text{Nitrogen consumed}} \times 100$$

where I is intake of nitrogen, F is fecal nitrogen while subjects are consuming a test protein, F_0 is endogenous fecal nitrogen when subjects are maintained on a nitrogen-free diet, U is urinary nitrogen while subjects are consuming a test protein, and U_0 is endogenous urinary nitrogen when subjects are maintained on a nitrogen-free diet.

Although NPU can be measured in humans through nitrogen balance studies in which two groups of well-matched experimental subjects are used, a more nearly accurate measurement is made on experimental animals through direct analysis of the animal carcasses. In either case, one experimental group is fed the test protein, while the other group receives an isocaloric, protein-free diet. When experimental animals are used as subjects, their carcasses can be analyzed for nitrogen directly (total carcass nitrogen, or TCN) or indirectly at the end of the feeding period. The indirect measurement of nitrogen is made by water analysis. Given the amount of water removed from the carcasses, an approximate nitrogen content can be calculated. NPU involving animal studies is calculated from the following equation:

$$\text{NPU} = \frac{\text{TCN on test protein} - \text{TCN on protein-free diet}}{\text{Nitrogen consumed}}$$

Proteins of higher quality typically cause a greater retention of nitrogen in the carcass than poor-quality proteins and thus have a higher NPU.

Net Dietary Protein Calories Percentage

The net dietary protein calories percentage (NDpCal%) can be helpful in the evaluation of human diets in which the protein to calorie ratio varies greatly. The formula is as follows: NDpCal% = Protein kcal/Total kcal intake $\times$ 100 $\times$ NPU_{op}, where NPU_{op} is NPU when protein is fed above the minimum requirement for nitrogen equilibrium.

Protein Information on Food Labels

Food labels are required to indicate the amount (quantity) of protein in grams and the % Daily Value for protein in a serving of food. As previously mentioned, the protein efficiency ratio (PER) is used to calculate the % Daily Value for infant formulas and baby foods. The U.S. Food and Drug Administration (FDA) specifies the use of the milk protein casein as a standard for comparison of protein quality based upon the PER. Specifically, for infant formulas and baby foods, if a test protein has a protein quality equal to or better than that of casein—that is, if the PER is ≥2.5—then 45 g of protein is considered equivalent to 100% Daily Value. If a test protein is lower in quality than casein—that is, if the PER is <2.5—then 65 g of protein is needed to provide 100% Daily Value. For foods other than baby foods, the protein digestibility corrected amino acid score (PDCAAS) method is used to establish the protein quality for % Daily Value on food labels. Specifically, 50 g of protein is considered sufficient if the food protein has a PDCAAS equal to or higher than that of milk protein (casein). However, 65 g of protein is needed if the protein is of lower quality than milk protein.

Assessing Protein and Amino Acid Needs

To prevent deficiencies, people need to achieve adequate intakes of energy and protein as well as other essential nutrients. Two techniques—nitrogen balance and indicator amino acid oxidation—are commonly used to assess the adequacy of protein and amino acid intakes.

Nitrogen Balance/Nitrogen Status

Nitrogen balance studies involve the evaluation of dietary nitrogen intake and the measurement and summation of nitrogen losses from the body. They can be conducted when subjects consume a diet with a protein (nitrogen) intake that is at or near a predicted adequate amount, less than (including protein-free nitrogen) a predicted adequate amount, or greater than a predicted adequate amount. This technique or modified versions of it are often used with hospitalized patients to determine whether protein intake is adequate.

To determine nitrogen balance or status, nitrogen intake and output must be assessed. Assessment of nitrogen intake is based upon protein intake. Protein contains approximately 16% nitrogen. Thus, to calculate grams of nitrogen consumed from grams of protein, we can do the following calculation: $0.16 \times$ protein ingested (measured in g) = nitrogen (measured in g). Expressed alternately, ingested protein (g)/6.25 = ingested nitrogen (g). So, for example, 70 g of protein intake provides 11.2 g of nitrogen. To reverse the calculations and convert grams nitrogen into grams of protein: protein (g) = nitrogen (g) $\times$ 100/16, or protein (g) = nitrogen (g) $\times$ 6.25.

Nitrogen losses are measured in the urine (U), feces (F), and skin (S). For example, in the urine, nitrogen is found mainly as urea but also as creatinine, amino acids, ammonia, and uric acid. In the feces, nitrogen may be found as amino acids and ammonia. To calculate nitrogen balance/status, nitrogen losses are summed and then subtracted from nitrogen intake (In). Thus, nitrogen balance/status = In $-$ [$(U - U_e) + (F - F_e) + S$]. The subscript e (in U_e and F_e) in the equation stands for *endogenous* (also called obligatory) and refers to losses of nitrogen that occur when the subject is on a nitrogen-free diet.

In clinical settings, nitrogen losses are often estimated. Fecal and insensible (including skin, nail, hair) losses of nitrogen are thought to account for about 1 g of nitrogen each for a total of 2 g. Urinary losses of nitrogen are measured either as total urinary nitrogen (UN), which gives the most accurate value, or as urinary urea nitrogen (UUN). If urinary urea nitrogen is measured, 2 g of nitrogen is usually added to this value to account for the urinary losses of other nitrogenous compounds such as creatinine, uric acid, ammonia, and so on. Thus, nitrogen balance/status = [protein intake (g)/6.25] $-$ [UN + 2 g], whereby the 2 g accounts for the fecal and insensible nitrogen losses, or nitrogen balance/status = [protein intake (g)/6.25] $-$ [UUN + 2 g + 2 g], whereby the first 2 g accounts for the losses in the urine of nonurea nitrogen compounds and the other 2 g accounts for the fecal and insensible nitrogen losses.

Nitrogen balance studies have been criticized for overestimating true nitrogen retention rates in the body because of incomplete collection or measurement of losses. In addition, nitrogen balance does not necessarily mean amino acid balance; that is, a person may be in nitrogen balance but in amino acid imbalance. The method often used in clinical settings to estimate losses can be inaccurate if the individual has larger than normal fecal nitrogen losses (as with diarrhea) or insensible nitrogen losses (as with excessive losses from skin with burns or fever).

Indicator Amino Acid Oxidation

Studies assessing protein and amino acid requirements have relied on the indicator amino acid oxidation technique. This method involves feeding test amino acids individually to a person in graded amounts in the presence of an indicator amino acid. The amounts of the test amino acid that are provided include quantities below, at, and above the expected requirement. The method is based upon a few principles, including (1) if a test amino acid is not provided, oxidation of the indicator amino acid will be maximal and protein synthesis will be minimal; (2) at an intake above the expected requirement of the test amino acid, oxidation of the indicator amino acid will diminish; and (3) at an intake that is the requirement for the test amino acid, oxidation of the indicator amino acid will be fairly constant. Thus, changes in the oxidation of the indicator amino acid reflect metabolism of the limiting amino acid in the body since if one amino acid is limiting for protein synthesis, other amino acids (including the indicator amino acid) would be "extra" and would need to be oxidized. Additionally, any "losses" of the amino acid associated with digestion, absorption, and cellular metabolism are accounted for. Most studies have relied on (1-^{13}C) phenylalanine in the presence of excess tyrosine, lysine, and leucine as the indicator amino acid. The technique has enabled the examination of the requirements for protein as well as the essential amino acids and some conditionally essential amino acids.

Recommended Protein and Amino Acid Intakes

Protein and amino acid requirements of humans are influenced by age, body size, and physiological state, as well as by the level of energy intake. Multiple studies using multiple methods, especially indicator amino acid oxidation, nitrogen balance studies, and the factorial method, have been used over the years to determine the protein and amino acid needs of adults. At present, the Estimated Average Requirement for protein for adults (men and women age 19 years and older) is 0.66 g of protein per kg of body weight, or 105 mg of nitrogen per kg of body weight per day [20]. This value represents the lowest continuing dietary protein intake necessary to achieve nitrogen equilibrium or a zero nitrogen balance in a healthy adult [20]. The Recommended Dietary Allowance (RDA) for protein for adults is 0.8 g of protein per kg of body weight per day [20].

The protein RDAs for children, adolescents, and adults, including women during pregnancy and lactation, are provided on the inside cover of this book. Instead of RDAs, the recommendations for protein for infants from birth to 6 months of age are given as an Adequate Intake (AI). The AI was derived from data from infants fed human milk as the primary nutrient source for the first 6 months [20].

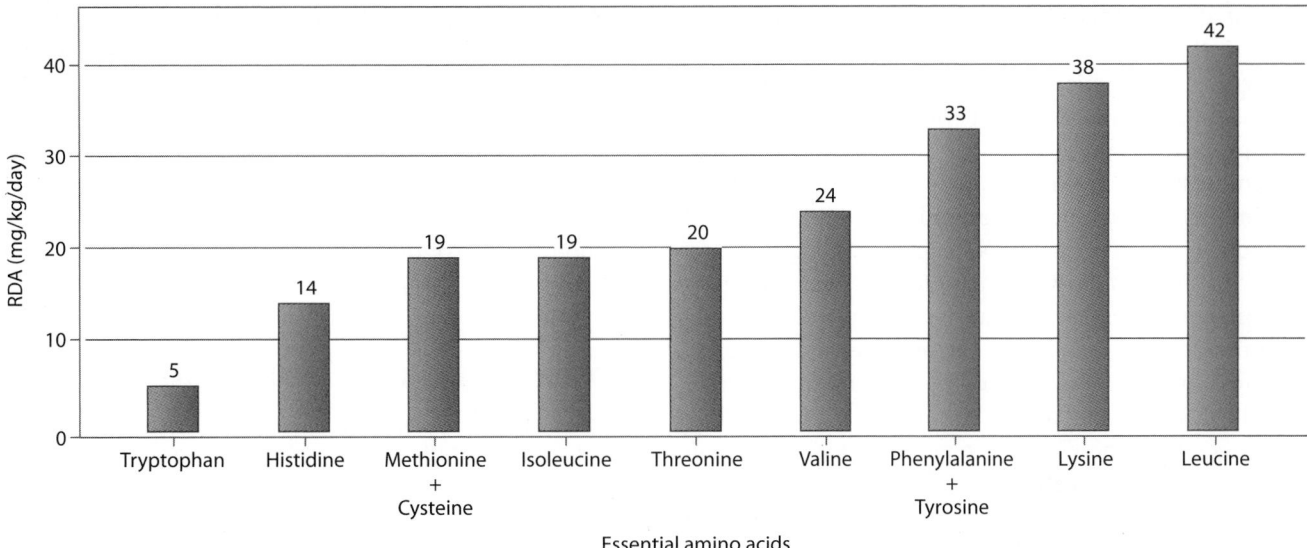

Figure 6.42 Recommended Dietary Allowances for indispensable amino acids for adults.

Source: Dietary Reference Intakes for Energy, Carbohydrate, Fiber, Fat, Fatty Acids, Cholesterol, Protein, and Amino Acids. Food and Nutrition Board, Institute of Medicine, Washington DC, National Academic Press, 2005, p. 680. Reprinted with permission from the National Academies Press.

In addition to recommendations for protein intake, RDAs for the indispensable amino acids have also been established. These recommendations, based upon a variety of methods including amino acid balance and indicators of amino acid oxidation studies, are shown in Figure 6.42. The reader is directed to the Dietary Reference Intakes for Energy, Carbohydrate, Fiber, Fat, Protein and Amino Acids [20] for in-depth information on the methods used in determining the recommendations for the amino acids and protein.

No Tolerable Upper Intake Level for protein or any of the amino acids has been established. The long-term effects of the ingestion of a diet supplying >35% of kilocalories from protein have not been well investigated. Only a few population groups routinely ingest high-protein diets. Weight lifters and body builders, for example, often ingest up to 3 g of protein/kg body weight, higher than the recommendation of about 1.2 to 1.8 (or up to 2) g of protein/kg body weight for athletes. Thus, intakes of 300 g of protein per day are not uncommon among some athletes [21].

Whether high-protein diets are detrimental to health is controversial. The most commonly cited hazards include increased risk of dehydration and possible kidney and bone damage. Dehydration, caused by the need to excrete large amounts of urea and other nitrogenous wastes from protein catabolism, can be prevented with appropriate fluid consumption. Renal damage in people with no prior history of renal problems has not been widely reported. Effects on bone vary; some studies suggest catabolic effects, and others suggest anabolic effects. The catabolic effects of a high-protein diet on bone are most commonly attributed to the generation of large amounts of acids from the

dietary protein, although other mechanisms have been proposed.

The effects of an acidic ash load are briefly reviewed here. Acidic as well as alkaline ash is produced in the body in varying amounts, based upon the foods consumed. For example, eating milk, yogurt, and fruits and vegetables produces more alkaline ash than acidic ash. In contrast, ingestion of meat, fish, eggs, cheese and, to a lesser extent, most grain products generate more acidic ash. Most of the acids generated by these protein-rich foods are thought to arise from oxidation of the sulfur-containing amino acids. Soft drinks (consumed in large quantities), however, also provide considerable amounts of acids (especially phosphoric acid) that are absorbed into the body. Excess acids in the body are excreted in the urine; however, the pH of the urine can only go so low—usually not less than about 4.5. A low-grade metabolic acidosis (in the blood) is thought to be generated by the production of relatively large amounts of acids from the ingestion of large amounts of high-protein foods and the presence of inadequate amounts of bicarbonate and other substances (derived largely from fruit and vegetable consumption) to buffer the acids. If the kidneys cannot completely excrete the excess acid load, and in the absence of adequate fruit and vegetable intakes to supply buffers, the buffering is thought to occur at the expense of bone, which releases calcium, magnesium, and carbonate, among other compounds, to serve as the buffers. (See also the Chapter 11 Perspective.)

Alternately, high-protein diets have been shown to promote anabolic effects on bone and even reduce fracture risk in older people. Moreover, some studies have suggested that elderly women may need more protein (> 0.84 g of protein/kg body weight) than is currently recommended to optimize bone mass [22,23]. Various mechanisms for the anabolic effects of protein on bone have been proposed. Amino acids, for example, are needed for the synthesis of proteins in bones. Moreover, amino acids and diets high in protein stimulate insulinlike growth hormone I, which promotes bone growth. It has also been found that in most individuals, protein intake is associated with increased phosphorus and calcium intakes, which diminish calcium losses. Further, any decreases in serum calcium concentrations caused by increased protein-induced calcium losses would stimulate parathyroid hormone secretion, increase active vitamin D synthesis, and thus increase calcium absorption. Effects on the bone are then thought to depend (at least partially) on the amount of calcium in the diet and the body's ability to make these hormonal changes. Clearly, the relationship between protein and bone health requires additional study, as do the long-term effects of a high-protein diet on health.

To help guide decisions in choosing good sources of protein, the U.S. Department of Agriculture (USDA) published the Food Patterns and MyPlate, which include five major food groups. MyPlate is designed for the consumer and can be accessed at www.choosemyplate.gov. From this site, an individual can determine the appropriate amount of foods recommended from each of the food groups. The amounts vary based upon a person's gender and age. Generally, however, the recommended quantities for adults from the meat, poultry, fish, eggs, beans, nuts, and seed group range from 5 to 6.5 oz per day, and the recommended amount from the dairy group is 3 cups per day depending on gender and age. Foods ingested from these protein-rich food groups should also be low in fat. Grains also provide some protein. Choices from this group should be high in fiber and low in fat; recommended amounts from the grain group for adults range from 3 to 4 oz or the equivalent per day depending on gender and age. One slice of bread, 1 cup of ready-to-eat cereal, or ½ cup of cooked cereal, pasta, or rice is equal to 1 oz equivalent.

In addition to the RDA for protein, the Institute of Medicine has published an Acceptable Macronutrient Distribution Range for protein of 10% to 35% of energy intake. Use of this range is appropriate as long as the intake of energy is adequate. If, for example, a person only ingests 800 kcal per day, then 10% to 35% of energy as protein equals 80 to 280 kcal; since protein provides 4 kcal/g, this translates into 20 to 70 g of protein. An intake of 20 g of protein is not sufficient for an adult to maintain nitrogen balance; however, depending on the age, gender, and body weight of the individual, 70 g may be more than adequate.

Protein Deficiency/Malnutrition

Protein deficiency can occur in those ingesting inadequate protein with or without adequate energy (kcal). Kwashiorkor is one form of protein malnutrition whereby people typically ingest enough energy, usually as carbohydrate, but insufficient protein. Kwashiorkor is characterized by poor (inadequate) visceral protein status, which is manifested by below-normal concentrations of total protein, albumin, retinol-binding protein, and prealbumin (transthyretin) in the blood. Without enough of these visceral proteins in the blood, water diffuses out of the blood (the intravascular space) into interstitial (intercellular) spaces, causing edema (swelling). The edema usually appears first in the legs but may also be present in the face or more generalized all over the body. Body weight, muscle mass, and adipose (fat) mass may be normal in those with kwashiorkor. The condition is widely seen in developing countries but is also seen in persons who are hospitalized with conditions such as burns, sepsis, trauma, or following major surgery. In these situations, protein needs are exceptionally high, and if the patient fails to consume adequate protein, malnutrition ensues.

Marasmus is a second form of protein malnutrition. People with marasmus are typically extremely thin (emaciated or underweight) with wasted (depleted) muscle mass and adipose tissue. Bones are prominent in appearance and the skin often droops or hangs from the body. Indicators of visceral protein status are typically within the normal range or just below the normal range but not decreased to the extent seen in kwashiorkor. Marasmus typically results from a chronic (prolonged) period of insufficient energy and protein intakes.

SUMMARY

Proteins in foods become available for use by the body after they have been broken down into their component amino acids. Nine of these amino acids are considered essential; therefore, the quality of dietary proteins correlates with their content of these indispensable amino acids. In the body, proteins play many vital roles including functions in structural capacities and as enzymes, hormones, transporters, and immunological protectors, among other roles.

An important concept in protein metabolism is that of amino acid pools, which contain amino acids of dietary origin plus those contributed by the breakdown of body tissue. The amino acids comprising the pools are used in a variety of ways: (1) for synthesis of new proteins for

growth and/or replacement of existing body proteins; (2) for production of nonprotein nitrogen-containing compounds; (3) for oxidation as a source of energy; and (4) for synthesis of glucose, ketones, or fatty acids.

The liver is the primary site of amino acid metabolism, but no clear picture of the body's overall handling of nitrogen can emerge without considering amino acid metabolism in a variety of tissues and organs. Of particular significance are the metabolism of the branched-chain amino acids in the skeletal muscle, the role of the intestine in citrulline production, and the role of the kidneys in the production of dispensible amino acids, nitrogen-containing compounds, and glucose as well as the elimination of nitrogenous wastes.

Of the nonessential amino acids, glutamine, glutamate, and alanine assume particular importance because of the versatility in the overall metabolism of these amino acids. Glutamate and its α-keto acid make possible many crucial reactions in various metabolic pathways for amino acids. An appreciation for the functions performed by glutamine and glutamate and the numerous amino acids functioning as or used to synthesize neurotransmitters, biogenic amines, and neuropeptides makes one realize that the term "dispensable" as applied to many amino acids may be quite misleading.

References Cited

1. Rose W. The amino acid requirements of adult man. Nutr Abstr Rev. 1957; 27:631–43.
2. Mahe S, Roos N, Benamouzig R, et al. True exogenous and endogenous nitrogen fractions in the human jejunum after ingestion of small amounts of 15N-labeled casein. J Nutr. 1994; 124:548–55.
3. Adibi S, Gray S, Menden E. The kinetics of amino acid absorption and alteration of plasma composition of free amino acids after intestinal perfusion of amino acid mixtures. Am J Clin Nutr. 1967; 20:24–33.
4. Shoveller A, Stoll B, Ball R, Burrin D. Nutritional and functional importance of intestinal sulfur amino acid metabolism. J Nutr. 2005; 135:1609–12.
5. Mendez C, McClain C, Marsano L. Albumin therapy in clinical practice. Nutr Clin Prac. 2005; 20:314–20.
6. Rebouche CJ. Kinetics, pharmacoekinetics, and regulation of L-carnitine and acetyl L-carnitine metabolism. Ann NY Acad Sci. 2004; 1033:30–41.
7. Anonymous. L-Carnitine. Alt Med Rev. 2005; 10:42–50.
8. Mesa JLM, Ruiz JR, Gonzalez-Gross MM, et al. Oral creatine supplementation and skeletal muscle metabolism in physical activity. Sports Med. 2002; 32:903–44.
9. Brosnan JT, Brosnan ME. Creatine: endogenous metabolite, dietary and therapeutic supplement. Ann Rev Nutr. 2007; 27:241–61.
10. Volek J, Rawson E. Scientific basis and practical aspects of creatine supplementation for athletes. Nutr. 2004; 20:609–14.
11. Artioli GG, Gualano B, Smith A, et al. Role of β-alanine supplementation on muscle carnosine and exercise performance. Med Sci Sports Exerc. 2010; 42:1162–73.
12. Derave W, Everaert I, Beeckman S, Baguet A. Muscle carnosine metabolism and β-alanine supplementation in relation to exercise and training. Sports Med. 2010; 40:247–63.
13. Food and Nutrition Board. Dietary Reference Intakes for Thiamin, Riboflavin, Niacin, Vitamin B6, Folate, Vitamin B12, Pantothenic Acid, Biotin, and Choline. Washington, DC: National Academy Press. 1998 pp. 390–422.
14. Matthews DE, Marano MA, Campbell RG. Splanchnic bed utilization of glutamine and glutamic acid in humans. Am J Physiol. 1993; 264:E848–54.
15. Morris S. Arginine: beyond protein. Am J Clin Nutr. 2006; 83(suppl):S508–12.
16. Van de Poll M, Soeters P, Deutz N, et al. Renal metabolism of amino acids: its role in interorgan amino acid exchange. Am J Clin Nutr. 2004; 79:185–97.
17. Yudkoff M, Daikhin Y, Nissim I, et al. Brain amino acid requirements and toxicity: the example of leucine. J Nutr. 2005; 135:S1531–38.
18. Welle S, Nair K. Relationship of resting metabolic rate to body composition and protein turnover. Am J Physiol. 1990; 258:E990–98.
19. Behnke AR, Wilmore JH. Evaluation and Regulation of Body Build and Composition. Upper Saddle River, NJ: Prentice Hall. 1974.
20. Food and Nutrition Board. Dietary Reference Intakes for Energy, Carbohydrate, Fiber, Fat, Protein and Amino Acids. Washington, DC: National Academy Press. 2002.
21. Gleeson M. Interrelationship between physical activity and branched chain amino acids. J Nutr. 2005; 135:S1591–95.
22. Devine A, Dick I, Islam A, et al. Protein consumption is an important predictor of lower limb bone mass in elderly women. Am J Clin Nutr. 2005; 81:1423–28.
23. Alexy U, Remer T, Manz F, et al. Long-term protein intake and dietary potential renal acid load are associated with bone modeling and remodeling at the proximal radius in healthy children. Am J Clin Nutr. 2005; 82:1107–14.

Suggested Reading

Journal of Nutrition 2008 volume 138. 7th Amino Acid Assessment Workshop
Report of the DGAC on the Dietary Guidelines for Americans 2010. Part D. Section 4. Protein.

THE IMPACT OF STARVATION, METABOLIC STRESS, AND LOW-GRADE INFLAMMATION ON BODY PROTEINS AND PROTEIN METABOLISM

In the healthy adult, protein synthesis approximately balances protein degradation. However, with starvation, sepsis (the presence of a pathogenic microorganism or its toxin in the blood and/or body tissues), and injury (including surgery, trauma, and burns), protein synthesis and protein degradation are not in balance. Further, the imbalance that occurs with sepsis or injury greatly exceeds that found in fasting (starvation) due to the metabolic stress that accompanies sepsis and injury but not starvation. This Perspective reviews the impact that starvation and metabolic stress, and to a lesser extent low-grade inflammation, have on body proteins and protein metabolism.

STARVATION

In starvation or when food is not consumed for prolonged periods, protein synthesis decreases. This decrease occurs because of both a reduction in mRNA needed for the translation of proteins and a decreased rate of peptide bond formation or RNA "activity." Even proteins with very rapid turnover, such as plasma proteins, are synthesized at a rate 30% to 40% below normal. In muscle, protein synthesis rates drop even lower. However, protein degradation rates decrease concurrently so that in chronic starvation daily nitrogen losses become quite small, about 4 to 5 g urinary nitrogen per day in most normal-weight individuals.

These changes in protein turnover with starvation result largely from alterations in hormone concentrations. In particular, insulin production decreases sharply. In addition, muscle and adipocytes become somewhat resistant to insulin's action so that whatever insulin is circulating is ineffective in promoting cellular nutrient uptake for protein synthesis and lipogenesis. Decreased insulin activity, coupled with increased synthesis of counter-regulatory hormones such as glucagon as well as catecholamines like epinephrine and glucocorticoids like cortisol, promotes fatty acid mobilization from adipose tissue, production of ketones, and proteolysis. Cortisol, in particular, promotes catabolism of muscle protein to provide substrates for gluconeogenesis. However, with prolonged starvation, cortisol and tri-iodothyronine (T_3, a thyroid hormone) secretion diminish; decreased T_3 in turn lowers the body's metabolic rate and thus energy needs.

In the initial stages or first few days of fasting or starvation, glycogen in the liver is depleted. Muscles undergo proteolysis. Urinary 3-methylhistidine excretion increases to reflect myofibrillar protein catabolism. Muscles undergoing proteolysis also release into the blood a mixture of amino acids containing relatively high alanine and glutamine concentrations. Alanine is a preferred substrate for gluconeogenesis and serves to stimulate the secretion of the gluconeogenic hormone glucagon. Alanine released from muscle is taken up by the liver, where the nitrogen is removed and converted to urea for excretion by the kidney and where the pyruvate can be used to make glucose by way of the gluconeogenic pathway. Glucose is also made in the liver from recycled lactate and pyruvate (the Cori cycle) and from glycerol released from adipose tissue lipolysis. Glucose formed in the liver may be released into the blood for cellular uptake and metabolism. Glutamine released from muscles circulates in the blood for uptake and metabolism primarily by the gastrointestinal tract and, over time, especially by the kidneys.

As fasting or starvation continues, tissues continue to use fatty acids and glucose for energy but also begin to use ketones formed in the liver from fatty acid oxidation. A decrease in protein catabolism (and thus urea synthesis) and gluconeogenesis occurs concurrently with the brain's and other tissues' adaptation to ketones as a source of energy. Acidosis increases, however, as ketone production accelerates. Consequently, more glutamine is directed to the kidneys (and away from other organs) for maintenance of acid-base balance. In the kidneys, the amino groups from the glutamine are used to produce ammonia. Ammonia can combine with hydrogen ions and be excreted in the urine to help correct the acidosis. The carbon skeleton from the glutamine is used in the kidneys to make glucose by gluconeogenesis. After about 5 to 6 weeks of fasting, splanchnic glucose production totals about 80 g per day with 10 to 11 g of glucose per day synthesized from ketones, 35 to 40 g per day from recycled lactate and pyruvate, 20 g per day from glycerol, and 15 to 20 g from amino acids (mostly alanine) released from muscle [1].

Figure 1a illustrates how adaptation to starvation allows the conservation of body protein. Fatty acids are shown generating ketones that are then used for energy by muscle. The use of the ketones means that less glucose is needed and allows the sparing of lean body mass. In other words, because less carbohydrate (glucose) is required by the body, less protein must be broken down to supply amino acids for gluconeogenesis. Amino acids resulting from proteolysis of muscle tissue can be used for the synthesis of crucial visceral proteins, which have more rapid turnover rates than muscle.

METABOLIC STRESS

Figure 1b depicts substrate use with metabolic stress, a hypermetabolic, catabolic state that occurs in response to sepsis, injury/trauma, and some diseases. In hypermetabolic states, basal metabolic rate (metabolism) is elevated above normal. The severity and length (or degree) of hypermetabolism typically correlates with the severity of the condition. For example, with minor surgery or injury, the rise in metabolism (and the catabolic state that also occurs) may last less than a week, whereas with severe burns or multiple traumatic injuries, it may last several months.

Like starvation, metabolic stress results in the degradation of body tissues. Adipose tissue undergoes lipolysis. However, with metabolic stress, the fatty acids generated from lipolysis do not produce ketones because ketogenesis is inhibited by insulin. Without the use of ketones, body proteins, especially those from white fast-twitch muscle, continue to be degraded to supply amino acids, which are used for the synthesis of glucose (gluconeogenesis) and more critical acute phase proteins (discussed in later paragraphs) [2]. Coupled with the metabolic stress-induced increase in muscle catabolism is a decrease in amino acid uptake and protein synthesis in muscle. Muscle cachexia, characterized by muscle wasting and weakness, results. With metabolic stress, urinary 3-methylhistidine excretion increases, reflecting increased protein catabolism, and overall urinary nitrogen losses frequently total 30 g or more per day. Each gram of nitrogen lost can be translated into the breakdown of *approximately 30 g* of *hydrated lean tissue* (whereby 1 g nitrogen = 6.25 g protein; muscle is about 80% water, so 80% of 30 g = 24 g, and 30 g muscle = 24 g water + 6.25 g protein). In metabolic stress, the body systems prioritize wound repair and host defense at the expense of body tissues, in essence gambling that convalescence or a return to health will occur before tissue depletion threatens survival.

The differences in substrate use between starvation and metabolic stress result in part from differences in hormone concentrations. Figure 2 demonstrates the endocrine response to metabolic stress. When these changes are combined with a diagnosis of sepsis and specific changes in heart and respiration rates, blood pressure, body temperature, and white blood cell counts, the term *systemic inflammatory response syndrome (SIRS)* may be used. As shown in Figure 2, with metabolic stress, glucocorticoids (primarily cortisol), catecholamines (e.g., epinephrine), insulin, and glucagon

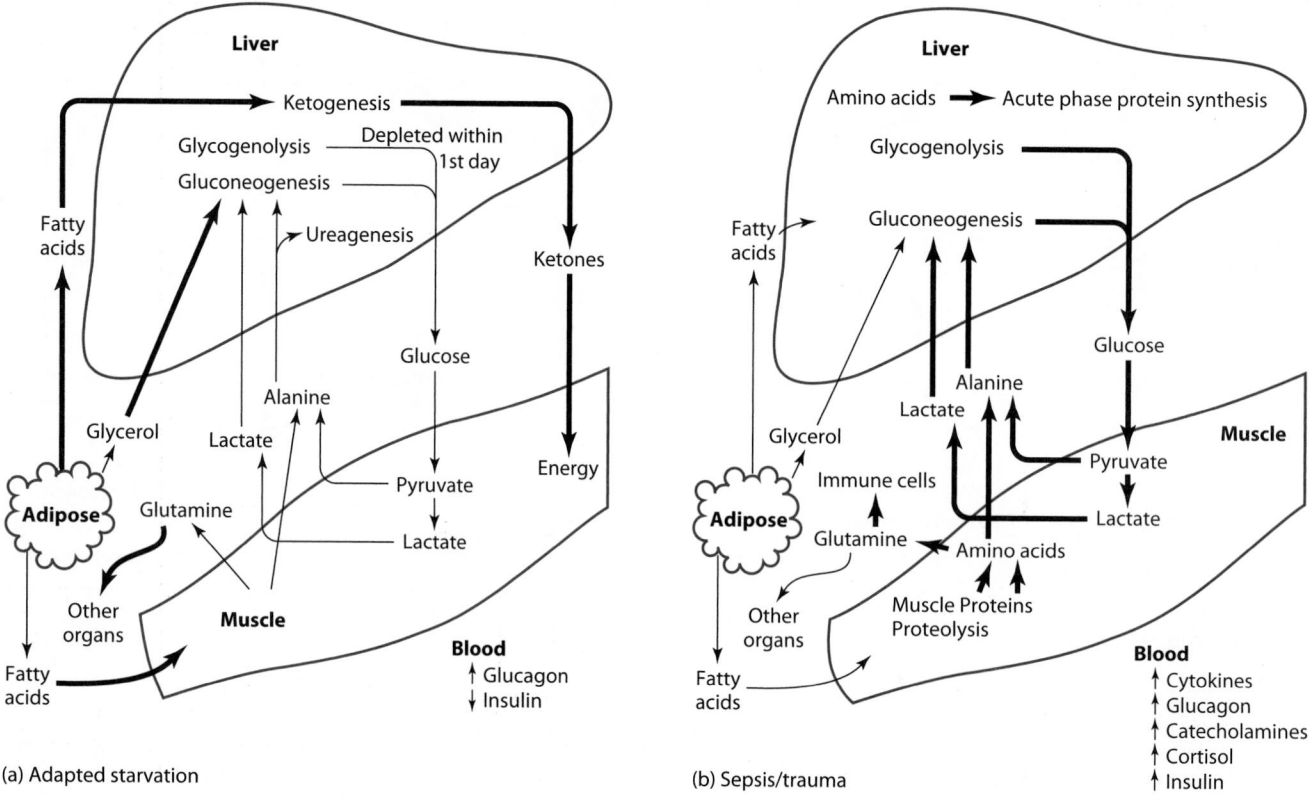

Figure 1   Substrate utilization during (a) adapted starvation and (b) sepsis/trauma. Note: Increased responses are shown by heavy black arrows.

release increase. However, the body's tissues become resistant to insulin action, and hyperglycemia (high blood glucose concentration) persists despite the presence of insulin. In addition, blood cortisol concentrations may remain elevated for prolonged periods and promote ongoing proteolysis and hyperglycemia in conditions such as extensive trauma. Additional hormonal changes associated with metabolic stress include the release of aldosterone and antidiuretic hormone. Aldosterone promotes renal sodium and fluid reabsorption, thus increasing blood volume. Antidiuretic hormone (ADH) inhibits diuresis (urination), also increasing blood volume. Both aldosterone and ADH help diminish fluid losses and restore circulation if it has been depressed by shock or as a result of fever, burns, and/or hemorrhage associated with injury or surgery.

In addition to differing hormonal responses, the release of cytokines in response to metabolic stress contributes to differences in substrate use as compared to starvation. Cytokines, low–molecular-weight peptides that evoke a number of varied reactions in the body, are produced mainly by immune system cells. Three cytokines—interleukin-1 (IL-1), IL-6, and tumor necrosis factor (TNF)-α—mediate many of the changes in hormone concentrations, such as increased cortisol, as well as changes in protein metabolism, including the acute phase response, that occur with metabolic stress and to a lesser extent with low-grade inflammation. During the acute phase response, selected proteins, especially muscle, are preferentially degraded (by the proteasomal system), whereas other proteins are selectively synthesized. The synthesis of proteins such as albumin, retinol-binding protein, and prealbumin that are normally produced by the liver and released into the plasma is decreased during metabolic stress, while the synthesis of another group of proteins—called acute phase reactant or response proteins—by the liver, macrophages, lymphocytes, and fibroblasts increases considerably. Some examples of the acute phase response proteins and their functions include:

- C-reactive protein, a protein that stimulates phagocytosis and activates complement proteins, which are needed for antibody-induced destruction of microorganisms; concentrations rise dramatically in response to inflammation, including that caused by infection or injury

- orosomucoid (α 1 acid glycoprotein), a protein with unclear functions but thought to be important in wound healing and immunomodulatory functions

- serum amyloid A, proteins with different isoforms resembling apolipoproteins, and which displace apoprotein A1 on high-density lipoproteins during an acute phase response; they are thought to recruit immune cells to inflammatory sites in the body

- fibrinogen, a protein that contributes to blood viscosity and can be converted to fibrin by thrombin to promote blood clotting; increased plasma fibrinogen may increase arterial thromboembolism (blood clot formation and dislodgement) risk

- fibrinonectin, a glycoprotein functioning in cell adhesion and wound healing

- haptoglobin, a protein that binds hemoglobin that has been released into the blood due to red blood cell hemolysis and inhibits microbial use of iron

- ceruloplasmin, a copper-containing protein with the ability to scavenge free radicals and with oxidase activity to promote iron oxidation and thus inhibit microbial iron use

- α2 macroglobulin, a protease inhibitor that, for example, inhibits blood coagulation and fibrinolysis

In addition to the synthesis of these proteins, more metallothionein (a zinc-containing protein) and ferritin (an iron-containing protein) are made in the liver with sepsis and inflammation. Consequently, hepatic zinc and iron concentrations increase, while plasma zinc and iron concentrations decrease. Such changes diminish the likelihood of microorganisms utilizing the body's zinc and iron for their own proliferation.

INFLAMMATION

Inflammation, specifically low-grade systemic inflammation, occurs with several chronic conditions, especially central/visceral obesity. The low-grade inflammatory state is thought to result from elevations in some of the same cytokines as those produced in metabolic stress, such as IL-1, IL-6, and TNF-α, but also interleukin (IL)-8 and interferon (IFN)-γ. However, with obesity, the adipose tissue and the stroma vascular

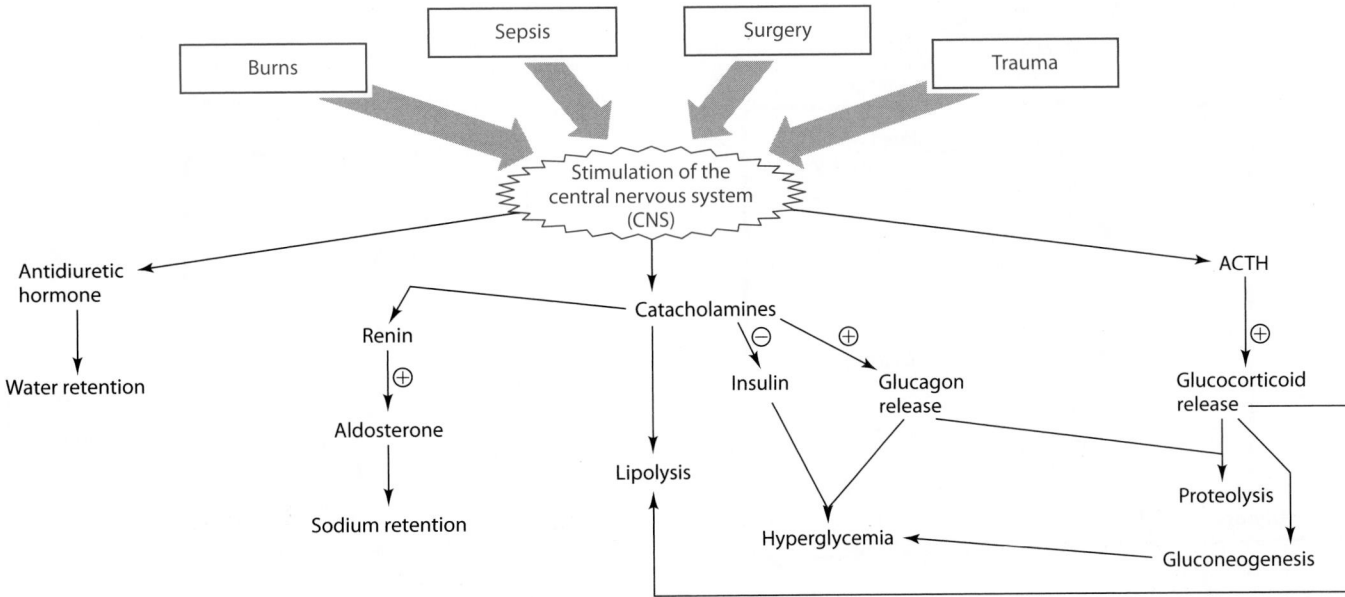

Figure 2 Response to metabolic stress.

fraction, a group of cells—including pre-adipocytes, fibroblasts, macrophages, and histocytes, among others—associated with white adipose tissue play a major role. These cells and tissues secrete cytokines as well as growth factors and adipokines (molecules secreted by white adipose tissue, such as resistin, visfatin, adiponectin), which either directly or indirectly promote inflammation. Moreover, macrophages that become embedded within the adipose tissue also induce inflammation. Obesity-induced inflammation is related mechanistically to chronic, low-grade sepsis [3] and results in up-regulation of systemic immunity and some of the same metabolic effects as found in those with metabolic stress (see Figure 1B). Serum concentrations of several acute phase reactant proteins, including plasma fibrinogen, orosomucoid (α1 acid glycoprotein), and C-reactive protein, are elevated with inflammation; concentrations of C-reactive protein may be 10-fold greater than normal in those with obesity [3].

While a discussion of the nutrition support for starvation, metabolic stress, and inflammation is beyond the scope of this text, it is important to note that inadequate nutrient intakes diminish the immune, antioxidant defense, and acute phase responses. Further, inadequate nutrient intakes can result in the atrophy of intestinal mucosa, which increases the likelihood of translocation of bacteria and toxins from the intestinal tract lumen into the blood. Research is focused on the development of specialized nutrition products rich in immunomodulating nutrients such as omega-3 fatty acids; phytochemicals like polyphenols, resveratrol, and catechins; and vitamin D, among other nutrients, to improve recovery from metabolic stress and inflammation.

References Cited

1. Cahill GF. Fuel metabolism in starvation. Ann Rev Nutr. 2006; 26:1–22.
2. Wray C, Mammen J, Hasselgren P. Catabolic response to stress and potential benefits of nutrition support. Nutr. 2002; 18:971–77.
3. Cave MC, Hurt RT, Frazier TH, et al. Obesity, inflammation, and the potential application of pharmaconutrition. Nutr Clin Prac. 2008; 23:16–34.

Suggested Readings

Bistrian B. Systemic response to inflammation. Nutr Rev. 2007; 65:S170–72.

Berger MM, Chiolero RL. Antioxidant supplementation in sepsis and systemic inflammatory response syndrome. Crit Care Med. 2007; 35:S584–90.

Levi M, Keller TT, van Gorp E, Cate H. Infection and inflammation and the coagulation system. Cardiovasc Res. 2003; 60:26–39.

7

INTEGRATION AND REGULATION OF METABOLISM AND THE IMPACT OF EXERCISE AND SPORT

CHAPTERS 3, 5, AND 6 FEATURED carbohydrate, lipid, and protein metabolism at the level of the individual cell, with emphasis on metabolic pathways common to nearly all eukaryotic cells. Those chapters also discussed how the pathways are regulated at the level of regulatory enzymes by substrate availability, allosteric mechanisms, and covalent modifications such as phosphorylation.

For their significance to be fully appreciated, metabolic pathways—and the specific metabolic roles of different organs and tissues—must be viewed in the context of the whole organism. Therefore, in this chapter we examine (1) how the major organs and tissues interact through integration of their metabolic pathways, (2) homeostasis of energy and the control between catabolism and anabolism, (3) hormonal regulation of these metabolic processes in maintaining homeostasis, and (4) examples of the body's ability to maintain homeostasis under the special circumstances of fasting, refeeding, and exercise. The Perspective at the end of the chapter discusses what happens when the control of these pathways falters, leading to "metabolic syndrome." The individual pathways are not reproduced again in this chapter. When appropriate, the reader is referred to pertinent sections in previous chapters where the pathways are described. A brief section on sports nutrition is included at the end of this chapter to demonstrate adaptation to special needs. The dynamics of substrate use in supplying energy for physical exercise provide a practical example of how the various metabolic pathways interrelate. Skeletal muscle, which represents about 43% of body mass by weight, uses a disproportionate amount of the body's energy reserves during exercise.

The interrelationship among carbohydrates, lipids, and proteins has been alluded to in the previous chapters. Each of these energy-producing nutrients can be metabolized to CO_2 and H_2O. The macronutrients are involved in reactions that are anabolic or catabolic and contribute to growth. Generally, anabolic reactions require energy and NADPH, and catabolic reactions produce energy (ATP, NADH, and $FADH_2$). The growth of the organism can be looked upon as the accumulation of macromolecules.

INTERRELATIONSHIP OF CARBOHYDRATE, LIPID, AND PROTEIN METABOLISM

If ingested in sufficient amounts, any of the three energy-producing nutrients—carbohydrate, fat, and protein (amino acids)—can provide the body with its needed energy on a short-term basis. (Alcohol is also an

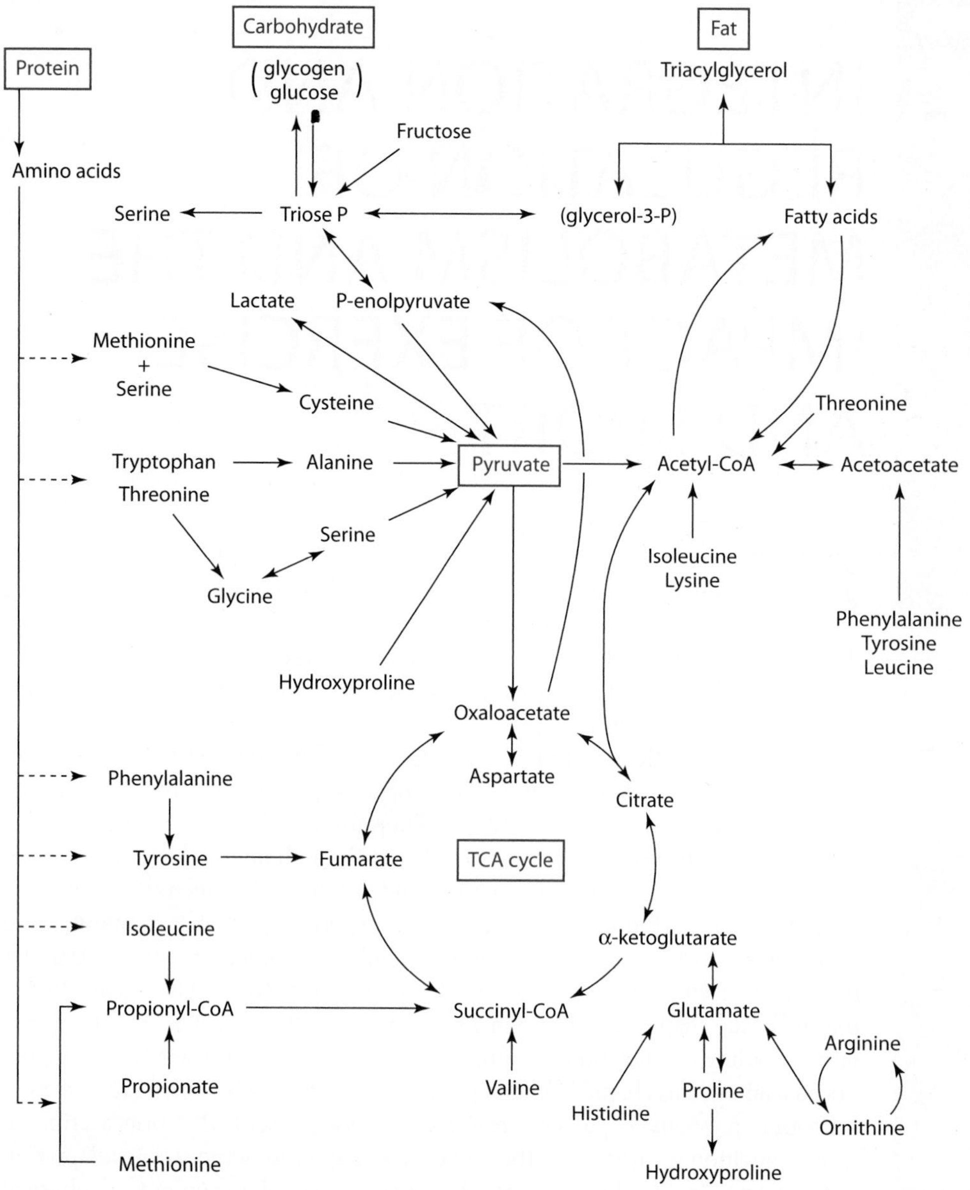

Protein

Carbohydrate
(glycogen)
glucose

Fat
Triacylglycerol

Amino acids

Fructose

Serine ← Triose P → (glycerol-3-P)　Fatty acids

Lactate　P-enolpyruvate

Methionine + Serine

Cysteine

Tryptophan → Alanine → Pyruvate → Acetyl-CoA ↔ Acetoacetate

Threonine

Threonine

Serine

Isoleucine
Lysine

Glycine

Phenylalanine
Tyrosine
Leucine

Hydroxyproline

Oxaloacetate

Aspartate

Citrate

Phenylalanine

Tyrosine → Fumarate

TCA cycle

α-ketoglutarate

Isoleucine

Propionyl-CoA → Succinyl-CoA　Glutamate

Arginine

Propionate

Valine　Histidine　Proline

Ornithine

Methionine

Hydroxyproline

Figure 7.1 Interconversion of the macronutrients.

energy-producing nutrient, but it is not considered a normal part of the diet and will not be considered in this discussion.) Within certain limitations, anabolic interconversion among the nutrients also occurs. For example, as explained in Chapter 6 and shown in Figure 7.1, certain amino acids can be synthesized in the body from carbohydrate or fat, and, conversely, most amino acids can serve as precursors for carbohydrate or fat synthesis. An overview of the metabolic interconversions among nutrients is given in Figure 7.1. Not evident from the figure, but important to recall, is that the tricarboxylic acid (TCA) cycle is an amphibolic pathway, meaning that it not only functions in the oxidative catabolism of carbohydrates, fatty acids, and amino acids but also provides precursors for many biosynthetic pathways, particularly gluconeogenesis (Figure 3.32). Along with pyruvate, several TCA cycle intermediates—including α-ketoglutarate,

succinate, fumarate, and oxaloacetate—can be formed from the carbon skeletons of certain amino acids and can function as gluconeogenic precursors.

MACRONUTRIENT INTERMEDIATES INTERCONVERSIONS

The fact that animals can be fattened on a predominantly carbohydrate diet is evidence of the apparent ease by which carbohydrate can be converted to fat. However, human lipogenesis from glucose is tightly regulated and requires energy sources and NADPH. A major factor in weight gain is the phosphorylation of key enzymes involved at the branch points in carbohydrate metabolism, which is controlled by the cellular concentrations of ATP,

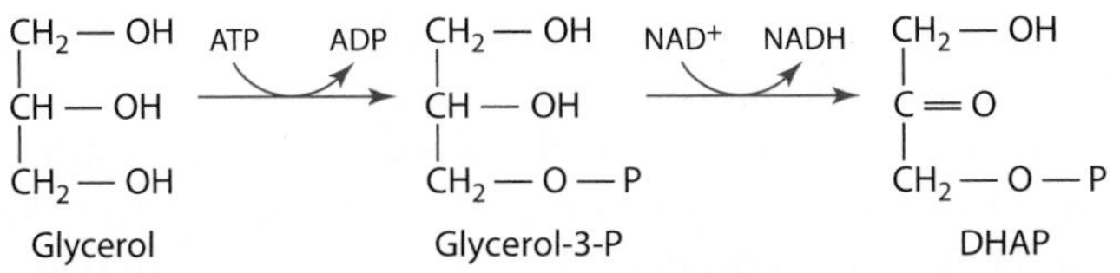

$$CH_2-OH \xrightarrow[\text{ATP} \quad \text{ADP}]{} CH_2-OH \xrightarrow[\text{NAD}^+ \quad \text{NADH}]{} CH_2-OH$$

$$CH-OH \qquad CH-OH \qquad C=O$$

$$CH_2-OH \qquad CH_2-O-P \qquad CH_2-O-P$$

Glycerol   Glycerol-3-P   DHAP

Figure 7.2 Phosphorylation and oxidation of glycerol to dihydroacetone phosphate (DHAP).

ADP, and AMP. One of the consequences of this enzymatic phosphorylation is the reduction of lipolysis rather than direct carbohydrate lipogenesis [1]. This topic is covered more extensively in a later section.

Glucose is the precursor for the glycerol of triacylglycerol (TAG) in adipose tissue. It can be formed from dihydroxyacetone phosphate (DHAP), a three-carbon intermediate in glycolysis (Figures 3.17, 7.2). Reduction of DHAP by glycerol-3-phosphate dehydrogenase and NADH produces glycerol-3-phosphate. The fatty acid components of TAG in adipose tissue can come from the diet, from adipose tissue (via lipolysis), or from the liver, where they are synthesized and packaged for delivery to adipocytes by VLDL or LDL. TAG is synthesized by the reaction of the glycerol-3-phosphate with CoA-activated fatty acids (Figure 5.30). Recall that muscle and adipose tissue lack the glycerol kinase that can phosphorylate glycerol directly and must obtain the glycerol-3-phosphate through glycolysis.

Key to metabolism and energy homeostasis is the fate of pyruvate and acetyl-CoA: whether they will be oxidized for energy or be stored. One option for pyruvate is the dehydrogenase complex that translocates pyruvate from the cytosol into the mitochondria while simultaneously decarboxylating it to acetyl-CoA. The acetyl-CoA can be oxidized to CO_2 and H_2O to produce ATP by the TCA cycle. Another fate of pyruvate is for it to be reduced in the cytosol to lactic acid. The lactate can be oxidized in the muscle or used for gluconeogenesis in the liver. Most of the acetyl-CoA is produced in the mitochondria through the β-oxidation of fatty acids. If it is to be involved in anabolic reactions, the acetyl-CoA has to be translocated back to the cytosol across the mitochondrial membrane, which is not permeable to it. Therefore, the acetyl-CoA in the mitochondria combines with oxaloacetic acid to form citrate (as in the TCA cycle), to which the mitochondrial membrane is freely permeable. The citrate moves into the cytosol and can break down again to oxaloacetic acid and acetyl-CoA. The acetyl-CoA may undergo a carboxylation reaction catalyzed by acetyl-CoA carboxylase to form malonyl-CoA, the first step of fatty acid synthesis (Figures 5.28 and 7.3).

While, as described previously, carbohydrate can be converted into both the glycerol and the fatty acid components of TAG, only the glycerol portion of TAG can be converted to carbohydrate. The conversion of fatty acids into carbohydrate is not possible because *the pyruvate*

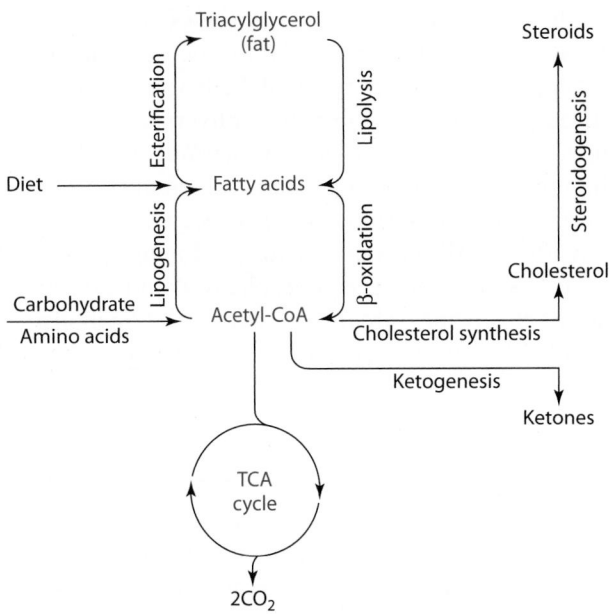

Figure 7.3 Overview of lipid metabolism, emphasizing the central role of acetyl-CoA.

dehydrogenase reaction is not reversible. This fact prevents the direct conversion of acetyl-CoA, the sole catabolic product of even-numbered-carbon fatty acids, into pyruvate for gluconeogenesis. In addition, gluconeogenesis from acetyl-CoA as a TCA cycle intermediate cannot occur, because for every two carbons in the form of acetyl-CoA entering the TCA cycle, two carbons are lost by decarboxylation in early reactions of the cycle (Figure 3.18). Therefore, there can be no net conversion of acetyl-CoA to pyruvate or to the gluconeogenic intermediates of the cycle. Consequently, acetyl-CoA produced from whatever source must be used for energy, lipogenesis, cholesterol synthesis, or ketogenesis (Figure 7.3).

Although fatty acids that have an even number of carbons are degraded exclusively to acetyl-CoA and therefore are not glucogenic (gluconeogenic) for the reasons mentioned, fatty acids that possess an odd number of carbon atoms are partially glucogenic. Fatty acids with an odd number of carbons can be partially converted to glucose because propionyl-CoA ($CH_3-CH_2-COSCoA$), ultimately formed by β-oxidation, is carboxylated and rearranged to succinyl-CoA, a glucogenic TCA cycle intermediate (Figure 5.26). Fatty acids with an odd number of carbon atoms are not common in the diet.

Metabolism of the amino acids gives rise to a variety of amphibolic intermediates, some of which produce glucose (glucogenic), while others produce ketone bodies (ketogenic) by their conversion to acetyl-CoA or acetoacetyl-CoA. Only the amino acids leucine and lysine are purely ketogenic. The dispensable (nonessential) glucogenic amino acids can be converted to carbohydrate, but like the ketogenic amino acids, they can also be converted (indirectly) into fatty acids by undergoing oxidation to acetyl-CoA. Fatty acids cannot be converted into the glucogenic amino acids for the same reason that fatty acids cannot be converted into glucose—namely, the irreversibility of the pyruvate dehydrogenase reaction. Although entirely possible, the conversion of the glucogenic amino acids into fat is rather uncommon. Only when protein is supplying a high percentage of calories would glucogenic amino acids be expected to be used in fat synthesis. All the amino acids producing acetyl-CoA directly—isoleucine, threonine, phenylalanine, tyrosine,* lysine, and leucine—are indispensable. The catabolism of the individual amino acids is covered in Chapter 6.

ENERGY HOMEOSTASIS

The body needs a constant supply of energy; thus, the homeostatic mechanisms available tend to protect against extended periods of fasting rather than periods of excessive energy intake. The interconversion of the energy-producing nutrients is skewed toward providing the organism with an energy source in a form that can be easily stored and accessed when it is needed (fat), thereby providing for times when food is not readily available. Energy released by the catabolism of the major nutrients must be shared by the energy-requiring synthetic pathways discussed earlier. On reaching the cells, the energy-producing nutrients can be catabolized to produce energy that is trapped in molecules with high phosphate transferring potential such as ATP, creatine phosphate, and so on; those with reductive energy including NADH, NADPH, and $FADH_2$; or both. Alternatively, the energy-producing nutrients may be synthesized into more complex organic compounds or macromolecules that become cellular components. For synthesis of a cellular component to occur, however, chemical energy must be provided. Therefore, when the cell places priority on synthesizing a particular component, another energy-producing material must be catabolized. The common energy pool within a cell is finite, and all anabolic and endergonic processes compete for this energy. When a liver cell is producing glucose by gluconeogenesis, for example, it cannot be synthesizing lipids and proteins at the same time. Instead, some of the existing cellular proteins or lipids are hydrolyzed, and the resulting amino acids or fatty acids are oxidized to generate the NADH and ATP needed for gluconeogenesis. Likewise, when hepatic de novo lipogenesis occurs, glucose must be used to produce the NADPH and ATP necessary for the conversion of acetyl-CoA to fatty acids.

There are a several points of regulation to control whether a cell or organ is producing energy (catabolism)

or is in the synthetic mode (anabolism). As discussed earlier, one key intermediate is acetyl-CoA. If energy is needed, the pyruvate from glycolysis is sent to the mitochondria, decarboxylated to acetyl-CoA, and oxidized via the TCA cycle to produce ATP through oxidative phosphorylation (Figures 3.18 and 3.29).

In addition to releasing energy, the mitochondrial processes are crucial for many other metabolic sequences:

- CO_2 produced by oxidation of acetyl-CoA is a source of cellular carbon dioxide for carboxylation reactions that initiate fatty acid synthesis and gluconeogenesis. This CO_2 also supplies the carbon of urea and certain portions of the purine and pyrimidine rings (Figures 6.7, 6.27, and 6.31).

- The TCA cycle provides common intermediates that provide the cross-linkages between lipid, carbohydrate, and protein metabolism, as illustrated in Figure 7.1. Particularly notable intermediates are α-ketoglutarate and oxaloacetate. Another interrelationship, not shown in Figure 7.1, is that between heme and an intermediate of the TCA cycle, succinyl-CoA. The initial step in heme biosynthesis is the formation of α-aminolevulinic acid from "active" succinate and glycine (Figure 13.6).

- TCA cycle intermediates—citrate and malate—intermesh with lipogenesis. Citrate can move from the mitochondria into the cytosol, where citrate lyase cleaves it into oxaloacetate and acetyl-CoA, the initiator of fatty acid synthesis. Malate, in the presence of $NADP^+$-linked malic enzyme, may provide a portion of the $NADPH^+$ required for reductive stages of fatty acid synthesis.

AMP-Activated Protein Kinase

ATP-producing and -consuming processes must remain in balance [2]. This is accomplished by regulatory systems that include AMP-activated protein kinase (AMPK). It is activated by an increasing AMP:ATP ratio (high AMP and low ATP), which signifies low energy. This can be caused by metabolic stresses that interfere with ATP production such as hypoxia or increased ATP utilization that occurs with muscle contraction. The lack of available glucose can also cause AMPK activation, so AMPK can function as a glucose sensor. When active, this protein kinase phosphorylates key enzymes involved in ATP formation. It switches on catabolic pathways that generate ATP and switches off ATP-consuming pathways such as the synthesis of lipids, glucose, glycogen, and proteins.

AMPK and Catabolic Pathways

AMPK activates a transporter protein in the cell that is involved in the translocation of GLUT4 to the membrane, which increases the uptake of glucose by hepatocytes and adipocytes. AMPK stimulates glycolysis

---

* Tyrosine is formed by hydroxylation of phenylalanine; therefore, its carbon skeleton cannot be synthesized in the body but must be obtained from food.

by phosphorylating 6-phosphofructokinase-2, which produces 2,6-bisphosphate, a powerful inhibitor to fructose-1,6-bisphosphatase, which is involved in gluconeogenesis. AMPK phosphorylates and inactivates acetyl-CoA carboxylase-2 (Chapter 3). This is an isoform of acetyl-CoA carboxylase that produces malonyl-CoA in the mitochondrial intermembrane space. Malonyl-CoA is an inhibitor of fatty acid uptake into the mitochondria via the carnitine:palmitate-CoA transferase-1 system (Figure 5.23). Since the inhibitor of fatty acid uptake is blocked, the result is the stimulation of fatty acid oxidation.

AMPK also switches off some anabolic enzymes by direct phosphorylation. Examples are HMG-CoA involved in cholesterol synthesis and glycogen synthase, the enzyme involved in glycogen synthesis. AMPK inhibits protein synthesis. A less immediate effect of AMPK is the expression of certain catabolic enzymes, which it achieves by phosphorylating some transcription factors and coregulators [2].

The role of AMPK is so central to energy homeostasis that a drug that activates AMPK in the liver, muscle, and vascular system has been developed. This medication, metformin, is the drug of choice to treat type 2 diabetes. Metformin appears to translocate GLUT4 to the cell surface by an insulin-independent mechanism, possibly the same mechanism that causes translocation of GLUT4 during exercise.

AMPK is key to the regulation of a number of biological systems that are designed to regulate whole-body energy balance and that go beyond just decreasing anabolism and increasing catabolism. For instance, leptin, a hormone released by adipose tissue to signal that the body has adequate energy stores, has different effects depending upon the tissue. In the muscle leptin stimulates AMPK, which increases catabolism, whereas in the hypothalamus leptin inhibits AMPK, which results in the suppression of appetite.

Malonyl-CoA, a Key Signaling Molecule

Malonyl-CoA, whose intermembrane space formation is inhibited by AMPK as discussed previously, plays a central role in energy homeostasis in its own right [3]. Malonyl-CoA and acetyl-CoA are part of a rapid energy cycle. If energy is not needed by the cell (i.e., the ATP:ADP ratio is very high), the acetyl-CoA will be transferred back to the cytosol from the mitochondria and carboxylated to form malonyl-CoA, which is the first step of fatty acid and sterol synthesis (Figures 5.28, 5.30, and 5.33). Malonyl-CoA is synthesized from acetyl-CoA and CO_2 in a reaction catalyzed by the enzyme acetyl-CoA carboxylase (ACC; Figure 5.28), and is decarboxylated back to acetyl-CoA by the enzyme malonyl-CoA decarboxylase (MCD). This cycle is rapid, and the size of the malonyl-CoA cellular pool appears to be determined by the activities of these opposing enzymes. In lipogenic tissues such as the liver, adipose tissue, and lactating mammary glands, malonyl-CoA is a cosubstrate for the cytosolic fatty synthase system for the de novo synthesis of palmitic acid (Chapter 5).

Malonyl-CoA is also involved in the elongation reactions of fatty acids in the ER.

There are two isoforms of ACC: ACC-1, which is thought to be the provider of malonyl-CoA for fatty acid synthesis and elongation, and ACC-2, which is located in the intermembrane space of the mitochondria and is inhibited by AMPK. Malonyl-CoA is an inhibitor of carnitine:palmitate transferase-2. The removal of this inhibition (by inhibiting malonyl-CoA synthesis) permits the transfer of fatty acids into the mitochondria and stimulates the β-oxidation of fatty acids to produce ATP. During the transition from fed to fasting, liver fatty acid metabolism is transitioned from de novo synthesis to β-oxidation. Returning to the fed state reverses this transition [3].

In cardiac muscle 50% to 80% of the energy is derived from fatty acids. Fatty acids provide less energy following consumption of a high-carbohydrate meal and more following a high-fat meal. The amount of malonyl-CoA in skeletal muscle is increased by glucose and insulin, resulting in a decrease in β-oxidation of fatty acids due to the inactivation of AMPK, which causes inhibition of the enzyme carnitine:palmitate transferase-2. Malonyl-CoA is also thought to function as one of the signals for β-cells of the pancreas to secrete insulin in response to elevated glucose blood levels. The elevated malonyl-CoA levels inhibit the transfer of fatty acids into the mitochondria, and the increased fatty acid levels in the cytosol act as a coupling factor for insulin secretion.

Malonyl-Co is also associated with the restraint of food intake. It acts through the hormone leptin released by adipose tissue to signal that TAG storage in adipose is adequate. This will be discussed in Chapter 8 under the section on the control of food intake.

THE CENTRAL ROLE OF THE LIVER IN METABOLISM

Each tissue and organ of the human body has a specific function that is reflected in its anatomy and metabolic activity. For example, skeletal muscle uses metabolic energy to perform mechanical work, the brain uses energy to pump ions against concentration gradients to transfer electrical impulses, and adipose tissue serves as a depot for stored fat, which on release provides fuel for the rest of the body. Central to all these processes is the liver. It plays the key role of processor and distributor in metabolism, furnishing by way of the bloodstream a proper combination of nutrients to all other organs and tissues. The liver thus warrants special attention in a discussion of tissue-specific metabolism.

Figures 7.4, 7.5, and 7.6 illustrate the fate of glucose-6-phosphate, amino acids, and fatty acids (respectively) in the liver. In these figures, anabolic pathways are shown

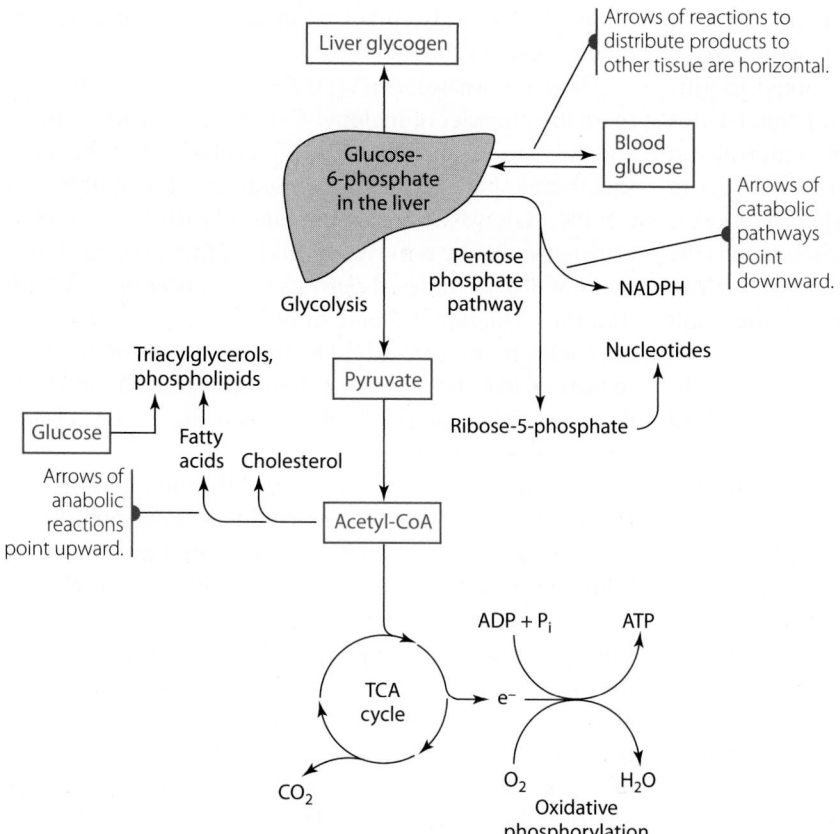

Figure 7.4 Metabolic pathways for glucose-6-phosphate in the liver.

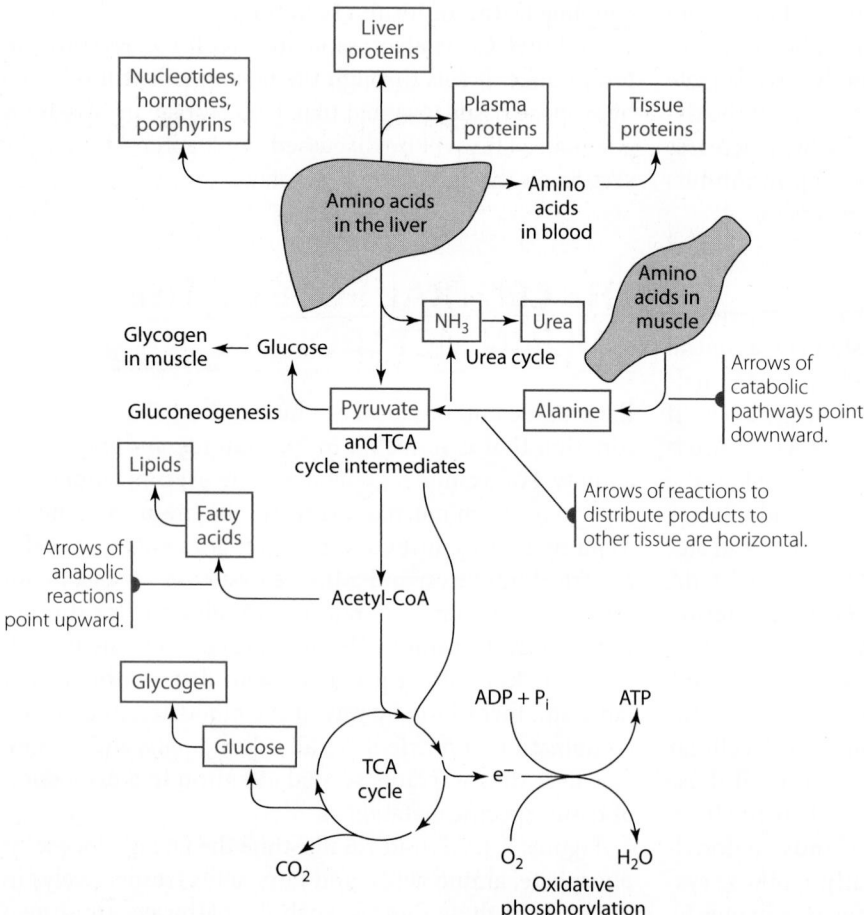

Figure 7.5 Pathways of amino acid metabolism in the liver.

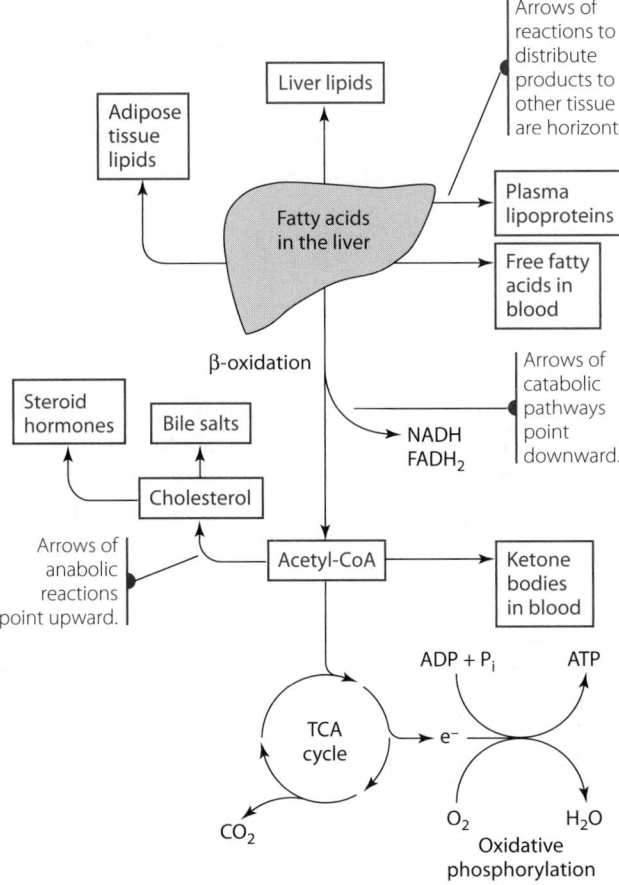

Figure 7.6 Pathways of fatty acid metabolism in the liver.

pointing up; catabolic pathways are pointing down; and distribution to other tissues is running horizontally. The pathways indicated are described in detail in Chapters 3, 5, and 6, which deal with carbohydrate, lipid, and protein metabolism, respectively.

Glucose entering the hepatocytes is phosphorylated by glucokinase to glucose-6-phosphate. Other dietary monosaccharides (fructose, galactose, and mannose) are also phosphorylated and rearranged to glucose-6-phosphate. Figure 7.4 shows the possible metabolic routes available to glucose-6-phosphate. Liver glycogenesis likely relies primarily on newly synthesized glucose derived from gluconeogenic precursors delivered to the hepatocytes from peripheral tissues as a substrate, rather than preformed glucose directly (Figure 3.13). This finding is referred to again in the following section.

Figure 7.5 reviews the particularly active role of the liver in amino acid metabolism. The liver is the site of synthesis of many different proteins, both structural and plasma-borne, from amino acids. Amino acids also can be converted in the liver into nonprotein products such as nucleotides, hormones, and porphyrins. Catabolism of amino acids can take place in the liver, where most are transaminated and degraded to acetyl-CoA and other TCA cycle intermediates. These substances in turn can be oxidized

for energy or converted to glucose or fat. Glucose formed from gluconeogenesis can be transported to muscle for use by that tissue. Newly synthesized fatty acids can be transported to adipose tissue for storage or used as fuel by muscle. Hepatocytes are the exclusive site for the formation of urea, the major excretory form of amino acid nitrogen.

The fate of fatty acids entering the liver is outlined in Figure 7.6. Fatty acids can be assembled into liver triacylglycerols or released into the circulation as plasma lipoproteins. In humans, most fatty acid synthesis takes place in the liver rather than in adipocytes. Adipocytes store triacylglycerols that arrive from the liver, primarily in the form of plasma VLDLs, and are released via lipoprotein lipase's action on chylomicrons. Under most circumstances, fatty acids are the major fuel supplying energy to the liver by oxidation. The acetyl-CoA that cannot be used for energy can be used for the formation of the ketone bodies, which are important fuels for certain peripheral tissues such as the brain and heart muscle, particularly during periods of prolonged fasting.

TISSUE-SPECIFIC METABOLISM DURING THE FED-FAST CYCLE

Carbohydrate and Lipid Metabolism

The best way to appreciate the interrelationship of metabolic pathways and the involvement of different organs and tissues in metabolism is to gain an understanding of the fed-fast cycle. The human typically eats specific meals followed by periods of not eating. Food consumption is often 100 times greater than basic caloric needs during the short period of time spent eating the meal, allowing humans to survive from meal to meal without nibbling continuously. Because glucose is a major fuel for tissues, it is important that glucose homeostasis be maintained, whether the person has just consumed food or is in a fasting state. If the period since the last meal is short (less than 18 hours), the mechanisms used to maintain glucose homeostasis are different from those used if the fasting state is prolonged. During prolonged fasts, other fuels gain importance, as discussed in the Chapter 6 Perspective. The extent to which different organs are involved in carbohydrate and fat metabolism varies within the fed-fast cycles that underlie the eating habits of the human being. When energy consumption exceeds expenditures, the excess calories are stored as glycogen and fat, which can be used as needed. A fed-fast cycle can be divided into four states, or phases:

- the fed state, which lasts about 3 hours after a meal is ingested

- the postabsorptive or early fasting state, which occurs from about 3 hours to about 12 to 18 hours following the meal

- the fasting state, which lasts from about 18 hours up to about 2 days without additional intake of food
- the starvation state or long-term fast, a fully adapted state of food deprivation that lasts as long as several weeks

Clearly, in a normal eating routine only the fed and postabsorptive (early fasting) states apply. The time frames of the phases cited are only approximate and are strongly influenced by factors such as activity level, the caloric value and nutrient composition of the meal, and the subject's metabolic rate.

The Fed State

Figure 7.7 illustrates the disposition of glucose, fat, and amino acids among the various tissues during the fed state. The red blood cells (RBCs) do not have mitochondria and therefore cannot oxidize fatty acids or glucose aerobically; they can oxidize glucose only anaerobically and produce lactate. The central nervous system (CNS) has no metabolic mechanisms by which glucose or fatty acids can be converted to energy stores. It cannot make glycogen or store triacylglycerols. Glucose available to these tissues is oxidized immediately to produce energy. In the liver, in contrast, some glucose can be converted directly to glycogen. Liver glycogen is synthesized indirectly from gluconeogenic precursors (pyruvate, alanine,

and lactate) returning to the liver from the periphery rather than directly from dietary glucose entering the liver by way of the portal vein (see Chapter 3). This preferential use of gluconeogenic precursors has been attributed to the low phosphorylating activity of the liver at physiological concentrations of glucose. A likely source of lactate for the liver is the RBCs, as indicated in Figure 7.7.

The liver is the first tissue to have the opportunity to use dietary glucose. In the liver, glucose can be converted to glycogen. When available glucose or its gluconeogenic precursors exceed the glycogen storage capacity of the liver, the excess glucose can be metabolized in a variety of ways, as shown in Figure 7.4 and in somewhat more detail in Figure 7.7. The conversion of glucose to glycogen and fatty acids is important because both represent the storage of glucose carbon. The potential conversion of excess glucose to fatty acids is particularly crucial because these fatty acids, along with those removed from the chylomicrons and VLDL by lipoprotein lipase, can be stored in the adipose tissue, thereby providing a ready source of fuel for most body tissues during the postabsorptive and fasting states. The conversion of glucose to fatty acids appears to occur only if energy intake exceeds energy expenditure.

Because liver glucokinase has a low K_m and is not fully active at physiological concentrations, some dietary glucose bypasses the liver and circulates to other tissues. The

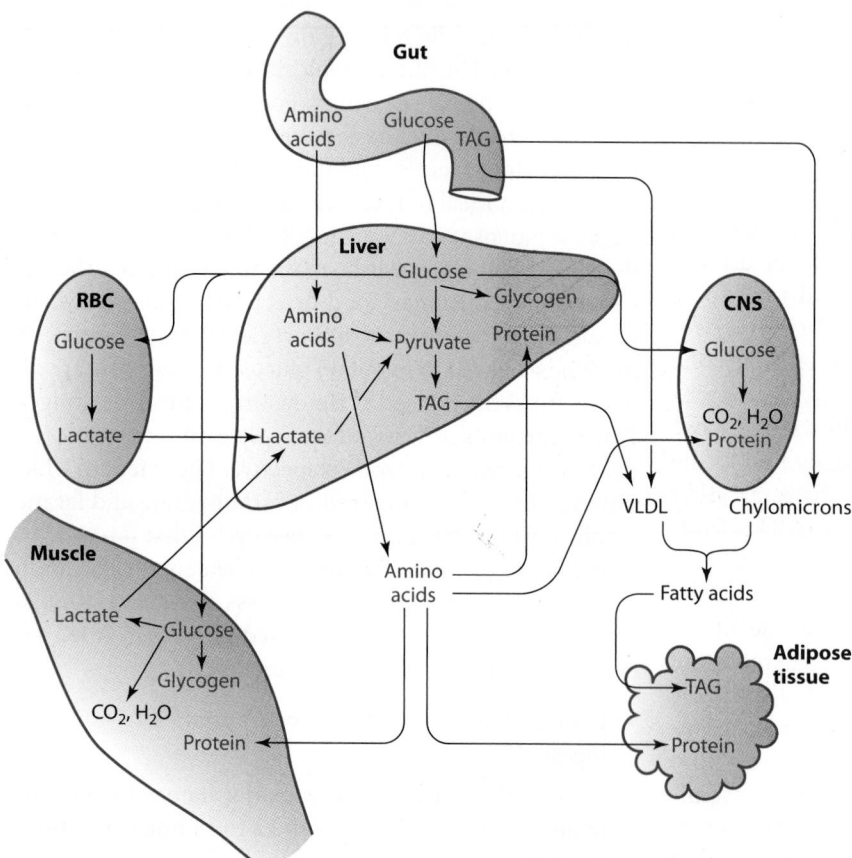

Figure 7.7 Disposition of dietary glucose, amino acids, and fat in the fed state.

brain and the central nervous system are almost solely dependent on glucose as an energy source during the fed and postabsorptive states. Other major users of glucose include:

- the RBCs, which, lacking mitochondria, convert glucose by way of the glycolytic pathway to lactate for the small amount of energy the cell requires and also use glucose as a source of NADPH through the pentose phosphate pathway

- adipose tissue, which can use glucose to some extent as a precursor for both the glycerol and the fatty acid components of triacylglycerols (although most TAG are synthesized by the liver and transported to the adipose tissue)

- muscle, which uses glucose for the synthesis of glycogen and for the production of energy

With the exception of the RBCs, all the tissues included in Figure 7.7 actively catabolize glucose for energy by glycolysis and the TCA cycle.

In considering fat delivery to the tissues, it is necessary to differentiate between dietary and endogenous fat. Dietary fat, except for short-chain fatty acids, enters the lymphatic system as chylomicrons, which are promptly acted upon by lipoprotein lipase from the vascular endothelium, releasing free fatty acids and glycerol (Chapter 5). Chylomicron remnants remaining from this hydrolysis are taken up by the liver, and their lipid contents are transferred to the very-low-density lipoprotein (VLDL) fraction. Endogenous fatty acids are made into TAG in the liver and excreted into the blood by exocytosis. Adipose tissue and other nonhepatic tissues take up the fatty acids from the lipoprotein particles following lipolysis (Chapter 5). In the adipocytes, fatty acids are reesterified with glycerol to form triacylglycerols and are stored as such as large fat droplets within the cells.

The Postabsorptive or Early Fasting State

With the onset of the postabsorptive state, tissues can no longer derive energy directly from ingested glucose or other ingested macronutrients but instead must begin to depend on other sources of fuel (Figure 7.8). During the short period of time marking this phase (a few hours after eating), hepatic glycogenolysis is the major provider of glucose to the blood, which serves to deliver it to other tissues for use as fuel. When glycogenolysis is occurring, the synthesis of glycogen and triacylglycerols in the liver is diminished, and the de novo synthesis of glucose (gluconeogenesis) begins to help maintain blood glucose levels.

Lactate, formed in and released by RBCs and muscle tissue, becomes an important carbon source for hepatic gluconeogenesis. The glucose-alanine cycle, in which carbon in the form of alanine returns to the liver from

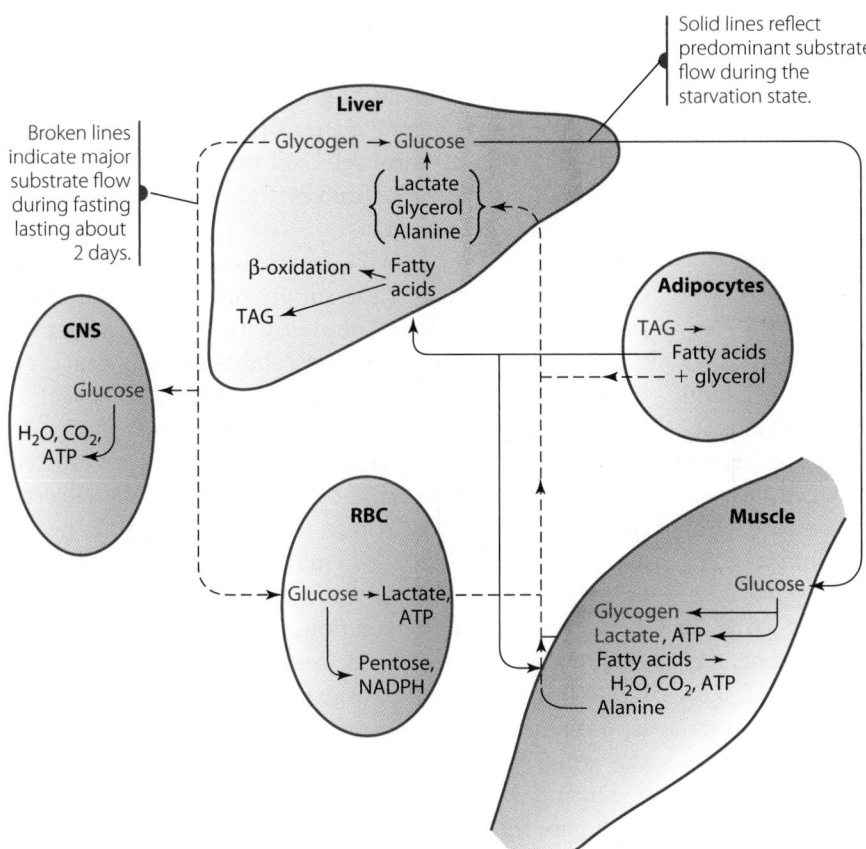

Figure 7.8 The primary postabsorption flow of substrates among the liver, CNS, adipose tissue, muscle, and red blood cells.
Source: Modified from Zakim D, Boyer T. eds., *Hepatology: A Textbook of Liver Disease*, 4th ed., Philadelphia: WB Saunders. Copyright Elsevier, 2003.

muscle cells, also becomes important. The alanine is then converted to pyruvate by the transfer of the amino group to α-ketoglutarate as the first step in the gluconeogenic conversion of alanine in the liver. Alanine cannot be converted to glucose in the muscle. In the postabsorptive state, glucose provided to the muscle by the liver comes primarily from the recycling of lactate and alanine and to a lesser extent from hepatic glycogenolysis. Muscle glycogenolysis provides glucose as fuel only for muscle cells in which the glycogen is stored, because muscle lacks the enzyme glucose-6-phosphatase, which converts glucose-6-phosphate to free glucose. Once phosphorylated in the muscle, glucose is trapped there and cannot leave except as three-carbon units of lactate or alanine.

The brain and other tissues of the CNS are extravagant consumers of glucose, oxidizing it for energy and releasing no gluconeogenic precursors in return. At rest, the brain uses about 20% of the available energy even though it is only about 2% of the body by weight. Mental activity does not increase energy utilization by the brain [4]. The rate of glucose use in the postabsorptive state is greater than the rate of glucose production by gluconeogenesis, and the stores of liver glycogen begin to diminish rapidly. In the course of an overnight fast, nearly all reserves of liver glycogen and most muscle glycogen have been depleted. Figure 7.8 shows the shifts of metabolic pathways that occur in the tissues during the postabsorptive state.

The Fasting State

The postabsorptive state evolves into the early fasting state after 18 to 48 hours of no food intake. Particularly notable in the liver is the de novo glucose synthesis (gluconeogenesis) that occurs in the wake of glycogen depletion (Figure 7.9). Amino acids from muscle protein breakdown provide the chief substrates for gluconeogenesis, although the glycerol from lipolysis and the lactate from anaerobic metabolism are used to some extent.

The shift to gluconeogenesis during prolonged fasting is mediated by the increased secretion of the hormone glucagon and the glucocorticosteroid hormones and low insulin levels in response to low levels of blood glucose. Proteins are hydrolyzed in muscle cells at an accelerated rate to provide the glucogenic amino acids. Of all the amino acids, only leucine and lysine cannot contribute at all to gluconeogenesis because they are ketogenic; however, as noted previously, these amino acids released by muscle protein hydrolysis serve a purpose as well. Because they are converted into ketones—that is, acetyl-CoA, acetoacetyl-CoA, acetoacetate, acetone, and β-hydroxybutyrate—they allow the brain, heart, and skeletal muscles to adapt to using these substrates if the nutritive state continues to deteriorate into a state of long-term fast or starvation.

The early fasting state is accompanied by large daily losses of nitrogen through the urine, in keeping with the high rate of breakdown of muscle protein and the synthesis of glucose through hepatic gluconeogenesis.

The Starvation State

If the fasting state persists and progresses into a starvation state (often referred to as a long-term fast), a metabolic fuel shift occurs again, this time in an effort to spare body protein. This new priority is justified by the vital physiological importance of body proteins. Proteins that must be conserved for life to continue include antibodies, which are needed to fight infection; enzymes, which catalyze life-sustaining reactions; and hemoglobin, which is necessary for the transport of oxygen to tissues. The protein-sparing shift at this point is from gluconeogenesis to lipolysis as the fat stores become the major supplier of energy. Fat stores, deposited when more calories were consumed than expended, are large in most people. The blood level of fatty acids increases sharply, and fatty acids become the primary fuel for the heart, liver, and skeletal muscle, which oxidize them for energy. The brain cannot use fatty acids for energy because they cannot cross the blood-brain barrier and instead adapts to using ketone bodies for energy. During starvation, two-thirds of the biological fuel for the brain comes from β-hydroxybutyrate and acetate [4]. The shift to fat breakdown also releases a large amount of glycerol, which replaces amino acids as the major gluconeogenic precursor, ensuring a continued supply of glucose as a fuel for RBCs. The kidney takes over the major role of producing glucose by gluconeogenesis. At this stage of starvation (several weeks), the visceral production of glucose is about 80 g/day: about 10 to 11 g/day from synthesis of glucose from ketone bodies, 35 to 40 g from gluconeogenesis from lactate and pyruvate, 20 g from glycerol released through lipolysis, and the remaining 15 to 20 g from hydrolyzed proteins' amino acids, mostly alanine [4].

Eventually, the use of TCA cycle intermediates for gluconeogenesis depletes the supply of oxaloacetate. Low levels of oxaloacetate, coupled with rapid production of acetyl-CoA from fatty acid catabolism, cause acetyl-CoA to accumulate, favoring formation of acetoacetyl-CoA and ketone bodies. Ketone body concentration in the blood then rises (ketosis) as these fuels are exported from the liver, which cannot use them. They are delivered through the bloodstream to the skeletal muscle, heart, and brain, which oxidize them instead of glucose. As long as ketone bodies are maintained at a high concentration by hepatic fatty acid oxidation, the need for glucose and gluconeogenesis is reduced, thereby sparing valuable protein. Figure 7.9 illustrates the changes in energy metabolism that occur in various tissues during the fasting and starvation states.

During this time the kidney becomes a major supplier of glucose through gluconeogenesis, using glycerol, glutamine, and α-ketoglutarate as substrates. The kidney also

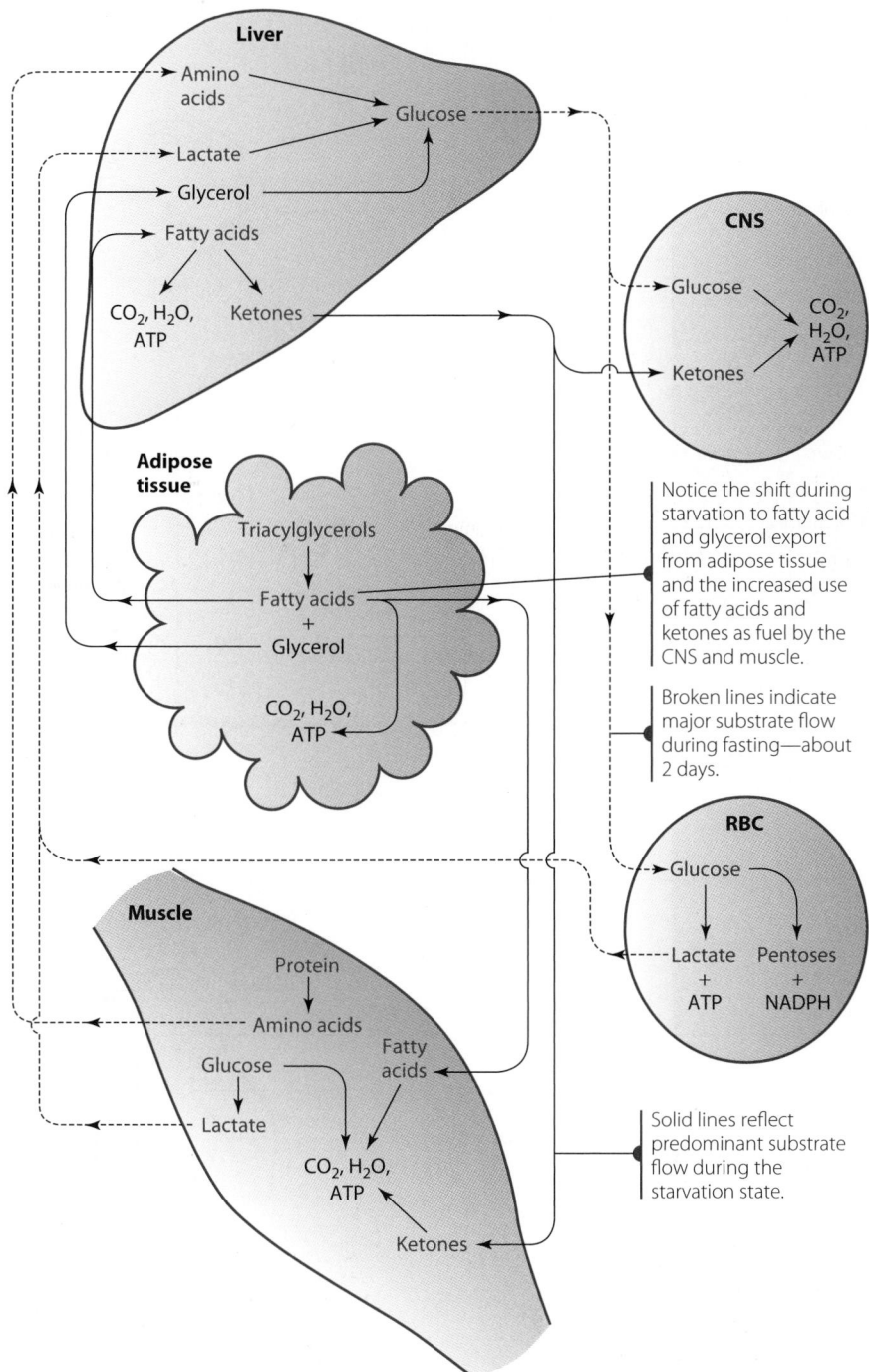

Notice the shift during starvation to fatty acid and glycerol export from adipose tissue and the increased use of fatty acids and ketones as fuel by the CNS and muscle.

Broken lines indicate major substrate flow during fasting—about 2 days.

Solid lines reflect predominant substrate flow during the starvation state.

Figure 7.9 Flow of substrates among the liver, CNS, adipose tissue, muscle, and red blood cells during fasting and starvation states.

produces NH_3 that helps neutralize the organic acids that are part of the ketone bodies. NH_3 is excreted as NH_4^+ in the urine.

Survival time in starvation depends mostly on the quantity of fat stored before starvation. Stored triacylglycerols in the adipose tissue of a person of normal weight and adiposity can provide enough fuel to sustain basal metabolism for about 3 months. A very obese adult probably has enough fat calories stored to endure a fast of more than a year, but physiological damage and even death could result from the accompanying extreme ketosis. When fat reserves are gone, the body begins to use essential protein, leading to the loss of liver and muscle function.

Amino Acid Metabolism

Organ interactions in amino acid metabolism, illustrated in Figure 7.10, are largely coordinated by the liver. The pathways shown undergo regulatory adjustments after consumption of a meal containing protein. In the fed state, absorbed amino acids pass into the liver, where the fate of most of them is determined in relation to needs of the body. Amounts in excess of need are degraded.

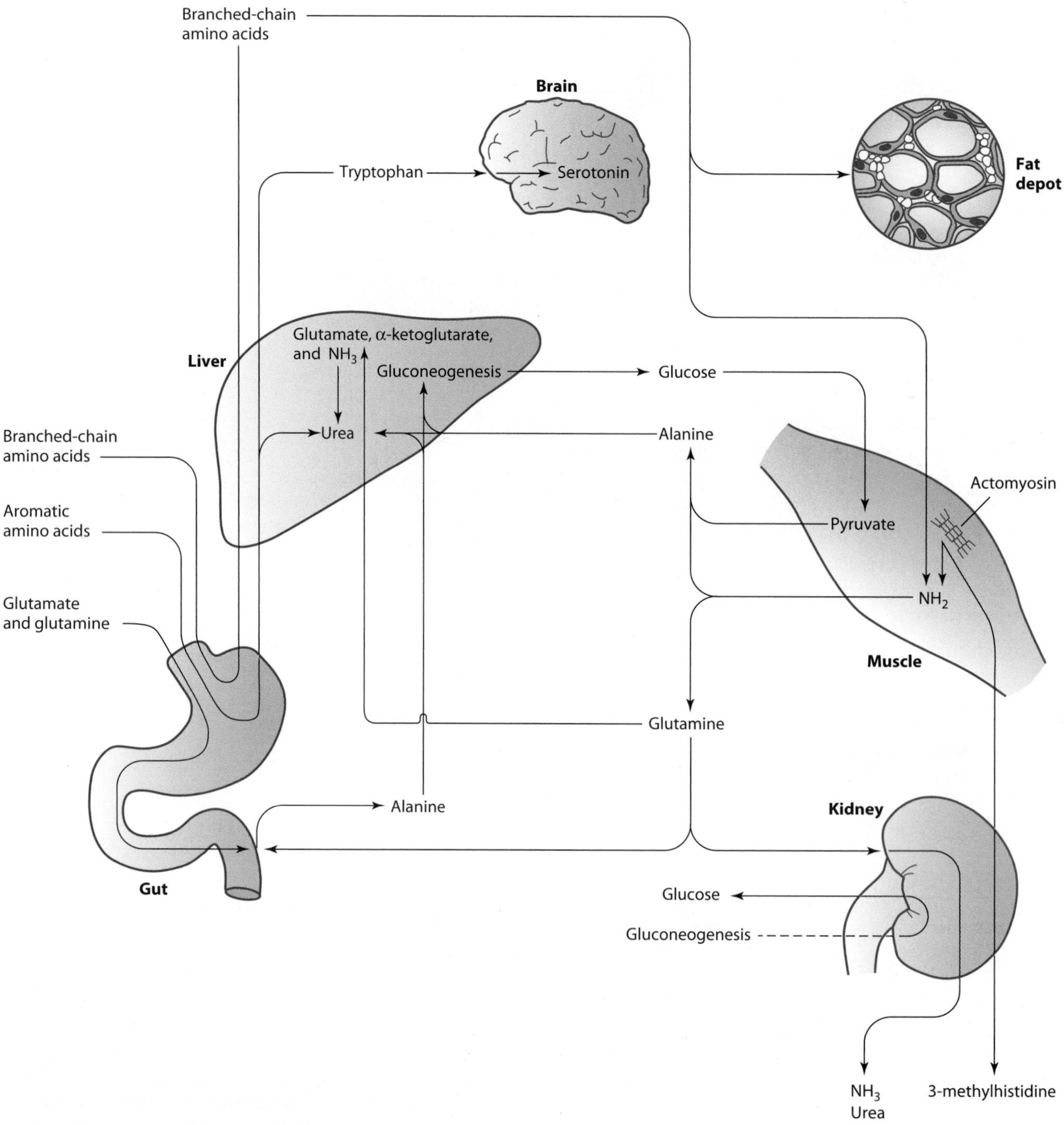

Figure 7.10   Interchanges of selected amino acids and their metabolites among body organs and tissue.

Source: Modified from Munro, H.N., Metabolic Integration of Organs in Health and Disease, 'Journal of Parenteral and Enteral Nutrition' 1982, 6; 4:271–279. Copyright © 1982 by Sage Publications. Reprinted by permission of SAGE Publications.

Only the branched-chain amino acids (BCAAs; leucine, isoleucine, and valine) are not regulated by the liver according to the body's needs. Instead, the BCAAs pass to the nonhepatic tissue, primarily to the muscles and adipose tissue, where they may be metabolized. Of particular interest is the fate of the BCAAs that reach the muscle. These amino acids are usually greatly in excess of the amount needed for muscle protein synthesis. The excess is believed to be used to synthesize the dispensable amino acids needed for the increase in protein synthesis that occurs after a protein meal. In the late fasting state the branched-chain amino acids do not leave the muscle after protein hydrolysis and are metabolized within the muscle. The nitrogen is released into the blood as glutamine or alanine [4].

The liver is the site of urea synthesis, the primary mechanism for disposing of the excess nitrogen derived from amino acids used for energy or gluconeogenesis. (Chapter 6 [see Figure 6.34] describes urea formation and the metabolism of glutamate, glutamine, and α-ketoglutarate.) The liver is active in removing the nitrogen from amino acids and uses the a-keto acids (amino acids from which the amine group has been removed) as the chief substrate. During fasting, gluconeogenesis becomes an important metabolic pathway in regulating plasma glucose levels, and even more nitrogen is available for excretion. Kidney gluconeogenesis is accompanied by the formation and excretion of ammonia.

The importance of the liver to muscle function during the fasting state or during very vigorous exercise is exemplified in the alanine-glucose cycle (Figure 6.35). During periods of fasting or strenuous exercise, the muscle breaks down protein to amino acids. The nitrogen from the amino acids is transaminated to α-ketoglutarate (formed in the TCA cycle) to make glutamic acid. The α-amino group from glutamic acid is then transaminated to pyruvate (formed from glycolysis) to make alanine. The alanine enters the bloodstream and is transported to the liver, where it again transaminates its amino group to α-ketoglutarate. Alanine is converted to pyruvate, and α-ketoglutarate is converted to glutamic acid. This cycle serves several functions. It removes the nitrogen from muscle during a period of high proteolysis and transports it to the liver in the form of alanine. This process also transfers the carbon structure of pyruvate to the liver, where it can be made into glucose through gluconeogenesis. The synthesized glucose can be transported back to the muscle and used for energy by that tissue. The glucose-alanine cycle also acts as a carrier of amino-nitrogen from intestinal mucosal cells to the liver during periods of amino acid absorption.

Glutamine also plays a central role in transporting and excreting amino acid nitrogen. Many tissues, including the brain, combine ammonia, released primarily by the glutamate dehydrogenase reaction, with glutamate to form glutamine. The reaction is catalyzed by glutamine synthetase. In the form of glutamine, ammonia can then be carried to the liver or kidneys for excretion as urea or ammonium ion, respectively. In those tissues, glutamine is acted upon by the enzyme glutaminase, releasing the ammonia for excretion and re-forming glutamate. Figure 7.10 gives an overview of organ cooperation in these and other aspects of glutamine and other amino acid metabolism. See Chapter 6 for a more detailed discussion of amino acid metabolism in general.

As stated previously, the kidney is a major site of glucose synthesis (gluconeogenesis) during starvation [4,5]. The quantity of glucose produced by the kidney exceeds the amount of glutamine available to the kidney. During the postabsorptive state (overnight fast), the kidney contributes about 20% of glucose by gluconeogenesis. The substrates glutamine, glycerol, and alanine account for about a third of the amount released; the source of the remainder has not yet been explained but may be lactate [6].

SYSTEM INTEGRATION AND HOMEOSTASIS

Integration of the metabolic processes, as outlined in the preceding sections, allows the "constancy of the internal milieu" of humans and other multicellular organisms that was described by the French physiologist Claude Bernard over a century ago. This integration of metabolism at the cellular and the organ and tissue levels, which is essential for the survival of the entire organism, receives its direction from body systems. The integration of body systems makes possible communication among all parts of the body.

Three major systems direct activities of the cells, tissues, and organs to ensure their harmony with the whole organism: the nervous, endocrine, and vascular systems.

The nervous system is considered the primary communication system because it not only has receiving mechanisms to assess the body's status in relation to its environment but also has transmitting processes to relay appropriate commands to various tissues and organs. The nervous system can inform the body of conditions such as hunger, thirst, pain, and lack of oxygen. This information allows organs to adjust to external changes and may initiate appropriate behavior by the whole organism. The nervous system can be compared to an elaborate system of wires connecting from the source of message initiation (the brain) to the place where message reception has its needed effect (peripheral tissue).

The endocrine system also carries messages to the organs of the body by way of highly specialized substances called hormones. The endocrine system depends upon the vascular system to carry messages to target tissues.

The vascular system can be thought of as a plumbing system with flexible pipes. When the heart contracts, the pipes expand with the increased pressure and then shrink as the heart goes into the diastolic phase. The vascular system is the primary transport mechanism for the body, not only delivering specialized chemical substances but also carrying oxygen, organic nutrients, and minerals from the external environment to cells throughout the body. The vascular system transports the waste products of metabolism from the cells, carrying them to the lungs, skin, and kidneys for elimination.

The concentration of solutes in the blood must be regulated within a narrow range. Among the most prominent sentinel cells that monitor and regulate solute concentration are those that synthesize and secrete hormones. Although hormone synthesis and secretion occur primarily in the endocrine system, considerable overlap exists between the endocrine system and the CNS. With the discovery of a variety of neuropeptides and recognition of the hormonal action of many of these peptides, it has become apparent that the CNS and the endocrine system are functionally interdependent. Tissues and cells that respond to hormones are called the target tissues and target cells of the hormones. These hormone-responsive cells have been preprogrammed by the process of differentiation to respond to the presence of hormones by acting in a predictable way. Not only do hormone-responsive cells respond to hormones through specific signaling-receptors, but their metabolic pathways also can be affected by the concentration of available substrates. Hormone-responsive cells live in a complex and continually changing environment of biological fuels, waste products, and ions. Their ultimate response to these changes is the net result of both hormonal and nonhormonal information brought to them by the extracellular fluids in which they are bathed. The response of the endocrine system to this information is discussed in the next section.

Endocrine Function in Fed State

Endocrine organs are distributed throughout the body, and most are involved primarily with nutrient ingestion—that is, the gastrointestinal (GI) tract. Interspersed among the absorptive and exocrine secretory cells of the upper GI tract are the highly specialized endocrine cells. These cells present a sensor face to the lumen and secrete granule-stored hormones into the bloodstream. Each of these cells is stimulated to secrete hormones by a different combination of chemical messages. Chemical messages include, for example, glucose, amino acids, fatty acids, and alkaline or acidic pH. Hormones secreted by these stimulated GI cells (GIP, CCK, gastrin, secretin; see Table 2.2) then enter the bloodstream and sensitize appropriate cells of the endocrine pancreas for response to the approaching nutrients. The primary action of the GI hormones, secreted in response to a mixed diet, is to amplify the response of the pancreatic islet β-cells to glucose (see Chapter 2).

Insulin Signaling

Insulin is the major anabolic hormone that impacts glucose, lipid, and amino acid synthesis and storage (Figure 7.11). Insulin regulates the uptake of glucose in muscle and adipose tissue and inhibits gluconeogenesis in the hepatic tissue. These two functions are important in the regulation of blood glucose levels, as they control glucose production in the liver and the uptake of glucose by the two largest tissues in the body, muscle and adipose tissue. Insulin also stimulates the storage or synthesis of the energy-producing nutrients. It stimulates glycogen synthesis from glucose, lipogenesis (synthesis of TAG), and protein synthesis. As an anabolic hormone, it inhibits lipolysis, glycogenolysis, and proteolysis (protein breakdown) [7]. These actions of insulin on the direction of energy metabolism during the fed state are illustrated in Figure 7.7.

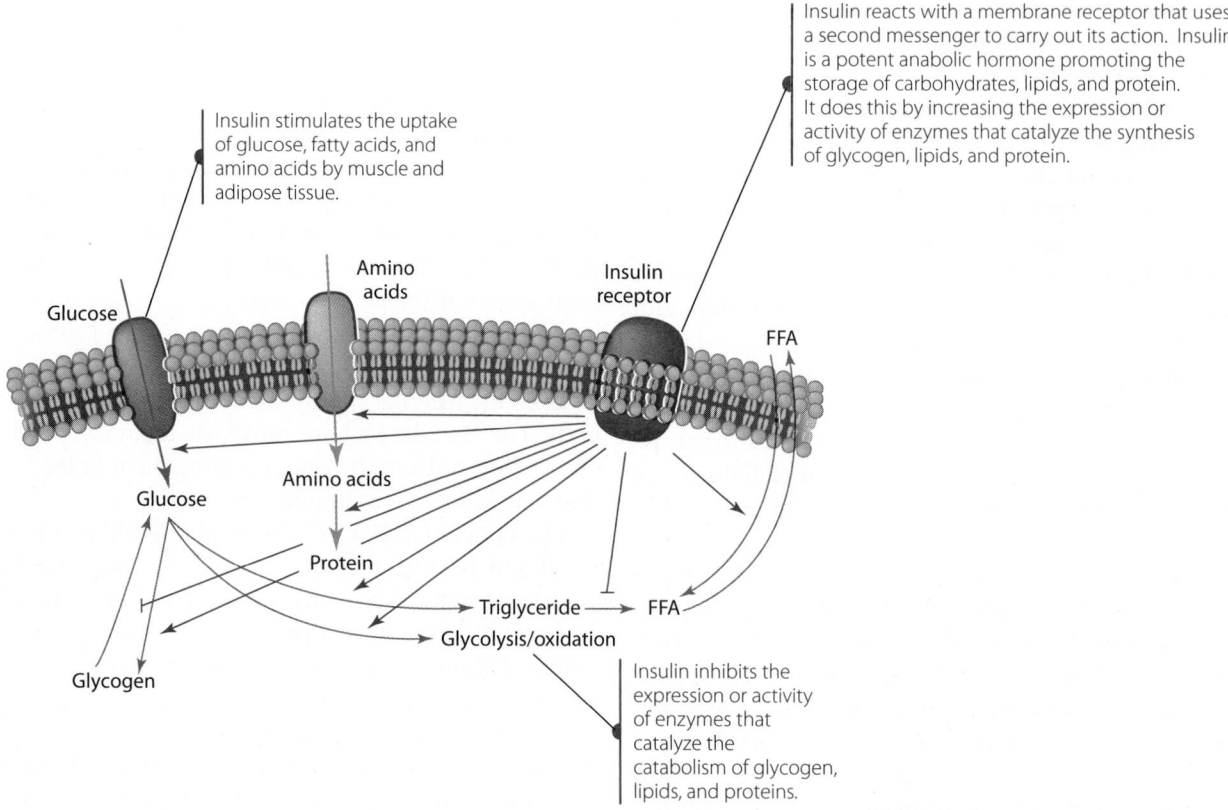

Insulin stimulates the uptake of glucose, fatty acids, and amino acids by muscle and adipose tissue.

Insulin reacts with a membrane receptor that uses a second messenger to carry out its action. Insulin is a potent anabolic hormone promoting the storage of carbohydrates, lipids, and protein. It does this by increasing the expression or activity of enzymes that catalyze the synthesis of glycogen, lipids, and protein.

Insulin inhibits the expression or activity of enzymes that catalyze the catabolism of glycogen, lipids, and proteins.

Figure 7.11 Insulin regulation of metabolism. Abbreviation: FFA = free fatty acids.

Insulin resistance or deficiency results in dysregulation of these processes. Insulin resistance is discussed in more detail in the Perspective on metabolic syndrome at the end of this chapter.

In the past few years much has been learned about signaling receptors on cell membranes. Most are protein-tyrosine kinases (PTKs) that phosphorylate tyrosine residues in a protein to activate them for additional phosphorylations. Some signaling receptors use G-protein receptor sites (as discussed in Chapter 1). As part of the signaling, inositol phospholipids are phosphorylated and they become second messengers. Some PTKs also phosphorylate serine and threonine residues in specific domains of the proteins. (A domain is a region within a protein containing specific amino acid sequences that participates in the signaling reactions.) Some hormones or cytokines also activate phosphorylases that control the signal's action and the length of the action. Cell signaling is complex in that the receptor initiates a cascade of reactions that are often designated by initials in research papers and textbooks. Researchers do not always use the same abbreviations for the same reaction or protein when reporting on cell signaling, which makes the process more difficult to follow for the reader. An overview of the insulin receptor will be described here because of its importance in controlling metabolism. Details of other signaling receptors are available in biochemistry and cell biology textbooks [8,9].

The insulin receptor site on the cell membrane is somewhat unique in the family of receptors. The receptor protein is a tetramer and composed of two α- and two β-chains. The α-chain is extracellular and contains the insulin binding site, as illustrated in Figure 7.12. The β-chain has an extracellular region, a transmembrane region, and an intracellular region. The α- and β-chains are bound together with disulfide bonds. Two of these α-β-chains complexes are held together by additional disulfide bonds connecting the α-chains to make a tetramer.

A single molecule of insulin binds to the α-chain, which induces a conformational change leading to the auto-phosphorylation of specific tyrosine residues within the β-chain. This activates the phosphorylation of a series of proteins that are attached to the receptor (Figure 7.13). One such group of proteins called the insulin-substrate proteins-1-4 (IRS1-4) serves as substrates of the insulin receptor tyrosine kinase. IRS proteins attach to one of the phosphorylated tyrosine residues in the PTK domain of the insulin receptor and stabilize the structure. The IRS proteins serve as docking sites for several other proteins, including phosphatidylinositol-3-kinase, which phosphorylates phosphatidylinositol-3-phosphates, which act as second messengers [9]. In the sequential process of phosphorylations, a protein (called Akt or PKB) is phosphorylated, which stimulates glucose uptake into skeletal muscle. In the liver Akt phosphorylates a cytoplasmic transcription factor. The resulting lack of the unphosphorylated transcription factor in the cytoplasm causes the nuclear transcription factor to dissociate from the coactivator and block the transcription of the enzymes required for gluconeogenesis. The result of this is a reduction in gluconeogenesis in the liver.

The action of insulin is modulated by a group of protein-tyrosine phosphatases that can dephosphorylate the insulin-receptor proteins and thereby terminate the signal. The generation of phosphatidylinositol-3-phosphate is blunted by phosphatases. Because the phosphorylated inositol serves as a second messenger, insulin signaling halts when this compound is dephosphorylated. Phosphorylation of tyrosine can be inhibited when serine residues are first phosphorylated by proteins stimulated by inflammatory cytokines, which cause insulin resistance (lack of response to insulin). Two additional proteins, Shc and Gab-1, are adaptor molecules that are part of a regulatory unit that activates small G proteins by binding to nucleotide exchange factors. Gab-1 and Shc are substrates of insulin-receptor tyrosine kinase. The proteins are involved in a mitogen-activated protein (MAP)-kinase pathway (cell proliferation and differentiation), which mediates a variety of extracellulary derived signals to the cytosol and nucleus. The signaling from insulin causes a cascade of proteins to be phosphorylated. These phosphorylations are expressed in developing

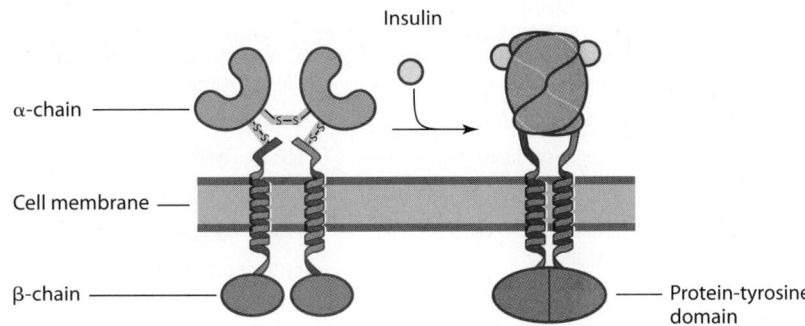

Figure 7.12 Insulin receptor activation. An inactive insulin receptor appears on the left. The receptor is a tetramer consisting of two α- and two β-chains. On the right, the receptor binds with a single insulin molecule, causing conformational changes in the β-chains, which activates the tyrosine kinase domain.

Source: Modified from Garrett & Grisham, Biochemistry, 4e. © Cengage Learning 2009.

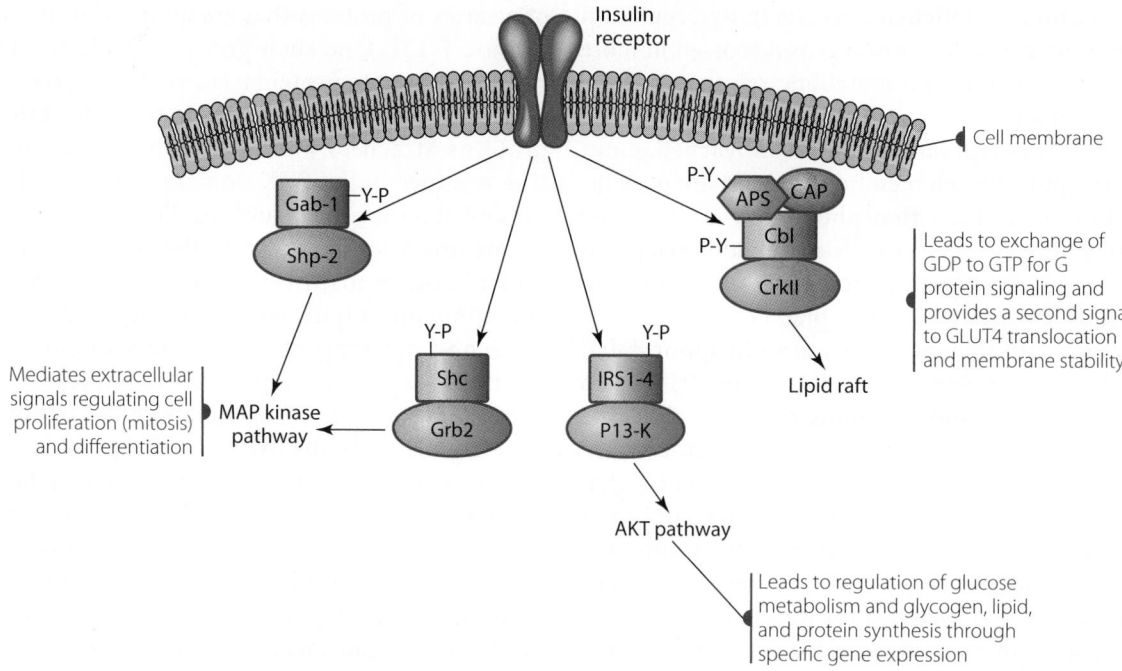

Figure 7.13 An overview of substrates of the insulin protein-tyrosine kinase. See text for details.

Source: Modified from Garrett & Grisham, Biochemistry, 4e. © Cengage Learning 2009.

adipocytes and are involved in regulating cell proliferation and differentiation [10].

The action of insulin has been examined to determine if there is a difference in response in men and women. As discussed in Chapter 8, there is a large difference in the ratio of fat-free mass to fat mass between men and women. Women typically have considerably higher body fat and lower lean body mass than men. These studies are ongoing, but at the present time it appears that women are more sensitive to insulin with regards to glucose metabolism in the liver and muscle. There is no difference in insulin's effect on lipolysis between men and women, and data are insufficient to determine whether there is a difference in the regulation of triacylglycerol and protein metabolism [11].

The human genome codes for over 90 different protein-tyrosine kinase receptors, which make up cell membrane receptors for a wide variety of ligands. Most contain only a single α-β-chain receptor kinase and many are G-protein-coupled receptors (Chapter 1).

Insulin's effects can be categorized, based upon the length of time it takes for action to occur, as (1) very fast, occurring in a matter of seconds; (2) fast, occurring in minutes; (3) slower, occurring in minutes to several hours; or (4) slowest, occurring only after several hours or even days. An example of a very fast action of insulin is membrane changes stimulated by the hormone. These changes occur in adipocytes and muscle cells where glucose entry depends upon membrane transport (see the "Glucose Transporters" section in Chapter 3). The fast action of insulin involves the activation or inhibition of

many enzymes, with anabolic actions accentuated. For example, insulin stimulates glycogenesis, lipogenesis, and protein synthesis while it inhibits opposing catabolic actions. Several metabolic effects of insulin and the corresponding target enzymes involved are listed in Table 7.1. Insulin favors glycogenesis through the activation of a phosphatase that dephosphorylates phosphorylase and glycogen synthase. This dephosphorylation activates glycogen synthetase while inhibiting the phosphorylase that initiates glycogenolysis. The fast effect of insulin on protein synthesis is not as clear-cut as its influence on lipogenesis and glycogenesis, and appears to be related to the availability of amino acids.

One slower action of insulin involves a further regulation of enzyme activity. This regulation is accomplished through the selective induction or repression of enzyme synthesis. The induced enzymes are the key rate-limiting enzymes for anabolic reaction sequences, whereas the repressed enzymes are crucial to the control of opposing catabolic reactions. An example of selective induction is

Table 7.1 Metabolic Effects of Insulin and Its Action on Specific Enzymes

Metabolic Effect	Target Enzyme
↑ Glucose uptake (muscle)	↑ Glucose transporter
↑ Glucose uptake (liver)	↑ Glucokinase
↑ Glycogen synthesis (liver, muscle)	↑ Glycogen synthase
↓ Glycogen breakdown (liver, muscle)	↓ Glycogen phosphorylase
↑ Glycolysis, acetyl-CoA production (liver, muscle)	↑ Phosphofructokinase-1
	↑ Pyruvate dehydrogenase complex
↑ Fatty acid synthesis (liver)	↑ Acetyl-CoA carboxylase

the effect of insulin on glucokinase activity. Insulin increases the synthesis of glucokinase by promoting transcription of the glucokinase gene. Another slower action of insulin is its stimulation of cellular amino acid influx. The slowest effect of insulin is its promotion of growth through mitogenesis (MAP kinase pathway) and cell replication. The passage of a cell through its various phases before it can replicate is a relatively slow process that requires 18 to 24 hours to complete.

Insulin Resistance

Much controversy persists regarding insulin insensitivity but, based on current evidence, insulin resistance results in hyperinsulinemia (increased blood insulin levels). The pancreas apparently releases more insulin in an effort to maintain normal blood glucose levels. The insulin insensitivity, combined with the elevated insulin levels, results in either elevated fasting blood glucose levels, glucose intolerance, or both. The insensitivity to insulin is primarily seen in muscle and adipose tissue (see Chapters 3 and 5 for details). Within insulin-resistant muscle, insulin loses its ability to stimulate glucose uptake; in adipose tissue, it no longer inhibits free fatty acid release. These observations can explain the elevated blood glucose and free fatty acid levels that accompany insulin resistance.

The liver and kidney retain their sensitivity to insulin, and the elevated insulin levels stimulate liver triacylglycerol (TAG) synthesis. As a consequence of the elevated TAG synthesis and the VLDL-TAG synthesis and secretion, fasting serum triacylglycerol and VLDL-TAG levels are increased. TAG levels in the liver also increase, resulting in nonalcoholic fatty liver disease. The kidney responds to the elevated insulin levels by increasing renal sodium retention and decreasing uric acid clearance. This response results in an increased prevalence of essential hypertension and higher plasma uric acid concentrations among those with insulin resistance.

Weight Loss and Insulin Insensitivity

Not all overweight or obese people have insulin resistance. Therefore, weight loss will not reduce the risk for cardiovascular disease (CVD) in all obese people equally. No simple test exists to determine who is insulin resistant and who is not. Fasting insulin levels, fasting plasma glucose levels, and triacylglycerol-HDL-C ratios have all been used as indicators for insulin resistance, with varying degrees of success. Considerable evidence demonstrates that if a person loses weight, insulin sensitivity improves. Fortunately, the hyperinsulinemia does not prevent weight from being lost. (Energy balance and the merits of different weight-loss diets are covered in Chapter 8.) Notably, variations in the macronutrient content of isocaloric diets have little effect on insulin sensitivity. One common weight-loss strategy is to lower the lipid content of the diet and replace it with carbohydrate.

The problem with a low-fat, high-carbohydrate diet for a person with insulin resistance, however, is that the additional carbohydrate requires more insulin to be secreted from the pancreas to maintain glucose homeostasis. If the person is insulin resistant, and the pancreas has the capacity, insulin levels will be elevated further.

The increasing prevalence of overweight and obesity makes the study of metabolic syndrome, insulin resistance, and obesity an important consideration for those studying nutrition. The investigation of the effectiveness of changing diet, lifestyle, and exercise patterns in decreasing mortality and morbidity in people with metabolic syndrome as they age will be an active area of research and practice for the future.

Growth Hormone

Growth hormone (GH) affects metabolism within adipose tissue, the liver, and skeletal muscle. Most of the effects of growth hormone are on carbohydrate and lipid metabolism. In adipose tissue, GH stimulates lipolysis, which results in an increase in fatty acids in circulation. This lipolytic action occurs predominantly in the visceral adipose tissue and to a lesser extent in the subcutaneous adipose tissue. The lipolysis that occurs is depot specific because GH stimulates hormone-sensitive lipase in the visceral adipose tissue. GH also suppresses glucose uptake in adipose tissue by an unknown mechanism.

In the liver, GH increases TAG uptake by inducing the expression of lipoprotein lipase and hepatic lipase. In the muscle, GH stimulates triacylglycerol uptake by inducing the expression of lipoprotein lipase. The additional TAG can be oxidized or stored intramuscularly. Growth hormone appears to antagonize the action of insulin in both carbohydrate and protein metabolism, though the mechanisms are not completely understood. Growth hormone has a net anabolic effect on protein metabolism. GH promotes insulin resistance, though the mechanism is again unknown [12].

Endocrine Function in Postabsorptive or Fasting State

Metabolic adjustments that occur in response to food deprivation operate on two time scales: acutely, measured in minutes (e.g., adjustments operating in a postabsorptive state), and chronically, measured in hours and days (adjustments occurring during fasting or starvation). In contrast to the fed state, in which insulin is the hormone primarily responsible for directing energy metabolism, the body deprived of food requires a variety of hormones to regulate its fuel supply.

Figure 7.8 depicts the postabsorptive state, in which hepatic glycogenolysis provides some glucose to the body while increased use of fatty acids for energy decreases the glucose requirement of cells. Also, gluconeogenesis is initiated, with latic acid, glycerol, and alanine serving as primary substrates.

Hepatic glycogenolysis is initiated through the actions of glucagon, which is secreted by the α-cells of the pancreas, and of epinephrine and norepinephrine, which are synthesized primarily in the adrenal medulla and the sympathetic nerve endings, respectively. Epinephrine is considerably more potent in stimulating glycogenolysis than is norepinephrine, which functions mainly as a neurotransmitter. Epinephrine and norepinephrine are called the catecholamine hormones because they are derivatives of the aromatic alcohol catechol. Although they influence hepatic glycogenolysis somewhat, the catecholamines exert their effect primarily on the muscles. The action of glucagon and the catecholamines is mediated through cAMP and protein kinase phosphorylation. (This mechanism is described in the section on glycogenolysis in Chapter 3; see also Figure 3.16.) Through the action of glucagon on the liver, phosphorylase and glycogen synthetase are phosphorylated, in direct opposition to the action of insulin. Consequently, phosphorylase is activated and glycogen synthetase is inhibited. As a result, glycogen is broken down, giving rise to glucose-6-phosphate, which then can be hydrolyzed by the specific liver phosphatase (glucose-6-phosphatase) to produce free glucose. The free glucose can then enter the bloodstream to maintain blood glucose levels.

Muscle glycogenolysis, in contrast, stimulated by the catecholamines, provides glucose only for use by the particular muscle in which the glycogen has been stored. Phosphorylated glucose cannot cross the cell membrane. Muscle tissue lacks glucose-6-phosphatase and cannot release free glucose into the circulation. The catecholamines, however, raise blood glucose levels indirectly by stimulating the secretion of glucagon and inhibiting the uptake of blood glucose by the muscles.

Glycogenolysis can occur within minutes and thus meets an acute need for raising the blood glucose level. However, because so little glycogen is stored in the liver (~60–100 g), blood glucose cannot be maintained this way over a prolonged period. The content of total muscle glycogen is ~350 g. Twelve to 18 hours following a meal, liver glycogen levels are very low. As mentioned previously, gluconeogenesis in the liver is a major supplier of glucose during fasting. Lactate, glycerol, alanine, and other amino acids are the primary precursors. Gluconeogenesis is fostered by the same hormones that initiate glycogenolysis (glucagon and epinephrine), but the amino acids needed as substrates are made available through the action of the glucocorticoids secreted by the adrenal cortex. Glucocorticoid hormones stimulate gluconeogenesis. Alanine, generated in the muscle from other amino acids and from pyruvate by transamination, not only serves as the principal gluconeogenic substrate but also acts as

a stimulant of gluconeogenesis through its effect on the secretion of glucagon. In fact, alanine is the prime stimulator of glucagon secretion by α-cells that have been sensitized to the action of alanine by the glucocorticoids.

Low levels of circulating insulin not only decrease the use of glucose but also promote lipolysis and a rise in free fatty acids. Contributing to this effect is the increase in glucagon during the fasting period. Glucagon raises the level of cAMP in adipose cells, and the cAMP then activates a hormone-sensitive lipase that hydrolyzes stored triacylglycerols. The muscles, inhibited from taking up glucose by the catecholamines, begin to use fatty acids as the major source of energy. This increased use of fatty acids by the muscles represents an important adaptation to fasting. Growth hormone and the glucocorticoids foster this adaptation because they, like the catecholamines, inhibit in some manner the use of glucose by the muscles.

As starvation is prolonged, less and less glucose is used, thereby reducing the amount of protein that must be catabolized to provide substrate for gluconeogenesis. As glucose use decreases, hepatic ketogenesis increases and the brain adapts to the use of ketones (primarily β-hydroxybutyrate) as a partial source of energy. After 3 days of starvation, about one-third of the energy needs of the brain are met by ketones. With prolonged starvation, ketones become the major fuel source for the brain. Under conditions of continued carbohydrate shortage, ketones are oxidized by the muscles in preference not only to glucose but also to fatty acids. During starvation, the use of ketones by the muscles as the preferred source of energy spares protein, thereby prolonging life. Although Figure 7.9 depicts fuel metabolism during starvation, it does not show some of the adjustments in energy substrates that occur when starvation is prolonged. These adjustments are shown in Table 7.2. As mentioned previously, the duration of starvation compatible with life depends to a large degree upon depot fat status.

Table 7.2 Fuel Metabolism in Starvation

Fuel Exchanges and Consumption	Amount Formed or Consumed in 24 hours (g)	
	Day 3	Day 40
Fuel Use by the Brain		
Glucose	100	40
Ketones	50	100
Fuel Mobilization		
Adipose tissue lipolysis	180	180
Muscle protein degradation	75	20
Fuel Output of the Liver		
Glucose	150	80
Ketones	150	150

Source: Adapted from Stryer L. Biochemistry. 3rd ed. New York: Freeman. 1988 p. 640.

SPORTS NUTRITION

Humans have courted the challenge of athletic performance and competition since the days of the early Greeks. The science of nutrition emerged much later, spurred by the expanding knowledge of metabolism and the biochemistry on which it is based. Because the energy for physical performance must be derived from nutrient intake, it was only a matter of time before these areas of interest would be linked. The heavy emphasis on the enhancement of health and physical performance in today's society has led sports nutrition to emerge as an important science. Nutrition, as a means of positively affecting physical performance, has become a topic of great interest to all those involved in human performance, the scientist as well as the athlete and athletic trainer.

The human body converts the potential energy of nutrients to usable chemical energy, part of which drives muscle contraction, a process fundamental to athletic prowess. Fluctuations in the body's demand for energy—for example, changes in exertion level among resting, mild exercise, and strenuous exercise—are accompanied by shifts in the rate of catabolism of the different stored forms of nutrients. It follows that an understanding of sports nutrition requires an understanding of the integration of the metabolic pathways that furnish the needed energy. In this respect, therefore, the energy demands of sport resemble the fed-fast cycle described earlier in this chapter, so a discussion of sports nutrition at this point in the text seems appropriate.

Biochemical Assessment of Physical Exertion

To fully understand sports nutrition, we need to examine different types of skeletal muscle. A more detailed discussion of this topic can be found in an exercise physiology or general physiology text (such as [13,14]). Muscle generally is classified as one of three distinct types, each emphasizing a different metabolic pathway: Type I, Type IIa, and Type IIx. Type I muscle fibers are also called slow oxidative fibers, slow-twitch fibers, or even red muscle. Type I fiber contains a large number of mitochondria and therefore is oxidative and red in color. Type I fibers are capable of oxidizing glucose to CO_2 and H_2O and carrying out β-oxidation of fatty acids. These fibers typically contain higher concentrations of myoglobin and are surrounded by more capillaries than other fiber types. The speed of contraction is considered slow. Type I fibers are used for aerobic endurance events. Type IIx fibers are sometimes called fast-twitch fibers or fast-glycolytic fiber, and are the fastest to contract. Type IIx fibers have fewer mitochondria, have an active glycolytic pathway, and are white in appearance. This type of muscle is used primarily for short-duration anaerobic events and power events. Type IIa muscle can be considered a hybrid of types I and IIx muscle fibers—as it evidences some characteristics of both—and is also called intermediate fibers or fast-oxidative glycolytic fibers. Endurance training can make type IIa muscle act more like type I muscle, whereas strength training or sprint training can make it more closely resemble type IIx.

Much more could be said about the muscle types and their response to nervous system stimulation and training, but this brief description provides sufficient information to foster an understanding of the resemblance of sports nutrition to the fed-fast cycle. The proportion (relative number) of each type of muscle fibers a person has is defined by genetics. Training can make modest changes in muscle fiber type; however, because some sports rely on a specific muscle type, some people are genetically better suited for a specific type of sport activity based on their muscle type makeup. Interestingly, women have more type I muscle than men. The result of this difference is that, under usual conditions of long-term aerobic exercise, women burn lipid at higher percentages of VO_2 max than do men. Further details on how the duration and intensity of activity and physical condition influence which muscle types are used and which metabolic energy pathways are active are discussed later in this chapter.

To understand how the muscle types relate to physical exercise at the cellular level, we need to examine two common measurements used by the exercise physiologist [13]: the respiratory quotient (RQ) and the maximal oxygen consumption (VO_2 max). The respiratory quotient is called the respiratory exchange ratio (R or RER) by exercise physiologists. RQ is the ratio of CO_2 production to O_2 consumption ($RQ = CO_2/O_2$). Typical RQs for carbohydrate, fat, and protein are 1.0, 0.70, and 0.82, respectively. The respiratory quotient (RQ) has served for nearly a century as the basis for determining the relative participation of carbohydrates and fats in exercise [13]. A newer generation of procedures (e.g., the isotope infusion method) has been developed to measure the relative contribution of substrates to energy supply during exercise. The isotope infusion method is more expensive and time consuming than measuring RQ, and is used more often for research than clinically. RQ is discussed more fully in Chapter 8.

It is assumed that no proteins are oxidized for energy during short-duration activity. Over longer periods, the amount of protein being oxidized can be estimated from the amount of urinary nitrogen excreted, and the remainder of the metabolic energy must be made up of a combination of carbohydrate and fat. Should the principal fuel source shift from mainly fat to carbohydrate, the RQ correspondingly increases, and a shift from carbohydrate to fat lowers the RQ. The RQ for a typical American diet is about 0.8—representing a mix of fat and carbohydrate. Tables (Chapter 8) that permit the estimation of the relative percentage of either carbohydrate or fat being used as a metabolic fuel based upon the RQ at any given time are available. During the past 25 years, however, the determination of the biological fuels being used has been advanced by invasive techniques such as arteriovenous measurements and the use of needle biopsies to quantify tissue stores of the energy nutrients. These measurements are used clinically to evaluate elevated rates of metabolism.

The concept of maximum oxygen uptake (VO_2 max) is fundamental. As work increases in intensity, the volume of oxygen taken up by the body also increases. The VO_2 max is defined as the point at which a further increase in the intensity of the exercise no longer results in an increase in the volume of oxygen uptake. The intensity level of a particular workload is most commonly expressed in terms of the percentage of the VO_2 max that it induces. As we discuss later, the metabolic pathway that supplies energy for work is determined by the availability of metabolic energy (carbohydrate or lipid) and oxygen as well as by the duration of the activity and the conditioned state of the person performing the work. As a person goes from an untrained state to a trained state, the VO_2 max increases. Isotope infusion can be used to quantify the contribution of the major energy substrates, plasma glucose and fatty acids, and muscle triacylglycerols and glycogen to energy expenditure during exercise. It involves the intravenous infusion of stable isotope (e.g., ^{2}H deuterium)–labeled glucose, palmitate, and glycerol during periods of rest and exercise. Monitoring the uptake of infused labeled glucose and palmitate and knowing whole-body substrate oxidation allows the contributions of muscle triacylglycerol and glycogen to the overall energy supply to be estimated, by measuring the stable isotope in the resulting CO_2 and H_2O [13].

Energy Sources during Exercise

The hydrolysis of the terminal phosphate group of ATP ultimately provides the energy for conducting biological work. In terms of physical performance, the form of work that is of greatest interest is the mechanical contraction of skeletal muscles. Physical exertion depends upon a reservoir of ATP, which is in an ever-changing state of metabolic turnover. Whereas ATP is consumed by physical exertion, its stores are supplemented by the metabolic pathways discussed next and are repleted during periods of rest. The key to optimizing physical performance lies in nutritional strategies that maximize cellular levels of stored nutrients as fuels for ATP production. Three energy systems supply ATP during different forms of exercise [15]:

- the ATP-CP (creatine phosphate) system
- the lactic acid system (anaerobic glycolysis)
- the aerobic system (aerobic glycolysis, TCA cycle, and β-oxidation of fatty acids)

The ATP-CP (Creatine Phosphate) System

The ATP-CP system is a cooperative system in muscle cells using the high-energy phosphate bond of creatine phosphate (CP) together with ATP (Chapter 3). When the body is at rest, energy needs are fulfilled by aerobic catabolism (see the "The Aerobic System" section in this chapter) because the low demand for oxygen can easily be met by oxygen exchange in the lungs and by the oxygen carried to the muscle by the cardiovascular system. (The ATP-CP system also operates continuously during this time, though at a slow pace.) If physical activity is initiated, the energy requirements of contracting muscle are met by existing ATP. However, stores of ATP in muscle are limited, providing enough energy for only a few seconds of maximal exercise. As ATP levels diminish, they are replenished rapidly by the transfer of high-energy phosphate from creatine phosphate to form ATP in the ATP-CP system (Figure 3.22). The muscle cell concentration of CP is only four to five times greater than that of ATP, and therefore most energy furnished by this system is diminished after the first 15 to 25 seconds of strenuous exercise. As the ATP-CP system is exhausted, the lactic acid system (anaerobic glycolysis) picks up to produce more ATP. Performance demands of high intensity and short duration such as weightlifting, 100-m sprinting, some positions in football, and various short-duration field events benefit most from the ATP-CP and lactic acid systems. Lower-intensity activity may allow a person to use the combined ATP-CP and lactic acid systems for several minutes.

The Lactic Acid System

This system involves the glycolytic pathway, which produces ATP through substrate phosphorylation by the incomplete breakdown of glucose anaerobically into 2 mol of lactate in skeletal muscle. The sources of glucose are primarily muscle glycogen and, to a lesser extent, circulating glucose. The system can generate ATP quickly for high-intensity exercise. As pointed out in Chapter 3, the lactic acid system is not efficient from the standpoint of the quantity of ATP produced. However, because the process is so rapid, the small amount of ATP is produced quickly.

The lactate produced by this system rapidly crosses the muscle cell membrane into the bloodstream, from which it can be cleared by other tissues (including the liver) for aerobic production of ATP or gluconeogenesis. If the rate of production of lactate exceeds its rate of clearance, blood lactate accumulates. The quantity of lactate released at the initiation of a strenuous activity is low, but when it accumulates, it lowers the pH of the blood and is one cause of fatigue. Under such circumstances, exercise cannot be continued for long periods.

The lactic acid system is engaged to provide a rapid source of energy. When an inadequate supply of oxygen prevents the aerobic system from furnishing sufficient

ATP to meet the demands of exercise, the lactic system will continue to function for a brief time, resulting in what is called "oxygen debt." Although the lactic acid system is operative as soon as strenuous exercise begins, it becomes the primary supplier of energy only after CP stores in the muscle are depleted, which occurs after about 15 to 25 seconds at maximal energy output. As a backup to the ATP-CP system, the lactic acid system becomes important in high-intensity anaerobic power events that last from about 20 to 75 seconds, such as sprints of up to 800 m and swimming events of 100 or 200 m. During these events the anaerobic system (lactic acid system) and the aerobic system each supply about 50% of the energy at maximal energy output [15].

The Aerobic System

The aerobic system involves the TCA cycle, through which carbohydrates, fats, and some amino acids are completely oxidized to CO_2 and H_2O. During the initiation of maximal exercise, glucose and fatty acids provide nearly all of the aerobic energy, with both intracellular triacylglycerols and plasma fatty acids contributing to the overall energy supply. The aerobic system is highly efficient from the standpoint of the quantity of ATP produced. Because oxygen is necessary for the system to function, a person's VO_2 max becomes an important factor in performance capacity. Contributing to the VO_2 max are the cardiovascular system's ability to deliver blood (which carries the oxygen, glucose, and fatty acids) to exercising muscle, pulmonary ventilation, oxygenation of hemoglobin, and release of oxygen from hemoglobin

at the muscle. Matching these contributors to the cellular need for oxygen in exercising muscle is complex because low efficiency of any of them becomes rate limiting for long-term exercise at maximal outputs. The aerobic system is the predominant supplier of energy for forms of exercise lasting longer than 2 or 3 minutes, depending upon the intensity of the exercise. Many types of exercise or sports meet these criteria: for example, distance running, distance swimming, and cross-country skiing, just to name a few of the endurance feats [15].

Current thinking is that the three energy systems do not simply take turns serially but function simultaneously to meet the demands of exercise as it begins and continues. All systems function at all times, and though at any one time one predominates, the others participate to varying degrees. The interaction of the ATP-CP, lactic acid, and aerobic systems over the course of the first 2 minutes of exercise is shown in Figure 7.14. To summarize, the primary supplier of energy for activity is the ATP-CP system during the first 15 to 25 seconds of a strenuous aerobic activity; the lactic acid system between 25 and 75 seconds after initiation; and the aerobic systems for events lasting longer than 2 minutes. Of course the actual system that supplies energy depends upon the conditioning of the athlete and the intensity of the activity.

Fuel Sources during Exercise

Carbohydrate, fat, and protein are the macronutrients that provide the fuel for energy transformation in the muscle. At rest, and during normal daily activities, fats are the primary source, providing 80% to 90% of energy.

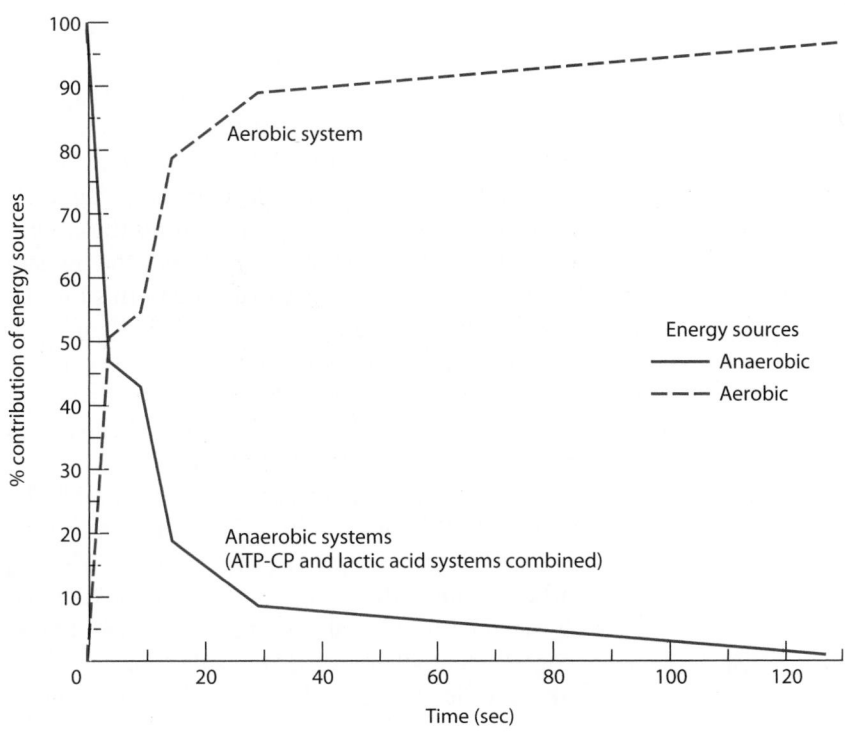

Figure 7.14 Primary energy sources for initiation of strenuous activity.

Source: Adapted from Fox, E.L., Bowers, R.W., Foss, M.I., *The Physiological Basis for Exercise and Sports*, 3rd ed., Dubuque, IA: Brown and Benchmark, 1989, p. 37. Reproduced with permission of The McGraw-Hill Companies.

During the resting state carbohydrates provide 5% to 18% of energy, and protein provides 2% to 5% [16].

During exercise, the oxidation of amino acids contributes only minimally to the total amount of ATP used by working muscles. Significant breakdown of amino acids occurs only toward the end of a long endurance event, when carbohydrate (glycogen) stores are somewhat depleted. Amino acids can be transaminated to form alanine from pyruvate. The alanine is transported to the liver and is a primary substrate for gluconeogenesis. This process is termed the glucose-alanine cycle or Cori cycle and is described in Chapter 3. The carbon skeleton of some amino acids can be oxidized directly in the muscle. During exercise, the four major endogenous sources of energy are:

- muscle glycogen
- plasma glucose
- plasma fatty acids
- intramuscular triacylglycerols

The extent to which each of these substrates contributes energy for exercise depends upon several factors, including:

- the intensity and duration of exercise
- the level of exercise training
- initial muscle glycogen levels
- supplementation with carbohydrates through the intestinal tract during exercise

This section describes the relationship between these factors and the "substrate of choice" for energy supply [17]. A graphical representation of the contribution of these substrates at 25%, 65%, and 85% VO₂ max is shown in Figure 7.15.

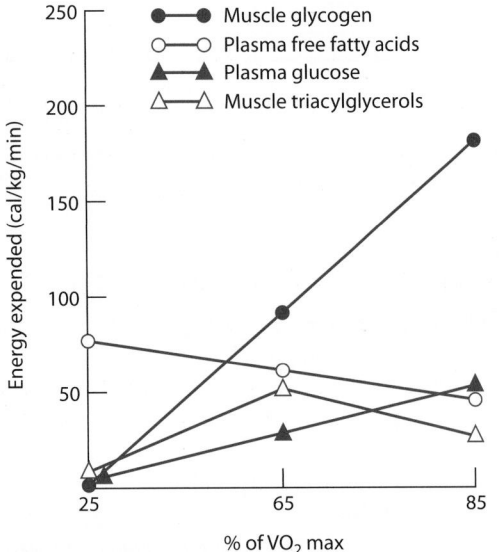

Figure 7.15 Contribution of the four major substrates to energy expenditure after 30 minutes of exercise at 25%, 65%, and 85% VO₂ max.

Exercise Intensity and Duration

In the fasting state, much of the energy required for low-intensity exercise (2–30% VO₂ max) is derived from muscle triacylglycerols and plasma fatty acid oxidation, with a small contribution from plasma glucose. The pattern does not change significantly over a period of up to 2 hours at this exercise level, which is equivalent to walking. During this time, the consumed plasma fatty acids are replaced by fatty acids mobilized from the large triacylglycerol stores in adipocytes throughout the body. However, as exercise intensity increases to 65% and on up to 85% VO₂ max, fewer adipocyte fatty acids are released into the plasma, resulting in a decreased concentration of plasma fatty acids. This decrease occurs despite a continuing high rate of lipolysis in adipocytes. The decreased replacement of plasma fatty acids from fat stores at higher levels of exercise has been attributed to insufficient blood flow and albumin delivery of fatty acids from adipose tissue into the systemic circulation [17]. Since glycerol is still being released from the adipocyte, fatty acids must become trapped in adipose tissue and accumulate there during high levels of exercise [16]. A rapid rise in plasma fatty acid levels occurs following exercise of high intensity (85% VO₂ max).

With moderate-intensity exercise (~65% VO₂ max) equivalent to running for 1 to 3 hours, total fat oxidation increases, despite the reduced rate of return of adipose fatty acids into the circulation. This increase is attributed to an increase in the oxidation of muscle triacylglycerols. In fact, as shown in Figure 7.15, plasma fatty acids and muscle triacylglycerols contribute equally to energy expenditure at this level of exertion in endurance-trained athletes. Within the exertion range of 60% to 75% VO₂ max, however, fat cannot be oxidized at a rate sufficiently rapid to provide needed energy, and therefore nearly half of the required energy must be furnished by carbohydrate oxidation. Note that fatty acids have only two oxygen molecules, compared to carbohydrates' equal number of oxygen and carbon molecules. This characteristic means that fatty acid catabolism requires the cardiovascular system to deliver more oxygen. Also, the transfer of fatty acids into mitochondria is slow, and this may be a rate-limiting event. The result is that when tissue oxygen levels become low or high-intensity exercise calls for a large quantity of energy, carbohydrate becomes a more favored substrate. Fatty acids are the favored substrates for intensities of up to about 50% VO₂ max.

As exercise intensity increases to 85% VO₂ max, the relative contribution of carbohydrate oxidation to total metabolism increases sharply (Figure 7.15). At 85% VO₂ max, carbohydrate in the form of blood glucose (derived from glycogenolysis of hepatic glycogen stores) and muscle glycogen essentially becomes the sole supplier of energy. Like muscle glycogen, the concentration of blood glucose falls progressively during prolonged, strenuous exercise. This decrease occurs because glucose uptake by working muscle (independent of insulin) may increase to as much as 20-fold or more above resting levels, while hepatic glucose output decreases with exercise duration. Interestingly, however, hypoglycemia is not always observed at exhaustion, particularly at exercise intensities >70% VO_2 max. Hypoglycemia following liver glycogen depletion apparently can be postponed by an inhibition of glucose uptake and accelerated gluconeogenesis in the liver, using the glycerol produced in lipolysis, and by lactate and pyruvate (which was carried to the liver as alanine) produced by the glycolytic activity of the working muscles.

Accompanying high rates of carbohydrate catabolism is a rise in the production of lactate, which accumulates in muscle and blood. This increase in lactate is particularly evident in situations of oxygen debt, in which insufficient oxygen to complete the oxidation of pyruvate to CO_2 and H_2O instead favors its reduction to lactate.

Fatigue

Muscle fatigue has a variety of causes, some of which are related to substrate availability. For example, fatigue occurs when the supply of glucose is inadequate, such as with muscle glycogen depletion or hypoglycemia. Thus, the consumption of glucose may temporarily delay fatigue. As muscle fatigue begins to set in, the person must reduce workload intensity to a level that matches his or her ability to oxidize fat predominantly, possibly as low as 30% VO_2 max. The reason for this limitation, and thus the dependence of muscle upon carbohydrate as an energy source, is not fully understood. However, traditional thinking is that the limitation may be based on two factors: (1) oxidation of fatty acids is limited by the enzyme carnitine acyltransferase (CAT), which catalyzes the transport of fatty acids across the mitochondrial membrane; and (2) CAT is known to be inhibited by malonyl-CoA. When availability of carbohydrate to the muscle is high, fatty acid oxidation may be reduced by the inhibition of CAT by glucose-derived malonyl-CoA [17,18].

Level of Exercise Training

Endurance training increases an athlete's ability to perform more aerobically at the same absolute exercise intensity. Several factors aid in this increase. First, endurance-trained muscle exhibits an increase in the number and size of mitochondria. Cardiovascular and lung capacity also increase, and type I muscle hypertrophies. The activity of oxidative enzymes in endurance-trained subjects has been shown to be 100% greater than in untrained subjects at 65% VO_2 max. Endurance training also results in an increased use of fat as an energy source during submaximal exercise. In skeletal muscle, fatty acid oxidation inhibits glucose uptake and glycolysis. For this reason, the trained athlete benefits from the carbohydrate-sparing effect of enhanced fatty acid oxidation during competition because muscle glycogen and plasma glucose are depleted more slowly. This effect largely accounts for the training-induced increase in endurance for exercise over a prolonged period.

Trained athletes have been reported to have lower plasma fatty acid concentrations and exhibit less adipose tissue lipolysis than untrained counterparts do at similar exercise intensity. This finding suggests that the primary source of fatty acids used by the trained athlete is intramuscular triacylglycerol stores, rather than adipocyte triacylglycerols. After exercise, the intramuscular triacylglycerols are replaced, utilizing plasma fatty acids supplied by lipolysis within adipocytes. This process can result in shrinking the size of the adipose tissue.

Endurance training appears to result in an increased capacity for muscle glycogen storage. Therefore, the trained athlete benefits not only from a slower use of muscle glycogen (as explained earlier) but also from the capacity to have higher glycogen stores at the onset of competition.

Initial Muscle Glycogen Levels

The ability to sustain prolonged moderate-to-heavy exercise largely depends upon the initial content of skeletal muscle glycogen, and the depletion of muscle glycogen is the single most consistently observed factor that contributes to fatigue. High muscle glycogen levels allow exercise to continue longer at a submaximal workload. Even in the absence of carbohydrate loading (see the following section), a strong positive correlation exists between initial glycogen level and time to exhaustion, level of performance, or both during exercise periods that last more than 1 hour. The correlation does not apply at low levels of exertion (25–35% VO_2 max), or at high levels of exertion for short periods, because glycogen depletion is not a limiting factor under these conditions. It has been suggested that the importance of initial muscle glycogen stores is related to the inability of glucose and fatty acids to cross the cell membrane rapidly enough to provide adequate substrate for mitochondrial respiration [16].

Carbohydrate Supplementation (Supercompensation)

When muscle glycogen was identified as the limiting factor for the capacity to exercise at intensities requiring 70% to 85% VO_2 max, dietary manipulation to maximize glycogen stores followed naturally. The most popular subject for research of this nature has been the marathon runner or cross-country skier because of the prolonged physical taxation of these events and the fact that the athlete's performance is readily measurable by the time required

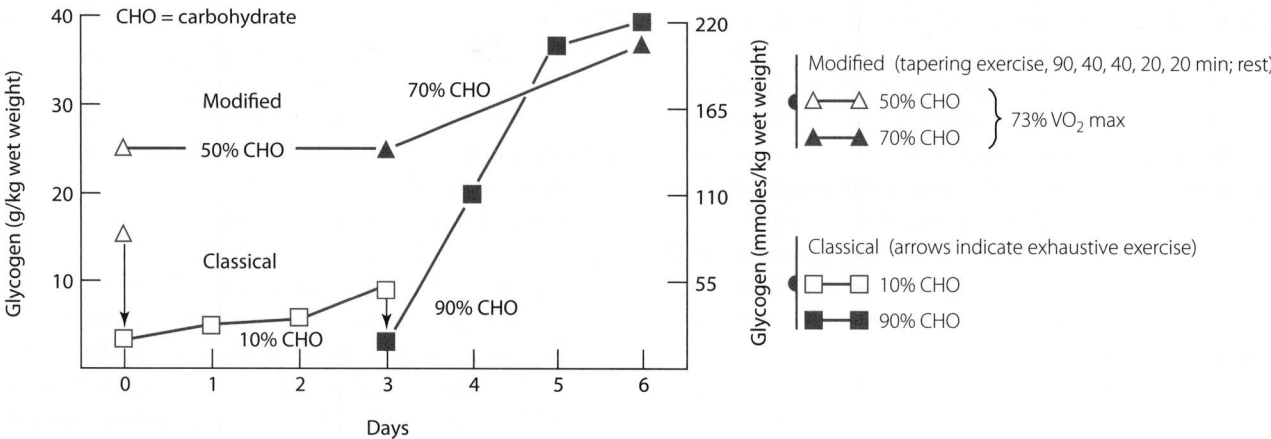

Figure 7.16 Schematic representation of the "classical" and modified regimens of muscle glycogen supercompensation.

Source: From Sherman, W.M., Carbohydrate, muscle glycogen, and muscle glycogen supercompensation, In 'Ergogenic Aids in Sport' by Williams, M.H., Champaign, IL: Human Kinetics Publishers, 1983, p. 14. Reprinted by permission.

to complete the course. The major dietary concern to emerge in the endurance training of marathon runners was how to elevate muscle glycogen to above-normal (supercompensated) levels. In sporting vernacular, maximizing glycogen content by dietary manipulation is referred to as carbohydrate loading.

The classical regimen for carbohydrate loading resulted from investigations in the late 1960s by Scandinavian scientists [19]. This regimen involved two sessions of intense exercise to exhaustion to deplete muscle glycogen stores, separated by 2 days of a low-carbohydrate diet (<10%) to "starve" the muscle of carbohydrate. This interval was followed by 3 days of a high-carbohydrate diet (>90%) and rest. The event would be performed on day 7 of the regimen. On completion of this regimen, muscle glycogen levels approached 220 mmol/kg wet weight (expressed as glucose residues), more than double the athlete's resting level. However, because of various undesirable side effects of the classical regimen, such as

irritability, dizziness, and a diminished exercise capacity, a less stringent regimen of diet and exercise has evolved that produces comparably high muscle glycogen levels.

In the modified regimen, runners perform tapered down exercise sessions over the course of 5 days, followed by 1 day of rest. During this time, 3 days of a 50% carbohydrate diet are followed by 3 days of a 70% carbohydrate diet, generally achieved by consuming large quantities of pasta, rice, or bread. The modified regimen, which can increase muscle glycogen stores 20% to 40% above normal, has been shown to be as effective as the classical approach, with fewer adverse side effects [20].

Figure 7.16 illustrates graphically the amount of muscle glycogen formed as a result of each regimen. Predictably, the supercompensation of muscle glycogen by either approach has been shown to improve performance in trained runners during races of 30 km and longer. It did not improve performance in shorter races (<21 km) because glycogen depletion is not the limiting factor in such events.

SUMMARY

Animal survival depends on a constant internal environment maintained through specific control mechanisms. Controls, operative at all levels (cellular, organ, and system), integrate energy metabolism and allow the body to adapt to a wide variety of environmental conditions. Primary among the mechanisms of adaptation is the regulation of metabolism through the cooperative input of the nervous, endocrine, and vascular systems. In the normal operation of these systems, metabolic pathways may be stimulated, maintained, or inhibited, depending upon the conditions imposed on the body. A pointed example of metabolic adaptation is the shift that occurs in substrate use and metabolic pathways in answer to changes in the body's nourishment status (i.e., fed, fasting, and starvation states).

Energy homeostasis is maintained by regulation through protein kinases. Protein-tyrosine kinases are part of the signaling system involving insulin and other hormones. Insulin is the primary anabolic hormone. A number of hormones including glucagon, growth hormone, and the catacholamines are involved in the regulation of catabolic processes.

The physical stress of exercise and sports presents an interesting challenge to the regulatory capacity of the body to provide the additional energy needed by exercising muscles. Substrates fueling this energy include plasma free fatty acids, plasma glucose, muscle glycogen, and muscle triacylglycerols, and their use varies according to the intensity and duration of the exercise.

References Cited

1. Kolditz CI, Langin D. Adipose tissue llipolysis. Curr Opin Clin Nutr Metab Care. 2010; 13:377–81.
2. Hardie DG. Sensing of energy and nutrients by AMP-activated protein kinase. Am J Clin Nutr. 2011; 93:S891–96.
3. Saggerson D. Malonyl-CoA: a key signaling molecule in mammalian cells. Annu Rev Nutr. 2008; 253–72.
4. Cahill, GF Jr. Fuel metabolism in starvation. Annu Rev Nutr. 2006; 26:1–22.
5. Cano N. Bench-to-bedside review: glucose production from the kidney. Critical Care. 2002; 6:317–21.
6. Meyer C, Stumvoll M, Dostou J, et al. Renal substrate exchange and gluconeogenesis in normal postabsorptive humans. Am J Physiol Endocrinol Metab. 2002; 282:E424–34.
7. Saltiel AR. Insulin signalling and the regulation of glucose and lipid metabolism. Nature. 2001; 414:799–806.
8. Garrett RH, Grisham CM. Biochemistry. 4th ed. Boston, MA: Brooks/Cole. 2010.
9. Karp G. Cell and Molecular Biology: concepts and Experiments. 6th ed. Hoboken, NY: John Wiley & Sons. 2010.
10. Saltiel AR. Putting the brakes on insulin signaling. N Engl J Med. 2003; 349:2560–62.
11. Magkos F, Wang X, Mittendorfer B. Metabolic actions of insulin in men and women. Nutr. 2010; 26:686–93.
12. Vijayakumar A, Novosyadlyy R, Wu YJ, et al. Biological effects of growth hormone on carbohydrate and lipid metabolism. Growth Horm IGF Res. 2010; 1–14.
13. Powers SK, Howley ET. Exercise Physiology: theory and Application to fitness and Performance. 6th ed. New York. 2007 pp. 52–72.
14. Sherwood L. Human Physiology: from Cells to Systems. 7th ed. Belmont CA: Brooks/Cole. 2010.
15. Gastin PB. Energy system interaction and relative contribution during maximal exercise. Sports Med. 2001; 31:725–41.
16. Coyle EF. Substrate utilization during exercise in active people. Am J Clin Nutr. 1995; 61:S968–79.
17. Spriet LL, Watt MJ. Regulatory mechanism in the interaction between carbohydrate and lipid oxidation during exercise. Acta Physiol Scand. 2003; 178:443–52.
18. Kiens B. Skeletal muscle lipid metabolism and insulin resistance. Physiol Rev. 2006; 86:205–43.
19. Bergstrom J, Hultman E. A study of the glycogen metabolism during exercise in man. Scand J Clin Lab Invest. 1967; 19:218–28.
20. Ivy JL. Dietary strategies to promote glycogen synthesis after exercise. Can J Appl Physiol. 2001; 26 (suppl):S236–45.

Suggested Readings

Benardot D. Nutrition for Serious Athletes. Champaign, IL: Human Kinetics, 2000.

A practical book that examines specific sports activities and provides nutritional strategies for improved performance.

Coyle EF. Substrate utilization during exercise in active people. Am J Clin Nutr. 1995; 61 (suppl):S968–79.

A useful review of the hierarchy of substrates as they are used for energy release in exercise.

McArdle WD, Katch FL, Katch VL. Sports and Exercise Nutrition. 3rd ed. Philadelphia: Lippincott Williams & Wilkins, 2009.

A textbook that covers the science behind nutrition in exercise.

Williams MH. Nutrition for Health, Fitness and Sport. 8th ed. New York: McGraw Hill, 2007.

An easy-to-read, well-documented textbook that covers nutritional aspects of exercise.

Driskell JA, Wolinsky I. (Eds.). Nutritional Concerns in Recreation, Exercise and Sport. Boco Raton, FL: CRC Press. 2009.

A thorough treatment of what is known and what is not in sports nutrition.

Web Sites

www.nal.usda.gov

National Agricultural Library at USDA; then click on Food and Nutrition

www.umass.edu/cnshp/index.html

Center for Nutrition in Sport and Human Performance at the University of Massachusetts

www.cdc.gov/nccdphp/dnpa

Centers for Disease Control and Prevention, Division of Nutrition, Physical Activity, and Obesity

www.ajcn.org

American Journal of Clinical Nutrition

www.gssiweb.com

Gatorade Sports Science Institute

www.beverageinstitute.org

The Coca-Cola Company Beverage Institute for Health and Wellness

METABOLIC SYNDROME

A syndrome is not a specific disease entity but a clustering of factors that occur together more often than expected based upon chance alone, and whose cause is often uncertain. Metabolic syndrome (MetS)—a pandemic that has developed in close parallel with the worldwide pandemic of obesity—fulfills this definition. Metabolic syndrome refers to a clustering of a group of risk factors for cardiovascular disease (CVD), chronic kidney disease, and type 2 diabetes.

Diabetes mellitus is an abnormality in glucose homeostasis. In type 1 diabetes, the abnormality is caused by complete or near-complete insulin deficiency, which is likely caused by autoimmune reactions that destroy the insulin-releasing β-cells of the pancreas. Type 2 diabetes is a relative insulin deficiency, a mismatch between insulin production and insulin requirements. There is no single cause for type 2 diabetes; rather, a number of primary genetic and environmental insults appear to be involved, and manifestations range from severe insulin resistance to limited insulin secretion (or some combination). Unlike type 1 diabetes, which is little influenced by genetic predisposition, type 2 diabetes has a strong genetic component (predisposition often accounts for greater than 90% of risk), though it does not result from a single gene modification [1].

The definition of MetS, which has also been referred to as insulin resistance syndrome or syndrome X, has evolved over the years. Various professional disease-related national and regional societies have communicated various criteria for diagnosis, with the most common distinction being the criteria for evaluating central (abdominal) obesity, a key component of the syndrome. Recently, however, an international group of representatives from the National Heart, Lung, and Blood Institute; the American Heart Association; the World Heart Federation; the International Atherosclerosis Society; and the International Association for the Study of Obesity met and agreed upon the criteria for clinical diagnosis. Diagnosis of MetS requires that an individual exhibit at least three of the five conditions listed in Table 1 [2].

Abdominal obesity has consistently been recognized as a symptom of the syndrome. Because some representatives at the meeting to determine diagnostic criteria preferred the use of waist circumference to assess for central obesity whereas others preferred body mass index (BMI), cut points were defined specifically for each population. The agreed upon criterion is a waist circumference of 102 cm (about 40 in) for men or 88 cm (about 35 in) for women in the United States and Canada. This is equivalent to a BMI of about 30 kg/m^2. Other countries use lower cut points for waist circumference to define central obesity. The additional criteria for diagnosing MetS are elevated TAG, reduced HDL-C, elevated blood pressure, and elevated fasting glucose. (If a drug is being used to treat any of these conditions, that condition is considered to be present.) The prevalence of MetS among U.S. adults is about 35% [2]. When the lower cut points for central obesity are used, the prevalence is slightly greater.

There has been considerable debate about the usefulness of MetS as either a predictor of future disease or a practical clinical tool that identifies patients in need of treatment [3]. Metabolic syndrome holds promise as a predictor of disease: it is associated with a 2-fold increase in risk for CVD, CVD-related mortality, myocardial infarction (MI; the blockage of an artery of the heart, causing necrosis of the heart muscle), and stroke. MetS is associated with a 1.5-fold increase in risk of all-cause mortality [4]. Still to be determined, however, is whether a diagnosis of MetS is a better predictor of risk than the sum of the individual risk factors for each disease. According to a recent meta-analysis of 87 prospective observational studies including more than 950,000 subjects, this question has not yet been answered [4]. This study also concluded that patients with MetS but without type 2 diabetes still had an increased risk for CVD-related mortality, MI, and stroke, and that women with MetS had a significantly higher risk than men.

The increase in the prevalence of metabolic syndrome parallels the increase in the prevalence of worldwide obesity. Though the definition of MetS has been controversial, there now appears to be international agreement, with alternate measures of central obesity for different population groups. This standard definition of MetS benefits both the researcher and the clinician. Employment of a common definition allows the researcher to utilize methods such as meta-analysis when he or she studies the epidemiology of the syndrome, the risk of morbidity and mortality, and/or the effectiveness of prevention and treatment programs in diverse population groups. For clinicians, it is important to identify the syndrome so that all components can be comprehensively treated. The effectiveness of the treatment in altering the patient outcome is of interest to the clinical researcher. MetS is also important to those interested in nutrition because one of the primary treatments is the modification of diet and lifestyle. Research has demonstrated that if MetS is identified in its earlier stages, it can be reversed with adherence to a weight-loss and aerobic exercise program resulting in loss of as little as 7% of body weight [1]; a weight loss of 10% or more provides an even better outcome. Reversal of MetS means that the individual is no longer classified as having the syndrome, and that some of the signs of inflammation are also reduced. These improvements contrast with the later stages of type 2 diabetes, which is likely to progress until serious complications develop.

References Cited

1. Magkos F, Yannakoulia, Chan JL, Mantzoros CS. Management of the metabolic syndrome and type 2 diabetes through life style modification. Annu Rev Nutr. 2009; 29:233–56.

2. Alberti, KGMN, Eckel RH, Grundy SM, et al. Harmonizing the metabolic syndrome: a joint interim statement of the International Diabetes Federation Task Force on Epidemiology and Prevention; National Heart, Lung, and Blood Institute; American Heart Association; World Heart Federation; International Atherosclerosis Society; and International Association for the Study of Obesity. Circulation. 2009; 120:1640–45.

3. Tenebaum A, Fisman E. "The metabolic syndrome . . . is dead": these reports are an exaggeration. Cardiovascular Diabetology. 2011; 10:11–15.

4. Mottillo S, Filion KB, Genest J, et al. The metabolic syndrome and cardiovascular risk. J Am Coll Cardiology. 2010; 56:1113–32.

Table 1 Criteria for Clinical Diagnosis of the Metabolic Syndrome

Measure	Categorical Cut Points
Elevated waist circumference	102 cm (40 in for men)
	88 cm (35 in for women)
Elevated triacylglycerols*	≥ 150 mg/dL
Reduced HDL-C*	< 40 mg/dL (1.0 mmol/L) in males
	< 50 mg/dL (1.3 mmol/L) in females
Elevated blood pressure*	Systolic ≥130 and/or diastolic ≥85 mm Hg
Elevated fasting glucose*	≥ 100 mg/dL

* Drug treatment for elevated condition is an alternate indicator.
Source: Modified from Alberti, KGMN, Eckel RH, Grundy SM, et al. Harmonizing the metabolic syndrome: a joint interim statement of the International Diabetes Federation Task Force on Epidemiology and Prevention; National Heart, Lung, and Blood Institute; American Heart Association; World Heart Federation; International Atherosclerosis Society; and International Association for the Study of Obesity. Circulation. 2009;120:1640–45 to show cut points for U. S. and Canada.

8 BODY COMPOSITION, ENERGY EXPENDITURE, AND ENERGY BALANCE

BODY WEIGHT AND COMPOSITION ARE important areas in the study of nutrition. The current rapid increase in the prevalence of obesity in this country is making headlines. Government, medical, public health, and nutrition professionals are examining the etiology and developing strategies to stop or reverse this trend of increased obesity. This chapter explores what we should weigh, our body composition, and how to determine the proportions of fat mass and fat-free mass. The chapter also addresses the balance between energy intake and expenditure as well the impact of energy imbalance on our weight and body composition. Understanding the influences of genetics and hormones that regulate our appetite, weight, and body composition will assist in developing and implementing interventions.

BODY WEIGHT: WHAT SHOULD WE WEIGH?

Recognition of body weight as an indicator of health status is probably universal and as old as humanity itself. In fact, in 1846 English surgeon John Hutchinson published a height-weight table based upon a sample of 30-year-old Englishmen and urged that future census taking include such information, which he believed to be valuable in promoting health and detecting disease [1]. Today, scientists and health professionals recognize that the risk of many diseases—including heart disease, stroke, diabetes mellitus, hypertension, osteoarthritis, infertility, and some cancers (breast, endometrial, colon, and kidney)—increases with excess body fat. Because body fat is so difficult to measure, body weight is a good proxy in the nonathletic population. Furthermore, a low body weight may indicate malnutrition or an eating disorder and may pose risks for other diseases, such as osteoporosis. What represents too much weight or too little weight for a given height? Unfortunately, recommendations from health experts vary. This chapter covers some of the currently accepted approaches to weight assessment.

Body Mass Index

Body mass index (BMI), first described in the 1860s and known as Quetelet's Index, is at present one of the most accepted approaches to assessing appropriate weight for a given height. The body mass index is considered an indication of body adiposity but does not measure body fat. BMI is calculated from a person's height and weight as shown in this formula:

$$\text{Body mass index} = \frac{\text{Weight}}{\text{Height}^2}$$

with weight measured in kilograms (kg) and height measured in meters (m) and raised to a power of 2. BMI is expressed in units of kg/m^2.

Body mass index is considered a good index of total body fat in both men and women and has generally replaced calculations of percent relative body weight and percent ideal body weight (see the "Formulas" section) for classifying people as underweight or overweight. For adults, classification of weight based upon BMI by the National Institutes of Health [2–4] is presented in Figure 8.1 and is based upon the following criteria:

- BMI < 18.5 kg/m^2, underweight (with < 16 suggesting a possible eating disorder)
- BMI 18.5 to 24.9 kg/m^2, healthy/low health risks
- BMI 25 to 29.9 kg/m^2, overweight and associated with increased risk of disease
- BMI 30 to 34.9 kg/m^2, obese (grade 1) and associated with further increased risk of disease
- BMI 35 to 39.9 kg/m^2, obese (grade 2) and associated with higher risk of disease
- BMI $\geq$ 40 kg/m^2, extremely or morbidly obese (grade 3)

BMI is also used to assess weight in children, but through comparison to population standards for sex and age. BMI changes with age in healthy children, as demonstrated by the body mass index growth curve for boys and girls 2 to 20 years of age shown in Figure 8.2. A BMI <5th percentile is underweight, a healthy weight is equivalent to a BMI between the 5th and 85th percentiles, BMIs between the 85th and 95th percentiles are classified as overweight, and a BMI > 95th percentile is considered obese [5]. Body weight and recumbent length for boys and girls under 2 years of age are assessed using growth charts similar to those in Figure 8.2 from the Centers for Disease Control and Prevention (CDC). These charts provide percentiles of weight for recumbent length.

Using the formula to calculate the BMI of a 5-foot, 11-inches (or 71-inches) man weighing 165 lb would involve two conversions before plugging numbers into the BMI formula. First, to convert weight in pounds (lb) to weight in kilograms (kg), divide by 2.2 (because there are 2.2 lb per 1 kg): 165 lb ÷ 2.2 lb/kg = 75 kg. Next, convert height in feet and inches to meters (m). Because there are 39.37 inches/m, divide the man's height of 71 inches by 39.37 inches/m to get 1.803 m. With weight in kilograms and height in meters, the formula can be used: BMI = 75 kg ÷ (1.803 m)^2 = 75 kg ÷ 3.25 m^2 = 23.1 kg/m^2.

Although the body mass index is a valuable tool for assessing weight, like many other methods it does not determine body fatness. Thus, people such as athletes may

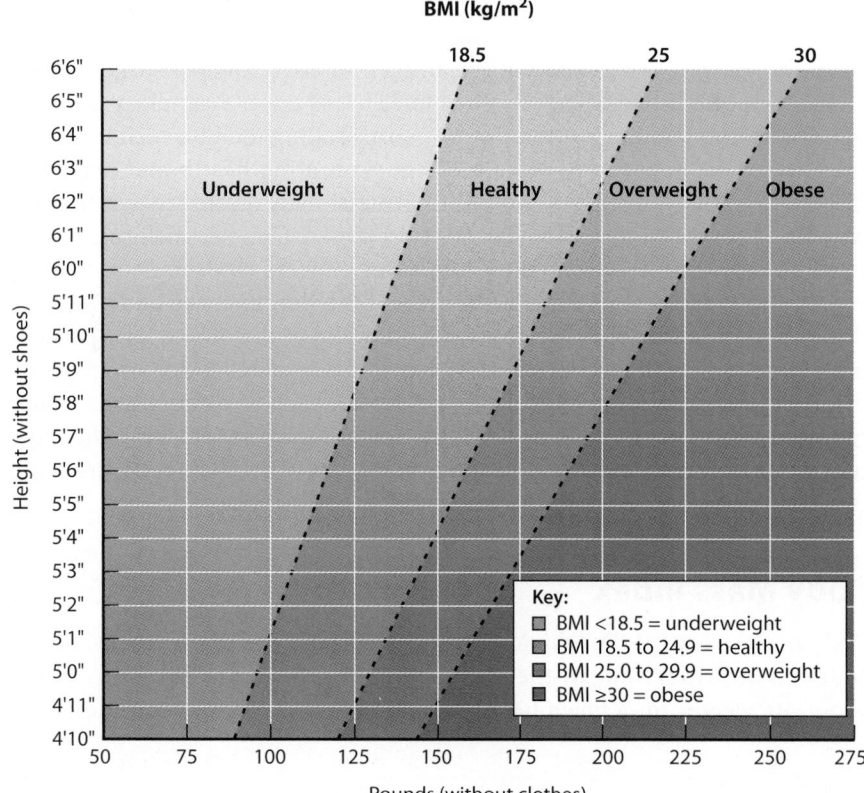

Figure 8.1 BMI values used to assess weight.
Source: U.S. Department of Agriculture and Human Services, Nutrition and Your Health: Dietary Guidelines for Americans. Washington, DC, 2000, p. 7.

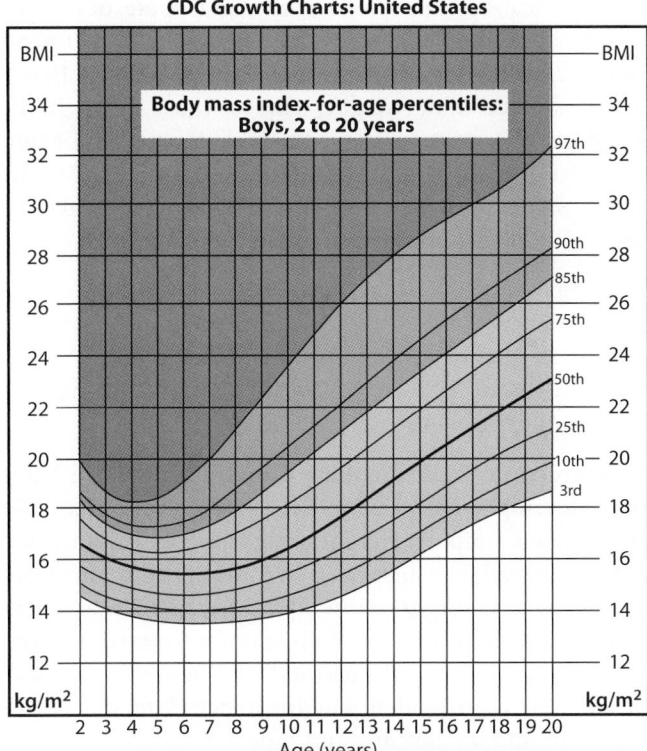

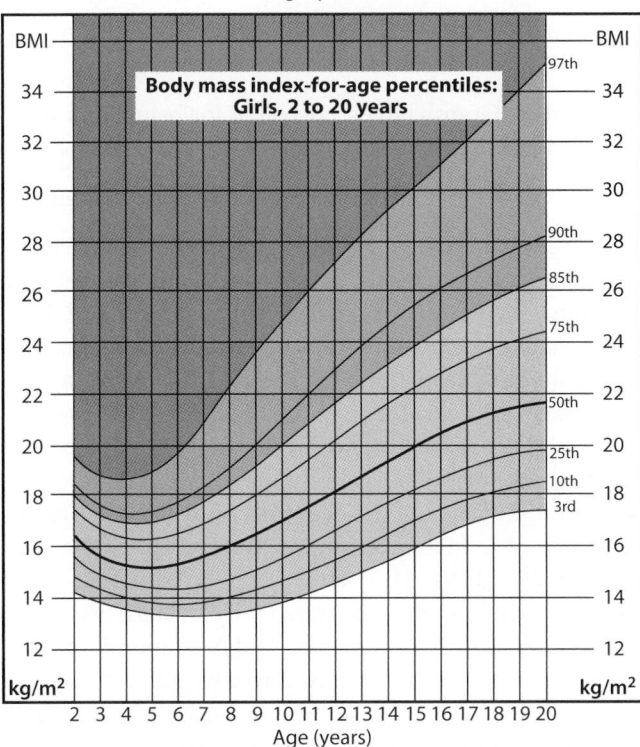

Figure 8.2 Example of growth curves (2 to 20 years): boys' and girls' body mass index-for-age percentiles.

Source: http://www.cdc.gov/growthcharts/.

have large amounts of lean body mass and a high BMI (and thus be considered overweight or obese by classification) but have a low percentage of body fat. The relationship between BMI and body fat has been shown to vary among different age, sex, and race/ethnic groups.

Formulas

Based upon comparisons between ideal body weight (IBW) equations along with published height-weight tables and the body mass index, the BMI that corresponds to "ideal body weight" is 22 kg/m^2 [6]. In addition to the body mass index, other formulas are available to calculate IBW. One of the more popular formulas is that by Devine [7,8]:

$$\text{IBW for men} = 50 \text{ kg} + 2.3 \text{ kg/inch} > 5 \text{ foot}$$
$$\text{IBW for women} = 45 \text{ kg} + 2.3 \text{ kg/inch} > 5 \text{ foot}$$

These formulas have been modified somewhat and converted into the following familiar empirical formulas for those with a medium-size body frame:

$$\text{IBW for men} = 110 \text{ lb} + 5 \text{ lb/inch} > 5 \text{ foot}$$
$$\text{IBW for women} = 100 \text{ lb} + 5 \text{ lb/inch} > 5 \text{ foot}$$

A slightly modified formula for men is also used:

$$\text{IBW for men} = 106 \text{ lb} + 6 \text{ lb/inch} > 5 \text{ foot}$$

The Devine formula usually includes a range of 10% below and above the calculated ideal weight to allow for differences in weight from a small or a large frame, respectively. Frame size traditionally is assessed using either of two methods based upon measurements of wrist or elbow breadth and height. The method of determining the elbow breadth is shown in Figure 8.3. In addition, the frame index 2 considers not only elbow breadth and height but also age and gender. The frame index 2 value is determined by the following formula:

$$\text{Frame index 2 value} = \frac{\text{Elbow breadth}}{\text{Height}} \times 100$$

with elbow breadth measured in millimeters (mm) and height measured in centimeters (cm) [9]. Once calculated, a person's frame index 2 value is compared with age-based values (shown in Table 8.1) to determine small, medium, or large frame size.

Table 8.1 Classification of Frame Size Based on Frame Index 2 Values

Age (yrs)	Male			Female		
	Small	Medium	Large	Small	Medium	Large
18.0–24.9	<38.4	38.4 to 41.6	>41.6	<35.2	35.2 to 38.6	>38.6
25.0–29.9	<38.6	38.6 to 41.8	>41.8	<35.7	35.7 to 38.7	>38.7
30.0–34.9	<38.6	38.6 to 42.1	>42.1	<35.7	35.7 to 39.0	>39.0
35.0–39.9	<39.1	39.1 to 42.4	>42.4	<36.2	36.2 to 39.8	>39.8
40.0–44.9	<39.3	39.3 to 42.5	>42.5	<36.7	36.7 to 40.2	>40.2
45.0–49.9	<39.6	39.6 to 43.0	>43.0	<37.2	37.2 to 40.7	>40.7
50.0–54.9	<39.9	39.9 to 43.3	>43.3	<37.2	37.2 to 41.6	>41.6
55.0–59.9	<40.2	40.2 to 43.8	>43.8	<37.8	37.8 to 41.9	>41.9
60.0–64.9	<40.2	40.2 to 43.6	>43.6	<38.2	38.2 to 41.8	>41.8
65.0–69.9	<40.2	40.2 to 43.6	>43.6	<38.2	38.2 to 41.8	>41.8

Source: This table was published in Matarese, L., Gottschlich, M., *Contemporary Nutrition Support Practice*, p. 37. Copyright Elsevier, 2003.

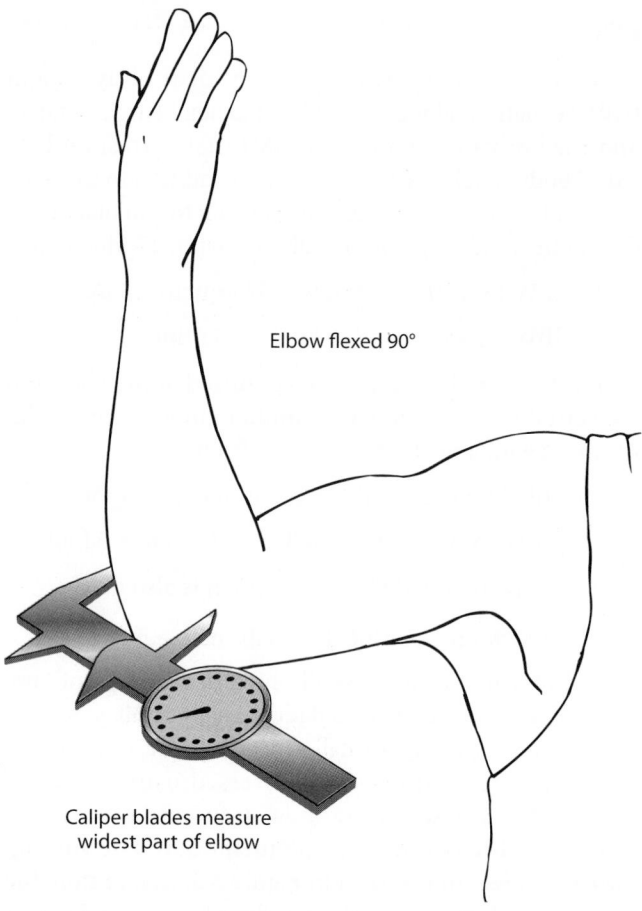

Elbow flexed 90°

Caliper blades measure
widest part of elbow

Upper arm parallel to floor

Figure 8.3 Measurement of elbow breadth. Extend your arm and bend the forearm upward at a 90° angle. Keep your fingers straight, and turn the inside of your wrist toward your body. Place the calipers on the two prominent bones on either side of the elbow. Measure the space between the bones with the caliper to the nearest 0.1 cm or 1/8 inch.

Using the formulas, a man who is 5 foot, 11 inches tall with a medium frame should weigh either 165 lb (110 + [5 × 11] = 165 lb) or 172 lb (106 + [6 × 11] = 172 lb), depending upon which formula is used. If the man has a small frame, ideal body weight would be 10% less than that calculated for a medium frame size (i.e., 165 lb − 16.5 lb = 148.5 lb or 172 lb − 17.2 lb = 154.8 lb, respectively). A female who is 5 foot 6 inches tall and has a large frame has an ideal body weight of 143 lb (100 + [5 × 6] = 130 lb + 13 lb [accounting for the 10% addition for the large frame size] = 143 lb).

Dividing a person's actual body weight by the ideal body weight calculated (from the Devine formula) for his or her estimated frame size gives a value called percentage ideal body weight, as shown:

$$\% \text{ IBW} = \frac{\text{Actual Body Weight}}{\text{Ideal Body Weight}} \times 100$$

Although largely replaced by use of the body mass index, calculation of percent IBW is another approach used for classification of people as overweight, obese, or underweight. For example, people whose body weight is 10% or more below the ideal for a given height (i.e., ≤90% IBW) are considered underweight, whereas those whose body weight is 10% or more above the ideal for a given height (i.e., ≥110% IBW) are considered overweight. People with a weight for height 20% or more above the ideal (i.e., ≥120% IBW) are considered obese.

Using the formula, a male with a medium frame who is 6 foot, 3 inches tall and weighs 260 lb would have a % IBW of 260 lb/(106 lb + [6 lb/inch + 15 inches]) × 100, or 260 lb/196 lb × 100 or 132.7%. At 132.7% IBW, this male would be considered obese.

Regression equations for estimating IBW also have been developed based upon the 1959 Metropolitan Life Insurance Company height-weight tables [1] and the ideal body weight tables used by Grant [10] in nutrition assessment. The regression equation is still used even though the Metropolitan Life Insurance Company tables have been replaced by the use of BMI. The equation based on the 1959 Metropolitan Life Insurance Company tables [11] (with indoor clothing and shoes) is:

$$\text{IBW (lb)} = -139.17 + 3.86(\text{height}) + 9.52(\text{frame}) + 5.01(\text{sex})$$

Based on Grant's tables, corrected for height and nude weight, the equation becomes:

$$\text{IBW (lb)} = -133.99 + 3.86(\text{height}) + 9.52(\text{frame}) + 3.08(\text{sex})$$

In these two equations, height is in inches. Values used for frame size are 1 for small, 2 for medium, and 3 for large. Values for sex are +1 for male and −1 for female.

Although measuring both height and weight is relatively easy and can serve as a screen for underweight, overweight, or obesity, no method (weight for height from tables, formulas, or body mass index) is necessarily a valid indicator of the degree of body fatness. The inadequacy of weight as a valid measure of fatness became clear in World War II when A. R. Behnke, a Navy physician, was able to demonstrate by hydrostatic weighing that several football players who had been found unfit for military service because of excessive weight actually had less body fat than controls of normal weight [12]. The excessive weight of these athletes resulted from hypertrophy of muscles rather than excessive adipose tissue [12]. Behnke's work rekindled interest in studying the composition of the human body, an interest that had lain dormant for about 50 years.

These methods for evaluating body weight in relation to height are useful clinically for broad classification, particularly for epidemiological studies, but they have their limitations. The BMI levels that are associated with the lowest all-cause and cardiovascular mortality vary with age: Optimum BMI tends to be higher for older adults compared with the young or middle-aged population [13]. Moreover, the increased risk for diseases with obesity is more associated with levels of body fat than with weight. BMI is correlated with body fat but does not measure it directly. Also, as discussed in Chapter 7, visceral (abdominal) fat is a greater risk factor for cardiovascular disease and stroke than subcutaneous fat. Methods that evaluate body fat will be examined later in this chapter, but body composition must be discussed first.

THE COMPOSITION OF THE HUMAN BODY

The chemical composition of the human body was first described in 1859 in a book that dealt with the chemical composition of food [14]. Analytic chemistry was a rapidly growing science at the time, and the chemical compositions of the different body tissues were compared with those of various foods. Additional chemical composition data from whole-body analysis of fetuses, children, and adults collected during the next few decades represent a direct (rather than indirect) measure of body composition [15–20].

The concept of the reference man and woman was developed in the 1970s [19]. These reference figures provide information on body composition based upon average physical dimensions and hence a frame of reference for comparisons. The characteristics of the reference man and woman are presented in Table 6.8. Recall (Table 6.8) that the reference man has 3% essential fat, 12% storage fat (for a total of 15% body fat), 44.8% muscle, 14.9% bone, and 25.3% other components. The reference woman has 12% essential fat, 15% storage fat (for a total of 27% body fat), 36% muscle, 12% bone, and 25% other components. Essential fat includes the fat that is associated with bone marrow, the central nervous system, internal organs, and the cell membranes. The essential fat in females also includes the fat in mammary glands and the pelvic region. These gender differences must be considered when body composition is evaluated. Normal changes in body composition associated with development and aging should also be accounted for; these are detailed in Chapter 6, in the "Changes in Body Mass with Age" section.

Body composition assessment typically involves the division of body tissues into "compartments" that are then measured. In this chapter, we focus on the two-compartment model, which includes fat mass (FM) and fat-free mass (FFM); and the four-compartment model, which in addition to FM and FFM includes bone mineral and total body water. These methods often measure the specific organs or the location of adipose tissue. The four-compartment model is considered the gold standard but requires special equipment to measure all of the components. The most frequently used methods to compare and evaluate body composition consider only two compartments, fat mass and fat-free mass. Fat mass consists mostly of triacylglycerols and other lipid components, with relatively small amounts of water or electrolytes. Fat-free mass is much more diverse. It is made up of muscle, bones, and the intra- and extracellular fluids. Muscle contains about 73% water. The differences in the properties of the two compartments—for example, variations in density (weight for a given volume), the ability to conduct an electrical current, the electrolyte content, and the X-ray density—form the basis for many of the methods of determining body composition.

METHODS FOR MEASURING BODY COMPOSITION

The choice of the method for measuring body composition depends upon the purpose, the number of individuals to be measured, age, and cost. Division of the body into components is used extensively for *in vivo* studies of body composition. The body can be analyzed in terms of its atomic elements—primarily carbon, oxygen, hydrogen, and nitrogen, which make up about 95% of body mass, along with about another 50 or so elements that make up the remaining 5%. Alternately, the body may be thought of from a nutritional or molecular perspective as consisting of water, protein, fat, carbohydrate, and minerals. Multicompartment models to assess body composition rely on calculations of these different nutrient components.

Commonly available methods are indirect and provide a means to calculate body components (direct measurement is accomplished only on cadavers). Although different procedures are available, accuracy varies not only with the equipment or method used but also with the technician. Several indirect methods of body composition assessment are reviewed in this section.

Systems using the two-component (FM and FFM) model include anthropometry, densitometry, ultrasound, total body water, and infrared interactance. At one time, densitometry (underwater weighing) was the one standard against which other indirect measurements of body composition were evaluated [14,18,20]. The basic assumption for methods dependent upon body density is that the densities of the fat mass and fat-free mass are constant. Fat mass includes essential and nonessential fat (triacylglycerols), whereas fat-free mass includes protein, water, carbohydrate (glycogen), and minerals [14,18]. Though the term *lean body mass* is often used synonymously with *fat-free mass*, lean body mass is a broader term since it also includes essential body fat [14,20].

Currently, the most accepted method for evaluating healthy adults is dual-energy X-ray absorptiometry (DXA), which is based on the difference in dual-energy X-rays of bone mineral, bone-free fat-free mass, and fat mass. This method is now commonly used for evaluating clinical populations. There are several additional methods for body composition assessment available, some based upon the two-component model and a few (including dual-energy X-ray and computerized tomography and magnetic resonance) based on the four-component model.

Anthropometry

Anthropometry estimates body composition through measurement at various circumference and skin fold (fat) sites. Skin varies in thickness from 0.5 to 2 mm [21]; thus, fat beneath the skin typically represents most of the skin fold measurement. The assumption is that a direct relationship exists between total body fat and fat deposited in depots just beneath the skin (i.e., subcutaneous fat). Skin fold measurements can be used in one of two ways:

- Scores from the various measurements can be added and the sum used to indicate the relative degree of fatness among subjects.

- Scores can be plugged into various mathematical regression equations developed to predict body density or to calculate percentage of body fat [20,22].

Five sites commonly used for measuring skin fold thickness are the triceps (measured on the back of the upper arm), subscapula (measured just below the tip of the scapula), suprailiac (measured above the hip bone), abdomen (measured 1 inch to the right of the umbilicus), and thigh (measured at the midpoint of the thigh, between the kneecap and the hip) [23,24]. Additional sites often include the pectoral (chest), midaxillary, and calf. Figure 8.4 shows the technique for measuring the back of the upper arm (triceps)—a vertical fold is measured at the midline of the upper arm halfway between the tip of the shoulder and the tip of the elbow. The right side of the body is used for most measurements if comparisons are being made to standards derived from data from U.S. surveys because such surveys typically measured the right side of subjects. Other locales such as the United Kingdom use the left side. The handedness of the subject affects skin fold measurements taken on the arm such that measurements on the dominant side exceed those on the nondominant side by 0.2 to 0.3 standard deviation units [25].

Bias associated with the side of the measurement, however, is less significant than error caused by measurement [25]. All measurements should be repeated at least two or three times, and the average should be used as the skin fold value. Measurement procedures and the use of formulas (see the next paragraph) contribute to procedure error. The precision of skin fold thickness measurements depends upon the skill of the anthropometrist; in general, a precision of within 5% can be obtained by a well-trained and experienced anthropometrist [26]. The use of anthropometry for predicting visceral fat content offers limited accuracy [27]. Nevertheless, the method is quite inexpensive compared with other techniques.

Several population-specific equations for calculating total body fat from skin fold sites have been developed. Equations developed by Katch and McArdle [23] for predicting total body fat in young (age 17–26 years) men and women from the triceps and subscapular skin folds are shown:

Young women: percent body fat = 0.55(A) + 0.31(B) + 6.13

Young men: percent body fat = 0.43(A) + 0.58(B) + 1.47

where A = triceps fat fold measured in millimeters and
B = subscapular fat fold measured in millimeters.

Measurements from multiple (at least three) sites are deemed better for overall subcutaneous fat assessment than measurements from only one or two sites [23].

Circumference or girth measurements also may be used to assess body fat. Typical sites of measurement include the abdomen, buttocks, right thigh, and right upper arm. As with skin fold measurements, body fat prediction equations utilizing circumferences have been developed that are age and gender specific.

Circumference measurements of the waist (abdominal circumference) and hips (gluteal circumference) also provide an index of regional body fat distribution and have been shown to correlate with visceral fat [27]. Waist measurements should be made below the rib cage and above the umbilicus in a horizontal plane at the narrow site, or the site of least circumference. Hip circumference should be measured at the site with the greatest circumference around the hips or buttocks. Soft tissue should not be compressed or indented during these measurements, and all measurements should be taken with the subject

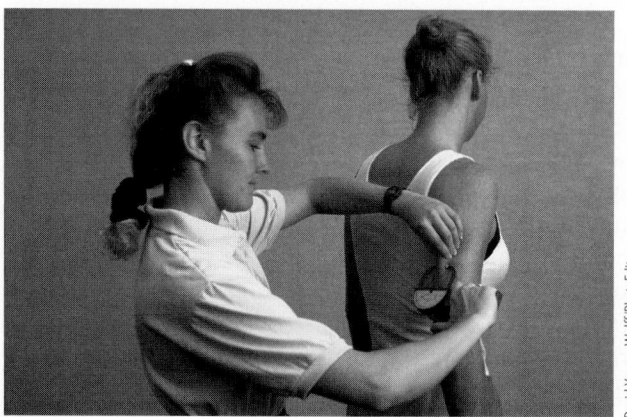

David Young-Wolff/PhotoEdit

Figure 8.4 Measuring triceps skin fold with a Lange caliper to estimate body fat.

standing. Reproducibility of circumference measurements is good with only a 2% error in measurement [27]. The ratio of waist to hip circumference is calculated following measurement of the subject's waist and hip. Ratios >0.8 inches (women) and >0.95 inches (men) are thought to indicate increased health risk. Waist circumferences >40 inches (men) and >35 inches (women), without comparison to hip circumference, also may be used to identify increased abdominal fat and thus increased risk for the development of obesity-associated conditions [28,29].

Other anthropometric measurements have been piloted in efforts to achieve results that are easy to obtain and to understand, with varying success. The most common measurement is the waist-hip ratio mentioned above. Another interesting ratio is called the Body Adiposity Index (BAI). This ratio was developed by identifying anthropometric measurements that correlated best with body fat. The researchers discovered that the hip circumference and height gave the largest correlation coefficient. It was determined that the best predictive equation is [29]:

$$BAI = \frac{\text{Hip circumference}}{(\text{Height})^{1.5}} - 18$$

where hip circumference is measured in centimeters and height in meters.

It is too early to determine if BAI will catch on and be useful, but it has been evaluated in several different population groups and successfully identified individuals with excessive visceral adiposity [30,31].

Densitometry/Hydrodensitometry

The principle of hydrostatic weighing on which densitometry or hydrodensitometry is based can be traced to the Greek mathematician Archimedes. He discovered that the volume of an object submerged in water is equal to the volume of water displaced by the object. The specific gravity or density of an object can be calculated by dividing the object's weight (wt) in air by its loss of weight in water. For example, for a person who weighs 47 kg in air and 2 kg underwater, 45 kg represents the loss of body weight and the weight of the water displaced. After an adjustment for the change in density of water at different temperatures is made, the volume of the person can be calculated. Figure 8.5 illustrates the apparatus for weighing under water. Correction for residual air volume in the lungs (RLV) and gas in the gastrointestinal tract (GIGV) must be made.

Body density is calculated using the following formula:

$$\text{Body density} = \frac{\text{Wt of body in air}}{\dfrac{\left(\dfrac{\text{Wt of body}}{\text{in air}} - \dfrac{\text{Wt of body}}{\text{underwater}}\right)}{\text{Density of water}} - RLV - GIGV}$$

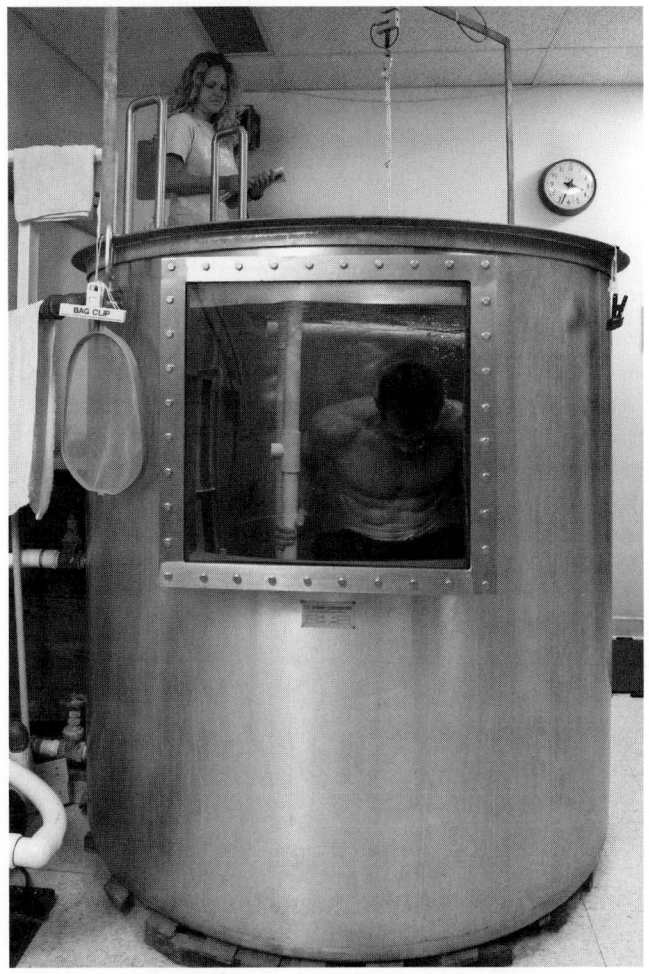

Figure 8.5 Apparatus for underwater weighing to determine body density.

Residual lung volume is thought to be about 24% of vital lung capacity. The volume of gas in the gastrointestinal tract is estimated to range from 50 to 300 mL. This volume typically is neglected, or a value of 100 mL may be used in calculations. The density or the weight of water is known for a wide range of temperatures and must be obtained for the calculation.

Calculating the density of the human body allows an estimation of body fat. At any known body density, estimating the percentage of body fat in an adult is possible using an equation derived by Siri [32]:

$$\text{Percentage of body fat} = \frac{495}{\text{Body Density}} - 450 \times 100$$

or an equation derived by Brozek [32]:

$$\text{Percentage of body fat} = \frac{457}{\text{Body Density}} - 414 \times 100$$

Calculations of body density are derived in part from the knowledge that the density of fat mass is 0.9 g/cm³ and that the density of fat-free mass is 1.1 g/cm³ (assuming fat-free mass is composed of about 20.5% protein, 72.4% water, and 7.1% bone mineral). Once the percentage of body fat has been calculated, the weight of the fat and the lean body mass can be estimated as follows [20]:

$$\text{Body weight} \times \text{percentage body fat} = \text{Weight of body fat}$$

$$\text{Body weight} - \text{weight of body fat} = \text{Lean body weight}$$

Various calculations for determining ideal or desirable body weight based upon body composition have been proposed, such as this formula [23]:

$$\text{Desirable body weight} = \frac{\text{Lean body weight}}{1 - \text{percent fat desired}}$$

Calculations would be as follows for a woman who weighs 200 lb, with a measured 40% of this weight as fat:

$$200 \text{ lb} \times 0.40 = 80 \text{ lb (fat weight)}$$

$$200 \text{ lb} - 80 \text{ lb} = 120 \text{ lb (lean body weight)}$$

Because the desirable amount of fat in females ranges from about 20% to 30%, a figure of 25% (0.25) is used in the following equation for the sample woman:

$$\text{Desirable body weight} = \frac{120}{1 - 0.25} = \frac{120}{0.75} = 160 \text{ lb}$$

Underwater weighing is considered a noninvasive and relatively precise method for assessment of body fat. The standard error of estimate of body fat using densitometry has been estimated at 2.7% for adults and about 4.5% for children and adolescents [23]. Measurements obtained by underwater weighing correlate well in broad populations with those obtained by other techniques. Some studies have reported some variations or underestimation of fat in specific groups when this method is compared with air displacement plethysmography and dual-energy X-ray absorptiometry (DEXA) [33–36]. The differences between underwater weighing and DEXA have not been fully explained but in part are due to discrepancies between assumed and measured lung volumes and bone mineral density. Limitations of underwater weighing include its relatively high equipment cost, the inability to measure gas volume in the gastrointestinal tract, its impracticality for large numbers of subjects, and the extreme cooperation and time required of subjects, who must be submerged and remain motionless for an extended time. Thus, the technique is not suitable for young children, older adults, or subjects in poor health. Additional limitations to its use include its assumption that density of lean body mass is relatively constant, when in fact bone density typically changes with age [36].

Air-Displacement Plethysmography

Another way to determine the volume of the body is with air-displacement plethysmography (ADP). In the commercially available apparatus shown in Figure 8.6 (Bod

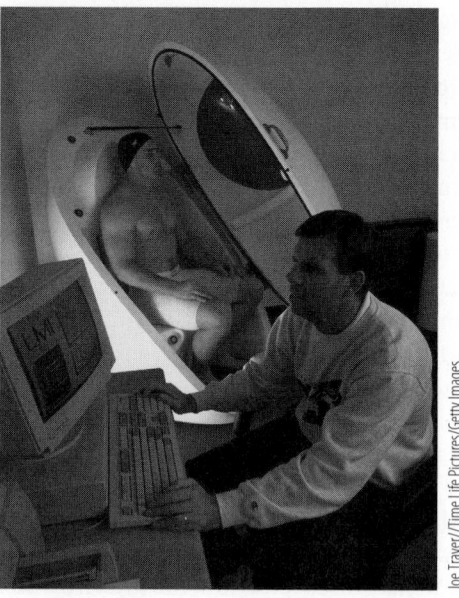

Figure 8.6 Air-displacement plethysmography determines body density by measuring the amount of air displaced.

Pod Life Measurements Inc.), the subject is seated in a sealed chamber of known volume, separated from a second chamber by a membrane. The instrument measures the change in pressure caused by the volume occupied by the person. The person is dressed in a tight-fitting bathing suit and wears a bathing cap (to displace pockets of air in the hair). The measurement takes only a few minutes to complete. The apparatus has an advantage in that it can measure the body composition in age groups that are not suitable for underwater weighing, such as the elderly or the very young. A similar instrument called the PEA POD is designed for infants and small children. Once the density of the body is obtained, the calculation of body composition is the same as with hydrodensitometry.

Absorptiometry

Photon Absorptiometry

Absorptiometry is an imaging technique that involves scanning the entire body or a portion of the body with a photon beam. Single-photon absorptiometry involves scanning the body with photons from ^{125}I (iodine) at a specific energy level. However, this technique does not allow accurate measurement at soft tissue sites. This problem has been eliminated with the development of dual-photon absorptiometry. In dual-photon absorptiometry, the radionuclide source is generally ^{153}Gd (gadolinium), and photons at two different energy levels are emitted. Bone mineral content as well as fat mass and fat-free mass may be estimated via dual-photon absorptiometry.

A three-dimensional photonic scanner has been used for accurate measurements of body shape and dimensions. Total or regional body volumes or dimensions can be obtained. These volumes have been compared with those obtained through underwater weighing and were found to be slightly greater [37].

Dual Energy X-ray Absorptiometry (DXA)

Dual energy X-ray absorptiometry (abbreviated DXA or DEXA), introduced in the late 1980s, involves scanning subjects with X-rays at two different energy levels and is illustrated in Figure 8.7. The subject lies on a table while an X-ray source beneath the table and the detector above the table pass across the subject's body. Attenuation of the beam of X-rays as it passes over the body is calculated by computer. Percentage of fat mass, bone-free fat-free mass, and bone mineral (total body or specific sites) can be calculated based on the restriction in the flux of the X-rays across the fat and the fat-free masses [26,37–40].

DXA is considered to be the gold standard technique for diagnosing osteoporosis and osteopenia and is a commonly used method for body composition measurements. It is widely available and entails relatively low X-ray exposure: 1% to 10% that of a chest X-ray [37]. Limitations to the use of absorptiometry include the expense of the equipment and the exposure of subjects to radiation. In addition, trained personnel are required to run the instrument and analyze the scans. DXA measurements are highly reproducible and correlate with other body composition assessment methods. The technique, however, is not accurate for people with metal implants, including, for example, pins or rods. The table on which the procedure is performed has a weight limit, and extremely obese people may have difficulty getting on it. This problem is being addressed by the

equipment manufacturers. For very large people, fat mass estimates are influenced by trunk thickness.

Computerized (Axial) Tomography (CAT or CT)

Computerized or computed (axial) tomography (CT or CAT), another imaging technique involving an X-ray tube and detectors aligned at opposite poles of a circular gantry, creates visual images and thus enables regional body composition (such as visceral organ mass, regional muscle mass, subcutaneous and internal fat, and bone density) to be determined. Subjects lie face up on a movable platform that passes through the instrument's circular gantry. Cross-sectional images of tissue are constructed by the scanner computer as the X-ray beam rotates around the person being assessed. Differences in X-ray attenuation are related to differences in the physical density of tissues [26]. The relative surface area or volume occupied by tissues (e.g., bone, adipose, and fat-free tissue) can be calculated from the images produced by the instrument. Results are highly reproducible [27]. CT scans can assess body fat distribution, distinguish trabecular and cortical bones, and measure a true body mass density [30,37]. However, CT has drawbacks as a composition assessment method: the excessively long exposure of subjects to ionizing radiation and the expense of purchasing and operating the equipment. Thus, this technique is used primarily for research purposes.

Magnetic Resonance Imaging (MRI)

Magnetic resonance imaging (MRI) is based upon the principle that when an external magnetic field is applied across the body, atomic nuclei behave like magnets—that is, the nuclei attempt to align with the field. The nuclei also absorb radio frequency waves directed into the body and in turn change their orientation in the magnetic field [26]. Abolishing the radio wave results in the emission of a radio signal by the activated nuclei, and this emitted signal is used to develop a computerized image. Magnetic resonance imaging is used to measure organ size and structure, body fat and fat distribution (subcutaneous, visceral, intra-abdominal), and muscle size, as well as body water contents. The technique is noninvasive and safe; however, the cost is high. Reproducibility of visceral fat area measured by magnetic resonance imaging is about 10% to 15% [27]. However, for assessment of adipose tissue distribution, MRI provided the least variability when compared to skin fold thickness, ^{40}K counting (see the section "Total Body Potassium"), bioelectrical impedance, total body water assessment with ^{18}O (see the "Total Body Water" section), and hydrostatic weighing [41]. MRI is considered to be the most accurate for the *in vivo* quantification

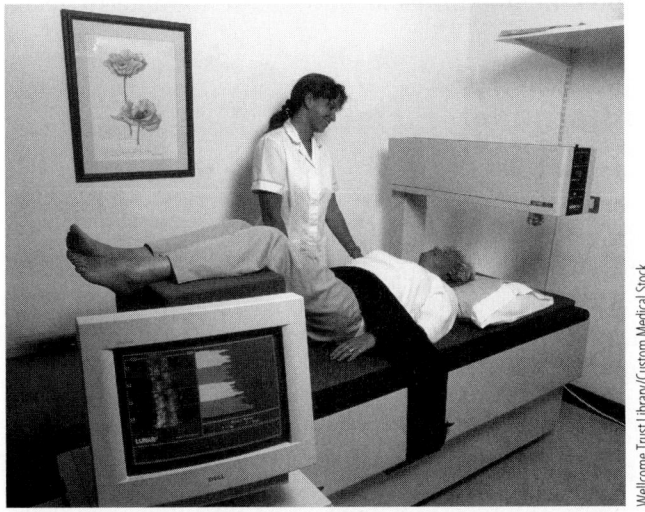

Wellcome Trust Library/Custom Medical Stock

Figure 8.7 Dual-energy X-ray absorptiometry (DEXA) uses two X-ray beams of different energy to determine fat-free mass, fat mass, and bone tissue.

of body composition [37]. MRI can quantify the distribution of adipose tissue into visceral, subcutaneous, and intramuscular deposits. Its limitations include its high cost and the difficulty in fitting large individuals within the field of view. Manufacturers are modifying the equipment so that it will accommodate larger people. Conventional MRI cannot determine lipids or water in skeletal muscle. These measurements require proton-magnetic resonance spectroscopy [37].

Bioelectrical Impedance Analysis (BIA)

Bioelectrical impedance analysis (BIA; Figure 8.8), also called bioelectrical impedance (BEI), is a commonly used technique based upon the two-compartment model that depends upon changes in electrical conductivity. The BIA measurement of electrical conductivity is made on the extremities and not on the whole body. Subjects lie face up on a bed, with their extremities away from the body. Electrodes are placed on the limbs in specific locations. An instrument generates a current or multiple electrical current frequencies that are passed through the body by means of the electrodes. Opposition to the electric current, called impedance, is detected and measured by the instrument. Impedance is the inverse of conductance. The lowest resistance value of a person is used to calculate conductance and predict lean body mass or fat-free mass. For example, muscle, organs, and blood, which have high water and electrolyte contents, are good conductors [42]. Tissues containing little water and electrolytes (such as adipose tissue) are poor conductors and have a high resistance to the passage of electrical current [42]. When multiple frequencies are used, the higher frequencies can estimate both intracellular and extracellular water because the higher-frequency current can penetrate cell membranes. At lower frequencies, the flow of the current is blocked, and the measured resistance indicates extracellular water [37].

Bioelectrical impedance is a safe, noninvasive, and rapid means to assess body composition. The equipment is portable and fairly easy to operate, although it is also relatively expensive. Bioelectrical impedance readings are affected by hydration and electrolyte imbalances. Thus, the technique is more useful for healthy subjects. Several bioelectrical impedance analysis prediction equations have been developed for various populations. The use of multifrequency BIA provides results that are in good agreement with other body composition methods because this technique estimates both total body water and extracellular water [37].

Ultrasonography or Ultrasound

Ultrasound provides images of tissue configuration or depth readings of changes in tissue density [26]. Electrical energy is converted in a probe to high-frequency ultrasonic energy. The ultrasonic energy is transmitted through the skin and into the body in the form of short pulses or waves. The waves pass through adipose tissue until they reach lean body mass. At the interface between the adipose and lean tissues, part of the ultrasonic energy is reflected back to the receiver in the probe and transformed to electrical energy. The echo is visualized on an oscilloscope. A transmission gel used between the probe and the skin provides acoustic contact. The equipment is portable, and the technique may provide information on the thickness of subcutaneous fat as well as the thickness of muscle mass. Reliability of the technique has improved to 91%, and accuracy is similar to that of skin fold measurements [43]. Ultrasound measurements of subcutaneous and visceral abdominal fat thickness in older adults correlate well with similar data obtained using the MRI technique, and represent an improvement over anthropometric techniques [44].

Infrared Interactance

Infrared interactance is based upon the principle that when material is exposed to infrared light, the light is absorbed, reflected, or transmitted depending upon the scattering and absorption properties of the material. To assess body composition, a probe that acts as an infrared transmitter and detector is placed on the skin. Infrared light of two wavelengths is transmitted by the probe. The signal penetrates the underlying tissue to a depth of 4 cm [26]. Infrared light also is reflected and scattered at the site from the skin and underlying subcutaneous tissues and detected by the probe. Estimates of body composition can be made by analyzing specific

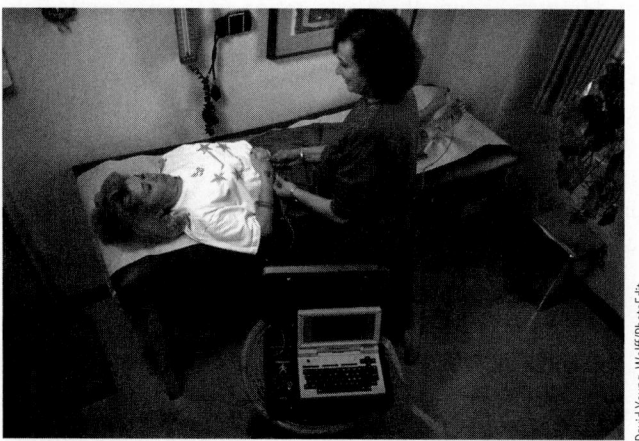

David Young-Wolff/PhotoEdit

Figure 8.8 Bioelectrical impedance (BIA) apparatus used to measure impedance and conductance.

characteristics of the reflected light. The method is safe, noninvasive, and rapid; however, overestimates of body fat in lean (<8% body fat) subjects and underestimates of body fat in obese (>30% body fat) subjects have been reported [45]. The accuracy of the technique requires further investigation. There are several reports in the literature describing the use of infrared interactance to monitor patients with chronic kidney disease, frequently to detect any deterioration of their lean body mass. A recent paper evaluating infrared interactance as a field test reported that its results correlated with those of DXA and bioelectrical impedance analysis. The infrared interactance procedure was not affected by skin color or fluid retention but had a larger variability than DXA; 44% of the calculated fat mass was within 3.5% of the DXA measurement [46].

Atomic Methods

Some methods of body composition assessment use an atomic perspective to quantify one or more components of the body and then use various calculations to determine the other body components. Measurements of body composition by assessment of total body water, total body potassium, or neutron activation analysis employ such an approach.

Total Body Water (TBW)

Quantification of total body water involves the use of isotopes of H—typically deuterium (D_2O), radioactive tritium (^3H_2O), or oxygen-18 (^{18}O)—and is based upon principles of dilution. Water can be labeled with any one of the three isotopes. The water containing a specific amount (concentration) of the isotope is then ingested or injected intravenously. Following ingestion or injection, the isotope distributes itself throughout the body water, which occupies about 73.2% of fat-free body mass. After a specified time period (usually 2 to 6 hours) for equilibration has elapsed, samples of body fluids (usually blood and urine) are taken. Losses of the isotope in the urine must be determined. If ^{18}O is used, breath samples are collected for analysis. Concentrations of the isotope in the breath or body fluids are determined by scintillation counters or other instruments.

The initial concentration (C_1) and volume (V_1) of the isotope given are equal to the final concentration of the isotope in the plasma (C_2) and the volume of total body water (V_2), expressed as $C_1V_1 = C_2V_2$. Thus, total body water (V_2) is equal to C_1V_1 divided by C_2. Once total body water has been determined, the percentage of lean body mass can be calculated: Fat-free mass equals total body water divided by 0.732. Body fat can be obtained by subtracting fat-free mass from body weight. A three-component model (consisting of total body water, body volume, and body weight) has been shown to measure changes in body fat as low as 1.54 kg in people [38]. Many studies, however, have shown that the degree of hydration varies considerably in the lean body tissue of apparently healthy people. Therefore, implications about total body fat derived from estimates of lean body mass based upon total body water may be misleading [36]. In addition, adipose tissue has been shown to contain as much as 15% water by weight [39]. Thus, extracellular fluid should be measured and subtracted from total body water to give an indication of intracellular water and thus of body cell mass.

Because total body water involves radiation exposure if ^3H is used, the method is not suitable for use with some subjects (such as children and pregnant women). ^{18}O is in itself expensive and requires expensive mass spectrometry equipment for its analysis. Deuterated water (D_2O) is relatively inexpensive to purchase but is expensive to measure [42].

Total Body Potassium

Total body potassium is also used to assess fat-free mass. Potassium is present within cells but is not associated with stored fat. About 0.012% of potassium occurs as ^{40}K, a naturally occurring isotope that emits a characteristic gamma ray. External counting of gamma rays emitted by ^{40}K permits determination of the amount of total body potassium; however, getting accurate counts of ^{40}K may be difficult because of external or background radiation. After measurement of potassium (^{40}K) radiation from the body, calculation of total body potassium from the data is required. Fat-free mass can be estimated from the total body potassium based upon any one of several conversion factors, which vary in men from 2.46 to 3.41 g potassium per kilogram fat-free mass and in women from 2.28 to 3.16 g potassium per kilogram fat-free mass [39]. Total body fat can be calculated by subtracting fat-free mass from body weight. Overestimation of fat mass in obese subjects has been reported with total body potassium [45]. The technique should not be used in people with potassium-wasting diseases.

Neutron Activation Analysis

Neutron activation analysis enables *in vivo* estimation of body composition, including total body concentrations of nitrogen (TBN), calcium (TBCa), chloride (TBCl), sodium (TBNa), and phosphorus (TBP), among other elements. A beam of neutrons is delivered to the person being assessed. The body's atoms (nitrogen, calcium, chloride, sodium, and phosphorus) interact with the beam of neutrons to generate unstable radioactive elements, which emit gamma-ray energy as they revert back to their stable forms. The specific energy levels correspond to specific elements, and the radiation's level of activity indicates the element's abundance [26].

Assessment of many body components may be conducted with neutron activation analysis. For example, measuring nitrogen makes lean body mass assessment possible, and subtracting lean body mass from total body water allows total body fat calculation [47–49]. Neutron activation analysis is noninvasive and provides reliable and reproducible data. However, the equipment is expensive and requires a skilled technologist, and subjects are exposed to considerable amounts of radiation. It is not a commonly used procedure.

Summary of Methods

Table 8.2 provides an overview of the methods described in this chapter as well as a few additional methods. In brief review, the methods available to assess lean body mass (LBM) or fat-free mass include neutron activation analysis, total body potassium, intracellular water (total body water minus extracellular water), and bioelectrical impedance analysis. Body fat may be assessed by anthropometry, densitometry, air-displacement plethysmography, dual-photon or energy X-ray absorptiometry, ultrasound, and infrared interactance. Adipose tissue typically is measured using computerized tomography, magnetic resonance imaging, and ultrasound. Bone mineral density may be assessed using single- or dual-photon absorptiometry or by dual energy X-ray absorptiometry [24,32,42].

ENERGY BALANCE

The body is in energy balance when the energy intake is equal to the energy output. Energy input (or intake) is simpler to define than energy output. Energy intake is the sum of the energy provided by all of the food and beverages consumed, and is derived from the oxidation or breakdown of carbohydrates, protein, fats, and alcohol in our bodies. Energy output is more complex; it includes the energy involved in the absorption, metabolism, and storage of the nutrients in the food we eat as well as the energy we spend as we breathe, our hearts beat, our bodies cool or warm, and we perform physical exercise. The regulation of food intake, expenditure of energy, and storage of energy is complex, and all aspects are not fully understood.

Consistent imbalance of energy results in either a gain or loss of body weight. If too little energy (calories) is consumed to balance energy expended, the amount of tissue in the body is reduced. The desired goal of a weight-reduction program is to lose adipose tissue, but other tissues such as muscle can also be lost. If the energy consumed exceeds expenditure, adipose stores are increased; and if the positive balance is large enough or continues for a long enough time, the person can become overweight or obese. An imbalance of just 10 kcal per day can result in the gain of 1 lb of adipose tissue per year or 10 lb per decade. Remember that obesity is defined as an excess of body fat and that we use body weight as a convenient proxy. For the nonathlete, body fat and body weight are well correlated.

For the past 30 years or so, prevalence of overweight and obesity has increased rapidly. This increase is considered to be an obesity epidemic (or a pandemic worldwide) by public health officials. Obesity is associated with an increased risk of morbidity and mortality. Conditions associated with being overweight or obese include hypertension, stroke, coronary artery disease, dyslipidemia, type 2 diabetes, sleep apnea, osteoarthritis, and numerous others. Energy balance is an area of utmost importance for those interested in the subject of nutrition and metabolism.

Prevalence of Obesity

Ongoing changes in body weight and composition are an innate characteristic of the maturation and aging process. These compositional changes occur throughout the life cycle, beginning with the embryo and extending through old age. Rapid growth entails not only an increase in body mass but also a change in the proportions of components making up this mass. Young adulthood is a period of relative homeostasis, but in some people, body composition can change. Following the more or less homeostatic period of young adulthood is the period of progressive aging, when some undesirable changes in body composition and often weight inevitably occur.

Obesity has been observed throughout history, but recently it has reached epidemic proportions [50]. The data on the prevalence of obesity in the United States has been mostly obtained from the National Health and Nutrition Examination Surveys (NHANES). NHANES surveys (once conducted intermittently, but now continuously) sample the U.S. population to permit prevalence calculations for a variety of nutrition and health parameters.

The prevalence of obesity (BMI $\geq$ 30) was stable from 1960 to 1980 [51]. During the NHANES I and II surveys, conducted during 1971 to 1974 and 1976 to 1980, respectively, just over 12% of men and 16% of women between 20 and 74 years of age were obese. In the NHANES III survey, conducted from 1988 to 1994, the rate of obesity jumped to 20.6% in men and 25.9% in women. Starting with the continuous surveys, all ages were sampled.

Table 8.2 Methods for Assessing Body Composition [31,35,38,39,44]

Anthropometry:	Skin fold thicknesses from a variety of locations, body weight, and limb circumferences can be used to calculate fat, fat-free mass, and muscle size. Measurements can be made in the field but require skilled technicians for accuracy. Skin folds can provide some information about regional subcutaneous fat as well as about total fat. Measurements may not be applicable to all population groups.
Densitometry:	Measurements of total body density through determination of body volume by underwater weighing, helium displacement, or combination of water displacement by body and air displacement by head. Measurements can be used to determine body density, which in turn allows calculation of percentage of body fat and fat-free mass.
(a) Underwater weighing:	Measurements are precise and were long considered the gold standard for determining body composition but must be conducted in the laboratory; subject cooperation is necessary for underwater weighing. The method is not suitable for young children or the elderly.
(b) Air-displacement plethysmography (ADP):	Values of body density obtained by ADP correlate well (though with some variability) with underwater weighing for most populations. With the commercial availability of equipment, ADP can be used for infants, young children, and the elderly.
Total body water (TBW):	Measured by dilution with deuterium (D_2O), tritium ($3H_2O$), or oxygen-18 (^{18}O). TBW is used as index of human body composition based on findings that water is not present in stored triglycerides but occupies an approximate average of 73.2% of the fat-free mass. A specified quantity of the isotope is ingested or injected; then, following an equilibration period, a sampling is made of the concentration of the tracer in a selected biological fluid. TBW (V_2) is calculated from the equation $C_1V_1 = C_2V_2$ where V_1 is the volume of the tracer given, C_1 is the amount of tracer given, and C_2 is the final concentration of tracer in the selected biological fluid. The extracellular fluid (ECF) can be estimated by a variety of methods. Subtracting ECF from TBW allows calculation of fat-free mass. This is a difficult procedure with limited precision, and the cost can be great, particularly when ^{18}O is used as the tracer.
Total body potassium:	^{40}K, a naturally occurring isotope, is found in a known amount (0.012%) in intracellular water and is not present in stored triacylglycerols. These facts allow fat-free mass to be estimated by the external counting of gamma rays emitted by ^{40}K. The instrument for counting ^{40}K is expensive and must be properly calibrated for precision. The method is limited to laboratories.
Urinary creatinine excretion:	Creatinine is the product resulting from the nonenzymatic hydrolysis of free creatine, which is liberated during the dephosphorylation of creatine phosphate. The preponderance of creatine phosphate is located in the skeletal muscle; therefore, urinary creatinine excretion can be related to muscle mass. Drawbacks to this method include large individual variability of creatinine excretion due to the renal processing of creatinine and the effect of diet. The creatine pool does not seem to be under strict metabolic control and is to some degree independent of body composition. Another technical difficulty is control of accurately limited 24-hour urine collections.
3-methylhistidine excretion:	3-methylhistidine has been suggested as a useful predictor of human body composition because this amino acid is located principally in the muscle and cannot be reused after its release from catabolized myofibrillar proteins (methylation of specific histidine residues occurs posttranslationally on protein). Some concern exists over the use of 3-methylhistidine as a marker of muscle protein because of the potential influence of nonskeletal (skin and gastrointestinal tract) muscle protein turnover on its excretory rate. Additional problems with this method are the need for consumption of a relatively controlled meat-free diet and complete and accurate urine collections.
Bioelectrical impedance analysis:	This method measures the electrical conductivity between extremities. Determinations of resistance and reactance are made, and the lowest resistance value for an individual is used to calculate conductance and to predict LBM. Equipment is portable and is a reliable method for large populations.
Absorptiometry	
(a) Dual-photon:	This method allows estimation of LBM as well as total bone mineral of the whole body. The body is scanned transversely in very small steps over its entire length by radiation from gadolinium-153 (^{153}Gd). This isotope emits two gamma rays of different energies; attenuation measurements at the two discrete photon energies allow quantification of bone mineral and soft tissue. The equipment required for dual-photon absorptiometry is expensive, complicated calibration is required, and data collected require complicated mathematical treatment.
(b) Dual X-ray photon:	Similar to dual-photon, this method involves scanning subjects at two different energy levels; however, X-rays are used instead of a radionuclide source. Radiation exposure to subjects is very low, and the procedure is relatively quick. This method appears to be the best choice for measuring bone mineral density.
Computerized tomography:	This method determines regional body composition. An image is generated by computerized processing of X-ray data. Fat, lean tissue, and bone can be identified by their characteristic density-frequency distribution. Information about regional fat distribution can be obtained; computerized tomography has been used to determine the ratio of intra-abdominal to subcutaneous fat in humans. The size of the liver, spleen, and kidney can be determined by computerized tomography. Both cost of the equipment and technical difficulties are great. This method is a laboratory procedure presently limited primarily to large medical centers.
Ultrasound:	Approach uses an instrument in which electrical energy is converted in a probe to high-frequency ultrasonic energy. Subsequent transmission of these sound waves through various tissues can be used to calculate tissue thickness. Method is frequently used to determine the thickness of subcutaneous fat layers. Large laboratory instruments and smaller portable equipment are available. Although data suggest a reasonable validity of method, its general use has been limited because the appropriate signal frequency of the probe has not been well defined and the needed constant pressure by the probe to the scan site is difficult to achieve. Changes in pressure from probe application can prejudice ultrasonic determination of adipose tissue thickness.
Infrared interactance:	Measurement of body fat is made at various sites on the extremities through use of short wavelengths of infrared light. The amount of fat can be calculated from the absorption spectra and used with a prediction equation to estimate TBF.
Magnetic resonance imaging:	This approach is based upon the fact that atomic nuclei can behave like magnets. When an external magnetic field is applied across a part of the body, each nucleus attempts to align with the external magnetic field. If these nuclei are simultaneously activated by a radio frequency wave, once the radio wave is turned off the activated nuclei will emit the signal absorbed; this emitted signal is used to develop images by a computer. This method has the capability of generating images in response to intrinsic tissue variables and of representing characteristics such as level of hydration and fat content. This method appears to have much potential, but both the cost of equipment and technical difficulties are great.
Neutron activation analysis:	This is the only technique currently available for measurement of multielemental composition of the human body. Low radiation doses produce isotopic atoms in tissues; the induced nuclides permit measurement of many elements, including nitrogen, calcium, phosphorus, magnesium, sodium, and chloride. Although precision of measurement is great, so are the technical difficulties and cost of equipment. This method of measuring body composition is limited to a few laboratories in this country and abroad.

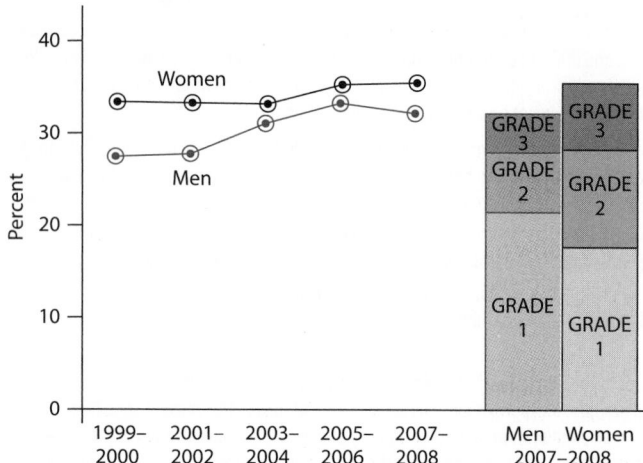

Figure 8.9 Prevalence of obesity between 1999–2000 and 2007–2008.
Source: Data from Flegal, K.M., Caroll, M.D., Ogden, C.L., Curtin, L.R., Prevalence and trends in obesity among U.S. adults, 1999–2008. J Am Med Assoc. 2010; 303:235–41.

Figure 8.9 shows the prevalence of obesity in adults over the age of 20 years and the distribution of obesity grades 1, 2, and 3 (defined previously in the "Body Mass Index" section) for 2007 to 2008. During 2007 to 2008, the overall obesity prevalence among men ≥20 years of age was 32.2%; 36.1% of these men were overweight, 21.5% grade 1 obese, 6.5% grade 2 obese, and 4.2% grade 3 obese. In the same NHANES cycle, the prevalence of obesity was 35.5% among women ≥20 years, with 28.6% overweight, 17.7% grade 1 obese, 10.6% grade 2 obese, and 7.2% grade 3 obese. Thus, in comparison, more men were overweight but more women were obese. For this cycle, the prevalence of overweight and obesity for non-Hispanic black and Hispanic individuals was around 80%, depending upon the specific age range [51]. Between 1999 and 2008, the prevalence of obesity increased for men but not for women.

Similar changes in the prevalence of obesity have been observed in people younger than 20 years of age [43]. Since 1980, for example, the obesity rate for school-age children has tripled [5]. As stated previously, children above the 95th percentile of BMI for age on standardized charts (Figure 8.2) are considered obese, and those between the 85th and 95th percentiles are considered overweight. The CDC [5] also reports data on those at or above the 97th percentile (there is no defined label for this group). The 2007 to 2008 NHANES cycle reported that 17.8% of boys and 15.9% of girls were obese. Interestingly, since the 1999 to 2000 survey cycle, there has been no increase in the linear trends of the prevalence among boys or girls after adjusting for race. Since the epidemic of childhood obesity began, a large number of programs and research projects to help better understand both the problem and potential solutions have been implemented. A recent review is available for the interested reader [53].

COMPONENTS OF ENERGY EXPENDITURE

Nutrition professionals need to know how to assess both body weight and composition as well as energy expenditure to determine nutrient needs and identify or prevent disease. Whether body weight is being maintained, increased, or decreased depends primarily upon the extent to which the energy requirements of the body (i.e., total energy expenditure) have been met or exceeded by energy intake. Total energy expenditure is composed primarily of:

- the resting energy expenditure (REE), or basal metabolic rate (BMR)
- the thermic effect of food (TEF)
- the energy expenditure of physical activity or exercise (EEPA)

A fourth component, thermoregulation, is sometimes included. The average division of energy expenditure among the components, each of which is described in the following sections, is shown in Figure 8.10.

Basal Metabolic Rate and Resting Energy Expenditure

Basal metabolic rate (BMR) represents the rate at which the body expends energy to sustain basic life processes such as respiration, heartbeat, renal function, and blood circulation. It also includes the energy needed to remain in an awake state because the measurements are usually made shortly after the person awakens. The word *basal*, as it is used in BMR, is often confused with the term *resting*; however, *basal* is more precisely defined than is *resting*. The measurement of oxygen consumed and carbon dioxide produced that is used in calculating energy expenditure is made under closely controlled and standardized

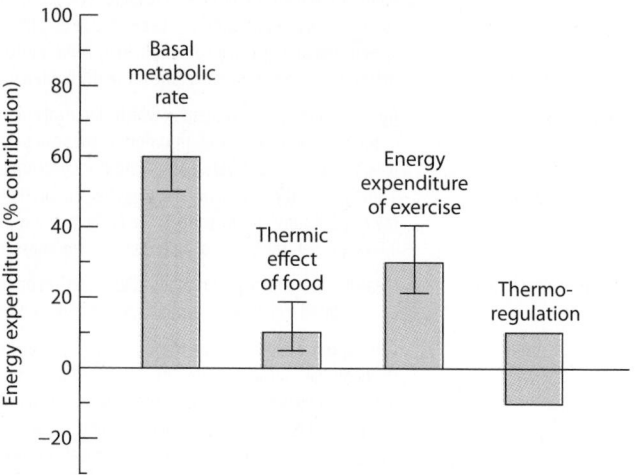

Figure 8.10 Components of energy expenditure and their approximate percentage contribution.

conditions. A person's basal metabolic rate is determined when he or she is in a postabsorptive state (i.e., no food intake for at least 12 hours), is lying down (supine), and is completely relaxed (motionless)—preferably very shortly after awakening from sleep in the morning. In addition, the temperature of the room in which the measurement takes place is made as comfortable as possible (thermoneutral) for the person. Any factors that could influence the person's internal work are minimized as much as possible. For most people, energy expenditure is slowest during sleep. BMR is usually converted to units of kcal/24 hours and called *basal energy expenditure* (BEE).

In contrast to BMR, resting metabolic rate (RMR) is measured when the person is at rest in a comfortable environment. Fasting for 12 hours is not required. Instead, the fast for RMR is usually about 2 to 4 hours. RMR usually is slightly higher (about 10%) than BMR because of its less stringent conditions of measurement [54]. RMR is thought to account for about 65% to 80% of daily total energy expenditure. BMR accounts for about 50% to 70% of daily total energy expenditure [55]. The term *resting energy expenditure* (REE) is used when RMR is extrapolated to units of kcal/24 hours [56].

Basal metabolism is a result of energy exchanges occurring in all cells of the body. The rate of oxygen consumption, however, is most closely related to the actively metabolizing cells, that is, the body's lean body mass or fat-free mass. In aging, for example, fat mass increases at the expense of fat-free mass, and BMR decreases. With maturation, the proportion of supporting structures (i.e., bone and muscle) increases more rapidly than does total body weight. Bone and muscle, though components of body cell mass, have a much lower metabolic activity at rest than organ tissues but much greater activity than adipose tissue. This difference in the rate of weight accretion between the less active and the more active components of mass means a decrease in the overall metabolic activity of cell mass and a concurrent decrease in BMR per unit of body weight. These changes that occur during maturation explain the lower REE of children as compared to very young infants (see Chapter 6).

A look at the metabolic activity among the different components of the cell mass in an adult male illustrates its variability. Under normal circumstances, about 5% to 6% of total body weight can be attributed to the weight of the brain, liver, heart, and kidney, whereas about 30% to 40% of body weight is attributable to muscle mass. At the same time, the metabolic activity of these vital organ tissues accounts for about 60% of basal oxygen consumption, whereas muscle mass accounts for only about 25%. Tissues such as bone, glands, intestine, and skin account for 33% of body weight and contribute 15% to 20% of metabolic activity. In contrast, fat usually accounts for at least 20% of body weight but contributes only 5% of metabolic activity. Thus, changes in BMR can occur whenever the proportions of body tissues change in relation to one another.

Thermic Effect of Food

A second component of energy expenditure is the thermic effect of food (i.e., the metabolic response to food), also called diet-induced thermogenesis, specific dynamic action, or the specific effect of food. The thermic effect of food represents the increase in energy expenditure associated with the body's processing of food, including the work associated with the digestion, absorption, transport, metabolism, and storage of energy from ingested food. The percentage increase in energy expenditure over BMR caused by the thermic effect of food has been estimated to range from about 5% to 30% [57].

Protein in foods has the greatest thermic effect, increasing energy expenditure 20% to 30%. Carbohydrates have an intermediate effect, raising energy expenditure 5% to 10%, and fat increases energy expenditure 0% to 5% [55]. The value most commonly used for the thermic effect of food is 10% of the caloric value of a mixed diet consumed within 24 hours [53,54]. The rise in metabolism following food consumption appears to reach a maximum about 1 hour after eating and is generally, but not always, absent 4 hours postprandial (after eating) [53]. Consequently, the thermic effect of food often is not included in calculations of total energy requirements.

Energy Expenditure of Physical Activity

The energy expenditure of physical activity (i.e., voluntary movement, including fidgeting) is the most variable of the components and also the only component that is easily altered. Although on average, physical activity accounts for about 20% to 40% of total energy expenditure, it can contribute considerably less in a truly sedentary person or much more in a very physically active person [54,56]. Factors impinging on energy expenditure during exercise, other than the activity itself, include the intensity, duration, and frequency with which the activity is performed; the body mass of the person; his or her efficiency at performing the activity; and any extraneous movements that may accompany the activity. In addition, oxygen consumption and thus energy expenditure can remain elevated for a short period of time after the exercise activity has stopped.

Thermoregulation

An additional component of energy expenditure that is of some importance is thermoregulation, also called adaptive, nonshivering, facultative, or regulatory thermogenesis. Thermoregulation refers to the alterations in metabolism necessary to maintain the body's core temperature. Changes in metabolism occur most often with changes in environmental temperature, especially below the comfort zone (zone of thermoneutrality), but can also occur with overfeeding, trauma, burns, and physical conditioning, among other situations [55]. For example, when temperatures decrease below the comfort zone and a person has not adjusted to the change by altering the thickness of the clothes he or she is wearing, energy expenditure increases to maintain or restore the body temperature to normal. The overall contribution of thermoregulation to energy needs is small, given that most people alter clothing as needed to maintain a comfortable body temperature.

ASSESSING ENERGY EXPENDITURE

Energy expenditure can be assessed through direct or indirect calorimetry, or the doubly labeled water method as well as with several calculations using derived formulas. Each of these methods of assessment is explained in the following sections.

Direct Calorimetry

Measurement of total energy expenditure can be determined by **direct calorimetry,** which measures the dissipation of heat from the body [58]. Heat dissipation—including both sensible heat loss and heat of water vaporization—is measured using an isothermal principle, a gradient-layer system, or a water-cooled garment [58]. Although the concept of direct calorimetry is relatively simple, direct measurement of body heat loss is expensive, cumbersome, and usually rather unpleasant for the subject or subjects involved. Direct calorimetry is seldom used and has been replaced by the indirect methods discussed in the following sections.

Indirect Calorimetry

Indirect calorimetry measures the consumption of oxygen and the expiration of carbon dioxide. Urinary nitrogen excretion should also be measured because for every 1 g of nitrogen excreted, about 6 L of oxygen are consumed and 4.8 L of carbon dioxide are produced [58,59]. Oxygen consumption and carbon dioxide production are measured using either portable equipment (Figure 8.11) that can be placed on a person, enabling collection and analysis of expired air and quantification of inspired air, or stationary equipment often referred to as a metabolic cart (Figure 8.12). The exchange of oxygen and carbon dioxide is proportional to metabolism.

The amount of energy expended can be calculated from the ratio of the carbon dioxide expired to the oxygen inhaled. This ratio is known as the respiratory quotient (RQ). Exercise physiologists use the term *respiratory exchange ratio* (R or RER). Examination of respiratory quotients provides meaningful information with respect to both energy expenditure and the biological substrate (carbohydrate or fat) being oxidized but no information about metabolism (substrate oxidation) within individual organs and tissues [58]. The next sections present a brief explanation of how the respiratory quotient is used to assess substrate oxidation and how it is used to determine energy expenditure.

The Respiratory Quotient and Substrate Oxidation

An RQ equal to 1.0 suggests that carbohydrate is being oxidized because the amount of oxygen required for the

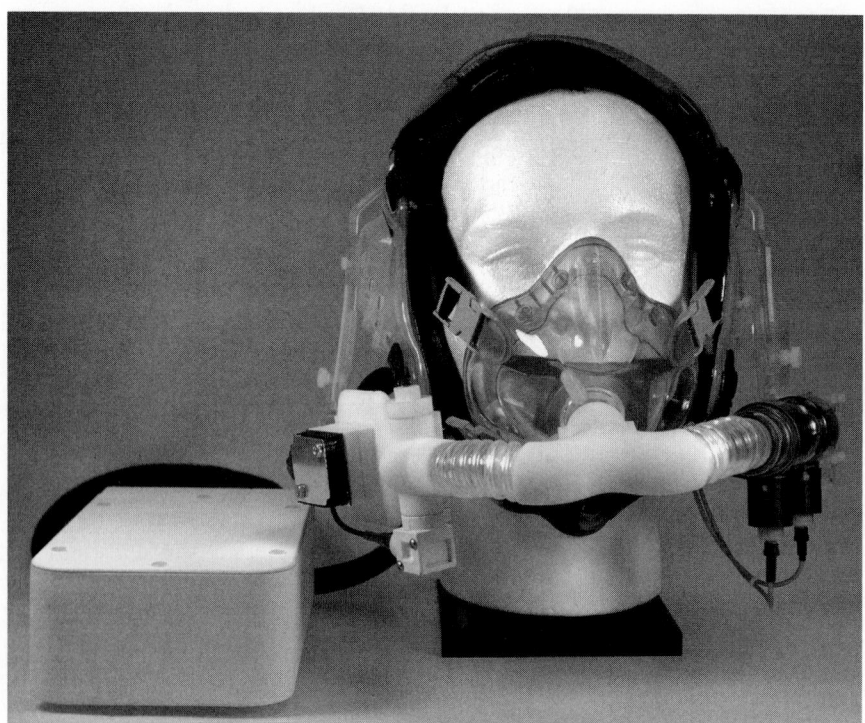

Photo courtesy of the NASA John H. Glenn Research Center

Figure 8.11 A portable device to measure oxygen consumption and carbon dioxide production. The headgear contains oxygen and carbon dioxide sensors on the left side and the flow sensor on the right side, all tethered to an electronics box (to the left of the headgear) that fits into a small wearable pack.

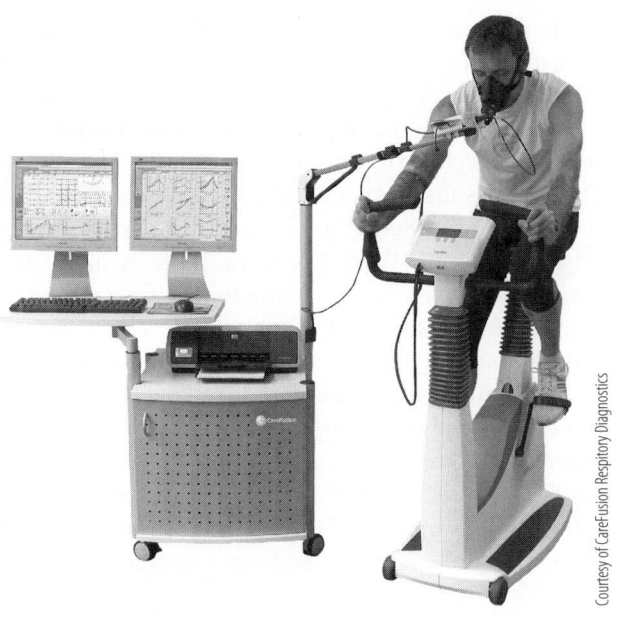

Courtesy of CareFusion Respitory Diagnostics

Figure 8.12 A metabolic cart (shown here with bicycle ergometer) measures oxygen consumption and CO_2 exhaled.

combustion of glucose equals the amount of carbon dioxide produced, as shown here:

$$C_6H_{12}O_6 + 6\,O_2 \longrightarrow 6\,CO_2 + 6\,H_2O$$

$$RQ = 6\,CO_2/6\,O_2 = 1.0$$

The RQ for a fat is <1.0 because fatty acids are a much less oxidized fuel source (fewer oxygen molecules). For example, a triacylglycerol such as tristearin, shown in the following reaction, requires 163 mol of oxygen and produces 114 mol of carbon dioxide per 2 tristearin molecules:

$$2\,C_{57}H_{110}O_6 + 163\,O_2 \longrightarrow 114\,CO_2 + 110\,H_2O$$

$$RQ = 114\,CO_2/163\,O_2 = 0.70$$

Calculating the RQ for protein oxidation is more complicated because metabolic oxidation of amino acids requires removing the nitrogen and some oxygen and carbon as urea, a compound excreted in the urine. Urea nitrogen represents a net loss of energy to the body, and only the remaining carbon chain of the amino acid can be oxidized in the body. The following reaction illustrates the oxidation of a small protein molecule into carbon dioxide, water, sulfur trioxide, and urea:

$$C_{72}H_{112}N_{18}O_{22}S + 77\,O_2 \longrightarrow 63\,CO_2 + 38\,H_2O$$
$$+ SO_3 + 9\,CO(NH_2)_2$$

$$RQ = 63\,CO_2/77\,O_2 = 0.818$$

The average figures 1.0, 0.7, and 0.8 are accepted as the representative RQs for carbohydrate, fat, and protein, respectively. The RQ for an ordinary mixed diet consisting of the three energy-producing nutrients is usually considered to be about 0.85. An RQ of 0.82 represents the metabolism of a mixture of 40% carbohydrate and 60% fat [32]. RQs that are actually computed from gaseous exchange and that come closer to 1.0 or nearer to 0.7 would indicate that more carbohydrate or fat, respectively, was being used for fuel. In clinical practice, an RQ < 0.8 suggests that a patient may be underfed, an RQ < 0.7 suggests starvation or ingestion of a low-carbohydrate or high-alcohol diet, and an RQ of 1.0 suggests that lipogenesis is occurring [58]. Occasionally the RQ value can be greater than 1. For instance, when you hyperventilate you exhale more CO_2 without using more O_2, resulting in an RQ greater than 1. This may also occur when the body is in acidosis, such as following exhaustive exercise when lactic acid builds up. $NaHCO_2$ neutralizes the lactic acid to form sodium lactate and carbonic acid (H_2CO_3). The carbonic acid is converted to CO_2 and H_2O and exhaled, which results in a loss of CO_2 that is not related to oxygen uptake.

The Respiratory Quotient and Energy Expenditure

Once the RQ has been computed from gaseous exchange, the calculation of energy expended is simple. Table 8.3 gives the caloric value for 1 L of oxygen and for 1 L of carbon dioxide, given various RQs. When the volume of oxygen or carbon dioxide in the exchange has been determined, the total caloric value represented by the exchange can be calculated. Determining the amounts of carbohydrate and fat being oxidized in the production of these calories is also possible.

> For example, if under standard conditions for the determination of BMR a person consumed 15.7 L of oxygen per hour and expired 12.0 L of carbon dioxide, the RQ would be 12.0/15.7, or 0.7643. From Table 8.3, the caloric equivalent for an RQ of 0.76 is 4.751 kcal for 1 L of oxygen or 6.253 kcal for 1 L of carbon dioxide. Based on the caloric equivalent for oxygen, calories produced per hour are 15.7 × 4.751, or 74.59 kcal. Based upon the caloric equivalent for carbon dioxide, calories produced per hour are 12.0 × 6.253, or 75.04 kcal. If we use 75 kcal/h as the caloric expenditure under basal conditions, the basal energy for the day would be about 1,800 kcal (75 kcal/h × 24 h). At this RQ of 0.76, fat is supplying almost 81% of energy expended (Table 8.3).

Because under ordinary circumstances the contribution of protein to energy metabolism is so small, the oxidation of protein is ignored in the determination of the so-called nonprotein RQ. If a truly accurate RQ is required, a minimal correction can be made by measuring the amount of urinary nitrogen excreted over a specified time period. As you have read, for every 1 g of nitrogen excreted, about 6 L of oxygen are consumed and 4.8 L of carbon dioxide are produced. The amount of oxygen and carbon dioxide exchanged in the release of energy from protein can then be subtracted from the total amount of measured gaseous exchange.

Table 8.3 Thermal Equivalent of O_2 and CO_2 for Nonprotein RQ

Nonprotein RQ	Caloric Value 1 L O_2	Caloric Value 1 L CO_2	Source of Calories Carbohydrate (%)	Fat (%)
0.707	4.686	6.629	0	100
0.71	4.690	6.606	1.10	98.9
0.72	4.702	6.531	4.76	95.2
0.73	4.714	6.458	8.40	91.6
0.74	4.727	6.388	12.0	88.0
0.75	4.739	6.319	15.6	84.4
0.76	4.751	6.253	19.2	80.8
0.77	4.764	6.187	22.8	77.2
0.78	4.776	6.123	26.3	73.7
0.79	4.788	6.062	29.9	70.1
0.80	4.801	6.001	33.4	66.6
0.81	4.813	5.942	36.9	63.1
0.82	4.825	5.884	40.3	59.7
0.83	4.838	5.829	43.8	56.2
0.84	4.850	5.774	47.2	52.8
0.85	4.862	5.721	50.7	49.3
0.86	4.875	5.669	54.1	45.9
0.87	4.887	5.617	57.5	42.5
0.88	4.899	5.568	60.8	39.2
0.89	4.911	5.519	64.2	35.8
0.90	4.924	5.471	67.5	32.5
0.91	4.936	5.424	70.8	29.2
0.92	4.948	5.378	74.1	25.9
0.93	4.961	5.333	77.4	22.6
0.94	4.973	5.290	80.7	19.3
0.95	4.985	5.247	84.0	16.0
0.96	4.998	5.205	87.2	12.8
0.97	5.010	5.165	90.4	9.58
0.98	5.022	5.124	93.6	6.37
0.99	5.035	5.085	96.8	3.18
1.00	5.047	5.047	100	0

Source: Adapted from McArdle, W.D., Katch, F.I., Katch, V.L., "Exercise Physiology", 2nd ed., p. 127 (Philadelphia: Lea & Febiger, 1986). Adapted by permission.

Measurement of the energy expended in various activities has also been made primarily through indirect calorimetry. The method for measuring gas exchange, however, differs from that used for determining BMR. The subject performing the activity for which energy expenditure is being determined inhales ambient air, which has a constant composition of 20.93% oxygen, 0.03% carbon dioxide, and 78.04% nitrogen. Air exhaled by the subject is collected in a spirometer (a device used to measure respiratory gases) and is analyzed to determine how much less oxygen and how much more carbon dioxide it contains compared with ambient air. The difference in the composition of the inhaled air and the exhaled air reflects the energy release from the body. A lightweight portable spirometer (Figure 8.11) can be worn during the performance of almost any sort of activity, and thus freedom of movement outside the laboratory is possible. In the laboratory, the Douglas bag was once routinely used to collect expired air, but it has been replaced by the metabolic cart (Figure 8.12).

Tables are available that list the kilocalories expended per kilogram body weight per minute or hour for a wide variety of activities. Table 8.4, an example of such a table, groups various broad activities together according to their average level of energy expenditure. This table incorporates the basal energy expenditure. To use this table to calculate the energy expended for a given activity by your body, multiply the kcal/lb or kg/min by your weight and then by the number of minutes spent performing the activity. Care must be taken in using tables of this type; note how time is measured (by the minute or hour) and whether the basal energy expenditure is included.

Doubly Labeled Water

The doubly labeled water method also enables assessment of total energy expenditure. $^2H_2$ (deuterium) and $^{18}O_2$ are stable isotopes of hydrogen and oxygen, respectively. In this technique, stable isotopes of water are given as $H_2^{18}O$ and as ^2H_2O (or as $^2H_2^{18}O_2$). The isotopes equilibrate throughout the water compartments in the body over about 5 hours. The labeled hydrogen can leave the body as water (^2H_2O) in sweat, urine, and pulmonary water vapor, while the labeled oxygen can leave the body as either labeled water (H_2O^{18}) or $C^{18}O_2$. The disappearance of the $H_2^{18}O$ and ^2H_2O is measured in the blood and urine for about 3 weeks. The disappearance of the $H_2^{18}O$ is representative of the flux of water (i.e., water turnover) and of the production rate of carbon dioxide. Because the $^2H_2$ can be excreted only as H_2O, the disappearance of the ^2H_2O represents water turnover alone. Thus, the difference between the disappearance rate of $H_2^{18}O$ and that of ^2H_2O corresponds to the production rate of carbon dioxide. To assess oxygen consumption, a food quotient (FQ) is calculated from diet records kept throughout the testing period. In subjects maintaining body weight, the food quotient is equal to the respiratory quotient. Oxygen consumption, and thus energy expenditure, can be calculated from the FQ and carbon dioxide production [60].

Use of the doubly labeled water method to assess total energy expenditure in free-living individuals produces accurate results that correlate well with those of indirect calorimetry. The one source of error in the technique lies with the use of food records, which may not necessarily be accurate, and with the calculation of oxygen consumption from the food quotient [54]. Other sources of errors and the validity of the assumptions are discussed in a review [60]. This method is now considered to be the gold standard for determining energy utilization. One primary drawback is the high cost of $^{18}O_2$.

Table 8.4 Energy Expended on Various Activities

The values listed in this table reflect both the energy expended in physical activity and the amount used for BMR. To calculate kcalories spent per minute of activity for your own body weight, multiply kcal/lb/min (or kcal/kg/min) by your exact weight and then multiply that number by the number of minutes spent in the activity. For example, if you weigh 142 pounds, and you want to know how many kcalories you spent doing 30 minutes of vigorous aerobic dance: $0.062 \times 142 = 8.8$ kcalories per minute; 8.8×30 minutes $= 264$ total kcalories spent.

Activity	kcal/lb/min	kcal/kg/min
Aerobic dance (vigorous)	.062	.136
Basketball (vigorous, full court)	.097	.213
Bicycling		
13 mph	.045	.099
15 mph	.049	.108
17 mph	.057	.125
19 mph	.076	.167
21 mph	.090	.198
23 mph	.109	.240
25 mph	.139	.306
Canoeing, flat water, moderate pace	.045	.099
Cross-country skiing		
8 mph	.104	.229
Gardening	.045	.099
Golf (carrying clubs)	.045	.099
Handball	.078	.172
Horseback riding (trot)	.052	.114
Rowing (vigorous)	.097	.213
Running		
5 mph	.061	.134
6 mph	.074	.163
7.5 mph	.094	.207
9 mph	.103	.227
10 mph	.114	.251
11 mph	.131	.288
Soccer (vigorous)	.097	.213
Studying	.011	.024
Swimming		
20 yd/min	.032	.070
45 yd/min	.058	.128
50 yd/min	.070	.154
Table tennis (skilled)	.045	.099
Tennis (beginner)	.032	.070
Vacuuming and other household tasks	.030	.066
Walking (brisk pace)		
3.5 mph	.035	.077
4.5 mph	.048	.106
Weight lifting		
light-to-moderate effort	.024	.053
vigorous effort	.048	.106
Wheelchair basketball	.084	.185
Wheeling self in wheelchair	.030	.066
Wii games		
bowling	.021	.046
boxing	.021	.047
tennis	.022	.048

Source: Rolfes, Pinna, Whitney, Understanding Normal & Clinical Nutrition, 9/e. © Cengage Learning.

Derived Formulas

The doubly labeled water technique has been used in humans only since the 1980s; in contrast, estimating rather than measuring basal metabolic rate or resting energy expenditure has been the practice among clinicians since about 1925. Many different methods for estimating energy needs have been used over the years [61]. Estimations have been based upon body surface area, body weight, and calculations from regression equations that incorporate the person's gender, age, weight, and height. Such estimates have been shown to correlate with measurements from indirect calorimetry or from doubly labeled water.

The derived regression equations most often used to estimate RMR in the clinical setting are those derived by Mifflin and St. Jeor [62]. A review by an Academy of Nutrition and Dietetics evidence working group compared the ability of several regression equations to accurately predict RMR within 10% of that measured in both nonobese and obese adults. The Mifflin–St. Jeor equations were determined to be best able to predict RMR within 10% of that measured in 82% of the cases. Mifflin and St. Jeor developed separate equations to predict REE (kilocalories per day) in men and women based upon weight in kilograms (W), height in centimeters (H), and age in years (A):

Men: $\text{REE} = (10 \times W) + (6.25 \times H) - (5 \times A) + 5$

Women: $\text{REE} = (10 \times W) + (6.25 \times H) - (5 \times A) - 161$

The earliest equation that is still being used was developed by Harris and Benedict in 1919, based upon indirect calorimetry [63], and only slightly modified. The Harris-Benedict equations were originally published as predictive of BMR; however, because the data used to formulate them were collected under resting conditions, they actually estimate RMR. These equations are listed here:

Men: $\text{RMR} = 66.5 + (13.7 \times W) + (5.0 \times H) - (6.8 \times A)$

Women: $\text{RMR} = 655.1 + (9.56 \times W) + (1.85 \times H) - (4.7 \times A)$

A female who is 35 years old, weighs 125 lb (56.82 kg), and is 5 foot, 5 inches tall (165.1 cm) would have a RMR of 1,339 kcal (using the Harris-Benedict equation) and an RMR of 1,264 kcal (using the Mifflin–St. Jeor equation).

The various equations used to calculate energy expenditure are reevaluated regularly in scientific literature. Reevaluations have shown that predicted values for RMR are often higher than the actual expenditure and may not be applicable to all people (e.g., those who are obese) [61]. Thus, one must be alert to the literature for recent findings and recognize the limitations and implications of the use of the various equations.

Using the Mifflin–St. Jeor or Harris-Benedict equations, among other formulas mentioned, provides information on a person's resting energy needs. To determine total energy needs for a particular person, the energy required for physical activity must be added to the energy needed for basal needs. Depending upon the type, duration, intensity, and frequency of physical activity, energy needs for physical activity may vary from about 20% to 70% or more of basal metabolism. Activity factors can be multiplied by basal energy calculations to address the energy needs of physical activity.

> Using the formulas, for example, a person with resting energy needs of 1,580 kcal who does little activity (i.e., is sedentary) may expend only about 20% more kilocalories per day being physically active and thus would require 1,580 kcal resting + (1,580 kcal × 0.20 activity) = 1,580 kcal resting + 316 kcal activity = 1,896 kcal. This calculation also may be written as 1,580 kcal resting × 1.20 activity factor = 1,896 kcal. Energy needed for the thermic effect of food is not included in many equations used to calculate total energy needs, but when it is used, a value of 10% of resting energy needs is usually used. Thus, using the preceding example and including the thermic effect of foods (TEF) in the calculation, a person with resting energy needs of 1,580 kcal would need another 1,580 kcal resting × 0.10 TEF = 158 kcal for TEF. Total energy needs would be 1,580 kcal + 316 kcal + 158 kcal, or 2,054 kcal.

Based upon data on total daily energy expenditure measured by the doubly labeled water method, the Food and Nutrition Board has developed several equations to calculate estimated energy requirements (EER). For an adult, "the estimated energy requirement is defined as the dietary energy intake that is predicted to maintain energy balance in a healthy adult of a defined age, gender, weight, height, and level of physical activity consistent with good health" [56,64].

Formulas to calculate the estimated energy requirements for adults follow:

$$\text{Adult men: EER} = 662 - (9.53 \times \text{age}) + \text{PA} (15.91 \\ \times \text{weight} + 539.6 \times \text{height})$$

$$\text{Adult women: EER} = 354 - (6.91 \times \text{age}) + \text{PA} (9.36 \\ \times \text{weight} + 726 \times \text{height})$$

where age is in years, weight is in kilograms (kg), and height is in meters (m). PA in the equation refers to physical activity coefficients and varies with the level of activity and gender. PA values for different physical activity levels are given in the following table.

PA Values for Different Physical Activity Levels [56]				
Gender	Sedentary	Low Active	Active	Very Active
Men	1.00	1.11	1.25	1.48
Women	1.00	1.12	1.27	1.45

The appropriate PA value should be inserted into the EER equation to calculate total energy expenditure.

These formulas apply to adults with healthy body weights (BMI of 18.5–25 kg/m^2) who are not pregnant or lactating.

REGULATION OF BODY WEIGHT AND COMPOSITION

Earlier, you read that the prevalence of obesity is increasing rapidly to what some public health experts are calling an epidemic. Recall that the goal of weight maintenance is to balance energy intake with energy expenditure. Weight maintenance is a lofty goal, but regulating food and beverage intake and energy expenditure is very complex, and this goal is not easy to achieve. Energy intake and energy expenditure clearly do not correlate over a short period of time such as a day or two. Equally clearly, however, their correlation over an extended period of time, such as a week to a few months to years, is excellent. If you consume as little as 10 kcal per day more than you expend, you gain about a pound a year (or 10 lb a decade).

The literature and the lay press have suggested many causes for the alarming increase in obesity, ranging from the huge portion sizes at fast-food restaurants, to the high percentage of fat in the diet, and the ready availability of high-fructose corn syrup and other caloric sweeteners. Each of these so-called causes may contribute, but no simple answer exists. The increased prevalence of obesity has been brought about by a combination of many physiological, psychological, and environmental factors, all of which interact and contribute to the overweight and obesity problem. Though obesity clearly is a result of an energy imbalance, some have pointed out that obesity involves more than this [65]. Besides those causes mentioned, other factors such as certain drugs, viruses, and toxins have been shown to be important in developing obesity in experimental animals. The importance of these factors has not been shown in humans, however.

This section covers some of the principles of regulating energy intake, storing excess energy, and losing body weight. Many of the regulatory factors have been discovered relatively recently, and the full story is not yet known. Because of the enormous scope of the problem and the economic effects of its health consequences, this is an active area for research. This section prepares the reader to put the results of this new research into context as they are released.

Genetic Influences

Our body shape and size have a strong genetic component. More than 127 candidate genes are associated with human obesity phenotypes. Every chromosome except the Y chromosome has one or more loci (the area on a chromosome that codes for a protein) [66]. A defect in some of these genes (such as those that involve the melanocortin receptor) can result directly in a person becoming obese. The melanocortin receptor is involved in the control of appetite and is covered later in this chapter.

Uncoupling proteins (covered in Chapter 5) also can play a role in developing obesity. Remember that uncoupling proteins are present in brown fat and uncouple phosphorylation (ATP synthesis) from electron transport. Some polymorphisms produce alleles that result in greater weight gain in times of positive energy balance [66].

The heritability of body weight and composition also has been shown by studies of body-weight changes in response to overfeeding or energy restriction in pairs of identical twins. The individuals who shared the same genes responded in a similar manner, whereas some pairs of twins gained or lost weight more easily than others [67].

Awareness of the influence of genetics on body weight has led to a hypothesis that in general terms suggests that we each have a genetically predetermined body weight. If we go over that weight, we eat less (or exercise more), and if we go under that weight, we eat more. Obviously our environment can override the set point, or we would not be having an explosion in the prevalence of obesity. The large increase in the prevalence of obesity cannot be explained by genetics alone [67]. Nonetheless, the set point has been one of the concepts used to explain the difficulty in successfully dieting and maintaining the weight loss for several years. Ninety-five percent of people who diet to lose weight gain back all or more within 5 years [65].

Hormonal Influences

For the set-point theory to be valid, a mechanism must exist for controlling our food intake, both on a meal-to-meal basis and in the longer term. Numerous circulating hormones and steroids produced by the body influence appetite and food intake by their actions on the hypothalamus, the brainstem, and the autonomic nervous system. The hormones are secreted by the gastrointestinal tract, pancreas, and fat cells [68]. The area of the hypothalamus that is considered the center for fuel sensing and feeding control is called the **arcuate nucleus.** Two groups of neurons with opposing actions are produced in the arcuate nucleus. The first group manufactures neurotransmitters of the melanocortin family, primarily melanocyte-stimulating hormone (MSH), which works by binding to a brain receptor. These neurons suppress hunger through release of these **anorexigenic** (appetite-inhibiting) peptides. The other group of neurons in the arcuate nucleus produces neuropeptide Y (NPY) and agouti-related proteins. Agouti-related proteins, which are potent stimulators of appetite, act indirectly by inhibiting the appetite-suppressing actions of MSH. There are several redundant mechanisms for long-term energy balance and shorter-term food intake. Each will be discussed separately and are summarized in Table 8.5.

Leptin

Leptin is a hormone secreted by white adipose tissue that interacts with the hypothalamus to reduce hunger. The level of leptin is correlated with fat stores; the more triacylglycerol the adipocyte contains, the more leptin it produces. During starvation, the leptin level drops. Specific leptin receptors in the arcuate nucleus of the

Table 8.5 Agents of Energy Regulation

Agent	Site of Production	Stimulus	Action	Comments
Leptin	White adipose tissue	Levels increase with overfeeding or increased adipose tissue. Levels decrease with starvation or reduced adipose tissue.	Decreases the urge to eat and increases physical activity to produce a negative energy balance.	Leptin resistance reported in the obese.
Ghrelin	Stomach and duodenum	Levels increase between meals and decrease after a meal and when absorption begins.	Stimulates hunger and food intake. Promotes digestion and is a secretagogue for growth hormone.	Only orexigenic hormone.
Adiponectin	Adipocytes	Levels increase with decreased fat mass. Levels decrease with increased fat mass.	Protects against insulin resistance, glucose intolerance, and dyslipidemia.	No role in food intake.
Cholecystokinin (CCK)	Intestine	Levels increase during and after a meal.	Suppresses appetite and promotes satiety.	
PYY	Small and large intestine	Levels rapidly increase after a meal. Levels are low in a fasting state.	Suppresses appetite in the long term.	May influence weight loss following surgery.
Insulin	β-cells of pancreas	Levels increase with elevated blood glucose levels.	Suppresses hunger and stimulates the deposition of triacylglycerols in adipose tissue, which stimulates leptin.	Role of insulin in the regulation of appetite is not well defined.
Glucocorticoids	Adrenal glands	Levels controlled by hypothalamus and stress.	Excess glucocorticoids stimulate appetite and low levels lead to anorexia.	

hypothalamus bind leptin to suppress the release of neuropeptide Y and agouti-related peptide and to stimulate the release of MSH, which works to suppress hunger. The effect of leptin, then, is to control the level of stored body fat. As the level of body fat decreases, the amount of leptin secreted is reduced, and hunger is not repressed as much. In contrast, as the body fat level increases, the leptin level increases, and energy intake is reduced. It has been theorized that the leptin mechanism was important for survival during the plenty/famine cycles of our ancestors.

This mechanism works well in normal-weight people. In overweight people, however, the receptors in the hypothalamus become defective, and increased leptin levels fail to suppress hunger [68]. The elucidation of the action of leptin is hoped to be an important tool in the treatment of obesity, but this has yet to be fully realized. Leptin administration to individuals with genetic disorders that cause low leptin production (a condition that causes wasting of adipose stores and triggers metabolic responses that resemble starvation) can correct these conditions. In contrast, very obese individuals generally have high levels of leptin (about 10% of obese individuals have low levels) but do not respond with decreased food intake; instead, these obese individuals develop leptin resistance [69]. The concept of leptin resistance is important because in the majority of cases of obesity, increased leptin levels fail to bring about weight loss even though the leptin receptor is intact. The mechanism of this resistance is not fully understood. One theory is that part of the resistance is due to the inability of leptin to reach the receptor. Another hypothesis is that cytokine receptors inhibit the full cascade of reactions that occur when the leptin receptor is stimulated, which limits its actions. (Recall the discussion of the cascade of reactions that are a result of insulin binding with its receptor in Chapter 7.) This is an area of active investigation.

Ghrelin

Another important hunger signal that was identified after leptin was discovered is a hormone produced by the stomach and duodenum, called **ghrelin.** Ghrelin secretion rises between meals when the stomach is empty. This hormone reacts with receptors in the same area of the hypothalamus as leptin to stimulate the release of neuropeptide Y and agouti-related protein, which increase food intake. As a meal is consumed and absorption begins, ghrelin secretion rapidly diminishes, and hunger is reduced. The half-life of ghrelin in the serum is only about 30 minutes [68,70]. Ghrelin is the only circulating agent that stimulates the **orexigenic** neurons that produce NPY and agouti proteins, which also promote digestion by stimulating gastric acid secretion and gastric motility. Ghrelin also functions as a **secretagogue** to stimulate the

release of growth hormone (GH). GH secretion promotes nutrient incorporation into muscle and other tissue. The active form of ghrelin appears to be the peptide that has been acylated with octonoic acid (an 8-carbon acid) [71].

Other Regulatory Appetite Signals

- **Adiponectin.** Adiponectin is an adipocyte-derived hormone that plays a role in energy homeostasis. Plasma adiponectin levels decrease with obesity and increase with weight loss. It is negatively correlated with body fat. Based upon animal experimentation, adiponectin levels appear to be protective against insulin resistance [68].

- **Cholecystokinin.** An antagonistic hormone that regulates the urge to eat is cholecystokinin (CCK), produced in the intestine. CCK secretion rises during and after a meal and produces satiety (suppresses hunger). CCK is secreted following a meal to reduce appetite, which promotes satiety [68].

- **PYY.** A recently discovered peptide hormone secreted by the small and large intestine called PYY suppresses the appetite for a longer time, about 12 hours. PYY levels are low in the fasting state and rapidly increase following a meal. PYY levels are elevated following bariatric surgery and produce prolonged satiety that may be related to part of the weight loss following the surgery [68].

- **Insulin.** Insulin is another hormone that suppresses hunger. Insulin stimulates the deposition of triacylglycerols in adipose tissue, which stimulates the release of leptin. Insulin is also thought to enter the brain and act directly on the leptin receptors of the hypothalamus to suppress the release of neuropeptide Y and MSH. The exact role of insulin in regulating appetite is not well defined [68].

- **Glucocorticoids.** Glucocorticoids are derived from the adrenal gland. Cortisol deficiency that occurs in primary adrenal failure leads to anorexia. Excess glucocorticoids can cause hyperphagia [68].

The interested reader should see the article by Flier and Maratos-Flier listed under Suggested Readings for an overview of the control of food intake.

Positive Energy Balance

As stated earlier in this chapter, weight changes are brought about by an imbalance in energy. Chapter 7 covered the integration of the metabolism of carbohydrate, protein, and fat. The primary nutrients contributing to energy are alcohol (when present), carbohydrate, and fat in that order. When alcohol is consumed, the liver converts it to two-carbon units (acetate). The acetate is transported to the peripheral tissue, such as muscle, for oxidation. The acetate is not converted to fatty acids in the liver [72].

If alcohol is not involved, most of the body's energy comes from carbohydrate and fat. Carbohydrate (glucose) is first used for energy. When the body's energy needs are met, glucose is used to synthesize glycogen until these stores are filled. If glucose is being used for energy, fewer fatty acids are being oxidized. (Remember the regulation of the TCA cycle, described in Chapter 3.) If fatty acids are not being oxidized, fewer are needed, so less lipolysis takes place.

Only when the quantity of carbohydrate exceeds the total energy needs does de novo synthesis of fatty acids occur. The newly synthesized fatty acids are made into triacylglycerols, transported from the liver by VLDL, and taken up by the adipocytes. When sufficient carbohydrate is consumed to meet or exceed energy needs, very few fatty acids are oxidized for energy [72]. No tissue is solely dependent on fatty acids for energy, though heart muscle oxidizes them preferentially. Because the dietary fatty acids found in triacylglycerols are not used for energy, they are taken up by the adipocytes and stored as triacylglycerol without using much metabolic energy. This fact is demonstrated by the fatty acid profile of storage fat, which resembles the fatty acid profile of the diet and not that of de novo synthesized fatty acids. The conversion of either glucose or amino acids to fatty acids is inefficient and requires considerable metabolic energy. Both glucose and amino acids must be converted first to acetyl-CoA; then the acetyl-CoA units are synthesized into fatty acids. Both steps require energy.

If the energy imbalance continues, the adipocytes in the body become enlarged (hypertrophy). In the process called hyperplasia, new adipocytes can also be produced to accept the additional triacylglycerol. The number of fat cells increases most rapidly in late childhood and early puberty whenever a positive energy balance exists, but hyperplasia can occur later in life as well. Obese people have more, and larger, fat cells than normal-weight people. If body fat is lost, the number of fat cells does not decrease; they just get smaller.

Negative Energy Balance

Each year many people "go on diets" for the purpose of losing weight. Actually, the goal should be to lose adipose tissue and to retain fat-free mass. Depending upon the nature of the caloric restriction and the level and type of exercise, both body fat and fat-free mass may be lost. Limited information is available on the proportion of fat and muscle lost on different weight-loss regimes.

Losing weight (body fat) requires a negative energy balance over an extended period of time. Exercise alone is generally considered to be less effective than calorie restriction with exercise [73,74]. In a systematic review of weight-loss programs lasting at least 6 months, the authors concluded that moderate weight loss (5–10 kg) that consists of both fat mass and fat-free mass can be achieved by calorie restriction alone [74]. If exercise is added to the weight-loss program, however, some or all of the fat-free mass can be spared. Most studies have used an aerobic exercise component, and in those that combined calorie restriction with exercise, most of the weight lost was fat mass and very little (0–1.5 kg) was fat-free mass. The few studies reviewed by [74] that included resistance training reported small losses or even a gain in fat-free mass.

Research has also explored the relationship between diet composition and weight loss. What percentages of macronutrients should these diets contain, and should micronutrient intakes vary from general recommendations? Some controversy remains as to whether a weight-reduction (calorie-restricted) diet should be low in fat, high in carbohydrate, and moderate in protein; or moderately high in protein and fat and relatively low in carbohydrates [75–85]. In short-term programs lasting up to about 12 weeks, diets moderately high in protein (about 25% of calories) and low in carbohydrates (about 40% of calories or less) with the balance of calories from fat produce greater weight loss. However, in longer-term studies that last a year or more, the amount of weight lost is about the same with no major differences due to the distribution of the macronutrients. High-protein diets reduce the amount of fat-free mass lost [74].

The high-protein diets are often recommended to be ad lib rather than carefully planned to restrict intake. Because the high-protein diet produces greater satiety, however, the individual actually consumes fewer calories. There are several explanations suggested for the effectiveness of these diets. First, compared to the other macronutrients, protein provides a greater feeling of satiety for a longer period of time; second, the thermogenesis from protein is likewise greater; and third, because fat-free mass is preserved the basal metabolism is maintained. It has also been shown that carbohydrate restriction has a more favorable impact on the risk factors that constitute metabolic syndrome than adoption of a high-carbohydrate, low-fat diet [77].

One reason that diets moderately high in protein and low in carbohydrates result in a greater weight loss in the first few weeks is the greater loss of body water due to lower glycogen stores. If the carbohydrate content is less than about 40 g per day, ketosis is likely to occur. This would allow some ketone bodies to be exhaled from the lungs and excreted in urine. This is not thought to be a large contribution to the weight loss.

SUMMARY

Public health estimates of what we should weigh are based upon body mass index. However, BMI does not evaluate body composition. With an accurate measure of height, weight, and skin folds from selected areas of the body, the percentage of body fat can be determined. Then, by difference, lean body mass can be estimated. Certain skin fold or circumference measurements, as well as use of more elaborate equipment such as DEXA and bioelectrical impedance analysis, can also provide some information about distribution of body fat, a factor that may be even more important to health than percentage of total body fat.

Despite the differences in the various body components that have been noted among individuals and populations, the component that shows the greatest variability is clearly the one over which we have the most control—total body fat. Although changes in energy balance produce weight changes, the extent of these changes varies from person to person. One of the greatest problems in predicting energy needs centers around estimations of energy expenditure. Energy expenditure has three defined components: basal metabolic rate, thermic effect of foods, and the effect of exercise or physical activity, none of which is constant.

The prevalence of overweight and obesity has increased rapidly over the past 30 years and is now considered to be reaching epidemic proportions among children and adults. Among children, the prevalence appears to have leveled off for the past decade, though it has not fallen. Morbidity and mortality from hypertension, stroke, coronary artery disease, dyslipidemia, type 2 diabetes, sleep apnea, and numerous other weight-related conditions are likely to increase because of the high prevalence of overweight and obesity in the U.S. population.

Body shape and size have a strong genetic component. Defects in certain genes have been shown to cause obesity. For instance, a defect in the gene that codes for the uncoupling protein can cause a change in basal metabolism. The hypothalamic sites that control appetite are also genetically controlled. Appetite is regulated by opposing hormones such as ghrelin, which stimulates appetite, and CCK, leptin, and insulin, which suppress hunger.

Each year, many people attempt to lose weight. An active area of research is examining the efficacy and safety of energy-deficient diets that have different proportions of the macronutrients. The size of the caloric deficit appears to be more important to weight loss than the composition of the diet when weight-loss programs are adhered to for more than a year. Weight loss has been reported with moderate-protein/low-carbohydrate/high-fat diets and high-carbohydrate/low-fat diets.

References Cited

1. Weigley ES. Average? Ideal? Desirable? A brief review of height-weight tables in the United States. J Am Diet Assoc. 1984; 84:417–23.
2. National Institutes of Health. Clinical Guidelines on the Identification, Evaluation, and Treatment of Overweight and Obesity in Adults. Bethesda, MD: National Institutes of Health, National Health, Lung, and Blood Institute. 1998.
3. Abernathy RP, Black DR. Healthy body weights: an alternative perspective. Am J Clin Nutr. 1996; 63(suppl3):S448–51.
4. Sandowski S. What is the ideal body weight? Family Practice. 2000; 17:348–51.
5. Ogden CL, Caroll MD, Curtin LR, Flegal KM. Prevalence of high body mass index in US children and adolescents: 2007–2008. J Amer Med Assoc. 2010; 303:242–49.
6. Shah B, Sucher K, Hollenbeck CB. Comparison of ideal body weight equations and published height-weight tables with body mass index tables for healthy adults in the United States. Nutr Clin Pract. 2006; 21:312–19.
7. Devine BJ. Gentamicin therapy. Drug Intell Clin Pharm. 1974; 8:650–55.
8. Robinson J, Lupklewicz S, Palenik L, et al. Determination of ideal body weight for drug dosage calculations. Am J Hosp Pharm. 1983; 40:1016–19.
9. Frisancho AR. Anthropometric standards for the assessment of growth and nutritional status. Ann Arbor, MI: University of Michigan Press. 1990 p. 28.
10. Grant A, DeHoog S. Anthropometry. In: Nutritional Assessment and Support, 3rd ed. Seattle: Grant. 1985 p. 11.
11. Giannini VS, Giudici RA, Merrill DL. Determination of ideal body weight. Am J Hosp Pharm. 1984; 41:883–87.
12. Behnke AR, Feen BG, Welham WC. The specific gravity of healthy men. JAMA. 1942; 118:495–98.
13. Heiat A. Impact of age on definition of standards for ideal weight. Prev Cardiol. 2003; 6:104–07.
14. Friis-Hansen B. Body composition in growth. Pediatrics. 1971; 47:264–74.
15. Mitchell HH, Hamilton TS, Steggerda FR, Bean HW. The chemical composition of the adult human body and its bearing on the biochemistry of growth. J Biol Chem. 1945; 158:625–37.
16. Widdowson EM, McCance RA, Spray CM. The chemical composition of the human body. Clin Sci. 1951; 10:113–25.
17. Forbes RM, Cooper AR, Mitchell HH. The composition of the adult human body as determined by chemical analysis. J Biol Chem. 1953; 203:359–66.
18. Clarys JP, Martin AD, Drinkwater DT. Gross tissue weights in the human body by cadaver dissection. Hum Biol. 1984; 56:459–73.
19. Behnke AR, Wilmore JH. Evaluation and Regulation of Body Build and Composition. Englewood Cliffs, NJ: Prentice Hall. 1974.
20. Brozek J, Grande F, Anderson JT, Keys A. Densitometric analysis of body composition: revision of some quantitative assumptions. Ann NY Acad Sci. 1963; 110:113–40.
21. Clarys JP, Martin AD, Drinkwater DT, Marfell-Jones MJ. The skinfold: myth and reality. J Sports Sci. 1987; 5:3–33.
22. Sinning WE, Dolny DG, Little KD, et al. Validity of "generalized" equations for body composition analysis in male athletes. Med Sci Sports Exerc. 1985; 17:124–30.
23. McArdle WD, Katch FI, Katch VL. Exercise Physiology: Energy Nutrition, & Human Performance, 7th ed. Philadelphia: Lippincott Williams & Wilkins. 2010.

24. Harrison GG, Buskirk ER, Carter JEL, et al. Skinfold thicknesses and measurement technique. In: Lohman TG, Roche AF, Martorell R, eds. Anthropometric Standardization Reference Manual. Champaign, IL: Human Kinetics Publishers. 1988 pp. 55–80.

25. Martorell R, Mendoza F, Mueller WH, Pawson IG. Which side to measure: right or left. In: Lohman TG, Roche AF, Martorell R, eds. Anthropometric Standardization Reference Manual. Champaign, IL: Human Kinetics Publishers. 1988 pp. 87–91.

26. Lukaski HC. Methods for the assessment of human body composition: traditional and new. Am J Clin Nutr. 1987; 46:537–56.

27. van der Kooy K, Seidell JC. Techniques for the measurement of visceral fat: a practical guide. Internl J Obesity. 1993; 17:187–96.

28. Flegal KM, Shepherd JA, Looker AC, et al. Comparisons of percentage body fat, body mass index, waist circumference and waist-stature ratio in adults. Am J Clin Nutr. 2009; 89:500–08.

29. Camhi SM, Bray GA, Bouchard C, et al. The relationship of waist circumference and BMI to visceral, subcutaneous, and total body fat: sex and race differences. Obesity. 2011; 19:402–08.

30. Bergman RN, Stefanovski D, Buchanan TA, et al. A better index of body adiposity. Obesity. 2010; 19:1083–89.

31. Barreira TV, Harrington DM, Stainano AE, et al. Body adiposity index, body mass index and body fat in white and black adults. J Am Med Assoc. 2011; 306:828–30.

32. Siri WE. Gross composition of the body. In: Lawrence JH, Tobias CA, eds. Advances in Biological and Medical Physics. New York: Academic Press. 1956 pp. 239–80.

33. Vescovi JD, Zimmerman SL, Miller WC, et al. Evaluation of Bod Pod for estimating percentage body fat in a heterogeneous group of adult humans. Eur J Appl Physiol. 2001; 85:326–32.

34. Bosy-Westphal A, Mast M, Eichhorn C, et al. Validation of air-displacement plethysmography for estimation of body fat mass in healthy elderly subjects. Eur J Nutr. 2003; 42:207–16.

35. Holmes JC, Gibson AL, Cremades JG, Mier CM. Body-density measurement in children: the Bod Pod verses hydrodensitometry. Internat J Sport Nutr Exerc Metabol. 2011; 21:240–47.

36. Pace N, Rathbun EN. Studies on body composition, III: the body water and chemically combined nitrogen content in relation to fat content. J Biol Chem. 1945; 158:685–91.

37. Lee SY, Gallagher D. Assessment methods in human body composition. Curr Opin Clin Nutr Metab Care. 2008; 11:566–72.

38. Jebb AS, Murgatroyd PR, Goldberg GR, et al. In vivo measurement of changes in body composition: description of methods and their validation against 12-d continuous whole-body calorimetry. Am J Clin Nutr. 1993; 58:455–62.

39. Jensen MD. Research techniques for body composition assessment. J Am Diet Assoc. 1992; 92:454–60.

40. Genant H, Engelke K, Fuerst T, et al. Noninvasive assessment of bone mineral and structure: state of the art. J Bone Min Res. 1996; 11:707–30.

41. Fuller MF, Fowler PA, McNeill G, Foster MA. Imaging techniques for the assessment of body composition. J Nutr. 1994; 124:S1546–50.

42. Heymsfield SB, Matthews D. Body composition: research and clinical advances. JPEN. 1994; 18:91–103.

43. Fanelli MT, Kuczmarski RJ. Ultrasound as an approach to assessing body composition. Am J Clin Nutr. 1984; 39:703–09.

44. Rolfe EDL, Sleigh A, Finucane FM, et al. Ultrasound measurements of visceral and subcutaneous abdominal thickness to predict abdominal adiposity among older men and women. Obesity. 2010; 18:625–631.

45. Garrow JS. New approaches to body composition. Am J Clin Nutr. 1982; 35:1152–58.

46. Bross R, Chandramohan G, Kovesdy CP, et al. Comparing body composition assessment tests in long-term hemodialysis patients. Am J Kidney Dis. 2010; 55:885–96.

47. Andres R. Mortality and obesity: the rationale for age-specific height-weight tables. In: Andres R, Bierman EL, Hazzard WR, eds. Principles of Geriatric Medicine. New York: McGraw-Hill. 1985 pp. 311–18.

48. Cohn SH, Vartsky D, Yasumura S, et al. Indexes of body cell mass: nitrogen versus potassium. Am J Physiol. 1983; 244:E305–10.

49. Cohn SH, Vaswani AN, Yasumura S, Ellis KJ. Improved models for determination of body fat by in vivo neutron activation. Am J Clin Nutr. 1984; 40:255–59.

50. Ogden CL, Yanovski SZ, Carroll MD, Flegal KM. The epidemiology of obesity. Gastroenterol. 2007; 132:2087–2102.

51. Flegal KM, Caroll MD, Ogden CL, Curtin LR. Prevalence and trends in obesity among US adults: 1999–2008. J Am Med Assoc. 2010; 303:235–41.

52. Biro FM, Wien M. Childhood obesity and adult morbidities. Am J Clin Nutr. 2010; 91:S1499–1505.

53. Han JC, Lawlor DA, Kimm SYS. Childhood obesity. Lancet. 2010; 375:1737–48.

54. Institue of Medicine, Food and Nutrition Board. Dietary Reference Intakes for Energy, Carbohydrate, Fiber, Fat, Fatty Acids, Cholesterol, Protein, and Amino Acids. Washington, DC. National Academies Press. 2005 pp. 119–21.

55. Ravussin E, Bogardus C. A brief overview of human energy metabolism and its relationship to essential obesity. Am J Clin Nutr. 1992; 55:S242S–45.

56. Food and Nutrition Board. Dietary Reference Intakes for Energy, Carbohydrates, Fiber, Fat, Protein, and Amino Acids. Washington, DC: National Academy Press. 2002.

57. Horton ES. Introduction: an overview of the assessment and regulation of energy balance in humans. Am J Clin Nutr. 1983; 38:972–77.

58. Jequier E, Acheson K, Schutz Y. Assessment of energy expenditure and fuel utilization in man. Ann Rev Nutr. 1987; 7:187–208.

59. Westerterp KR. Food quotient, respiratory quotient, and energy balance. Am J Clin Nutr. 1993; 57:S759–65.

60. Schoeller D. Measurement of energy expenditure in free-living humans by using doubly labeled water. J Nutr. 1988; 118:1278–89.

61. Frankenfield D, Roth-Yousey L, Compher C. Comparison of predictive equations for resting metabolic rate in healthy nonobese and obese adults: a systematic review. J Am Diet Assoc. 2005; 105:775–89.

62. Mifflin MD, St Jeor ST, Hill LA, et al. A new predictive equation for resting energy expenditure in healthy individuals. Am J Clin Nutr. 1990; 51:241–47.

63. Harris J, Benedict F. A Biometric Study of Basal Metabolism in Man. Publication 279. Washington, DC: Carnegie Institution. 1919.

64. Institute of Medicine, Food and Nutrition Board. Dietary Reference Intakes for Energy, Carbohydrate, Fiber, Fat, Fatty Acids, Cholesterol, Protein, and Amino Acids. Washington, DC: National Academies Press. 2005.

65. Bray GA, Champagne CM. Beyond energy balance: there is more to obesity than kilocalories. J Am Diet Assoc. 2005; 105:S17–23.

66. Loos RJF, Rankinen T. Gene-diet interactions on body weight changes. J Am Diet Assoc. 2005; 105:S29–34.

67. Rankinen T, Zuberi A, Chagnon YC, et al. The human obesity gene map: the 2005 update. Obesity. 2006; 14:529–644.

68. Coll AP, Farooqi IS, O'Rahilly S. The hormonal control of food intake. Cell. 2007; 129:251–62.

69. Gautron L, Elmquist JK. Sixteen years and counting: an update on leptin and energy balance. J Clin Invest. 2011; 121:2087–93.

70. Varela L, Vazquez MJ, Cordido F, et al. Ghrelin and lipid metabolism: key partners in energy balance. J Mol Endocrinol. 2011; 46:R43–63.

71. Castaneda TR, Tong J, Datta R, et al. Ghrelin in the regulation of body weight and metabolism. Frontiers in Neuroendocrinology. 2010; 31:44–60.

72. Hellerstein MK. De novo lipogenesis in humans: metabolic and regulatory aspects. Eur J of Clin Nutr. 1999; 53:S53–65.

73. Abete I, Astrup A, Martinez JA, et al. Obesity and the metabolic syndrome: role of different dietary macronutrient distribution patterns and specific nutritional components on weight loss and maintenance. Nutr Rev. 2010; 68:214–31.

74. Weinheimer EM, Sands LP, Campbell WW. A systematic review of the separate and combined effects of energy restriction and exercise on fat-free mass in middle-aged and older adults: implications for sarcopenic obesity. Nutr Rev. 2010; 68:375–88.

75. Shai I, Schwarzfuchs D, Henkin W, et al. Weight loss with a low-carbohydrate, Mediterranean, or low-fat diet. N Engl J Med. 2008; 359:229–41.

76. Sacks FM, Bray GA, Carey VJ, et al. Comparison of weight-loss diets with different compositions of fat protein, and carbohydrates. N Engl J Med. 2009:360:859–73.

77 Volek JS, Phinney SD, Forsythe CE, et al. Carbohydrate restriction has a more favorable impact on the metabolic syndrome than a low fat diet. Lipids 2009; 44:297–309.

78. Golay A, Allaz AF, Morel Y, et al. Similar weight loss with low- or high-carbohydrate diets. Am J Clin Nutr. 1996; 63:174–78.

79. Johnston CS, Tjonn SL, Swan PD. High-protein, low-fat diets are effective for weight loss and favorably alter biomarkers in health adults. J Nutr. 2004; 134:586–91.

80. Klein S. Clinical trial experience with fat-restricted vs. carbohydrate-restricted weight-loss diets. Obesity Res. 2004; 12:S141–44.

81. Dansinger ML, Gleason JA, Griffith JL, et al. Comparison of the Atkins, Ornish, Weight Watchers, and Zone diets for weight loss and heart disease risk reduction. JAMA. 2005; 293:43–53.

82. Gardner CD, Kiazand A, Alhassan S, et al. Comparison of the Atkins, Zone, Ornish, and LEARN diets for change in weight and related risk factors among overweight premenopausal women: the A to Z Weight Loss Study: a randomized trial. JAMA. 2007; 297:969–77.

83. Segal-Isaacson CJ, Johnson S, Tomuta V, et al. A randomized trial comparing low-fat and low-carbohydrate diets matched for energy and protein. Obesity Res. 2004; 12:S130–40.

84. Douketis JD, Macie C, Thabane I, Williamson DF. Systematic review of long-term weight loss studies in obese adults: clinical significance and applicability to clinical practice. Int J Obesity. 2005; 29:1153–67.

85. Schoeller DA, Buchholz AC. Energetics of obesity and weight control: does diet composition matter? J Am Diet Assoc. 2005; 105:S24–28.

Suggested Reading

Flier FS, Maratos-Flier E. What fuels fat? Scientific American. 2007; 297:72–83.

Nordmann AJ, Nordmann A, Briel M, et al. Effects of low-carbohydrate vs low-fat diets on weight loss and cardiovascular risk factors. Arch Int Med. 2006; 285–93.

Hession M, Rolland C, Kulkarni U, Wise A, Broom J. Management of obesity: systematic review of randomized controlled trials of low-carbohydrate vs. low-fat/low-calorie diets in the management of obesity and its comorbidities. Obesity Reviews. 2008; 10:36–50.

EATING DISORDERS

Few things can create as large a sensation in the media as a new weight-reduction diet guaranteed to remove unwanted fat. The authors of the sensational new diet are interviewed on television talk shows, the news media give publicity to the new diet (and its authors), and the book promoting the new and revolutionary diet joins its companions on the shelves of all bookstores. The fact that the new diet book has so many companions on the bookshelves attests to the fact that none of these "new and revolutionary" diets is successful in helping people reduce weight and keep it off. Nevertheless, following some sort of weight reduction diet appears to be a way of life among many Americans, particularly women.

The desire of girls and women to be thin has a foundation: the ideal female body image is dictated to a large extent by movie and television celebrities, fashion models, and beauty pageant contestants. Society considers thin to be healthy. In fact, although more recent winners of the Miss America pageant have body mass indices at the lower end of the normal range, many of the pageant winners during the 1970s and 1980s were considered undernourished, having body mass indices between 16.9 and 18.5 kg/m^2 [1,2]. Children as young as 9 years of age have been reported curtailing their food intake to avoid becoming fat [3]. A female's body size too often affects her self-worth and self-esteem. Body image distress results when people become dissatisfied with their weight, and, if people believe that their weight and shape are central to their self-worth as a person, an eating-disorder mindset often ensues [4]. Dieting behavior or weight loss is often the initial event in the development of eating disorders.

While reports of the prevalence of eating disorders are thought to be underestimated, about 1 million men and between 7 and 10 million women in the United States are estimated to have eating disorders [5]. About 10% of eating disorders are diagnosed in children under the age of 10 years, while 86% are diagnosed during the teen years [6]. The incidence of eating disorders, particularly in male athletes and in 15- to 24-year-old females, has increased over the last several decades [7,8].

Although a new system for categorizing eating disorders has been proposed, the American Psychiatric Association's *Diagnostic and Statistical Manual of Mental Disorders*, fourth edition (DSM-IV), is commonly used to define eating disorders [9,10]. The main eating disorder categories listed in DSM-IV are anorexia nervosa, bulimia nervosa, and eating disorder not otherwise specified. This third category includes all other disorders affecting eating.

ANOREXIA NERVOSA

Being too thin is dangerous, even deadly. Anorexia nervosa is a chronic, relapsing illness for many individuals. Of the many psychiatric disorders, anorexia nervosa possesses the highest mortality rate; if left untreated, up to one-fifth of people with the condition die, often before 30 years of age, and many, despite treatment, die from eating disorder–related complications or suicide [11–14].

Anorexia nervosa, described over 100 years ago as a loss of appetite caused by a morbid mental state, is actually misnamed because its victims do not typically experience a loss of appetite. People with anorexia nervosa have a distorted body image and an irrational fear of weight gain. This distorted body image is a perception that they are fat even though they are extremely thin. Further, anorectics are extremely critical of their body as a whole and often more critical about selected body areas (such as thighs, stomach, etc.). Thus, they become obsessed with weight loss and relentlessly pursue thinness, often eating diets providing less than 800 kcal per day.

Eating patterns of people with anorexia nervosa mostly fall into one of two categories: the restricting type or the binge eating–purging type. Anorectics with the restricting type eat to a very limited extent without regularly inducing vomiting or misusing laxatives or diuretics. People with the binge eating–purging type alternate between restricting food intake and bouts of binge eating or purging behavior

with laxative or diuretic misuse or self-induced vomiting [9]. However, in addition to these controlled eating behaviors, anorectics often exercise excessively to further weight loss efforts, to prevent possible weight gain, and to try to correct perceived imperfections in body size and shape. Exercise is considered excessive if its postponement is accompanied by intense guilt or when it is undertaken solely to influence weight or shape [15].

Some of the diagnostic criteria for anorexia nervosa (Table 1) based on DSM-IV include refusal to maintain body weight at or above minimally normal weight for age and height (e.g., at least 85% of expected weight for height; or, from the International Classification of Diseases, a body mass index of at least 17.5 kg/m^2), intense fear of gaining weight or being fat, and **amenorrhea** (absence of at least three consecutive menstrual cycles) [9,10,16]. Self-worth based on weight or shape, preoccupation with food, and abnormal food consumption patterns are also typical of those with anorexia nervosa [16].

The causes of anorexia nervosa are unknown, but the disease is thought to be multifactorial. Genetic vulnerability as well as anxiety, obsessive-compulsive personality disorders, and perfectionism traits are typically present in those who develop anorexia nervosa [16–21]. Anorectics also may exhibit depression and substance abuse [16–21]. In addition, those who develop anorexia nervosa often have a poor self-image and want to please others because their perceived

Table 1 Diagnostic Criteria for 307.1 Anorexia Nervosa

A. Refusal to maintain body weight at or above a minimally normal weight for age and height (e.g., weight loss leading to maintenance of body weight less than 85% of that expected; or failure to make expected weight gain during period of growth, leading to body weight less than 85% of that expected).

B. Intense fear of gaining weight or becoming fat, even though underweight.

C. Disturbance in the way in which one's body weight or shape is experienced, undue influence of body weight or shape on self-evaluation, or denial of the seriousness of the current low body weight.

D. In postmenarcheal females, amenorrhea, i.e., the absence of at least three consecutive menstrual cycles. (A woman is considered to have amenorrhea if her periods occur only following hormone, e.g., estrogen, administration.)

Specify type:

Restricting Type: during the current episode of anorexia nervosa, the person has not regularly engaged in binge-eating or purging behavior (i.e., self-induced vomiting or the misuse of laxatives, diuretics, or enemas)

Binge-Eating/Purging Type: during the current episode of anorexia nervosa, the person has regularly engaged in binge-eating or purging behavior (i.e., self-induced vomiting or the misuse of laxatives, diuretics, or enemas)

Source: Reprinted with permission from the *Diagnostic and Statistical Manual of Mental Disorders*, Fourth Edition, Text Revision, Copyright 2000. American Psychiatric Association.

self-worth is heavily dependent upon the words and actions of others (such as teachers, coaches, or instructors). Other traits associated with the development of this eating disorder include issues concerning food and body weight, issues concerning relationships with oneself and with others, conflict regarding maturation, and problems with separation, sexuality, self-esteem, and compulsivity [16,22–24].

The initial weight loss of the anorectic may not always result from a deliberate decision to diet; initial weight loss may occur unintentionally, for example, as the result of the flu or a gastrointestinal disorder [25]. However, following the initial weight loss, whatever its cause, additional diet restriction (and excessive exercise) is deliberate. Weight loss or control of body weight becomes the overriding goal in life, especially during stressful periods when pressures become overwhelming. The anorectic learns the caloric contents of foods and the energy expenditure associated with various activities. Because anorectics have such a disturbed body image and such an intense fear of becoming fat, they may continue starving themselves to emaciation and even death should intervention be delayed too long.

The effects of anorexia nervosa on the body are similar to the effects of hypometabolic states (such as starvation, protein-calorie malnutrition, or **marasmus**) and affect all parts of the body. Table 2 lists some potential consequences of anorexia nervosa. Growth and development slow. Adipose tissue, lean body mass, and bone mass are lost. Organ mass may be lost, and organ function may become impaired. Loss of heart muscle can weaken the heart and cause, among other serious complications, an irregular heartbeat or a prolonged QT interval (the QT interval is the time that it takes for the heart to contract and refill with blood; with a prolonged QT interval, the heart takes longer to recharge between beats in preparation for the next heartbeat). The gastrointestinal tract atrophies such that peristalsis is slowed, gastric emptying is delayed, and intestinal transit time is lengthened. The secretion of digestive enzymes and of digestive juices also is diminished. Constipation often results, along with abdominal distention after eating just small amounts of food. Hormone and nutrient levels in the blood become altered. Skin typically becomes dry, hair loss from the head occurs while **lanugo**-type (soft woolly) hair may appear on the sides of the face and arms, and body temperature drops. A long-term consequence of the bone loss that occurs with anorexia nervosa is osteopenia and ultimately osteoporosis, which occurs much earlier in those who have (or have had) anorexia nervosa than in those who have not had the condition [26–28].

Treatment of anorexia nervosa is multidisciplinary (involving a physician, dietitian, nurse, psychologist, psychiatrist, and family therapist, among others) and may be accomplished through outpatient or inpatient care, depending upon the severity of the condition. Assessment for inpatient treatment generally includes an evaluation of the person's mental status, how much the person is eating, current weight (inpatient treatment is warranted if weight is <25–30% of ideal), speed of weight loss, motivation and adherence to treatment, family support, purging behavior,

Table 2 Some Potential Medical Complications of Anorexia Nervosa

Gastrointestinal
  Gastric distention
  Constipation

Cardiovascular
  Heart muscle atrophy
  Bradycardia
  Hypotension
  Arrhythmias
  Mitral valve prolapse
  Peripheral edema

Endocrine/Metabolic
  Amenorrhea
  Hypothermia

Hematologic
  Anemia

Skeletal
  Stress fractures
  Premature osteoporosis

Muscle
  Depleted muscle mass

Brain
  Abnormal electrical activity
  Confusion

and comorbid complications, especially those affecting the heart [11,23]. Whether the patient is treated as an inpatient or as an outpatient, goals for the patient's health are established, often with a written contract signed by the patient as well as by members of the health care team.

Summaries of treatment outcomes for anorexia nervosa show that ~40% to 50% recover completely, ~30% improve, 20% to 25% continue to experience chronic problems with the condition, and another 10% to 15% die from medical complications, suicide, or malnutrition [13,14,29,30]. Mortality typically is highest among people who have sustained severe weight loss, who have had the condition for a prolonged duration, and who developed the condition at an older age [23,29,31].

BULIMIA NERVOSA

Bulimia nervosa, another eating disorder, is a condition characterized by recurring binge eating coupled with self-induced vomiting and misuse of laxatives, diuretics, or other medications to prevent weight gain. Binge eating is marked by a sense of lack of control over eating during the binge episode [22]. A binge is defined as eating an amount of food larger than most people would eat during a similar time period and under similar circumstances [9]. Bulimia denotes a ravenous appetite (or "ox hunger") associated with powerlessness to control eating [25]. Criteria [9] for the diagnosis of bulimia nervosa are given in Table 3.

Bulimia occurs primarily in young women, especially college-age women who are of normal weight or slightly overweight. The typical bulimic, rather than being overly concerned with losing weight and becoming very thin (like the person with anorexia nervosa), seeks to be able to eat without gaining weight [25]. Other factors associated with the development of bulimia include a history of sexual abuse, psychoactive substance abuse or dependence, a family history of depression or alcoholism, obsessive-compulsive disorder, negative self-evaluation, and a high use of escape-avoidance coping [21,22,29,32].

Table 3 Diagnostic Criteria for 307.51 Bulimia Nervosa

A. Recurrent episodes of binge eating. An episode of binge eating is characterized by both of the following:
  (1) eating, in a discrete period of time (e.g., within any 2-hour period), an amount of food that is definitely larger than most people would eat during a similar period of time and under similar circumstances.
  (2) a sense of lack of control over eating during the episode (e.g., a feeling that one cannot stop eating or control what or how much one is eating).

B. Recurrent inappropriate compensatory behavior in order to prevent weight gain, such as self-induced vomiting; misuse of laxatives, diuretics, enemas, or other medications; fasting; or excessive exercise.

C. The binge eating and inappropriate compensatory behaviors both occur, on average, at least twice a week for 3 months.

D. Self-evaluation is unduly influenced by body shape and weight.

E. The disturbance does not occur exclusively during episodes of anorexia nervosa.

Specify type:

Purging Type: during the current episode of bulimia nervosa, the person has regularly engaged in self-induced vomiting or the misuse of laxatives, diuretics, or enemas.

Nonpurging Type: during the current episode of bulimia nervosa, the person has used other inappropriate compensatory behaviors, such as fasting or excessive exercise, but has not regularly engaged in self-induced vomiting or the misuse of laxatives, diuretics, or enemas.

Source: Reprinted with permission from the *Diagnostic and Statistical Manual of Mental Disorders*, Text Revision, Copyright 2000. American Psychiatric Association.

Table 4 Some Potential Medical Complications of Bulimia Nervosa

Gastrointestinal	**Cardiovascular**
Erosion of the teeth	Arrhythmias
Dental caries	
Sore throat	**Respiratory and Skeletal**
Swollen parotid glands	Aspiration pneumonia
Esophageal rupture or tears	Rib fracture
Stomach tear	
Gastroesophageal reflux disease	**Endocrine/Metabolic**
Constipation	Irregular menses or amenorrhea
Cathartic colon	Electrolyte imbalance

Bulimia often starts with dieting attempts in which hunger feelings get out of control. These dieting attempts, usually based upon food abstinence or excessive food restriction, lead to binge eating. Once binge eaters discover that they can undo the consequences of their overeating by vomiting the ingested food, they begin to binge not only when they are hungry but also when they are experiencing any distressing emotion [25,29]. Most binge eating is done privately in the afternoon or evening, with an intake of about 3,500 kcal; purging behaviors reduce retention of energy to about 1,200 kcal [33–35]. Favorite foods for binging usually are dessert and snack foods very high in carbohydrates.

Diagnosis is usually dependent upon self-reported symptoms or on treatment for related problems or conditions. Conditions that may develop as the result of bulimia are listed in Table 4. The gastrointestinal tract is greatly affected by repeated vomiting and the use of laxatives. Repeated vomiting also causes other problems, including skin lesions or calluses on the dorsal side of the hands (especially over the joints), severe dental erosion, swollen enlarged neck glands (due to salivary or parotid gland enlargement), reddened eyes, headache, and fluid and electrolyte imbalances. Laxative misuse may exacerbate fluid and electrolyte losses and, when coupled with vomiting, may lead to heart arrhythmias and heart failure. The presence of lesions or calluses on the hands (due to the scraping of teeth against the skin while self-inducing vomiting), the swollen neck glands, and the frequent trips to the bathroom after meals often are recognized by health professionals and family or friends and facilitate detection and diagnosis of the problem.

The treatment of bulimia, like that of anorexia nervosa, is multidisciplinary. Goals typically focus on eliminating binge-purge behaviors, normalizing eating habits, maintaining weight, and resuming normal menses, if they are affected [29]. The patient is most likely to be hospitalized with problems such as electrolyte imbalance, drug (e.g., laxatives, diuretics) dependence, severe depression, or suicidal tendencies [29]. The prognosis of those suffering from bulimia nervosa is generally more favorable than for those with anorexia nervosa; over 50% of those with bulimia nervosa fully recover or achieve good outcomes, while fewer than 10% have poor outcomes [36].

BINGE EATING DISORDER

The American Psychiatric Association's *Diagnostic and Statistical Manual of Mental Disorders* includes a provisional eating disorder diagnosis, binge eating disorder, which is not associated with purging as in bulimia nervosa [9]. Binge eating disorder is characterized by binge eating at least twice a week for at least a 6-month period with no compensatory behaviors. The binge eating episode typically involves eating (usually with a general sense of lack of control) large amounts of highly energy-dense foods (such as dessert and snack food type items) more rapidly than normal, and continues despite the individual feeling uncomfortably full. Subtypes of the disorder are mainly distinguished by whether the binge precedes dieting or whether dieting precedes the binge eating [37]. Factors associated with binge eating include repeated exposure to negative comments about eating, shape, and weight; depression; negative self-evaluation; and vulnerability to obesity [38]. For those with a binge eating disorder, food often provides comfort and a sense of emotional well-being, especially if the person is feeling stressed, anxious, unhappy, or depressed [39,40]. Thus, the binge usually occurs when the person is not physically hungry but is emotionally unhappy. The binge usually happens in private because of embarrassment, and following the binge, feelings of disgust, guilt, and depression are common.

DISORDERED EATING

Eating disorders (Table 5) other than anorexia nervosa, bulimia nervosa, and binge eating disorder are categorized by the American Psychiatric Association as eating disorders not otherwise specified [9]. The characteristics of those with disordered eating are similar to those of individuals with anorexia nervosa and bulimia nervosa and include fear of being fat, restrained eating, binge eating, purging behavior, and distorted body image; however, people with disordered eating do not meet the criteria for anorexia nervosa or bulimia nervosa (Tables 1 and 3). Disordered eating is likely more common than anorexia and bulimia nervosa, and is seen in both males and females, especially female athletes, where it often exists as part of the female athlete triad.

The Female Athlete Triad

The female athlete triad, first described in 1992 and defined as the combination of disordered eating, amenorrhea, and osteopenia, is described as a complex interrelationship between menstrual status, bone health, and energy availability [41]. The condition appears most often in women participating in sports in which physique and body image are important and extra body weight is undesirable. While all female athletes are considered at risk, women most at risk include long-distance runners, figure skaters, gymnasts, ballet dancers, swimmers, and divers [8,29,42,43].

Inadequate energy intakes among athletes may be related to disordered eating—with an estimated prevalence of 10% to 20% in athletes—or simply to a failure to meet the high energy needs of the sport (unassociated with disordered eating) [22]. Amenorrhea is experienced by the majority (over 50%) of female athletes (versus only 2–5% of women in the general population) [42]. The causes of amenorrhea in athletes, as in women with eating disorders, are not clearly understood. They are thought to relate to synergistic effects of excessive amounts of physical activity and training, constant stress or anxiety, low amounts of body fat, weight fluctuations, and poor diet, especially an extreme energy (caloric) deficit [41,44,45]. The effect of these various factors

Table 5 307.50 Eating Disorder Not Otherwise Specified

The Eating Disorder Not Otherwise Specified category is for disorders of eating that do not meet the criteria for any specific Eating Disorder. Examples include

1. For females, all of the criteria for anorexia nervosa are met except that the individual has regular menses.

2. All of the criteria for anorexia nervosa are met except that, despite significant weight loss, the individual's current weight is in the normal range.

3. All of the criteria for bulimia nervosa are met except that the binge eating and inappropriate compensatory mechanisms occur at a frequency of less than twice a week or for a duration of less than 3 months.

4. The regular use of inappropriate compensatory behavior by an individual of normal body weight after eating small amounts of food (e.g., self-induced vomiting after the consumption of two cookies).

5. Repeatedly chewing and spitting out, but not swallowing, large amounts of food.

6. Binge-eating disorder: recurrent episodes of binge eating in the absence of the regular use of inappropriate compensatory behaviors characteristic of bulimia nervosa.

Source: Reprinted with permission from the *Diagnostic and Statistical Manual of Mental Disorders*, Fourth Edition, Text Revision, Copyright 2000. American Psychiatric Association.

is to evoke changes in the release of hormones such as follicular stimulating and luteinizing hormones that then lead to diminished release of estrogen and progesterone (among other hormones), which in turn can cause amenorrhea. The amenorrhea—more specifically, the diminished serum estrogen concentrations—in turn negatively impact the skeletal system, similar to what is observed in those with anorexia nervosa [27]. Premature bone loss, inadequate bone formation, or both with resulting low bone mass, stress fractures, and other orthopedic problems are common among female athletes; in fact, over 50% of athletes with amenorrhea have low bone mass or bone densities at least one standard deviation below the mean [29,45,46]. High levels of cortisol in the blood, common in athletes, and extensive training regimens also can contribute to bone loss along with poor energy and nutrient (especially vitamin D and calcium) intakes [26–28]. Some of the American College of Sports Medicine's recommendations for the prevention and treatment of the female athlete triad emphasize optimizing energy and nutrient availability and providing medications, as needed, to improve bone health and for psychological problems, although the full reversal of low bone mineral density is thought to be unlikely [41].

SUMMARY

The early identification and treatment of the female athlete triad as well as eating disorders is crucial if serious complications are to be avoided. Just as obesity is associated with increased risk for a variety of diseases, eating disorders are associated with a multitude of risks, including death. Combating eating disorders is difficult; not only must the victims be treated, but the values of society, including images of beauty, must also be rehabilitated [47].

References Cited

1. Rubinstein S, Caballero B. Is Miss America an undernourished role model? JAMA. 2000; 283:1569.

2. Byrd-Bredbenner C, Murray J. A comparison of the anthropometric measurements of idealized female body images in media directed to men, women, and mixed gender audiences. Top Clin Nutr. 2003; 18:117–29.

3. Pugliese MT, Lifshitz F, Grad G, et al. Fear of obesity. N Engl J Med. 1983; 309:513–18.

4. Devlin M, Zhu A. Body image in the balance. JAMA 2001; 286:2159.

5. Association of Anorexia Nervosa and Associated Disorders (ANAD). http://www.anad.org/get-information/about-eating-disorders/general-information/Accessed September 9, 2011.

6. Ross CC. The importance of nutrition as the best medicine for eating disorders. Explore. 2007; 3:153–57.

7. Hoek HW, Van Hoeken D. Review of the prevalence and incidence of eating disorders. Int J Eat Disord. 2003; 34:384–86.

8. Glazer JL. Eating disorders among male athletes. Curr Sports Med Rep. 2008; 7:332–37.

9. American Psychiatric Association. Diagnostic and Statistical Manual of Mental Disorders, 4th ed., text revision. Washington, DC. 2000.

10. Crow S, Peterson CB. Refining treatments for eating disorders. Am J Psychiatry. 2009; 166:266–67.

11. Anzai N, Lindsey-Dudley K, Bidwell R. Inpatient and partial hospital treatment for eating disorders. Child Adoles Psych Clin N Am. 2002; 11:279–309.

12. Powers P, Santana C. Childhood and adolescent anorexia nervosa. Child Adol Psych Clin. 2002; 11:219–35.

13. Steinhausen H. The outcome of anorexia nervosa in the 20th century. Am J Psychiatry. 2002; 159:1284–93.

14. Birmingham CL, Su J, Hlynsky JA, et al. The mortality rate from anorexia nervosa. Int J Eat Disord. 2005; 38:143–46.

15. Mond J, Hay P, Rodgers B, Owen C. An update on the definition of excessive exercise in eating disorder research. Int J Eat Disord. 2006; 39:147–53.

16. Bulik CM, Reba L, Siega-Riz A, Reichborn-Kjennerud T. Anorexia nervosa: definition, epidemiology, and cycle of risk. Int J Eat Disord. 2005; 37:S2–S9.

17. Godart NT, Flament MF, Perdereau F, Jeammet P. Comorbidity between eating disorders and anxiety disorders: a review. Int J Eat Disord. 2002; 32:253–70.

18. Steinhausen HC. Outcome of eating disorders. Child Adolesc Psychiatr Clin North Am. 2009; 18:225–42.

19. Jordan J, Joyce PR, Carter FA, et al. Specific and nonspecific comorbidity in anorexia nervosa. Int J Eat Disord. 2008; 41:47–56.

20. Kaye WH, Bulik CM, Thornton L, et al. Comorbidity of anxiety disorders with anorexia and bulimia nervosa. Am J Psychiatry. 2004; 161:2215–21.

21. Anderluh MB, Tchanturia K, Rabe-Hesketh S, Treasure J. Childhood obsessive-compulsive personality traits in adult women with eating disorders: defining a broader eating disorder phenotype. Am J Psychiatry. 2003; 160:242–47.

22. American Dietetic Association. Position of the American Dietetic Association: Nutrition intervention in the treatment of anorexia nervosa, bulimia nervosa, and other eating disorders. J Am Diet Assoc. 2006; 106:2073–82.

23. Mehler P. Diagnosis and care of patients with anorexia nervosa in primary care settings. Ann Intern Med. 2001; 134:1048–59.

24. Keel PK, Klump KL, Miller KB, et al. Shared transmission of eating disorders and anxiety disorders. Int J Eat Disord. 2005; 38:99–105.

25. Casper RC. The pathophysiology of anorexia nervosa and bulimia nervosa. Ann Rev Nutr. 1986; 6:299–316.

26. Katzman D. Osteoporosis in anorexia nervosa: a brittle future. Curr Drug Targets CNS & Neurolog Dis. 2003; 2:11–15.

27. Mehler PS, MacKenzie TD. Treatment of osteopenia and osteoporosis in anorexia nervosa: a systematic review of the literature. Int J Eat Disord. 2009; 42:195–201.

28. Misra M. Long-term skeletal effects of eating disorders with onset in adolescence. Ann NY Acad Sci. 2008; 1135:212–18.

29. Walsh J, Wheat M, Freund K. Detection, evaluation, and treatment of eating disorders. J Gen Intern Med. 2000; 15:577–90.

30. Treasure J, Schmidt U. Anorexia nervosa. Clin Evid. 2002; 7:824–33.

31. Brown J, Mehler P, Harris R. Medical complications occurring in adolescents with anorexia nervosa. West J Med. 2000; 172:189–93.

32. Johnson J, Cohen P, Kasen S, Brook J. Childhood adversities associated with risk for eating disorders or weight problems during adolescence or early adulthood. Am J Psychiatry. 2002; 159:394–400.

33. Muuss RE. Adolescent eating disorder: bulimia. Adolescence. 1986; 21:257–67.

34. Mitchell JE, Pyle RL, Eckert ED. Frequency and duration of binge-eating episodes in patients with bulimia. Am J Psychiatry. 1981; 138:835–36.

35. Kaye WH, Weltzin TE, Hsu LK, et al. Amount of calories retained after binge eating and vomiting. Am J Psychiatry. 1993; 50:969–71.

36. Fichter MM, Quadflieg N. Six year course of bulimia nervosa. Int J Eat Disord. 1997; 22:361–84.

37. Manwaring JL, Hilbert A, Wilfley D, et al. Risk factors and patterns of onset in binge eating disorder. Int J Eat Disord. 2006; 39:101–07.

38. Fairburn CG, Doll HA, Welch SL, et al. Risk factors for binge eating disorder: a community based, case-control study. Arch Gen Psychiatry. 1998; 55:425–32.

39. Masheb RM, Grilo CM. Emotional overeating and its association with eating disorder psychopathology among overweight patients with binge eating disorder. Int J Eat Disord. 2006; 39:141–46.

40. Stein R, Kenardy J, Wiseman C, et al. What's driving the binge in binge eating disorder? a prospective examination of precursors and consequences. Int J Eat Disord. 2007; 40:195–203.

41. American College of Sports Medicine. The female athlete triad. Med Sci Sport Exerc. 2007; 39:1867–82.

42. Hobart J, Smucker D. The female athlete triad. Am Fam Physician. 2000; 61:3357–64.

43. Golden N. A review of the female athlete triad (amenorrhea, osteoporosis and disordered eating). Int J Adolesc Med Health. 2002; 14:9–17.

44. Sabatini S. The female athlete triad. Am J Med Sci. 2001; 322:193–95.

45. Kleposki R. The female athlete triad: a terrible trio implications for primary care. J Am Acad Nurs. 2002; 14:26–31.

46. Sanborn C, Horea M, Siemers B, Dieringer K. Disordered eating and the female athlete triad. Clin Sports Med. 2000; 19:199–213.

47. Martin JB. The development of ideal body image perceptions in the United States. Nutr Today. 2010; 45:98–110.

Web Sites

www.nationaleatingdisorders.org

www.nimh.nih.gov/publicat/eatingdisorders.cfm

http://www.anad.org/get-information/about-eating-disorders/general-information/

Suggested Readings

Attia E. Anorexia nervosa: current status and future directions. Ann Rev Med. 2010;61:425-35.

Ferriter C, Ray LA. Binge eating and binge drinking: an integrative review. Eat Behav. 2011;12:99-107.

Nutrition in Clinical Practice. 2010;25:101-59. Several articles in this issue are devoted to disordered eating.

Treasure J, Claudino AM, Zucker N. Eating disorders. Lancet. 2010;375:583-93.

9 WATER-SOLUBLE VITAMINS

THE EARLY PART OF THE 20TH CENTURY was the most exciting era in the history of nutrition science. It was during this time that the discovery of vitamins, or "accessory growth factors," began. Researchers found that for life and growth, animals required something more than a chemically defined diet consisting of purified carbohydrate, protein, fat, minerals, and water. The first of these dietary essentials to be discovered was an antiberiberi substance isolated from rice polishings by Casimir Funk, a Polish biochemist. Funk gave it the name vitamine because the substance was an amine and necessary for life (*vita* means "life" in Latin). Very shortly thereafter McCollum and Davis extracted a factor from butter fat that they called fat-soluble A to distinguish it from the water-soluble antiberiberi substance. These two essential factors became known as vitamine A and vitamine B.

Much of the initial research used to identify vitamins relied on the historical method, which seeks to explain the cause of past events and to interpret current happenings on the basis of these findings. Sources of information for the historical researcher are primarily documentary, existing in the form of written records and accounts of past events as well as literary productions and critical writings. The researcher relies, if possible, only on primary data, that is, data that are "firsthand" and therefore minimally distorted by the channels of communication. Generally, information gathered by historical research does not need to be analyzed by any form of statistical treatment or data analysis. A brief history of each vitamin's discovery is presented at the start of its section.

As each additional vitamin was discovered, it was assigned a letter. The *e* on *vitamine* was dropped to give the general name *vitamin* because only a few of the essential substances were found to be amines. As the chemical structure of a vitamin became known through its isolation and synthesis, it was given a chemical name. Each chemical name assigned was assumed to apply only to one substance, with one specific activity. We now know that a vitamin may have a variety of functions, and that vitamin activity may be found in several closely related compounds, known as vitamers. An excellent example of this range of activity is vitamin A, which has several seemingly unrelated functions and encompasses not only retinol but also retinal and retinoic acid.

Vitamins are organic compounds with regulatory functions that are required in the diet if the species (humans) is unable to synthesize them. Thus, vitamins are considered essential. Moreover, because these substances must be supplied by the diet, their discovery often came about because of their absence in the diet. Although the clinician should be able to recognize the deficiency syndrome caused by a lack of a particular vitamin, in a country with an abundant and varied food supply such as the United States, the nutrition professional should think in terms of what a specific vitamin does rather than what disease it prevents. Unfortunately, relating the function of the vitamin directly to its deficiency syndrome is often impossible.

Vitamins, for the most part, are not related chemically and differ in their physiological roles. The broad classifications of water-soluble vitamins and fat-soluble vitamins are made because of certain properties common to each group. The body handles the water-soluble vitamins differently from the way it handles the fat-soluble vitamins (which are discussed in Chapter 10). They are absorbed into portal blood, in contrast to fat-soluble vitamins, and, with the exception of cobalamin (vitamin B_{12}), they cannot be retained for long periods by the body. Any storage of water-soluble vitamins that occurs results from their binding to enzymes and transport proteins. Water-soluble vitamins are excreted in the urine whenever plasma levels exceed renal thresholds.

With the exception of vitamin C, water-soluble vitamins are members of the B complex. Most of the B-complex group can be further divided according to general function: energy releasing or hematopoietic. Other vitamins cannot be classified this narrowly because of their wide range of functions. Figure 9.1 shows the classification of water-soluble vitamins.

In this chapter, discussions of the various vitamins are grouped similarly. Each vitamin is considered (when precise information is available) in terms of structure, sources, absorption (also digestion where applicable), transport, storage, functions and mechanisms of action, metabolism and excretion, Recommended Dietary

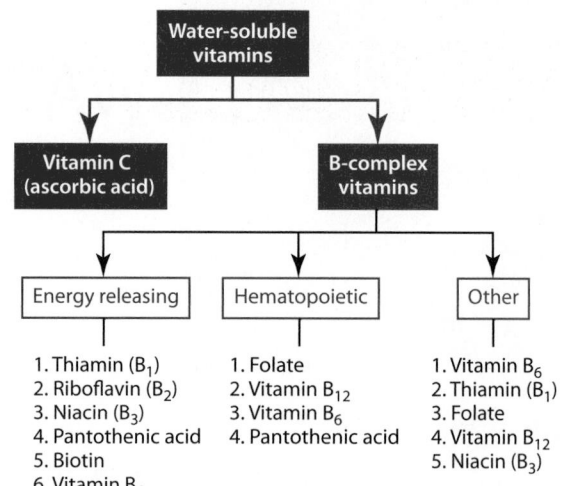

Figure 9.1 The water-soluble vitamins.

Allowance or Adequate Intake, deficiency, toxicity, and assessment of nuriture. Specific interrelationships with other nutrients are also noted for selected vitamins. Table 9.1 contains a summary of the coenzyme form(s), functions, deficiency syndrome, those at risk for deficiency, sources, and **Recommended Dietary Allowance (RDA)** or **Adequate Intake (AI)** of each of the water-soluble vitamins. The inside front book cover provides

Table 9.1 The Water-Soluble Vitamins: Functions, Deficiency Syndromes, Food Sources, Recommended Intake, and Individuals at Risk for Deficiency

Vitamin	Main Coenzyme(s)	Biochemical or Physiological Function(s)	Deficiency Syndrome or Symptoms	Good Food Sources	RDA* or AI†	Some Conditions and/ or Individuals at Risk for Deficiency
Thiamin (vitamin B_1)	Thiamin diphosphate (TDP) or thiamin pyrophosphate (TPP)	Oxidative decarboxylation of α-keto acids and 2-keto sugars	*Beriberi*, muscle weakness, anorexia, tachycardia, enlarged heart, edema	Yeast, pork, sunflower seeds, legumes	1.1 mg* 1.2 mg	Alcoholism, elderly, malabsorptive conditions
Riboflavin (vitamin B_2)	Flavin adenine dinucleotide (FAD); flavin mononucleotide (FMN)	Electron (hydrogen) transfer reactions	*Ariboflavinosis*, cheilosis, glossitis, hyperemia and edema of pharyngeal and oral mucous membranes, angular stomatitis, photophobia	Beef liver, meats, eggs, yogurt, ricotta cheese, nonfat milk	1.1 mg* 1.3 mg	Alcoholism, trauma, hypermetabolic conditions
Niacin (vitamin B_3) (nicotinic acid, nicotinamide)	Nicotinamide adenine dinucleotide (NAD); nicotinamide adenine dinucleotide phosphate (NADP)	Electron (hydrogen) transfer reactions	*Pellagra*, diarrhea, dermatitis, mental confusion or dementia	Tuna, beef liver, veal, chicken, beef, halibut, peanut butter	14 mg* 16 mg	Alcoholism, malabsorptive conditions, Hartnup disease
Pantothenic acid	Coenzyme A (CoA)	Acyl transfer reactions	Deficiency very rare; numbness and tingling of hands and feet, vomiting, fatigue	Widespread in foods	5 mg†	Alcoholism, malabsorptive conditions
Biotin	Carboxybiotinyl lysine	CO_2 transfer/ carboxylation reactions	Deficiency very rare; anorexia, nausea, glossitis, depression, dry scaly dermatitis	Synthesized by microflora of digestive tract; liver, soybeans, eggs	30 μg†	Excessive raw egg ingestion, alcoholism, malabsorptive conditions
Vitamin B_6 (pyridoxine, pyridoxal, pyridoxamine)	Pyridoxal phosphate (PLP)	Transamination and decarboxylation reactions	Dermatitis, glossitis, convulsions	Steak, navy beans, potato, salmon, banana, whole grains	1.3 mg*	Elderly, alcoholism, use of certain medications

(Continued)

Table 9.1 The Water-Soluble Vitamins: Functions, Deficiency Syndromes, Food Sources, Recommended Intake, and Individuals at Risk for Deficiency (*Continued*)

Vitamin	Main Coenzyme(s)	Biochemical or Physiological Function(s)	Deficiency Syndrome or Symptoms	Good Food Sources	RDA* or AI†	Some Conditions and/ or Individuals at Risk for Deficiency
Folate	Derivatives of tetrahydrofolic acid: 5, 10-methylene THF, 10-formyl THF, 5-formimino THF, 5, 10-methylenyl THF, 5-methyl THF	One-carbon transfer reactions	*Megaloblastic anemia*, diarrhea, fatigue, depression, confusion	Brewer's yeast, spinach, asparagus, turnip greens, lima beans, beef liver, fortified grain products	400 μg*	Alcoholism, malabsorptive conditions, use of certain medications
Vitamin B_{12} (cobalamin)	Methylcobalamin, adenosylcobalamin	Methylation of homocysteine to methionine; conversion of methylmalonyl-CoA to succinyl-CoA	*Megaloblastic anemia*, degeneration of peripheral nerves	Meat, fish, shellfish, poultry, milk	2.4 μg*	Elderly, strict vegetarians, pernicious anemia, some disorders affecting stomach and ileum
Ascorbic acid (vitamin C)	None	Antioxidant; hydroxylating enzymes involved in synthesis of collagen, carnitine, norepinephrine	*Scurvy*, hyperkeratosis of hair follicles, psychological manifestations, retarded wound healing, bleeding gums, spontaneous rupture of capillaries	Papaya, orange juice, cantaloupe, broccoli, Brussels sprouts, green peppers, grapefruit juice, strawberries	75 mg* 90 mg	Elderly, alcoholism, smoking

the Dietary Reference Intakes (DRIs), when available, for all nutrients and for all age groups.

Several different types of research methodologies are used to arrive at the DRIs for the different nutrients. The experimental method (also sometimes called the control group–experimental group design) is frequently used and involves two or more population groups, with the subjects of each group matched as closely as possible in characteristics to the subjects of the other group(s). One group serves as a control and is not exposed to any extraneous change. The experimental group is exposed to the alteration under study (such as an insufficient amount of a vitamin provided in the diet), and whatever change(s) (such as deficiency symptoms) is noted in this group relative to the subjects of the control group is presumed to be caused by the extraneous variable(s). The experimental method can also use just one group, a method sometimes called a pretest-posttest approach. In its simplest form, a group of subjects is evaluated (pretest), subjected to the experimental variable (test), and reevaluated (posttest). In so-called crossover studies, another common approach, the standard experimental method (with separate control and experimental groups) is performed twice. After the initial phase, in which the experimental group is subjected to the variable and differences in the findings are noted, the subjects switch groups: The original control group is exposed to the variable, thus becoming the experimental group, and the original experimental group becomes the unexposed control group. This approach corrects for any inherent differences in the two groups that might confound the experimental data.

In short, the experimental method is based on cause and effect. It involves intervention on the part of the researcher, who introduces a variable and records its effect.

Experimental research designs enable the investigator to control or manipulate one or more variables, designated as dependent or independent, in an effort to examine the relationship between the variables. The independent variable is the variable controlled or manipulated (such as the insufficient amount of the vitamin provided in the diet) by the investigator. The dependent variable (i.e., the deficiency symptoms) occurs as the result of the influence of the independent variable. The experimental design is one of the most common methodologies employed and encountered in nutrition literature, including many of the studies used to determine the DRIs for water-soluble and fat-soluble vitamins.

DRIs represent quantitative approximations of nutrient needs for the purpose of planning and assessing the diets of healthy people. DRIs include RDAs as well as AIs, Tolerable Upper Intake Levels (ULs), and **Estimated Average Requirements (EARs)**. RDAs represent the average daily dietary intake level that is sufficient to meet the nutrient requirements of about 97% of healthy people. They are based on EARs, which are the amounts of nutrients thought to meet the nutrient requirements of 50% of the healthy people in a specified age and gender group. RDAs are set higher than EARs by either two standard deviations or a coefficient of variation for the EAR. The intake of a nutrient is likely inadequate if it is significantly less than the EAR. Further, an intake above the EAR but less than the RDA may still be inadequate. AIs are provided for nutrients instead of RDAs when scientific data are insufficient to calculate the EARs. AIs are based on nutrient intake levels of healthy people (with adequate nutritional status), and are typically thought to exceed the requirement for the nutrient. Thus, nutrient intakes are likely adequate if they equal or exceed the AI, but may or may not be adequate if they are less than the AI. If nutrient intakes are above the RDA but less than the UL, then they are likely to be adequate. ULs provide the highest intake level for a nutrient that is unlikely to cause any risk of adverse health to almost all people in the age- or gender-specified groups. ULs are viewed as maximum amounts for those consuming fortified foods or supplements in large quantities. For some nutrients, the UL is not known, but the lack of a UL does not mean that large doses of the nutrient are harmless.

Suggested Reading

McCollum EV. A History of Nutrition. Boston: Houghton Mifflin. 1957.
Lanska DJ. Historical aspects of the major neurological vitamin deficiency disorders: the water soluble vitamins. Handbook of Clinical Neurology. 2010; 95:445–76.

VITAMIN C (ASCORBIC ACID)

Vitamin C (also known as ascorbic acid or, at physiological pH in its ionized form, as ascorbate or ascorbate anion after the loss of a hydrogen) was isolated in 1928, and its structure was determined in 1933. But this vitamin's deficiency disorder—referred to as scurvy—had been prevalent for centuries. Some of the most notable stories are those of the British sailors who frequently died from scurvy on sea voyages. It was a physician that eventually found that sucking the juice from a lime was protective, and in the late 1790s and early 1800s British sailors at sea began receiving limes (resulting in the nickname "limey" for the sailors) in an effort to prevent scurvy outbreaks. Szent-Györgyi (1928) and King (1932) are considered co-discoverers of vitamin C. Szent-Györgyi, who isolated the vitamin, and Haworth, who determined its structure, were awarded the Nobel prize in 1937 for their vitamin C work.

Vitamin C exists as both a D- and L-isomer; however, it is the L-isomer of the vitamin that is biologically active in humans. The human being is one of the few mammals unable to synthesize vitamin C, a six-carbon compound derived from glucose. Animals unable to synthesize the vitamin include primates, fruit bats, guinea pigs, and some birds. The inability to make vitamin C results from the lack of gulonolactone oxidase, the last enzyme in the vitamin C synthetic pathway (shown in Figure 9.2).

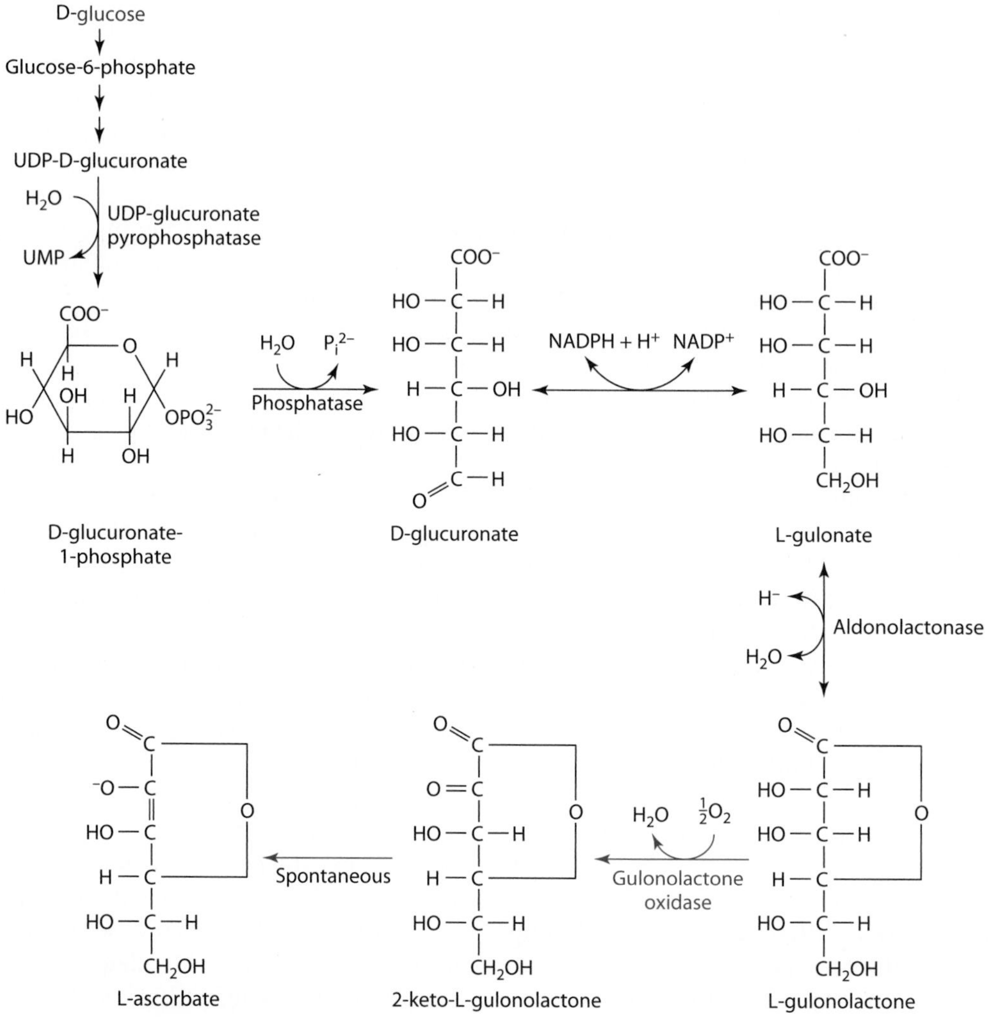

Figure 9.2 Synthesis of ascorbic acid. Humans lack the gulonolactone oxidase that catalyzes the final enzymatic reaction.

Sources

Food sources of vitamin C include primarily fruits and vegetables. Excellent sources of the nutrient are asparagus, papaya, oranges, orange juice, cantaloupe, cauliflower, broccoli, brussels sprouts, green peppers, grapefruit, grapefruit juice, kale, lemons, and strawberries. Of these foods, citrus products are commonly cited as significant sources, supplying about 70 to 80 mg of vitamin C per serving. One cup strawberries provides 90 mg of vitamin C; a medium kiwi, 75 mg; 1 cup of cantaloupe, 68 mg; and 1 banana or ½ cup pineapple, 12 mg. A small potato or ½ cup Brussels sprouts, broccoli, or cauliflower provides about 30 to 40 mg of vitamin C. Fortified breakfast cereals also contribute some vitamin C to the diet. A cup of Froot Loops®, for example, provides 25% of the Daily Value (which is 60 mg), or about 15 mg of vitamin C.

In foods, vitamin C is found mostly as ascorbic acid, but small amounts of vitamin C's oxidized form (with two electrons and two protons removed), called dehydroascorbic acid, also may be present. Supplements typically supply vitamin C as free ascorbic acid, calcium ascorbate, sodium ascorbate, and ascorbyl palmitate. Ester-C® contains calcium ascorbate, dehydroascorbate (the ionic form of dehydroascorbic acid), and some vitamin C metabolites. Rose hip (*Rosa*), a seed capsule found in roses, also contains vitamin C and is used commercially in vitamin C supplements. Neither Ester-C® nor vitamin C from rose hips appears to be superior to other vitamin C sources.

Vitamin C is destroyed by heat, light, oxidation, and alkaline solutions but is stable in acidic solutions. Thus, cooking and storage may reduce the vitamin C content of foods. Further, ingesting large amounts of iron or copper with vitamin C may result in the oxidative destruction of the vitamin in the digestive tract, yielding diketogulonic acid and other products without vitamin C activity.

Digestion, Absorption, Transport, and Storage

Vitamin C does not require digestion prior to being absorbed into intestinal cells. Absorption of ascorbic acid (but not dehydroascorbic acid) across the intestinal cell brush border occurs throughout the small intestine, including the ileum, assisted by sodium-dependent vitamin C transporters (SVCT) 1 and 2. SVCT1 is the main carrier responsible for intestinal vitamin C absorption. SVCT1 enables intestinal absorption of the vitamin in excess of cell needs, but is down-regulated by ascorbic acid, which limits the absorption of superphysiological doses.

The dehydroascorbic acid that is found in foods or that may be formed if ascorbic acid is oxidized in the gastrointestinal tract is absorbed by glucose transporters (GLUT), mainly GLUT 1 and 3. However, once it is absorbed, the dehydroascorbic acid is rapidly reduced back (recycled) to ascorbic acid by the enzyme dehydroascorbic acid reductase. Glutathione (GSH), which is required for the reduction of dehydroascorbic acid and thus spares vitamin C, is oxidized (to GSSG) in the process as shown in Figure 9.3. NADPH and the dithiol glutaredoxin also can be used instead of GSH to reduce the dehydroascorbic acid.

Over a range of usual vitamin C intakes (30–180 mg/day) from food, vitamin C absorption is about 70% to 90%. Absorption of the vitamin decreases with increased intake; for example, 16% is absorbed at high intakes (~12 g) versus

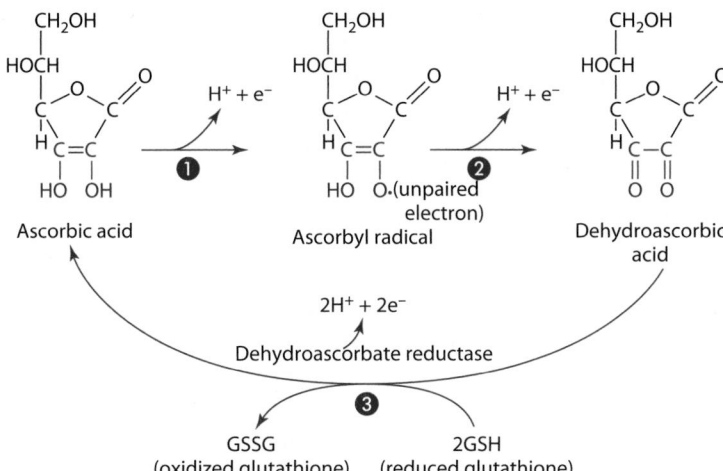

❶ During the oxidation of ascorbic acid, a free radical called ascorbyl radical (also called semidehydroascorbic acid radical, ascorbate free radical, ascorbyl, monodehydroascorbate radical) is formed but has a short half-life and reacts poorly with oxygen, so it does not form reactive oxygen species.
❷ Oxidation of the radical forms of vitamin C.
❸ Dehydroascorbic acid can be reduced to ascorbic acid with hydrogens provided by the reduced form of glutathione (GSH).

Figure 9.3 The interconversion of ascorbic acid and dehydroascorbic acid.

98% absorbed at low intakes ($<$20 mg). At intakes above 1 g, less than 50% of vitamin C is typically absorbed. From the intestinal cells, vitamin C diffuses through anion channels into extracellular fluid and enters the plasma by way of the capillaries.

Ascorbic acid and dehydroascorbic acid are transported in the blood primarily in free form; however, only small amounts of dehydroascorbic acid are found due to its rapid cellular uptake. Normal plasma ascorbic acid concentrations range from about 0.4 to 1.7 mg/dL; higher plasma vitamin C concentrations can be achieved with intravenous administration of the vitamin than with oral intake. Ascorbic acid uptake into body cells such as those of the liver and kidneys occurs by SVCT1. SVCT2 is also present in most metabolically active tissues with the exceptions of skeletal muscle and lungs. Dehydroascorbic acid uptake into cells utilizes GLUT transporters.

Tissue concentrations of vitamin C usually exceed plasma concentrations, with the magnitude dependent upon the specific tissue. The vitamin C content of white blood cells, for example, can be as much as 80 times greater than plasma concentrations. The highest concentrations of vitamin C are found in the adrenal and pituitary glands (with each possessing ~30–50 mg/100 g of wet tissue) as well as in the eyes, brain, and white blood cells. Intermediate levels of vitamin C are found in the liver, spleen, heart, kidneys, lungs, pancreas, and muscle. In absolute terms based on total weight, the liver contains the most vitamin C. The maximal vitamin C pool is estimated at about 2 g. Intakes of about 100 to 200 mg of vitamin C per day have been shown to produce plasma concentrations of about 1.0 mg/dL and to maximize the body pool. Intakes of 1.25 g of vitamin C generated a peak plasma vitamin C concentration of 2.37 mg/dL [2].

Functions and Mechanisms of Action

Despite its uncomplicated structure, vitamin C has complex functional roles in the body. Vitamin C is required in several reactions involved in body processes, including collagen synthesis, carnitine synthesis, tyrosine synthesis and catabolism, and neurotransmitter synthesis. More specifically, the enzymes catalyzing these various reactions contain a mineral (copper or iron) cofactor; vitamin C functions as a reducing agent (antioxidant) to maintain the iron and copper atoms in the metalloenzymes in the reduced state. In addition to its role as a reducing agent in enzymatic reactions, vitamin C functions as an important antioxidant in the body. Each of these processes, as well as some additional roles of vitamin C, is reviewed in this section.

Collagen Synthesis

Vitamin C functions in a number of hydroxylation reactions. Three hydroxylation reactions requiring vitamin C are necessary for the synthesis of collagen, a structural protein found in skin, bones, dentine, tendons, and cartilage (connective tissue) and made up of three polypeptide chains that are synthesized by fibroblasts. Collagen is initially made as tropocollagen, which consists of a triple helix of polypeptide chains twisted around each other and linked by hydrogen bonds to form a coil. After these tropocollagen chains are made, the vitamin C–dependent hydroxylation reactions occur posttranslationally and allow aggregation and further cross-linking of the chains. Prolyl 4-hydroxylase and prolyl 3-hydroxylase (also called dioxygenases) catalyze the hydroxylations of specific proline residues on newly synthesized chains. Proline and hydroxyproline provide more rigidity to the collagen. Lysine hydroxylation by lysyl hydroxylase (also called dioxygenase) results in the formation of hydroxylysyl residues, which provide for attachment to carbohydrate moieties and which allow for additional posttranslational modifications, such as glycosylation and phosphorylation, to further strengthen the collagen. Additionally, a copper–, but not vitamin C–, dependent oxidation reaction between collagen chains occurs for added strength.

The role of vitamin C in the hydroxylation reactions relates to the iron cofactor that is part of prolyl hydroxylases and lysyl hydroxylase. During the reactions, the hydroxylases incorporate one atom of O_2 into the product, and the second atom of O_2 into the cosubstrate α-ketoglutarate to form the new carboxyl group of succinate (Figure 9.4). During these reactions, the iron cofactor in the enzymes is oxidized; that is, it is converted from a ferrous ($^{2+}$) state to a ferric ($^{3+}$) state. Vitamin C functions as the reductant, thereby reducing the iron back to its ferrous state ($^{2+}$) in the prolyl and lysyl hydroxylases.

Although these reactions may seem simple, normal development and maintenance of skin, tendons, cartilage, bone, and dentine depend on an adequate supply of vitamin C. Also, the basement membrane lining the capillaries, the "intracellular cement" holding together the endothelial cells, and the scar tissue responsible for wound healing all require the presence of vitamin C for their formation and maintenance.

Carnitine Synthesis

Vitamin C is involved in two reactions required for the synthesis of carnitine, a nonprotein, nitrogen-containing compound essential for the transport of long-chain fatty acids from the cell cytosol into the mitochondria for β-oxidation. Carnitine is made from the amino acid lysine, which has been methylated using S-adenosyl methionine. The reactions in carnitine synthesis involving vitamin C are hydroxylations similar to those for proline and lysine hydroxylation. Vitamin C functions as a reducing agent, specifically reducing the iron atom from the ferric state (Fe^{3+}) back to the ferrous state (Fe^{2+}) for the reactions catalyzed by trimethyllysine hydroxylase and 4-butyrobetaine hydroxylase (see Figure 6.23).

Proline

Hydroxyproline

α-ketoglutarate   Succinate

Lysine ——— Lysyl hydroxylase ———→ Hydroxylysine

O_2

Fe^{2+} Fe^{3+}

CO_2

Dehydroascorbate   Ascorbate ❶

❶ Ascorbate acts as a reducing agent to convert the oxidized iron atom (Fe^{3+}) back to its reduced state (Fe^{2+}) in the enzymes lysyl hydroxylase and prolyl hydroxylase, which incorporate one atom of oxygen (*) in the hydroxyl group of the product and the other in succinate.

Figure 9.4 Ascorbate functions in the hydroxylation of peptide-bound proline and lysine in the synthesis of collagen.

Tyrosine Synthesis and Catabolism

Tyrosine is synthesized in the body from the amino acid phenylalanine. Tyrosine synthesis requires the hydroxylation of phenylalanine by the iron-dependent enzyme phenylalanine monooxygenase (also called hydroxylase). The reaction occurs in the liver and the kidneys and requires the cosubstrate tetrahydrobiopterin, which gets oxidized in the reaction. Vitamin C is needed to regenerate tetrahydrobiopterin from oxidized dihydrobiopterin (see Figure 6.10).

In another hydroxylation reaction in tyrosine catabolism, vitamin C is a preferred reductant for copper, a cofactor for the enzyme para (p)-hydroxyphenylpyruvate hydroxylase (also called dioxygenase). This enzyme converts para (p)-hydroxyphenylpyruvate to homogentisate, as shown in Figure 6.10 and here.

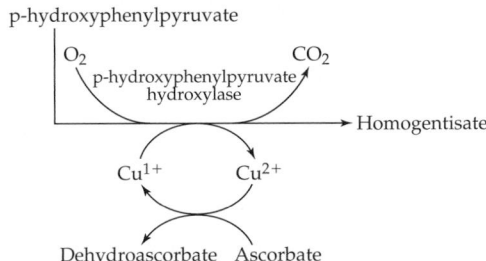

p-hydroxyphenylpyruvate

O_2 CO_2

p-hydroxyphenylpyruvate
hydroxylase

———→ Homogentisate

Cu^{1+} Cu^{2+}

Dehydroascorbate   Ascorbate

Lastly, in tyrosine catabolism (Figure 6.10), vitamin C functions as the reductant as homogentisate is converted to 4-maleylacetoacetate by the iron-dependent enzyme homogentisate dioxygenase. Defects in this enzyme result in the disorder alkaptonuria. Alkaptonuria is characterized by an accumulation of homogentisic acid in the body (leading to painful joints) and in body fluids such as

urine. The condition is notable because when the urine is exposed to air, the homogentisic acid, and thus the urine, turns black.

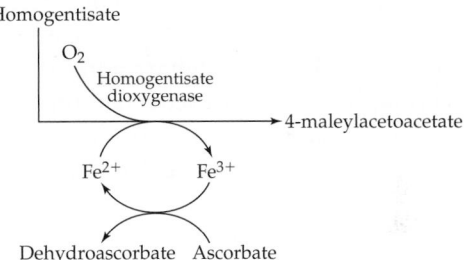

Homogentisate

O_2

Homogentisate
dioxygenase

———→ 4-maleylacetoacetate

Fe^{2+} Fe^{3+}

Dehydroascorbate   Ascorbate

Neurotransmitter Synthesis

Vitamin C is also involved in neurotransmitter synthesis. As with the synthesis of carnitine and collagen, vitamin C reduces mineral cofactors that get oxidized in some of the reactions needed for the synthesis of neurotransmitters, such as norepinephrine. Additionally, vitamin C serves to reduce cosubstrates such as tetrahydrobiopterin, which get oxidized during the synthesis of other neurotransmitters such as serotonin.

Norepinephrine Norepinephrine (a catecholamine) is generated from the hydroxylation of the side chain of dopamine in a vitamin C–dependent reaction. The reaction is catalyzed by dopamine monooxygenase, which contains eight copper atoms and is found primarily in the adrenal glands but also in the nervous system (Figure 6.10). The copper atoms in the enzyme are thought to act as intermediates, accepting electrons from ascorbic acid as they are reduced to cuprous ions (Cu^{1+}) and subsequently transferring these electrons to oxygen as they are reoxidized back to cupric ions (Cu^{2+}).

Serotonin Vitamin C, tetrahydrobiopterin, and oxygen are also involved in the hydroxylation of tryptophan for the synthesis of the neurotransmitter serotonin (5-hydroxytryptamine) in the brain (Figure 6.11). Tryptophan hydroxylase, also called monooxygenase, catalyzes the first step in serotonin synthesis, whereby tryptophan is converted to 5-hydroxytryptophan in a tetrahydrobiopterin-dependent reaction. Vitamin C may help regenerate the cosubstrate tetrahydrobiopterin from dihydrobiopterin. Subsequently, 5-hydroxytryptophan is decarboxylated in a vitamin B_6–dependent reaction to generate serotonin.

Other Neurotransmitters and Hormones Vitamin C also serves as a reductant, keeping the copper atom in peptidylglycine α-amidating monooxygenase in its reduced state, as shown in Figure 9.5. Although most of the substrate peptides for this enzyme have a terminal glycine residue, the enzyme is also active with peptides terminating in other amino acids. Many of the amidated peptides resulting from this reaction are active as hormones, hormone-releasing factors, or neurotransmitters. Examples include bombesin or gastrin-releasing peptide (GRP), calcitonin, cholecystokinin (CCK), thyrotropin, corticotropin-releasing factor, gastrin, growth hormone–releasing factor, oxytocin, and vasopressin. The enzyme is found in neuroendocrine cells of the pituitary, adrenal, and thyroid glands and in the brain. As a reductant for the required amidating enzyme, vitamin C assumes important, although indirect, roles in many regulatory processes.

Microsomal Metabolism

A group of enzymes makes up a microsomal metabolizing system that functions mostly in liver microsomes and reticuloendothelial tissues to inactivate both endogenous and exogenous substances. Endogenous substrates include various hormones like aldosterone and cortisol, and steroids such as cholesterol. For example, cholesterol

7α-hydroxylase, found in the microsomes of the liver, is required for the initial step in the synthesis of bile acids from cholesterol. Vitamin C plays an undefined role in this hydroxylation.

Exogenous substrates for the microsomal metabolizing system are usually xenobiotics. *Xenos* means "stranger" in Greek, and **xenobiotics** are foreign chemicals such as drugs, carcinogens, pesticides, food additives, pollutants, or other noxious compounds. The reactions needed to metabolize these substances usually involve hydroxylations followed by conjugations or methylations to produce polar metabolites for excretion. The hydroxylation reactions are catalyzed by monooxygenases or cytochrome P-450 mixed-function oxidases and require oxygen as well as reducing agents such as vitamin C and NAD(P)H. The exact role of vitamin C, however, has not been established.

Antioxidant Activity

In addition to vitamin C's roles in collagen, carnitine, and neurotransmitter synthesis and in microsomal metabolism, vitamin C functions in a general capacity as a reducing agent or electron donor and thereby has antioxidant activity or functions. Ascorbic acid (which can be thought of as hydrogen ascorbate) acts as a reducing agent in aqueous solutions such as the blood and within cells. Stated slightly differently, vitamin C is an antioxidant in that it reverses oxidation. Reducing agents or antioxidants such as vitamin C may reverse oxidation by donating electrons and hydrogen ions. Vitamin C's two hydroxyl groups and carbonyl group facilitate its ability to act as a hydrogen or electron donor. Ascorbate (AH^-) is the ionized form—that is, the form of vitamin C that results when a proton (hydrogen) has dissociated from ascorbic acid, as in a solution or with donation of hydrogen. The reduction potential of vitamin C is such that it readily donates electrons/hydrogen ions to regenerate other antioxidants, such as vitamin E and glutathione, and to reduce free reactive oxygen and nitrogen radicals. Free radicals, which

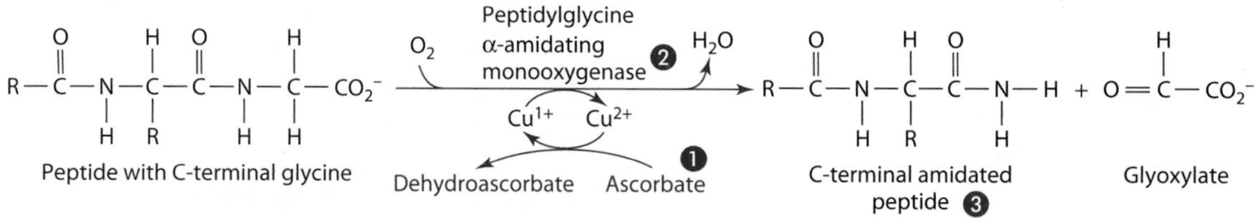

① Vitamin C functions as a reducing agent to convert copper that has become oxidized during the reaction back to a reduced (Cu^{1+}) form.

② The enzyme cleaves the carboxyl-terminal residue on the peptide substrate. The residue is released as glyoxylate.

③ Many of the amidated peptides are active hormones, hormone-releasing factors, or neurotransmitters, as discussed in the text.

Figure 9.5 Amidation of peptides with C-terminal glycine requires vitamin C.

are formed during normal cellular metabolism, exist independently and contain one or more unpaired electrons in an outer orbital surrounding the nucleus of the atom. Vitamin C reduces these radicals including:

- hydroxyl radical ($^{\bullet}OH$), a very reactive oxygen-centered radical
- hydroperoxyl radical ($HO_2^{\bullet}$), an oxygen-centered radical
- superoxide radical ($O_2^{\bullet}$), an oxygen-centered radical
- alkoxyl radical ($RO^{\bullet}$), an oxygen-centered radical
- peroxyl radical ($RO_2^{\bullet}$), an oxygen-centered radical

Hydrogen peroxide (H_2O_2), a nonradical because it has no unpaired electrons in its orbital, is an example of a reactive oxygen species that, like hypochlorous acid (HOCl) and singlet oxygen ($^1O_2$), is scavenged by vitamin C. Two reactive nitrogen species, peroxynitrite radicals and nitric oxide radicals, also may be reduced by vitamin C.

Once formed, free radicals and reactive species attack cellular nucleic acids in DNA, polyunsaturated fatty acids in phospholipids, and amino acids in proteins. Ascorbic acid has been shown to interact with these radicals in the aqueous phase before they initiate damage, especially to cell lipids. Furthermore, ascorbic acid appears to be superior to other water-soluble antioxidants. The ability of plasma antioxidants to protect lipids against peroxidation has been shown to be: vitamin C = thiols > bilirubin > uric acid > vitamin E [1]. When vitamin C reacts with $^{\bullet}OH$, $O_2^{\bullet}$, or H_2O_2, the radicals or reactive oxygen species are converted to water, while vitamin C is oxidized. The role of vitamin C and other antioxidants as a defense against oxidative damage to cells is discussed in the Perspective at the end of Chapter 10.

As an antioxidant, vitamin C provides electrons/hydrogens and becomes oxidized in the process. Regenerating ascorbic acid or ascorbate anion from the ascorbyl radical is crucial. To accomplish this regeneration, two ascorbyl radicals may react to form ascorbic acid and dehydroascorbic acid; this is especially likely in situations with high levels of oxidant stress. Alternately, reductases, found in most tissues, can reduce the ascorbyl radical and dehydroascorbic acid to ascorbic acid. Niacin and thiols such as dihydrolipoic acid, glutathione, and thioredoxin also assist in vitamin C regeneration. Reactions involved in the regeneration of vitamin C are shown in the Perspective for Chapter 10.

Pro-Oxidant Activity

Paradoxically, vitamin C also may act as a pro-oxidant. Vitamin C can reduce transition metals—for example, cupric ions (Cu^{2+}) to cuprous (Cu^{1+}) and ferric ions (Fe^{3+}) to ferrous (Fe^{2+})—while itself becoming oxidized, as shown here:

$$\text{Ascorbate anion } (AH^-) + Fe^{3+} \text{ or } Cu^{2+} \longrightarrow$$
$$\text{Ascorbyl radical } (A^{\bullet}) + Fe^{2+} \text{ or } Cu^{1+}$$

The products—Fe^{2+} and Cu^{1+}—generated from these reactions can cause cell damage by generating reactive oxygen species and free radicals. Examples of some of these reactions include:

$$Fe^{2+} \text{ or } Cu^{1+} + H_2O_2 \longrightarrow Fe^{3+} \text{ or } Cu^{2+} + OH_2 + {}^{\bullet}OH$$
$$Fe^{2+} \text{ or } Cu^{1+} + O_2 \longrightarrow Fe^{3+} \text{ or } Cu^{2+} + O_2^{\bullet}$$

It is important to note that vitamin C reacts with *free* ferric or cupric ions. Yet, in the body, iron and copper are both *bound* to various proteins (i.e., not free) to minimize the likelihood of such interactions. In addition, although vitamin C appears to act as a pro-oxidant to promote lipid and cellular damage, such activity has been shown only *in vitro* and at high (nonphysiological) concentrations [2,3].

Other Functions

Many other diverse biochemical functions for vitamin C have been proposed. Possible functions for vitamin C include roles in collagen gene expression; synthesis of bone matrix, proteoglycans, fibronectin, and elastin; regulation of cellular nucleotide (cAMP and cGMP) concentrations; and immune function, including complement synthesis. Experimental evidence supporting these functions varies considerably, and the mechanism by which vitamin C may be involved is generally unclear. Much attention also has been directed toward vitamin C and its possible effects on diseases ranging from the common cold to cancer and heart disease, among others.

Colds Colds, affecting the average adult about two to six times each year, are caused most often by viruses including adenovirus, rhinovirus, coronavirus, and respiratory syncytial virus, among others. The ability of vitamin C to enhance immune system functions by promoting chemotaxis and proliferation of some immune cells like macrophages and lymphocytes, increasing the activity of natural killer cells, and destroying histamine (associated with some of a cold's symptoms) provides a theoretical basis for the use of vitamin C in the prevention and treatment of colds. Numerous studies, involving tens of thousands of individuals, have been conducted over the last several decades to examine the effectiveness of vitamin C in cold prevention and treatment. Unfortunately, ingestion of high doses (1–2 g per day) of vitamin C has not been shown to prevent the common cold or to reduce its symptoms. However, *regular* vitamin C use (up to 1 g per day) appears to modestly reduce the duration of symptoms by about 3% to 13% in adults [4,5].

Cancer Epidemiological studies provide evidence that increased intakes of fruits and vegetables are associated with a decreased risk of some cancers. The association between vitamin C intake (usually 80–200 mg) and a protective effect against cancer is generally stronger with cancers of the oral cavity, pharynx, esophagus, stomach, lung, breast, and colon. However, not all studies show protective effects, and clinical trials providing vitamin C to prevent or treat cancer overwhelmingly show no overall benefits. Future trials providing vitamin C intravenously in high doses are hoped to generate more positive findings [6].

Cardiovascular Disease Many (but not all) epidemiological and prospective studies report that increased fruit and vegetable intakes, vitamin C intake, and/or plasma vitamin C concentrations are associated with a decreased risk of heart disease. It is suspected that vitamin C's antioxidant abilities may inhibit low-density lipoprotein (LDL) oxidation, which in turn can diminish plaque formation associated with heart disease. Vitamin C also may be helpful because it decreases monocyte adhesion to endothelial cells lining blood vessels; adhesion represents one of the first steps in atherogenesis and is followed by monocyte migration into the arterial intima (the innermost layer of blood vessels), transformation into macrophages, and uptake of oxidized cholesterol in LDL. With continued accumulation of oxidized LDL, macrophages develop into foam cells, and over time fatty streaks develop. Vitamin C, alone and with vitamin E, is thought to help prevent heart disease by scavenging reactive species/free radicals before they reach and initiate oxidative damage to cells. The vitamins are also thought to reduce thrombotic potential and vascular reactivity. Vitamin C may also play beneficial roles in preventing heart disease by enhancing type IV collagen generation in endothelial cells, preventing endothelial cell apoptosis, enhancing endothelial cell function, and inhibiting smooth muscle cell proliferation. Yet, studies providing supplements of vitamin C and other antioxidants typically have not reported beneficial effects in the prevention of heart disease [7].

Eye Health It has been suggested that vitamin C is beneficial in diminishing the risks of age-related macular degeneration and cataracts, both major causes of blindness, especially in older people. The macula, found in the center of the retina, maintains central vision. Behind the retina is the choroid, which contains blood vessels. In age-related macular degeneration (dry form), cellular debris called drusen accumulates between the retina and the choroid, and in the wet (exudative) form of the condition, abnormal blood vessels grow under the macula. In both forms of age-related macular degeneration, there is a loss of vision in the center of the visual field because of damage to the retina. The condition makes reading and recognition of faces difficult, although peripheral vision remains relatively unaffected. Unfortunately, vitamin C taken alone or with other antioxidant nutrients does not appear to affect the development of age-related macular degeneration [8–10]; however, supplementation with vitamin C (500 mg), vitamin E (400 IU), beta-carotene (15 mg), zinc (80 mg),

and copper (2 mg) (as used in the Age-Related Eye Disease Study) may slow the progression of the condition, as suggested in one study [11].

A cataract affects the lens of the eye, causing it to become cloudy. The lens (which functions to focus light onto the retina and adjust eye focus) is made up of over a million lens fiber cells. These cells have a high protein content (especially the protein α-crystallin) and, unlike other tissues, the proteins in the lens do not turn over. α-crystallin functions to maintain optical clarity by removing damaged proteins from the lens. However, with age, the activity and concentration of α-crystallin diminish. This change results in the accumulation and aggregation of abnormal proteins in the lens. In addition, with aging, the concentrations of antioxidants diminish and lead to oxidative damage in the eye including lipid peroxidation and protein cross-linking. The damaged proteins aggregate and precipitate, causing the lens to become cloudy and causing vision to become impaired. Because oxygen and oxyradicals are thought to contribute to the development of cataracts, and because vitamin C functions as an antioxidant, it is logical that vitamin C may help in the prevention of cataracts. Studies, however, have examined primarily multivitamin (not just vitamin C) supplementation and risk of cataracts, and while some of these studies, especially those providing long-term supplementation, have suggested benefits, others have not [10,12–20].

Interactions with Other Nutrients

One of vitamin C's most notable interactions is with the mineral iron in the gastrointestinal tract. Vitamin C enhances the absorption of nonheme iron either by reducing iron to a ferrous (Fe^{2+}) state from a ferric (Fe^{3+}) state or by forming a soluble complex with the reduced iron in the alkaline pH of the small intestine. Vitamin C's benefits are thought to be maximized at about 75 mg. It is commonly suggested that individuals, especially if iron deficient, consume vitamin C–rich foods such as orange juice when ingesting nonheme iron-rich foods to promote the iron's absorption.

Metabolism and Excretion

As vitamin C intakes increase, plasma vitamin C concentrations increase but reach an upper limit as renal handling of the vitamin shifts from active saturable reabsorption by SVCT1 carriers in the renal tubules to a renal threshold in which the maximum reabsorption of the vitamin is achieved. The renal reabsorption threshold occurs at a plasma vitamin C concentration of about 1.3 to 1.8 mg/dL. At vitamin C intakes of about 500 mg, all vitamin C is usually excreted [21].

Vitamin C may be excreted intact or may be oxidized to dehydroascorbic acid. Oxidation occurs primarily in the liver but also to some extent in the kidneys. Oxidation of dehydroascorbic acid begins with hydrolysis (opening) of the ring structure to yield 2,3-diketogulonic acid, which possesses no vitamin C activity and can be excreted in the urine or further hydrolyzed (Figure 9.6). When further hydrolyzed, diketogulonic acid is cleaved by separate pathways either into a variety of five-carbon sugars (xylose, xylonate, and lyxonate) or into the four-carbon sugar threonic acid and oxalic acid. Oxalic acid is excreted in the urine, and its urinary concentration does not appear to vary with vitamin C intakes up to about 200 mg [22]. The four- and five-carbon sugars can be converted into cellular compounds or be oxidized and excreted as CO_2 and water. Other urinary vitamin C metabolites include 2-O-methyl ascorbate, ascorbate 2-sulfate, and 2-ketoascorbitol.

Recommended Dietary Allowance

Current requirements for adult men and women for vitamin C intake, based on nearly maximizing tissue concentrations and minimizing urinary excretion of the vitamin, are 75 mg and 60 mg, respectively [23]. Vitamin C's Recommended Dietary Allowance (RDA) for adult men and women is 90 mg and 75 mg, respectively [23]. During pregnancy and lactation, recommendations for vitamin C increase to 100 mg and 120 mg, respectively [23]. Further, because smoking accelerates the depletion of the body's ascorbic acid pool, it is recommended that smokers consume an added 35 mg of vitamin C daily [23].

Deficiency: Scurvy

Inadequate intakes of vitamin C result in the deficiency condition **scurvy**. Scurvy is typically manifested when the total body vitamin C pool falls below about 300 mg and plasma vitamin C concentrations drop to < 0.2 mg/dL [3,24]. This situation may develop in as little as 1 month with vitamin C intakes less than 10 mg daily. Scurvy is characterized by a multitude of signs and symptoms. Initial symptoms include fatigue and malaise that may be associated with impaired carnitine synthesis. The impaired hydroxyproline and hydroxylysine synthesis leads to problems with formation of collagen's triple helix structure and thus diminished vascular wall strength and other defects in body structures rich in collagen. Some of the more notable signs and symptoms are enlarged, hyperkeratotic hair follicles, especially on the arms, legs, and buttocks; "corkscrew"-shaping of hair; small, red skin discolorations caused by ruptured small blood vessels (called **petechiae**) along with easy bruising (characterized by ecchymoses—purple discolorations of the skin due to ruptured blood vessels—and purpurae—dark red to purple spots on the skin due to hemorrhage); impaired wound and fracture healing; and joint pain (arthralgia). Oral changes include swollen, bleeding, necrotic gums; sublingual hemorrhages; and loose and decaying teeth. Scurvy is fatal if untreated. The four Hs—*hemorrhagic* signs, *hyperkeratosis* of hair follicles, *hypochondriasis* (psychological manifestation), and *hematologic* abnormalities (associated with impaired collagen synthesis and iron absorption)—are often used as a mnemonic device for remembering scurvy signs.

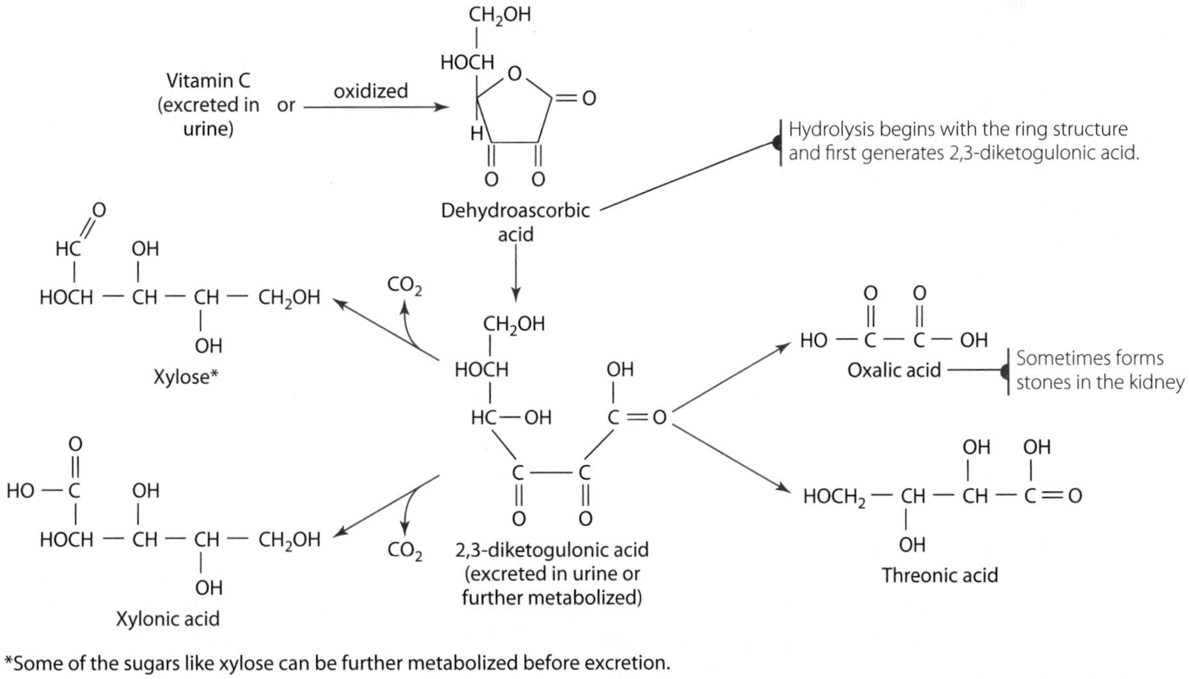

Figure 9.6 Vitamin C and the formation of its metabolites excreted in the urine.

Scurvy is usually treated with vitamin C doses of about 100 to 300 mg daily until symptoms are gone, which usually takes about 3 months.

Although scurvy is rare in the United States, low vitamin C status has been observed in the elderly, especially if institutionalized, and among smokers. People who have poor diets, especially if coupled with alcoholism or drug abuse, are likely to be deficient. People with malabsorption disorders may exhibit diminished intestinal absorption of the vitamin, and those with conditions such as diabetes mellitus and some cancers are at risk due to increased vitamin C turnover.

Toxicity

Daily intakes of up to 2 g of vitamin C are routinely consumed without adverse effects [2,25]. Because vitamin C absorption is saturable and dose dependent, more vitamin C is absorbed, and thus toxicity is theoretically more likely, if several large (1 g) doses of the vitamin are ingested throughout the day than if the same amount is ingested as one single dose. The most common side effect from the ingestion of large amounts (2 g) of the vitamin is gastrointestinal problems characterized by abdominal pain and osmotic diarrhea. The osmotic diarrhea occurs when the unabsorbed vitamin C in the intestinal tract is metabolized by bacteria within the colon. Based on this side effect, a Tolerable Upper Intake Level of 2 g of vitamin C has been recommended [22].

Two other side effects reported from the use of large amounts of vitamin C are thought to affect (if at all) only selected populations. These side effects include increased risk of kidney stones (nephrolithiasis) for those with renal disease and iron toxicity for those with disorders of iron metabolism. The idea that high intakes increase risk of kidney stones, either oxalic acid or uric acid in content, is based upon vitamin C's metabolism, which generates oxalic acid, a common constituent of kidney stones. However, although doses of up to 10 g of vitamin C have been shown to increase oxalate excretion, the amount of oxalate excreted (generally < 50 mg) typically remains within a normal, safe range [25]. Nevertheless, some suggest that people predisposed to calcium oxalate kidney stones avoid high doses ($\geq$500 mg) of vitamin C [25]. Furthermore, because of interactions in the kidney between vitamin C and uric acid, which also is a constituent of kidney stones, it is also advised that people with uric acid kidney stones avoid ingesting large doses of the vitamin. Specifically, vitamin C competitively inhibits the renal reabsorption of uric acid, thereby increasing uric acid excretion and acidifying the urine to promote precipitation of uric acid crystals and uric acid kidney stones. The actual clinical importance of uricosuria (high levels of uric acid in the urine) with regard to stone formation, however, is unknown [25].

In addition to increasing the probability of kidney stones, chronic high doses of vitamin C are also purported to be unsafe for people with disorders involving iron metabolism, including people with **hemochromatosis, thalassemia,** and **sideroblastic anemia** [25]. However, others contend that pro-oxidant effects of vitamin C on mobilization of iron stores do not occur *in vivo* [26].

The issue of systemic conditioning to high intakes of vitamin C is currently deemed doubtful. Although scurvylike symptoms were reported in a few people on abrupt withdrawal of large intakes of vitamin C, the reports are anecdotal. Further substantiation of conditioned (also called rebound) scurvy is needed before recommendations can be made [26].

Excessive vitamin C excretion can interfere with some clinical laboratory tests. Vitamin C in the urine, for example, may act as a reductive agent and thus interfere with diagnostic tests using redox chemistry such as those used to test for glucose in the urine (for diabetes testing) or for blood in the feces (for gastrointestinal tract bleeding testing).

Assessment of Nutriture

Plasma vitamin C concentrations respond to changes in dietary vitamin C intakes and thus are used to assess recent vitamin C intake; however, white blood cell (leukocyte) content of the vitamin better reflects body stores. Plasma concentrations of vitamin C below 0.2 mg/dL are considered to be deficient. Concentrations associated with tissue saturation are about 1.0 mg/dL, and those typically found with recommended intakes range from about 0.6 to 0.8 mg/dL [22]. Leukocyte vitamin C concentrations of 10 μg/10^8 or less are considered deficient [22,23].

References Cited for Vitamin C

1. Stadtman E. Ascorbic acid and oxidative inactivation of proteins. Am J Clin Nutr. 1991; 54:S1125–28.
2. Padayatty S, Sun H, Wang Y, et al. Vitamin C pharmacokinetics: implications for oral and intravenous use. Ann Intern Med. 2004; 140:533–37.
3. Levine M, Wang Y, Padayatty S, Morrow J. A new recommended dietary allowance of vitamin C for healthy young women. Proc Natl Acad Sci. 2001; 98:9842–46.
4. Douglas RM, Hemila H, D'Souza R, et al. Vitamin C for preventing and treating the common cold. Cochrane Database Systematic Reviews. 2004;(4), CD000980.
5. Hemila H, Chalker E, Douglas B. Vitamin C for preventing and treating the common cold. Cochrane Database of Systematic Reviews. 2007;(3), CD000980.
6. Levine M, Espey MG, Chen Q. Losing and finding a way at C: new promise for pharmacologic ascorbate in cancer treatment. Free Radic Biol Med. 2009; 47:27–29.
7. Farbstein D, Kozak-Blickstein A, Levy AP. Antioxidant vitamins and their use in preventing cardiovascular disease. Molecules. 2010; 5:8098–8110.
8. Fletcher AE, Bentham GC, Agnew M, et al. Sunlight exposure, antioxidants and age-related macular degeneration. Arch Ophthalmol. 2008; 126:1396–1403.

9. Chong E, Wong TY, Kreis AJ, et al. Dietary antioxidants and primary prevention of age related macular degeneration: systematic review and meta-analysis. BMJ. 2007; 335:755–62.

10. Chiu C, Taylor A. Nutritional antioxidants and age-related cataract and maculopathy. Exp Eye Res. 2007; 84:229–45.

11. Age-related Eye Disease Study Research Group. A randomized placebo-controlled clinical trial of high dose supplementation with vitamins C and E, β carotene, and zinc for age-related macular degeneration and vision loss. Arch Ophthalmol. 2001; 119:1417–36.

12. Jacques PF, Taylor A, Moeller S, et al. Long-term nutrient intake and 5-year change in nuclear lens opacities. Arch Ophthalmol. 2005; 123:517–26.

13. Mares-Perlman JA, Lyle BJ, Klein R, et al. Vitamin supplement use and incident cataracts in a population-based study. Arch Ophthal. 2000; 118:1556–63.

14. Tan AG, Mitchell P, Flood VM, et al. Antioxidant nutrient intake and the long-term incidence of age-related cataract: the Blue Mountains Eye Study. Am J Clin Nutr. 2008; 87:1899–1905.

15. Chylack LT, Brown NP, Bron A, et al. The Roche European American Cataract Trial (REACT): a randomized clinical trial to investigate the efficacy of an oral antioxidant micronutrient mixture to slow progression of age-related cataract. Ophthalmic Epid. 2002; 9:49–80.

16. Christen WG, Glynn RJ, Sesso HD, et al. Age-related cataract in a randomized trial of vitamins E and C in men. Arch Ophthalmol. 2010; 128:1397–1405.

17. Gritz DC, Srinivasan M, Smith SD, et al. The antioxidants in prevention of cataracts study: effects of antioxidant supplements on cataract progression in South India. Br J Ophthalmol. 2006; 90:847–51.

18. Ferrigno L, Aldigeri R, Rosmini F, et al. Associations between plasma levels of vitamins and cataract in the Italian-American clinical trial of nutritional supplements and age-related cataract (CTNS): CTNS report #2. Ophthalmic Epid. 2005; 12:71–80.

19. Agte V, Tarwadi K. The importance of nutrition in the prevention of ocular disease with special reference to cataract. Ophthalmic Res. 2010; 44:166–72.

20. Fernandez MM, Afshari NA. Nutrition and the prevention of cataracts. Curr Opin Ophthal. 2008; 19:66–70.

21. Padayatty S, Katz A, Wang Y, et al. Vitamin C as an antioxidant: evaluation of its role in disease prevention. J Am Coll Nutr. 2003; 22:18–35.

22. Levine M, Cantilena-Conry C, Wang Y, et al. Vitamin C pharmacokinetics in healthy volunteers: evidence for a recommended requirement. Proc Natl Acad Sci. 1996; 93:3704–09.

23. Food and Nutrition Board. Dietary Reference Intakes for Vitamin C, Vitamin E, Selenium, and Carotenoids. Washington, DC: National Academy Press. 2000 pp. 95–185.

24. Jacob RA, Sotoudeh G. Vitamin C function and status in chronic disease. Nutr Clin Care. 2002; 5:66–74.

25. Massey LK, Liebman M, Kynast-Gales SA. Ascorbate increases human oxaluria and kidney stone risk. J Nutr. 2005; 135:1673–77.

26. Hathcock J. Vitamins and minerals: efficacy and safety. Am J Clin Nutr. 1997; 66:427–37.

Suggested Reading

Baron JH. Sailors' scurvy before and after James Lind: a reassessment. Nutr Rev. 2009; 67:315–32.

De Luca LM, Norum KR. Scurvy and cloudberries: a chapter in the history of nutritional sciences. J Nutr. 2011; 141:2101–05.

THIAMIN (VITAMIN B₁)

The need for thiamin was first recognized in the late 1800s by a Dutchman, C. Eijkman, when it was discovered that fowl fed a diet of cooked, polished rice (devoid of the outer germ and bran layers and containing primarily the endosperm) developed neurologic problems (now

called beriberi). The substance initially called thiamine that corrected the problems was later isolated from rice bran in 1912 by Casmir Funk. The vitamin's structure (discovered by R. Williams from the United States) was not determined until about the mid 1930s. Figure 9.7 shows the structure of thiamin (vitamin B₁), which consists of a pyrimidine ring and a thiazole moiety (meaning one of two parts) linked by a methylene (CH_2) bridge. The thiazole moiety contains a sulfur atom.

Sources

Thiamin is widely distributed in foods. Meats (especially pork) are rich in this vitamin. Pork loin, for example, provides about 0.65 mg of thiamin/3-oz serving; beef and beef liver contain about 0.07 mg and 0.26 mg of thiamin/3-oz serving, respectively. Salmon contains about 0.23 mg/3 oz. Legumes and grain products (whole, fortified, or enriched), cereals, and breads are also good sources of thiamin. Black beans provide 0.4 mg of thiamin/cup, whole-grain wheat bread (1 slice) provides 0.08 mg of thiamin, enriched white bread about 0.11 mg of thiamin/slice, and enriched spaghetti has 0.29 mg/cup. Bran cereal with raisins and Cheerios® (1 cup) both provide 25% of the Daily Value (1.5 mg), or about 0.38 mg of thiamin. Other good sources of the vitamin include yeast, wheat germ, and soy milk. Most thiamin in the American diet comes from products that have been enriched; such products also contribute to the riboflavin, niacin, and iron contents of the diet. In supplements, thiamin is found mainly as thiamin hydrochloride or thiamin mononitrate salt.

Thiamin is destroyed (primarily at the methylene bridge) in an alkaline environment (pH of 8 or above) and by heat. Thus, cooking thiamin-rich foods in water will promote loss of the vitamin.

Digestion, Absorption, Transport, and Storage

Thiamin exists in a free (nonphosphorylated) form in plant foods. However, in animal products, 95% of thiamin occurs in a phosphorylated form, primarily thiamin diphosphate (TDP), also called thiamin pyrophosphate (TPP),

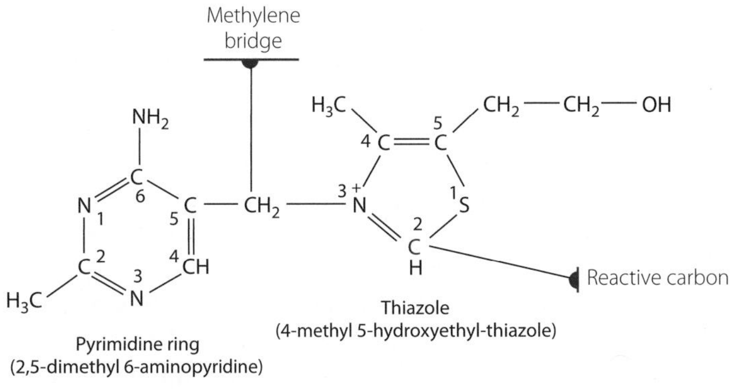

Figure 9.7 Structure of thiamin.

with lesser amounts (5%) as thiamin monophosphate (TMP) and thiamin triphosphate (TTP). Digestion of these phosphorylated forms must occur for thiamin to be absorbed. Intestinal phosphatases are responsible for this digestion, specifically hydrolyzing the phosphates from the thiamin di-, mono- and triphosphates prior to absorption. Thus it is free thiamin that is absorbed into the intestinal cells.

Absorption of thiamin from foods is thought to be high. Occasionally, however, antithiamin factors may be present in the diet. For example, thiaminases found in raw fish catalyze the cleavage of thiamin, destroying the vitamin. These thiaminases are thermolabile, so cooking fish renders the enzymes inactive. Other antithiamin factors include polyhydroxyphenols such as tannic, chlorogenic, and caffeic acids. Polyhydroxyphenols, which are thermostable, are found in coffee, tea, betel nuts, and certain fruits and vegetables such as blueberries, black currants, Brussels sprouts, and red cabbage. These polyhydroxyphenols inactivate thiamin by an oxyreductive process that destroys the thiazole ring; the destructive process can be facilitated by the presence of divalent minerals such as calcium and magnesium. Thiamin destruction may be prevented, however, by the presence of reducing compounds such as vitamin C and citric acid.

Absorption of thiamin occurs primarily in the jejunum and ileum, with lesser amounts absorbed in the duodenum. Absorption of thiamin is both active and passive, depending upon the amount of the vitamin presented in the intestine. With high thiamin intakes (2.5 mg or more), absorption is predominantly by passive diffusion. At physiological concentrations, thiamin absorption is mediated by two thiamin transporters, ThTr1 and ThTr2, which have been identified in a variety of tissues including the intestine and kidneys, and are thought to exchange thiamin for H$^+$ ions as part of an antiport carrier system [1–3]. Active, sodium-dependent, and sodium-independent carrier-mediated thiamin transport also have been suggested [4,5]; however, defects in the gene SLC19A2, which codes for ThTr1, have been shown to cause thiamin deficiency [2] and thus suggest ThT1 is largely responsible for intestinal thiamin absorption.

While it is free thiamin that is absorbed, thiamin may be phosphorylated within the intestinal cell. Thiamin enters the blood from the enterocytes via transport across the basolateral membrane by ThTr1. Alcohol inhibits the intestinal expression of ThT1 and ThT2, and thus thiamin absorption.

Thiamin is typically found in the plasma in its free (unphosphorylated) form, bound to albumin, or as TMP; it is only free thiamin or TMP that is thought to be able to cross cell membranes to enter cells. About 90% of the thiamin in the blood is present within the blood cells as TDP (formed within the cell), with smaller amounts of free thiamin and TMP. Transport of vitamin into the red blood cells is thought to occur by facilitated diffusion, whereas transport into other tissues requires energy.

The human body contains approximately 30 mg of thiamin, with relatively high but still small concentrations found (stored) in the liver, skeletal muscles, heart, kidneys, and brain. In fact, skeletal muscles are thought to contain about half of the body's thiamin. Thiamin's half-life is estimated at about 10 to 20 days.

Following absorption, most free thiamin is taken up by the liver and phosphorylated to its TDP coenzyme form; this reaction requires energy and is catalyzed by thiamin pyrophosphokinase, an enzyme found in most body tissues. About 80% of the total thiamin in the body exists as TDP.

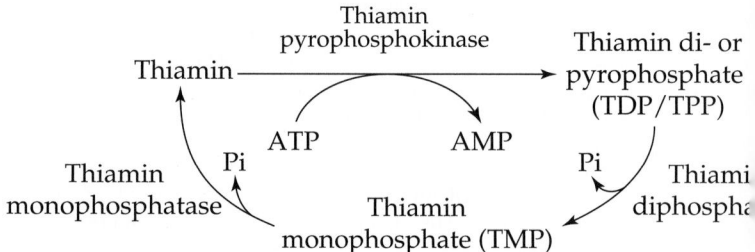

About 10% of thiamin is found in the body tissues as TTP. TTP is synthesized by action of a TDP-ATP phosphoryl transferase that phosphorylates TDP.

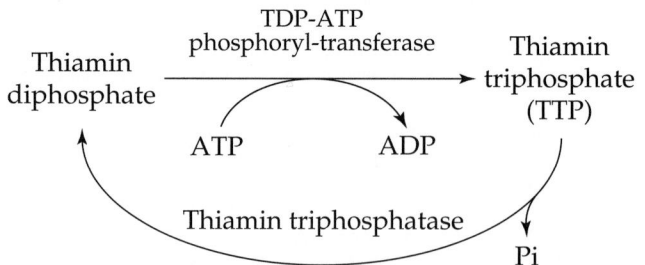

TTP, as well as TDP and TMP, are found in small amounts in muscle and organs, including the brain, heart, liver, and kidneys. Hydrolysis or dephosphorylation of thiamin's phosphorylated forms also occurs in tissues throughout the body. The terminal phosphate on the TTP is hydrolyzed by thiamin triphosphatase to yield TDP, and TDP can be converted to TMP by thiamin diphosphatase, which cleaves the terminal phosphate on TDP. TMP can be then converted to free thiamin by thiamin monophosphatase.

Functions and Mechanisms of Action

Thiamin plays essential coenzyme and noncoenzyme roles in the body, including these:

- energy transformation (a coenzyme role)
- synthesis of pentoses and nicotinamide adenine dinucleotide phosphate (NADPH; also a coenzyme role)
- membrane and nerve conduction (in a noncoenzyme capacity)

Each of these three roles is discussed in this section.

Coenzyme Roles

As TDP, thiamin functions in energy transformation as a coenzyme of the pyruvate dehydrogenase complex, the α-ketoglutarate dehydrogenase complex, and the branched-chain α-keto acid dehydrogenase complex. In addition, TDP serves as a coenzyme for transketolase needed for the synthesis of NADPH and pentoses. The reactions are shown as an overview in Figure 9.8 and discussed in detail in the next section.

Energy Transformation Thiamin as TDP functions as a coenzyme necessary for the oxidative decarboxylation of pyruvate, α-ketoglutarate, and the three branched-chain amino acids isoleucine, leucine, and valine. These reactions are instrumental in generating energy (ATP). Inhibition of the reactions, especially for pyruvate and α-ketoglutarate, prevents synthesis of ATP and of the acetyl-CoA needed for the synthesis of fatty acids, cholesterol, and other important compounds. Inhibition also results in the accumulation of pyruvate, lactate, and α-ketoglutarate.

The steps that occur in the oxidative decarboxylation of pyruvate to form acetyl-CoA, shown in Figure 9.9, require a multienzyme complex known as the pyruvate

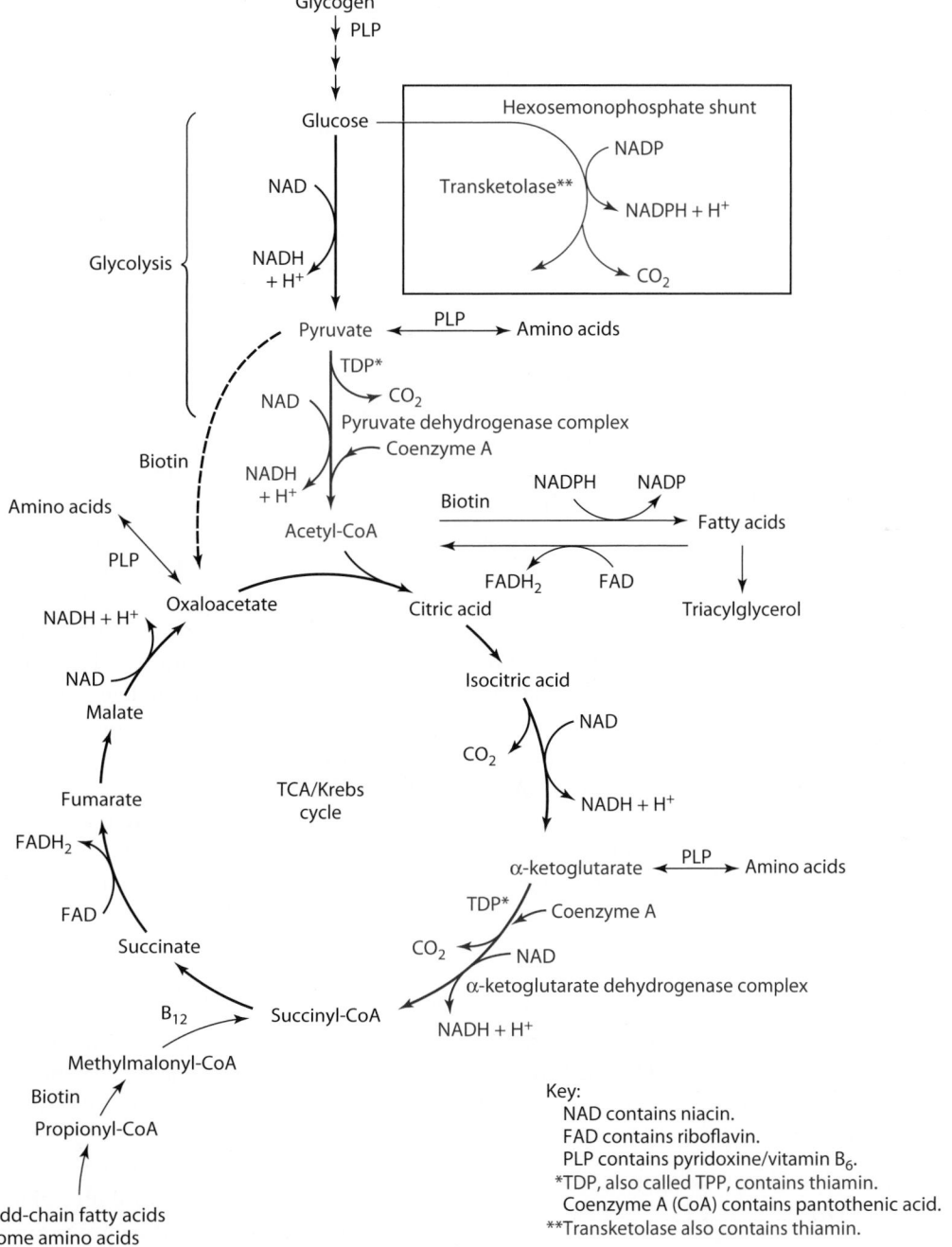

Figure 9.8 Various vitamin cofactors and their action sites in energy metabolism. The role of thiamin as TDP is shown by an asterisk.

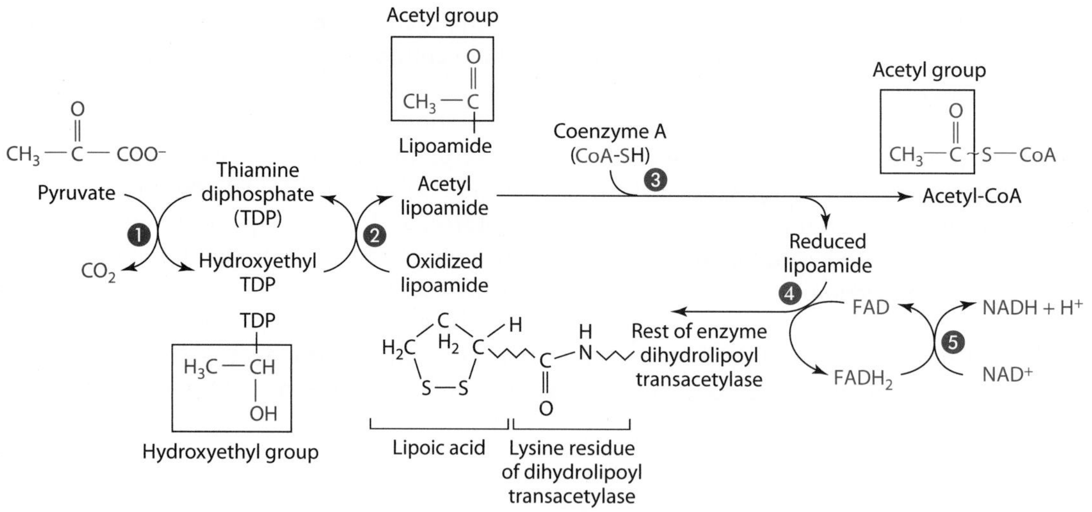

1 CO_2 is removed from pyruvate and the rest of the compound (hydroxyethyl) attaches to TDP to form hydroxyethyl TDP.

2 The hydroxyethyl group is transferred to oxidized lipoamide, which consists of lipoic acid attached by an amide link (CO-NH) to a lysine residue of the enzyme dihydrolipoyl transacetylase. With the transfer of the hydroxyethyl group acetyl lipoamide is generated.

3 Acetyl lipoamide reacts with coenzyme A (CoA-SH) to form acetyl-CoA and reduced lipoamide.

4 Reduced lipoamide is oxidized by the flavo (FAD)-dependent enzyme dihydrolipoyl dehydrogenase.

5 The reduced flavo ($FADH_2$) protein is oxidized by NAD^+, which then transfers reducing equivalents to the respiratory chain.

Figure 9.9 The oxidative decarboxylation of pyruvate by the pyruvate dehydrogenase complex.

dehydrogenase complex, which is bound to the mitochondrial membrane. Three enzymes make up this complex: a TDP-dependent pyruvate dehydrogenase; a lipoic acid–dependent dihydrolipoyl transacetylase; and an FAD-dependent dihydrolipoyl dehydrogenase. The roles of four vitamins—thiamin (TDP), riboflavin (FAD), niacin (NAD^+), and pantothenic acid (CoA-SH)—in this process are described briefly and shown in Figures 9.9 and 9.10. ATP and Mg^{2+} also are required.

In the first reaction (Figure 9.10), the carbon 2 atom between the nitrogen and sulfur atoms in the thiazole ring of TDP ionizes to form a carbanion, which then combines with the 2-carbonyl group of pyruvate, α-ketoglutarate, and other α-keto acids, forming a covalent bond. After forming the adduct (attachment) between pyruvate and TDP, pyruvate dehydrogenase (the first enzyme of the complex) catalyzes the removal of pyruvate's COO group to form hydroxyethyl-TDP (Figure 9.9). The hydroxyethyl group is then transferred to oxidized lipoamide (which is bound to the second enzyme, dihydrolipoyl transacetylase), forming acetyl lipoamide. The acetyl lipoamide then reacts with coenzyme A to form acetyl-CoA and reduced lipoamide. Lipoamide is oxidized by the third enzyme, dihydrolipoyl dehydrogenase, which requires FAD. NAD^+ oxidizes $FADH_2$. Thus, the overall reaction is:

$$\text{Pyruvate} + NAD^+ + \text{CoA} \longrightarrow \text{Acetyl-CoA} +$$
$$\text{NADH} + H^+ + CO_2$$

The decarboxylation of α-ketoglutarate by the α-ketoglutarate dehydrogenase complex and the decarboxylation of the branched-chain keto acids by the branched-chain α-ketoacid dehydrogenase complex are similar to that of pyruvate. The α-ketoglutarate dehydrogenase complex decarboxylates α-ketoglutarate and forms succinyl-CoA. Decarboxylation of the branched-chain α-keto acids, which arise from the transamination of valine, isoleucine, and leucine, is an oxidative process that also requires thiamin as TDP (see Figure 6.36). Failure to oxidize the α-keto acids of leucine, isoleucine, and valine causes both the branched-chain amino acids and their α-keto acids to accumulate in blood and other body fluids. Such changes are characteristic of maple syrup urine disease (MSUD), an inborn error of metabolism that results from insufficient branched-chain α-keto acid dehydrogenase enzyme complex activity. People with MSUD must limit their consumption of protein-containing foods to curtail intakes of leucine, isoleucine, and valine. Medical foods devoid of these three amino acids provide most nutrients for those with MSUD.

Synthesis of Pentoses and NADPH Thiamin as TDP also functions as a loosely bound prosthetic group of transketolase, a key cytosolic enzyme in the pentose phosphate pathway (hexose monophosphate shunt). This is the pathway in which sugars of varying chain lengths are interconverted (Figure 3.30). It is found in several tissues but is especially active in the liver. The pentose phosphate pathway is essential for the generation of pentoses for nucleic acid synthesis and of NADPH, which is needed, for example, for fatty acid synthesis. TDP forms a carbanion that transfers

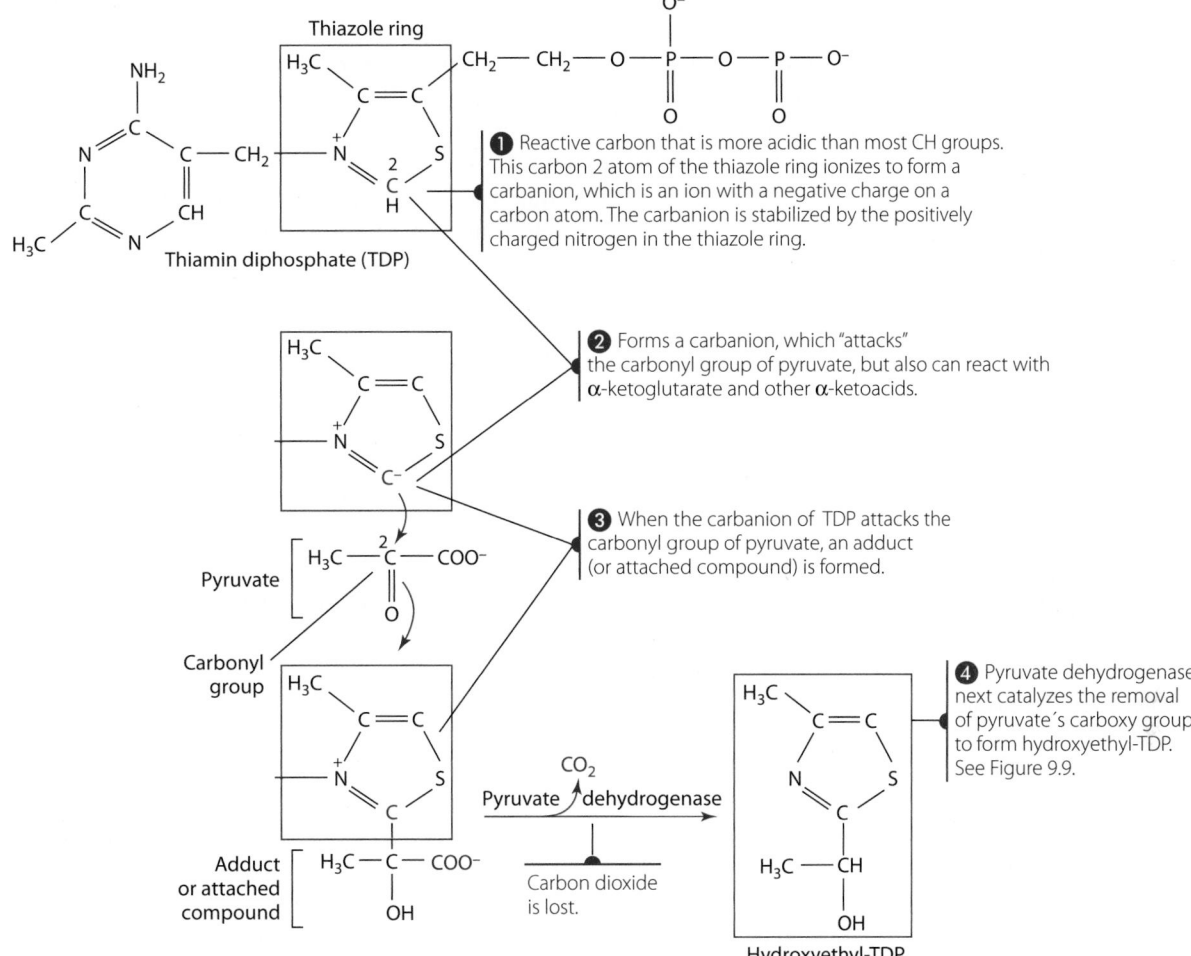

Figure 9.10 The first steps in the decarboxylation of pyruvate by thiamin diphosphate.

an activated aldehyde from a donor ketose substrate to an acceptor—in this case, xylulose. Transketolase hydrolyzes the carbon-to-carbon bond in xylose-5-P, sedoheptulose-7-P, and fructose-6-P (i.e., ketoses) and transfers the two-carbon fragment (carbons 1 and 2 of the ketoses) to an aldose receptor. The transketolase-catalyzed reactions are Mg^{2+} dependent and can be written as follows:

Transketolase

xylulose 5-P + ribose 5-P ⟷ Sedoheptulose 7-P + glyceraldehyde 3-P

Transketolase

xylulose 5-P + erythrose 4-P ⟷ Glyceraldehyde 3-P + fructose 6-P

Noncoenzyme Roles: Membrane and Nerve Conduction

In addition to its coenzyme roles, thiamin, likely as TTP, is involved in nervous system function. The vitamin is released in response to nervous system stimulation, and changes in electrical activity occur with the use of thiamin antagonists. In nerve membranes, thiamin is thought to activate chloride transport. Thiamin, as TTP, also may be involved in nerve impulse transmission by regulating sodium channels and in phosphorylation of proteins.

Metabolism and Excretion

Thiamin, TMP, and TDP in excess of tissue needs and storage capacity may be excreted intact, or catabolized prior to urinary excretion. Degradation of thiamin begins with cleavage of the vitamin into its pyrimidine and thiazole moieties. The two rings are then further catabolized, generating 20 or more metabolites including, for example, 4-methyl thiazole 5-acetic acid and 2-methyl 4-amino 5-pyrimidine carboxylic acid.

Recommended Dietary Allowance

Recommendations for thiamin intake are based upon the results of numerous metabolic studies examining urinary excretion, changes in erythrocyte transketolase activity, and thiamin intake data. The Recommended Dietary Allowance (RDA) for thiamin for adult men is 1.2 mg/day and for adult women is 1.1 mg/day; the requirements for men and women are 1.0 mg/day and 0.9 mg/day, respectively

[6]. Differences in thiamin needs between men and women are based upon differences in body size and energy needs. Thiamin recommendations with pregnancy and lactation increase to 1.4 mg/day and 1.5 mg/day, respectively [6]. The inside front cover of the book provides additional RDAs for thiamin for other age groups.

Deficiency: Beriberi

Despite the known functional roles of thiamin at the cellular level, it has as yet been impossible to explain all the pathophysiological manifestations that are associated with the thiamin deficiency **beriberi** (*beri* means "weakness"), of which there are three types. Dry beriberi, found predominantly in adults, results from a chronic low thiamin intake, especially if coupled with a high carbohydrate intake. Dry beriberi is characterized by muscle weakness and wasting, especially in the lower extremities, and peripheral neuropathy. The neuropathy consists of symmetrical sensory and motor nerve conduction problems mostly affecting the distal parts of the limbs (i.e., the ankles, feet, wrists, and hands). A symmetrical foot drop may be present and is usually associated with tenderness of the calf muscles. Wet beriberi, a second type of thiamin deficiency, results in more extensive cardiovascular system involvement than dry beriberi; cardiomegaly (enlarged heart), rapid heart beat (tachycardia), right-side heart failure with respiratory involvement, and peripheral edema are common symptoms. The third type, acute beriberi, occurs mostly in infants. Acute beriberi is associated with anorexia, vomiting, lactic acidosis (the lack of thiamin, which is needed to convert pyruvate to acetyl-CoA, causes pyruvate to be converted to lactic acid; the lactic acid then accumulates, causing acidosis), altered heart rate, and cardiomegaly. Use of parenteral nutrition devoid of thiamin or containing excessive amounts of glucose can cause acute thiamin deficiency within a few weeks.

In the United States and other developed countries, thiamin deficiency is often associated with alcoholism. People with alcohol dependency are particularly prone to thiamin deficiency because of decreased food consumption (and thus thiamin intake), increased requirements for the vitamin because of liver damage (decreased liver function impairs TDP formation and, consequently, vitamin use), and decreased thiamin absorption. The thiamin deficiency often seen in those with alcoholism may be associated with a neurologic disorder called Wernicke's encephalopathy [7]. Symptoms of Wernicke's encephalopathy include **ophthalmoplegia** (paralysis of the ocular muscles), **nystagmus** (constant, involuntary eyeball movement), **ataxia** (impaired muscle coordination), loss of recent memory, and confusion. Without treatment, brain damage (referred to as Wernicke-Korsakoff syndrome) may result. Administration of thiamin intravenously or intramuscularly (100–500 mg over 30 minutes for 3 days) is important in treatment for those with Wernicke's encephalopathy, as it allows plasma thiamin concentrations to reach sufficient levels for transport across the blood-brain barrier [8,9].

Thiamin deficiency also is fairly prevalent in people with congestive heart failure; the higher prevalence is thought to be attributable to low thiamin intakes and increased urinary thiamin losses secondary to diuretic use. Treatment consists of therapeutic oral (~100 mg or more) or intravenous (~50 mg or more) doses of thiamin.

Other populations, including the elderly, are also at risk for thiamin deficiency. People with diseases that impair the vitamin's absorption (i.e., some gastrointestinal tract cancers, liver disease, inflammatory bowel diseases) and those with increased needs such as individuals with some cancers are also at greater risk of developing deficiency. Treatment of thiamin deficiency usually requires 15 to 250 mg of thiamin given intramuscularly or intravenously, or therapeutic oral thiamin hydrochloride in doses of 5 to 30 mg daily for one month or longer depending on the severity of the deficiency.

Toxicity

No Tolerable Upper Intake Level has been established for thiamin, and no side effects have been reported from oral intakes of 500 mg daily. Such pharmacological levels of thiamin are used in treating some inborn errors of metabolism such as MSUD. Other metabolic diseases that may respond to large doses of the vitamin are thiamin-responsive megaloblastic anemia and thiamin-responsive lactic acidosis. Although the role of thiamin in correcting anemia is not clear, in lactic acidosis large doses of thiamin increase hepatic pyruvate dehydrogenase activity, thereby decreasing pyruvate conversion to lactic acid as more pyruvate is decarboxylated to acetyl-CoA for entry into the TCA cycle. However, thiamin given in amounts of 100 times recommendations intravenously or intramuscularly has been associated with headache, convulsions, cardiac arrhythmia, and anaphylactic shock, among other signs [6].

Assessment of Nutriture

Thiamin status can be assessed by measuring thiamin in the blood or urine and by measuring erythrocyte transketolase activity in hemolyzed whole blood. Urinary thiamin excretion decreases with decreased thiamin status and is also correlated with intake. Urinary thiamin excretion <40 μg/day or <27 μg/g creatinine suggests thiamin deficiency. The activity of transketolase, the thiamin-dependent enzyme of the pentose phosphate pathway, is measured after the addition of thiamin to the incubation medium to assess status. An increase in transketolase activity of >25% indicates thiamin deficiency; an increase in activity of 15% to 25% suggests marginal status; and an increase of <15% suggests adequate status. Transketolase concentrations of <120 nmol/L also have been used to indicate deficiency; concentrations of 120 to 150 nmol/L suggest marginal thiamin status.

References Cited for Thiamin

1. Ganapathy V, Smith S, Prasad P. SLC19: the folate/thiamine transporter family. Eur J Physiol. 2004; 447:641–46.
2. Subramanian V, Marchant J, Parker I, Said H. Cell biology of the human thiamine transporter-1 (hTHTR1): intracellular trafficking and membrane targeting mechanisms. J Biol Chem. 2003; 278:3976–84.
3. Oishi K, Barchi M, Au AC, et al. Male infertility due to germ cell apoptosis in mice lacking the thiamin carrier. Tht1. Dev Biol. 2004; 266:299–309.
4. Said HM. Recent advances in carrier-mediated intestinal absorption of water soluble vitamins. Ann Rev Physiol. 2004; 66:419–46.
5. Dudeja P, Tyagi S, Gill R, Said H. Evidence for carrier-mediated mechanism for thiamine transport to human jejunal basolateral membrane vesicles. Dig Dis Sci. 2003; 48:109–15.
6. Food and Nutrition Board. Dietary Reference Intakes for Thiamin, Riboflavin, Niacin, Vitamin B$_6$, Folate, Vitamin B$_{12}$, Pantothenic Acid, Biotin, and Choline. Washington, DC: National Academy Press. 1998 pp. 58–86.
7. Butterworth RF. Thiamin deficiency and brain disorders. Nutr Res Rev. 2003; 16:277–83.
8. Sechi G, Serra A. Wernicke's encephalopathy: new clinical settings and recent advances in diagnosis and management. Lancet Neurol. 2007; 6:442–55.
9. Francini-Pesenti F, Brocadello F, Manara R, et al. Wernicke's syndrome during parenteral feeding: not an unusual complication. Nutrition. 2009; 25:142–46.

Suggested Reading

Bettendorff L, Wins P. Thiamin diphosphate in biological chemistry: new aspects of thiamin metabolism, especially triphosphate derivatives acting other than as cofactors. FEBS Journal. 2009; 276:2917–25.

RIBOFLAVIN (VITAMIN B$_2$)

In 1917 scientists discovered riboflavin (vitamin B$_2$), which was originally called vitamin G in the United States. Kuhn and coworkers are credited with determining its structure along with Szent-Györgyi and Wagner-Jaunergy in 1933. The name *riboflavin* signifies the presence of a ribose-like side chain (ribo) and its yellow color (*flavus* means "yellow" in Latin). Riboflavin consists of a flavin molecule (isoalloxazine ring) with a ribitol (sugar alcohol) side chain attached. The structures of riboflavin and its two coenzyme derivatives, FMN (flavin mononucleotide) and FAD (flavin adenine dinucleotide), are shown in Figure 9.11.

Sources

Riboflavin is found in a wide variety of foods, but especially those of animal origin. Milk and milk products such as cheeses are thought to contribute the most to dietary riboflavin intakes. A cup of nonfat milk provides about 0.45 mg of riboflavin, while an ounce of cheese provides 0.08 to 0.11 mg, depending on the variety. Plain low-fat yogurt contains 0.48 mg/cup. Eggs are also a good source, containing about 0.26 mg of riboflavin/egg. Meat and legumes provide riboflavin in significant quantities. Legumes provide about 0.05 mg per half-cup serving. Meats contain about 0.1 to 0.25 mg/3-oz serving; liver is exceptionally rich, with about 2 to 3 mg/3-oz serving. Green vegetables like spinach (0.2 mg of riboflavin per half-cup serving) represent fairly good riboflavin sources. Fruits and cereal grains are minor contributors of dietary riboflavin. Refined grains are enriched with riboflavin because during the milling of grains the removal of the bran and germ layers results in the loss of most (about two-thirds) of its riboflavin. Wheat bran cereal with raisins (1 cup) provides 25% of the Daily Value, which is 1.7 mg, or about 0.42 mg of riboflavin.

The form of riboflavin in food varies. Free or protein-bound riboflavin is found in milk, eggs, and enriched breads and cereals. In most other foods, the vitamin occurs as one or the other of its coenzyme derivatives FMN or FAD, although phosphorus-bound riboflavin and amino acid–bound FAD are also found in some foods.

Riboflavin can be destroyed with exposure to sunlight (one reason milk is usually not sold in glass bottles); even photo (light) therapy, used to treat neonatal hyperbilirubinemia, causes riboflavin destruction. The vitamin is fairly resistant to heat, oxidation, and acid.

Digestion, Absorption, Transport, and Storage

The riboflavin that is found in foods attached noncovalently to proteins must be digested or "freed" from the protein prior to absorption; this process is accomplished by the action of hydrochloric acid secreted within the stomach and by gastric and intestinal enzymatic hydrolysis of the protein. The riboflavin in foods as FAD, FMN, and riboflavin phosphate must also be freed prior to absorption. FAD pyrophosphatase converts FAD to FMN, and FMN in turn is converted to free riboflavin by FMN phosphatase.

$$\text{FAD} \xrightarrow{\text{FAD pyrophosphatase}} \text{FMN} \xrightarrow{\text{FMN phosphatase}} \text{Riboflavin}$$

Other intestinal phosphatases, such as nucleotide diphosphatase and alkaline phosphatase, are thought to hydrolyze riboflavin from riboflavin phosphate.

Not all bound riboflavin is hydrolyzed and available for absorption. A small amount (~7%) of FAD is covalently bound to either of two amino acids, histidine or cysteine. Thus, following consumption of foods with FAD bound to either of these amino acids, the proteins are degraded; however, the riboflavin remains bound to the

Riboflavin

Ribitol

Flavin
or
Isoalloxazine

Flavokinase

ATP
Mg²⁺ or Mn²⁺
ADP

Flavin mononucleotide (FMN)
(coenzyme)

FAD synthetase

ATP
Mg²⁺ or Mn²⁺
PP$_i$

Pyrophosphate

FMN

AMP

Flavin adenine dinucleotide (FAD)
(coenzyme)

Figure 9.11 Structures of riboflavin and its coenzyme forms.

histidine or cysteine residues. Should absorption of the histidine- or cysteine-bound riboflavin occur, it cannot function in the body and the complex gets excreted unchanged in the urine [1].

Free riboflavin is absorbed by a saturable, energy-dependent, sodium-independent carrier (riboflavin transporter 2, abbreviated RFT2), primarily in the proximal small intestine [2]. When large amounts of the vitamin are ingested, riboflavin may be absorbed by diffusion. The presence of bile facilitates absorption. Alcohol impairs riboflavin digestion and absorption [3].

About 95% of riboflavin intake from foods is absorbed, up to a maximum of about 25 mg, where absorption plateaus and plasma concentrations peak [1].

On absorption into the intestinal cells, riboflavin is phosphorylated to form FMN, a reaction catalyzed by flavokinase and requiring ATP, as shown here and in Figure 9.11.

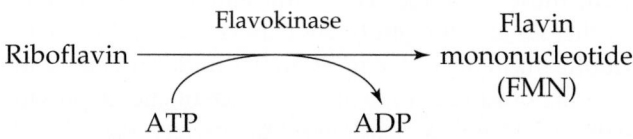

At the serosal membrane of the intestinal cell, most FMN is probably dephosphorylated by a nonspecific alkaline phosphatase to riboflavin, which enters portal blood for transport to the liver. The vitamin is carried to the liver, where it is converted again to FMN by flavokinase and to its other predominant flavoenzyme in tissues, FAD, by FAD synthetase (shown here and in Figure 9.11).

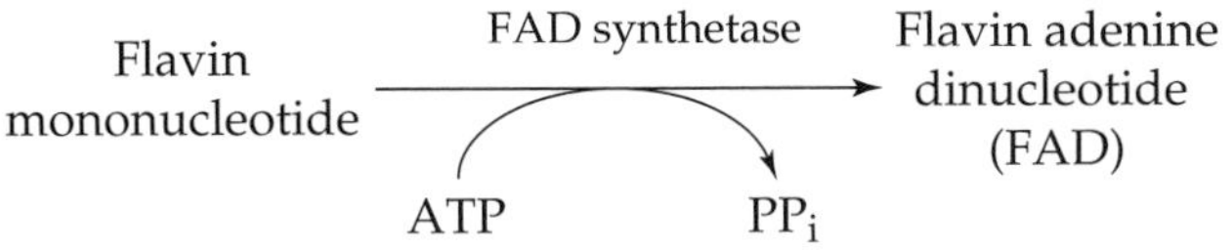

$$\text{Flavin mononucleotide} \xrightarrow[\text{ATP} \quad \text{PP}_i]{\text{FAD synthetase}} \text{Flavin adenine dinucleotide (FAD)}$$

Most flavins are found in the blood as riboflavin (50%), although FMN (10%) and FAD (40%) also may be present. Riboflavin, FMN, and FAD are transported in the plasma by a variety of proteins, including albumin, fibrinogen, and globulins (principally immunoglobulins). Albumin appears to be the primary transport protein. Immunoglobulins have been shown to use riboflavin to activate the antibody-catalyzed water oxidation pathway in which singlet oxygen ($^1O_2$, which is derived from, e.g., activated white blood cells) and water react to form hydrogen peroxide [4]. Hydrogen peroxide assists in the destruction of foreign antigens, although it is also destructive to human cells.

Regardless of the form in which the vitamin reaches the tissues, free riboflavin is the form that traverses most cell membranes, primarily by a carrier-mediated process requiring a riboflavin-binding protein. Some riboflavin carriers in some tissues such as the liver appear to be regulated by calcium or calmodulin [2]. Diffusion also may contribute to cellular riboflavin uptake when concentrations of the vitamin are high.

Riboflavin is found in small quantities in a variety of tissues. The greatest concentrations are found in the liver, kidneys, and heart. It is estimated that the body stores enough riboflavin to meet the body's needs for about 2 to 6 weeks.

Within cells, riboflavin is converted to its coenzyme forms by flavokinase and FAD synthetase, both of which are widely distributed in tissues, especially the liver, spleen, small intestine, kidneys, and heart. FMN is the major form (~60–95%) present in cells, followed by FAD (~5–20%). Synthesis of FMN and FAD appears to be influenced by endproduct inhibition and hormones including ACTH, aldosterone, and the thyroid hormones, all of which accelerate the conversion of riboflavin into its coenzyme forms, apparently by increasing the activity of flavokinase. Once synthesized, the flavin coenzymes become bound to apoenzymes. FMN and FAD function as prosthetic groups for enzymes called flavoproteins that are involved in oxidation-reduction reactions.

Functions and Mechanisms of Action

FMN and FAD function as coenzymes for a wide variety of oxidative enzyme systems and remain bound to the enzymes during the oxidation-reduction reactions. Flavins can act as oxidizing agents because of their ability to accept a pair of hydrogen atoms. The isoalloxazine ring is reduced by two successive one-electron transfers with the intermediate formation of a semiquinone free radical, as shown in Figure 9.12. Reduction of the isoalloxazine ring yields the reduced forms of the flavoprotein, which can be found in $FMNH_2$ and $FADH_2$.

Flavoproteins

Flavoproteins exhibit a wide range of redox potentials and therefore can play a wide variety of roles in intermediary metabolism. Some of these roles are listed here.

- The role of flavoproteins in the *electron transport chain* is illustrated in Figures 3.25 and 3.28.
- In vitamin B_6 metabolism (seen later in Figure 9.36), *pyridoxine phosphate oxidase*—which converts pyridoxamine phosphate (PMP) and pyridoxine phosphate (PNP) to pyridoxal phosphate (PLP), the primary coenzyme form of vitamin B_6—is dependent upon FMN.
- *L-amino oxidase* uses FMN in the dehydrogenation of L-amino acids to imino acids.
- In the *oxidative decarboxylation of pyruvate* (Figure 9.9) and α-ketoglutarate, FAD serves as an intermediate electron carrier, with NADH being the final reduced product.

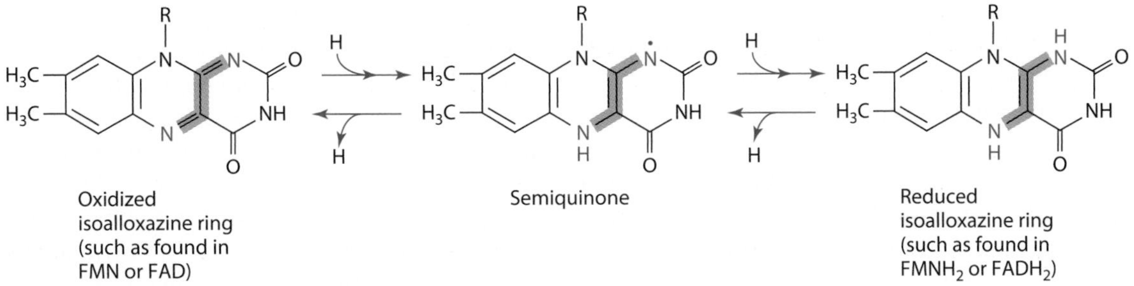

Figure 9.12 Oxidation and reduction of isoalloxazine ring.

- *Succinate dehydrogenase* is an FAD flavoprotein that removes electrons from succinic acid to form fumarate, and that forms $FADH_2$ from FAD (Figure 3.26). The electrons are then passed into the electron transport chain by coenzyme Q (Figure 3.25).

- In fatty acid beta-oxidation, *acyl-CoA* dehydrogenases require FAD (Figure 5.24). Supplements of riboflavin (50–150 mg/day) have been shown to improve enzyme activity in some individuals with acyl-CoA dehydrogenase deficiencies secondary to genetic mutations in the enzyme.

- *Sphinganine oxidase,* in sphingosine synthesis, requires FAD.

- As a coenzyme for an oxidase such as *xanthine oxidase,* FAD transfers electrons directly to oxygen with the formation of hydrogen peroxide. Xanthine oxidase, which contains both iron and molybdenum, is necessary for purine catabolism (see the section on molybdenum in Chapter 13).

- Similarly, *aldehyde oxidase* using FAD reacts with aldehydes such as pyridoxal (vitamin B_6)—to form pyridoxic acid—and retinal (a form of vitamin A)—to produce retinoic acid—while also passing electrons to oxygen and generating hydrogen peroxide.

- Synthesis of an *active form of folate,* 5-methyl THF, requires $FADH_2$ (shown later in Figure 9.28).

- A step in *the synthesis of niacin from tryptophan* that is catalyzed by kynureninase monooxygenase requires FAD (see Figure 9.15).

- In *choline catabolism,* several enzymes such as choline dehydrogenase, dimethylglycine dehydrogenase, and sarcosine (also called monomethylglycine) dehydrogenase require FAD.

- Some neurotransmitters (such as dopamine) and other amines (tyramine and histamine) require FAD-dependent *monoamine oxidase* for metabolism.

- Reduction of the oxidized form of glutathione (GSSG) to its reduced form (GSH) is also dependent upon FAD-dependent *glutathione reductase.* This reaction forms the basis of one assay used to assess riboflavin status (see the "Assessment of Nutriture" section).

- *Erol and sulfhydryl oxidases* are FAD dependent and help to form disulfide bonds involved in the structure or folding of selected secretory proteins. Impaired oxidative folding and subsequently impaired secretion of proteins have been observed with riboflavin deficiency [5].

- *Thioredoxin reductase* is a flavo (FAD) enzyme that contains selenocysteine at its active site and transfers reducing equivalents from NADPH through its bound FAD to reduce disulfide bonds within the oxidized form of thioredoxin. The enzyme works as part of a complex set of reactions with ribonucleotide reductase (which contains thiol groups), as shown here:

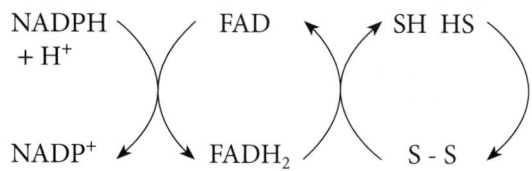

Thioredoxin reductase
(a flavoenzyme)

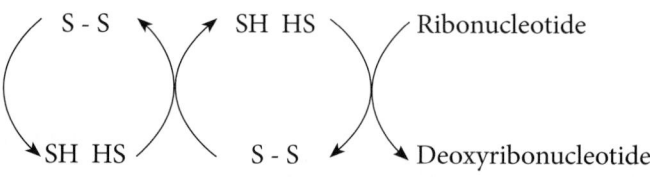

Thioredoxin   Ribonucleotide
or glutaredoxin   reductase

- *Ribonucleotide reductase* catalyzes the conversion of ribonucleotides to deoxyribonucleotides (such as dADP, dGDP, dCDP, and dUDP; see Figure 6.28), which are needed for DNA synthesis. In the reaction, the sulfhydryl groups in ribonucleotide reductase become oxidized, forming a disulfide bond. Thioredoxin (or glutaredoxin—a small protein like thioredoxin) provides electrons (H), but upon donation becomes oxidized itself (containing a disulfide bond). The flavoenzyme thioredoxin reductase (or glutaredoxin reductase), which also contains sulfhydryl groups, reduces the thioredoxin (or glutaredoxin). NADPH then reduces the thioredoxin reductase (or glutaredoxin reductase) to eliminate the disulfide bond and regenerate the sulfhydryl groups.

Metabolism and Excretion

Riboflavin and its metabolites are excreted primarily in the urine. It is the free riboflavin (i.e., not bound to proteins in the plasma) that is filtered by the glomerulus and excreted in the urine. Most riboflavin ($\sim$60–70%) is excreted intact in the urine in amounts $>$120 μg/day or 80 μg/g creatinine with adequate riboflavin intake. Metabolites arise from tissue degradation of covalently bound flavins as well as from degradation of the vitamin. The metabolites present in the greatest concentrations in the urine include 7α- and 8α-hydroxymethyl riboflavin, 8α-sulfonyl riboflavin, 10-hydroxyethyl flavin, and riboflavinyl peptide ester. Riboflavin bound to cysteine and histidine also may be found in the urine if absorbed in such form from the gastrointestinal tract or if generated in body cells from the degradation of flavoenzymes such as succinate dehydrogenase and monoamine oxidase [1]. Futher, some metabolites formed in the intestinal tract by the bacterial degradation of the vitamin also may be absorbed, but then are excreted in the urine [1]. Only small amounts of riboflavin are lost in the feces. Fecal riboflavin metabolites arise from the catabolism of riboflavin by intestinal bacteria.

Unlike that of other vitamins, the urinary excretion of riboflavin is often noticeable within a couple of hours following oral ingestion of the vitamin. Riboflavin is a fluorescent yellow compound. Thus, following riboflavin intake in a quantity such as 1.7 mg (similar to that found in a supplement), the urine color deepens from a typical light yellow to a brighter, orangish yellow.

Recommended Dietary Allowance

The RDAs for riboflavin have been estimated through various studies involving urinary excretion of riboflavin, the relationship of dietary intake to clinical signs of deficiency, and the activity of erythrocyte glutathione reductase. Recommendations for riboflavin for adult men and women are 1.3 mg/day and 1.1 mg/day, respectively; the requirements for adult men and women are 1.1 mg and 0.9 mg, respectively [1]. With pregnancy and lactation, recommendations for daily riboflavin intake increase to 1.4 mg and 1.6 mg, respectively [1]. The inside front cover of the book provides additional RDAs for riboflavin for other age groups.

Deficiency: Ariboflavinosis

An acute deficiency of riboflavin, sometimes called ariboflavinosis, rarely occurs in isolation but most often is accompanied by other nutrient deficits. No clear riboflavin deficiency disease has been characterized; however, clinical symptoms of deficiency after about 3 to 4 months of inadequate intake include painful lesions or fissures on the outside of the lips (cheilosis) and corners of the mouth (angular stomatitis); inflammation of the tongue (glossitis), which may appear smooth and magenta in color; red or bloody (hyperemia) and swollen (edema) mouth/oral cavity; an inflammatory skin condition, seborrheic dermatitis (associated with the secretion of a waxy substance found noticeably around the nose or nasolabial fold); anemia; and peripheral nerve dysfunction (neuropathy), among other signs. Severe deficiency of riboflavin may diminish the synthesis of the coenzyme form of vitamin B_6 and the synthesis of niacin from tryptophan. Studies in cell cultures have found that riboflavin deficiency can result in protein and DNA damage and arrest cells in the G1 phase of the cell cycle [5]. Treatment of deficiency usually requires about 10 to 20 mg of riboflavin daily until symptoms resolve.

Because of limited dietary intake and diminished absorption, people consuming excess alcohol are at risk of deficiency. The deficiency condition also remains fairly common in developing countries. Because riboflavin metabolism is altered with thyroid disease, and riboflavin excretion is enhanced with diabetes mellitus, trauma, and stress, people with these conditions are at risk for deficiency. Tricyclic medications used to treat depression inhibit riboflavin absorption. Poor riboflavin status in people who have a homozygous mutation ($677C \longrightarrow T$) in methylene tetrahydrofolate reductase further increases plasma homocysteine concentrations, a risk factor for heart disease; see the Perspective at the end of this chapter for a further discussion of this enzymatic mutation. Lastly, some individuals with defects in acyl-CoA dehydrogenases may benefit from riboflavin supplements, which in some cases improve enzyme activity.

Toxicity

Toxicity associated with large oral doses of riboflavin has not been reported, and no Tolerable Upper Intake Level for riboflavin has been established [1]. Trials using large amounts (400 mg) of the vitamin have shown it to be effective in treating migraine headaches without side effects, although more studies are needed [6].

Assessment of Nutriture

The most sensitive method for determining riboflavin nutriture is to measure the activity of the FAD-dependent enzyme erythrocyte glutathione reductase, which catalyzes the following reaction:

$$NADPH + H^+ + GSSG \longrightarrow NADP^+ + 2GSH$$

In this reaction, glutathione in its oxidized form is designated GSSG, and in its reduced form, GSH. In cases of a riboflavin deficiency or marginal riboflavin status, the activity of glutathione reductase is limited, and less NADPH is used to reduce the oxidized glutathione. *In vitro* enzyme activity in terms of "activity coefficients" (AC) is determined both with and without the addition of FAD to the medium. Activity coefficients represent a ratio of the enzyme's activity with FAD to the enzyme's activity without FAD. When the addition of FAD stimulates enzyme activity to generate an AC of 1.2 to 1.4, riboflavin status is considered low; an AC > 1.4 suggests riboflavin deficiency. Conversely, if FAD is added and AC is < 1.2, then riboflavin status is considered acceptable. In addition to the use of glutathione reductase activity, the activity of a FMN-dependent enzyme, pyridoxamine phosphate oxidase, needed for interconversions of vitamin B_6 coenzyme forms, also appears to be a biomarker of riboflavin status. Cellular riboflavin concentrations and urinary riboflavin excretion also are used to assess status. Cellular riboflavin concentrations $< 10\ \mu g/dL$ and urinary riboflavin excretion $< 19\ \mu g/g$ creatinine (without recent riboflavin intake) or $< 40\ \mu g$ per day are indicative of deficiency.

References Cited for Riboflavin

1. Food and Nutrition Board. Dietary Reference Intakes for Thiamin, Riboflavin, Niacin, Vitamin B_6, Folate, Vitamin B_{12}, Pantothenic Acid, Biotin, and Choline. Washington, DC: National Academy Press. 1998 pp. 87–122.
2. Said HM. Recent advances in carrier-mediated intestinal absorption of water soluble vitamins. Ann Rev Physiol. 2004; 66:419–46.
3. Pinto J, Huang Y, Rivlin R. Mechanisms underlying the differential effects of ethanol upon the bioavailability of riboflavin and flavin adenine dinucleotide. J Clin Invest. 1987; 79:1343–48.
4. Nieva J, Kerwin L, Wentworth A, et al. Immunoglobulins can utilize riboflavin (vitamin B_2) to activate the antibody-catalyzed water oxidation pathway. Immunol Letters. 2006; 103:33–38.
5. Manthey K, Rodriguez-Melendez R, Hoi J, Zempleni J. Riboflavin deficiency causes protein and DNA damage in HepG2 cells, triggering arrest in G1 phase of the cell cycle. J Nutr Biochem. 2006; 17:250–56.
6. Woolhouse M. Migraine and tension headaches: a complementary and alternative medicine approach. Australian Fam Physician. 2005; 34:647–51.

Suggested Reading

Henriques BJ, Olsen RK, Bross P, Gomes CM. Emerging roles for riboflavin in functional rescue of mitochondrial β-oxidation flavoenzymes. Curr Med Chem. 2010; 17:3842–54.

NIACIN (VITAMIN B₃)

Like thiamin, which was discovered through its deficiency disorder beriberi, niacin (also called vitamin B_3) was discovered through the condition pellagra in humans and a similar condition, called black tongue, in dogs. In fact, the vitamin was once called the anti–black tongue factor because of its effect in dogs. In humans, pellagra was once especially prevalent in the southeastern United States where corn (which contains a relatively unavailable form of niacin) was a main dietary staple in the early 1900s. It was not until about 1937 that Elvehjem isolated the vitamin, which was shown then to cure both pellagra and black tongue. The vitamin was named niacin in the early 1940s.

Niacin, however, is a generic term for nicotinic acid and nicotinamide (also called niacinamide), which both provide vitamin activity. Structurally, nicotinic acid is pyridine 3-carboxylic acid, whereas nicotinamide is nicotinic acid amide (Figure 9.13).

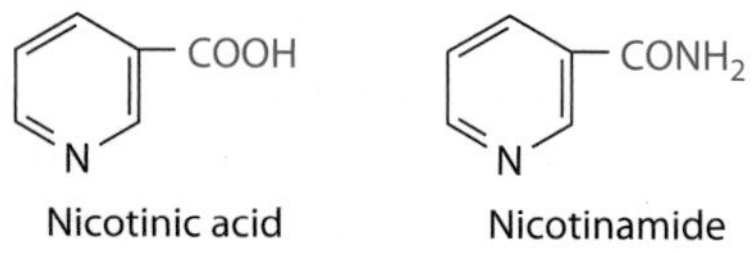

Sources

The best sources of niacin include most fish and meats. A 3-oz serving of tuna or halibut provides about 11.3 mg or 6.1 mg of niacin, respectively. Beef and pork contain about 4.5 to 7.2 mg of niacin/3 oz; a 3-oz chicken breast provides 11.8 mg, and 3 oz of white turkey meat contains about 5.7 mg of niacin. Beef liver is especially rich, with about 15 mg of niacin/3-oz serving. Veal provides about 8.9 mg of niacin/3-oz serving. Enriched cereals and bread products, whole grains, fortified cereals, seeds, and legumes also contain appreciable amounts of niacin. A cup of spaghetti provides 2.3 mg of niacin, while enriched white or brown rice has about 1.3 mg of niacin/½ cup. A slice of enriched white bread contains 1.1 mg of niacin, and 1 cup of Cheerios® provides 25% of the 20 mg Daily Value, or 5 mg. Peanut butter (2 tablespoons) has 4.3 mg of niacin. Niacin is also found in coffee and tea, and in lesser amounts in green vegetables and milk. In coffee, a compound called trigonelline is converted to niacin by heat (such as with coffee bean roasting) and acid.

Niacin is generally found as nicotinamide in supplements but may be present in several forms in foods. In animal foods, niacin occurs mainly as nicotinamide and the nicotinamide nucleotides—nicotinamide adenine dinucleotide (NAD) and nicotinamide adenine dinucleotide phosphate (NADP). Figure 9.14 shows the structures of NAD and NADP. In their oxidized forms, NAD and

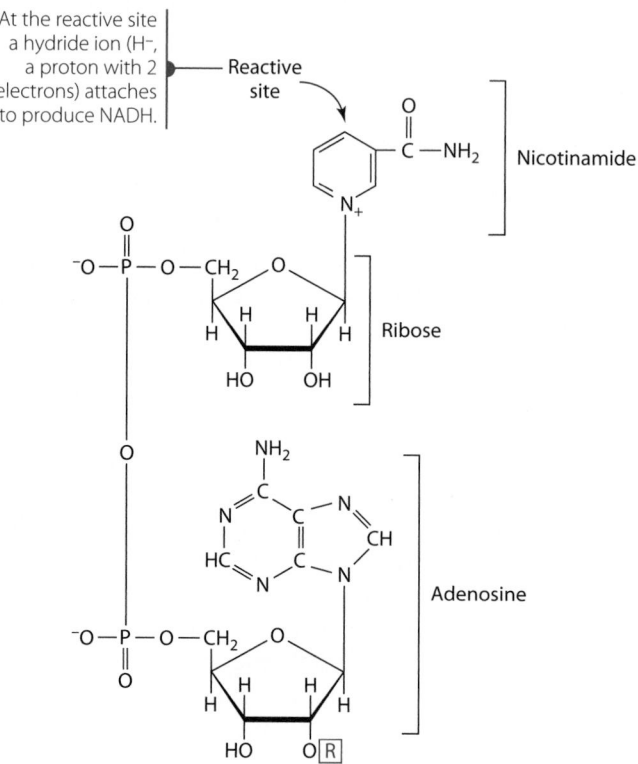

At the reactive site a hydride ion (H^-, a proton with 2 electrons) attaches to produce NADH.

R = H for NAD⁺ (nicotinamide adenine dinucleotide)

R = PO_3^{2-} for NADP⁺ (nicotinamide adenine dinucleotide phosphate)

Figure 9.14 The structures of NAD and NADP.

Figure 9.13 Nicotinic acid and nicotinamide.

Nicotinic acid

Nicotinamide

NADP possess a positive charge and therefore may alternatively be written NAD^+ and $NADP^+$. In plant foods, niacin is present mainly as nicotinic acid. Niacin in foods is fairly stable; minimal losses of the vitamin result from cooking or storage.

In addition to being present as nicotinic acid, nicotinamide, NAD, and NADP in foods, niacin may be bound covalently to complex carbohydrates and called niacytin, or it may be bound to small peptides and called niacinogens. This bound form of niacin is found primarily in corn but also in wheat and some other cereal products. Chemical treatment with bases such as lime water can improve the availability of some bound niacin. Some niacin also may be released from niacytin on exposure to gastric acid. However, only about 10% of the niacin from maize is thought to be available for absorption.

In addition to dietary sources of niacin, niacin may be synthesized in the liver and some other tissues from the amino acid tryptophan. This biosynthetic pathway, which provides an important contribution to the niacin needs of the body, is depicted in Figure 9.15. Only about 3% of the tryptophan that is metabolized follows the pathway. An estimated 1 mg of niacin is produced from ingestion of 60 mg of dietary tryptophan (see the RDA section for niacin to understand how this synthesis is accounted for in niacin recommendations). Riboflavin (FAD), vitamin B_6 (PLP), and iron are required in some of the reactions, and thus deficiency of these nutrients, along with other dietary factors such as poor tryptophan and energy intakes, can impair niacin synthesis.

Digestion, Absorption, Transport, and Storage

Digestion of NAD and NADP is needed to enable the absorption of niacin. A pyrophosphatase is required for phosphate hydrolysis off NADP. The NAD is then hydrolyzed by glycohydrolase and releases free nicotinamide.

$$\text{NAD and NADP} \xrightarrow{\text{Glycohydrolase}} \text{Nicotinamide}$$

Nicotinamide and nicotinic acid can be absorbed in the stomach, but they are more readily absorbed in the small intestine by sodium-dependent, carrier-mediated (facilitated) diffusion. At high concentrations (as with 3–4 g pharmacological doses), niacin is absorbed almost completely by passive diffusion in the intestine.

In the plasma, niacin is found primarily as nicotinamide, but also as nicotinic acid. Up to about one-third of nicotinic acid in the plasma is bound to plasma proteins. From the blood, nicotinamide and nicotinic acid move across cell membranes by simple diffusion; however, nicotinic acid transport into the kidney tubules and red blood cells requires a carrier, and uptake into the brain is energy dependent.

Nicotinamide serves as the primary precursor of NAD, which is synthesized in all tissues. Nicotinic acid also may be used to synthesize NAD, but this reaction occurs primarily in the liver. Phosphorylation of NAD by NAD kinase using ATP generates NADP (Figure 9.15). These

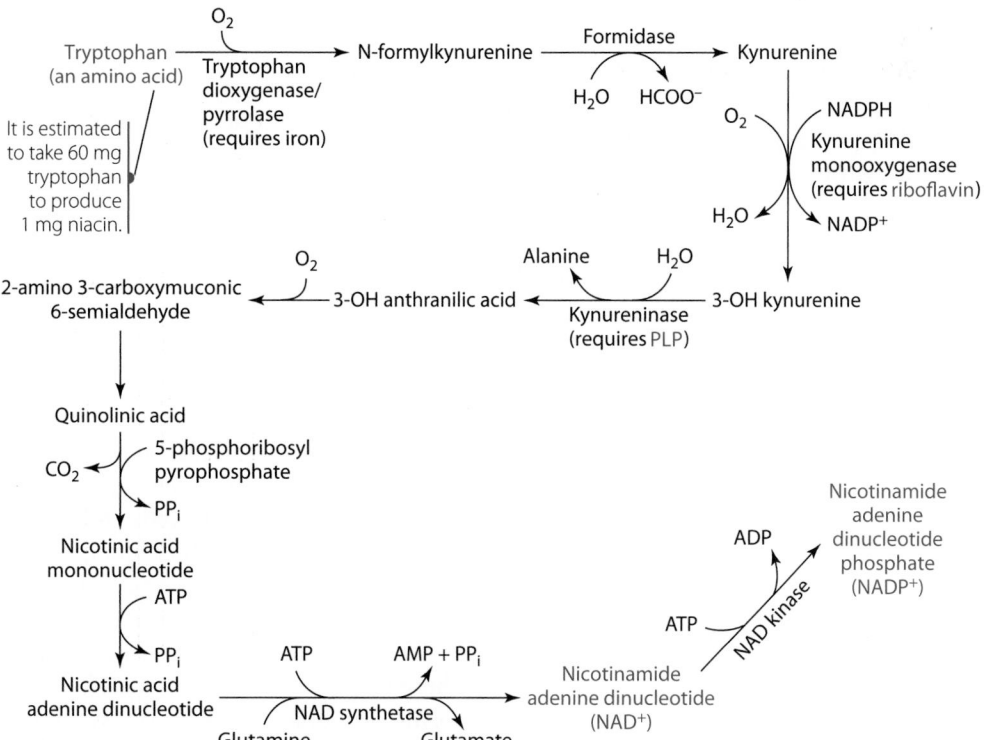

Figure 9.15 NAD$^+$ and NADP$^+$ synthesis from the amino acid tryptophan.

reactions may be reversed, converting NADP to NAD, and NAD to nicotinamide, which then is available for transport to other tissues.

As NAD or NADP, the vitamin is trapped within the cell. Intracellular concentrations of NAD typically predominate over those of NADP. In the liver, excess niacin and tryptophan are converted to NAD, which is stored in small amounts not bound to enzymes. NAD is found primarily in its oxidized form (NAD^+), whereas NADP is found in cells mainly in its reduced form (NADPH).

Functions and Mechanisms of Action

Approximately 200 enzymes, primarily dehydrogenases, require the coenzymes NAD and NADP, which act as a hydrogen donor or electron acceptor. Figure 9.16 demonstrates the oxidation-reduction that may occur in the nicotinamide moiety of the coenzymes. In addition to its coenzyme roles, niacin functions in nonredox roles as a donor of adenosine diphosphate ribose.

Coenzymes

Although NAD and NADP are similar and undergo reversible reduction in the same way, their functions in the cell are different. The major role of NADH, formed from NAD, is to transfer its electrons from metabolic intermediates through the electron transport chain (Figure 3.25), thereby producing ATP. NADPH, in contrast, acts as a reducing agent in many biosynthetic pathways such as fatty acid, cholesterol, and steroid hormone synthesis and also in other pathways. NAD and NADP coenzymes are tightly bound to their apoenzymes and can easily transport hydrogen atoms from one part of the cell to another. Reactions in which they participate occur both in the mitochondria and in the cytosol.

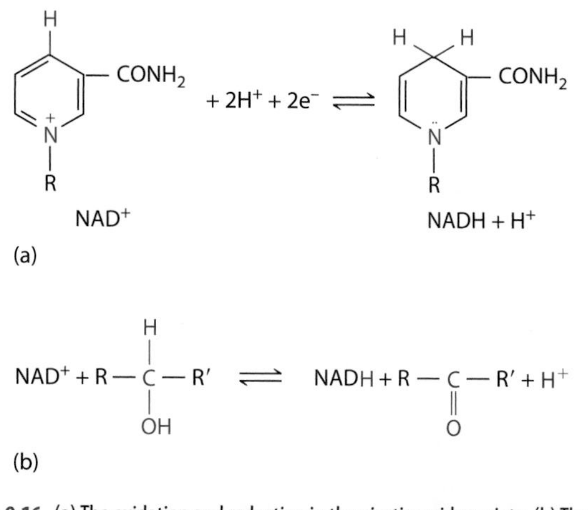

Figure 9.16 (a) The oxidation and reduction in the nicotinamide moiety. (b) The role of NAD in dehydrogenation reactions. One H of the substrate goes to NAD.

Oxidative reactions in which NAD participates and is reduced to NADH (and in turn can be transferred to the electron transport chain for ATP generation) include:

- glycolysis (Figure 3.17)
- oxidative decarboxylation of pyruvate to acetyl-CoA (Figure 9.9)
- oxidation of acetyl-CoA in the TCA cycle (Figure 3.18)
- β-oxidation of fatty acids (Figure 5.24)
- oxidation of ethanol (Figure 5.36)

In addition to its roles in energy metabolism, NAD is also required by aldehyde dehydrogenase for catabolism of vitamin B_6 as pyridoxal to its excretory product, pyridoxic acid.

NADP is reduced to NADPH. This reaction occurs as part of the pentose phosphate pathway (Figure 3.30) and the mitochondrial membrane malate aspartate shuttle (Figure 3.21). The NADPH produced in these reactions is used in a variety of reductive biosynthetic processes, including:

- fatty acid synthesis (Figure 5.30)
- cholesterol and steroid hormone synthesis
- proline synthesis (Figure 6.33)
- deoxyribonucleotide (precursors of DNA) synthesis (Figure 6.28)
- glutathione, vitamin C, and thioredoxin regeneration
- folate coenzyme synthesis (dihydrofolate [DHF], tetrahydrofolate [THF], 5-methyl THF, and 5,10-methylene THF; Figure 9.28 later in this chapter)

Nonredox Roles

NAD acts as a donor of adenosine diphosphate ribose (ADP-ribose) for both the posttranslational modification of proteins associated with chromosomes and the formation of cyclic ADP-ribose. There are several types of ADP-ribosylation reactions; these reactions generally control cellular processes such as DNA repair, replication, and transcription; G-protein activity; chromatin structure; and intracellular calcium signaling [1]. Mono ADP-ribosyl transferases (sometimes abbreviated ARTs) transfer one (mono) ADP-ribose from NAD to various acceptor proteins found on cell surfaces or outside cells. For example, a substrate for ART1 is defensin, an antimicrobial peptide made by immune system cells and thus important in the immune response [2]. Other mono ADP-ribosyl transferases are found within cells or attached to cell membranes and function to modify proteins typically involved in cell regulation of the cell cytoskeleton and cell signaling. Poly ADP-ribose polymerases (PARP) transfer several (*poly* > 200) polymers of branched ADP-riboses from NAD onto various target proteins. PARP-1, the most abundant of 5 polymerases, binds to DNA strand breaks. This interaction leads to NAD use, and poly ADP-ribose formation [1]. Targets for the transferases generally include various chromosomal proteins. The proteins also function in DNA repair and replication as well as in cell differentiation [2,3]. Cyclic ADP-ribose, generated by NAD glycohydrolases, is thought to function in certain cells as a second messenger involved in control of ryanodine receptors and in mobilization of calcium from intracellular stores, especially in neurons [2,3].

Metabolism and Excretion

NAD and NADP undergo degradation in cells by glycohydrolase to form ADP-ribose and nicotinamide. The released nicotinamide is then methylated and oxidized in the liver into a variety of products that are excreted in the urine. The primary metabolites of nicotinamide are N′ methyl nicotinamide (sometimes abbreviated NMN and representing ~20–30% of niacin metabolites) and N′ methyl 2-pyridone 5-carboxamide (also called 2-pyridone and representing ~40–60%). Small amounts of N′ methyl 4-pyridone carboxamide (called 4-pyridone) also may be present. Nicotinic acid is metabolized mainly to N′ methylnicotinic acid. Little free nicotinic acid or nicotinamide is excreted, as both compounds are actively reabsorbed from the glomerular filtrate.

Recommended Dietary Allowance

Recommendations for niacin intake include calculations of niacin derived from the amino acid tryptophan, with about 60 mg of tryptophan estimated to generate 1 mg of niacin. Total niacin thus is provided to the body as nicotinic acid and nicotinamide and from tryptophan. The term *niacin equivalent* (NE) is used to account for the provision by tryptophan.

Although recommendations are given in niacin equivalents, food composition tables report only preformed niacin. A rough estimate of niacin equivalents from a protein can be made by assuming that 10 mg of tryptophan are provided for every 1 g of high-quality (complete) protein in the diet; that is, 1 g of complete, high-quality protein = 10 mg of tryptophan. This estimate means that an intake of 60 g of complete protein, for example, would provide 600 mg of tryptophan (10 mg tryptophan/1 g protein × 60 g protein = 600 mg tryptophan). Then, because it takes 60 mg of tryptophan to generate 1 mg of NE, 600 mg of tryptophan would generate 10 NEs (600 mg tryptophan × 1 mg NE/60 mg tryptophan = 10 NEs). The average U.S. diet usually contains about 900 mg of tryptophan daily, and tryptophan provides about 50% of niacin intake in the United States [4].

Information used in estimating niacin requirements and recommendations has come from several studies, including human depletion and repletion studies as well as other studies with primarily urinary metabolites of niacin serving as indicators to base requirements and recommendations. The RDAs for niacin for adult men and women are 16 mg of niacin equivalents and 14 mg of niacin equivalents/day, respectively [5]. Estimated requirements are 12 mg and 11 mg of niacin for adult men and women, respectively. With pregnancy and lactation, the RDA for niacin increases to 18 mg and 17 mg of niacin equivalents, respectively [5]. The inside front cover of the book provides additional RDAs for niacin for other age groups.

Deficiency: Pellagra

A deficiency of niacin results in the condition known as **pellagra** (*pelle* means "skin" and *agra* means "rough" in Italian). The four Ds—*dermatitis, dementia, diarrhea,* and *death*—are often used as a mnemonic device for remembering its signs. The dermatitis is similar to sunburn at first and appears on areas exposed to the sun, such as the face and neck, and on extremities such as the back of the hands, wrists, elbows, knees, and feet. The presence of the dermatological changes on the neck is sometimes called Casal's collar or necklace. Neurological manifestations include headache, apathy, loss of memory, peripheral neuritis, paralysis of extremities, confusion, disorientation, and dementia or delirium. Gastrointestinal manifestations include glossitis, cheilosis, angular stomatitis, nausea, vomiting, and diarrhea. If it is untreated, death occurs. Treatment requires about 500 mg of nicotinamide daily for several weeks.

A niacin deficiency or diminished niacin status can result from the use of several medications and from malabsorptive conditions. The antituberculosis drug isoniazid, for example, binds with vitamin B₆ as PLP and thereby reduces PLP-dependent kynureninase activity required for niacin synthesis. Mercaptopurine, a drug used in cancer treatment, inhibits NAD phosphorylase. Malabsorptive disorders (chronic diarrhea, inflammatory bowel diseases, some intestinal cancers, and Hartnup disease) may impair niacin and/or tryptophan absorption to increase the likelihood of niacin deficiency. Finally, people who consume excessive amounts of alcohol typically have poor food, and thus vitamin, intakes and are at risk for niacin deficiency.

Toxicity

Large doses of nicotinic acid (up to 6 g/day in divided doses) are used to treat hypercholesterolemia (high blood cholesterol). These pharmacological doses have been shown to significantly lower total serum cholesterol, triacylglycerols, and low-density lipoproteins (LDLs) and increase high-density lipoproteins (HDLs). Although the mechanisms of action are not fully understood, niacin appears to act in multiple ways to improve serum lipids. The vitamin acts through several receptors including G-protein coupled receptors, activation of ATP synthetase in the liver, and NADPH and direct enzyme inhibitions [6]. Niacin (when given in pharmacologic doses) inhibits lipolysis in adipose tissue and decreases hepatic VLDL synthesis and secretion from the liver and LDL production. Niacin also inhibits diacylglycerol acyltransferase in the liver to diminish triacylglycerol synthesis and by both direct and indirect means increases HDL cholesterol concentrations [6].

Despite the therapeutic benefits of nicotinic acid, some undesirable side effects are associated with its use as a drug, especially in certain forms and in doses of typically 1 g or more per day. Some of these side effects are vasodilatory, mediated in part by histamine release, including uncomfortable flushing and redness along with burning, itching (pruritus), tingling, and headaches. Gastrointestinal problems include heartburn, nausea, and possibly vomiting. Liver injury (hepatic toxicity), high blood uric acid concentrations (hyperuricemia) and possibly gout, and high blood glucose concentrations (hyperglycemia) also may occur [6,7].

Newer extended-release forms of nicotinic acid with fewer side effects are available; however, hepatic toxicity, headaches, and gastrointestinal distress may still result. Nicotinamide in large doses does not exhibit toxic effects, but neither does it reduce blood lipids. Nicotinamide, however, is sometimes used topically to reduce inflammation in the treatment of one form of acne (acne vulgaris). In addition, the vitamin has been used orally in the treatment of another skin condition, necrobiosis lipoidica, which is characterized by reddish-brown bruise-like markings most often on the lower legs. Over time the lesions become yellowish in color and atropic plaques develop; the condition, although fairly rare, is most often seen in those with diabetes mellitus.

Because of the vasodilatory effects associated with supplemental niacin, a Tolerable Upper Intake Level for adults for niacin (both nicotinic acid and nicotinamide) from supplements and from fortified foods has been set at 35 mg/day [5]. For those being treated for hyperlipidemia, the benefits of nicotinic acid as a cholesterol-lowering agent must be weighed against its potential toxic effects.

Assessment of Nutriture

Several methods are employed to assess niacin status. Most methods involve measurement of one or more urinary metabolites of the vitamin. Urinary excretion of <0.8 mg/day of N′ methyl nicotinamide and of <0.5 mg of N′ methyl nicotinamide/1 g of creatinine are suggestive of poor (deficient) niacin status [8]. Marginal niacin status is suggested by urinary amounts in the range of 0.5 to 1.59 mg of N′ methyl nicotinamide/1 g of creatinine, while levels in excess of 1.6 mg reflect adequate status [8]. This ratio, however, has been criticized as being difficult

to interpret because of multiple influences on urinary creatinine excretion. It usually is employed during a period of 4 to 5 hours after a 50 mg test dose of nicotinamide. Another ratio employed to assess niacin status is that of urinary N′ methyl 2-pyridone 5-carboxamide (2-pyridone) to N′ methyl nicotinamide (NMN). Although a ratio of <1 is found with niacin deficiency, this ratio is not thought to be sensitive enough to detect marginal niacin intakes and may better reflect dietary protein adequacy as opposed to niacin status [8].

In addition to measurement of urinary metabolites, serum or red blood cell indicators are used to assess niacin status. NAD concentrations and the ratio of NAD to NADP (<1.0) in erythrocytes have been used. In plasma, concentrations of 2-pyridone drop below the detection level with low niacin intakes and thus may be used as an index of niacin status [8].

References Cited for Niacin

1. Kirkland JB. Poly ADP-ribose polymerase-1 and health. Exp Biol Med. 2010; 235:561–68.
2. Corda D, DiGirolamo M. Functional aspects of protein mono-ADP-ribosylation. EMBO J. 2003; 22:1953–58.
3. Kirkland JB. Niacin status impacts chromatin structure. J Nutr. 2009; 139:2397–2401.
4. Food and Nutrition Board. Dietary Reference Intakes for Energy, Carbohydrates, Fiber, Fat, Protein and Amino Acids. Washington, DC: National Academy Press. 2002.
5. Food and Nutrition Board. Dietary Reference Intakes for Thiamin, Riboflavin, Niacin, Vitamin B$_6$, Folate, Vitamin B$_{12}$, Pantothenic Acid, Biotin, and Choline. Washington, DC: National Academy Press. 1998 pp. 123–49.
6. Al-Mohaissen MA, Pun SC, Fohlich JJ. Niacin: from mechanisms of action to therapeutic uses. Medicinal Chem. 2010; 10:204–17.
7. Robinson A, Sloan H, Arnold G. Use of niacin in the prevention and management of hyperlipidemia. Prog Cardiovasc Nurs. 2001; 16:14–20.
8. Gibson RS. Principles of Nutritional Assessment. New York: Oxford University Press. 2005 pp. 562–68.

PANTOTHENIC ACID

Pantothenic acid's essentiality was not discovered until 1954, although the vitamin had been isolated in about 1931 by R. J. Williams and its structure determined in 1939. Structurally, pantothenic acid (once called vitamin B$_5$) consists of β-alanine and pantoic acid joined by a peptide bond/amide linkage and is shown at the top of Figure 9.17. The vitamin is used to form a part of coenzyme A (the A referring to acetylation), as shown in Figure 9.18. It was F. Lipmann who, in 1957, won the Nobel prize for his work showing that coenzyme A facilitated biological acetylation reactions.

Sources

The Greek word *pantos* means "everywhere," and the vitamin pantothenic acid, as its name implies, is found widely distributed in nature. Because this vitamin is present

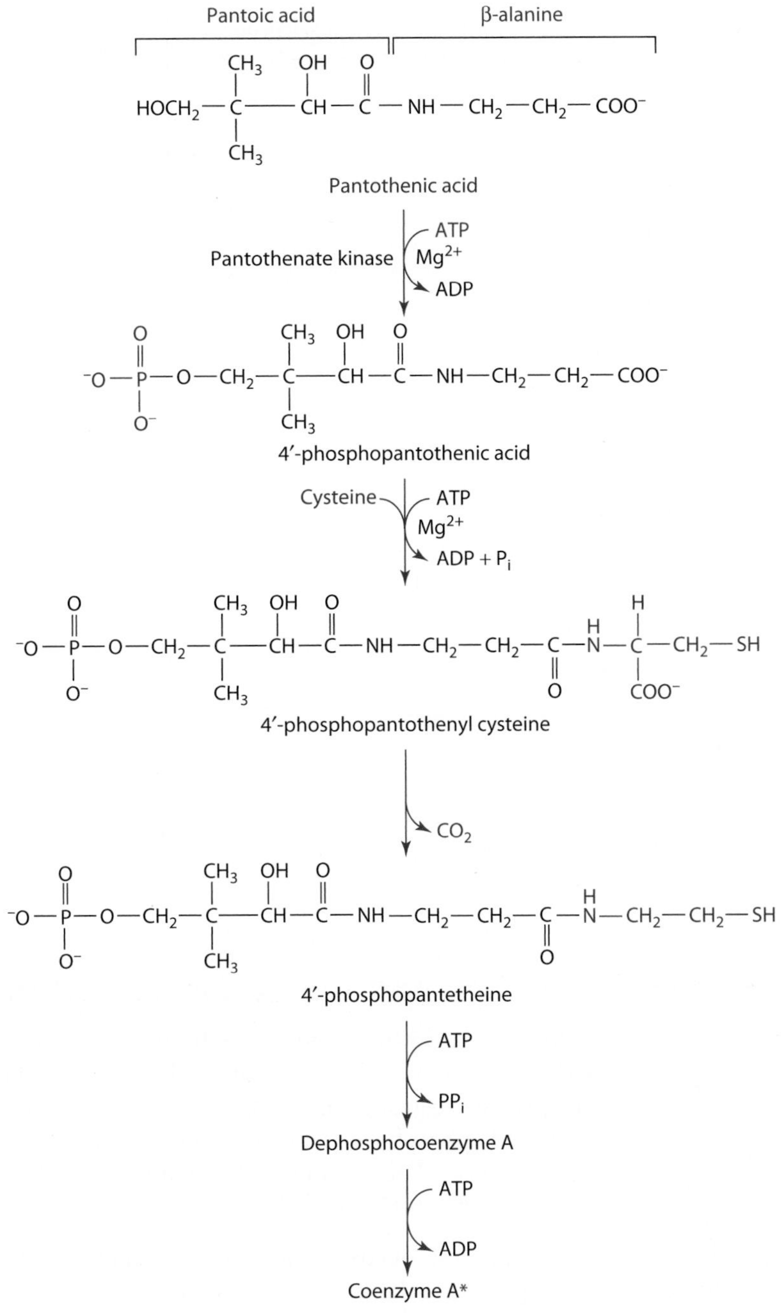

Pantoic acid | β-alanine

CH₃ OH O
HOCH₂—C——CH—C—NH—CH₂—CH₂—COO⁻
CH₃

Pantothenic acid

Pantothenate kinase ⟨ ATP Mg²⁺ → ADP ⟩

O
‖
⁻O—P—O—CH₂—C——CH—C—NH—CH₂—CH₂—COO⁻
O⁻   CH₃ OH O
      CH₃

4′-phosphopantothenic acid

Cysteine ⟨ ATP Mg²⁺ → ADP + Pᵢ ⟩

O   CH₃ OH O   H
‖   ‖ |
⁻O—P—O—CH₂—C——CH—C—NH—CH₂—CH₂—C—N—C—CH₂—SH
O⁻   CH₃   O   COO⁻

4′-phosphopantothenyl cysteine

⟨ → CO₂ ⟩

O   CH₃ OH O   H
‖   ‖ |
⁻O—P—O—CH₂—C——CH—C—NH—CH₂—CH₂—C—N—CH₂—CH₂—SH
O⁻   CH₃   O

4′-phosphopantetheine

⟨ ATP → PPᵢ ⟩

Dephosphocoenzyme A

⟨ ATP → ADP ⟩

Coenzyme A*

*Structure shown in Fig. 9.18

Figure 9.17 Synthesis of coenzyme A from pantothenic acid.

in virtually all plant and animal foods, a deficiency is unlikely. Good sources of the vitamin are meats (particularly liver with 5 to 6 mg of pantothenic acid/3-oz serving and chicken with 1.0 mg/3-oz serving), egg yolk, yogurt (1.3 mg/cup), legumes, whole-grain cereals, potatoes, mushrooms (1.8 mg/½ cup), broccoli, and avocados, among other foods. Royal jelly from bees also provides large amounts (about 0.5 mg/g) of pantothenic acid. The Daily Value for pantothenic acid is 10 mg. In supplements, pantothenic acid is usually found as calcium pantothenate or as panthenol, an alcohol form of the vitamin. Most adults in the United States consume about 4 to 7 mg pantothenic acid per day. The vitamin is easily destroyed with

heating and freezing. It is stable when dry and in solution at a neutral pH but destroyed in acidic and alkaline solutions. The refining of grains decreases their pantothenic acid content by as much as 75%.

Digestion, Absorption, Transport, and Storage

Pantothenic acid occurs in foods in free and bound forms. About 85% of the pantothenic acid in food occurs bound as a component of coenzyme A, abbreviated CoA. During digestion, CoA is hydrolyzed in the gastrointestinal tract lumen in several steps to

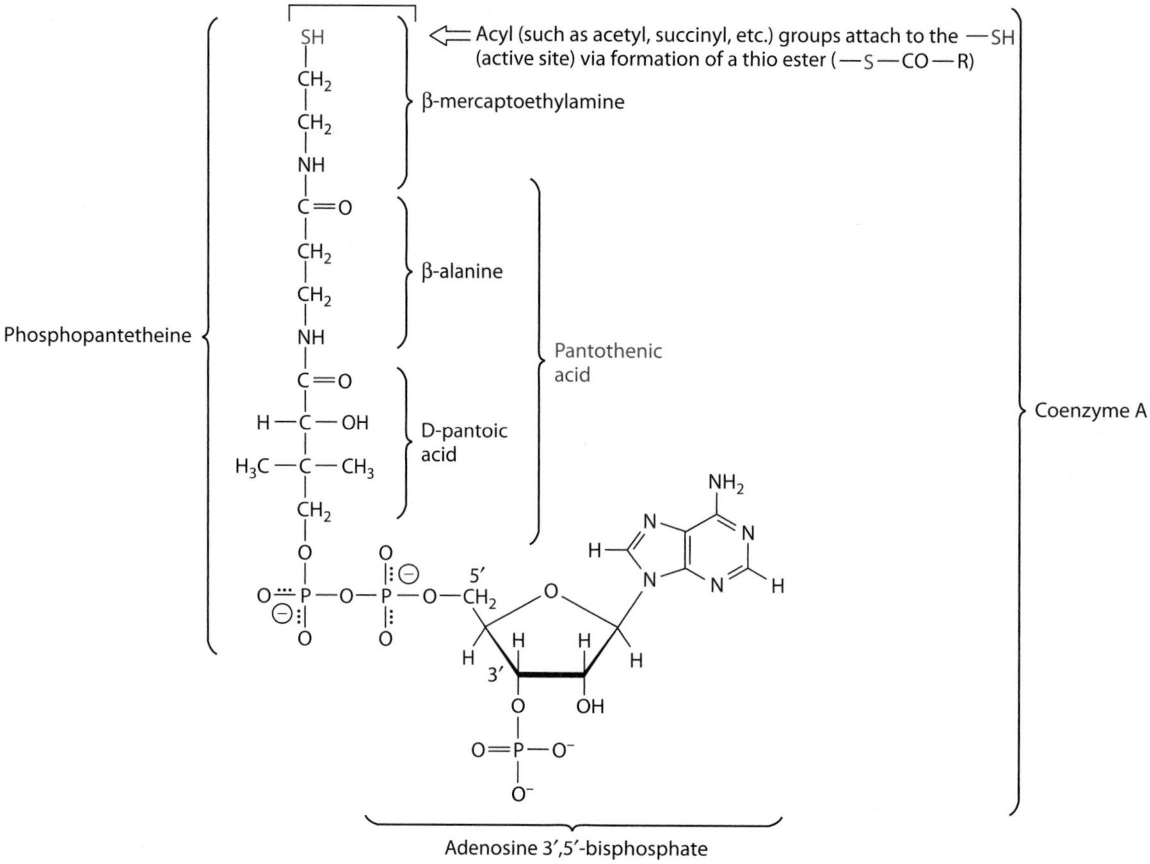

Figure 9.18 Structure of coenzyme A and identification of components.

4′-phosphopantetheine, which is then dephosphorylated to pantetheine. This later compound is subsequently converted to pantothenic acid.

Pantothenic acid is absorbed principally in the jejunum by passive diffusion when present in high concentrations and by a sodium-dependent multivitamin transporter (SMVT) when present in low concentrations [1]. Pantothenic acid shares the intestinal multivitamin transporter with biotin (another B vitamin) and lipoic acid. Panthenol is also absorbed and converted to pantothenic acid. Approximately 50% (range 40–61%) of the ingested pantothenic acid is absorbed [2]. However, pantothenic acid absorption decreases to about 10% when vitamin ingestion approaches 10 times the recommended intake in pill form.

From the intestinal cell, pantothenic acid enters portal blood for transport to the liver and other body cells. Pantothenic acid is found free in the blood, primarily within the red blood cells. The uptake of the vitamin into organs is dependent upon the same SMVT carrier as is found in the intestine. Pantothenic acid, 4-phosphopantothenic acid, and pantetheine all may be found within cells. Most pantothenic acid is used to synthesize or resynthesize CoA, which is found in fairly high concentrations in the liver, adrenal gland, kidneys, brain, and heart.

Functions and Mechanisms of Action

Pantothenic acid functions in the body as a component of the acylation factors, CoA and 4′-phosphopantetheine (the prosthetic group for acyl carrier protein). The synthesis of 4′-phosphopantetheine and CoA which requires pantothenic acid, the amino acid cysteine, and ATP is depicted in Figure 9.17 and outlined hereafter.

- The synthesis of coenzyme A starts with the rate-limiting phosphorylation of pantothenic acid by pantothenate kinase to form 4′-phosphopantothenic acid. ATP and Mg^{2+} are required for this reaction, which occurs in the cytosol.

- Next, in another ATP- and Mg^{2+}-requiring reaction in the cytosol, cysteine reacts with the 4′-phosphopantothenic acid to form 4-phosphopantothenylcysteine. A peptide bond is formed between the carboxyl group of the 4′-phosphopantothenic acid and the amino group of cysteine by the enzyme phosphopantothenylcysteine synthase.

- Third, a carboxyl group from the cysteine moiety is removed by phosphopantothenylcysteine decarboxylase to generate 4′-phosphopantetheine in the cytosol.

- Next, an adenylation occurs in the mitochondrial inner membrane whereby ATP reacts with the

4′-phosphopantetheine; adenosine monophosphate (AMP) is added to the 4′-phosphopantetheine to form dephosphocoenzyme A with the release of pyrophosphate.

- Last, phosphorylation with ATP of the 3′-hydroxyl group of the dephosphocoenzyme A produces CoA. This reaction also occurs in the mitochondrial inner membrane.

The synthesis of CoA is inhibited by acetyl-CoA, malonyl-CoA, and propionyl-CoA as well as by other, longer-chain acyl-CoAs. CoA metabolism has been reviewed in depth by Robishaw and Neely [3]. Figure 9.18 shows the structure of CoA. Note from this figure that CoA contains several components, including phosphopantetheine and adenosine 3′,5′-bisphosphate. The figure also shows the active site where CoA binds to acyl groups through the formation of a thio ester $\overset{O}{\overset{\|}{(-S-C-R)}}$ with carboxylic acids. CoA can in turn transfer these groups, typically 2 to 13 carbons in length, as needed for various cellular reactions. Examples of some carboxylic acids carried by CoA include:

- acetic acid (two carbons)
- malonic acid (three carbons)
- propionic acid (three carbons)
- methylmalonic acid (four carbons)
- succinic acid (four carbons)

These carboxylic acids arise in the body during metabolism, and some can be obtained exogenously by ingesting food. For example, propionic acid is found naturally in some fish and also is derived from the catabolism of several amino acids, including methionine, threonine, and isoleucine, and from the catabolism of odd-chain fatty acids. As another example, succinic acid is found as an intermediate in the TCA cycle.

Coenzyme A

Pantothenic acid, as part of CoA, participates extensively in nutrient metabolism, including degradation reactions resulting in energy production and synthetic reactions for the production of many vital compounds. In addition to its role in nutrient metabolism, CoA acetylates nutrients, including sugars and proteins among others. Some of the specific reactions and processes involving CoA are presented next.

The metabolism of carbohydrate, lipids, and protein (energy-producing nutrients) relies to varying degrees on CoA. For example, a crucial reaction in nutrient metabolism is the conversion of pyruvate to acetyl-CoA, which condenses with oxaloacetate to introduce acetate for oxidation during the TCA cycle (Figure 9.8). Acetyl-CoA, the common compound formed from the three energy-producing nutrients, holds the central position in the

transformation of energy. Pantothenic acid thus joins the B vitamins thiamin, riboflavin, and niacin in the oxidative decarboxylation of pyruvate (Figure 9.9). These same vitamins also participate in the oxidative decarboxylation of α-ketoglutarate to succinyl-CoA, a TCA cycle intermediate and compound used with the amino acid glycine to synthesize heme.

In lipid metabolism, CoA is important in the synthesis of cholesterol, bile salts, ketone bodies, fatty acids, and steroid hormones. For example, in cholesterol and ketone body synthesis, acetyl-CoA and acetoacetyl-CoA react to form the key intermediate HMG-CoA (Figure 5.34). Condensation of acetyl-CoA with activated CO_2 to form malonyl-CoA represents the first step in fatty acid synthesis (Figure 5.28). Moreover, phospholipid and sphingomyelin production from phosphatidic acid and sphingosine, respectively, also use acyl-CoA.

Pantothenic acid as CoA is involved in the acetylation (donation of the long-chain fatty acids or acetate) of some proteins and sugars as well as some drugs. The acetylation of the proteins by CoA occurs posttranslationally and in turn affects protein functions, activity, and location. For example, acetylation of some proteins and peptides prolongs half-life, thereby delaying the degradation of the protein, while acetylation of some enzymes results in either activation or inactivation. Other proteins that may undergo acetylation include microtubules of the cell's cytoskeleton as well as histones and other DNA-binding proteins. Microtubules, made from polymerization of α- and β-tubulin dimers, appear to be stabilized by acetylation and destabilized when deacetylated. Choline is acetylated to form the neurotransmitter acetylcholine. Also, aminosugars such as glucosamine and galactosamine are acetylated by CoA to form N-acetyl glucosamine and N-acetyl galactosamine, respectively. These acetylated aminosugars in turn may function structurally in the cell, for example, to provide recognition sites on cell surfaces or to direct proteins for membrane functions, among other roles.

Acyl Carrier Protein (ACP)

Pantothenic acid as part of 4′-phosphopantetheine also functions as the prosthetic group for acyl carrier protein, a component of the fatty acid synthase complex. The sulfhydryl group in the 4′-phosphopantetheine prosthetic group binds and transfers acyl groups to another sulfhydryl group located in the enzyme complex. These two groups are located close to each other so that the acyl chain being synthesized can be transferred between them. Fatty acid synthesis is discussed further in Chapter 5.

Metabolism and Excretion

Pantothenic acid does not appear to undergo metabolism prior to excretion. The vitamin is excreted intact primarily in the urine, with only small amounts excreted in the feces. No metabolites of the vitamin have been identified in the urine or feces. Urinary excretion of pantothenic acid usually ranges from about 1 to 8 mg/day.

Adequate Intake

The Adequate Intake (AI) recommendation for adults for pantothenic acid is 5 mg [3]. AIs for pantothenic acid of 6 mg/day and 7 mg/day are suggested for women during pregnancy and lactation, respectively [3]. The inside front cover of this book provides AIs for pantothenic acid for other age groups.

Deficiency: Burning Feet Syndrome

Burning feet syndrome is characterized by numbness of the toes and a sensation of burning in the feet. The condition is exacerbated by warmth and diminished with cold and is thought to result from pantothenic acid deficiency. The syndrome can be corrected with calcium pantothenate administration. Other symptoms of deficiency include vomiting, fatigue, weakness, restlessness, and irritability. A metabolic inhibitor of pantothenic acid, omega methylpantothenate, has been used in studies to induce low pantothenate status in humans.

Deficiency of pantothenic acid is thought to occur more often in conjunction with multiple nutrient deficiencies, as in malnutrition. Some conditions that may increase the need for the vitamin include alcoholism, diabetes mellitus, and inflammatory bowel diseases. Increased excretion of the vitamin has been observed in people with diabetes mellitus. Absorption is likely to be impaired with inflammatory bowel diseases. Intake of the vitamin typically is low in people with excessive alcohol intake.

Toxicity

Pantothenic acid toxicity has not been reported to date in humans. Intakes of about 10 g of pantothenic acid as calcium pantothenate daily for up to 6 weeks have caused no problems [2]. However, intakes of about 15 to 20 g have been associated with mild intestinal distress, including diarrhea [2].

Assessment of Nutriture

Blood pantothenic acid concentrations < 100 mg/dL are thought to reflect low dietary pantothenic acid intakes; however, blood concentrations do not correlate well with changes in dietary pantothenic acid intake and status. Urinary pantothenic acid excretion is considered to be a better indicator of status, with excretion of < 1 mg/day considered indicative of poor status.

References Cited for Pantothenic Acid

1. Said HM. Cellular and molecular aspects of human intestinal biotin absorption. J Nutr. 2009; 139:158–62.
2. Food and Nutrition Board. Dietary Reference Intakes for Thiamin, Riboflavin, Niacin, Vitamin B_6, Folate, Vitamin B_{12}, Pantothenic Acid, Biotin, and Choline. Washington, DC: National Academy Press. 1998 pp. 357–73.
3. Robishaw J, Neely J. Coenzyme A metabolism. Am J Physiol. 1985; 248:E1–9.

BIOTIN

Biotin's discovery was based upon research investigating the cause of what was called egg white injury. Eating raw eggs was known to result in hair loss, dermatitis, and various neuromuscular problems. Szent-Györgyi in 1931 found a substance (now called biotin) in liver that could cure and prevent the condition. It was not until about 10 years later (the early 1940s) that Kogl (from Europe) and du Vigneaud and colleagues (from the United States) determined biotin's structure. Biotin consists structurally of two rings—an ureido ring joined to a thiophene ring—with an additional valeric acid side chain (Figure 9.19). Biotin was once called vitamin H (the H refers to *haut* in German and means "skin") as well as vitamin B_7.

Sources

In addition to being made by intestinal bacteria living within the colon, biotin is found widely distributed in foods. Good food sources include liver (beef, about 31 μg), soybeans, and egg yolk (about 4 μg), as well as cereals (Cheerios® and Frosted Flakes®, 0.03 and 0.04 μg/serving), legumes, and nuts (peanuts 4.9 μg, almonds 1.3 μg/serving) [1]. Canned salmon provides about 3.7 μg/serving [1]. The Daily Value for biotin is 30 μg. Within many foods, biotin is found either bound covalently to protein or as biocytin (also called biotinyllysine), which consists of biotin bound to the amino acid lysine (Figure 9.20).

Avidin, a glycoprotein in raw egg whites, irreversibly binds biotin in what has been suggested as the tightest noncovalent bond found in nature. This binding in turn prevents biotin absorption. Yet, because avidin is heat

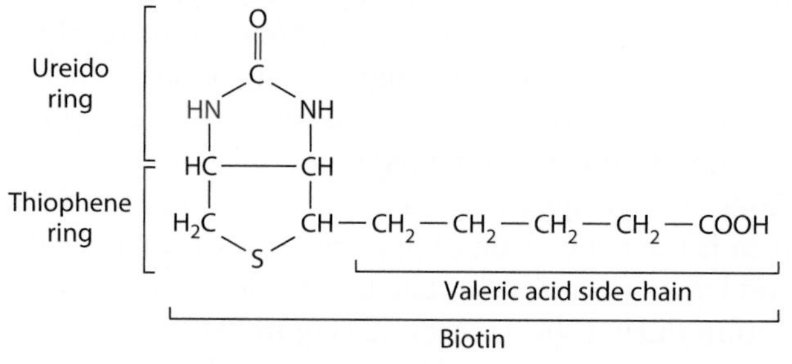

Figure 9.19 The structure of biotin.

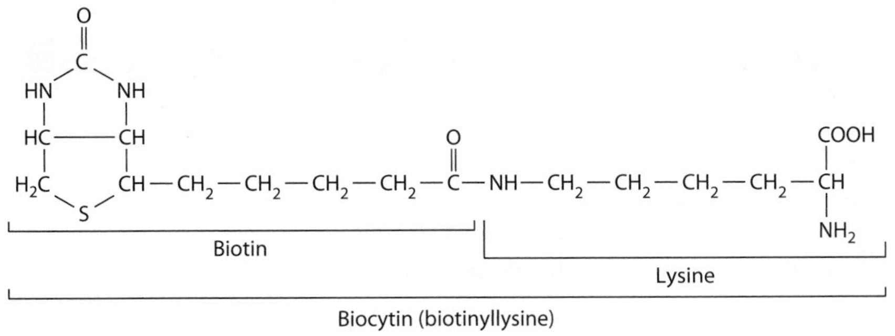

Figure 9.20 The structure of biocytin, also called biotinyllysine.

labile (unstable with heat), eating cooked egg whites does not compromise biotin absorption.

Digestion, Absorption, Transport, and Storage

Protein-bound biotin requires digestion by enzymes prior to absorption. Proteolysis by pepsin and intestinal proteases yields free biotin, biotinyl peptides, or biocytin. Biotinyl peptides are further hydrolyzed by other proteases or peptidases within the small intestine, and biocytin is further hydrolyzed by biotinidase. Biotinidase is found on the intestinal brush border membrane as well as in pancreatic and intestinal juices secreted into the small intestine. The enzyme hydrolyzes the biocytin to release free biotin and lysine in the intestine. Some undigested biocytin may be absorbed intact by peptide carriers and subsequently hydrolyzed by biotinidase present in plasma and in most other body cells.

Biotinidase is active over a wide pH range, and its activity is expressed in multiple cellular locations including the nucleus. At a more acidic pH, biotinidase cleaves biocytin to produce biotin and lysine, or cleaves covalently bound biotin from any biotinyl peptides that have been released as biotinylated proteins are degraded. The enzyme also cleaves biotin from histones. At a more alkaline pH, the enzyme itself becomes biotinylated while also generating free lysine; in other words, the biotinidase enzyme becomes attached to the biotin that was previously part of biocytin. Biotinidase deficiency (first discovered in 1983) is caused by an autosomal recessive inborn error of metabolism. Should infants and children with the disorder go untreated, a biotin deficiency, among other problems, develops. Some clinical features associated with the genetic disorder include developmental delays, dermatitis, alopecia (hair loss), seizures, ataxia, aciduria, and acidosis.

Free biotin is absorbed nearly completely, primarily in the proximal small intestine [2,3]. Biotin that is synthesized by colonic bacteria is absorbed in the proximal and midtransverse colon; however, bacterially made biotin cannot totally meet the biotin needs of humans [2]. Alcohol inhibits biotin absorption in both the small intestine and colon.

The mechanism of biotin absorption varies with intake. Biotin absorption occurs by passive diffusion with consumption of pharmacologic doses (as is needed with some genetic disorders). With physiological biotin intakes, biotin absorption across the brush border membrane of the small intestine and across the colon cell membranes is carrier mediated and sodium dependent. The main carrier for biotin found in the small intestine as well as the liver (among other tissues) also transports pantothenic acid and lipoic acid and is called the sodium-dependent multivitamin transporter (SMVT) [2]. SMVT transcription is regulated by cell biotin concentrations. With high cellular biotin, an enzyme called holocarboxylase synthetase (discussed further under enzyme roles) translocates to the nucleus, where it biotinylates specific histones at the promoter site of the SMVT gene and suppresses transcription of the vitamin transporter gene. Transport of biotin across the basolateral membrane of the enterocyte is SMVT carrier mediated, but not sodium dependent [2].

Biotin is found in the plasma mostly (~80%) in a free, unbound state, with lesser amounts bound to plasma proteins, including albumin, α- and β-globulins, and biotinidase, which has two binding sites for the vitamin and arises from hepatic secretion [4]. Biotin uptake into the liver, and probably other tissues, is thought to involve SMVT as well as monocarboxylate transporter (MCT) 1 for blood mononuclear (and possibly other) cells. Biotin is stored in small quantities in the muscle, liver, and brain.

Functions and Mechanisms of Action

Biotin functions in cells as a coenzyme. In addition, biotin functions in noncoenzyme capacities including possible roles in cell proliferation and gene expression.

Coenzyme Roles

For coenzyme functions within cells, biotin is covalently bound to each of four carboxylases (Table 9.2). The attachment of biotin to these enzymes occurs in two steps and is catalyzed by the enzyme holocarboxylase synthetase, which is found in both the cell cytosol and mitochondria. In the first step of biotinylation of the

Table 9.2 Biotin-Dependent Enzymes

Enzyme	Role	Significance
Pyruvate carboxylase	Converts pyruvate to oxaloacetate	Replenishes oxaloacetate for TCA cycle Necessary for gluconeogenesis
Acetyl-CoA carboxylase	Forms malonyl-CoA from acetate	Commits acetate units to fatty acid synthesis
Propionyl-CoA carboxylase	Converts propionyl-CoA to methylmalonyl-CoA	Provides mechanism for metabolism of some amino acids and odd-numbered chain fatty acids
β-methylcrotonyl-CoA carboxylase	Converts β- methylcrotonyl-CoA to β-methylglutaconyl-CoA	Allows catabolism of leucine and certain isoprenoid compounds

carboxylases, biotin reacts with ATP in a Mg^{2+}-dependent reaction to form biotinyl adenosine monophosphate (also called activated biotin) and pyrophosphate. In the second step, the activated biotin reacts with any of four apocarboxylases to form a holoenzyme carboxylase (sometimes called holocarboxylases or biotinylated carboxylases) with the release of AMP. A mutation in holocarboxylase synthetase, as was first discovered in 1981, or in any of the four biotin-dependent carboxylases negatively impacts metabolism and is manifested in the first month of life by vomiting, lethargy, aciduria, hypotonia, and acidosis.

The four biotinylated carboxylases, which are synthesized by holocarboxylase synthetase, are pyruvate carboxylase, acetyl-CoA carboxylase, propionyl-CoA carboxylase, and β-methylcrotonyl-CoA carboxylase.

Table 9.2 lists these enzymes and their roles in metabolism. Knowles [5] provides detailed information on the mechanism of action of the biotin-dependent enzymes.

Each biotinylated carboxylase is a multisubunit enzyme to which biotin is attached by an amide linkage. Specifically, the carboxyl terminus of biotin's valeric acid side chain is linked to the ε amino group of a specified lysine residue in the carboxylase apoenzyme, as shown in Figure 9.21 [6]. The chain connecting biotin and the apoenzyme is long and flexible, allowing the biotin to move from one active site of the carboxylase to another. One active site on the apoenzyme generates the carboxybiotin enzyme, and the other transfers the activated carbon dioxide (as HCO_3^-) to a reactive carbon on the substrate. Figure 9.22 illustrates the formation of the CO_2-biotin-enzyme complex.

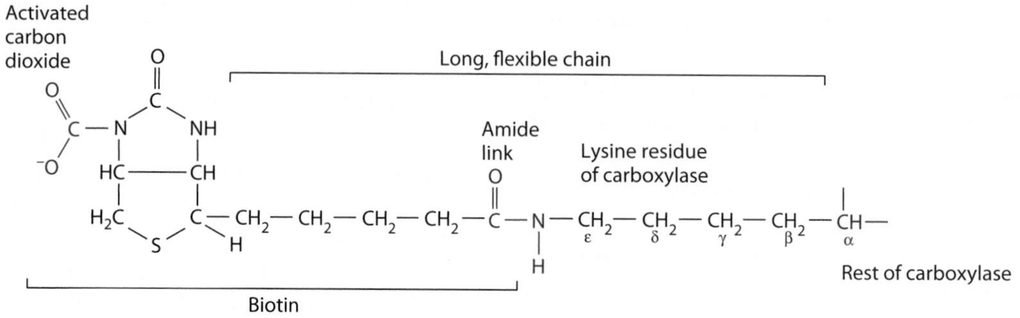

Figure 9.21 Biotin bound to the lysine residue of carboxylase and functioning as a carrier of activated CO_2.

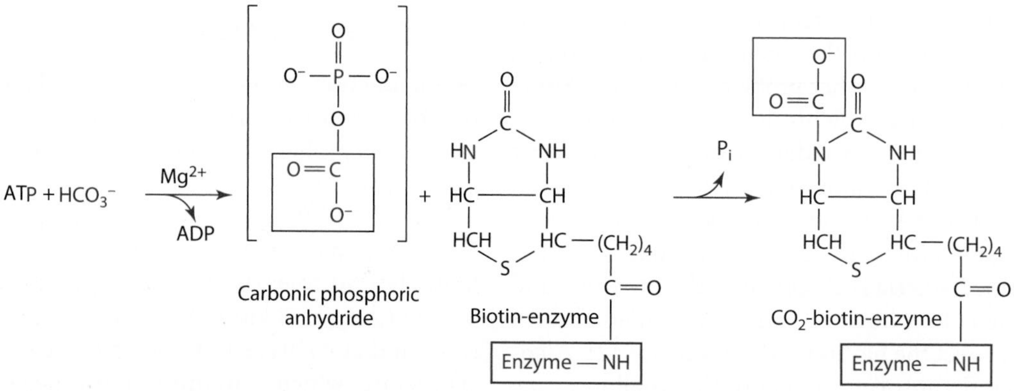

Figure 9.22 The formation of the CO_2-biotin-enzyme complex.

Pyruvate Carboxylase Pyruvate carboxylase is a particularly important enzyme because of its regulatory function. Specifically, pyruvate carboxylase (a mitochondrial enzyme) catalyzes the carboxylation of pyruvate to form oxaloacetate (Figure 9.23). For its activation, pyruvate carboxylase requires the presence of acetyl-CoA as well as ATP and Mg^{2+}. Acetyl-CoA serves as an allosteric activator, and its presence indicates the need for increased amounts of oxaloacetate. If the cell has a surplus of ATP, the oxaloacetate is then used for gluconeogenesis. However, if the cell is deficient in ATP, the oxaloacetate enters the TCA cycle on condensation with acetyl-CoA.

Acetyl-CoA Carboxylase The importance of biotin in energy metabolism is further exemplified by its role in the initiation of fatty acid synthesis—that is, the formation of malonyl-CoA from acetyl-CoA by the regulatory and rate-limiting enzyme acetyl-CoA carboxylase (see Figure 5.28). This enzyme (found in both the mitochondria and the cytosol) is allosterically activated by citrate and isocitrate, and inhibited by long-chain fatty acyl-CoA derivatives. ATP and Mg^{2+} are required for the reaction.

Propionyl-CoA Carboxylase Propionyl-CoA carboxylase (a mitochondrial enzyme) is important for the catabolism of the amino acids isoleucine, threonine, and methionine, each of which generates propionyl-CoA. Propionyl-CoA also arises from the catabolism of odd-number–chain fatty acids found, for example, in some fish. Propionyl-CoA carboxylase catalyzes the carboxylation of propionyl-CoA to D-methylmalonyl-CoA (Figure 9.24). The reaction requires ATP and Mg^{2+}. Deficient or defective propionyl-CoA carboxylase activity causes the genetic disorder propionic acidemia, characterized by the accumulation of propionyl-CoA, which is then shifted into an alternate metabolic pathway. This alternate pathway results in increased production and urinary excretion of 3-hydroxypropionic acid (3HPA) and methylcitrate (MCA).

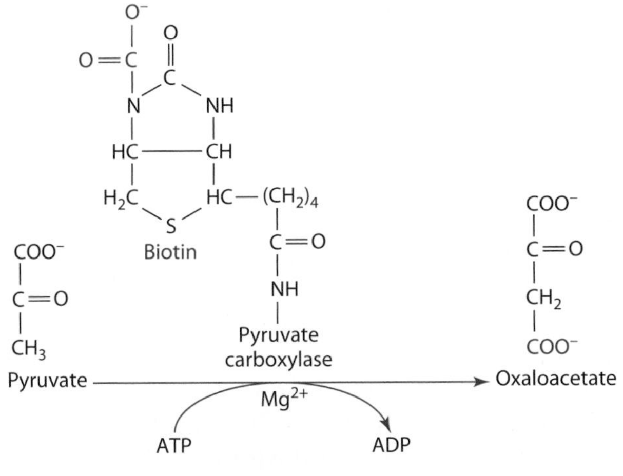

Figure 9.23 The role of biotin in the synthesis of oxaloacetate from pyruvate.

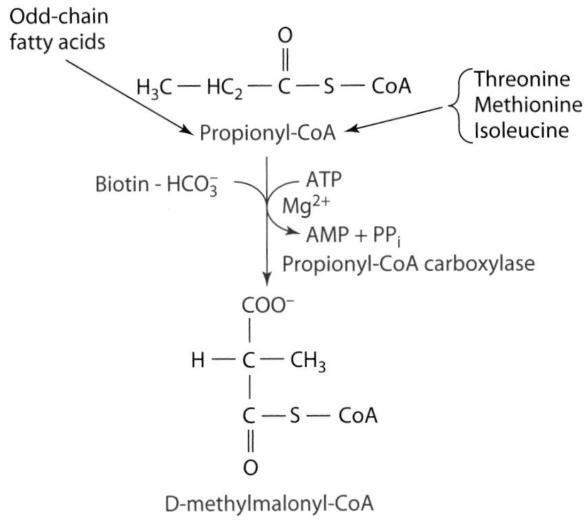

Figure 9.24 The role of biotin in the oxidation of propionyl-CoA.

β-methylcrotonyl-CoA Carboxylase β-methylcrotonyl-CoA carboxylase is important in the catabolism of the amino acid leucine. During leucine catabolism (Figures 6.36 and 9.25), β-methylcrotonyl-CoA is formed. This compound is carboxylated in an ATP-, Mg^{2+}-, and biotin-dependent reaction by β-methylcrotonyl-CoA carboxylase to form β-methylglutaconyl-CoA, which is further catabolized to generate acetoacetate and acetyl-CoA. Deficient β-methylcrotonyl-CoA carboxylase activity causes the accumulation of β-methylcrotonyl-CoA, which is then shunted into an alternate metabolic pathway. This alternate pathway results in increased production and urinary excretion of 3-hydroxyisovaleric acid (3-HIA), 3-methylcrotonylglycine (3MCG), and isovalerylglycine (IVG). Increased 3-HIA and decreased biotin concentrations in the urine are indicative of biotin deficiency [5].

Noncoenzyme Roles

Although the coenzyme role of biotin is well characterized, other possible roles of biotin are less known and investigated. Some of these roles are reviewed briefly in this section.

Biotinylation of Proteins and Gene Expression Biotin influences multiple cellular functions through biotinylation of proteins, especially nonhistone and histone proteins. Histones, of which there are five classes—H1, H2A, H2B, H3, and H4—are small proteins that group together and are found bound to or associated with DNA and thus chromatin. DNA base pairs are wrapped in the histones, which when tightly packed together minimize access to gene promoter sequences. Modification of the histones, however, can open up the "packing." Histones consist of a flexible amino (also called N) terminus (often called the histone tail) and a globular domain. It is the tail section of the histones that can be covalently modified (e.g., by biotinylation, acetylation, and methylation).

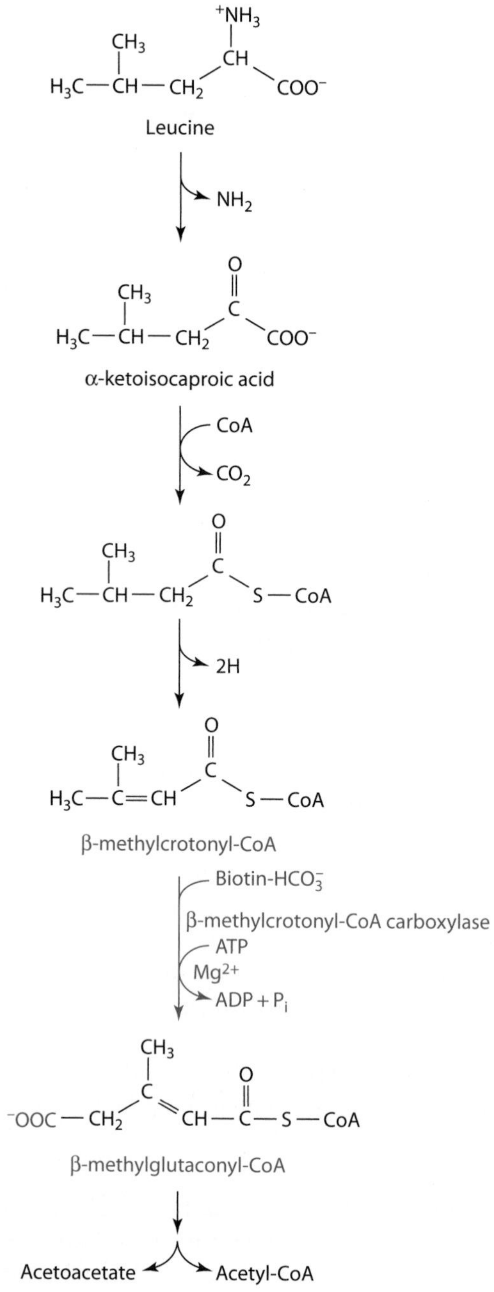

CH$_3$
H$_3$C—CH—CH$_2$—CH(^+NH$_3$)—COO$^-$

Leucine

↓ ⤙ NH$_2$

CH$_3$
H$_3$C—CH—CH$_2$—C(=O)—COO$^-$

α-ketoisocaproic acid

↓ ⤙ CoA ⤚ CO$_2$

CH$_3$
H$_3$C—CH—CH$_2$—C(=O)—S—CoA

↓ ⤚ 2H

CH$_3$
H$_3$C—C=CH—C(=O)—S—CoA

β-methylcrotonyl-CoA

↓ ⤙ Biotin-HCO$_3^-$
β-methylcrotonyl-CoA carboxylase
⤙ ATP
Mg^{2+}
⤚ ADP + P$_i$

CH$_3$
$^-$OOC—CH$_2$—C=CH—C(=O)—S—CoA

β-methylglutaconyl-CoA

↓

Acetoacetate ⤙⤚ Acetyl-CoA

Figure 9.25 The role of biotin in leucine catabolism.

This modification causes the histones to "uncoil" and thus creates pores through which transcription factors can enter to reach DNA and activate gene promoter sequences. Some of the biotin-dependent transcription factors and cell signals that are involved in gene expression include biotinyl-AMP and cGMP, nuclear factors (NF)-κB, transcription factors Sp1 and Sp3, and receptor tyrosine kinases [7–9]. The attachment of biotin to histones is mediated by holocarboxylase synthetase and biotinidase. The biotinidase becomes biotinylated (i.e., forms biotinyl biotinidase) from the biotin moiety of biocytin and then transfers the biotin moiety to the histones to form biotinylated histones at an alkaline pH.

Over 2,000 human genes depend upon biotin for expression. Effects of biotin on gene expression have been demonstrated in animal and *in vitro* studies. Specifically, biotin appears to be necessary for the transcription of some genes and for the translation of some mRNAs [10–14]. For example, biotin stimulates the expression (transcription) of glucokinase but inhibits the expression of phosphoenolpyruvate carboxykinase [7,12]. Biotin also increases mRNA levels of 6-phospho-fructokinase when given to biotin-deficient rats, and mRNA levels of holocarboxylase synthetase are reduced with biotin deficiency and then increased in response to biotin supplementation [12].

Cell Cycle Biotin is required for cells to progress normally through the cell cycle. Studies show that mononucleated blood cells at the G1, S, G2, and M phases of the cell cycle displayed significantly more biotinylated histones versus quiescent cells [8,9]. Further, deficiency of biotin appears to cause cells to arrest in the G1 phase.

Metabolism and Excretion

Catabolism of the biotin holocarboxylases by proteases yields biotin oligopeptides and ultimately biocytin. The biocytin is then typically degraded by biotinidase to yield lysine and free biotin. While the biotin is usually further degraded, small amounts of intact biotin and biocytin may appear in the urine. In the catabolism of biotin, only small amounts of metabolites are formed from oxidation of the sulfur in biotin's ring; these metabolites include biotin sulfoxide and biotin sulfone. Most of the metabolites arise from the degradation of biotin's valeric acid side chain by β-oxidation. The main metabolites following catabolism of this side chain are bisnorbiotin and tetranorbiotin and, to a lesser degree, derived metabolites such as bisnorbiotin methyl ketone and tetranorbiotin methyl ketone. Biotin metabolites, some of which are shown in Figure 9.26, are excreted in the urine. Smoking appears to accelerate biotin catabolism in women [15].

Biotin that has been synthesized by intestinal bacteria but not absorbed is excreted in the feces. Very little dietary biotin that has been absorbed is excreted in feces [2].

Adequate Intake

Because intestinally synthesized biotin is not sufficient to maintain normal biotin status, humans need to obtain biotin from the diet. An Adequate Intake (AI) recommendation for adults of 30 μg of biotin per day has been suggested [16]. Adequate Intakes for biotin of 30 μg and 35 μg per day are suggested for women during pregnancy and lactation, respectively [16]. The inside front cover of this book provides additional AIs for biotin for other age groups.

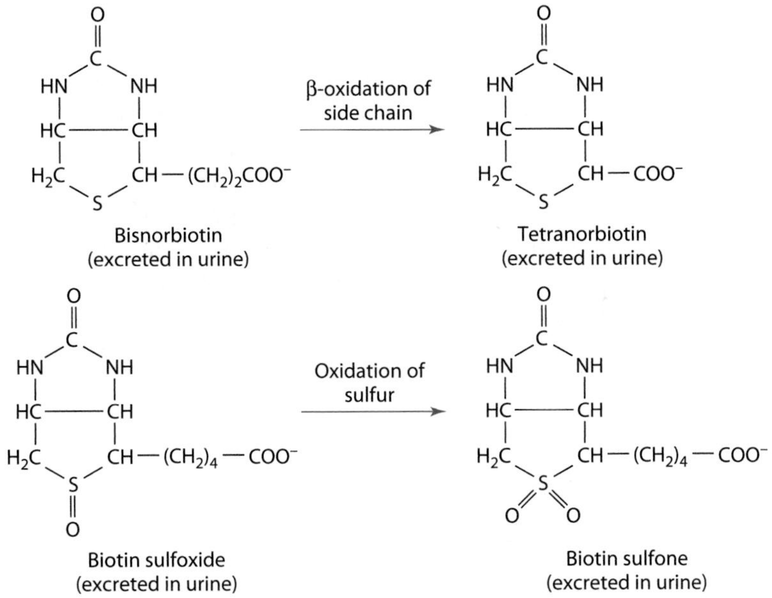

Figure 9.26 Selected metabolites from biotin degradation.

Deficiency

Because some biotin is synthesized by intestinal bacteria and absorbed, biotin deficiency in humans is rare. Nonetheless, it can occur, especially in those with a genetic mutation such as a biotinidase deficiency. Some of the neurologic symptoms associated with a biotin deficiency include lethargy, paresthesia in extremities (an abnormal sensation which may feel like pins and needles or numbness), hypotonia (reduced muscle tone), depression, and hallucinations. The most notable cutaneous symptom is a red, scaly dermatitis found around the eyes, nose, and mouth. In addition, anorexia, nausea, alopecia (hair loss), and muscle pain may occur. Death may result if biotin deficiency goes untreated. Therapeutic doses of up to 10 mg of biotin daily are used to treat a deficiency.

Biotin deficiency or poor biotin status may be present in selected populations. People who ingest raw eggs in excess amounts are likely to develop biotin deficiency because of impaired biotin absorption. Impaired biotin absorption also may occur with gastrointestinal disorders such as inflammatory bowel disease or in chronic consumers of excessive alcohol, which decreases biotin absorption. Biotin status has been shown to decline in some women during pregnancy [6] and in those on anticonvulsant drug therapies such as phenobarbital, phenytoin, or carbamazepine. People with genetic defects involving biotinidase and holocarboxylase synthetase activities develop biotin deficiency unless treated with pharmacologic doses of biotin. Biotin supplements in amounts of 5 to 10 mg daily are used to treat biotinidase deficiency, and doses of 40 to 100 mg of biotin daily are needed for those with holocarboxylase synthetase deficiency.

Toxicity

Toxicity from biotin use has not been reported, and no Tolerable Upper Intake Level has been established [16]. Fairly large doses (100 mg or more) of biotin have been given daily, without side effects, to people with inherited disorders of biotin metabolism. Use of biotin as a hair and skin conditioning agent in cosmetics has also been shown to be safe [17].

Assessment of Nutriture

The evaluation of biotin in the blood and urine is used most often to assess biotin status. Normal plasma biotin concentrations range from about 215 to 750 pg/mL. Low plasma concentrations of biotin, however, have not been shown to accurately reflect intake or status [16].

Decreased urinary biotin excretion (<6 μg/day or <200 pg/mL) and increased urinary excretion of 3-hydroxyisovaleric acid and 3-hydroxyisovaleryl carnitine, generated from altered metabolism of β-methylcrotonyl-CoA, are sensitive and early indicators of biotin deficiency [6,16,18]. Normal 3-hydroxyisovaleric acid excretion is < 0.2 μmol/mg of creatinine. A diet devoid of biotin can result in decreased plasma biotin concentrations and in reduced biotin excretion in about 2 to 4 weeks [19].

References Cited for Biotin

1. Staggs CG, Sealey WM, McCabe BJ, et al. Determination of the biotin content of select foods using accurate and sensitive HPLC/avidin binding. J Food Compost Anal. 2004; 17:767–76.
2. Said HM. Cellular and molecular aspects of human intestinal biotin absorption. J Nutr. 2009; 139:158–62.
3. Subramanya SB, Subramanian VS, Kumar JS, et al. Inhibition of intestinal biotin absorption by chronic alcohol feeding: cellular and molecular mechanisms. Am J Physiol Gastrointest Liver Physiol. 2011; 300:G494–501.

4. Mock D, Malik M. Distribution of biotin in human plasma: most of the biotin is not bound to protein. Am J Clin Nutr. 1992; 56:427–32.

5. Knowles J. The mechanism of biotin-dependent enzymes. Ann Rev Biochem. 1989; 58:195–221.

6. Stratton SL, Horvath TD, Bogusiewicz A, et al. Urinary excretion of 3-hydroxyisovaleryl carnitine is an early and sensitive indicator of marginal biotin deficiency in humans. J Nutr. 2011; 141:353–58.

7. Pacheo-Alvarez D, Solorzano-Vargas R, Del Rio A. Biotin in metabolism and its relationship to human disease. Arch Med Res. 2002; 33:439–47.

8. Stanley J, Griffin J, Zempleni J. Biotinylation of histone in human cells: effects of cell proliferation. Eur J Biochem. 2001; 268:5424–29.

9. Zempleni J. Uptake, localization, and noncarboxylase roles of biotin. Ann Rev Nutr. 2005; 25:175–96.

10. Peters DM, Griffin JB, Stanley JS, et al. Exposure of UV light causes increased biotinylation of histones in Jurkat cells. Am J Physiol Cell Physiol. 2002; 283:C878–84.

11. Kothapalli N, Sarath G, Zempleni J. Biotinylation of K12 in histone H4 decreases in response to DNA double-strand breaks in human jar choriocarcinoma cells. J Nutr. 2005; 135:2337–42.

12. Chauhan J, Dakshinamurti K. Transcriptional regulation of the glucokinase gene by biotin in starved rats. J Biol Chem. 1991; 266: 10035–38.

13. Solorzano-Vargas R, Pacheco-Alvarez D, Leon-Del-Rio A. Holocarboxylase synthetase is an obligate participant in biotin-mediated regulation of its own expression and of biotin-dependent carboxylases mRNA levels in human cells. Proc Nutr Acad Sci. 2002; 99:5325–30.

14. Rodriguez-Melendez R, Cano S, Mendez S, Velazquez A. Biotin regulates the genetic expression of holocarbxylase synthetase and mitochondrial carboxylases in rats. J Nutr. 2001; 131:1909–13.

15. Sealey W, Teague A, Stratton S, Mock D. Smoking accelerates biotin catabolism in women. Am J Clin Nutr. 2004; 80:932–35.

16. Food and Nutrition Board. Dietary Reference Intakes for Thiamin, Riboflavin, Niacin, Vitamin B$_6$, Folate, Vitamin B$_{12}$, Pantothenic Acid, Biotin, and Choline. Washington, DC: National Academy Press. 1998 pp. 374–89.

17. Fiume M. Final report on the safety assessment of biotin. Internl J Toxicology. 2001; 20(suppl4):1–12.

18. McMahon R. Biotin metabolism and molecular biology. Ann Rev Nutr. 2002; 22:221–39.

19. Lewis B, Rathman S, McMahon R. Dietary biotin intake modulates the pool of free and protein-bound biotin in rat liver. J Nutr. 2001; 131:2310–15.

Suggested Reading

Symposium: advances in the understanding of the biological role of biotin at the clinical, biochemical, and molecular level. J Nutr. 2009; 139:152–70.

FOLATE

Folate's and vitamin B$_{12}$'s discoveries resulted from the search to cure the disorder megaloblastic anemia, a problem in the late 1870s and early 1880s. As with many of the other vitamins, eating liver was shown to cure the condition. Mitchell and colleagues are credited with folate's discovery in 1941.

The terms *folate* and *folic acid* are not interchangeable. *Folic acid* refers to the oxidized form of the vitamin *found in fortified foods and in supplements*. *Folate* refers to the reduced form of the vitamin *found naturally in foods and in biological tissues*. The Latin word *folium* means "leaf," and the word *folate* from Italian means "foliage."

Folate is composed of three parts, all of which must be present for vitamin activity. Figure 9.27 shows the structure of folate. As shown in the figure, 2-amino-4-hydroxpteridine, also called pteridine or pterin, is conjugated by a methylene group (—CH$_2$—) to para-aminobenzoic acid (PABA) to form pteroic acid. The carboxy group of PABA is peptide-bound to the amino group of glutamic acid to form folate, which is also called pteroylglutamic acid or pteroylmonoglutamic acid. In the body, metabolically active folate has multiple glutamic acid residues attached. Although humans can synthesize all three components of the vitamin, they do not have the conjugase enzyme necessary for the coupling of the pterin molecule to PABA to form pteroic acid.

Sources

Good food sources of folate include mushrooms and green vegetables such as spinach (131 μg/½ cup), Brussels sprouts, broccoli (92 μg/½ cup), asparagus (127 μg/½ cup), turnip and collard greens (~75 μg/½ cup), and okra. Additional good sources of the vitamin are peanuts, legumes (especially pinto with 155 μg/½ cup, black with 130 μg/½ cup, and lima and kidney beans), lentils (160 μg/½ cup), fruits (especially strawberries and oranges) and their juices, and liver. A banana, orange, or ¼ cantaloupe provides about 20 to 30 μg of folate.

Raw foods are typically higher in folate than cooked foods because of folate losses incurred with cooking. Folate is destroyed by heat, oxidation, and exposure to ultraviolet light. It is also reduced by 50% to 80% with food processing and preparation. Thus, consuming folate-rich foods raw or after cooking them quickly in little water can help to minimize loss of the vitamin.

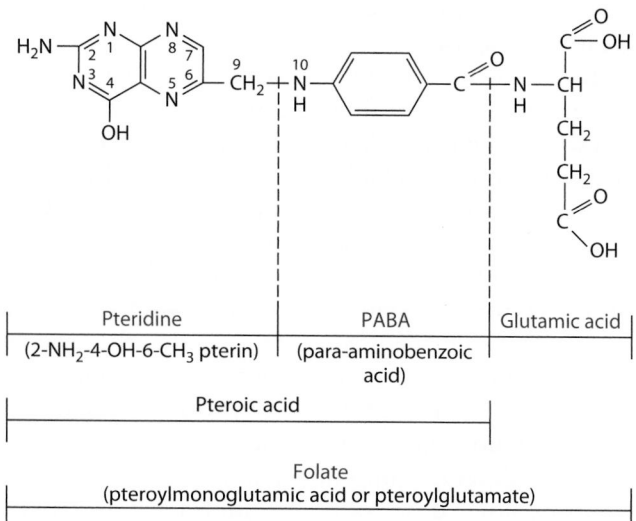

Figure 9.27 Structural formula of folate. Folate is made up of pteridine, which is conjugated by a methylene group (—CH$_2$—) to PABA, forming pteroic acid. The carboxy group (—CO—) of PABA is peptide bound to the amino group (—NH—) of glutamic acid to form the monoglutamate form of folate.

Fortification of flours, grains, and cereals with folic acid (140 μg of folic acid per 100 g of product) was initiated in 1998. Thus, fortified cereals, breads, and grain products now represent major sources of the vitamin. Enriched white bread provides 2.5 to 3 μg/slice, and fortified oatmeal provides 100 μg/cup. Bran cereal with raisins has 25% of the Daily Value of 400 μg, or 100 μg folate. Some juices are also fortified with folic acid. Because of this fortification program more Americans are meeting recommendations for folate intakes.

Folate in foods exists primarily in the reduced form, and it usually contains up to nine glutamic acid residues (versus the one glutamic acid shown in Figure 9.27) attached to PABA. The principal pteroylpolyglutamates in foods are 5-methyl tetrahydrofolate (THF) and 10-formyl THF, although over 150 different forms of folate have been reported. In supplements and in fortified foods, folic acid is provided as pteroylmonoglutamate, the most oxidized and stable form of the vitamin. As a supplement, folic acid is almost completely bioavailable (especially if consumed on an empty stomach). When fortified foods are consumed with natural sources of folate, the vitamin is about 85% bioavailable.

Generally, folate bioavailability from a mixed diet is thought to be about 50%, although it may range from 10% to 98% [1,2]. Variations in intestinal pH, genetic variations in enzymatic activity needed for folate digestion, dietary constituents such as inhibitors, and the food matrix influence bioavailability. Because of the difference in the efficiency of folate absorption from foods versus folic acid from supplements and fortified grain products, folate equivalents are used in recommendations for dietary folate intakes (see the "Recommended Dietary Allowances" subsection in this section).

Digestion, Absorption, Transport, and Storage

Before the polyglutamate forms of folate in foods can be absorbed, they must be digested to the monoglutamate form. This hydrolysis or deconjugation is performed by at least two folylpoly γ-glutamyl/glutamate carboxypeptidases (FGCP), also referred to as pteroylpolyglutamate hydrolases or conjugases. These enzymes exhibit separate activities in the jejunum, one soluble (from pancreatic juice and bile), and the other bound to the enterocyte's brush border membrane. The brush border carboxypeptidase is a zinc-dependent exopeptidase that stepwise cleaves the polyglutamate into monoglutamate. Zinc deficiency impairs carboxypeptidase activity and diminishes digestion and thus absorption of folate [3]. Alcohol ingestion and inhibitors in foods such as legumes, lentils, cabbage, and oranges also diminish enzyme activity to impair digestion of the vitamin's polyglutamate forms and thus

inhibit folate absorption. Folic acid in fortified foods and supplements does not need to undergo digestion because it already is present in the monoglutamate form.

The main carrier system responsible for transporting folate as well as 5-methyl THF into intestinal cells is the proton-coupled folate transporter (PCFT). This high-affinity folate carrier is found mostly in the duodenum, but also in the upper jejunum. While this transporter has also been shown to serve as a heme carrier protein, it is not thought to be of physiological significance for heme transport in humans. Because defects in PCFT result in hereditary folate malabsorption and severe folate deficiency, PCFT is thought to be the primary transporter of folate into intestinal cells [4]. PCFT-mediated folate absorption may be reduced in alkaline environments but enhanced in acidic conditions.

Within the intestinal cell, folic acid and folate are reduced to dihydrofolate (DHF), which is then reduced to generate THF (Figure 9.28). The reduction to THF occurs stepwise through the action of NADPH-dependent dihydrofolate reductase, a cytosolic enzyme (Figure 9.28). Four hydrogens are added at positions 5, 6, 7, and 8. Folate-binding proteins are thought to transport folate within cells. Transport of folate across the enterocyte's basolateral membrane to enter the blood is active and carrier dependent, likely involving multidrug resistance protein (MRP) 3 [4]. Folate is found in portal circulation as folate and 5-methyl THF, although dihydrofolate and formylated forms are also present; all forms are as mono- and not polyglutamates.

The uptake of folate into the liver and other tissues is carrier mediated. Reduced folate carriers (RFC), which are ubiquitously expressed, deliver folate from systemic circulation into many cells. Proton-coupled folate transporter, which is also expressed on many tissue membranes including the liver, kidneys, and spleen, among others, also is responsible for folate uptake into some tissues. Lastly, three folate receptors (FRα, β, or γ), which have been identified on the cell surfaces of some tissues, are thought to mediate uptake [4].

Within liver cells, THF is found as THF (~33%), converted to 5-methyl THF (~33%), and converted to either 5- or 10-formyl THF (~33%). Bound to these various folates are four to eight glutamate residues. Folylpolyglutamate synthetase, found in a variety of body tissues, catalyzes the ATP-dependent additions of the glutamates, which are usually added one at a time to the monoglutamate. Addition of these glutamate residues traps the folate in the cell. Before release into systemic blood, however, glutamate residues are removed from folate polyglutamates by hydrolases.

In systemic blood, folate is found as a monoglutamate either free (~1/3) or bound to proteins (~2/3), including albumin, α-2 macroglobulin, and a high-affinity folate-binding protein, which is thought to represent a soluble

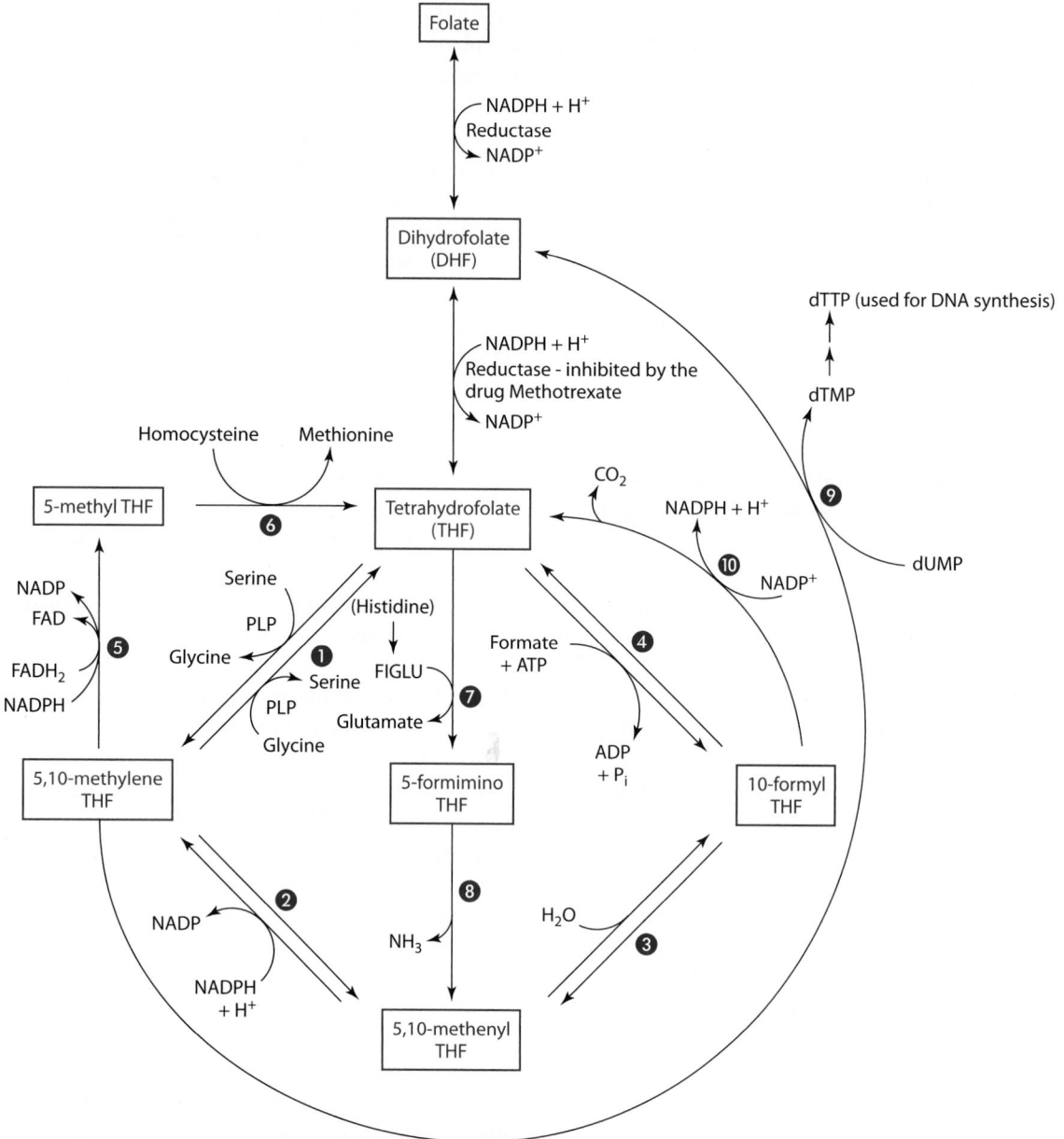

Enzymes involved in interconversions of coenzyme forms of THF:

1 Serine hydroxymethyltransferase (coenzyme-PLP) - folate accepts carbon units as 5,10-methylene from serine resulting in 5, 10-methylene THF and glycine generation; the reverse reaction also occurs.

2 Methylene THF dehydrogenase - interconversions between coenzyme forms of folate; the generation of 5,10-methylene THF from 5, 10-methenyl THF is important given the roles of 5,10-methylene THF in serine synthesis and pyrimidine synthesis.

3 Cyclohydrolase - interconversion between coenzyme forms of folate. The production of 10-formyl THF is especially important for purine synthesis.

4 Formate-activating enzyme - interconversions between coenzyme forms of folate. 10-formyl THF is especially important for purine synthesis.

5 Methylene-THF reductase - the generation of 5-methyl THF is essential for methionine synthesis from homocysteine.

6 Methionine synthetase (coenzyme-B$_{12}$) - see Figure 9.30 for details on this reaction.

7 Formiminotransferase - folate accepts a formimino group from FIGLU and facilitates the final step in histidine catabolism.

8 Cyclodeaminase - interconversion between coenzyme forms of folate.

9 Thymidylate synthetase - 5,10-methylene THF provides the formaldehyde group for this reaction needed for pyrimidine synthesis.

10 10-formyl THF dehydrogenase - interconversion between coenzyme forms of folate.

Figure 9.28 Interconversions of coenzyme forms of tetrahydrofolate (THF).

form of the cell membrane-derived folate receptor. The major forms of folate found in systemic blood are THF, 5-methyl THF, and 10-formyl THF. Red blood cells contain more folate than does plasma; however, red blood cell folate is attained during erythropoiesis. In other words, folate is not taken up by mature red blood cells. Thus, red blood cell folate concentrations represent an index of longer-term (2–3 months) folate status than does plasma.

Total body folate levels range from about 11 to 28 mg [5], with about one-half stored in the liver. The main storage forms are the polyglutamate forms of THF and 5-methyl THF. Storage occurs in association with intracellular folate-binding proteins.

Folate is found in both the cytosol and mitochondria of cells, where it functions as a coenzyme or cosubstrate to accept and donate one-carbon units. The availability of folate to crucial tissues where rapid cell division is occurring appears to be regulated when folate is limited. The mechanisms of this regulation are unclear but may involve changes in the rate of synthesis of polyglutamates and the release of folate monoglutamates from less metabolically active tissues to the liver, which then redistributes the folate to the actively proliferating cells through unknown processes.

Functions and Mechanisms of Action

THF functions as a coenzyme in both the mitochondria and cytosol to accept single- or one-carbon groups (generated typically from amino acid metabolism) at specific positions (N5 and/or N10) on the pteridine ring. These THF derivatives then serve as donors of one-carbon units in a variety of synthetic reactions, including amino acid, purine, and pyrimidine synthesis.

The coenzyme forms of folate are interconvertible (as shown in Figure 9.28), except that 5-methyl THF cannot be converted directly back to 5,10-methylene THF. Genetic polymorphisms in some of the folate-dependent enzymes have been identified. Several mutations in FAD-dependent methylene THF reductase (sometimes abbreviated MTHFR), which converts 5,10-methylene THF to 5-methyl THF, have been identified. Such mutations impair 5-methyl THF formation and thus reduce remethylation of homocysteine (see the Perspective at the end of this chapter for further information on this mutation).

The THF derivatives, their one-carbon units, and the oxidation states are illustrated as follows:

5- and 10-formyl THF	$O{=}CH$	Formate
5-formimino THF	$-HC{=}NH-$	Formate
5,10-methenyl THF	${=}CH-$	Formate
5,10-methylene THF	$-CH_2-$	Formaldehyde
5-methyl THF	$-CH_3$	Methanol

The formyl derivatives represent the most oxidized forms of folate, and 5-methyl THF is the most reduced form. Table 9.3 provides an overview of some of the metabolic roles of folate.

Amino Acid Metabolism

Folate is involved in the metabolism of several amino acids, including histidine, serine, glycine, and methionine.

Table 9.3 Forms of Folate and Their Metabolic Roles in the Body

Folate Form	Roles
10-formyl THF	**Folate transfers formate as 10-formyl THF for purine synthesis:**
	5-phosphoribosylglycinamide ribonucleotide (GAR) conversion to 5-phosphoribosyl formylglycinamide (FGAR) by glycinamide ribonucleotide transformylase and
	5-phosphoribosyl 5-amino 4-imidazole carboxyamide ribonucleotide (AICAR) conversion to 5-phosphoribosyl 5-formamido 4-imidazole carboxamide ribonucleotide (FAICAR) by aminoimidazolecarboxamide ribonucleotide transformylase
5, 10-methylene THF	**Folate transfers formaldehyde as 5,10-methylene for pyrimidine synthesis:**
	Deoxyuridine monophosphate (dUMP) conversion to deoxythymidine monophosphate (dTMP) by thymidylate synthetase
	Folate receives formaldehyde for serine degradation/glycine synthesis:
	Serine conversion to glycine by serine hydroxymethyltransferase
	Folate receives formaldehyde for glycine degradation:
	Glycine conversion to carbon dioxide and ammonium by the glycine cleavage system
	Folate receives formaldehyde for glycine synthesis:
	Dimethylglycine and its catabolic product sarcosine are degraded to glycine by dimethylglycine dehydrogenase and sarcosine dehydrogenase, respectively
5-formimino THF	**Folate receives a formimino group in histidine degradation:**
	Formiminoglutamate (FIGLU) conversion to glutamate by formiminotransferase
5-methyl THF	**Folate provides a methyl group for methionine synthesis:**
	Homocysteine conversion to methionine by methionine synthase

Histidine The final reaction in histidine catabolism requires THF. Histidine catabolism begins with deamination of the amino acid to generate urocanic acid, which undergoes further metabolism to yield formiminogluta-mate (FIGLU). The formimino group is removed from FIGLU with the help of formiminotransferase to generate glutamate. THF receives the formimino group to yield 5-formimino THF, as shown here and in Figure 9.29.

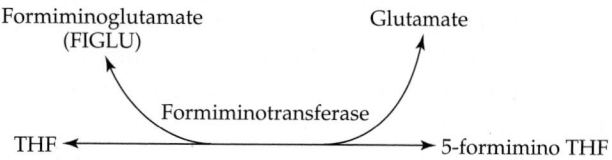

This reaction can be used as a basis for determining folate deficiency. In the diagnostic procedure, subjects are given an oral histidine load, and FIGLU excretion is measured in the urine. With adequate folate (THF), FIGLU is converted to glutamate, and little to no FIGLU appears in the urine. With a folate deficiency, FIGLU accumulates in the blood and is excreted in higher than normal concentrations in the urine.

Serine and Glycine Serine represents a major source of one-carbon units for use in folate reactions. The enzyme serine hydroxymethyltransferase, which requires vitamin B_6 as pyridoxal phosphate (PLP) for activity and is found in the cytosol and mitochondria in all tissues, especially the liver and kidneys, transfers a one-carbon unit from serine to THF to generate glycine and 5,10-methylene THF.

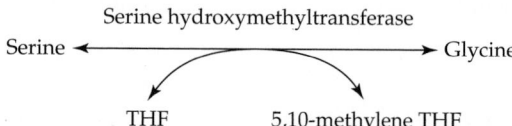

The conversion of serine to glycine is reversible. However, the direction of the reaction varies among tissues; some tissues, such as the kidneys, generate more serine, whereas others generate more glycine.

Some additional reactions involving glycine metabolism also require folate. Glycine degradation, for example, requires THF, as shown here.

$$Glycine \xrightarrow[\text{NAD}^+ \quad \text{NADH} + \text{H}^+]{\text{THF} \quad \text{5,10-methylene THF}} CO_2 + {}^+NH_4$$

Glycine synthesis from choline degradation also involves folate. Choline is catabolized in the liver in a NAD^+-dependent reaction to form betaine and NADH + H^+. Betaine, also called trimethylglycine, functions as a methyl donor that provides methyl groups to compounds such as homocysteine through a methyltransferase. Removal of the methyl group from betaine, which is oxidized primarily in the liver and kidneys, generates dimethylgly-cine. The dimethylglycine undergoes further metabolism to generate sarcosine (also called monomethylglycine) in a reaction catalyzed by dimethylglycine dehydrogenase. Sarcosine dehydrogenase converts sarcosine to glycine, with THF functioning as the carbon acceptor, forming 5,10-methylene THF. Riboflavin as FAD also is required.

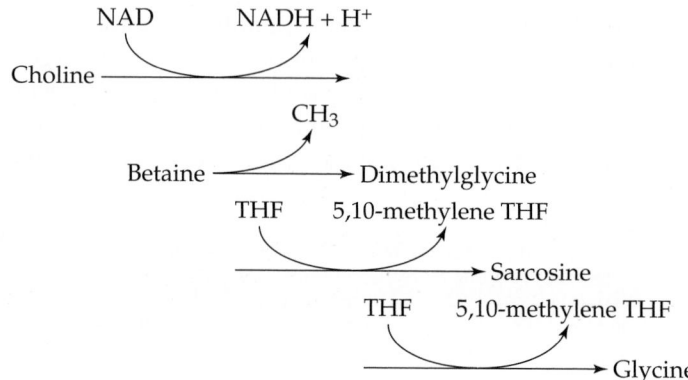

Figure 9.29 The role of folate in histidine catabolism.

In addition to its synthesis from choline, betaine is found in the diet in both animal and plant foods. Estimated betaine intake ranges from about 1 to 2.5 g per day. Folic acid supplementation appears to increase betaine concentrations [6], and betaine supplements reduce plasma homocysteine concentrations in those with elevated blood levels [7].

Methionine Methionine regeneration from homocysteine also involves folate as 5-methyl THF. Before this regeneration is addressed, a brief review of the conversion of methionine to homocysteine (discussed also in more detail in Chapter 6) may be helpful. As shown in Figure 9.30, methionine is converted initially to S-adenosyl methionine (SAM) in an ATP-requiring reaction catalyzed by methionine adenosyl transferase. The removal of the methyl group from SAM results in the formation of S-adenosyl homocysteine (SAH). Removal of the adenosyl group from SAH yields homocysteine.

Folate is needed for the remethylation of homocysteine to form methionine. This reaction, which occurs when SAM concentrations are low, requires folate as 5-methyl THF as a methyl donor and vitamin B_{12} in the form of methylcobalamin as a prosthetic group for methionine synthase (also called homocysteine methyltransferase). For methionine synthase to transfer a methyl group from 5-methyl THF to homocysteine, cobalamin must be tightly bound to the enzyme. While bound to methionine synthase, cobalamin picks up the methyl group from 5-methyl THF to generate methylcobalamin and THF. Methylcobalamin then serves as the methyl donor for converting homocysteine to methionine. These reactions are shown in Figure 9.30 and are broken down into steps to facilitate understanding in the "Functions and Mechanisms of Action" section under vitamin B_{12}.

SAM is an important compound, serving as a methyl donor in many reactions in the body. For example, DNA and RNA methylation, myelin maintenance, neural

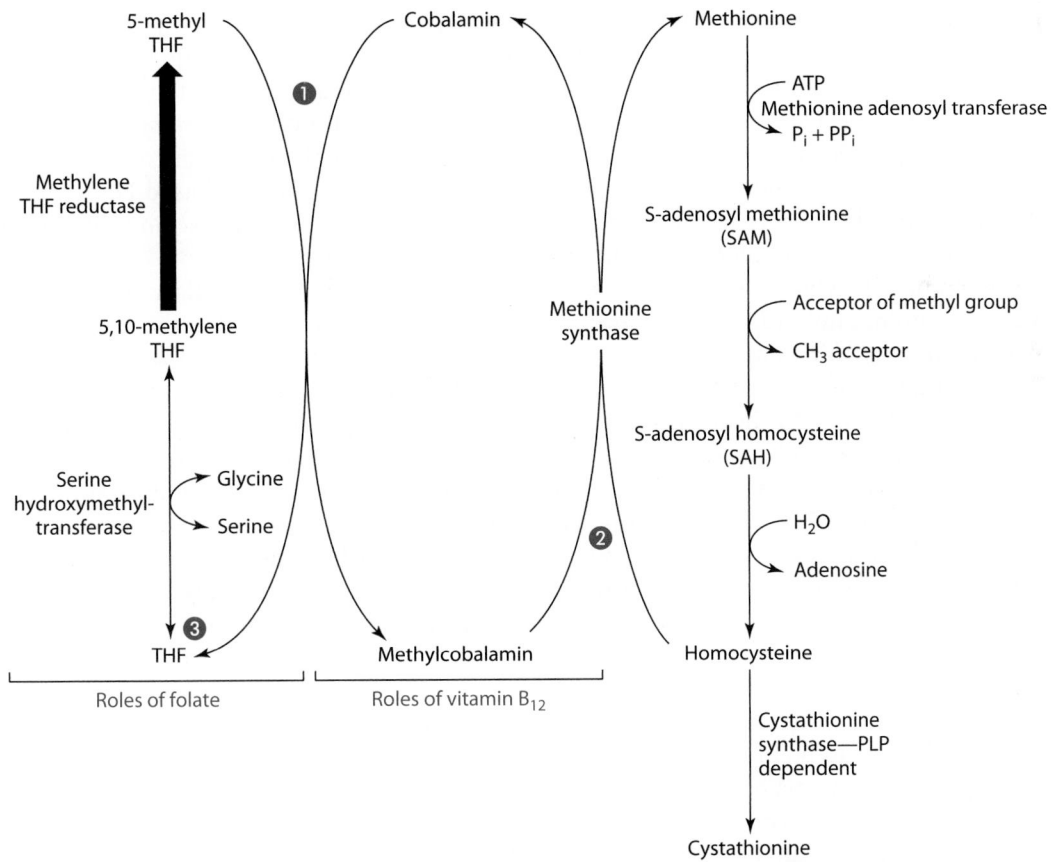

❶ Cobalamin, which is bound to the enzyme methionine synthase, picks up the methyl group on 5-methyl THF, forming THF and methylcobalamin.

❷ Methylcobalamin, which is still bound to the enzyme methionine synthase, gives the methyl group to homocysteine, which then forms methionine and reforms cobalamin.

❸ THF must be reconverted to 5-methyl THF for the reaction to proceed again. This process requires two reactions catalyzed first by serine hydroxymethyl transferase to generate 5,10-methylene THF. Second, methylene THF reductase converts 5,10-methylene THF to 5-methyl THF, which can once again donate its methyl group to cobalamin.

Figure 9.30 The resynthesis of methionine from homocysteine, showing the roles of folate and vitamin B_{12}.

function, and polyamine, carnitine, and catecholamine synthesis, among other processes, are dependent upon methylation reactions using SAM. SAM concentrations in part regulate methionine metabolism, including the remethylation of homocysteine to methionine. SAM concentrations increase with increased methionine. Higher SAM concentrations stimulate the transsulfuration pathway in which homocysteine is converted, in an irreversible reaction, to cystathionine by vitamin B_6–dependent cystathionine synthase (Figure 9.30) and ultimately is converted to cysteine. Higher SAM concentrations (as well as the endproduct 5-methyl THF) inhibit methylene THF reductase, which converts 5,10-methylene THF to 5-methyl THF. This inhibition decreases 5-methyl THF availability to decrease remethylation of homocysteine.

Possible Relationships with Diseases The roles of folate and vitamin B_{12} in the conversion of homocysteine to methionine, along with the role of vitamin B_6 in the conversion of homocysteine to cystathionine (Figure 9.30), continue to receive considerable attention. The attention results because low intakes of these three vitamins, especially folate, are inversely associated with plasma homocysteine concentrations, and elevated plasma homocysteine concentrations ($>15\ \mu mol/L$) are associated with premature heart disease, occlusive vascular disease, and cerebral (i.e., stroke) and peripheral vascular diseases.

The mechanisms by which hyperhomocysteinemia increases vascular disease risk have not been elucidated, but it may act by impairing endothelial function, promoting the growth of smooth muscle cells leading to vascular lesions, promoting an autoimmune response, and/or promoting platelet adhesiveness and clotting, among other hypotheses. A 5 $\mu mol/L$ increase in serum homocysteine concentrations increases the risk for heart disease by as much as 20% to 30% [8]. Folic acid supplementation in people with hyperhomocysteinemia improves endothelial function. Supplementation of folic acid, vitamin B_{12}, and vitamin B_6 in people (both healthy and with heart disease) with hyperhomocysteinemia normalizes or reduces blood homocysteine concentrations but does not consistently diminish the risk of cardiovascular events or stroke [9–12].

Another condition possibly linked to poor folate status is dementia, including Alzheimer's dementia [13]. Memory and abstract thinking appear to be influenced by folate. Cognitive dysfunction and dementia have been shown to correlate with plasma homocysteine concentrations, which in turn are influenced in part by folate status [14].

Folate deficiency or poor folate status is suspected in the development (initiation) of some cancers, especially colon cancer but also lung and other gastrointestinal cancers [15]. Folate deficiency in cells and tissues may alter gene expression to promote cancer. Folate deficiency–induced breaks in chromosomes are thought to result from hypomethylation of DNA—that is, decreased DNA

methylation (especially of tumor suppression genes)—and/or increased DNA strand breaks (associated with misincorporation of uridylate for thymidylate in DNA caused by folate deficiency, as discussed in the next section) [16]. Polymorphisms in methylenetetrahydrofolate reductase can decrease the likelihood for colorectal cancers, as discussed in more detail in the Perspective at the end of this chapter. In addition, cancer may be promoted with folate deficiency due to instability of DNA and altered gene transcription.

Purine and Pyrimidine Synthesis/Nucleotide Metabolism

The involvement of THF derivatives in purine and pyrimidine synthesis makes folate essential for DNA synthesis and cell division. The synthesis of cells with short life spans, such as enterocytes and red blood cells (erythrocytes), is particularly affected if folate is inadequate.

In pyrimidine synthesis, thymidylate synthetase uses 5,10-methylene THF to convert deoxyuridine monophosphate (dUMP) to thymidylate (dTMP) and dihydrofolate (DHF) (Figures 6.28 and 9.28). The folate provides formaldehyde as 5,10-methylene THF. dTMP is required for DNA synthesis; the reaction is rate limiting to DNA replication. Inadequate folate restricts this conversion and normal cell cycle progression, causing intracellular uracil accumulation, misincorporation of uracil into DNA, and ultimately increased DNA strand breakage. Both thymidylate synthetase and dihydrofolate reductase (which converts DHF to THF) are especially active in cells, including tumor cells, undergoing division. The drug methotrexate is used in the treatment of some cancers and psoriasis, among other conditions, because it binds to dihydrofolate reductase's active site to prevent resynthesis of THF needed for actively dividing cells. Such effects help to diminish tumor growth.

In purine synthesis (see Figures 6.29 and 6.30), folate as 10-formyl THF provides formate in two reactions needed for purine (adenine and guanine) ring formation. Purine-ring carbon atom 2 is acquired by formylation of 5-phosphoribosyl 5-amino 4-imidazole carboxamide ribonucleotide (AICAR) by aminoimidazolecarboxamide ribonucleotide transformylase. Purine ring carbon 8 is also acquired by 10-formyl THF, which donates the formyl group to 5-phosphoribosylglycinamide, also called glycinamide ribotide (GAR), to form 5-phosphoribosyl formylglycinamidine ribotide (FGAR) in a reaction catalyzed by glycinamide ribonucleotide transformylase.

Interactions with Other Nutrients

A synergistic relationship exists between folate and vitamin B_{12}. This relationship, whereby without vitamin B_{12} the methyl group from 5-methyl THF cannot be removed and thus is trapped, is sometimes called the methyl-folate trap. The following sequence of events leads to the methyl-folate trap (tracing the reactions shown in Figures 9.28 and 9.30 is helpful). Serine donates single-carbon units through conversion to glycine, and in the process THF is converted to 5,10-methylene THF. The 5,10-methylene THF is readily reduced by a reductase to 5-methyl THF. 5-methyl THF is required for methionine synthesis from homocysteine. Methyl groups are transferred by the enzyme methionine synthase from 5-methyl THF to vitamin B_{12}. Adequate vitamin B_{12} must be present for the activity of methionine synthase. The addition of the methyl group to vitamin B_{12} generates methylcobalamin, which serves as the methyl donor for converting homocysteine to methionine. Without vitamin B_{12} to accept the methyl group from 5-methyl THF, the 5-methyl THF accumulates and is trapped, and THF is not regenerated. Thus, the cells have folate but not in a form that can be used for DNA synthesis. With adequate vitamin B_{12} status, the THF resulting from the methionine resynthesis can be used to make the forms of folate needed for DNA synthesis, including 10-formyl THF (which is needed for purine synthesis) and 5,10-methylene THF (which is needed for thymidylate synthesis).

Metabolism and Excretion

Folate is excreted from the body in both the urine and the feces. Within the kidneys, folate-binding proteins present in the renal brush border coupled with tubular reabsorption of the vitamin help the body retain needed folate. Excess folate is excreted in the urine with some folate excreted intact and some catabolized in the liver prior to excretion. Oxidative cleavage of folate is thought to occur between C9 and N10 of polyglutamate forms of the vitamin. This cleavage generates para-aminobenzoyl polyglutamate and pteridine. All but one of the glutamate residues are then hydrolyzed, and usually the compound is acetylated to form the major urinary metabolite N-acetyl para-aminobenzoyl glutamate. Smaller amounts of para-aminobenzoyl glutamate also are found in the urine.

In addition to urinary losses, folate (up to about 100 μg) is secreted by the liver into the bile. Most of this folate, however, is reabsorbed with enterohepatic recirculation, so vitamin losses in the feces are minimal. Folate of microbial origin, however, may appear in the feces in relatively high amounts.

Recommended Dietary Allowance

The recommendations for folate intake consider its bioavailability as well as several indices of nutriture in its determination. Folate requirements are estimated at 320 μg per day [5]. Recommendations for folate are provided as dietary folate equivalents (DFE), which account for the high bioavailability of folic acid taken as supplements versus the lower bioavailability of folate in foods. The RDA for adults for folate is 400 μg DFE per day, although some studies suggest that increased body size and MTHFR mutations may alter needs [5,17]. One DFE is equal to 1 μg of food folate, 0.6 μg of folic acid from a supplement or fortified food consumed with a meal, or 0.5 μg of folic acid from a supplement taken without food (empty stomach) [5]. Stated alternately, DFE = μg food folate + (1.7 × μg folic acid); the definition is based on the assumption that the bioavailability of folic acid supplemented in foods is greater than folate found naturally in foods by a factor of 1.7, while that of synthetic folic acid, when ingested on an empty stomach, is two times as much [5].

Because of evidence that folic acid supplementation during the periconceptional period of pregnancy may reduce the incidence of neural tube defects, the Centers for Disease Control and Prevention (CDC) suggests 400 μg of synthetic folic acid/day for women capable of becoming pregnant [18]. Foods that are good sources of folate (that is, that provide ≥ 10% of the 400 μg Daily Value or at least 40 μg/serving) are permitted by the U.S. Food and Drug Administration (FDA) to make the health claim "Healthful diets with adequate folate may reduce a woman's risk of having a child with a neural tube (brain or spinal cord) defect" [19]. RDAs for folate of 600 μg and 500 μg of DFE per day are suggested for pregnancy and lactation, respectively [5]. Additional RDAs for folate for other age groups are provided on the inside front cover of the book.

Deficiency: Megaloblastic Macrocytic Anemia

Folate deficiency results in megaloblastic macrocytic anemia—the release into circulation of red blood cells that are fewer than normal in number as well as large and immature. Other signs and symptoms of the condition include fatigue, weakness, headaches, irritability, difficulty concentrating, shortness of breath, and heart palpitations.

The deficiency is characterized initially (within a month if the diet is devoid of folate) by low plasma folate. Red blood cell folate concentrations diminish after about 3 to 4 months (remember red blood cells live about 90–120 days) of low folate intake. After approximately 4 to 5 months, rapidly dividing cells such as those in the gastrointestinal tract and blood become megaloblastic. Mean cell volume (MCV) increases, and hypersegmentation (increased lobes) of white blood cells (neutrophils) occurs, along with decreased blood cell counts. The treatment of the deficiency usually requires 1 to 5 mg folate daily.

Megaloblastic macrocytic anemia, also called megaloblastic anemia, is relatively common in the United States. It may result from a deficiency of either folate or vitamin B_{12}, both of which disrupt DNA synthesis (replication) and thus cell division. As discussed under the functions of folate, the 10-formyl THF coenzyme form of folate is needed for purine synthesis, and the 5,10-methylene THF coenzyme form is needed for thymidylate synthesis. Without folate, these compounds are not made, and DNA synthesis becomes impaired. In the bone marrow, precursor red blood cells exhibit deranged DNA synthesis and defective cell maturation and division, resulting in abnormally large (macrocytic) and immature red blood cells (megaloblasts) with shortened life spans. Over time, the megaloblasts steadily increase in number in the blood while the numbers of healthy red blood cells decrease in the blood. These changes diminish the blood's oxygen carrying capacity. Figure 9.31 reviews the formation and maturation of erythrocytes.

The impaired DNA synthesis is also evident in other body cells, especially those of the gastrointestinal tract, which also normally exhibit rapid turnover. Folate deficiency is associated with a bright red tongue, and the shortening of the villi's height and thinning of the layers of the gastrointestinal tract. The latter two changes may result in impaired nutrient absorption and diarrhea.

Some conditions associated with an increased need for folate intake include excessive alcohol ingestion (which inhibits folate digestion and thus absorption) and malabsorption disorders such as inflammatory bowel diseases. Several medications also affect folate. The diuretic furosemide, used to treat hypertension, decreases intestinal folate absorption. Folate deficiency has been observed in people taking diphenylhydantoin or phenytoin, anticonvulsants used to treat epilepsy. Folate and phenytoin each inhibit the gastrointestinal cellular uptake of the other. Methotrexate, used to treat rheumatoid arthritis and some cancers, among other conditions, binds to dihydrofolate reductase and thus prevents THF synthesis. Other drugs, including cholestyramine (used to treat high blood cholesterol concentrations) and sulfasalazine (used to treat inflammatory bowel diseases), have also been shown to interact with folate to create folate deficiency.

Other populations that appear to have an increased need for folate include those with the genetic polymorphisms in enzymes involved in folate metabolism such as the MTHFR 677C $\longrightarrow$ T variant (see the Perspective at the end of this chapter). Finally, because inadequate folate status in women increases the risk of neural tube defects in infants, specific recommendations are provided for women capable of becoming pregnant, as discussed in the section on Recommended Dietary Allowances. Folic acid supplements taken before or about the time of

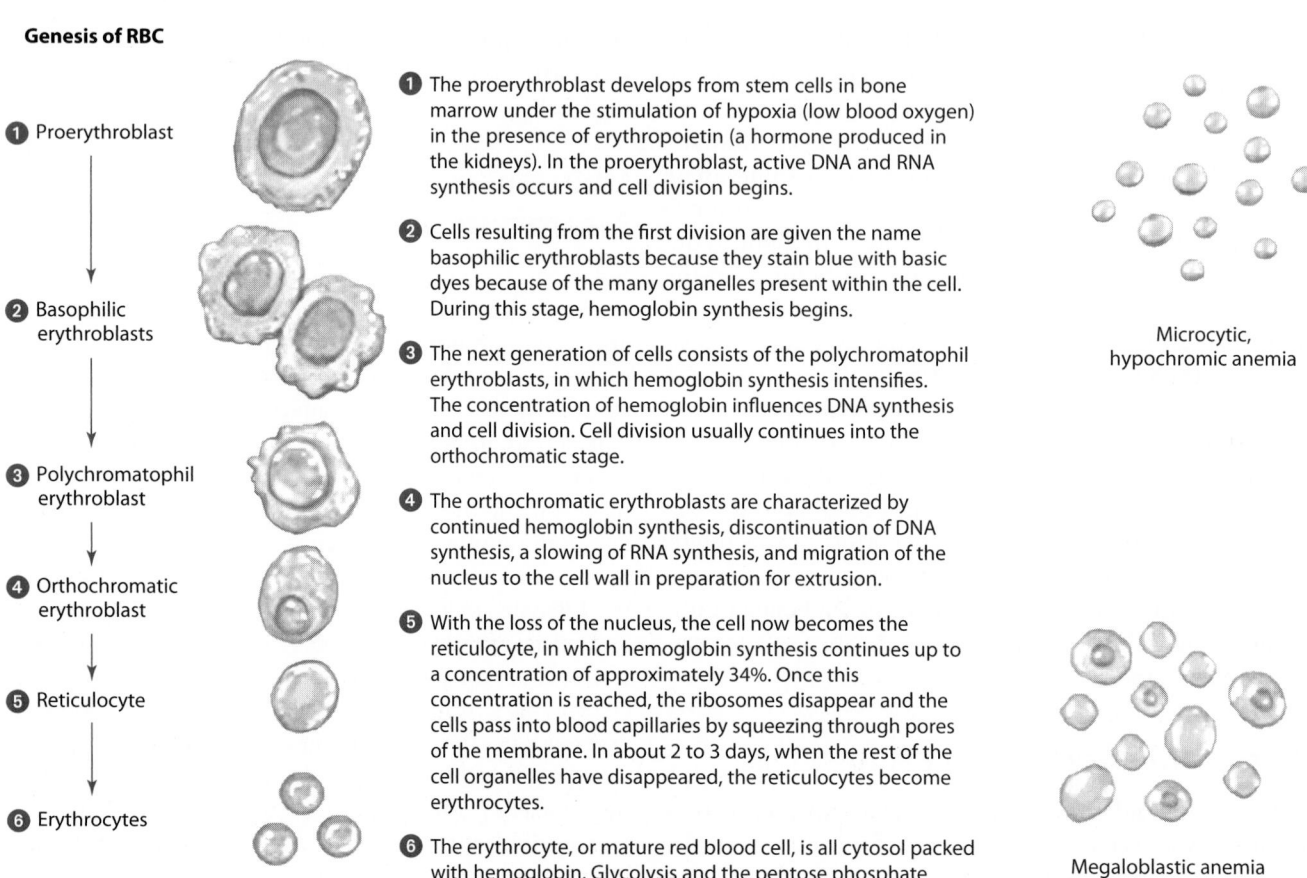

Genesis of RBC

1. Proerythroblast
2. Basophilic erythroblasts
3. Polychromatophil erythroblast
4. Orthochromatic erythroblast
5. Reticulocyte
6. Erythrocytes

1. The proerythroblast develops from stem cells in bone marrow under the stimulation of hypoxia (low blood oxygen) in the presence of erythropoietin (a hormone produced in the kidneys). In the proerythroblast, active DNA and RNA synthesis occurs and cell division begins.

2. Cells resulting from the first division are given the name basophilic erythroblasts because they stain blue with basic dyes because of the many organelles present within the cell. During this stage, hemoglobin synthesis begins.

3. The next generation of cells consists of the polychromatophil erythroblasts, in which hemoglobin synthesis intensifies. The concentration of hemoglobin influences DNA synthesis and cell division. Cell division usually continues into the orthochromatic stage.

4. The orthochromatic erythroblasts are characterized by continued hemoglobin synthesis, discontinuation of DNA synthesis, a slowing of RNA synthesis, and migration of the nucleus to the cell wall in preparation for extrusion.

5. With the loss of the nucleus, the cell now becomes the reticulocyte, in which hemoglobin synthesis continues up to a concentration of approximately 34%. Once this concentration is reached, the ribosomes disappear and the cells pass into blood capillaries by squeezing through pores of the membrane. In about 2 to 3 days, when the rest of the cell organelles have disappeared, the reticulocytes become erythrocytes.

6. The erythrocyte, or mature red blood cell, is all cytosol packed with hemoglobin. Glycolysis and the pentose phosphate pathway (hexose monophosphate shunt) are the only metabolic pathways occurring in the erythrocyte.

Microcytic, hypochromic anemia

Megaloblastic anemia

Figure 9.31 Genesis and maturation of the red blood cells (left); red blood cells characteristic of microcytic and megaloblastic anemias (right).

conception reduce the risk of neural tube defects; however, the mechanism(s) by which folate plays a role in the etiology of neural tube defects is unclear [20].

Toxicity

A Tolerable Upper Intake Level for adults of 1,000 μg (1 mg) for synthetic folic acid in supplements or from fortified foods (not natural foods) has been suggested based upon the ability of folate to mask the neurological manifestations of vitamin B_{12} deficiency [5]. Folic acid supplements can alleviate the megaloblastic anemia caused by a vitamin B_{12} deficiency, but the neurological damage caused by the deficiency progresses undetected and is irreversible (see the deficiency section for vitamin B_{12}). Folate intakes of 15 mg (i.e., 15 times the Tolerable Upper Intake Level) have been associated with insomnia, malaise, irritability, and gastrointestinal distress [5,21,22]. Additionally, intakes of supplemental folic acid in amounts ranging typically from about 0.8 mg up to about 5 mg have been shown to increase cancer risk and cancer mortality [16]. Some of the proposed mechanisms for the observed effects include increased uracil misincorporation and methylation (inactivation) of tumor suppression genes. Such findings may lead to a re-evaluation of the level of folic acid fortification in foods in the United States.

Assessment of Nutriture

Folate status is most often assessed by measuring folate concentrations in the plasma, serum, or red blood cells. Serum or plasma folate levels reflect recent dietary intake; thus, true deficiency must be interpreted through repeated measures of serum or plasma folate. Serum folate concentrations < 6.8 nmol/L (3 μg/L) typically suggest deficiency [5,23,24]. Red blood cell folate concentrations are more reflective of folate tissue status than is serum folate and represent vitamin status at the time the red blood cells were synthesized [5,24]. Red blood cell folate concentrations < 305 nmol/L (140 ng/mL) suggest folate deficiency; however, concentrations are also lowered with a vitamin B_{12} deficiency [5,24,25].

Formiminoglutamate (FIGLU) excretion may also be used to measure folate nutriture because folate as THF must be available for the formimino group to be removed from FIGLU and glutamate to be formed (Figure 9.29). FIGLU excretion is measured in a 6-hour urine collection after ingestion of 2 to 5 g oral L-histidine. Normal FIGLU excretion is <35 μM/day in folate-adequate adults, whereas with folate deficiency it rises to > 200 μM/day [23]. A deficiency of vitamin B_{12}, however, also elevates FIGLU excretion.

The deoxyuridine suppression test, another method for assessing folate status, measures the availability of folate for thymidine synthesis. In this test, the activity of thymidylate synthetase is measured in cultured lymphocytes

or bone marrow cells. The reaction catalyzed by thymidylate synthetase is dependent on folate and, indirectly, on vitamin B_{12}; therefore, the change in activity elicited by adding one or the other vitamin allows the deficiency to be identified. In other words, if a person were folate deficient, adding folate—but not vitamin B_{12}—would normalize enzyme activity. Likewise, if a person were vitamin B_{12} deficient, adding vitamin B_{12}—and not folate—would normalize thymidylate synthetase activity. In the case of a deficiency of both vitamins, enzyme activity could be normalized only by adding both vitamins [23].

A functional marker of folate and vitamin B_{12} deficiencies is elevated plasma homocysteine concentrations. Remember, both vitamins are required for the remethylation of homocysteine to methionine. With deficiency of either vitamin, plasma homocysteine concentrations become elevated.

References Cited for Folate

1. McNulty H, Pentieva K. Folate bioavailability. Proc Nutr Soc. 2004; 63:529–36.
2. Hannon-Fletcher M, Armstrong N, Scott J, et al. Determining bioavailability of food folates in a controlled intervention study. Am J Clin Nutr. 2004; 80:911–18.
3. Pfeffer C, Rogers L, Bailey L, Gregory J. Absorption of folate from fortified cereal grain products and of supplemental folate consumed with or without food determined using a dual label stable isotope protocol. Am J Clin Nutr. 1997; 66:1388–97.
4. Zhao R, Diop-Bove N, Visentin M, Goldman ID. Mechanisms of membrane transport of folates into cells and across epithelia. Ann Rev Nutr. 2011; 31:177–201.
5. Food and Nutrition Board. Dietary Reference Intakes for Thiamin, Riboflavin, Niacin, Vitamin B_6, Folate, Vitamin B_{12}, Pantothenic Acid, Biotin, and Choline. Washington, DC: National Academy Press. 1998 pp. 196–305.
6. Melse-Boonstra A, Holm P, Ueland P, et al. Betaine concentration as a determinant of fasting total homocysteine concentrations and the effect of folic acid supplementation on betaine concentrations. Am J Clin Nutr. 2005; 81:1378–82.
7. Craig SAS. Betaine in human nutrition. Am J Clin Nutr. 2004; 80:539–49.
8. Wald DS, Law M, Morris JK. Homocysteine and cardiovascular disease: evidence on causality from a meta-analysis. BMJ. 2002; 325:1202–09.
9. Abraham JM, Cho L. The homocysteine hypothesis: still relevant to the prevention and treatment of cardiovascular disease? Clin J Med 2010; 77:911–18.
10. Manolescu BN, Oprea E, Farcasanu IC, et al. Homocysteine and vitamin therapy in stroke prevention and treatment: a review. Acta Biochimica Polonica. 2010; 57:467–77.
11. DeBree A, Miero LA, Draijer R. Folic acid improves vascular reactivity in humans: a meta-analysis of randomized, controlled trials. Am J Clin Nutr. 2007; 86:610–07.
12. Marti-Carvajal AJ, Sola I, Lathyris D, Salanti G. Homocysteine lowering interventions for preventing cardiovascular disease. Cochrane Database Syst Rev. 2009; CD006612.
13. Ravaglia G, Forti P, Maioli F, et al. Homocysteine and folate as risk factors for dementia and Alzheimer disease. Am J Clin Nutr. 2005; 82:636–43.
14. Selhub J. Folate, vitamin B_{12} and vitamin B_6 and one carbon metabolism. J Nutr Hlth Aging. 2002; 6:39–42.
15. Su LJ, Arab L. Nutritional status of folate and colon cancer risk. Ann Epidemiol. 2001; 11:65–72.

16. Mason JB. Folate, cancer risk, and the Greek god, Proteus: a tale of two chameleons. Nutr Rev. 2009; 67:206–12.

17. Winkels RM, Bouwer IA, Verhoef P, et al. Gender and body size affect the response of erythrocyte folate to folic acid treatment. J Nutr. 2008; 138:1456–61.

18. Centers for Disease Control and Prevention (CDC). Recommendations for the use of folic acid to reduce the number of cases of spina bifida and other neural tube defects. MMWSR. 1992; 41:1–7.

19. FDA Labeling and Nutrition. www.fda.gov/food/LabelingNutrition/default.htm

20. Blom HJ, Smulders Y. Overview of homocysteine and folate metabolism. With special reference to cardiovascular disease and neural tube defects. J Inherit Metab Dis. 2011; 34:75–81.

21. Rogovik AL, Vohra S, Goldman RD. Safety considerations and potential interactions of vitamins: should vitamins be considered drugs? Ann Pharmacother. 2010; 44:311–24.

22. Drazkowski J, Sirven J, Blum D. Symptoms of B_{12} deficiency can occur in women of child-bearing age supplemented with folate. Neurology. 2002; 58:1572–73.

23. Gibson RS. Principles of nutritional assessment. New York: Oxford University Press. 2005 pp. 595–615.

24. Pfeiffer CM, Caudill SP, Gunter EW, et al. Biochemical indicators of B vitamin status in the US population after folic acid fortification. Am J Clin Nutr. 2005; 82:442–50.

25. Green R. Indicators for assessing folate and vitamin B_{12} status and for monitoring the efficacy of intervention strategies. Food Nutr Bull. 2008; 29(suppl):S52–63.

Suggested Readings

Bailey LB, Rampersaud GC, Kauwell GP. Folic acid supplements and fortification affect the risk for neural tube defects, vascular disease and cancer: evolving science. J Nutr. 2003; 133:S1961–68.

Cortese C, Motti C. MTHFR gene polymorphism, homocysteine and cardiovascular disease. Pub Hlth Nutr. 2001; 4:493–97.

Fairfield KM, Fletcher R. Vitamins for chronic disease prevention in adults. JAMA. 2002; 287:3116–26.

Friso S, Choi S-W. Gene-nutrient interactions and DNA methylation. J Nutr. 2002; 132:S2382–87.

Klerk M, Verhoef P, Clarke R, et al. MTHFR 677 C → T polymorphism and risk of coronary heart disease: a meta analysis. JAMA. 2002; 288:2023–31.

Malouf M, Grimley EJ, Areosa SA. Folic acid with or without vitamin B_{12} for cognition and dementia. Cochrane Database Syst Rev. 2003; (4):CD004514.

Olney RS, Mulinare J. Trends in neural tube defect prevalence, folic acid fortification, and vitamin supplement use. Semin Perinatol. 2002; 26:2777–85.

Shea TB, Lyons-Weiler J, Rogers E. Homocysteine, folate deprivation and Alzheimer neuropathology. J Alzheimer's Dis. 2002; 4:261–67.

VITAMIN B₁₂ (COBALAMIN)

Vitamin B_{12} (also called cobalamin) was the last vitamin to be discovered. It was isolated in 1948 by Smith (from England) and by Rickes and others (from the United States). Its structure was discovered by Hodgkin; however, Minot and Murphy in 1926 showed that eating large amounts of liver could help correct pernicious anemia associated with deficiency of the vitamin. It took about two decades to identify the vitamin in liver.

Vitamin B_{12} is considered a generic term for a group of compounds called corrinoids because of their corrin nucleus. The vitamin consists of a macrocyclic ring made of four reduced pyrrole rings linked together. In the ring's center is an atom of cobalt (Co) to which is attached, at almost right angles, the nucleotide 5,6-dimethylbenzimidazole. Also attached to the cobalt atom in vitamin B_{12} is one of the following:

Group Attached	Resulting Compound
—CN	Cyanocobalamin
—OH	Hydroxocobalamin
—H₂O	Aquo- or hydrocobalamin
—NO₂	Nitrocobalamin
—5'-deoxyadenosyl	5'-deoxyadenosylcobalamin
—CH₃	Methylcobalamin

The structure of cyanocobalamin is shown in Figure 9.32. Only two of these cobalamins, 5'-deoxyadenosyl-cobalamin (subsequently called adenosylcobalamin) and methylcobalamin, are active as coenzymes in humans.

Sources

Dietary sources of vitamin B_{12} come primarily from animal products, which have derived their cobalamins from microorganisms. Any vitamin B_{12} found in plant foods probably could be traced either to contamination with microorganisms from manure or, in the case of legumes, to

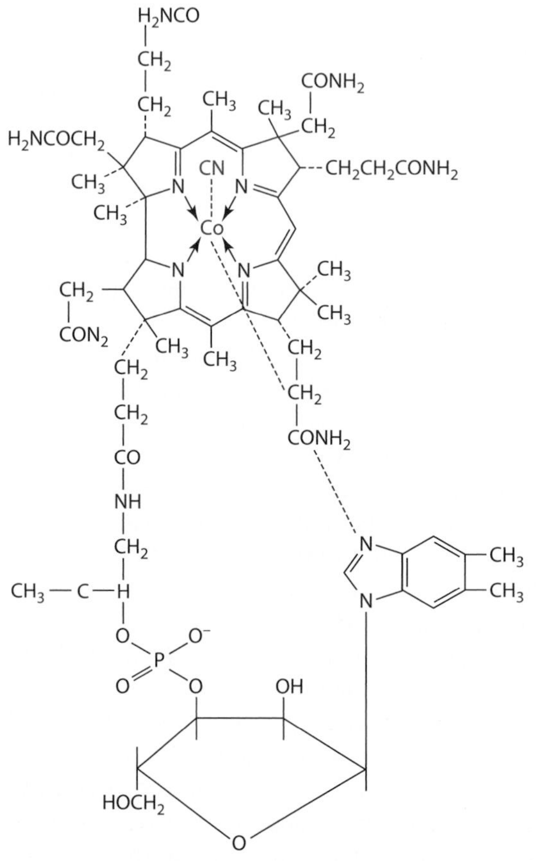

Figure 9.32 The structure of vitamin B_{12} (cyanocobalamin).

the presence of nitrogen-fixing bacteria in the plant root nodules [1].

The best sources of vitamin B_{12} are meat and meat products (beef steak, 1.35 μg/3 oz; pork loin, 0.65 μg/3 oz), poultry (~0.28 μg/3 oz), fish (cod, 0.9 μg/3 oz; salmon, 2.6 μg/3 oz), shellfish (especially clams, 84 μg/3 oz; oysters, 30 μg/3 oz), and eggs (0.6 μg/egg); the cobalamins in these products are predominantly adenosyl- and hydroxocobalamins. Milk (1.0 μg/cup) and milk products such as cheese, cottage cheese (0.7 μg/½ cup), and yogurt (0.9 μg/cup) contain less of the vitamin, mainly as methyl- and hydroxocobalamins; however, dairy products may provide a more highly bioavailable form of the vitamin than meats [2]. Bioavailability of vitamin B_{12} from meals ranges from about 40% to 89% [3]. Cyanocobalamin is found in few foods naturally but is present in tobacco. Plant-derived foods, such as ready-to-eat cereals and soymilk, are sometimes fortified with the vitamin. Bran cereal with raisins (1 cup) contains 25% of the 6 μg Daily Value, or 1.5 μg of vitamin B_{12}. Cyanocobalamin and hydroxocobalamin are the forms commercially available in, for example, vitamin preparations. The vitamin is fairly stable and is resistant to light, heat, and oxidation.

Digestion, Absorption, Transport, and Storage

The digestion and absorption of vitamin B_{12} are believed to proceed according to the scheme depicted in Figure 9.33. Ingested cobalamins must be released from the proteins/polypeptides to which they are linked in foods. This digestion usually occurs through the actions of the gastric proteolytic enzyme pepsin and hydrochloric acid in the stomach.

Next, vitamin B_{12} binds to an R protein that is found in saliva and gastric juice; the binding occurs prior to or just after the vitamin's release from food proteins in the stomach or duodenum. R proteins are thought to protect vitamin B_{12} from bacterial use. Within the alkaline environment of the small intestine, the R protein is hydrolyzed by pancreatic proteases, and free vitamin B_{12} is released. After release from the R protein, vitamin B_{12} (all forms) binds to intrinsic factor (IF), a glycoprotein that is synthesized by gastric parietal cells but escapes enzymatic catabolism.

The vitamin B_{12}–IF complex travels from the duodenum to the ileum, where it interacts with a protein receptor (called cubilin, IF receptor, or cubam). Cubilin then interacts with another protein, amnionless, which facilitates cubilin's attachment to the ileal cell's plasma membrane; another protein, megalin, also may be involved. Binding of the vitamin B_{12}–IF complex to the receptor triggers active endocytotic internalization. Defects in either of the receptor's subunits have been shown to result in vitamin B_{12} malabsorption [4]. Vitamin B_{12} is absorbed throughout the ileum, especially the distal third [1].

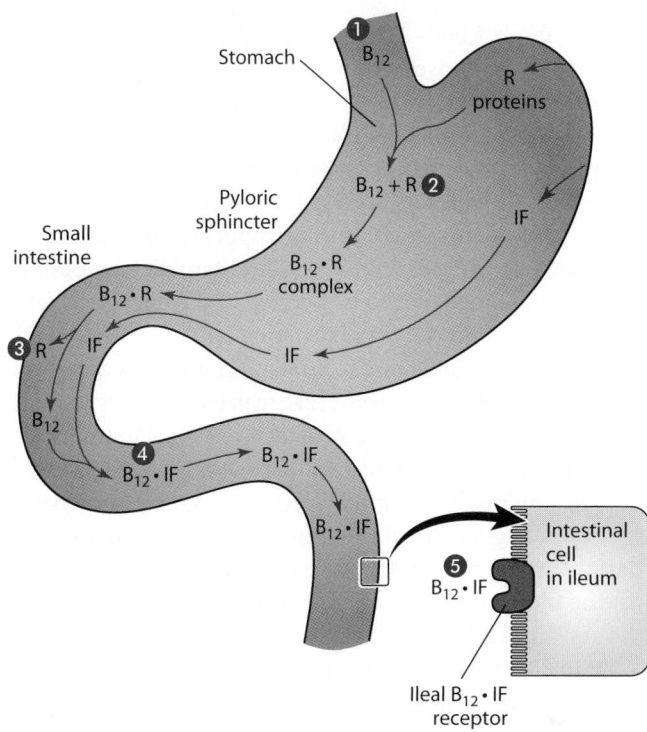

1. Vitamin B_{12} is released from food

2. Vitamin B_{12} binds to R proteins found in saliva and gastric juice

3. Within the small intestine R protein is digested to release vitamin B_{12}

4. Vitamin B_{12} binds intrinsic factor (IF) forming a complex in the small intestine

5. The vitamin B_{12}—IF complex binds to a receptor on enterocytes in the ileum and gets internalized by endocytosis

Figure 9.33 Vitamin B_{12} absorption.

Within the enterocyte, the vitamin is released from the IF complex. Next, in or before it is transported across the ileum's basolateral membrane, vitamin B_{12} binds to the protein transcobalamin II for transport in portal blood.

Several conditions can interfere with this absorptive process. Destruction of gastric parietal cells causing an absence of intrinsic factor results in malabsorption of the vitamin, a condition called pernicious anemia. An inability to release food-bound cobalamin so that it may bind to intrinsic factor is sometimes referred to as food cobalamin malabsorption; this inability often occurs in older individuals. Pancreatic insufficiency and Zollinger-Ellison syndrome result in a more acidic intestinal pH, which can impair the release of vitamin B_{12} from R protein; B_{12} preferentially binds to R proteins versus IF in an acidic environment. These conditions, among others, diminish the vitamin's absorption and increase a person's risk for deficiency, as discussed in more detail under the section on deficiency.

Intrinsic factor–mediated intestinal absorption of vitamin B_{12} is saturated at about 1.5 to 2.0 μg of vitamin B_{12} per meal [3]. Although most vitamin B_{12} is absorbed by this process, about 1% to 3% of intake may be absorbed by passive diffusion, especially when pharmacological doses (about 1,000–2,000 μg) of vitamin B_{12} are ingested, as needed for those with pernicious anemia. Overall absorption of vitamin B_{12} is 50% (range: ~11–65%), with decreased absorption efficacy as intake increases [5]. Absorption of free cyanocobalamin in people with healthy gastrointestinal tracts does not diminish with aging [6,7].

Enterohepatic circulation is important in vitamin B_{12} nutriture, accounting in part for the vitamin's long biological half-life. The vitamin is excreted in the bile; however, it can bind to IF in the small intestine and be reabsorbed in the ileum. Enterohepatic recirculation provides about 3 to 8 μg of the vitamin per day. Thus, malabsorption syndromes not only decrease absorption of ingested cobalamin but also interfere with its enterohepatic circulation, thereby increasing the amount of vitamin B_{12} required to meet body needs.

Following its absorption, the vitamin appears in circulation in about 3 to 4 hours. Peak levels of the vitamin in the blood typically are not reached for another 4 to 8 hours. In the blood, methylcobalamin comprises about 60% to 80% and adenosylcobalamin perhaps up to 20% of total plasma cobalamin. Other forms of cobalamin in the blood include cyanocobalamin and hydroxocobalamin.

Metabolism of the various forms of the vitamin occurs within cells. Hydroxocobalamin, for example, may undergo cytosolic methylation to generate methylcobalamin or may undergo reduction and subsequent reaction with ATP in the mitochondria to yield adenosylcobalamin. Cyanocobalamin is typically converted to aquo- or hydroxocobalamin, among other forms. However, individuals with an inherited cobalamin C defect exhibit impaired conversion of cyanocobalamin into either of the two coenzymes due to a defect in cyanocobalamin decyanase, which catalyzes the removal of the cyano group from cyanocobalamin.

Vitamin B_{12} circulates in the blood bound to transporter proteins, transcobalamin (TC) and haptocorrin (HC)-like proteins. TC, also more commonly referred to as TCII, is made in many body cells including enterocytes and is the main protein that carries newly absorbed cobalamin, in a one-to-one ratio, from the intestine into the blood and then to body tissues. About 20% to 30% of cobalamin is transported on TCII, which as holoTCII (i.e., the cobalamin-TCII complex) has a half-life of less than 2 hours. Two other proteins, related to haptocorrin and designated TCI and TCIII, also appear to participate in transport of vitamin B_{12}; however, the exact functions of these proteins are unknown. Much of vitamin B_{12} is transferred from TCII to TCI. TCI, which transports up to about 80% of vitamin B_{12}, is thought to function as a circulating storage form and may prevent bacterial use of the vitamin. TCIII may function in the delivery of cobalamin from peripheral tissues back to the liver.

A fairly common genetic mutation in TCII results in the substitution of cytosine (C) for guanine (G) at base pair 776 (written as TC 766C G). This substitution results in the insertion of arginine instead of proline, and in turn diminishes the protein's (TCII's) ability to bind and transport B_{12} to tissues. An estimated 20% of the population is homozygous for the GG variant, which is associated with low serum vitamin B_{12} and high serum homocysteine concentrations (a risk factor for heart disease) [8].

Uptake of vitamin B_{12} into tissues is receptor dependent. All tissues appear to have receptors for TCII, and nonspecific receptors have been shown to take up the TCI-B_{12} complex. The TCII-cobalamin complex, upon binding to TCII cell receptors, appears to enter cells by endocytosis with subsequent fusion to lysosomes that provide for proteolytic degradation of TCII and release of the vitamin within the cell cytosol. Chaperones, intracellular transport proteins, are thought to carry or escort the vitamin within the cell's various compartments and organelles.

Vitamin B_{12}, unlike other water-soluble vitamins, can be stored and retained in the body for long periods of time, even years; consequently, a deficiency may take 3 to 5 years to develop. About 2 to 4 mg of the vitamin is stored in the body, mainly (~50%) in the liver. Small amounts also are found in the muscle, bone, kidneys, heart, brain, and spleen and circulating in the blood as transcobalamins. Adenosylcobalamin represents about 70% of the body's vitamin B_{12} and is the primary storage form of the vitamin in the liver, red blood cells, kidneys, and brain. Methylcobalamin is the main form of the vitamin in the blood. Hydroxocobalamin and methylcobalamin are also stored, but to a lesser extent.

Functions and Mechanisms of Action

Two enzymatic reactions requiring vitamin B_{12} have been recognized in humans. One of these reactions requires methylcobalamin, whereas the other must have adenosylcobalamin.

The reaction requiring methylcobalamin as a coenzyme is the conversion of homocysteine into methionine (Figure 9.30). This reaction, which occurs in the cell's cytosol, is shown following this paragraph in a two-step process to facilitate understanding of the sequential nature of the reaction. First, to form the methylcobalamin needed in methionine synthesis, cobalamin bound to the methionine synthase (also called homocysteine methyltransferase) picks up the methyl group from 5-methyl tetrahydrofolate (THF), forming methylcobalamin bound to methionine synthase and THF.

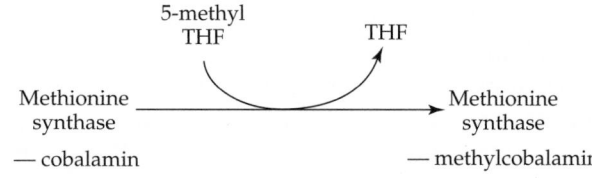

Next, methionine synthase releases the methyl group from its bound methylcobalamin for transfer to homocysteine, producing methionine and cobalamin. In this reaction, the transfer of the methyl group from methylcob(III)alamin results in the formation of cob(I) alamin. Cob(I)alamin, however, is easily oxidized and, with its oxidation, methionine synthase becomes inactive. Reactivation of methionine synthase is accomplished by the NADPH-dependent flavoenzyme methionine synthase reductase. Interestingly, polymorphisms in this reductase (causing reduced methionine synthase activity) have been linked with an increased risk of neural tube defects in individuals with suboptimal vitamin B_{12} status as well as in individuals with 5,10-methylene tetrahydrofolate reductase mutations.

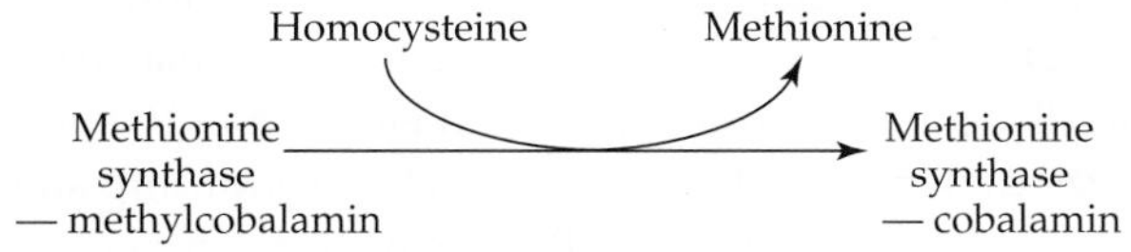

Because the formation of 5-methyl THF is irreversible, a vitamin B_{12} deficiency traps body folate in the 5-methyl form, in what is known as the methyl-folate trap hypothesis. This hypothesis helps explain in part the synergism between folate and vitamin B_{12} (see the "Interactions with Other Nutrients" subsection in the "Folate" section).

The second of the vitamin B_{12}–dependent reactions requires adenosylcobalamin for methylmalonyl-CoA mutase, which converts (rearranges the skeleton of) L-methylmalonyl-CoA to succinyl-CoA (Figure 9.34) in the cell's mitochondria. L-methylmalonyl-CoA is made from D-methylmalonyl-CoA, which in turn is generated from propionyl-CoA. Propionyl-CoA arises from the oxidation of methionine, isoleucine, and threonine and of odd-chain fatty acids. The conversion of propionyl-CoA to D-methylmalonyl-CoA is an ATP-, Mg^{2+}-, and

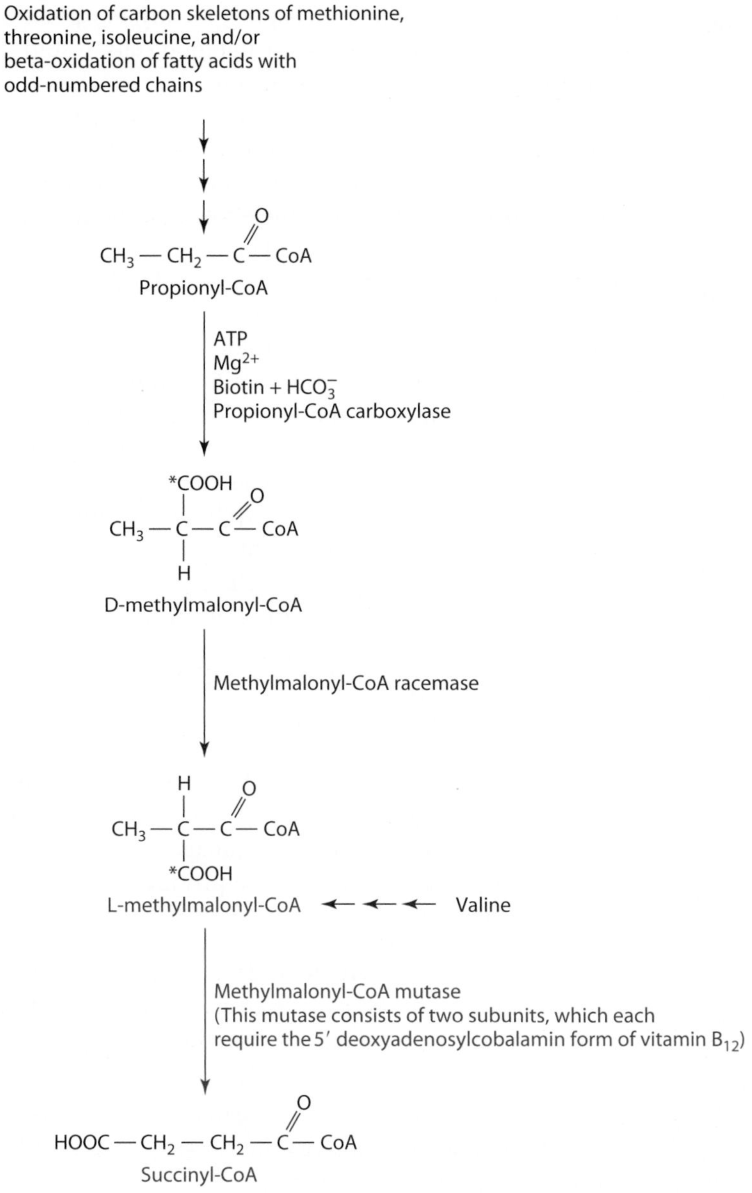

Homocysteine → Methionine

Methionine synthase — methylcobalamin ———→ Methionine synthase — cobalamin

Oxidation of carbon skeletons of methionine, threonine, isoleucine, and/or beta-oxidation of fatty acids with odd-numbered chains

$CH_3 — CH_2 — \overset{O}{\overset{\|}{C}} — CoA$
Propionyl-CoA

ATP
Mg^{2+}
Biotin + HCO_3^-
Propionyl-CoA carboxylase

$CH_3 — \overset{*COOH}{\underset{H}{\overset{|}{C}}} — \overset{O}{\overset{\|}{C}} — CoA$
D-methylmalonyl-CoA

Methylmalonyl-CoA racemase

$CH_3 — \overset{H}{\underset{*COOH}{\overset{|}{C}}} — \overset{O}{\overset{\|}{C}} — CoA$
L-methylmalonyl-CoA ← ← ← Valine

Methylmalonyl-CoA mutase (This mutase consists of two subunits, which each require the 5′ deoxyadenosylcobalamin form of vitamin B_{12})

$HOOC — CH_2 — CH_2 — \overset{O}{\overset{\|}{C}} — CoA$
Succinyl-CoA

Figure 9.34 Role of vitamin B_{12} in oxidation of L-methylmalonyl-CoA.

biotin-dependent reaction (previously discussed in the section on biotin; Figure 9.24). Methylmalonyl-CoA mutase (a dimer) requires two adenosylcobalamin molecules (one per subunit) to convert L-methylmalonyl-CoA to succinyl-CoA (Figure 9.34). With a deficiency of vitamin B_{12} or a genetic defect in the enzyme, mutase activity is impaired and methylmalonyl-CoA and methylmalonic acid, formed from hydrolysis of methylmalonyl-CoA, accumulate in body fluids. The response of serum methylmalonic acid to vitamin B_{12} depletion and repletion is useful in the diagnosis of vitamin B_{12} deficiency and in monitoring the response to treatment.

Metabolism and Excretion

Vitamin B_{12} undergoes little to no degradation prior to excretion. Turnover of the vitamin is approximately 0.1% (2 µg) per day, with most of the vitamin excreted (but reabsorbed) in the bile and only small amounts (<0.25 µg/day) lost in the urine. Trace dermal losses of vitamin B_{12} also may occur.

Recommended Dietary Allowance

Recommendations for vitamin B_{12} intake are based upon estimates of the vitamin's intake and turnover, and on amounts of the vitamin needed for the maintenance of normal serum vitamin indices and hematological status. The RDA for adults for vitamin B_{12} is 2.4 µg per day, although intakes of 4 to 7 µg per day have been recommended [9,10]. Increases of 0.2 µg and 0.4 µg per day above the RDA are suggested for women during pregnancy and lactation, respectively [5]. The requirement for the vitamin for adults is 2.0 µg/day [5]. People age 51 years and older are counseled to consume foods fortified with the vitamin or consume vitamin B_{12} supplements, because 10% to 30% of older people have changes to the gastrointestinal tract that limit their ability to absorb food-bound forms of the vitamin [5]. The inside front cover of the book provides additional recommendations for vitamin B_{12} intake for other age groups.

Deficiency: Megaloblastic Macrocytic Anemia

Deficiency of vitamin B_{12}, like that of folate, results in megaloblastic macrocytic anemia. A description of the development of this condition is provided in the folate deficiency section. The condition occurs with vitamin B_{12} because of the development of the methyl-folate trap, which is discussed in the "Folate" section in the "Interactions with Other Nutrients" subsection. Briefly, without vitamin B_{12}, folate coenzymes are reduced to 5-methyl folate and cannot be converted to the coenzyme forms 10-formyl THF and 5,10-methylene THF, which are needed for synthesis of the purine ring and thymidylate, respectively. Consequently, DNA synthesis becomes deranged, along with cell differentiation and maturation, and this negatively impacts cells, especially those with rapid turnover such as blood cells.

Manifestations of vitamin B_{12} deficiency occur in stages. Initially, serum vitamin B_{12} concentrations diminish; serum B_{12} concentrations, however, may remain normal until vitamin stores become depleted. Second, cell concentrations of the vitamin diminish, affecting the activities of both vitamin B_{12}–dependent enzymes. Third, DNA synthesis decreases and plasma homocysteine and methylmalonic acid concentrations increase. (Also note: Plasma homocysteine concentrations are inversely associated with plasma vitamin B_{12} concentrations and when elevated in the plasma are a risk factor for heart disease. The relationship among vitamin B_{12}, folate, vitamin B_6, plasma homocysteine concentrations, and heart disease is discussed in further detail in the "Folate" section of this chapter.) Finally, morphological and functional changes occur in blood cells, resulting in the megaloblastic macrocytic anemia.

Most of vitamin B_{12}'s deficiency signs and symptoms affect the body's hematologic and neurologic systems, although there is emerging evidence that deficiency of vitamin B_{12} may be involved in the etiology of neural tube defects in developing embryos [11]. Some hematological, among other, effects are anemia, low blood leukocyte and thrombocyte counts, skin pallor, fatigue, shortness of breath, and palpitations. Neurologic problems, which may be irreparable, are manifested by numbness in extremities, abnormal gait, increased loss of coordination, loss of a sense of relative position (proprioreception), loss of vibration sense or touch in the ankles and toes, swelling of myelinated fibers, and demyelination, along with irritability, memory loss, disorientation, psychosis, and dementia. The neurological problems, which occur in about 75% to 90% of those with vitamin B_{12} deficiency, are not responsive to folate therapy [5,12]. The cause(s) of the neuropathy is not clear but may be related to insufficient availability of S-adenosyl methionine (SAM); SAM is required for methylation reactions, which are essential to myelin maintenance and thus neural function. Other theories suggest it is an imbalance in cytokines and growth factors that causes myelin damage [13].

Vitamin B_{12} deficiency can be produced in several situations, such as with:

- *Inadequate intake*, which is most likely to occur in a strict vegetarian (vegan), especially in an infant or young child with minimal stores of the vitamin.

- *Impaired pancreatic exocrine function*, which decreases the pH of the intestinal tract (due to insufficient release of bicarbonate) and impairs the release of vitamin B_{12} from R proteins.

- *Impaired gastric function*, which may result from pernicious anemia or other gastric conditions and alters vitamin release and/or binding needed for absorption. Pernicious (which refers to death) anemia is an autoimmune condition in which the body produces antibodies that attack the gastric parietal and mucosal cells, causing destruction and atrophy in the body and fundus regions of the stomach. The destruction of the parietal cells causes diminished (hydrochlorhydria) or absent (**achlorhydria**) hydrochloric acid production and insufficient IF synthesis. Without IF, vitamin B_{12} cannot be absorbed. Further, with insufficient hydrochloric acid (as may also result from the use of some medications—H_2 blockers and proton pump inhibitors—for the treatment of ulcers and gastroesophageal reflux disease), vitamin B_{12} release from food protein is impaired, causing food cobalamin malabsorption. These conditions are especially prevalent in older individuals; the incidence of vitamin B_{12} deficiency in the elderly may be as high as 15%. Atrophic gastritis, characterized by a loss and inflammation of gastric cells, also diminishes acid production to impair vitamin absorption. Conversely, people with Zollinger-Ellison syndrome produce excessive quantities of gastric acid, which results in diminished intestinal pH and impaired release of vitamin B_{12} from R-proteins.

- *Impaired intestinal function*, especially if affecting the ileum, such as occurs with celiac disease and Crohn's disease, may decrease the absorptive surface and thus the vitamin receptors in the ileum to limit vitamin absorption.

- *Competition*. People with parasitic infections such as tapeworms may develop a vitamin B_{12} deficiency because the parasite uses the vitamin and consequently limits the vitamin's availability to the infected person. Similarly, the prolonged use of H_2 blockers and proton pump inhibitors (used to treat ulcers and gastroesophageal reflux disease) is associated with diminished absorption of vitamin B_{12} because of bacterial overgrowth. The intestinal bacteria over-grow in the more alkaline intestinal environment created when the medication diminishes acid production. Further, the bacteria use the vitamin B_{12} for their own growth, which limits its availability to and use by the individual.

- *Use of nitrous oxide* (an anesthetic agent), primarily in people who have poor vitamin B_{12} status, may result in deterioration of nervous system function, especially demyelination problems. Mechanisms by which nitrous oxide alters vitamin B_{12} metabolism and induces deficiency are under investigation [13].

Vitamin B_{12} deficiency due to inadequate intake of the vitamin is typically treated with up to 1 mg vitamin B_{12} for the first week or so, followed by slightly lower dosages for about one month. Treating pernicious anemia or deficiency secondary to malabsorption often requires monthly intramuscular injections of vitamin B_{12} in amounts of 500 to 1,000 μg or oral ingestion of pharmacologic amounts (2 mg) of the vitamin [5]. Vitamin B_{12} nasal sprays also are available. Nascobal®, for example, provides the vitamin as cyanocobalamin (500 μg/spray) in a nasal spray that is beneficial to people with malabsorptive disorders.

Toxicity

Although no clear toxicity from massive doses of vitamin B_{12} has been recorded, neither has any benefit been noted from an excessive intake of the vitamin by people with adequate vitamin status [5]. No Tolerable Upper Intake Level for vitamin B_{12} has been established [5].

Assessment of Nutriture

Vitamin B_{12} status may be assessed using several indices. Serum vitamin B_{12} concentrations, which include cobalamin bound to TCI, TCII, and TCIII, are commonly measured and reflect both intake and status. Increases in plasma holotranscobalamin TCII concentrations provide an indication of vitamin B_{12} absorption. Concentrations of vitamin B_{12} in the serum of < 200 pg/mL (based upon a radioassay method) are considered deficient, while those between 200 and 300 pg/mL suggest borderline deficiency [14]. However, because serum vitamin B_{12} concentrations can be maintained at the expense of tissues, a person may exhibit normal serum concentrations but have low tissue concentrations [12]. Thus, assessment that includes use of indices in addition to serum concentrations is beneficial.

Measurements of methylmalonyl-CoA or methylmalonic acid also are used to assess vitamin B_{12} status. Increased serum and urinary concentrations of these compounds result from insufficient vitamin B_{12}. Normally, no or only trace amounts of methylmalonic acid are excreted in the urine; however, with vitamin B_{12} deficiency, methylmalonic acid concentrations increase in the serum (greater than ~270 nmol/L) and excretion exceeds about 300 mg per day [12,14]. A breath test to assess vitamin B_{12} status has also been developed; carbon dioxide concentrations in the breath are measured following ingestion of labeled propionate. Deficiency of the vitamin is indicated by subnormal production of labeled carbon dioxide.

Other tests used to assess vitamin B_{12} nutriture include the deoxyuridine suppression test, discussed previously in the "Assessment of Nutriture" subsection of the "Folate" section, and the Schilling test. The Schilling test involves orally administering radioactive vitamin B_{12} and measuring urinary excretion of the vitamin. Below-normal urinary excretion of the vitamin suggests impaired absorption. In lieu of the Schilling test, the presence of antibodies to intrinsic factor and/or parietal cells may be directly measured in the blood as an indicator of an auto-immune response and pernicious anemia.

References Cited for Vitamin B$_{12}$

1. Seatharam B, Alpers D. Absorption and transport of cobalamin (vitamin B$_{12}$). Ann Rev Nutr. 1982; 2:343–69.
2. Sandberg D, Begley J, Hall C. The content, binding and forms of vitamin B$_{12}$ in milk. Am J Clin Nutr. 1981; 34:1717–24.
3. Watanabe F. Vitamin B$_{12}$ sources and bioavailability. Exp Biol Med. 2007; 232:1266–74.
4. He Q, Madsen M, Kilkenney A, et al. Amnionless function is required for cubilin brushborder expression and intrinsic factor-cobalamin (vitamin B$_{12}$) absorption in vivo. Blood. 2005;106:1447-53.
5. Food and Nutrition Board. Dietary Reference Intakes for Thiamin, Riboflavin, Niacin, Vitamin B$_6$, Folate, Vitamin B$_{12}$, Pantothenic Acid, Biotin, and Choline. Washington, DC: National Academy Press. 1998 pp. 306-56.
6. Carmel R. Cobalamin, the stomach and aging. Am J Clin Nutr. 1997; 66:750–59.
7. Van Asselt D, van den Broek W, Lamers C, et al. Free and protein-bound cobalamin absorption in healthy middle-aged and older subjects. J Am Geriatr Soc. 1996; 44:949–53.
8. von Castel-Dunwoody K, Kauwell G, Shelnutt K, et al. Transcobalamin 776C G polymorphism negative affects vitamin B$_{12}$ metabolism. Am J Clin Nutr. 2005; 81:1436–41.
9. Bor MV, von Castel-Roberts KM, Kauwell GPA, et al. Daily intake of 4 to 7 μg dietary vitamin B$_{12}$ is associated with steady concentrations of vitamin B$_{12}$ related biomarkers in healthy young population. Am J Clin Nutr. 2010; 91:571–77.
10. Bor MV, Lydeking-Olesen E, Moller J, Nexo E. A daily intake of approximately 6 μg vitamin B$_{12}$ appears to saturate all the vitamin B$_{12}$ related variable in Dannish postmenopausal women. Am J Clin Nutr. 2006; 83:52–58.
11. Thompson MD, Cole DE, Ray JG. Vitamin B$_{12}$ and neural tube defects: the Canadian experience. Am J Clin Nutr. 2009; 89:S697–701.
12. Beck W. Neuropsychiatric consequences of cobalamin deficiency. Adv Intern Med. 1991; 36:33–56.
13. Hathout L, El-Saden S. Nitrous oxide-induced B$_{12}$ deficiency myelopathy: perspectives on the clinical biochemistry of vitamin B$_{12}$. J Neurol Sci. 2011; 301:1–8.
14. Chatthanawaree W. Biomarkers of cobalamin (vitamin B$_{12}$) deficiency and its application. J Nutr Hlth Aging. 2011; 15:227–31.

Suggested Readings

Green R. Ins and outs of cellular cobalamin transport. Blood. 2010; 115:1476–77.
Jacobsen DW, Glushchenko AV. The transcobalamin receptor redux. Blood. 2009; 113:3–4.
Stover PJ. Vitamin B$_{12}$ and older adults. Current Opin Clin Nutr Metab Care. 2010; 13:24–27.

VITAMIN B$_6$

Vitamin B$_6$ was isolated in 1934 and its structure confirmed in 1939. Some of the initial research was aimed at correcting dermatitis in rats. Kuhn and Szent-Györgyi are credited with isolating the vitamin (which was called pyridoxine due to its structural homology to pyridine) in 1938 to correct the rat dermatitis. The pyridoxal and pyridoxamine forms of the vitamin were identified in the mid-1940s. Vitamin B$_6$ exists as six vitamers, the structural formulas of which are given in Figure 9.35. These vitamers are interchangeable and comparably active. Pyridoxine represents the alcohol form, pyridoxal the aldehyde form, and pyridoxamine the amine form. Each has a 5′-phosphate derivative.

Sources

All B$_6$ vitamers are found in food. Pyridoxine, the stablest of the compounds, and its phosphorylated form are found almost exclusively in plant foods. In some plants, some vitamin B$_6$ occurs in a conjugated form, pyridoxine-glucoside. Pyridoxal and pyridoxamine and their phosphorylated derivatives are found primarily in animal products, with sirloin steak, salmon, and the light meat of chicken being rich sources. For example, 3 oz of white and dark meat chicken provide 0.7 mg and 0.3 mg, respectively. Similarly, 3 oz of steak and ground beef provide 0.3 mg and 0.4 mg, respectively. Pork loin also contains 0.4 mg/3-oz serving. Salmon has about 0.5 mg/3-oz serving. Whole-grain

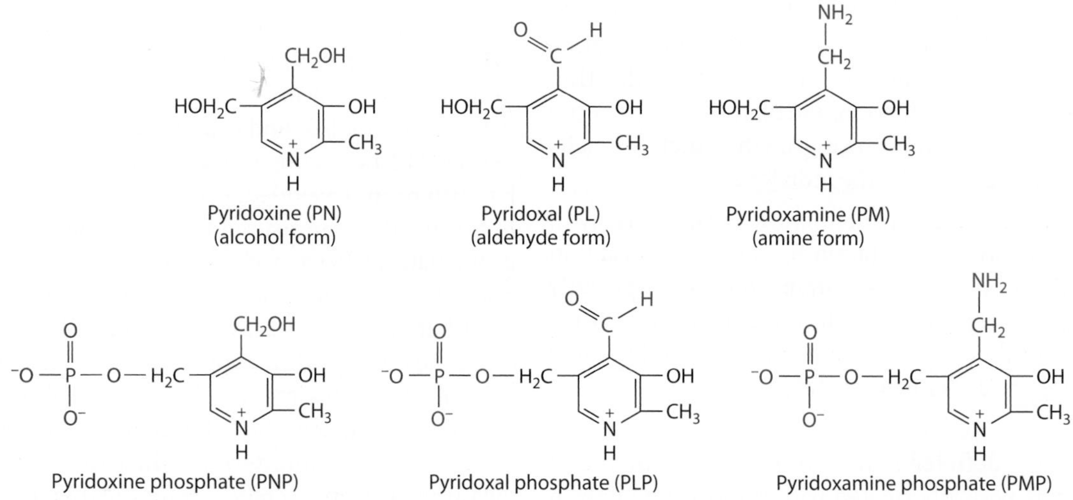

Figure 9.35 Vitamin B$_6$ structures.

products, vegetables, some fruits (e.g., bananas), and nuts as well as fortified cereals also represent major contributors of vitamin B_6 in the diet. A banana provides about 0.4 mg of the vitamin, and 1 oz of pecans has 0.06 mg. Cooked broccoli (½ cup) and cooked zucchini (½ cup) provide 0.16 and 0.07 mg, respectively, and a cup of raw carrots has 0.17 mg of vitamin B_6. A slice of whole-grain bread contains 0.1 mg. Cheerios® provides 25% of the Daily Value of 2 mg, or about 0.5 mg/1 cup. The form of vitamin B_6 in supplements is generally pyridoxine hydrochloride.

The bioavailability of vitamin B_6 from foods is influenced by the food matrix and by the extent and type of processing to which the foods are subjected. Much of the vitamin originally present in foods can be lost through prolonged heating (especially with sterilizing and canning), as well as with milling and refining of grains. Loss of the vitamin also may occur with food storage. The vitamin is fairly stable with cooking.

Digestion, Absorption, Transport, and Storage

For vitamin B_6 to be absorbed, the phosphorylated vitamers must be dephosphorylated. Alkaline phosphatase, a zinc-dependent enzyme found at the intestinal brush border, or other intestinal phosphatases, hydrolyze the phosphate from the phosphorylated vitamers to yield free pyridoxine (PN), pyridoxal (PL), or pyridoxamine (PM).

PL, PN, and PM are absorbed primarily in the jejunum by passive diffusion. At physiological intakes, the vitamin is absorbed rapidly in its free form; however, when the phosphorylated vitamers are ingested in high concentrations, some of these compounds may be absorbed without dephosphorylation. Absorption of some pyridoxine glucosides may also occur by passive diffusion, although mucosal glucosidase typically hydrolyzes the glucosides to free the vitamin. Overall absorption of vitamin B_6 furnished by the average U.S. diet is about 75%, with a range of about 61% to 92% [1].

Little metabolism of the vitamin occurs within the intestinal cell, although some PN may be converted to PNP and PLP. Most PN, PL, and PM are released directly into portal blood.

The liver is the main organ that takes up (by passive diffusion) and metabolizes newly absorbed vitamin B_6. Figure 9.36 shows these reactions and other interconversions of the B_6 vitamers. Unphosphorylated forms of the vitamin typically are phosphorylated by a kinase using ATP within the cytosol of the hepatocyte (liver cell) as well as other organs. PNP and PMP are then generally converted by the action of an FMN-dependent oxidase to the main vitamer PLP; the oxidase that catalyzes this reaction is dependent upon adequate riboflavin status and is found mainly in the liver and intestine and to lesser extents in the muscle, kidneys, brain, and red blood cells. Intracellular PLP concentrations are dependent, in

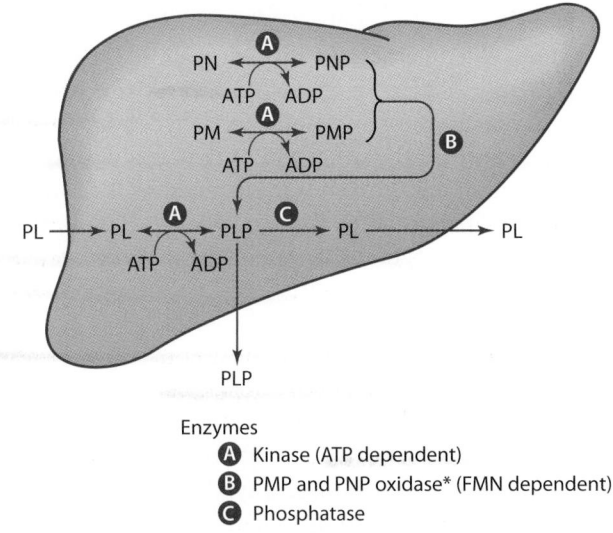

Enzymes
- **A** Kinase (ATP dependent)
- **B** PMP and PNP oxidase* (FMN dependent)
- **C** Phosphatase

*Oxidase is found mainly in the liver and enterocytes.

Figure 9.36 Vitamin B_6 metabolism in the liver.

part, upon the availability of binding proteins. With saturation of binding proteins, unbound PLP is hydrolyzed to PL, which is released into the blood for use by other tissues. From the liver, mostly PLP and PL, with smaller amounts of the other vitamers, are released into the blood for transport to extrahepatic tissues.

PLP is the main (60–90% of the total) form of the vitamin found in systemic blood. Most PLP in the plasma is bound to albumin. Other forms of the vitamin present in small amounts in the blood (also bound primarily to albumin) include PL, PN, PM, and PMP; unphosphorylated vitamers taken up by red blood cells are converted to PLP and bound to hemoglobin. Because only unphosphorylated vitamers may be taken up by other body tissues, PLP is typically hydrolyzed by alkaline phosphatase prior to cellular uptake.

Muscles represent the major (75–80%) storage site for the vitamin, which is found in the body in amounts ranging from about 40 to 185 mg. The liver stores about 5% to 10%. Most vitamin B_6 occurs in muscle as PLP bound to glycogen phosphorylase. Phosphorylation of the vitamin prevents its diffusion out of the cell, and the binding of the vitamin to protein prevents hydrolysis by phosphatases. Other tissues with substantial amounts of the vitamin are the brain, kidneys, and spleen; in these tissues the vitamin is found in a coenzyme form typically bound to enzymes.

Functions and Mechanisms of Action

The PLP coenzyme form of vitamin B_6 is associated with a vast number (>100) of enzymes, the majority of which are involved in amino acid metabolism. Vitamin B_6's noncoenzyme role affects gene expression.

Coenzymes

As a coenzyme in reactions involving amino acids, PLP, through the formation of a Schiff base (the product formed by an amino group and an aldehyde), labilizes all the bonds around the α-carbon of the amino acid. The specific bond that is broken is determined by the catalytic groups of the particular enzyme to which PLP is attached. The covalent bonds of an α-amino acid that can be made labile by its binding to specific PLP-containing enzymes are shown in Figure 9.37.

Some of the reactions involving amino acids that are catalyzed by PLP include transamination (which can also be catalyzed by PMP), dehydration (elimination)/deamination, decarboxylation, transulfhydration, transelenation, cleavage, racemization, and synthesis. In addition to its participation in reactions, vitamin B_6 functions by a different mechanism in the initial step of glycogen metabolism. Each of these types of reactions is discussed briefly.

Transamination Transamination reactions involve the transfer of an amino group ($^-NH_2$) from one amino acid to an α-ketoacid, and, like the deamination reactions discussed next, are important for the synthesis of nonessential amino acids and for the use of amino acid carbon skeletons for energy or glucose production. The most common aminotransferases for which PLP or PMP is a coenzyme are aspartic amino transferase (AST, also called glutamate oxaloacetate transaminase or GOT) and alanine aminotransferase (ALT, also called glutamate pyruvate transaminase or GPT) (see Figure 6.5 for the reactions catalyzed by these transaminases). Figures 9.38a and b show the two phases of transamination and demonstrate how the coenzyme forms a Schiff base. In the first phase, the corresponding α-keto acid of the amino acid is produced along with PMP. In the second phase, the transamination cycle is completed as a new α-keto acid substrate receives the amino group from the PMP. The corresponding amino acid is generated, along with regeneration of the PLP.

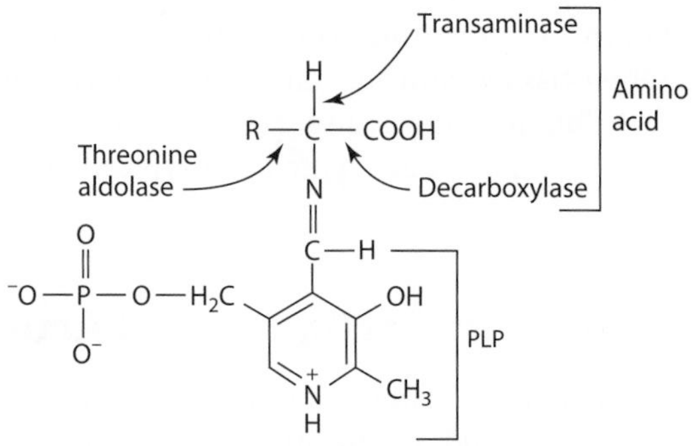

Figure 9.37 The covalent bonds of an acid that can be made labile by its binding to PLP-containing enzymes.

Dehydration (also called elimination) or Deamination PLP also participates in reactions in which an amino group is removed from a compound such as an amino acid and released as ammonia or ammonium ion. Such reactions may be called dehydration, elimination, or deamination reactions. Threonine dehydratase is an example of a PLP-dependent enzyme that is involved in such a reaction, specifically removing water and the amino group from the amino acid threonine; the reaction is shown in Figure 6.6.

Decarboxylation Decarboxylation reactions involve the removal of the carboxy (COO^-) group from an amino acid or other compound. Some examples of some common decarboxylation reactions include the formation of γ-aminobutyric acid (GABA) from glutamate (Figure 6.38), the production of serotonin from 5-hydroxytryptophan (Figure 6.39), and the synthesis of histamine from the amino acid histidine (Figure 6.14). Dopamine is formed following decarboxylation of dihydroxyphenylalanine, which is generated from the amino acid tyrosine (Figure 6.10).

Transulfhydration PLP is required for two enzymes catalyzing reactions in the transulfhydration pathway in which cysteine is synthesized from methionine. The two PLP-dependent enzymes in this pathway are cystathionine synthase and cystathionine lyase; both are shown in Figure 6.12, which depicts methionine transulfhydration and degradation.

Transelenation Similar to transulfhydration, selenomethionine may be converted through the transelenation pathway to selenocysteine (see Figure 13.16). γ-lyase, which is PLP dependent, directly cleaves the selenium from selenomethionine to generate selenide. Selenocysteine β-lyase, also PLP dependent, generates selenide from selenocysteine.

Cleavage An example of a cleavage reaction requiring PLP is the removal of the hydroxymethyl group from serine. In this reaction, PLP is the coenzyme for a transferase that transfers the hydroxymethyl group of serine to tetrahydrofolate (THF) so that glycine is formed (Figure 9.28).

Racemization PLP is required by racemases that catalyze the interconversion of D- and L-amino acids. Although such reactions are more prevalent in bacterial metabolism, some occur in humans.

Other Synthetic Reactions Vitamin B_6 is also necessary as a coenzyme in the first step in the synthesis of heme (Figure 13.6). PLP is required for aminolevulinic acid synthetase, which catalyzes the condensation, followed by decarboxylation, of glycine with succinyl-CoA to form

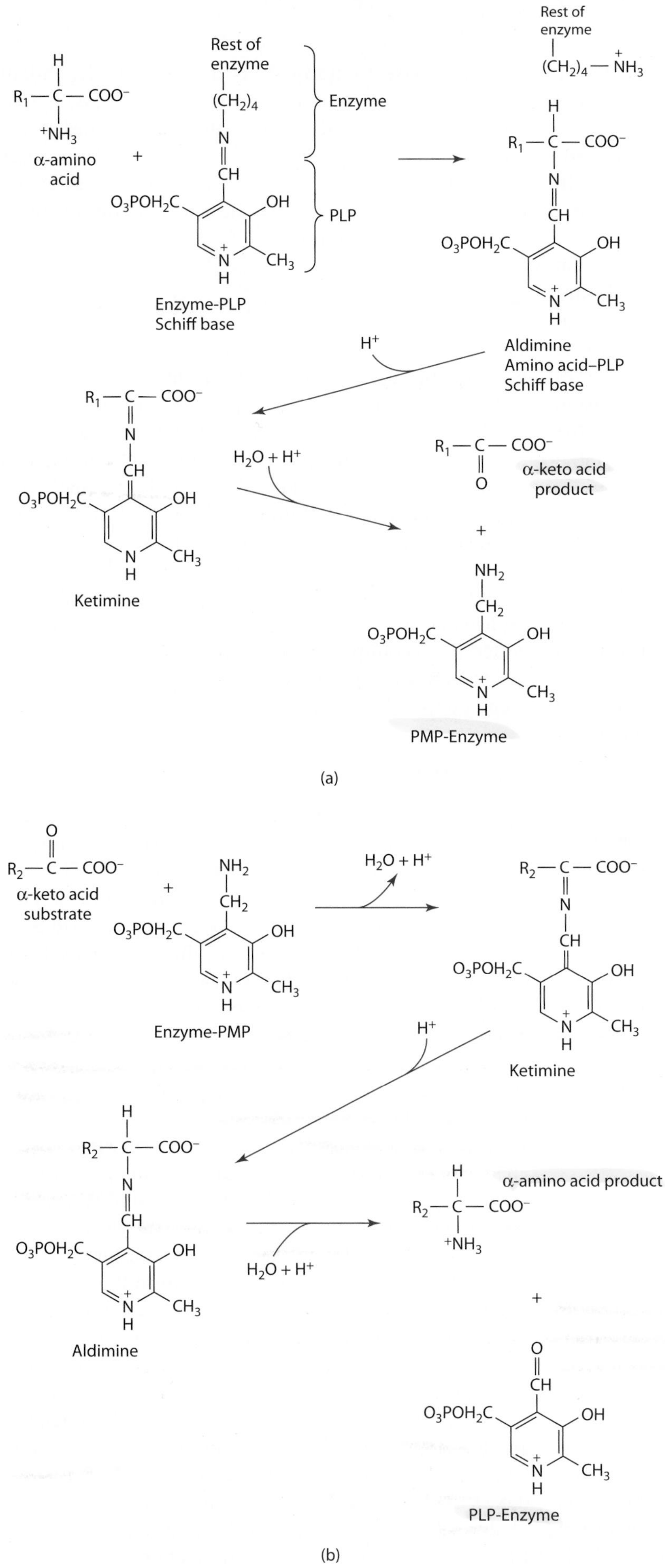

(a)

(b)

Figure 9.38 (a) The role of vitamin B_6 in transamination, phase 1. (b) The role of vitamin B_6 in transamination, phase 2.

aminolevulinic acid (ALA). ALA is used next to synthesize porphobilinogen (PBG), the parent pyrrole compound in porphyrin synthesis. Through a series of reactions, PBG is converted into protoporphyrin IX, which with the addition of Fe^{2+} by ferrochelatase forms heme. Defects in heme synthesis are evident in a vitamin B_6 deficiency as a microcytic anemia.

PLP functions as a cofactor for another condensation reaction necessary for sphingolipid synthesis. Specifically, the amino acid serine condenses with palmitoyl-CoA in a reaction catalyzed by a PLP-dependent transferase to form 3-dehydrosphinganine. This latter compound serves as a precursor for sphingolipids. In fatty acid metabolism, the PLP-dependent enzyme δ-6-desaturase catalyzes the synthesis of selected polyunsaturated fatty acids through desaturation of linoleic and γ-linolenic acids.

Niacin synthesis from tryptophan also requires an important PLP-dependent reaction. Specifically, kynureninase required for the conversion of 3-hydroxykynurenine to 3-hydroxyanthranilic acid requires vitamin B_6 (PLP) as a coenzyme (Figure 9.15).

Other compounds synthesized in the body in vitamin B_6-dependent reactions include carnitine, a nitrogen-containing nonprotein required for fatty acid oxidation (Figure 6.23), and taurine, a neuromodulatory compound generated during cysteine metabolism (Figure 6.12).

Glycogen Degradation The function of PLP in glycogen degradation is poorly understood. Glycogen is catabolized by glycogen phosphorylase to form glucose-1-PO_4 (Figure 3.15); vitamin B_6 is required for glycogen phosphorylase activity. The mechanism of action of the coenzyme appears to be different from that exerted with other enzymes. The phosphate of the coenzyme is believed to stabilize the compound and permit covalent bonding of the phosphate to form glucose-1-PO_4. Most vitamin B_6 found in muscle is present as PLP, which in turn is bound to glycogen phosphorylase. It is this role of the vitamin that is thought to account for the use of more than 50% of the body's vitamin B_6.

Noncoenzyme Role: Modulation of Gene Expression

Although the coenzyme roles of vitamin B_6 have been more thoroughly investigated, vitamin B_6 may be involved in gene expression. The vitamin has been shown to bind to DNA, and, in some cases, to modulate steroid hormone binding or transcription factor binding to regulatory regions on DNA [2].

Metabolism and Excretion

Little vitamin B_6 is excreted in the feces. 4-pyridoxic acid is the major metabolite of the vitamin and results from the oxidation of PL by either NAD-dependent aldehyde dehydrogenase, found in all tissues, or FAD-dependent aldehyde oxidases, found in the liver and kidneys. 4-pyridoxic acid is excreted in the urine and indicates recent vitamin intake, not vitamin stores. Ingesting large doses (100 mg) of the vitamin as PN results in urinary excretion of intact PN and 5-pyridoxic acid, and lower urinary 4-pyridoxic acid excretion.

Recommended Dietary Allowance

The RDA for vitamin B_6 for adult men age 19 to 50 years is 1.3 mg per day (requirement 1.1 mg) and for men age 51 years and older, 1.7 mg per day (requirement 1.4 mg) [1]. For adult women age 19 to 50 years, the RDA for vitamin B_6 is also 1.3 mg per day (requirement 1.1 mg), and for women age 51 years and older it is 1.5 mg daily (requirement 1.3 mg) [1]. With pregnancy and lactation, recommendations for vitamin intake increase to 1.9 mg and 2.0 mg, respectively [1]. Recommendations are based largely upon the maintenance of adequate plasma concentrations (at least 20 nmol/L) of the vitamin [1]. Some have suggested the recommendations need to be raised [3,4]. The inside front cover of the book provides additional recommendations for vitamin B_6 for other age groups.

Deficiency

Vitamin B_6 deficiency is relatively rare in the United States. In the 1950s, deficiency occurred in infants because of severe heat treatment of infant milk. The heat processing resulted in a reaction between the PLP and the ε amino group of lysine in the milk proteins to form pyridoxyl-lysine, which possesses little vitamin activity. Signs of vitamin B_6 deficiency (which can occur in as little as 2 to 3 weeks but may take up to ~2½ months) include a seborrheic rash on the face, neck, shoulders, and buttocks areas, weakness, fatigue, cheilosis, glossitis, and angular stomatitis, along with neurological problems such as confusion, peripheral neuropathy, and (especially in infants) seizures and convulsions. A hypochromic, microcytic anemia may also result due to impaired heme synthesis. Deficiency also impairs niacin synthesis from tryptophan, and inhibits metabolism of homocysteine, which may result in hyperhomocysteinemia, a risk factor for heart disease. While supplementation with vitamin B_6, folate, and vitamin B_{12} has been shown to lower plasma homocysteine concentrations, evidence showing lowered risk against heart disease is conflicting [5]. Deficiency of vitamin B_6 is usually treated with about 100 mg of the vitamin daily.

Groups particularly at risk for vitamin B_6 deficiency are the elderly, who may have a poor intake of the vitamin and may also have accelerated hydrolysis of PLP and oxidation of PL; and people who consume excessive amounts of alcohol (alcohol can impair the conversion of PN and PM to PLP, and the presence of acetaldehyde formed from alcohol metabolism enhances coenzyme degradation). People on a variety of drug therapies may also be at risk. For example, isoniazid used to treat tuberculosis interferes with vitamin activity. Penicillamine used to treat some autoimmune conditions and Wilson's disease inactivates the vitamin. Corticosteroids used to suppress the immune system promote the loss of the vitamin from the body, and anticonvulsants used to diminish seizures inhibit vitamin activity. Oral contraceptive use also may result in suboptimal vitamin B_6 status.

Toxicity

Pharmacological doses of vitamin B_6 have been advocated to prevent or treat a variety of states, including hyperhomocysteinemia, carpal tunnel syndrome, morning sickness, premenstrual syndrome, depression, and muscular fatigue. Although some beneficial results from megadoses of the vitamin have been noted in selected people, indiscriminate use of the vitamin is not without risk. Excessive pyridoxine use ($> \sim 200$ mg/day) causes sensory and peripheral neuropathy. Some symptoms include unsteady gait, tingling in the extremities, and impaired tendon reflexes. Intakes in excess of 2 g/day may cause paresthesia (tingling or numbness) in the feet and hands and impaired motor control or ataxia (loss of voluntary muscle control). High intakes also appear to cause degeneration of neurons (dorsal root ganglia) in the spinal cord, loss of myelination, and degeneration of sensory fibers in peripheral nerves [4]. The Tolerable Upper Intake Level for vitamin B_6 is 100 mg/day for adults to minimize the development of neuropathy [1].

Assessment of Nutriture

Plasma PLP concentrations are thought to be the best indicator of vitamin B_6 tissue stores, with plasma PLP $<$ 20 nmol/L suggestive of vitamin deficiency, concentrations of 20 to 30 nmol/L suggestive of marginal status, and adequacy indicated by plasma concentrations > 30 nmol/L [1]. Several other indices may be used in combination with plasma PLP concentration to assess vitamin B_6 nutriture. A commonly used functional test measures xanthurenic acid excretion following tryptophan loading (2 g or 100 mg of tryptophan/kg body weight). Abnormally high xanthurenic acid excretion is found in vitamin B_6 deficiency because 3-hydroxykynurenine, an intermediate in tryptophan metabolism, cannot lose its alanine moiety and be converted to 3-hydroxyanthranilic acid, as should occur (Figure 9.15). Instead, 3-hydroxykynurenine is converted to xanthurenic acid, which is excreted in the urine in greater than normal amounts—that is, > 25 mg/6 hours.

Urinary vitamin B_6 (measured over several days for a period of 1 to 3 weeks) and urinary 4-pyridoxic acid also have been used to assess the status of vitamin B_6. Urinary vitamin B_6 excretion of < 0.5 μM/day or < 20 μg/g creatinine and urinary 4-pyridoxic acid concentrations of ≤ 3.0 μM/day are thought to indicate deficiency [6]. Urinary 4-pyridoxic acid excretion, however, is considered to be a short-term indicator of vitamin B_6 status, and cutoff values are controversial [1].

Measuring transaminase activity before and after adding vitamin B_6 is an additional technique for determining vitamin B_6 nutriture, especially longer-term vitamin status. However, because of a variety of limitations with the assays, these tests are better used as an adjunct to other tests. The erythrocyte transaminase index examines the activity of glutamic oxaloacetic transaminase (abbreviated GOT or AST) and glutamic pyruvic transaminase (abbreviated GPT or ALT) after the addition of vitamin B_6. Deficient vitamin B_6 status is suggested by GOT/AST activity of $>$1.85 following the addition of the vitamin and by GPT/ ALT activity of $>$1.25 following the addition of the vitamin [6].

References Cited for Vitamin B_6

1. Food and Nutrition Board. Dietary Reference Intakes for Thiamin, Riboflavin, Niacin, Vitamin B_6, Folate, Vitamin B_{12}, Pantothenic Acid, Biotin, and Choline. Washington, DC: National Academy Press. 1998 pp. 150–95.
2. Oka T. Modulation of gene expression by vitamin B_6. Nutr Res Rev. 2001; 14:257–65.
3. Kwak H, Hansen C, Leklem J, et al. Improved vitamin B-6 status is positively related to lymphocyte proliferation in young women consuming a controlled diet. J Nutr. 2002; 132:3308–13.
4. Rogovik AL, Vohra S, Goldman RD. Safety considerations and potential interactions of vitamins: should vitamins be considered drugs? Ann Pharmacother. 2010; 44:311–24.
5. Marti-Carvajal AJ, Sola I, Lathyris D, Salanti G. Homocysteine lowering interventions for preventing cardiovascular events. Cochrane Database Syst Rev. 2009; CD006612.
6. Gibson RS. Principles of nutritional assessment. New York: Oxford University Press. 2005 pp. 575–94.

Suggested Reading

Hellmann H, Mooney S. Vitamin B_6: a molecule for human health? Molecules. 2010; 15:442–59.
Mooney S, Leuendorf J, Hendrickson C, Hellmann H. Vitamin B_6: a long known compound of surprising complexity. Molecules. 2009; 14:329–51.

GENETICS AND NUTRITION: THE EFFECT ON FOLIC ACID NEEDS AND RISK TO CHRONIC DISEASE, BY DR. RITA M. JOHNSON

"Genomic medicine holds the ultimate promise of revolutionizing the diagnosis and treatment of many illnesses." [1]

Since the completion of the Human Genome Project over 10 years ago, the research in genetics and its impact on disease risk has exploded. Academic libraries stock books and research-based journals about topics that were only a dream a decade ago. Books and articles about genetics and disease risk are widely available from libraries, bookstores, magazines, and the world-wide web. While interest in these findings continues to grow, in the past decade few advances directly related to humans and disease treatment have originated from the discovery of the human genome [2].

Similarly, the scientific literature and mass media also overflow with information about the relationship among food choices, an individual's genome, and disease risk. Nutrigenomics and nutrigenetics are increasingly discussed in the study of nutrition, and specialty career paths in these areas exist. The report *The Future of Nutrigenomics* states that an understanding of the interaction among our genes, our diets, and our individual differences will lead to both personalized nutrition and personalized medicine. In addition, the businesses that provide food and dietary supplements will change to meet these newly-identified individualized needs [3]. Nutrigenetics, a sub-study of nutrigenomics, studies the influence of a nutrient on a risk factor when the individual has a variation in the genetic code [4]. Nutrition professionals in the near future may need to both understand and practice nutrigenomics to provide evidence-based and individualized medical nutrition therapy for their clients' unique genetic traits [5].

Discoveries about folate metabolism provide an often-used example of nutrigenetics [6]. The identification of genetic variations in folate metabolism preceded the sequencing of the human genome, and these variations have been linked to neural tube defects, fetal malformations, coronary heart disease, colorectal cancer, dementia, and other health problems. The purposes of this perspective are to (1) describe the most common types of genetic variants in the enzyme methylene tetrahydrofolate reductase, (2) review the prevalence of the genetic variation in different ethnic groups, (3) briefly summarize the research that links these variants to disease risk, and (4) discuss the relationship between folic acid and choline requirements.

N⁵, N¹⁰ METHYLENE TETRAHYDROFOLATE REDUCTASE AND ITS GENETIC VARIANTS

As shown in Figures 9.28 and 9.30, methylene tetrahydrofolate reductase (abbreviated as MTHFR) catalyzes the unidirectional conversion of 5,10-methylene THF to 5-methyl THF. The activity of MTHFR, along with adequate amounts of NADPH and $FADH_2$, is essential to maintain the concentration of 5-methyl THF in the cell. As discussed in Chapter 9, 5-methyl THF provides the methyl group for the synthesis of methionine.

If MTHFR activity is low, intracellular 5-methyl THF concentrations will decrease and an impaired conversion of homocysteine to methionine will result. A lack of methionine results in a lack of the methyl groups necessary for reactions that include the methylation of RNA and DNA and the synthesis of carnitine, creatine, epinephrine, purines, and nicotinamide. At the same time, an accumulation of homocysteine is believed to increase risk for cardiovascular disease and dementias. Clearly, impairing the formation of 5-methyl THF has an effect on the body's ability to synthesize methylated products and remove homocysteine.

Many genetic variations of MTHFR have been reported. These variants are caused by substitutions in the DNA sequence that codes for the enzyme. When a variation is shared by more than 1% of the population, it is called a *genetic polymorphism* [6]. The genetic polymorphisms of MTHFR cause a decrease in its activity and the subsequent formation of 5-methyl THF. This Perspective discusses the most common MTHFR polymorphism, which is caused by a substitution of the nucleotide thymine (abnormal) for the nucleotide cytosine (normal) at position 677. Thus, the DNA contains a thymine when it should contain a cytosine. This polymorphism is abbreviated as MTHFR 677C ⟶ T or MTHFR 677C>T. The result of this alteration in the DNA sequence is that a molecule of valine (abnormal) is inserted into the amino acid sequence during the synthesis of MTHFR, instead of a molecule of alanine (normal) [7]. This polymorphism is an example of a single nucleotide polymorphism (SNP), pronounced "SNIP." More than 3.7 million SNIPs have been identified [8].

The MTHFR 677C ⟶ T variant can be heterozygous or homozygous. An individual with the heterozygous genotype, abbreviated 677CT, has one normal and one abnormal allele, while someone with the homozygous genotype, abbreviated 677TT or 677CC, has either two abnormal or two normal alleles, respectively [5,7]. The homozygous individual with two abnormal alleles (677TT) synthesizes MTHFR that is only 30% to 35% as active as that of the homozygous individual with the unaltered 677CC genotype, who is considered to have the normal or "wildtype" MTHFR activity [9,10]. Someone with the heterozygous (677CT) genotype exhibits 70% of the normal MTHFR activity [11].

The individual with the 677TT genotype may have an increased plasma homocysteine level and a decrease in the methylation reactions described above. Research has determined that these individuals have increased hypomethylation of DNA, lower serum and RBC folate levels, and an increased risk of neural tube defects [12]. This increased disease risk is less associated with the 677CT heterozygote, and most research has studied the 677TT homozygote. Since these polymorphisms in MTHFR were identified in the early 1990s, many researchers have investigated the folic acid needs of individuals who do not have normal MTHFR activity and the effect of intake on their individualized risk of chronic diseases. Thus, the identification of the 677C ⟶ T MTHFR polymorphism has implications related to the individualization of nutrition care.

ETHNIC DIFFERENCES IN GENETIC VARIATIONS IN MTHFR AND FOLATE NEEDS

Data from three studies show that the 677TT homozygous genotype is distributed by ethnic groups. Africans, African-Americans, and Asians (but not Japanese) have the lowest prevalence of less than 5%. The occurrence of the 677TT genotype in Northern Europeans, Japanese, and Caucasian Americans is between 9% and 14%. The greatest prevalence is reported in Italians (18%), Hispanics living in California (21%), Mexican women (18%), and Mexicans (36%) [9,10,13].

While the literature infers a differing risk for disease in those with the 677TT genotype, it is not clear that these individuals have greater folic acid requirements. Using a depletion/repletion design with Mexican women that had either the CC (normal), CT (heterozygote), or TT (homozygote) genotype, Guinotte et al. [11] measured serum folate, RBC folate, plasma homocysteine, and urinary folate excretion. The subjects all showed moderate folate deficiency after the 7-week depletion phase and returned to folate sufficiency after 7 weeks of repletion with 400 μg DFE/day, with no differences in plasma homocysteine. These data support the supposition that the RDA of 400 μg DFE met the needs of these subjects.

Not all research shares these findings, however. In a study of 126 healthy subjects with different MTHFR genotypes, the 677TT subjects had similar plasma folate, but higher plasma homocysteine levels than the CT or CC subjects when consuming a folate-rich diet that contained an average of 660 μg DFE/day [14]. These differences in plasma homocysteine levels disappeared when a folic acid supplement was added, boosting folate intake to an average of 814 μg DFE/day [14]. Based upon these data and the assumption that serum homocysteine reflects folate status, Ashfield-Watt et al. concluded that the 677TT subjects needed between 575 and 830 μg DFE/day.

Hung et al. [15] reported similar results in their study of 32 women with either the 677TT or 677CC genotype. With all folate coming from food, one group consumed 400 μg/d and the other 800 μg/d for 12 weeks. While the 677CC group had significantly higher serum folate and red blood cell folate and lower serum homocysteine than the 677TT group, the authors summarized that a diet containing 800 μg/d improves the folate status of both groups [15].

Solis et al. [16] also challenged the adequacy of the RDA of 400 μg DFE/d for individuals with the 677TT genotype. In a carefully controlled feeding study of male Mexican-Americans, 29 with the 677TT and 31 with the 677CC genotypes, a diet that provided 438 μg/d was consumed by the subjects for 12 weeks. Both groups started the study with mean folate status measures within normal values and not significantly different from one another. At the end of the study all subjects had decreased serum and red cell folate levels, but the 677TT subjects had significantly lower levels than the 677CC subjects. Similarly, plasma homocysteine levels were significantly different, with the 677CC subjects remaining relatively stable, while the 677TT subjects experienced a dramatic increase, with 23 of the 29 subjects having high plasma homocysteine levels. These data indicate that the RDA of 400 μg DFE/day does not meet the needs of Mexican-American men of either genotype [16].

Results from a large clinical trial of 932 northern Chinese women of child-bearing age showed that even after ingesting a folic acid supplement of 4000 μg/day for 6 months, 21% of the 327 subjects with the 677TT genotype had a high plasma homocysteine level (defined as > 10.4 μmol/L) [17]. Overall, the indicators of folate status of the 677TT subjects who received the supplement significantly increased (serum and red cell folate) or decreased (plasma homocysteine), but none reached the levels of the 677CC subjects. These results support the idea that these Chinese women with the 677TT genotype have much higher needs than others [17].

An analysis of data collected from 6793 NHANES III subjects, however, leads to different conclusions for the U.S. population [18]. NHANES III, conducted between 1991 and 1994, used a complicated subject selection process to choose a representative sample of Americans. Importantly, NHANES III occurred prior to the 1998 folic acid fortification of flour and grain products in the United States and Canada. The NHANES III data showed that there were no differences in serum folate between the 677TT and 677CC genotypes when folic acid intake exceeded 400 μg/d. Furthermore, when the authors divided folate intake into quintiles, the three quintiles of 677TT subjects that consumed $\geq$308 μg/day had mean serum homocysteine values that were within normal levels. These authors conclude that even before fortification, the combination of diet and supplemental folic acid was already protecting the 677TT individual and that fortification "may have attenuated the effect of the polymorphism" [18].

In conclusion, the MTHFR 677TT polymorphism has its greatest impact on folate status when folate and folic acid intakes are low and supplements are not taken. The fortification policies of the United States and Canada ensure that folic acid intake has increased since 1998.

MTHFR VARIATIONS AND RISK FOR CHRONIC DISEASE

Since the identification of the MTHFR polymorphisms, a great deal of research has investigated and reported risks for neural tube defects, cardiovascular disease, colorectal cancer, and dementias in people with poor folate status [12,19]. This research has an extra dimension when the MTHFR polymorphisms are also considered.

Neural Tube Defects (NTDs)
The impact of folic acid fortification in the United States, Canada, and other nations has been widely reported as beneficial. Different studies of the U.S. population ". . . reported an 11-20% decline in anencephaly and a 21-34% reduction in the occurrence of spina bifida . . ." [20, p 10]. Mills and Carter [21] reported that the Canadian health care system provided more complete data about neural tube defects and found a 50% reduction in NTDs after a folic acid fortification program similar to that in the U.S. was implemented.

Botto and Yang [13] pooled data from 15 studies from Europe and North America. They calculated the odds ratio of parents having the 677TT genotype to their children having an NTD and found a significant relationship. The increased risk is more related to the mother's genotype than the father's. But as discussed above, this increased risk does not mean that a woman with the 677TT genotype will automatically have poor folate status. A diet rich in folate and folic acid can normalize folate status in most people with the 677TT genotype. Thus, it is very important to include questions about specific folate-rich foods, folic acid-fortified foods, and folic acid supplements when assessing an individual's intake.

Coronary Heart Disease
While the increased risk for coronary heart disease (CHD) in individuals with hyperhomocysteinemia is well documented in case control studies, large prospective trials have not found the same relationship. It's not clear if hyperhomocysteinemia is a cause or a predictor of heart disease [22]. This uncertainty is reinforced by the general finding that individuals with the 677TT genotype have higher plasma homocysteine levels, but do not have a greater risk of cardiovascular disease. A meta-analysis of 80 studies including 26,000 subjects with the 677TT genotype and 31,813 677CC control subjects reported a small increase in the chances of 677TT subjects developing CHD. However, "This meta-analysis provides no evidence of a causal relation between homocysteine and heart disease risk in European, North American, and Australian populations" [23].

Dementias
If homocysteine accumulates inside cells, the cells will evict this metabolic oxidant into the bloodstream. Homocysteine crosses the blood-brain barrier and is theorized to be neurotoxic and cause increased oxidative stress [24]. Many people with dementias also have high serum homocysteine levels and these are positively correlated with lesions in the brain. Since research indicates that high plasma homocysteine is a risk factor for dementias and other cognitive problems (depression, psychosis), it logically follows that individuals with MTHFR genetic polymorphisms are at a greater risk. However, this relationship has not been verified [19,24].

Using a meta-analysis design, Ho, et al. [25] identified 1432 articles that met the search criteria, but used only 17 that provided enough data deemed necessary by the authors. They report that data from thousands of subjects do not support a causal relationship between high serum homocysteine and a later diagnosis of dementia. The genotype of the subjects is not mentioned. However, another meta-analysis that compared subjects with (n=672) and without (n=1038) vascular dementia (the most common type of dementia after Alzheimer's disease) noted their MTHFR 677C $\longrightarrow$ T genotype. Six studies included Caucasian subjects, while 5 were of Asian subjects. The overall odds ratio for vascular dementia among those with the 677TT genotype was 1.41, showing an increased risk, and the condition was significantly associated with the 677TT genotype for the Asian subjects [26].

Colorectal Cancer
Poor folate status is positively correlated with risk of colorectal cancer. This can be theoretically explained because a decrease in folate leads to DNA hypomethylation (due to a lack of 5-methyl THF, as shown in Figure 9.30) and increased uracil (instead of thymine) incorporation into DNA. In addition, DNA hypomethylation negatively affects gene expression. The presence of uracil increases the activity of DNA repair mechanisms, but the repair may not be totally effective. In summary, poor folate status increases the risk of cancer due to the combination of DNA hypomethylation and increased uracil incorporation [12].

But this seemingly straightforward relationship of poor folate status to an increased risk of colorectal cancer does not seem to hold when the MTHFR polymorphism is considered. The 677TT genotype, thought to increase risks for other diseases, may actually protect individuals from colorectal cancer. In a recent meta-analysis, Taioli et al. [27] sought to include all published and unpublished studies conducted since of the original report about MTHFR 677TT individuals' decreased risk of colon cancer. The 29 of the identified 199 articles that met the inclusion criteria for the study included 11,936 cases of colorectal cancer and 18,714 control subjects. Results from this statistical analysis showed that the 677TT genotype was related to a reduced risk of colorectal cancer, even when smoking, body mass index, and moderate alcohol intake (not alcohol abuse) were considered. When an odds ratio was calculated based upon ethnic groups, Whites and Asians with the 677TT genotype still had a reduced colorectal cancer risk, but Latinos and Blacks did not. This may be due to few studies being done in these two groups. These authors acknowledge the absence of information about the folic acid intake of any of the subjects.

Readers may wonder why this imbalance in thymine synthesis and DNA methylation might protect against colorectal cancer in the 677TT homozygote. Researchers state that the reported differences may be due to chance, but several meta-analyses share similar findings about this relationship. Perhaps the body's access to methyl groups, which are available from dietary methionine or choline, may explain the relationship.

THE RELATIONSHIP BETWEEN THE MTHFR 677C ⟶ T VARIANT AND CHOLINE STATUS

In 1998 the Institute of Medicine recognized the Adequate Intake (AI) of choline as between 425 and 550 mg/d for adults. Humans obtain choline by ingesting phosphatidlycholine (abundant in milk, liver, eggs, and peanuts) or through de novo synthesis. As shown in the illustration on the right column of page 348, the B vitamin choline is degraded to betaine, which functions as a methyl donor. In fact, the methyl group needed to convert homocysteine to methionine can come from either 5-methyl THF or betaine, as shown in Figure 6.12. How does good or poor choline status affect methylation reactions in people with the MTHFR 677C ⟶ T polymorphism?

Shin and co-authors [28] fed Mexican-American men with the 677TT (n = 29) or 677CC (n = 31) genotype a diet containing the RDA of folate combined with 300, 550, 1100, or 2200 mg/d of choline for 12 weeks. A variety of "functional biomarkers of 1-carbon metabolism" (p. 976) including plasma S-adenosylmethionine (SAM) and DNA methylation were measured. The results showed no difference in SAM levels, but the 677TT subjects needed 1100 or 2200 mg/d of choline to maintain DNA methylation and to prevent an increase in DNA damage. The authors acknowledge that their results do not automatically apply to health or a decrease in disease risk; they urge continued investigation into this relationship.

SUMMARY

This brief discussion about the effect of MTHFR polymorphisms currently has limited application to the general public for two reasons. First, there is currently little individualized genetic mapping of the population. A list of companies that do assay for the MTHFR variant is available from the Gene Tests page from the National Center for Biotechnology Information [29]. Second, the impact of an MTHFR polymorphism on an individual's health or on that of his/her children is not clear. This is especially true in the U.S. and Canada, where grain products are fortified with folic acid. However, research findings do strongly suggest that individuals with the 677TT MTHFR genotype should eat foods rich in folate, folic acid, and choline.

These two current limitations will decline with enhanced technology and continued research. Future nutrition professionals will probably consider MTHFR polymorphisms, among many other genetic traits, in their assessments and recommendations. Understanding how slight alterations in the human genome might affect nutrient needs and disease risk sheds light into the future provision of personalized nutrition care.

References

1. Collins, F., & McKusick, V.A. (2001). Implications of the Human Genome Project for medical science. *Journal of the American Medical Association, 285,* 540–544.

2. Varmus, H. (2010) Ten years on — the human genome and medicine. *New England Journal of Medicine, 362,* 2028–2029.

3. Life Sciences Research Office (2005). Life Sciences Research Office, Inc. Center for Emerging Issues in Science. *Report on: The future of nutrigenomics.* Bethesda, MD: Life Sciences Research Office.

4. The NCMHD Center of Excellence for Nutritional Genomics. Web site: http://nutrigenomics.ucdavis.edu/?page=Information/Glossary

5. Debusk, R.M., Fogarty, C.P., Ordovas, J.M., & Kornman, K.S. (2005). Nutritional genomics in practice: Where do we begin? *Journal of the American Dietetic Association, 105*(4), 589.

6. Nussman, R.L., McInnes, R.R., Willard, H.F. (2001). Genetics in medicine (6th ed.) Philadelphia, PA: W.B. Saunders Co, p 87.

7. Moyers, S., & Bailey, L. B. (2001). Fetal malformation and folate metabolism: Review of recent evidence. *Nutrition Reviews, 7,* 215–224.

8. Stover, P. J., & Garza, C. (2006). Polymorphisms: Effect on nutrient utilization and metabolism. In Shils, M, Shike, M., Ross, A. C., Caballero, B. & Cousins, R. J. (Eds.) *Modern nutrition in health and disease* (pp. 627–635). Baltimore, MD: Lippincott Williams & Wilkins.

9. Esfahani, S., Cogger, E.A., & Caudill, M.A. (2003). Heterogeneity in the prevalence of methlenetetrahydrofolate reductase gene polymorphisms in women in different ethnic groups. *Journal of the American Dietetic Association, 103*(2), 200–207.

10. Gueant-Rodriguez, R. M., Gueant, J. L., Debard, R., Thirion, S., Hong, L. X., Bornowicki, J. P., et al. (2006). Prevalence of methylenetetrahydrofolate reductase 677T and 1298C alleles and folate status: a comparative study in Mexican, West African, and European populations. *American Journal of Clinical Nutrition, 83,* 701–707.

11. Guinotte, C.L., Burns, M.G., Asume, J.A., Hata, H., Urrutia, T.F., Alamilla, A., et al. (2003). Methylenetetrahydrofolate reductase 677C → T variant modulates folate status response to controlled folate intakes in young women. *Journal of Nutrition, 133,* 1272–1280.

12. Rampersaud, G.C., Bailey, L.B., & Kauwell, G.P. (2002). Relationship of folate to colorectal and cervical cancer: Review and recommendations for practitioners. *Journal of the American Dietetic Association, 102*(9), 1273–1282.

13. Botto, L.D., & Yang, Q. (2000). Methylenetetrahydrofolate reductase (MTHFR) and birth defects. *American Journal of Epidemiology, 151*(9), 862–877.

14. Ashfield-Watt, P.A., Pullin, C.H., Whiting, J.M., Clark, Z.E., Moat, S.J., Newcombe, R.G., et al. (2002). Methylenetetrahydrofolate reductase 677C → T genotype modulates homocysteine responses to a folate-rich diet or a low-dose folic acid supplement: A randomized controlled trial. *American Journal of Clinical Nutrition, 76,* 180–186.

15. Hung, J., Yang, T.L., Urrutia, T.F., Li, R., Perry, C.A., Hata, H., et al. (2006). Additional food folate derived exclusively from natural sources improves folate status in young women with the MTHFR 677 CC or TT genotype. *Journal of Nutritional Biochemistry, 17*(11), 728.

16. Solis, C., Veenema, K., Ivanov, A.A., Tran, S., Li, R., Wang, W., et al. (2008). Folate intake at RDA levels is inadequate for Mexican American men with the Methylenetetrahydrofolate reductase 677TT genotype. *Journal of Nutrition, 138,* 67–72.

17. Crider, K. S., Zhu, J., Yang Q., Yang, T.P., Gindler, J., Maneval, D.R., et al. (2011). MTHFR 677C ⟶ T genotype is associated with folate and homocysteine concentrations in a large population-based, double-blind trial of folic acid supplementation. *American Journal of Clinical Nutrition, 93,* 1365–1372.

18. Yang, Q., Botto, L. D., Gallagher, M., Friedman, J. M., Sanders, C. L., Koontz, D. (2008). Prevalence and effects of gene-gene and gene-nutrient interactions on serum folate and serum total homocysteine concentrations in the United States: findings from the third National Health and Nutrition Examination Survey DNA Bank. *American Journal of Clinical Nutrition, 88,* 232–246.

19. Ames, B.N., Elson-Schwab, I., & Silver, E.A. (2002). High-dose vitamin therapy stimulates variant enzymes with decreased coenzyme binding affinity (increased Km): Relevance to genetic disease and polymorphisms. *American Journal of Clinical Nutrition, 75,* 616–658.

20. Mosley, B. S., Cleves, M. A., Siega-Riz, A. M., Shaw, G. M., Canfield, D., Waller, K., et al. (2009). Neural tube defects and maternal folate intake among

pregnancies conceived after folic acid fortification in the United States. *American Journal of Epidemiology, 169,* 9–17.

21. Mills, J. L., & Carter, T. C. (2009). Invited commentary: Preventing neural tube defects and more via food fortification? *American Journal of Epidemiology, 169,* 18–21.

22. Smulders, Y.M., & Blom, H.J. (2011). The homocysteine controversy. *Journal of Inherited and Metabolic Diseases, 34,* 93–99.

23. Lewis, S.J., Ebrahim, S., & Smith, G.D. (2005). Meta-analysis of MTHFR 677C → T polymorphism and coronary heart disease: Does totality of evidence support causal role for homocysteine and preventive potential of folate? *British Medical Journal, 331,* 7524.

24. Shea, T.B., Lyons-Weiler, J., & Rogers, E. (2002). Homocysteine, folate deprivation and Alzheimer neuropathology. *Journal of Alzheimer's Disease, 4,* 261–267.

25. Ho, R. C., Cheung, M. W., Fu, E., Win, H. H., Zaw, M. H., Nh, A., et al. (2011). Is high homocysteine level a risk factor for cognitive decline in elderly? A systematic review, meta-analysis, and meta-regression. *American Journal of Geriatric Psychiatry, 19,* 607–617.

26. Liu, H. , Yang, M., Li, G. M. Qiu, Y. Zheng, J., Du, X., et al. (2010). The MTHFR C677T polymorphism contributes to n increased risk for vascular dementia: a meta-analysis. *Journal of Neurological Sciences, 294,* 74–80.

27. Taioli, E., Garza, M. A., Ahn, Y. O., Bishop, D. T., Bost, J., Budai, B., et al. (2009). Meta- and pooled analyses of the methylenetetrahydrofolate reductase (MTHFR) C677T polymorphism and colorectal cancer: A HuGE-GSEC review. *American Journal of Epidemiology, 170,* 1207–1221.

28. Shin, W., Yan, J., Abratte, C.M., Vermeylen, F., & Caudill, M.A. (2010). Choline intake exceeding current dietary recommendations preserves markers of cellular methylation in a genetic subgroup of folate-compromised men. *Journal of Nutrition, 140*(5), 975–980.

29. National Center for Biotechnology Information. Web site: http://www.ncbi.nlm.nih.gov/sites/GeneTests/?db=GeneTests

FAT-SOLUBLE VITAMINS

THIS CHAPTER ADDRESSES EACH of the four fat-soluble vitamins—A, D, E, and K—and the carotenoids. The reader is referred to Chapter 9 for an overview of vitamins and information pertaining to the water-soluble vitamins. The absorption and transport of the fat-soluble vitamins, in contrast to those of the water-soluble vitamins, are closely associated with the absorption and transport of lipids. As with dietary lipids, optimal fat-soluble vitamin absorption requires the presence of bile salts. Similarly, fat-soluble vitamins are transported in the blood by chylomicrons. Moreover, the fat-soluble vitamins are stored in body lipids, although the amount stored varies widely among the four fat-soluble vitamins. Table 10.1 provides an overview of the discovery, function, deficiency syndrome, food sources, and Recommended Dietary Allowance (RDA) or Adequate Intake (AI) of each of the fat-soluble vitamins. The RDAs and AIs for all nutrients and for all age groups are provided on the inside front cover of the book.

VITAMIN A AND CAROTENOIDS

The term *vitamin A* (also called preformed vitamin A or retinoids) is generally used to refer to a group of compounds that possess the biological activity of all-*trans* retinol. The retinoids are structurally similar and include retinol, retinal, retinoic acid, and retinyl ester, as well as synthetic analogues. Structurally, retinoids contain a β-ionone ring and a polyunsaturated side chain, with either an alcohol group (retinol, Figure 10.1a), an aldehyde group (retinal, also called retinaldehyde, Figure 10.1b), a carboxylic acid group (retinoic acid, Figure 10.1c), or an ester group (retinyl ester [Figure 10.1d], such as retinyl stearate or palmitate [shown in Figure 10.1e]). The side chain is made up of four **isoprenoid** units with a series of conjugated double bonds. The double bonds may exist in a *trans* (as in all-*trans* retinol) or a *cis* configuration.

Vitamin A was initially found to be an essential growth factor in animal foods and was called fat-soluble A. McCollum and Davis, followed by Osborne and Mendel, are credited with its discovery in about 1915.

Carotenoids (often referred to as provitamin A) represent a group of compounds that are precursors of vitamin A. Although more than 600 carotenoids (lipid-soluble red, orange, and yellow pigments produced by plants) exist, fewer than 10% are thought to exhibit vitamin A activity. In other words, fewer than 60 can be converted to retinol. Structurally, carotenoids consist of an expanded carbon chain containing conjugated double bonds, usually, but not always, with an unsubstituted β-ionone ring at one or both ends of the chain. Three provitamin A carotenoids, which are found most often in the all-*trans* form but can occur as *cis* isomers, are β-carotene (Figure 10.1f), α-carotene

Table 10.1 The Fat-Soluble Vitamins: Discovery, Function, Deficiency Syndrome, Food Sources, and Recommended Dietary Allowance (RDA) or Adequate Intake (AI)

Vitamin	Discovery	Biochemical or Physiological Function	Deficiency Syndrome or Symptoms	Good Sources in Rank Order	RDA or AI
Vitamin A (retinol, retinal, retinoic acid) Provitamins Carotenoids, particularly β-carotene	McCollum (1915)	Synthesis of rhodopsin and other light receptor pigments; metabolites involved in growth, cell differentiation, bone development, and immune function	Poor dark adaptation, night blindness, xerosis, keratomalacia, Bitot's spots	Beef liver, dairy products, sweet potato, carrots, spinach, butternut squash, greens, broccoli, cantaloupe	900 μg RAE[a] 700 μg RAE[b]
Vitamin D Provitamins 7-dehydrocholesterol Vitamin D$_2$ (ergocalciferol) Vitamin D$_3$ (cholecalciferol)	McCollum (1922)	Regulator of bone mineral metabolism, blood calcium homeostasis, and cell differentiation, proliferation, and growth	Children: rickets Adults: osteomalacia	Synthesized in skin exposed to ultraviolet light; fortified milk	15–20 μg[c,d]
Vitamin E Tocopherols Tocotrienols	Evans and Bishop (1922)	Antioxidant	Myopathy, anemia, and neuropathy	Vegetable seed oils	15 mg α-tocopherol[c]
Vitamin K Phylloquinones Menaquinones	Dam (1935)	Activates blood-clotting factors by γ-carboxylating glutamic acid residues; carboxylates other proteins	Defective blood clotting	Synthesized by intestinal bacteria; green leafy vegetables, soy beans, beef liver	120 μg[a,e] 90 μg[b,e]

[a]Adult males
[b]Adult females
[c]Both males and females
[d]Varies with age for adults; see text
[e]Adequate intake

(Figure 10.1g), and β-cryptoxanthin (Figure 10.1h). Although not all carotenoids are vitamin A precursors, many carotenoids, such as lycopene (an open-chain analog of β-carotene; Figure 10.1i), and many oxycarotenoids (also called oxygenated carotenoids), such as canthaxanthin (Figure 10.1j), lutein (Figure 10.1k), and zeaxanthin, are thought to be of physiological importance to the body.

Sources

Both retinoids and carotenoids are found naturally in foods. Vitamin A is found primarily in selected foods of animal origin, especially liver; dairy products (including milk, cheese, and butter); eggs; fish, such as tuna (55 IU or 16.5 μg/3 oz), sardines (92 IU or 27.6 μg/3 oz), and herring (731 IU or 220 μg/3 oz); and fish oils, such as cod liver oil. Liver (3 oz beef) provides about 22,000 IU (6,600 μg) of vitamin A. An egg contains about 280 IU (84 μg) of vitamin A. Milk has about 500 IU (150 μg) of vitamin A/cup and cheddar and Swiss cheeses (1 oz) contain about 285 IU (85 μg) and 200 IU (60 μg) of vitamin A, respectively. Some products, such as margarine and breakfast cereals, may be fortified with vitamin A. Wheat bran cereal with raisins, for example, provides 15% of the Daily Value of vitamin A (which is 5,000 IU) or 750 IU

(225 μg) of vitamin A/cup, and margarine has 10% or 500 IU (150 μg) of vitamin A/tablespoon.

The main form of vitamin A in foods is as retinyl esters such as retinyl palmitate (Figure 10.1e). In pharmaceutical vitamin preparations, all-*trans* retinyl acetate and all-*trans* retinyl palmitate are commonly used. Aquasol A, a water-miscible form of the vitamin, is available for people with a fat malabsorptive disorder. Retinoids can undergo oxidation if exposed to varying degrees of, for example, oxygen, light, heat, and some metals.

Carotenoids are synthesized by a wide variety of plants and thus are found naturally in many fruits and vegetables. One of the most abundant carotenoids is β-carotene, which exhibits the greatest amount of provitamin A activity. Other common dietary carotenoids include α-carotene and β-cryptoxanthin (both provitamin A carotenoids) along with lycopene, lutein, and zeaxanthin. In general, yellow, orange, and red (brightly colored) fruits and vegetables such as carrots, watermelon, papayas, tomatoes, tomato products (ketchup, chili sauce, spaghetti sauce), squash, pink grapefruits, and pumpkins provide significant amounts of carotenoids. Green vegetables also contain some carotenoids, but the pigment is masked by (green) chlorophyll. Carrots typically represent a major source of both α- and β-carotene in American diets; ½ carrot provides about

4,550 μg of β-carotene. Other major dietary contributors of β-carotene include broccoli (725 μg β-carotene/½ cup cooked), cantaloupe (1,616 μg/½ cup), squash (136 μg/cup cooked), peas (600 μg/½ cup cooked), and spinach (5,660 μg/½ cup cooked). Fruits provide much of the dietary β-cryptoxanthin, and tomatoes, along with tomato sauces and watermelon, are good sources of dietary lycopene, a carotenoid that is red in color. Good sources of zeaxanthin include peppers (orange), corn, potatoes, and eggs. Broccoli, beets, kiwi fruit, and eggs provide some lutein. Canthaxanthin, a red-orange carotenoid, is found in plants as well as in fish and seafood such as sea trout and crustaceans. Meat and fish are not major sources of carotenoids, but because animals and fish feed on plants,

they can accumulate some carotenoids. Carotenoids also may be added to foods. β-carotene and canthaxanthin, for example, are approved by the Food and Drug Administration for use as food color additives.

Digestion and Absorption

Vitamin A, because it is bound to other food components, requires some digestion before it can be absorbed into the body (see Figure 10.2). Retinol, for example, is typically bound to fatty acid esters, the most common of which is retinyl palmitate (previously shown in Figure 10.1e). Furthermore, retinyl esters and carotenes in foods are often complexed with protein from which they must

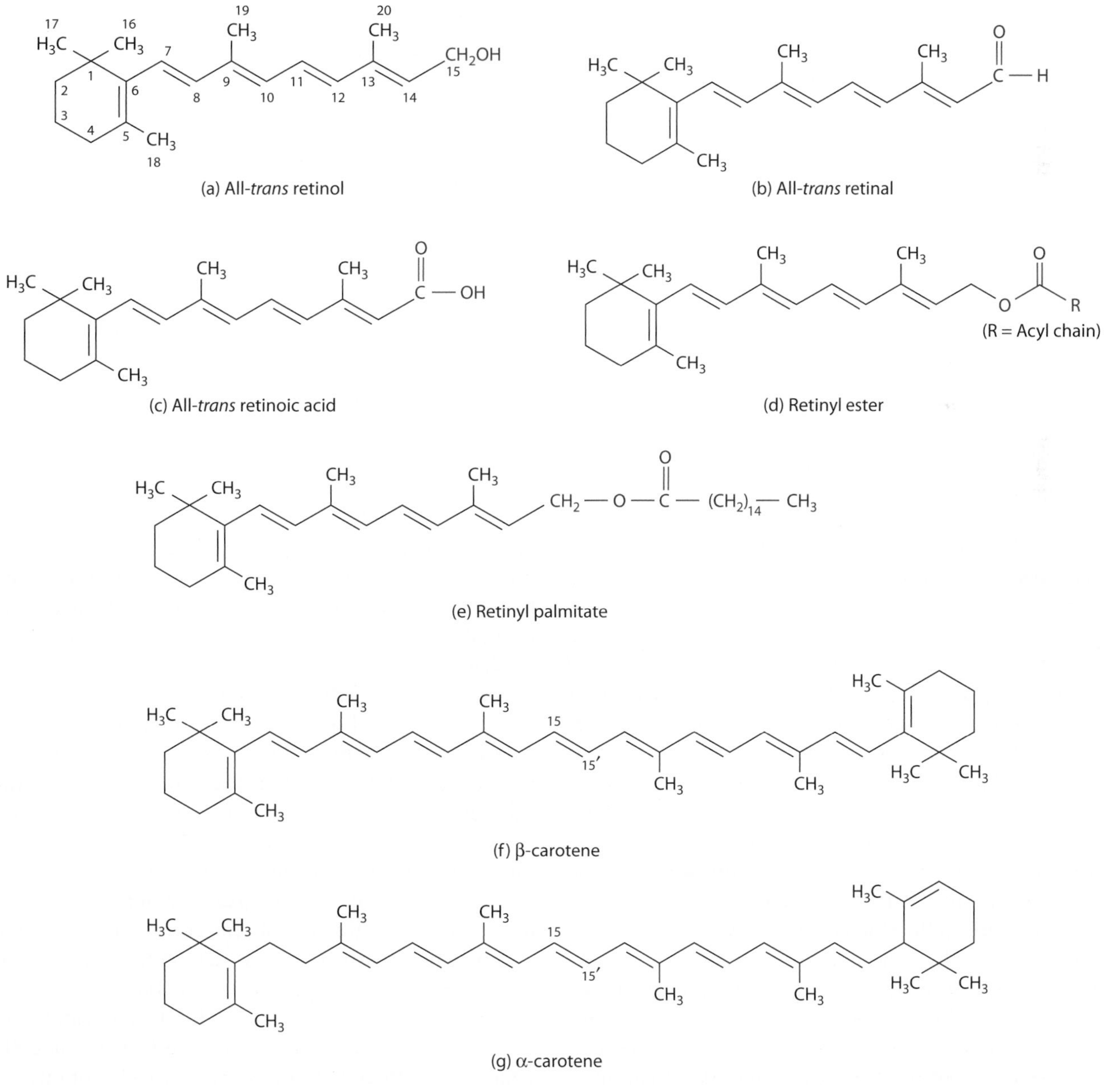

(a) All-*trans* retinol

(b) All-*trans* retinal

(c) All-*trans* retinoic acid

(d) Retinyl ester

(e) Retinyl palmitate

(f) β-carotene

(g) α-carotene

Figure 10.1 Vitamin A and carotenoid structures *(continued on next page)*.

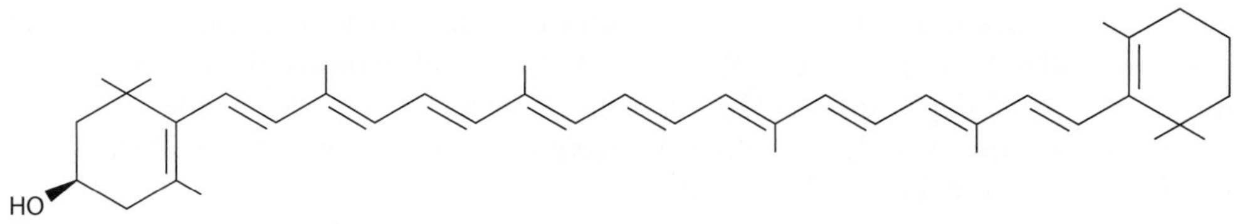

(h) β-cryptoxanthin

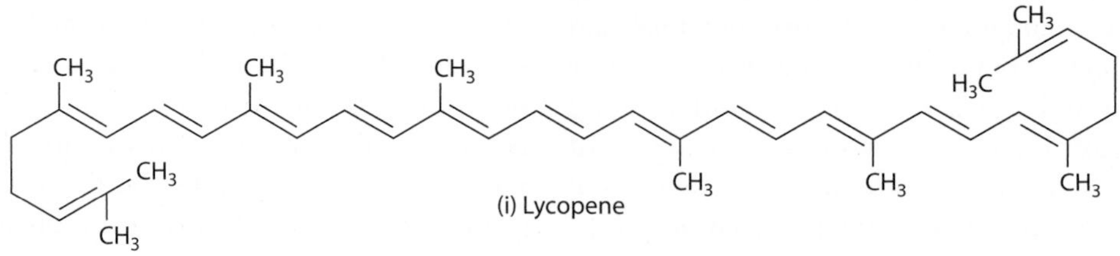

(i) Lycopene

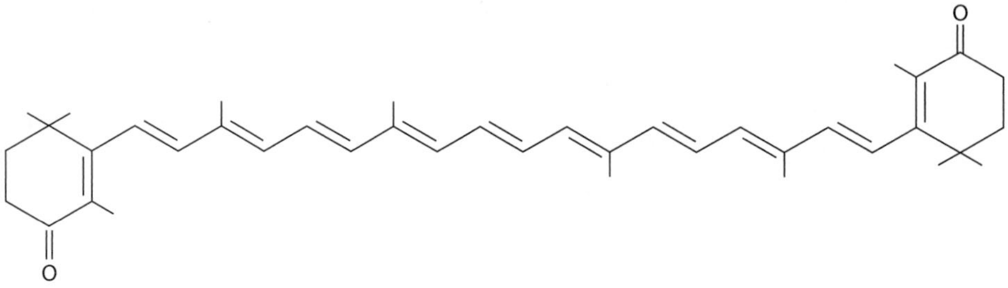

(j) Canthaxanthin

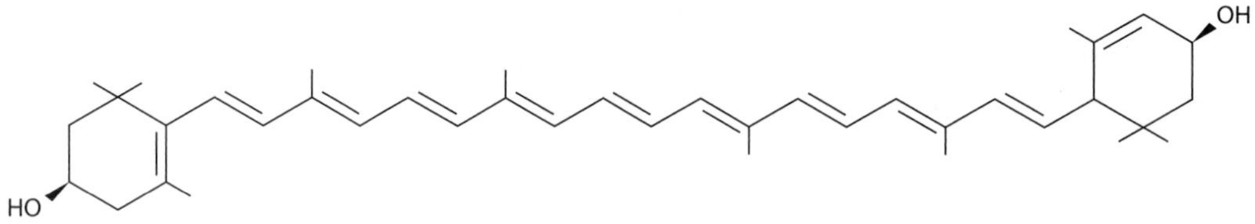

(k) Lutein

Figure 10.1 *(continued)* Vitamin A and carotenoid structures.

be released. Although heating plant foods weakens some complexes, such as protein-carotenoid complexes, enzymatic digestion is still required. Carotenoids and retinyl esters are initially hydrolyzed from protein by pepsin in the stomach. Because of their fat solubility, the freed (i.e., no longer bound to protein) retinyl esters and carotenoids typically coalesce, along with other lipids, to form fat globules in the stomach. These fat globules containing the vitamin are emptied into the duodenum, where bile is required to emulsify them (emulsification results in large fat globules being broken up into smaller droplets).

Proteolytic enzymes in the duodenum can hydrolyze any remaining protein-bound retinyl esters or carotenoids not freed in the stomach. Hydrolysis of retinyl and carotenoid esters by various hydrolases and esterases occurs at the same time that triacylglycerols, phospholipids, and cholesteryl esters are being hydrolyzed by pancreatic enzymes. Pancreatic lipase and pancreatic cholesterol ester hydrolase, secreted into the lumen of the small intestine, facilitate lipid and vitamin A digestion. Additionally,

enzymes such as retinyl ester hydrolase function on the intestinal brush border to digest the vitamin. Pancreatic hydrolases cleave shorter-chain retinyl esters, whereas intestinal brush border hydrolases act on longer-chain retinyl esters.

Micelles form within the lumen of the small intestine from bile salts, phospholipids, monoacylglycerol, and retinyl and carotenoid esters. The released or now free carotenoids and retinols in the small intestine remain solubilized in micellar solutions along with the other fat-soluble food components. The micellar solutions containing the carotenoids and vitamin A are absorbed by passive diffusion across the brush border membrane of the duodenum and jejunum and into the enterocyte. Carotenoids also may be absorbed by a carotenoid transporter, called scavenger receptor class B type 1 (SR-B1) [1,2].

The efficiency of absorption differs between vitamin A and carotenoids. Approximately 70% to 90% of dietary vitamin A is absorbed as long as the meal contains some (~10 g or more) fat [3]. Carotenoid absorption varies

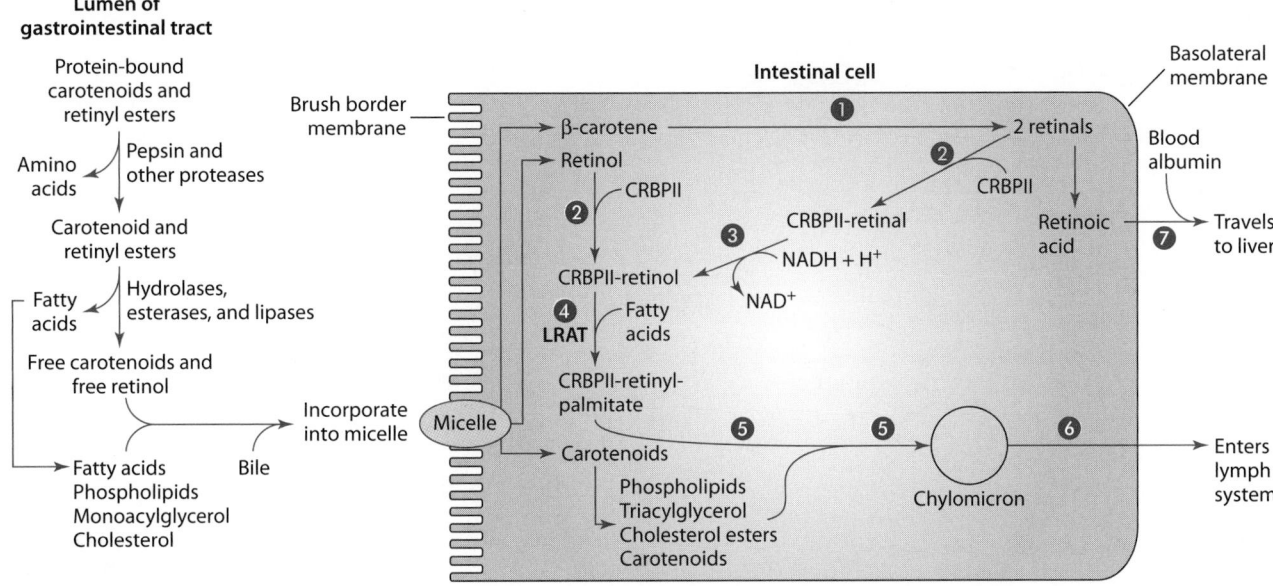

1. β-carotene is converted into two retinal molecules. See Figure 10.3 for details of this reaction.

2. Cellular retinol-binding protein (CRBP) II binds to both retinol and retinal in the intestinal cell.

3. Retinal, while attached to CRBPII, is reduced to retinol by retinal/retinaldehyde reductase to form CRBPII-retinol.

4. Lecithin retinol acyl transferase (LRAT) esterifies a fatty acid (palmitic acid) onto the CRBPII-bound retinol to form CRBPII-retinylpalmitate.

5. Retinyl esters are incorporated along with phospholipids, triacylglycerol, cholesterol esters, carotenoids, and apoproteins to form a chylomicron.

6. Chylomicrons leave the intestinal cell and enter the lymph system and ultimately the blood.

7. Retinoic acid can directly enter the blood, where it attaches to albumin for transport to the liver.

Figure 10.2 Digestion and absorption of carotenoids and vitamin A, and reesterification of retinol in the intestinal cell.

considerably, depending on food processing, but it is typically less than that of vitamin A. Carotenoid absorption ranges from about < 5% for carotenoids in uncooked vegetables or non–heat processed vegetable juices to about 60% if present as a pure oil or as part of an aqueous dispersion supplement [3,4]. Absorption of specifically β-carotene ranges from about 20% to 50%, while the absorption of other carotenoids is usually considerably less. Fiber (especially pectin) intake as well as excessive vitamin E consumption can diminish carotenoid absorption. Pectin appears to diminish absorption by interfering with micelle formation.

Within the enterocyte (and to some extent in the liver, adipose tissue, lungs, and kidneys, among other organs), some carotenoids, including α- and β-carotene and cryptoxanthin, undergo metabolism. The extent to which carotenoids are converted to retinoids is influenced by several factors, such as the vitamin A status of the person and the amounts and forms of the carotenoids consumed. For example, with higher vitamin A intake, receptor-mediated carotenoid absorption and conversion to vitamin A are decreased [2]. Additionally, as dietary β-carotene consumption increases, β-carotene conversion to vitamin

A decreases [5]. The synthesis of vitamin A (specifically all-*trans* retinal) from β-carotene within the enterocyte is accomplished by either noncentral cleavage by β-carotene 9′10′ dioxygenase, or hydrolysis by β-carotene 15,15′-mono-oxygenase (an iron-dependent oxygenase that is also found in the liver, lungs, kidneys, and retina) [6,7]. Noncentral cleavage generates several metabolites (alcohols, aldehydes, etc.), whereas mono-oxygenase activity converts one molecule of β-carotene into two molecules of retinal (Figures 10.2 and 10.3) [7]. However, up to about 15% of β-carotene may leave enterocytes intact (i.e., without oxidation to retinal). The efficiency of β-carotene conversion to retinal is estimated at about 50%. An estimated 12 μg of β-carotene or 24 μg of α-carotene or β-cryptoxanthin is required to produce 1 μg of retinol (which is generated from retinal, as discussed next).

Within enterocytes, retinoids also undergo metabolism (Figure 10.2). Retinal, produced from β-carotene or other carotenoids, is reduced by retinal/retinaldehyde reductase, an NADH-dependent enzyme, to retinol. Additionally, the vitamin must be reesterified to enable its incorporation into chylomicrons for release into the

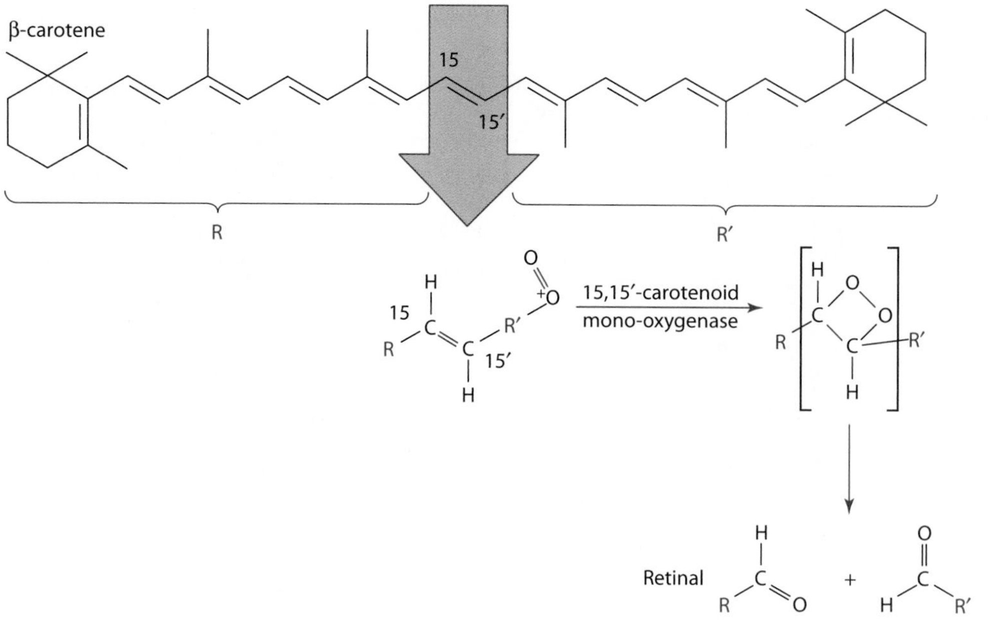

Figure 10.3 Cleavage of carotene to retinal.

blood. Retinol, whether formed by carotenoid oxidation or originating from dietary retinyl esters, follows one of two metabolic pathways for reesterification within the enterocyte. The primary pathway (Figure 10.2) involves cellular retinol-binding protein (CRBP) II, one of a group of low-molecular-weight lipid-binding proteins that help regulate retinol use in cells. CRBPII, present in the cytosol of the enterocyte, binds both retinol and retinal and directs the reduction of retinal to retinol and subsequent esterification to a fatty acid. CRBPII-bound retinol is esterified by lecithin retinol acyl transferase (LRAT) to form mainly retinyl palmitate, but also retinyl stearate, retinyl oleate, and retinyl linoleate, among others. LRAT specifically transfers sn-1 fatty acids from membrane-associated phosphatidylcholine to retinol that is bound to CRBPs. LRAT is thought to be the main enzyme responsible for esterification in the small intestine, liver, pigment epithelium of the retina, and likely other tissues [8]. The second, minor pathway for reesterification is by acyl-CoA retinol acyl transferase (ARAT). The fatty acids used to esterify retinol are not reflective of the fatty acid content of the meal consumed.

Additional metabolism of vitamin A also may occur within the enterocyte, as shown in Figure 10.4, and within other cells, as shown later in Figures 10.5 and 10.10. Retinol, for example, may be conjugated (especially in the liver but also in the intestine) to glucuronic acid to form retinoid β-glucuronide, which is excreted in the bile. In addition, some of the retinal may be irreversibly oxidized to retinoic acid within the intestinal cell. Some of this retinoic acid also may then be conjugated to glucuronic acid to form retinoyl β-glucuronide. Retinoyl β-glucuronide and retinoic acid, in contrast to retinol, can enter the circulation through the portal vein. Retinoic acid is transported in the plasma bound tightly to albumin (Figure 10.2). Retinoyl β-glucuronide concentrations in the plasma are typically low, but the metabolite appears to function in part like retinoic acid in tissues, where it promotes growth and cell differentiation, but does not bind to nuclear retinoic acid receptors. Retinol is also used within some (primarily extra-intestinal) tissues to produce 11-*cis* retinal that is needed for vision, and 9-*cis* retinoic acid that functions in gene expression, as discussed in more detail under the section on vitamin A's functions. All three retinoids—retinol, retinal, and retinoic acid—also may undergo metabolism, especially in the liver, by the cytochrome P-450 system to generate a variety of oxidized metabolites.

Transport, Metabolism, and Storage

To leave the enterocyte for transport to tissues, the newly formed retinyl esters, along with small amounts of unesterified retinol and any carotenoids that have been absorbed unchanged, are incorporated into chylomicrons, also containing cholesterol esters, phospholipid, triacylglycerols, and apoproteins. The presence of vitamin E within the enterocyte is thought to protect β-carotene from oxidation; however, if present in too high a concentration, vitamin E may inhibit carotenoid absorption [3]. The chylomicrons, once formed, enter first into the lymphatic system and then into general circulation (i.e., the blood) via the thoracic duct. Chylomicrons deliver retinyl esters, some unesterified retinol, and carotenoids to many extrahepatic tissues, including bone marrow, blood cells, spleen, muscle, lungs, kidneys, and adipose tissue. In fact, the adipose tissue, which takes up retinyl esters from chylomicrons, stores about 15% to 20% of the body's

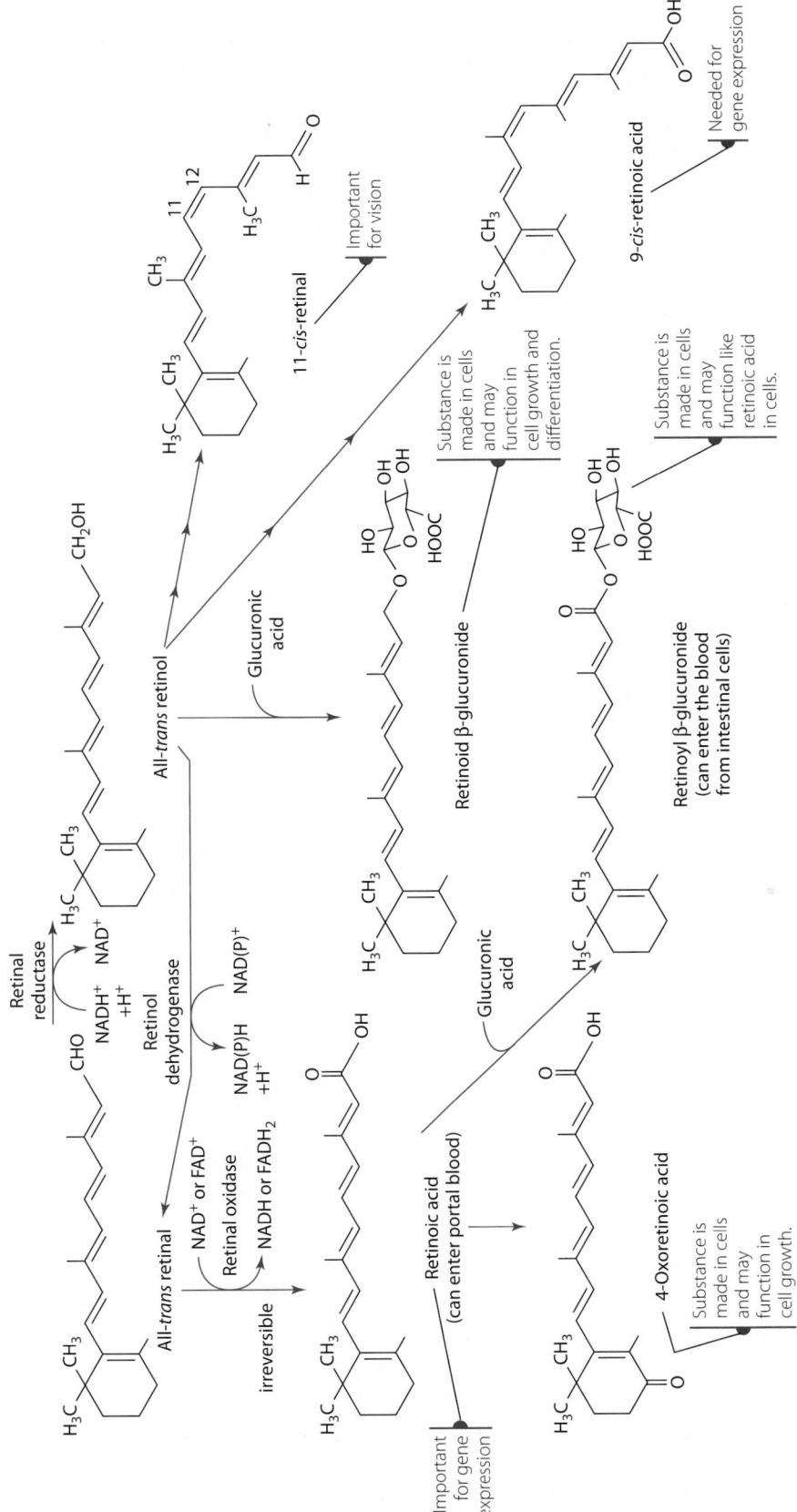

Figure 10.4 Retinoid metabolism.

vitamin A. Retinyl esters and carotenoids not taken up by peripheral tissue are transported to the liver as part of the chylomicron remnant. About 70% to 75% of chylomicron retinoids are cleared from circulation by the liver [9].

Carotenoids and vitamin A reaching the liver typically undergo additional metabolism. For example, carotenoids reaching the liver can follow three routes: cleavage, incorporation into and release as part of very-low-density lipoproteins (VLDLs) or other lipoproteins for transport to other tissues, and storage in the liver. The handling of retinyl esters that reach the liver is shown in Figure 10.5. However, most cells of the body are able to metabolize retinol generated from the retinyl esters through a number of metabolic pathways. The retinyl esters are hydrolyzed by a retinyl ester hydrolase following their uptake by the hepatic **parenchymal cells** (functional cells of an organ). Within the hepatic cell, retinol binds to a CRBP. CRBPs are found throughout the body. For example, CRBPI is present in all tissues but is found in especially high concentrations in the liver and kidneys. CRBPII is abundant in the intestine, especially the jejunum. CRBPIII is present in relatively high concentrations in the liver, skeletal muscle, kidneys, and heart; CRBPIV is mostly found in the heart, kidneys, and colon. As in the enterocyte, CRBPs in hepatic cells function both to help control cytosolic concentrations of free retinol and thus prevent its oxidation and to direct the vitamin, through a series of protein-protein interactions, to specific enzymes. CRBPs may also assist in the transfer of retinal across organelles for metabolism. As in the enterocyte, retinol metabolism (shown in Figure 10.5) includes possible esterification by enzymes such as LRAT if retinol is bound to CRBP, or ARAT if retinol is not bound to CRBP. Unbound CRBP concentrations are thought to inhibit LRAT and thereby prevent esterification for storage. CRBP-bound retinol also may be oxidized to retinal by NAD(P)H-dependent retinol dehydrogenase or phosphorylated to retinyl phosphate by ATP for glycoprotein functions.

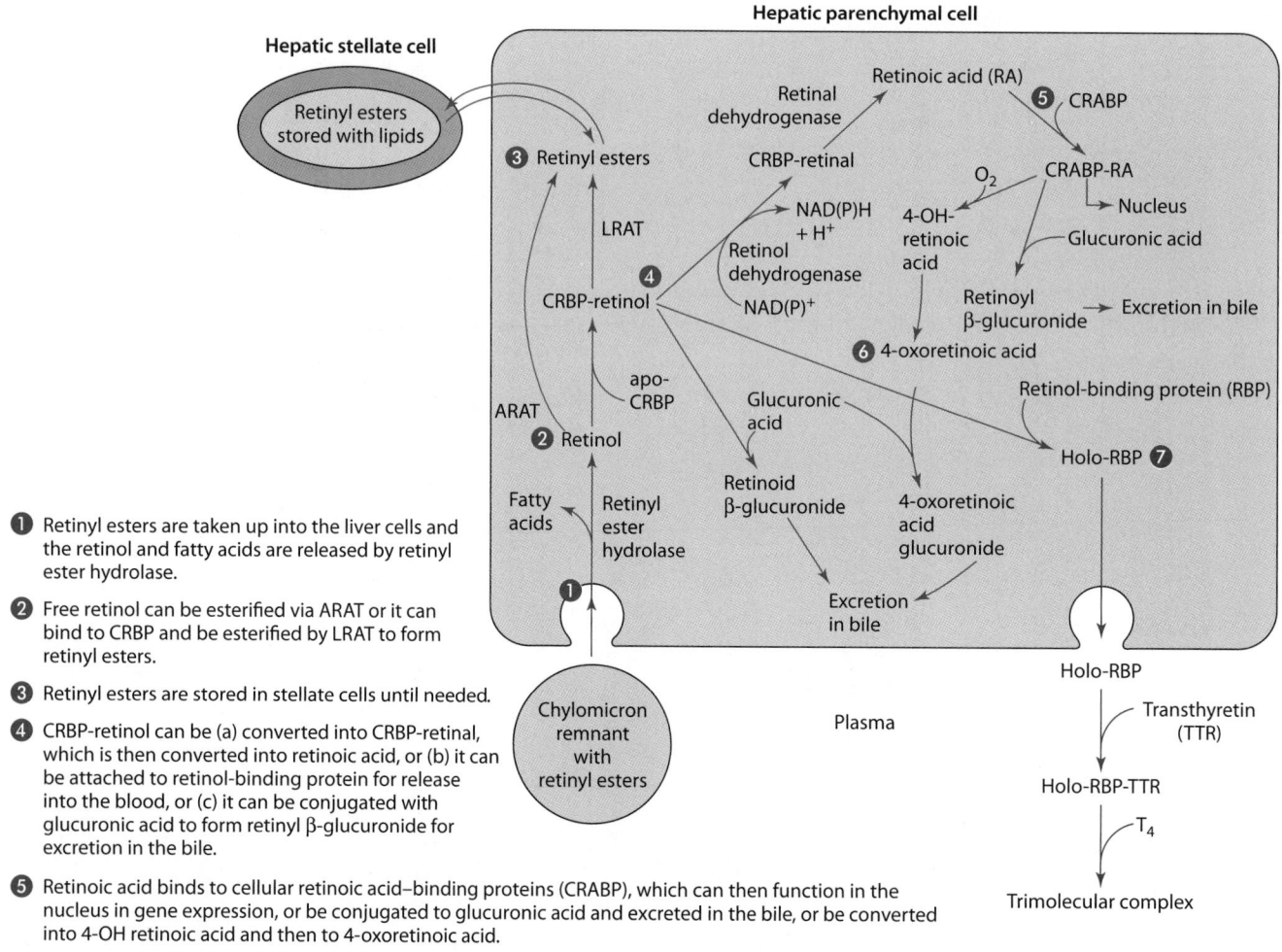

❶ Retinyl esters are taken up into the liver cells and the retinol and fatty acids are released by retinyl ester hydrolase.

❷ Free retinol can be esterified via ARAT or it can bind to CRBP and be esterified by LRAT to form retinyl esters.

❸ Retinyl esters are stored in stellate cells until needed.

❹ CRBP-retinol can be (a) converted into CRBP-retinal, which is then converted into retinoic acid, or (b) it can be attached to retinol-binding protein for release into the blood, or (c) it can be conjugated with glucuronic acid to form retinyl β-glucuronide for excretion in the bile.

❺ Retinoic acid binds to cellular retinoic acid–binding proteins (CRABP), which can then function in the nucleus in gene expression, or be conjugated to glucuronic acid and excreted in the bile, or be converted into 4-OH retinoic acid and then to 4-oxoretinoic acid.

❻ 4-oxoretinoic acid may function in cells like retinoic acid, or it may be conjugated to glucuronic acid for excretion in the bile.

❼ Retinol attaches to retinol-binding protein in the liver. The complex called holo-RBP is then released into the blood where it binds to transthyretin and thyroxine to form a trimolecular complex.

Figure 10.5 Vitamin A metabolism in the liver.

Retinol that has been esterified may be stored in the liver. Some storage of retinol occurs in the parenchymal cells, but about 80% to 95% of the retinol is stored in the liver in small perisinusoidal cells called **stellate cells** (also known as Ito cells), which constitute less than 15% of total liver cells. Note that retinoic acid does not accumulate in appreciable amounts in the liver or other tissues. In the stellate cells, vitamin A (retinol) is stored as retinyl esters (primarily retinyl palmitate, but also retinyl stearate, oleate, and linoleate) with lipid droplets. Hydrolases can release the retinol from its stores as needed for use. With adequate liver stores of vitamin A (minimum 20 μg of vitamin A per g of liver), plasma vitamin A concentrations remain fairly constant over a wide range of dietary intakes. When hepatic vitamin A concentrations are less than 20 μg of vitamin A per g of liver, plasma retinol concentrations usually decline; in contrast, hepatic concentrations in excess of 300 μg of vitamin A per g of liver cause plasma retinol concentrations to rise. Once hepatic stellate cells can accept no more retinol for storage, hypervitaminosis A (vitamin toxicity) occurs.

Retinol transport in the blood requires two specific proteins, retinol-binding protein (RBP) and transthyretin, also known as prealbumin and as thyroxine-binding globulin. Both proteins are synthesized by hepatic parenchymal cells. Initially, for hepatic release into the blood, one molecule of retinol released by a hydrolase from its ester form combines with one RBP to form holo-RBP (Figure 10.5). The synthesis of RBP depends not only on vitamin A but also on zinc and protein; RBP synthesis diminishes with inadequate protein, retinol, or zinc status. Holo-RBP (which contains the vitamin A bound in an interior, hydrophobic region of the complex) circulates in the blood attached to transthyretin, a tetrameric thyroid hormone transport protein (Figure 10.5). This holo-RBP-retinol-transthyretin ternary complex has a half-life of about 11 to 15 hours in the plasma. Blood/serum concentrations of the complex remain fairly constant even when total hepatic retinol concentrations vary greater than 15-fold [8]. Normal plasma retinol concentrations range from about 1.05 to 3 micromol/L (30–86 μg/dL) but decrease below normal with chronic consumption of inadequate vitamin A.

Uptake of retinol from the holo-RBP-retinol-transthyretin complex by tissues is not completely understood, but it is thought to be mediated by both cellular RBP receptors and by a receptor-independent mode, depending upon the specific tissue. Factors influencing uptake are not known but may involve CRBP concentrations or saturation, and the extent of intracellular retinol metabolism, among others. For receptor-dependent uptake, transthyretin is thought to dissociate as the RBP-retinol complex binds to the cellular RBP receptor. Cellular retinol uptake follows. Apo-RBP (with no retinol attached) is released back into the blood for reuse or degraded by the kidneys. Retinol appears to be recycled several times through RBP before being irreversibly oxidized. Some of the many tissues that use vitamin A from the complex include adipose tissue, skeletal muscle, lungs, kidneys, eyes, white blood cells, and bone marrow.

Carotenoids are also found in the blood and are transported as part of lipoproteins. Carotenoids such as β-carotene and lycopene concentrate in the hydrophobic core of lipoproteins for serum transport, whereas carotenoids with polar groups are found partly on the lipoprotein surface. β-carotene, α-carotene, and lycopene distribution among lipoproteins is similar: Low-density lipoproteins (LDLs) carry over half while high-density lipoproteins (HDLs) transport up to about one-quarter, and very-low-density lipoproteins (VLDLs) carry up to about 16% [10]. In contrast, lutein and zeaxanthin (polar carotenoids) are carried predominantly (53%) by HDLs but also by LDLs (31%) and VLDLs (16%) in a fasting state [10]. Serum carotene concentrations reflect recent intake and not body stores. The most common serum carotenoids are β-carotene, α-carotene, lycopene, lutein, zeaxanthin, and cryptoxanthin.

Uptake of carotenoids into target tissues differs from that of retinol. Carotenoids are taken up as part of the lipoprotein, with uptake mediated by specific apoprotein receptors found in a variety of tissues. Carotenoids, like vitamin A, are stored mainly in the liver and adipose tissue, but some specific tissues concentrate specific carotenoids. For example, the retina of the eye is relatively rich in lutein and zeaxanthin.

In contrast to retinol, which is mobilized from the liver for transport to other tissues, retinoic acid is thought to be produced from retinal in small amounts by individual cells and used within the cells. Within the cell cytosol, retinoic acid binds to cellular retinoic acid–binding proteins (CRABPs). CRABPs are thought to function in a capacity similar to that described for CRBPs. Although both CRBPs and CRABPs are often found in the same tissues, their relative distribution in the tissues differs. CRABPs solubilize retinoic acid, regulate cellular retinoic acid metabolism, and direct retinoic acid usage intracellularly. Metabolism of retinoic acid occurs in part through the cytochrome P-450 enzyme system CYP26, which is found in the liver and brain, among other tissues, and whose expression appears to be positively regulated by vitamin A [8]. This system also catalyzes the oxidation and glucuronidation of retinoic acid (shown in Figure 10.5) to generate polar metabolites such as 4-oxoretinoic acid, which appears to be involved along with retinoic acid in the synthesis of gap junction proteins needed for cell growth (see the "Growth" subsection in the "Functions and Mechanisms of Action" section for vitamin A).

Functions and Mechanisms of Action

Vitamin A

Vitamin A is recognized as being essential for vision as well as for cellular differentiation, growth, reproduction, bone development, and immune system functions. In the case of vision, it is the 11-*cis* retinal form that must bind to the protein opsin of visual pigments to mediate phototransduction (the process by which light is converted into electrical signals for the brain). For the other biological processes, it is all-*trans* retinoic acid and 9-*cis* retinoic acid that are needed. This section reviews each of these functions; the functions of the carotenoids are addressed in a later section.

Vision Several parts of the eye work together to ensure vision. For example, light enters the eye through the cornea, the outermost tissue that covers the front of the eye. The muscles of the iris adjust the size of the pupil in response to the dimness or brightness of the light. The light then passes through the lens and the vitreous humor (which shapes the eye) and hits the retina, the inner lining at the back of the eye. The retina contains specialized cells, called rods and cones, which act as photo- or light receptors. Cones are found near the center of the retina and function especially during the day in bright light. As darkness falls or light dims, the rods serve as the photo- or light receptors. Vitamin A is needed to form **rhodopsin** (a vitamin A–containing pigment protein) found in the rods. Rhodopsin is made up of vitamin A as 11-*cis* retinal and the protein opsin (Figure 10.6).

In basic terms (Figure 10.6), in a dim/dark environment, when a flash of light hits the retina, rhodopsin is cleaved. As the rhodopsin is cleaved, opsin is released, the

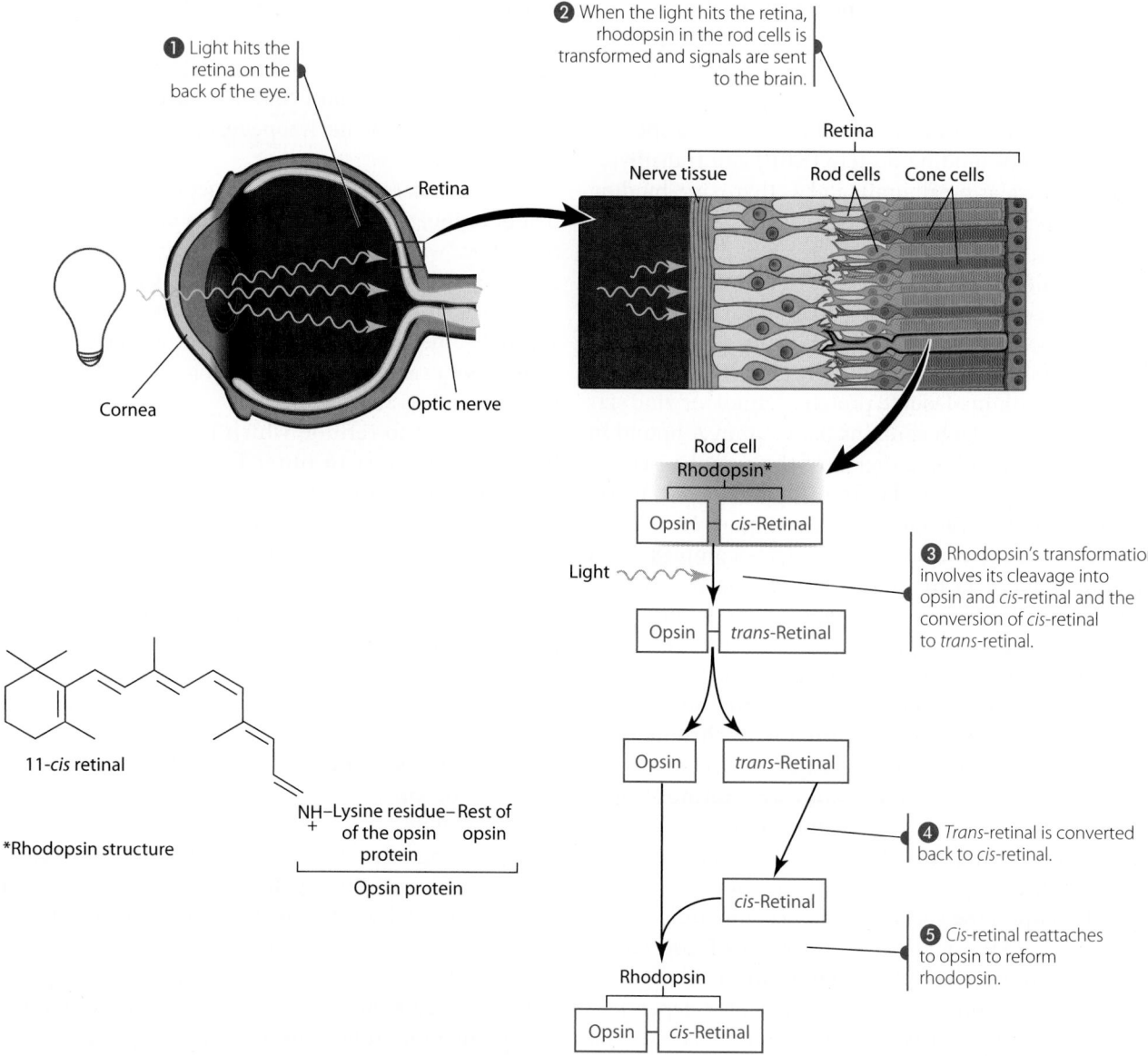

Figure 10.6 An overview of the role of vitamin A as a part of rhodopsin in vision.

Source: Beerman/McGuire, *Nutritional Sciences*, 1/e. © Cengage Learning.

cis-retinal is converted to *trans*-retinal, and signals are sent to the part of the brain involved with eyesight. To regain vision in the dark, the rhodopsin molecule must be remade using vitamin A as *cis*-retinal. The *trans*-retinal that is released is transported from the photoreceptor rod cells into the pigment epithelium of the retina, where it is converted back to *cis*-retinal. The *cis*-retinal is then transported back to the rod cell, where it reattaches to opsin to form rhodopsin. A failure or delayed recovery of vision in the dark following a light flash is called night blindness and may be caused by inadequate vitamin A.

Figure 10.7 shows the visual cycle (the formation and reformation of rhodopsin after its degradation) in more detail. This section focuses on how vitamin A is metabolized as part of the visual cycle. Retinol is transported to the retina in the blood as part of the holo-RBP-retinol-transthyretin complex. Following the binding of the complex to receptors on the pigment epithelium (a pigmented cell layer) adjacent to the photoreceptor rod cells (Figures 10.7 and 10.8), retinol enters the pigment epithelium cells and binds to CRBP. Much of the retinol is then converted by LRAT to all-*trans* retinyl esters, and some is isomerized into 11-*cis* retinyl esters. The all-*trans* retinyl esters in turn may be stored in the pigment epithelium and metabolized by an all-*trans* retinyl ester isomerohydrolase, as needed, to generate 11-*cis* retinol plus a fatty acid. Similarly, the 11-*cis* retinyl esters may be hydrolyzed, as needed, to 11-*cis* retinol and a fatty acid by retinyl ester hydrolase.

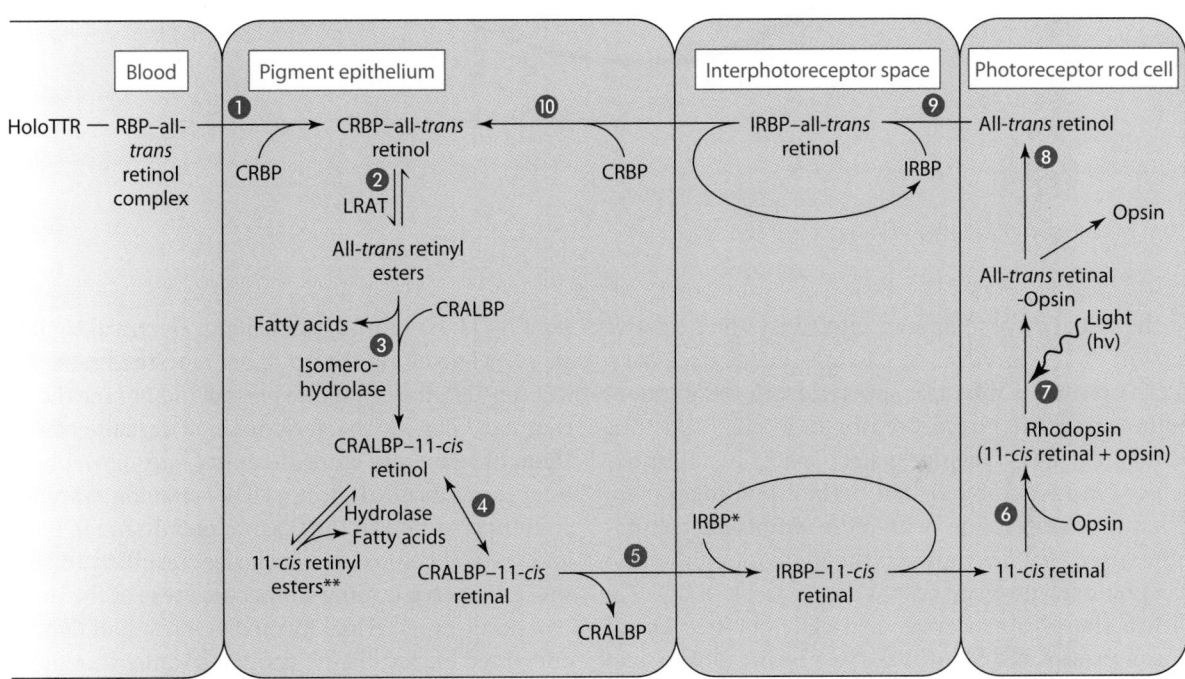

* IRBP: Interphotoreceptor retinol-binding protein.
** Stored until needed.

❶ All-*trans* retinol moves out of the blood [where it is found as part of a complex with transthyretin (TTR) and retinol-binding protein (RBP)] and into the pigment epithelium adjacent to the rod cell. In the pigment epithelium it attaches to CRBP (cellular retinol-binding protein).

❷ All-*trans* retinol is converted into all-*trans* retinyl esters by LRAT.

❸ All-*trans* retinyl esters are converted to 11-*cis* retinol, which is then attached to cellular retinal-binding protein (CRALBP).

❹ 11-*cis* retinol is converted to 11-*cis* retinal while attached to CRALBP.

❺ 11-*cis* retinal detaches from CRALBP and attaches to interphotoreceptor retinol-binding protein (IRBP) for transport across the interphotoreceptor space and into the photoreceptor rod cell. IRBP releases the 11-*cis* retinal upon delivery into the photoreceptor rod cell.

❻ 11-*cis* retinal attaches to opsin to form rhodopsin.

❼ Light hits the rod cell causing the cleavage of rhodopsin.

❽ All-*trans* retinal is first converted to all-*trans* retinol before being ultimately converted back to 11-*cis* retinal.

❾ All-*trans* retinol attaches to IRBP for transport across the interphotoreceptor space and into the pigment epithelium.

❿ All-*trans* retinol is released from IRBP and attaches CRBP in the pigment epithelium to enter the cycle again at ❷.

Figure 10.7 The visual cycle.

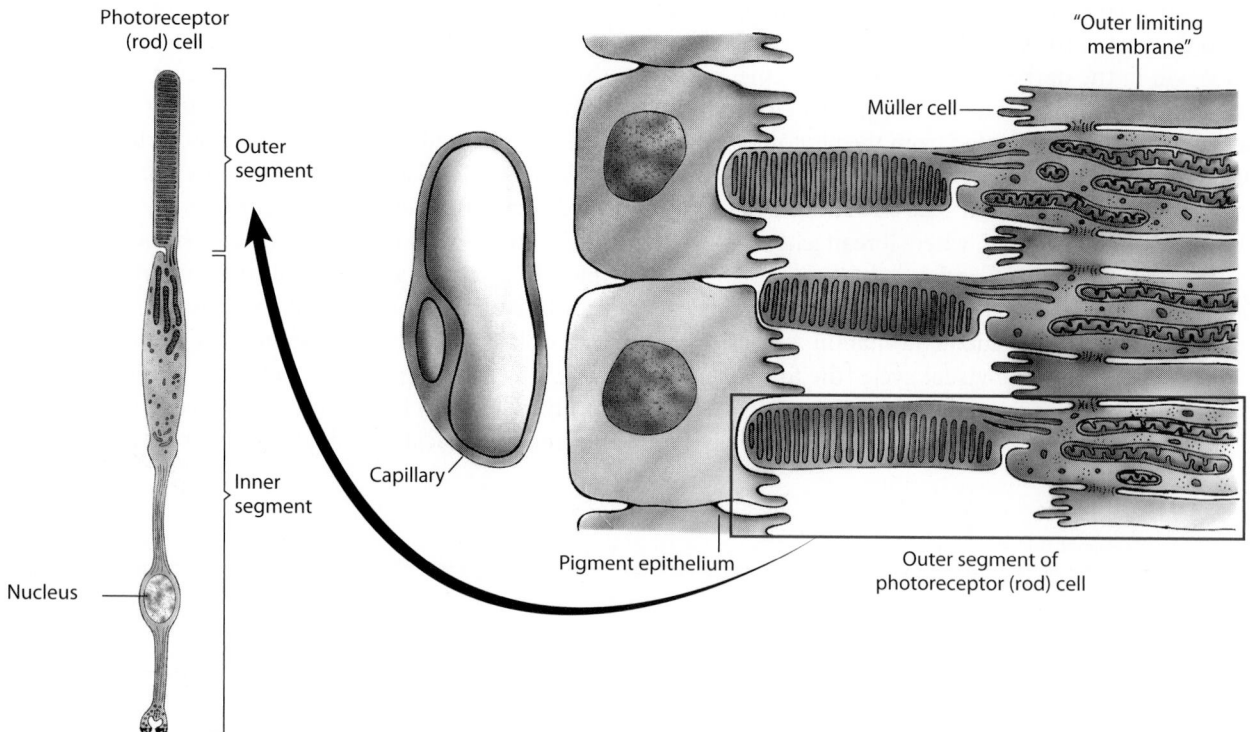

Figure 10.8 Photoreceptor (rod) cells, their structure, and their surroundings.

For the visual cycle to operate effectively, the oxidative conversion of 11-*cis* retinol to 11-*cis* retinal is necessary. The 11-*cis* retinal is next transported from the pigment epithelium into the photoreceptor rod cells (and thus across the interphotoreceptor matrix/space) by interphotoreceptor (also called interstitial) retinol-binding protein (IRBP); this protein resides within the retina's interphotoreceptor space that lies between the pigment epithelium and the photoreceptor rod cells.

Within the photoreceptor rod cells, 11-*cis* retinal binds as a protonated Schiff base to a lysine amino acid residue in the protein opsin (Figure 10.6) to produce the compound rhodopsin. Rhodopsin is embedded in disks located in the rod's outer segment, which is enclosed within a restricted compartment of the retina created by tight junctions between cells (Figure 10.8). The cells on the blood side are one layer thick and form the pigment epithelium. The "outer limiting membrane" is formed on the vitreal side of the photoreceptor cells by specific junctions between the photoreceptor cells and the Müller cells (Figure 10.8).

Within the photoreceptor cells, rhodopsin is able to detect small amounts of light, important for night vision. When a quantum of light (hv) hits the rhodopsin, changes occur in the vitamin A portion of the molecule such that 11-*cis* retinal is photoisomerized to generate all-*trans* retinal (Figures 10.6 and 10.7). The term *bleaching* is often used to describe this event because a loss of color occurs. A chain of events triggered by the absorption of

light by 11-*cis* retinal results in an electrical signal or impulse to and along the optic nerve to the brain. To transmit through the cell to the plasma membrane the message that light has hit the rhodopsin, a cascade of reactions thought to involve transducin (a G protein), phosphodiesterase, and cGMP occurs. This reaction cascade causes sodium channels in the plasma membrane to be blocked and the rod cell to hyperpolarize, resulting in signals by the optic nerve leading to specific areas of the brain.

The all-*trans* retinal formed as a result of light must be converted back to 11-*cis* retinal, and the rhodopsin must be regenerated. The steps for this conversion are thought to involve hydrolysis of all-*trans* retinal from the rhodopsin, reduction of all-*trans* retinal to all-*trans* retinol, and transport of all-*trans* retinol across the interphotoreceptor matrix and into the retinal pigment epithelium by IRBP (Figure 10.7). Within the pigment epithelium, the all-*trans* retinol may be metabolized as initially described—that is, in the same manner as upon uptake into the pigment epithelium—to repeat the visual cycle.

Gene Expression Two forms of vitamin A, all-*trans* retinoic acid and 9-*cis* retinoic acid (generated from retinol), regulate gene expression (Figure 10.9). Retinoic acid is thought to be transported into the nucleus by two intracellular lipid-binding proteins (iLBPs) found in the cell cytosol; these proteins in turn direct retinoic acid by binding to different nuclear receptors. Cellular retinoic acid–binding protein (CRABP) II, one iLBP, carries the

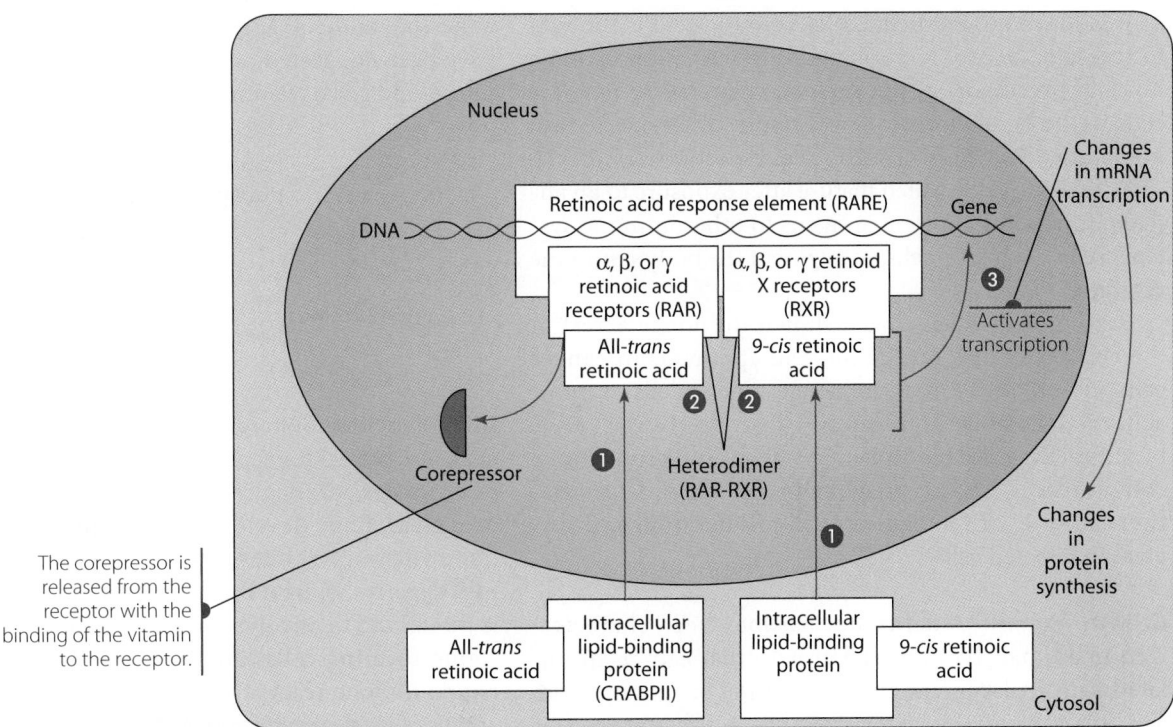

① All-*trans* or 9-*cis* retinoic acid moves into the nucleus of the cell bound to binding proteins.

② All-*trans* retinoic acid binds to retinoic acid receptors (RAR) and 9-*cis* retinoic acid binds to retinoid X receptors (RXR).

③ Binding of the vitamin to receptors on the DNA enhances the transcription of selected genes.

Figure 10.9 Hypothesized mode of action for retinoic acid on gene expression.

vitamin to nuclear retinoic acid receptors, while another iLBP called fatty acid–binding protein 5 transports the vitamin to nuclear peroxisome proliferator–activated receptors (PPAR) β/δ. All-*trans* retinoic acid binds and activates three isotypes (α, β, γ) of retinoic acid receptors (RAR) as well as PPAR β/δ; 9-*cis* retinoic acid binds and activates RAR as well as three isotypes (α, β, γ) of retinoid X receptors (RXR).

RXR and RAR are thought to be present together or with other nuclear receptors as part of a family (which may include vitamin D, thyroid hormone, steroid hormone, PPAR, or orphan receptors—with no known ligand) to form various **homodimers** or **heterodimers**. A homodimer is formed when two of the same receptors interact, such as RXR-RXR. A heterodimer is formed between two or more different receptors, such as RXR-RAR, VDR (vitamin D receptor)–RXR, RXR-PPAR, and RXR-TR (thyroid hormone receptor). These dimers are found as part of retinoic acid response elements (RARE) in the promoter regions of specific genes on DNA. When vitamin A is not present to bind the RARE, the dimer may be associated with corepressors to thus inhibit transcription activation. However, with vitamin A binding to the receptor, the receptor undergoes a conformational change that results in the release of the corepressors—and in some cases, the recruitment of coactivators—to promote the transcription of specific retinoic acid–regulated genes.

The genes affected by retinoic acid are mostly unknown but are thought to code for multiple proteins including enzymes and growth and transcription factors, among others, to impact a wide variety of cellular processes. Cell death, or apoptosis, is an example of a cellular process regulated in part by retinoic acid. The vitamin is delivered by CRABPII to the cell nucleus, where it binds to RAR within a retinoic acid response element on the DNA to upregulate the expression of caspase 9 and Bcl2, two proteins involved in the intrinsic apoptotic pathway (see Chapter 1 for further information on apoptosis).

Cellular Differentiation   Vitamin A, as retinoic acid, is needed by many cells for differentiation, the process by which an immature cell is transformed into a specific type of mature cell. Epithelial cells, found as part of our skin and in all internal body tracts, such as the respiratory, gastrointestinal, and urogenital tracts, are one example of cells that rely on vitamin A. Retinoic acid helps maintain both the normal structure and the functions of the epithelial cells. For example, retinoic acid directs the differentiation of **keratinocytes** (immature skin cells) into mature epidermal cells through interactions with nuclear chromatin and thus changes in gene expression. With vitamin A deficiency, keratin-producing cells replace mucus-secreting cells in many body tissues, especially the eyes, skin, gastrointestinal tract, and trachea.

In addition to epithelial cells, retinoic acid is thought to regulate the proliferation and differentiation of some myeloid precursor cells in the bone marrow. Progenitor cells in the bone marrow, for example, differentiate into immature dendritic cells with adequate retinoic acid [11]. The dendritic cells, which mature after exposure to an antigen, function to present antigens to other immune systems cells, such as T-cells, to augment the body's immune response.

Retinoids also have been shown to induce arrest of the cell cycle, differentiation, and apoptosis in cancer cells and other cell lines. In hematopoietic cells, retinoic acid mediates insulin receptor substrate (IRS) 1 levels by stimulating the binding of the ubiquitin-proteasomal complex to IRS 1; this attachment induces the degradation of IRS 1. IRS 1 regulates cell proliferation and survival in selected cells.

Growth Vitamin A deficiency has long been characterized in animals by impaired growth that can be stimulated with replacement by either retinol or retinoic acid. The mechanism(s) by which vitamin A affects growth is unclear. Moreover, the vitamin's ability to impact growth appears to be cell-specific, whereby it enhances proliferation and survival in some cells while, in others, it induces differentiation, cell cycle arrest, and/or apoptosis. Interactions between retinoic acid and RAR receptors, for example, can inhibit cell growth of some tumors. Alternately, retinoic acid interactions with PPARβ/δ stimulate cell growth and inhibit apoptosis. Another possible means by which growth is influenced may involve effects on gap junctions. Retinoic acid and 4-oxoretinoic acid, generated from retinoic acid, have been shown to increase the synthesis of a specific gap junction protein known as connexin 43 by stabilizing connexin 43 mRNA [12]. **Gap junctions**, cell-to-cell channels formed from connexin proteins, are important for the exchange of small signaling compounds and thus for cell-to-cell communication. A lack of gap junction communication results in uncontrolled cell growth, as can occur with cancer cells. Thus, vitamin A, in preserving this communication, plays a role in the control of cell growth.

Retinoic acid also may be able to modify cell surfaces, possibly by increasing glycoprotein synthesis at the gene level or by improving the attachment of glycoproteins to cell surfaces to induce cell adhesion. Retinol may also play a more direct role in glycoprotein synthesis. Retinyl phosphate (generated from retinol and ATP) can be converted to retinyl phosphomannose (also called mannosyl retinyl phosphate) in the presence of GDP mannose. Retinyl phosphomannose can in turn transfer the mannose to glycoprotein acceptors, which then become mannosylated glycoproteins. Such changes in the glycan portion of the glycoprotein can greatly affect differentiation of cells or tissues through their effects on cell recognition,

adhesion, and cell aggregation. These reactions (which have been suggested as a coenzyme role) involving vitamin A and glycosylation are shown here.

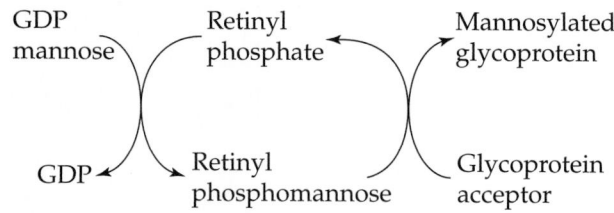

Other Functions Vitamin A, as retinol but not as retinoic acid, is essential for reproductive processes in both males and females, although the mechanism(s) of its action(s) is unclear. Bone development and maintenance also require vitamin A; either too much or too little of the vitamin negatively impacts bone mineral density. Vitamin A is thought to be involved in the regulation of **osteoblasts** (bone-forming cells) and/or **osteoclasts** (cells participating in bone resorption). Although the mechanism of action is unclear, vitamin A deficiency results in excessive deposition of bone by osteoblasts and reduced bone degradation by osteoclasts. Excess vitamin A, in contrast, stimulates osteoclasts and inhibits osteoblasts, decreasing bone mineral density and increasing fracture risk. Vitamin A appears to be involved in hematopoiesis, a function likely mediated by inhibition of erythropoiesis and alterations in iron distribution among tissues; iron-deficiency anemia is often observed in those with vitamin A deficiency. Several aspects of immune system function, both humoral and cell-mediated, also are influenced by vitamin A. Retinoic acid, produced in some immune cells such as antigen-presenting cells, stimulates phagocytic activity, cytokine production, and natural killer cell activity. Depletion studies suggest that vitamin A appears to be needed for T-lymphocyte function and for antibody response to viral, parasitic, and bacterial infections. Thus, people with vitamin A deficiency have an impaired ability to resist and fight infections. Another role of vitamin A, likely mediated by effects on gene expression, cell differentiation, and growth, is in morphogenesis/embryogenesis. Specifically, retinoic acid is thought to act as a morphogen in embryonic developments; nuclear retinoic acid receptors have been found in different cells during different times of development in the embryo.

Carotenoids

Carotenoids are thought to be present in the interior membranes of cells as well as in lipoproteins. Structurally, carotenoids possess an extended system (often nine or more) of conjugated double bonds that make them soluble in lipids and capable of quenching **singlet molecular oxygen** ($^1O_2$) and **free radicals** (atoms or molecules with one or more unpaired electrons). In other words, carotenoids function as antioxidants because they possess the ability to react with and quench free radical reactions in lipid membranes or compartments and possibly in solution. In addition to these antioxidant functions, studies with carotenoids suggest possible roles in cell proliferation, growth, and differentiation and in enhancing cell-mediated immune functions. The proposed antioxidant roles of carotenoids and their relationship to diseases are discussed first, followed by some of the other postulated roles of carotenoids.

Antioxidant Functions **Quenching** is a process by which electronically excited molecules or atoms, such as singlet molecular oxygen, are inactivated. Singlet molecular oxygen possesses higher energy and is more reactive than ground state molecular oxygen, which typically exists in triplet ($^3O_2$) rather than singlet ($^1O_2$) form. Singlet oxygen is generated from lipid peroxidation of membranes; transfer of energy from light (photochemical reactions); the respiratory, also called oxidative, burst occurring in some phagocytic cells (enzymatic reactions); and the dismutation of superoxides (spontaneous reaction). Singlet molecular oxygen readily reacts with organic molecules such as protein, lipids, and DNA and thus can damage cellular components unless removed. Carotenoids such as β-carotene or lycopene can react with (quench) singlet oxygen, and it is the conjugated double-bond systems within the carotenoids that permit the quenching. For example, β-carotene bound to lymphocytes taken from human blood directly quenches singlet molecular oxygen *in vitro*. Lycopene appears to have the highest rate constant (i.e., ability to react or complex) and is a more effective quencher of singlet oxygen than other carotenoids. The singlet oxygen ($^1O_2$) transfers its excitation energy and returns to the ground state ($^3O_2$), and the carotenoid receiving the energy enters an excited state. Resonance states in the excited carotenoid allow some stabilization. Carotenoids then release the energy in the form of heat and thus do not need to be regenerated like some other antioxidants (e.g., vitamins C and E).

$$^1O_2 + \beta\text{-carotene} \longrightarrow {}^3O_2 + \text{excited }\beta\text{-carotene}$$
$$\longrightarrow \beta\text{-carotene} + \text{heat}$$

In addition to quenching singlet oxygen, β-carotene and other carotenoids have the ability to react directly with radicals (radical scavenge), especially peroxyl radicals (O_2^{2-}), which cause lipid peroxidation. Such actions by carotenoids decrease circulating peroxides concentrations and reduce lipid peroxidation (thus helping to minimize damage to cells). Studies suggest that β-carotene works synergistically with vitamin E in scavenging radicals and inhibiting lipid peroxidation, although vitamin E has higher reactivity toward peroxyl radicals than does β-carotene. β-carotene is thought to function in the interior of the membrane, whereas vitamin E functions on

or at the surface of the membrane. Radical scavenging by carotenoids involves the donation of a hydrogen atom or an electron and results in the formation of a carotenoid radical. Electron delocalization over the carotenoid's conjugated double bond system stabilizes the carotenoid, but ultimately the carotenoid is decomposed.

Although most studies have focused on β-carotene, lycopene (in chemical assays) has been shown to be the strongest antioxidant [13]. In these *in vitro* assays, lycopene is followed in descending order by α-tocopherol (vitamin E), α-carotene, β-cryptoxanthin, zeaxanthin and β-carotene, and lutein [13]. Combinations of the carotenoids, however, especially lycopene and lutein, have been shown to work synergistically and thus are more effective than any one of the carotenoids by itself.

Because of the ability of carotenoids to react with free radicals and quench singlet oxygen, carotenoids are thought to be protective against several diseases. Some epidemiological studies have shown that people with high intakes of fruits and vegetables, which are also rich in carotenoids, and people with higher serum carotenoid concentrations have a lower incidence of diseases such as cataracts, age-related macular degeneration, and cardiovascular disease.

Carotenoids and Eye Health Age-related macular degeneration is a common cause of blindness in older people. The macula, found in the center of the retina, maintains central vision; this region can become damaged, as described in the "Eye Health" section under vitamin C in Chapter 9. Lutein and zeaxanthin, which are found in the macula, as well as β-carotene can inhibit the oxidation of cell membranes and thus may be protective against eye damage. While some studies have demonstrated that people in the highest quintile of intake of dietary carotenoids, especially lutein and zeaxanthin, and those with high serum lutein and zeaxanthin concentrations have significantly lower risk of macular degeneration, other studies have not [14–19]. After an extensive review, the Food and Drug Administration concluded (in 2006) that no credible evidence exists to allow a health claim for intake of lutein or zeaxanthin as a way to reduce risk of age-related macular degeneration [20]; new research since 2006 has not supported the use of carotenoids to diminish the risk of age-related macular degeneration.

Another cause of blindness in older individuals is cataracts, which affect the lens of the eye. As previously described in the "Vitamin C" section in Chapter 9, accumulation and aggregation of abnormal proteins in cells in the eye's lens (which functions to focus light onto the retina and adjust eye focus) cause the lens to become cloudy and vision to become impaired with cataracts. Free radicals are thought to contribute to the cataract's development, and because lutein and zeaxanthin are found in the eye and function as antioxidants, these carotenoids as well as β-carotene are purported to prevent and/or lower the risk of developing cataracts. Yet, while several studies have shown inverse correlations between high dietary intakes or plasma concentrations of lutein, zeaxanthin, and/or β-carotene and decreased risk of cataracts, according to the Food and Drug Administration there is not enough credible scientific evidence to recommend ingestion of carotenoids to lower the risk or slow the progression of cataracts [20–25].

Carotenoids and Heart Disease In the events associated with the development of atherosclerosis, the oxidation of cholesterol in LDLs increases the likelihood of a monocyte binding to and being taken into the blood vessel walls/endothelium (in comparison with native/unoxidized cholesterol). Monocytes, once present within the blood vessel endothelium, are called macrophages and continue to take up oxidized LDL cholesterol through a specific cell surface scavenger receptor and, when filled with cholesterol, become foam cells. Fatty streaks (an accumulation of foam cells) lead to atherosclerotic plaque in blood vessels and thus heart disease. Carotenoids, including β-carotene, lycopene, lutein, and α-carotene, are thought to prevent the oxidation of LDL cholesterol and other cell membrane lipids and thus prevent or slow the development of atherosclerosis. Supplementation with 800 IU of vitamin E; 1,000 mg of vitamin C; and 24 mg of β-carotene in people with coronary artery disease effectively reduces LDL susceptibility to oxidation [26]. Yet, the effectiveness of carotenoids alone in preventing or treating heart disease has not been established, and, at present, carotenoid supplementation is not recommended [27].

Cell Proliferation, Growth, and Differentiation Carotenoids inhibit cell proliferation and stimulate cell differentiation while also affecting growth. Lycopene, for example, inhibits the growth and proliferation of various cancer cells and induces cell differentiation. *In vitro*, canthaxanthin and β-carotene have been shown to inhibit carcinogen-induced neoplastic transformation as well as inhibit lipid oxidation in plasma membranes. As in their antioxidant roles, carotenoids appear to vary in their abilities to inhibit cell transformation. The mechanisms by which carotenoids carry out these roles are not clear, but some of their functions appear to be similar to those of the retinoids. For example, carotenoid-induced enhancement or induction of gap junction communication, similar to that of retinoic acid, has been proposed. Some carotenoids up-regulate the gene expression of connexin 43, a protein that enables connections (bridges) to form between cells, and in turn affects cell proliferation and growth [12]. Gap junction communications are inhibited in some cancer cells. Thus, the ability of carotenoids to protect this activity may be of significance in cancer prevention [28].

Carotenoids and Cancer Intervention trials using β-carotene have failed to show protective effects on health. More specifically, intervention trials providing 20 mg of β-carotene (BC) along with α-tocopherol (AT) in Finland (called the ATBC trial) or 30 mg of β-carotene and 25,000 IU of vitamin A (CARET trial) showed no benefit over a placebo in cancer prevention in asbestos-exposed workers and in people with a long history of smoking [29,30]. β-carotene taken with vitamin A even appeared to increase the risk of lung cancer and of mortality from cancer and heart disease in these high-risk populations (smokers and asbestos-exposed) [30]. These two intervention trials appear to suggest that β-carotene supplementation increases the risk of cancer; however, others suggest that the populations were at high risk for disease, with a long history of smoking (one pack or more cigarettes daily) or asbestos exposure along with alcohol consumption, and that only with these cofactors does β-carotene supplementation increase cancer risk [31,32]. Unfortunately, additional studies have not shown any beneficial effects from β-carotene supplementation in reducing the risk of cancer or mortality from cancer. The Institute of Medicine states that "beta-carotene supplements are not advisable for the general population" [4].

Carotenoids and Health Claims Health claims that are approved by the Food and Drug Administration are targeted at carotenoid-rich foods (fruits and vegetables) as well as grain products. These claims require the food to be low in fat and a good source of dietary fiber without fortification. An example model claim is "Low fat diets rich in fiber-containing grain products, fruits and vegetables may reduce the risk of some types of cancer, a disease associated with many factors" [33]. Another sample claim for fruits, vegetables, or grain products that are low in (saturated and total) fat and cholesterol and contain at least 0.6 g of soluble fiber per reference amount without fortification is "Diets low in saturated fat and cholesterol and rich in fruits and vegetables and grain products that contain some types of dietary fiber, particularly soluble fiber, may reduce the risk of heart disease, a disease associated with many factors" [33]. Another model claim— "Low fat diets rich in fruits and vegetables (foods that are low in fat and may contain dietary fiber, vitamin A, or vitamin C) may reduce the risk of some types of cancer, a disease associated with many factors"—has also been approved for fruits and vegetables that are a good source of vitamin A or C, or dietary fiber [33].

Interactions with Other Nutrients

Vitamin A and carotenoids interact with vitamins E and K. Excess dietary vitamin A intake interferes with vitamin K absorption. High β-carotene intake, in turn, may decrease plasma vitamin E concentrations.

Protein and zinc influence vitamin A status and transport. First, the activity of carotenoid dioxygenase, which cleaves β-carotene, is depressed by an inadequate protein intake. Second, overall vitamin A metabolism is closely related to protein and zinc status because the transport and use of the vitamin depend on two vitamin A–binding proteins and because zinc is required for protein synthesis as well as for alcohol dehydrogenase activity, which converts retinol to retinal. Impairments in the synthesis of retinol-binding protein and transthyretin have been shown to diminish retinol mobilization from the liver.

Iron metabolism is also interrelated with that of both carotenoids and vitamin A. Iron is a cofactor for 15,15′ mono-oxygenase, the enzyme responsible for the conversion of β-carotene into retinal. Vitamin A (likely as retinoic acid) also may directly affect iron absorption, metabolism, or storage or red blood cell differentiation. Vitamin A deficiency is associated with decreased incorporation of iron into red blood cells and diminished mobilization of iron from stores. Thus, vitamin A deficiency can be associated with iron-deficiency anemia, and in this situation supplementation of vitamin A (as opposed to supplementation with iron) improves indices of iron status.

Metabolism and Excretion

Vitamin A is excreted in both the urine and feces with the relative amounts varying based on vitamin intake. Urinary excretion of vitamin A metabolites usually accounts for up to about 60% of vitamin A excretion, and fecal excretion accounts for the remaining 40%; however, with higher intakes, fecal excretion generally exceeds urinary excretion [3]. For urinary excretion, retinol and retinoic acid are typically oxidized at the β-ionone ring and then conjugated to generate polar, water-soluble metabolites. Many of these metabolites, especially those that are short chain and acidic, are excreted by the kidneys. Small amounts of vitamin A, however, may be expired by the lungs as CO_2. Oxidized products of vitamin A that contain intact chains and have been conjugated to glucuronic acid, such as retinoic acid glucuronide and 4-oxoretinoic acid glucuronide (Figure 10.10), or to taurine are generally secreted into the bile for ultimate fecal excretion. Some polar vitamin A metabolites secreted into the bile, such as 4-oxoretinoic acid glucuronide, however, can be absorbed and returned to the liver through the enterohepatic circulation. This recycling mechanism helps to partially conserve the body's supply of vitamin A.

Carotenoids are metabolized, depending upon the individual carotenoid, into a variety of compounds for excretion. Carotenoid metabolites are excreted primarily into the bile for fecal elimination.

Recommended Dietary Allowance

Recommendations for vitamin A intake are expressed as retinol activity equivalents (RAE) to account for differences in the biological activities of the carotenoids. Older units of measure for vitamin A such as international units (IU) and retinol equivalents (RE) are still found in the literature, among other places. International units, for example, which may be found on food and supplement labels, do not account for differences in biological activities of the carotenoids. Conversion factors are: 1 IU vitamin A = 0.3 μg retinol from animal products = 3.6 μg β-carotene = 7.2 μg of other provitamin A carotenoids. The RAE equivalencies of retinol, β-carotene, and other provitamin A carotenoids are as follows: 1 RAE = 1 μg retinol = 12 μg β-carotene = 24 μg α-carotene or β-cryptoxanthin [3]. In other words, 12 times the amount of β-carotene or 24 times the amount of α-carotene or β-cryptoxanthin is needed to get the same effects as 1 μg of retinol.

The Recommended Dietary Allowance (RDA) for vitamin A is based upon the requirement plus twice the coefficient of variation (20%), with the value rounded to the nearest 100 μg [3]. The RDAs for vitamin A for adult men and women are 900 μg RAE (3,000 IU) and 700 μg

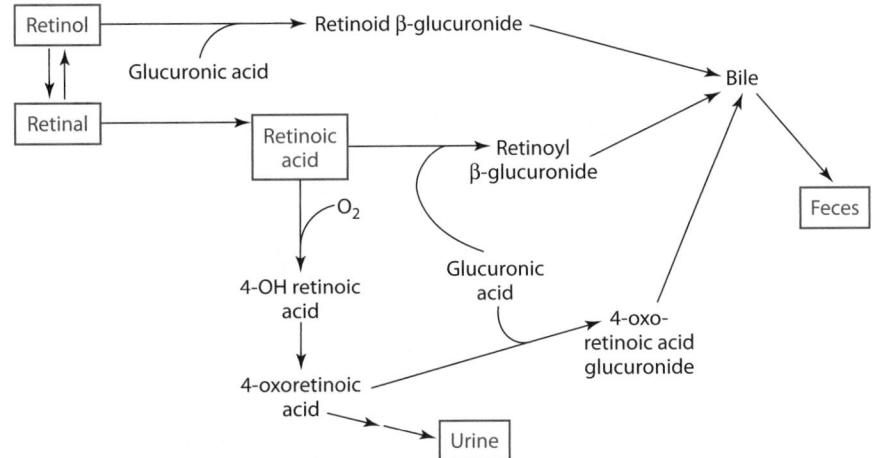

Figure 10.10 Metabolism of vitamin A, showing some excretory products that are secreted into the bile for removal from the body.

RAE (2,310 IU), respectively [3]. During pregnancy and lactation, the RDAs for vitamin A for adult women are higher, 770 μg RAE (2,565 IU) and 1,300 μg RAE (4,300 IU), respectively [3]. The requirements for vitamin A for adult men and women are 625 μg RAE and 500 μg RAE, respectively [3].

Deficiency

Vitamin A deficiency is less common in the United States than in developing countries, where inadequate intake occurs frequently in children under 5 years of age. In developing countries, increased mortality in children is associated with inadequate vitamin A stores as well as overt vitamin A deficiency.

Selected signs and symptoms of deficiency include anorexia, retarded growth, increased susceptibility to infections, obstruction and enlargement of hair follicles, keratinization of epithelial cells of the skin with accompanying failure of normal differentiation, and numerous ocular (eye) effects. Night blindness, which may be one of the first symptoms of vitamin A deficiency, results from impaired production of rhodopsin in the rod cells in the retina of the eye. Another sign affecting the eyes is **xerophthalmia,** which is characterized by dryness of the eye (because of inadequate mucus production) associated with the disappearance of goblet cells in the conjunctiva and the enlargement and keratinization of epithelial cells. Keratinization of the cornea's epithelial cells results in conjunctival and corneal xerosis (dryness) and Bitot's spots. **Bitot's spots** are small, white, foamy-looking accumulations of sloughed cells and secretions associated with keratinization of the conjunctiva. As the xerosis worsens, corneal scarring and ulcerations as well as keratomalacia (softening of the cornea) may occur; these may ultimately lead to corneal perforation and blindness. Treatment of a deficiency usually requires daily supplementation of 2,000 to 200,000 IU (606–60,600 μg RAE) of vitamin A depending upon the person's age and the severity of the deficiency.

Individuals with an increased need for vitamin A include people with malabsorptive disorders in which **steatorrhea** (excessive fat in the feces or fat malabsorption) occurs; fat malabsorption is most commonly found in those with conditions affecting the intestine, pancreas, liver, or gallbladder. Additionally, people with chronic nephritis (affecting the kidneys), acute protein deficiency, intestinal parasites, or acute infections may also become vitamin A deficient. Measles infections, for example, in developing countries are associated with high mortality. Measles is thought to depress vitamin A status (which may already be low in children in developing countries) by diminishing vitamin A intake, absorption, and use as well as by increasing urinary vitamin A excretion [34]. Vitamin A supplements are recommended by the World Health Organization and the United Nations Children's Fund for the routine treatment of measles in populations in which vitamin A deficiency is likely.

Toxicity: Hypervitaminosis A

The Tolerable Upper Intake Level (UL) for preformed vitamin A is 3,000 μg RAE (10,000 IU) per day [3]. Ingesting larger amounts (such as 50,000 IU) of vitamin A in a short time (even a single dose) may result in acute hypervitaminosis A. Symptoms of acute hypervitaminosis A include nausea, vomiting, double or blurred vision, increased intracranial pressure, headache, dizziness, skin desquamation, and muscle incoordination.

Chronic intake (daily for months or years) of lower doses (i.e., <50,000 IU) of vitamin A in excess of recommended amounts also can lead to hypervitaminosis A. For example, in adults, a chronic oral retinol intake in amounts as little as 3 to 4 times greater than the RDA can produce hypervitaminosis A, although generally a higher intake (about 10 or more times the RDA) is required to produce toxicity. Chronic vitamin A toxicity is manifested by a variety of maladies, including anorexia; dry, itchy skin with increased desquamation; alopecia (hair loss) and coarsening of the hair; ataxia; headache; bone and muscle pain; conjunctivitis and ocular pain; nausea; vomiting; abdominal pain; and liver damage. Additionally, an increased risk of bone fractures has been shown in those consuming vitamin A in amounts greater than 2,000 IU. Most manifestations of toxicity appear to subside gradually once excessive intake of the vitamin is discontinued.

Excessive intake of vitamin A in its natural form or in a synthetic form (as found in the oral acne treatment medications Accutane and Roaccutane [isotretinoin]) is also **teratogenic** (causes birth defects). For example, an oral intake of more than 4,500 μg RAE daily by pregnant women has been associated with an increased risk of malformations in infants born to the women [35]. Further, because the use of synthetic retinoids for acne by women in the early months of their pregnancy causes a number of birth defects among the infants born to these women, dermatologists prescribe contraceptives for patients in their childbearing years taking the drug.

The effects of hypervitaminosis A on the liver, the primary storage site for vitamin A, are multiple. They include fat-storing cell **hyperplasia** (excessive cell proliferation) and hyper trophy, fibrogenesis, sclerosis of veins, portal hypertension, and congestion in perisinusoid cells, which leads to hepatocellular damage and cirrhosis or a cirrhosislike hepatic disorder. Some toxic effects of excess vitamin A intake are thought to be mediated by changes in the regulation of vitamin A (retinoid) receptors in the nucleus and by effects on cell differentiation and growth, among other means. Another mechanism by which excess vitamin A is thought to exert toxic effects is related to its transport in the blood. When vitamin A intake is in large excess, serum retinol levels rise (often above 200 μg/dL, whereas normal is 30–86 μg/dL), and retinol is no longer transported exclusively by RBP but instead is carried as retinyl esters by plasma lipoproteins to the tissues. It has been suggested that when retinol is presented to the cell membranes in a form other than in an RBP complex, the released retinol produces toxic effects [3,10]. See Penniston and Tanumihardjo [36] for a review of the acute and chronic toxic effects of vitamin A.

Carotenoids, in contrast to vitamin A, appear to have few side effects. In fact, β-carotene is listed on the Generally Recognized as Safe (GRAS) list with the Food and Drug Administration for use as a dietary and nutrient supplement as well as for use as a colorant in foods, drugs, and cosmetics [37]. The most commonly cited problem with supplemental carotenoid use is hypercarotenosis, also called carotenodermia; this problem is most often seen in people ingesting about 30 mg or more of β-carotene daily for at least 1 to 2 months and with plasma β-carotene concentrations in excess of about 250 μg/dL. Hypercarotenosis results in a yellow discoloration of the skin, especially in the fat pads or fatty areas of the palms of the hands and soles of the feet. The condition usually disappears once the carotenoids are removed from the diet. No Tolerable Upper Intake Level has been established for β-carotene or other carotenoids [4], but excessive consumption of carotenoids may be detrimental to smokers [30–32] and possibly to nonsmokers; the effects are unknown at this time. Carotenoid supplements are not advised for the general public [4]; instead, the public is encouraged to consume at least 2½ cups of fruits and vegetables per day.

Assessment of Nutriture

Vitamin A status may be assessed in a variety of ways. To assess for night blindness, electrophysiological measurements, made by electroretinograms, directly measure the level of rhodopsin and its rate of regeneration in the eye. Other eye problems may be detected using conjunctival impression cytology, a histological method of assessment that involves examining morphological changes in the epithelial cells of the conjunctiva. A reduction in goblet cells and the derangement (enlargement and flattening) of epithelial cells in the conjunctiva suggest vitamin A deficiency.

Plasma retinol concentrations are frequently measured as a biochemical indicator of vitamin A status. Plasma retinol levels reflect status best if the person has exhausted his or her stores (primarily in the liver) of the vitamin, as with deficiency, or if the stores are filled to capacity, as with toxicity. Use of plasma retinol concentrations, however, also depends on the adequacy of dietary

energy, protein, and zinc because of their roles in the synthesis of retinol-binding protein. Moreover, use of plasma retinol is unreliable as an indicator of vitamin A status in people with infection or inflammation, both of which depress plasma vitamin concentrations. Plasma retinol concentrations less than ~20 μg/dL (0.7 μmol/L) are usually considered as deficient or marginal and suggestive of inadequate stores of the vitamin; although others suggest plasma retinol concentrations < 10 μg/dL (0.35 μmol/L) indicate deficiency, and 10 to 20 μg/dL (0.35–0.7 μmol/L) suggests marginal status [3,38]. Plasma retinol concentrations of 30 to 86 μg/dL (1.05–3 μmol/L) are thought to be adequate, and concentrations above 86 μg/dL (3 μmol/L) are thought to be excessive (toxic).

Adequacy of vitamin A stores in the liver can be assessed by the relative dose response (RDR) test or the modified relative dose response (MRDR) test. The RDR test involves measuring changes in plasma retinol concentration before and 5 hours after oral administration of retinyl esters (usually as acetate or palmitate). Blood is taken initially, vitamin A is ingested, and 5 hours later blood is taken again. Retinol concentrations of the blood are determined, and the difference in concentration is calculated and divided by the 5-hour concentration. RDR is then expressed as a percentage.

$$RDR (\%) = \frac{\text{5-hour plasma retinol} - \text{initial plasma retinol}}{\text{5-hour plasma retinol concentration}} \times 100$$

A % RDR equal to or greater than 20% suggests inadequate liver vitamin A stores [3,39]. The MRDR test involves measuring the ratio of 3,4 didehydroretinol to retinol in the blood after administering a single dose of 3,4 didehydroretinyl acetate. This test, unlike the RDR, requires that only one blood sample be taken, about 4 to 6 hours after the vitamin is ingested. An MRDR ratio at 5 hours of less than 0.04 in healthy adults indicates adequate vitamin status [40].

References Cited for Vitamin A

1. Harrison E. Mechanisms of digestion and absorption of dietary vitamin A. Ann Rev Nutr. 2005; 25:87–103.
2. Von Lintig J. Colors with functions: elucidating the biochemical and molecular basis of carotenoid metabolism. Ann Rev Nutr. 2010; 30:35–56.
3. Food and Nutrition Board, Institute of Medicine. Dietary Reference Intakes. Washington, DC: National Academy Press. 2001 pp. 82–161.
4. Food and Nutrition Board, Institute of Medicine. Dietary Reference Intakes. Washington, DC: National Academy Press. 2000 pp. 325–82.
5. Novotny JA, Harrison DJ, Pawlosky R, et al. β-carotene conversion to vitamin A decreases as the dietary dose increases in humans. J Nutr. 2010; 140:915–18.
6. Yeum K, Russell R. Carotenoid bioavailability and bioconversion. Ann Rev Nutr. 2002; 22:483–504.
7. Nagao A. Oxidative conversion of carotenoids to retinoids and other products. J Nutr. 2004; 134:S237–40.

8. Ross AC, Zolfaghari R. Regulation of hepatic retinol metabolism: perspectives from studies of vitamin A status. J Nutr. 2004; 134:S269–75.

9. Paik J, Vogel S, Quadro L, et al. Vitamin A: overlapping delivery pathways to tissues from the circulation. J Nutr. 2004; 134:S276–80.

10. Parker R. Absorption, metabolism, and transport of carotenoids. FASEB J. 1996; 10:542–51.

11. Hengesbach L, Hoag K. Physiological concentrations of retinoic acid favor myeloid dendritic cell development over granulocyte development in cultures of bone marrow cells in mice. J Nutr. 2004; 134:2653–59.

12. Sies H, Stahl W. Carotenoids and intercellular communication via gap junctions. Int J Vit Nutr Res. 1997; 67:364–67.

13. Sies H, Stahl W. Vitamin E and C, β-carotene, and other carotenoids as antioxidants. Am J Clin Nutr. 1995; 62(suppl):S1315–21.

14. SanGiovanni JP, Chew EY, Clemons TE, et al. The relationship of dietary carotenoid and vitamin A, E, and C intake with age-related macular degeneration in a case-control study: AREDS Report #22. Arch Ophthalmol. 2007; 125:1225–32.

15. Moeller SM, Parekh N, Tinker L, et al. Associations between intermediate age-related macular degeneration and lutein and zeaxanthin in the Carotenoids in Age-Related Eye Disease Study (CAREDS): Ancillary Study of the Women's Health Initiative. Arch Ophthalmol. 2006; 124:1151–62.

16. Flood V, Smith W, Wang JJ, et al. Dietary antioxidant intake and incidence of age-related maculopathy: the Blue Mountain Eye Study. Ophthalmology. 2002; 109:2272–78.

17. Cho E, Seddon JM, Rosner B, et al. Prospective study of intake of fruits, vegetables, vitamins and carotenoids and risk of age-related maculopathy. Arch Ophthalmol. 2004; 122:883–92.

18. Parisi V, Tedeschi M, Gallinaro G, et al. Carotenoids and antioxidants in age-related maculopathy Italian study: multifocal electroretinogram modifications after 1 year. Ophthalmology. 2008; 115:324–33.

19. Age-related Eye Disease Study Research Group: A randomized placebo-controlled clinical trial of high dose supplementation with vitamins C and E, β carotene, and zinc for age-related macular degeneration and vision loss. Arch Ophthalmol. 2001; 119:1417–36.

20. Trumbo PR, Ellwood KC. Lutein and zeaxanthin intakes and risk of age-related macular degeneration and cataracts: an evaluation using the Food and Drug Administration's evidence-based review system for health claims. Am J Clin Nutr. 2006; 84:971–74.

21. Christen WG, Liu S, Glynn RJ, et al. Dietary carotenoids, vitamins C and E, and risk of cataract in women: a prospective study. Arch Ophthalmol. 2008; 126:102–09.

22. Fernandez MM, Afshari NA. Nutrition and the prevention of cataracts. Curr Opin Ophthalmol. 2008; 19:66–70.

23. Chiu C, Taylor A. Nutritional antioxidants and age-related cataract and maculopathy. Exp Eye Res. 2007; 84:229–45.

24. Tan AG, Mitchell P, Flood VM, et al. Antioxidant nutrient intake and the long-term incidence of age-related cataract: the Blue Mountains Eye Study. Am J Clin Nutr. 2008; 87:1899–1905.

25. Chylack LT, Brown NP, Bron A, et al. The Roche European American Cataract Trial (REACT): a randomized clinical trial to investigate the efficacy of an oral antioxidant micronutrient mixture to slow progression of age-related cataract. Ophthalmic Epid. 2002; 9:49–80.

26. Mosca L, Rubenfire M, Mandel C, et al. Antioxidant nutrient supplementation reduces the susceptibility of low density lipoprotein to oxidation in patients with coronary artery disease. J Am Coll Cardiol. 1997; 30:392–99.

27. Voutilainen S, Nurmi T, Mursu J, Rissanen T. Carotenoids and cardiovascular health. Am J Clin Nutr. 2006; 83:1265–71.

28. Acevedo P, Bertram J. Liarozole potentiates the cancer chemopreventive activity of and the up-regulation of gap junctional communication and connexin 43 expression by retinoic acid and β-carotene in 10T1/2 cells. Carcinogenesis. 1995; 16:2215–22.

29. α-tocopherol, β-carotene (ATBC) Cancer Prevention Study Group: the effect of vitamin E and β carotene on the incidence of lung cancer and other cancers in male smokers. N Engl J Med. 1994; 330:1029–35.

30. Omenn G, Goodman G, Thomquist M, et al. Effects of a combination of β carotene and vitamin A on lung cancer and cardiovascular disease. N Engl J Med. 1996; 334:1150–55.

31. Omenn G, Goodman G, Thornquist M, et al. Risk factors for lung cancer and for intervention effects in CARET, the β-carotene and retinol efficacy trial. J Natl Cancer Inst. 1996; 88:1550–59.

32. Mayne S, Handelman G, Beecher G. β-carotene and lung cancer promotion in heavy smokers: a plausible relationship? J Natl Cancer Inst. 1996; 88:1513–15.

33. FDA Food and Labeling. www.fda.gov/Food/LabelingNutrition/LabelClaims/HealthClaimsMeetingSignificantScientificAgreementSSA/default.htm

34. Stephensen C. Vitamin A, infection, and immune function. Ann Rev Nutr. 2001; 21:167–92.

35. Mulholland CA, Benford DJ. What is known about the safety of multivitamin-multimineral supplements for the general healthy population. Am J Clin Nutr. 2007; 85(suppl):S318–22.

36. Penniston K, Tanumihardjo S. The acute and chronic toxic effects of vitamin A. Am J Clin Nutr. 2006; 83:191–201.

37. Life Sciences Research Office FDA Contract No. 223-75-2004. Evaluation of the Health Aspects of Carotene (β-carotene) as a Food Ingredient. Bethesda, MD: Federation of American Societies for Experimental Biology. 1979.

38. Craft N. Innovative approaches to vitamin A assessment. J Nutr. 2001; 131:S1626–30.

39. Russell R. The vitamin A spectrum: from deficiency to toxicity. Am J Clin Nutr. 2000; 71:878–84.

40. Tanumihardjo SA. Assessing vitamin A status: past, present and future. J Nutr. 2004; 134:S290–93.

Suggested Readings

Clagett-Dame M, DeLuca H. The role of vitamin A in mammalian reproduction and embryonic development. Ann Rev Nutr. 2002; 22:347–82.

Grune T, Lietz G, Palou A, et al. β-carotene is an important vitamin A source for humans. J Nutr. 2010; 140: S2268–85.

Hammond BR. Possible role for dietary lutein and zeaxanthin in visual development. Nutr Rev. 2008; 66:695–702.

Noy N. Between death and survival: retinoic acid in regulation of apoptosis. Ann Rev Nutr. 2010; 30:201–18.

Ribaya-Mercado JD, Blumberg JB. Vitamin A: is it a risk factor for osteoporosis and bone fracture? Nutr Rev. 2007; 65:425–38.

Sommer A. Vitamin A deficiency and clinical disease: an historical overview. J Nutr. 2008; 138:1835–39.

Vilhais-Neto GC, Pourquie O. Retinoic acid. Curr Biol 2008; 18:R191–92.

VITAMIN D

Through the years vitamin D (also known as calciferol) has been associated with skeletal growth and strong bones. This association arose because early in the 20th century it was shown that rickets, a childhood disease characterized by improper bone development, could be prevented by a fat-soluble factor D in the diet or by body exposure to ultraviolet light. Emphasis was placed on the dietary factor; therefore, any compound with curative action on rickets was designated as vitamin D. E. McCollum is credited with the vitamin's discovery.

Structurally, vitamin D is derived from a steroid and is considered to be a seco-steroid because one of its four rings is broken. Vitamin D contains three intact rings (A, C, and D) with a break between carbons 9 and 10 in the B ring (see the structure of previtamin D_3 in Figure 10.11). The two main forms of the vitamin (Figure 10.11), D_2 (also called ergocalciferol) and D_3 (also called cholecalciferol), differ in the structure of their side chains, but not in their general metabolism or functions in the body.

Sources

Dietary vitamin D, as D_3, is provided primarily by a small number of foods of animal origin. Liver, especially from beef (1 μg vitamin D/3 oz) and eggs (1.1 μg/egg) represent good sources of vitamin D_3. In addition, the vitamin is found in fatty fish (and their oils) including herring (2.4 μg/3 oz), salmon (11 μg/3 oz), tuna (1.7 μg/3 oz), and sardines (4.1 μg/3 oz). Cheeses (0.1–0.2 μg/oz) and butter (0.2 μg/tablespoon) contain small amounts of

vitamin D_3. A few foods of plant origin, such as shitake mushrooms (0.5 μg/½ cup cooked) provide some vitamin D as D_2. Yet, because so few foods in the United States contain much vitamin D, selected foods, including milk, yogurt, cheese, butter, and margarine as well as some orange juice, breads, and breakfast cereals, may be fortified with the vitamin, usually as D_3 but sometimes as D_2. In the United States, for example, milk and orange juice may be fortified with 2.5 μg (100 IU) of vitamin D_3/cup.

Most vitamin D supplements provide the vitamin as D_3. The Daily Value, used on food and supplement labels, for vitamin D is 400 IU. The vitamin D content of foods may be expressed as international units (IU) or μg, with 1 μg vitamin D = 40 IU or 1 IU = 0.025 μg vitamin D. Vitamin D in foods is fairly stable and thus not prone to cooking, storage, or processing losses.

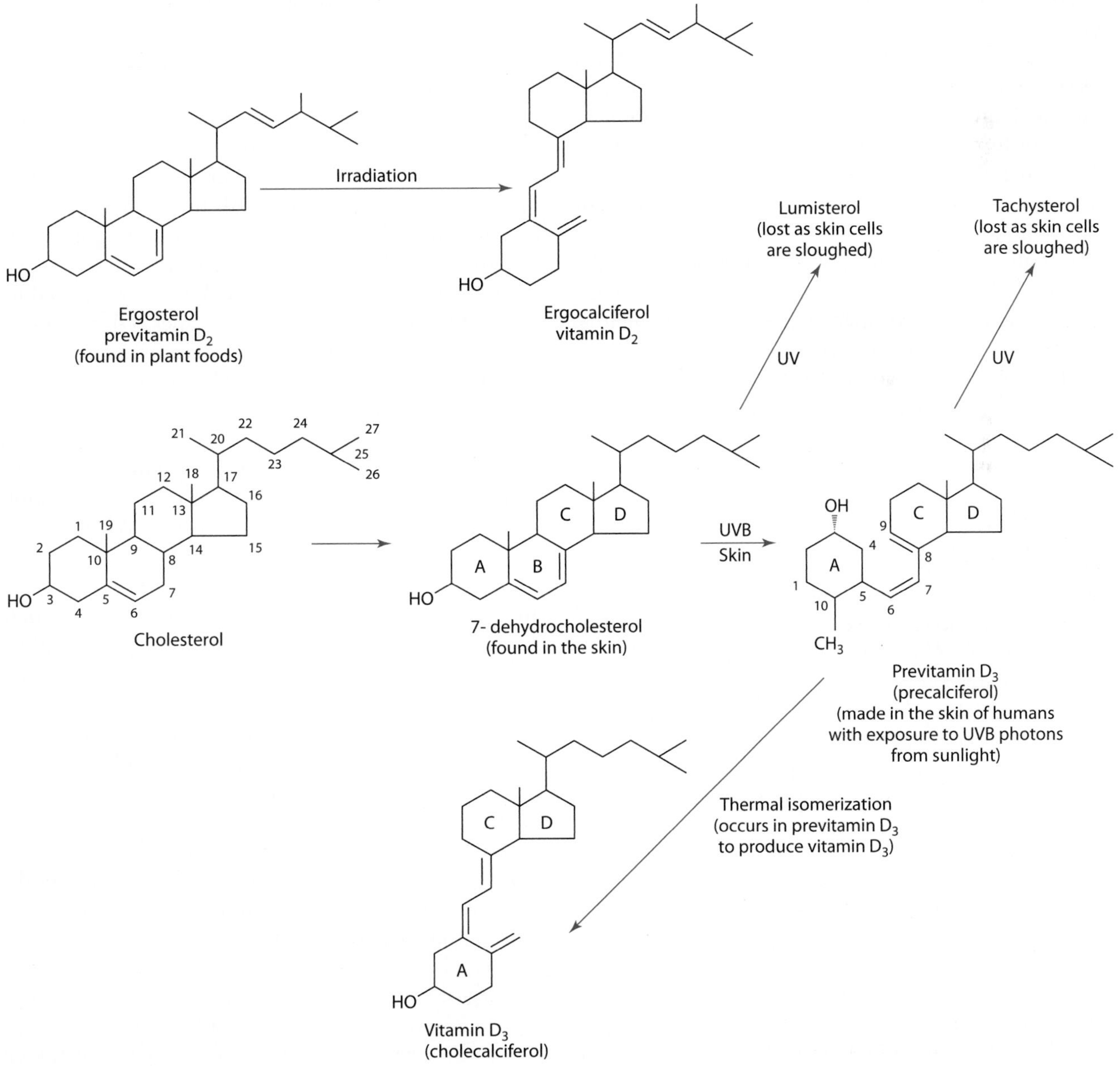

Figure 10.11 Production of ergocalciferol (vitamin D_2) and vitamin D_3 (cholecalciferol).

Another major source of vitamin D_3 is that made in the body from the steroid, 5,7-cholestradienol, commonly called 7-dehydrocholesterol (see Figure 10.11). Specifically, 7-dehydrocholesterol is synthesized in the skin's sebaceous glands and secreted onto the skin's surface, where it may be reabsorbed into the skin's various layers. It appears to be uniformly distributed throughout the epidermis and dermis. The conjugated set of double bonds (five to seven) in ring B of 7-dehydrocholesterol allows the absorption of specific wavelengths of light found in the ultraviolet range. Thus, during exposure to sunlight, ultraviolet B (UVB) photons (wavelength ~285–320 nm) penetrate into the epidermis and dermis. Some 7-dehydrocholesterol in the plasma membranes of skin cells absorbs the photons; this event causes ring B to open, forming previtamin D_3 (also called precholecalciferol). The unstable double bonds in previtamin D_3 are rearranged (a process also called thermal isomerization) over a period of several hours to a few days, resulting in the synthesis of vitamin D_3/cholecalciferol (Figure 10.11). Excess production of vitamin D_3 in the skin is prevented through the generation of inactive metabolites, especially lumisterol, which is also produced from 7-dehydrocholesterol in the presence of ultraviolet light, and tachysterol, which is generated by further irradiation of previtamin D_3.

This cutaneous production of vitamin D_3, which diffuses from the skin into the blood, represents a key source of the vitamin for many persons. Because neither lumisterol, tachysterol, nor previtamin D_3 has much affinity for vitamin D's main blood transport protein (vitamin D–binding protein), these compounds typically are lost as the skin sloughs off.

Absorption

Dietary vitamin D (both D_3 and D_2) requires no digestion and is absorbed from a micelle, in association with fat and with the aid of bile salts, by passive diffusion into the intestinal cell. About 50% of dietary vitamin D is absorbed. Although the rate of absorption is most rapid in the duodenum and jejunum, the largest amount of vitamin D is absorbed in the distal small intestine. Within the intestinal cell, vitamin D is incorporated primarily into chylomicrons, which then enter the lymphatic system with subsequent entry into the blood.

Transport, Metabolism, and Storage

Chylomicrons transport about 40% of vitamin D in the blood; some vitamin D may be transferred from the chylomicron to vitamin D–binding protein (DBP). Adipose tissue and muscle, among other tissues, take up

the vitamin from the chylomicrons, and chylomicron remnants deliver the remainder to the liver. Individuals with greater than normal amounts of body fat (as would be found in those who are overweight or obese) appear to store more of the vitamin in adipose tissue than those with normal weight and body fat. Thus, obese individuals with low vitamin D status likely need larger doses of the vitamin to reach appropriate serum concentrations than those who are of normal weight [1].

In contrast to vitamin D from the diet, vitamin D_3 that is made in the skin slowly diffuses from the skin into the blood and is picked up for transport by the hepatically synthesized DBP. About 60% of plasma vitamin D is bound to DBP for transport. The vitamin D bound to DBP is delivered primarily to the liver but may be picked up by other tissues, especially muscle and adipose tissue, before hepatic uptake. Thus, the difference in the transport mechanisms for the vitamin formed in the skin (i.e., going directly from the skin into the blood bound to DBP) and that absorbed from the digestive tract (i.e., incorporating into chylomicrons, entering the lymphatic system, and then entering the blood) affects the distribution of the vitamin in the body.

Vitamin D reaching the liver either by way of chylomicron remnants or by DBP must be hydroxylated by cytochrome P-450 hydroxylases to begin the generation of vitamin D's active form. Detailed reviews of these hydroxylases, which are collectively referred to as mixed-function oxidases (the enzymes reduce one atom of molecular oxygen to water and one to the hydroxyl group) and abbreviated CYP followed by numbers and letters, are available [2]. In the liver, 25-hydroxylase (primarily CYP2R1), which is NADPH-dependent, functions in the mitochondria to hydroxylate vitamin D at carbon 25 to form 25-OH (vitamin) D, also called calcidiol or 25-OH cholecalciferol (Figure 10.12). While the liver expresses most of the 25-hydroxylases, the enzyme is found in other organs, including the lungs, intestine, and kidneys. While the enzyme is largely unregulated, 25-hydroxylase is more efficient during periods of vitamin D deprivation than when normal amounts of the vitamin are available. With usual physiological intake, most vitamin D is converted to 25-OH D and released into the blood; however, with supraphysiological intake, more vitamin D is stored in the body's adipose tissue and then released as needed [3].

After its hepatic synthesis, most 25-OH D, which represents the main form of vitamin D in the body, is secreted from the liver and transported in the blood by DBP. Because little 25-OH D remains in the liver and very little is taken up by the extrahepatic tissues, the blood is the largest single pool (and represents the major storage site) of 25-OH D, which has a half-life of about 15 days to 3 weeks or more [4]. Other storage sites for the vitamin include adipose tissue, which contains primarily

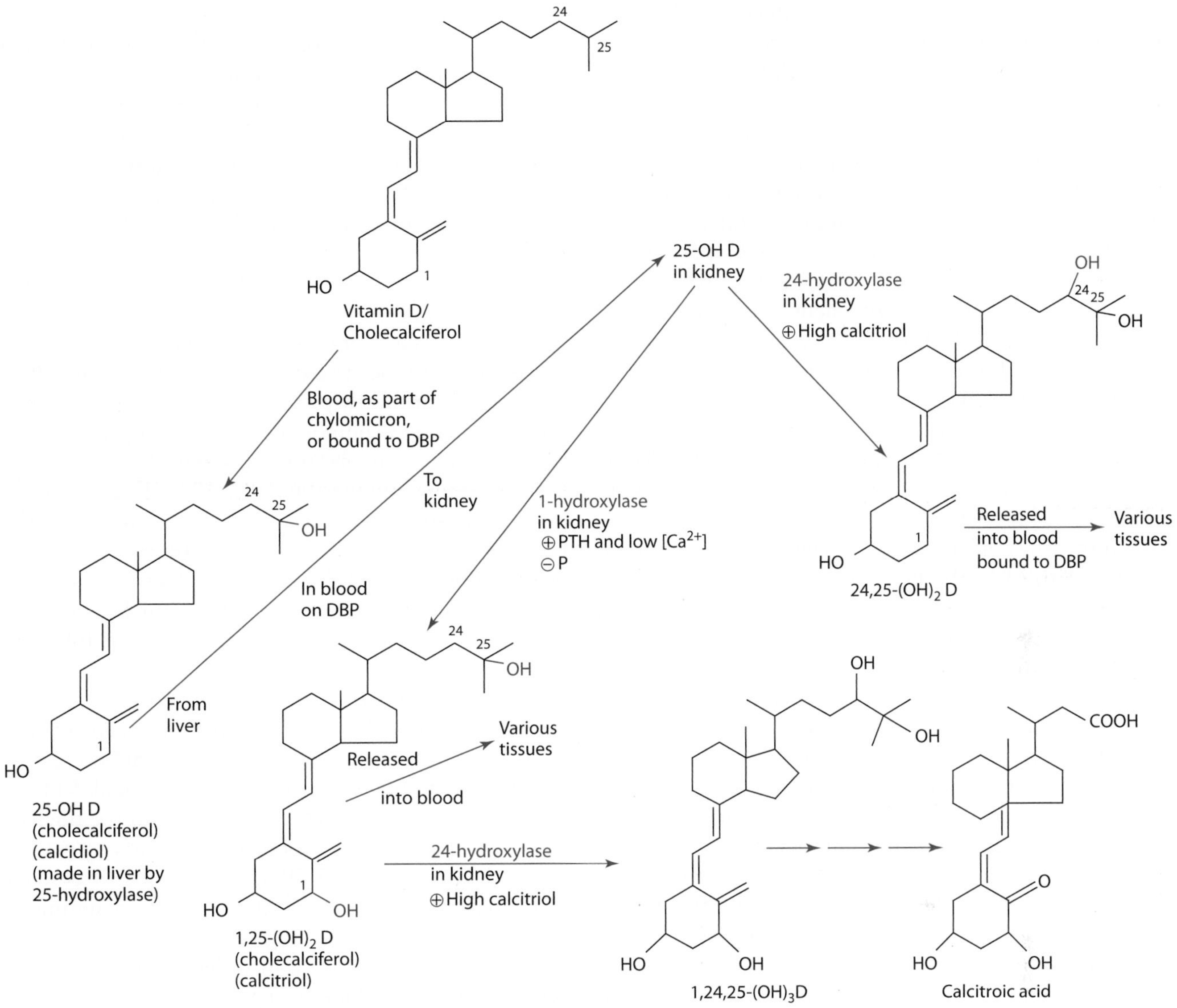

Figure 10.12 Hydroxylations of vitamin D.

(nonhydroxylated) vitamin D, and muscle, which contains both vitamin D and 25-OH D. Circulating 25-OH D concentrations reflect vitamin D status, which varies depending on both dietary vitamin D intake and sunlight exposure. Serum 25-OH D concentrations between about 30 and 40 ng/ml (75-100 nmol/L) are generally thought to be sufficient to maintain health [1].

From the blood, 25-OH D is taken up by tissues (mostly by the kidneys) in response to increased concentrations of parathyroid hormone (PTH). Specifically, the 25-OH D-DBP complex binds to a cubulin-megalin membrane receptor system on the kidneys' proximal tubule cell's plasma membrane to form a megalin-DBP-25-OH D complex. The complex is internalized by endocytosis into the cells, where the 25-OH D is released and is then hydroxylated at position 1 to form the vitamin's active form, 1,25-(OH)$_2$ (vitamin) D (also called calcitriol or 1,25 dihydroxycholecalciferol; Figure 10.12).

The 1-hydroxylase (CYP27B1), an NADPH-dependent mitochondrial enzyme, is expressed in the highest concentrations in the kidneys, but is also present in macrophages, skin, the intestine, and bone, among other tissues. Much of the calcitriol that is made in the kidneys is ultimately released into the blood for other tissues to use. However, many other tissues (besides the kidneys) are thought to use 25-OH D from the plasma to make their own calcitriol, provided that enough plasma 25-OH D is available.

The renal synthesis of calcitriol is tightly regulated by two hormones, PTH and fibroblast-like growth factor (FGF) 23, as well as other factors. PTH (secreted primarily when serum calcium concentrations are low but also to a lesser extent when serum phosphorus concentrations are low) stimulates the synthesis of the 1-hydroxylase, and thus the synthesis of calcitriol. In contrast, when FGF23 is secreted by osteocytes and osteoblasts, the synthesis of the enzyme (and thus calcitriol) is reduced. High serum concentrations of calcium (hypercalcemia) and phosphorus (hyperphosphatemia) also inhibit calcitriol synthesis. Additionally, the concentration of the enzyme's end product, $1,25\text{-}(OH)_2$ D (i.e., calcitriol), influences the enzyme's production by binding to a vitamin D response element (VDRE) on the promoter region of the 1-hydroxylase gene. Low concentrations of the end product stimulate 1-hydroxylase synthesis, while high concentrations inhibit 1-hydroxylase synthesis (thereby decreasing the vitamin's activation) and stimulate the production of another mixed-function oxidase, 24-hydroxylase. The 24-hydroxylase generates $24,25\text{-}(OH)_2$ D from the hydroxylation of 25-OH D, and $1,24,25\text{-}(OH)_3$ D from hydroxylation of $1,25\text{-}(OH)_2$ D (Figure 10.12); these 24-hydroxylation reactions represent steps in the vitamin's inactivation. These metabolites may be further oxidized to generate a variety of excretory products.

Vitamin D_2, although less frequently consumed, is metabolized in the body to calcitriol by the same 25-hydroxylase and 1-hydroxylase as vitamin D_3. The metabolism of D_2, however, produces additional metabolites not generated by D_3 and has been suggested to be less efficient in calcitriol production than D_3.

The calcitriol that is made in the kidneys is released into the blood, where it binds to DBP for transport. Thus, DBP serves to transport several forms of the vitamin to various target tissues. DBP's binding to calcitriol, however, is loose to facilitate the vitamin's release to tissues; this is in contrast to its tight binding of 25-OH D. Calcitriol in the blood has a half-life of about 2 to 6 hours; normal plasma calcitriol concentrations range from about 20 to 40 pg/mL, considerably lower than plasma 25-OH D concentrations. On reaching its target tissues, calcitriol is easily released from the DBP for cellular uptake.

Calcitriol's target tissues were once believed to be limited initially to the intestine, bone, and kidneys, but it is now known that receptors for the vitamin are found in many tissues including the heart, muscle, pancreas (β-cells), brain, skin, colon, prostate, breast, hematopoietic system, central nervous system, and immune system.

Functions and Mechanisms of Action

Calcitriol has several functions in the body. The mechanisms by which calcitriol performs these functions may be divided into two categories—nongenomic and genomic—although the details of these mechanisms have not been clearly elucidated. This section describes first the possible nongenomic, and then the genomic, mechanisms of action of the vitamin.

Many nongenomic actions of calcitriol are mediated by the activation of signal transduction pathways (also called intracellular signaling) linked to cell membranes. The binding of calcitriol to cell membrane receptors in selected tissues (especially intestine, parathyroid, liver, and pancreatic β-cells) triggers a series of events through signal transduction pathways to evoke relatively rapid (often within minutes or seconds) changes in some body processes. One such vitamin membrane receptor that has been identified and linked with these nongenomic actions of vitamin D is known as membrane-associated rapid response steroid-binding (MARRS) protein. The many actions initiated from these intracellular signaling pathways include increased calcium uptake, increased intracellular calcium concentration, and/or transcellular calcium flux in cells such as enterocytes, osteoblasts, adipocytes, and skeletal muscle. These cellular events are thought to be mediated primarily by the generation of second messengers and other compounds such as mitogen-activated protein (MAP) kinase, protein kinase C, cyclic AMP, tyrosine kinase, phospholipase C, diacylglycerol, inositol phosphate, and arachidonic acid. Additional details on possible vitamin D–mediated signal transduction pathways can be found in the article by Fleet [5]. Details of vitamin D–mediated nongenomic intestinal cell calcium uptake are discussed in the "Calcitriol and the Intestine" section.

Calcitriol also exerts its functions through genomic mechanisms of action (and thus regulates gene expression). Calcitriol's genomic mechanism of action is similar generally to that described for retinoic acid. Vitamin D appears to diffuse from the cytosol into the nucleus, where it (behaving like a hormone) binds to nuclear vitamin D receptors (VDRs; Figure 10.13). Nuclear VDRs have been found in over 30 organs, including the bone, intestine, kidneys, lungs, muscle, and skin. These nuclear VDRs are part of a so-called superfamily of receptors that also includes receptors for retinoic acid and thyroid and steroid hormones. VDRs usually exist as a heterodimer with another receptor (commonly retinoid X receptor—RXR) and are associated with specific DNA sequences called vitamin D response elements (abbreviated VDRE) that are found in the promoter regions of target genes. Additional comodulatory (either coactivator or corepressor) proteins may further interact with these regions to influence (enhance or inhibit) gene transcription. The mechanisms by which these comodulatory proteins function are mostly unknown, but they may help link the receptor to enzymes, such as RNA polymerase II, or to other components such as factors necessary for gene transcription [6]. Some of the comodulatory proteins are thought to include steroid receptor coactivators (SRC-1, SRC-2, and SRC-3), histone acetyl transferase, vitamin D–receptor interacting protein, and thyroid hormone–receptor interacting protein, among others [6,7].

In addition to its genomic interactions with VDRE on genes, calcitriol also appears to exert its effects through interactions with messenger (m)RNA to enhance or

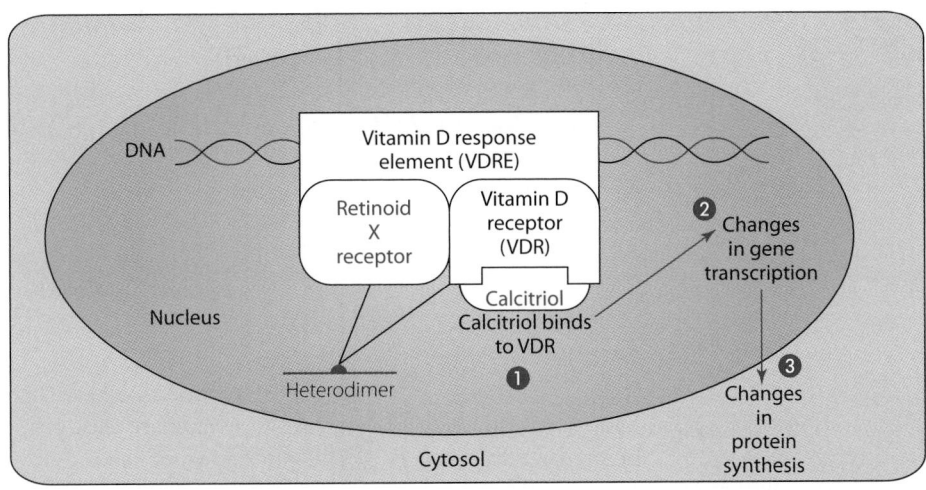

Figure 10.13 Proposed role of calcitriol bound to VDR on DNA in gene expression.

inhibit translation. The proteins that are ultimately generated from vitamin D's genomic actions are typically, but not exclusively, involved in calcium homeostasis and/or functions and include, for example, osteocalcin, osteopontin, 24-hydroxylase (CYP24), the epithelial transient receptor potential cation channel vanilloid-type subfamily member 6 (TRPV6), calbindin, and Ca^{2+}-ATPase. Over 50 genes appear to be regulated by calcitriol.

As suggested by its mechanisms of action, calcitriol affects several body processes. One of the most investigated roles of calcitriol relates to serum calcium homeostasis. This discussion will be followed by calcitriol's effects on phosphorus homeostasis; on cell differentiation, proliferation, and growth; and on muscle. Then some of calcitriol's others roles in the body will be discussed.

Serum Calcium Homeostasis—Actions to Increase Serum Calcium

Calcitriol synthesis is stimulated in response to changes in serum calcium concentrations and the release of PTH. Normal serum calcium concentrations range from about 8.5 to 10.5 mg/dL (2.12–2.62 mmol/L). **Hypocalcemia** (low serum calcium concentrations, i.e., <8.5 mg/dL) initially stimulates the secretion of PTH from the parathyroid gland through activation of calcium-sensing receptors. Vitamin D, when present in high concentrations, also influences PTH by interacting with VDRE in the promoter region of the PTH gene to inhibit its transcription. The PTH, in turn, travels to the kidneys, where it stimulates 1-hydroxylase to convert 25-OH D to calcitriol. Once synthesized, some calcitriol remains and functions within the kidneys, and some calcitriol is released into the blood bound to DBP. The vitamin then acts alone or with PTH on its other target tissues (the intestine and bone), causing serum calcium concentrations to rise back to within the normal range. The effects of calcitriol on its target tissues—intestine, kidneys, and bone—are discussed next and shown in Figure 10.14.

Calcitriol and the Intestine The primary function of calcitriol in the intestine is to increase the absorption of calcium (as well as phosphorus, as discussed later). The vitamin is believed to act through genomic and nongenomic mechanisms to exert its effects.

With respect to genomic effects on intestinal cell calcium absorption, calcitriol is transported into the enterocyte and carried into the nucleus, where it interacts with nuclear VDRs to directly regulate specific genes encoding for proteins involved in calcium uptake and transport. As the result of this interaction, selective DNA transcriptions occur that result in the biosynthesis of new mRNA molecules. These mRNA molecules are then translated on the endoplasmic reticulum into selected proteins. The proteins act at the brush border, in the cytosol, and at the basolateral membrane of the intestinal cells, especially in the duodenum and jejunum, to promote calcium absorption. For example, calbindin D9k, a calcium-binding protein in enterocytes, is synthesized in response to calcitriol's genomic actions. Calbindin D9k, which binds two calcium atoms, transports over 90% of calcium through the cytosol of enterocytes. Calcitriol also induces the expression of both basolateral membrane Ca^{2+}-ATPases and calcium channel transporters in enterocytes. For example, messenger RNA concentrations of TRPV6, a calcium channel transporter found in the brush border membrane of the duodenum, appear to be regulated by calcitriol. Thus, calcitriol first influences brush border membrane uptake of calcium through effects on calcium channels (TRPV6). Second, it enhances cellular calcium transport through stimulation of calbindin D9k synthesis, and finally, it enhances the extrusion of calcium across the basolateral membrane of the enterocyte and into the plasma by enhancing the synthesis of Ca^{2+}-ATPase pumps. Interestingly, however, in laboratory studies mice unable to make calbindin D9k or the calcium channel transporters exhibited adequate calcium absorption if provided with adequate dietary calcium intake [8]. Such findings suggest that other

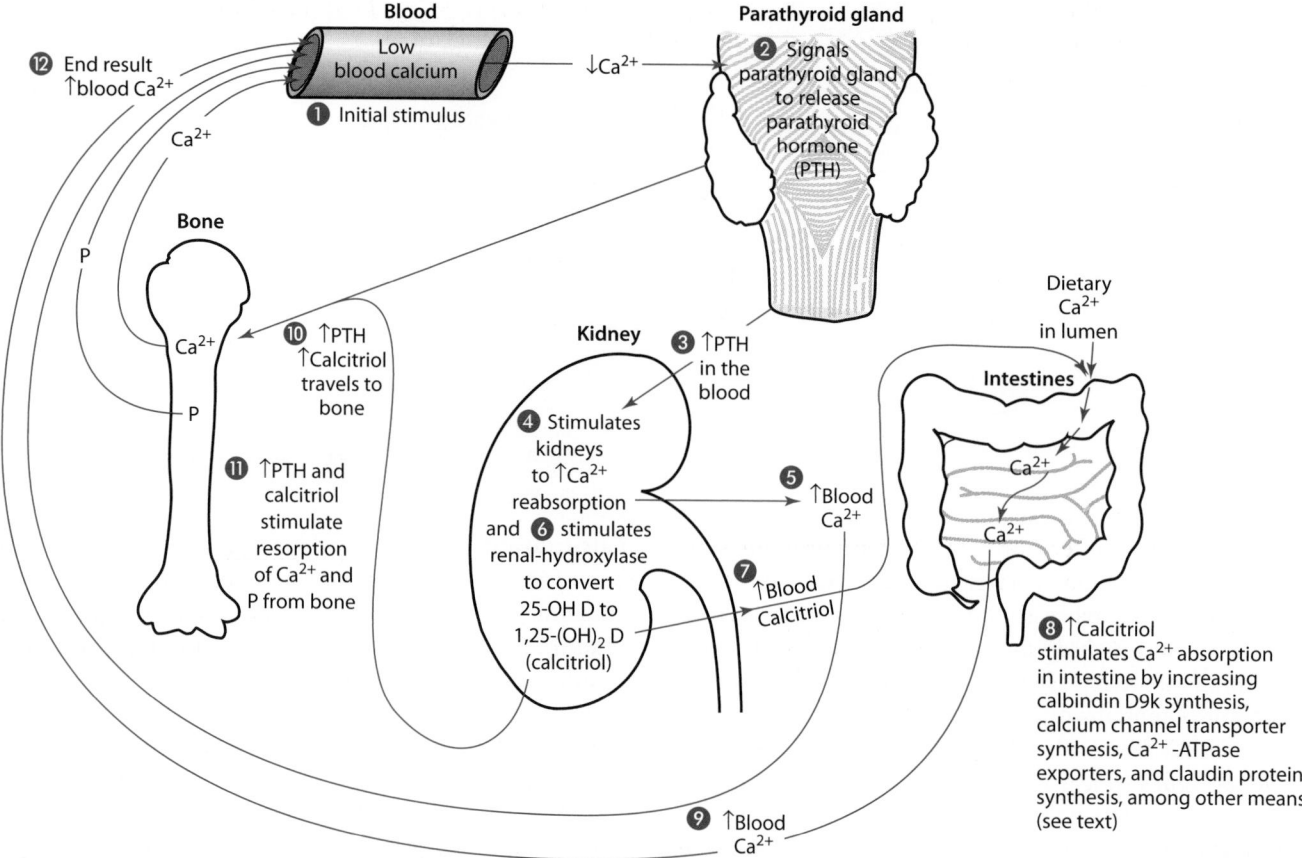

Figure 10.14 Calcitriol, 1,25 (OH)$_2$ D, synthesis and actions with parathyroid hormone (PTH).

absorptive mechanisms (such as paracellular absorption) for calcium are of significance.

Calcium may be absorbed in the intestine by paracellular (meaning occurring between the enterocytes) transport that is also regulated in part by vitamin D. Vitamin D enhances the expression of genes that code for a specific group of transmembrane proteins, called claudins, found in the tight junctions between cells, including those of the intestine. The synthesis of claudins 2 and 12, which have been shown to be essential for paracellular calcium absorption in the intestine, is activated by vitamin D [9].

A possible (but not well-defined) nongenomic process by which vitamin D may rapidly initiate intestinal calcium absorption is thought to involve calcitriol binding to a membrane-associated rapid response steroid-binding protein (MARRS) on the enterocyte's basolateral membrane. Maximal calcium absorption has been shown to correspond with serum 25-OH D concentrations of about 75 to 80 nmol/L (30–32 ng/mL); plasma PTH concentrations also rise significantly as serum 25-OH D concentration drop below about 75 nmol/L (30 ng/mL) [10].

Calcitriol and the Kidneys Calcitriol, along with PTH, functions to induce calcium reabsorption (Figure 10.14) in the kidneys. Specifically, PTH from the blood interacts

with receptors in the plasma membrane of renal (kidney) cells; this interaction ultimately leads to increased expression of 1-hydroxylase and subsequent synthesis of calcitriol. Calcitriol in turn exerts its genomic effects in the nucleus of renal cells to enhance gene expression of calbindin D28k, a larger form of the protein calbindin D9k that is found in the intestine. Calbindin D28k binds calcium and enhances its reabsorption in the kidney. Calcitriol also enhances the expression of another calcium channel protein, called TRPV5, and an ATP-dependent calcium transporter at the kidneys' basolateral membrane to enhance calcium reabsorption from the glomerular filtrate. These actions serve to increase the reabsorption of calcium back into blood, and thus to raise serum calcium concentrations to within a normal range.

Calcitriol and the Bone Elevated (above normal) blood PTH concentrations, along with calcitriol, direct the mobilization of calcium out of bone to help achieve a normal serum calcium concentration (Figure 10.14). More specifically, in the presence of high blood PTH and calcitriol, calcitriol interacts within the nucleus of mature osteoblasts to induce the expression of a cytokine called receptor activator of NFκβ ligand (RANKL). The RANKL released from the osteoblasts then interacts with the receptor protein

RANK, found on the cell surface of immature osteoclast precursors (also called pre-osteoclasts), to stimulate (via signal transduction) the differentiation, production, and maturation of the osteoclasts [11]. The mature osteoclasts in turn release hydrochloric acid, alkaline phosphatase, collagenase, and other hydrolytic enzymes and substances, which dissolve and catabolize (eat away at) the bone matrix. The net effect of these (bone demineralization) actions is an increase in serum calcium (and phosphorus) concentrations at the expense of the bone.

Serum Calcium Homeostasis—Actions to Decrease Serum Calcium

Although calcitriol is not thought to be directly involved in decreasing serum calcium concentrations should they rise above normal (hypercalcemia), calcitriol is indirectly involved through effects on PTH. Elevations in the serum concentrations of both calcitriol and ionized serum calcium decrease PTH production through long and short feedback loops as well as via down-regulation by fibroblast growth factor 23 (FGF 23). The long feedback loop is indirect, resulting from elevated serum ionized calcium's inhibitory effect on the parathyroid gland's secretion of PTH. The short feedback loop is direct: Calcitriol decreases the transcription of the gene for preparathyroid hormone, by interacting with the VDR in the parathyroid gland and influencing the regulatory region of the PTH gene. In addition, with above-normal elevations in serum calcium concentrations, calcitonin (a hormone produced by parafollicular endocrine clear [C] cells of the thyroid gland) is released. Calcitonin blocks calcium and phosphorus mobilization from bones by inhibiting osteoclast activity. In addition, it inhibits the tubular resorption of calcium (as well as phosphorus), leading to increased urinary calcium excretion. Further, but in contrast to their detrimental effects when present in high concentrations, calcitriol and PTH, when present in low concentrations, may promote bone anabolism and mineralization.

Phosphorus Homeostasis

Calcitriol affects phosphorus homeostasis by acting on the same target organs as when maintaining calcium homeostasis. In the intestine, calcitriol is thought to increase the activity of brush border alkaline phosphatase, which hydrolyzes phosphate ester bonds to free the phosphorus and thus enable its absorption. Calcitriol also regulates the number of carriers responsible for the sodium-dependent absorption of phosphorus at the brush border membrane of intestinal cells (especially of the jejunum and ileum). In bone, calcitriol promotes the resorption of phosphorus out of bone and into the blood. These actions serve ultimately to increase serum phosphorus concentrations. In the kidneys, calcitriol enhances phosphorus resorption in the distal tubules. However, excess phosphorus is excreted in the urine in response to PTH.

Cell Differentiation, Proliferation, and Growth

The local presence of the calcitriol within many non–calcium regulating tissues is thought to help maintain normal cell growth, differentiation, and proliferation and, in some tissues, prevent malignancy (by down-regulating cancer cell growth and inducing apoptosis if needed) [12]. Vitamin D typically promotes differentiation and inhibits proliferation in tissues. Some examples of cells affected by vitamin D include premyeloid white blood cells and stem cells, which differentiate into macrophages and monocytes in the presence of adequate calcitriol. Calcitriol also induces cell differentiation of stem cell monocytes in the bone marrow, which become mature osteoclasts. Vitamin D's ability to stimulate skin epidermal cell differentiation while inhibiting proliferation has been applied in the treatment of psoriasis (a disorder marked by enhanced proliferation and failed differentiation of keratinocytes). Specifically, calcitriol binds to VDRs in keratinocytes to alter the expression of regulatory proteins that serve to inhibit proliferation of the epidermis and induce normal differentiation in those with psoriasis.

Other mechanism(s) by which vitamin D affects aspects of cell differentiation, proliferation, and growth are not clear but are likely related to effects on genes coding for various regulatory factors, including ones that control cell growth and death. Calcitriol, for example, slows cell cycle progression by inhibiting key regulators of the transition from the gap (G)1 phase to the synthesis (S) phase of the cell cycle [13]. The vitamin also affects cell growth by altering concentrations of regulatory proteins involved in apoptosis such as caspases and bcl-2.

Calcitriol and Muscle

Muscle dysfunction (myopathy) is well documented in individuals with vitamin D deficiency. The most commonly reported problems include muscle weakness and pain, difficulty rising from a squatting or sitting position, difficulty walking (especially up stairs), and increased falls. Biopsies of muscle in those with vitamin D deficiency show atrophy of primarily type II (fast-twitch) muscle fibers (note that it is these fibers that are utilized to prevent falls). Vitamin D supplementation, in those with deficiency, in turn increases the type II muscle fiber area and diameter, as well as the synthesis of muscle cytoskeletal proteins such as calmodulin needed for muscle contraction. In muscle, calcitriol is thought to function through genomic mechanisms to enhance calcium uptake and thus intracellular calcium concentrations. Specifically, the vitamin is thought to increase the transcription of genes for calcium ATPase pumps (that actively transport calcium into the sarcoplasmic reticulum and sarcolemma), and for voltage-sensitive calcium channels. Such changes in intracellular calcium concentrations are important for contraction and relaxation of muscle. Calcitriol is also thought to modulate muscle contractility through non-genomic mechanisms. For example, through binding to cell surface receptors, calcitriol activates second messenger pathways to rapidly increase intracellular calcium concentrations by promoting calcium release from intracellular stores. Additionally, through second messenger pathways, calcitriol enhances myogenesis, cell proliferation, differentiation, and apoptosis.

Other Roles

Vitamin D is also purported to have roles in regulating blood pressure and diminishing risk of heart disease. The vitamin suppresses renin gene expression and thus diminishes the production of angiotensin II, thereby lowering blood pressure [14,15]. Vitamin D (when present as 25-OH D in the blood in concentrations greater than 75 nmol/L or 30 ng/mL) appears to decrease low-density lipoprotein concentrations and raise high-density lipoprotein concentrations [16], which may decrease risk of heart disease. Suboptimal serum 25-OH D concentrations have been associated with increased risk of heart disease; however, the efficacy of vitamin D supplementation for risk reduction is yet undetermined [17].

Some autoimmune conditions, including rheumatoid arthritis, Crohn's disease, multiple sclerosis, and type 1 diabetes mellitus, have been linked with inadequate vitamin D status. Protective effects against developing some of these diseases also have been found with the use of vitamin D supplements in amounts up to about 50 μg (2,000 IU) daily [18,19]. These findings are thought to be linked (at least partially) with vitamin D's role in immunity. Activated T- and B-cells express VDRs, as do antigen-presenting dendritic cells, monocytes, macrophages, and cytotoxic T-cells. Many of these cells also produce calcitriol. Vitamin D has been shown to enhance antibody synthesis from activated B-cells and phagocytosis by macrophages [12,18]. Vitamin D also regulates the expression and production of several cytokines; for example, the inflammatory cytokines interleukin (IL)2 and IL12 are down-regulated in response to vitamin D [20]. Additionally, production of antimicrobial peptides, such as cathelicidin (needed to help fight the infective agent that causes tuberculosis), is a function of local production of calcitriol, which in turn up-regulates production of these proteins [21].

Vitamin D also appears to play a role in pancreatic β-cell protection and insulin secretion. Insulin secretion has been negatively related to serum 25-OH D concentrations, whereas insulin sensitivity has been positively associated with serum 25-OH D concentrations [20]. It has been suggested that calcitriol influences β-cell calcium concentrations in a yet undefined way to affect insulin synthesis and secretion. The vitamin has been shown to improve β-cell function and marginally improve blood glucose control in individuals at high risk for diabetes [22].

Interactions with Other Nutrients

Discussion of vitamin D metabolism is impossible without noting the interrelationships among this vitamin/hormone and calcium, phosphorus, and vitamin K. The relationship with calcium is shown in Figure 10.14 and explained in the two serum calcium homeostasis sections. Calcitriol's impact on phosphorus homeostasis is presented in the "Phosphorus Homeostasis" section. The interaction of calcitriol and vitamin K–dependent proteins is discussed in the "Vitamin K and Bone" section.

Metabolism and Excretion

Calcitriol hydroxylation at carbon 24 generates the metabolite $1,24,25\text{-}(OH)_3$ D (Figure 10.12), which may be further oxidized to $1,25\text{-}(OH)_2$ 24-oxo D. Subsequent reactions, including side-chain cleavage, yield the major end product calcitroic acid (Figure 10.12), which, along with other vitamin D metabolites also formed after hydroxylation, oxidation, and conjugation, is excreted through the bile in the feces. Thus, little (<30%) vitamin D is excreted via the urine.

Recommended Dietary Allowance

An RDA for vitamin D was published for the first time in 2010 [1]. The recommendations, which assume minimal sun exposure, suggest an intake of 600 IU (15 μg) of vitamin D for children (age 1 year and older), adolescents, and adults including women who are pregnant or lactating. Recommended intakes increase to 800 IU (20 μg) of vitamin D for adults older than 70 years of age. Requirements are estimated at 400 IU (10 μg) for these age groups. Sufficient amounts of vitamin D are thought to be obtainable by exposure to sunlight for about 5 to 15 minutes between about 10 A.M. and 3 P.M. during spring, summer, and fall [18]. In the continental United States, about 1.5 IU of vitamin D/cm^2/hour during the winter and about 6 IU/cm^2/hour during the summer can be synthesized in the skin [23]. It is estimated that with full body exposure to the sun, fair-skinned individuals generate about 10,000 to 20,000 IU vitamin D in 15 to 30 minutes [1]. However, at higher latitudes (above about 35°) and during winter months, the UVB photon path length is longer, and fewer UVB photons reach the surface of the earth, resulting in less vitamin D production in the skin. In addition to latitude and season of the year, time of day affects UVB exposure; pollution, glass in windows, and clothing block UVB light. Further, in older people, diminished organ function and 7-dehydrocholesterol content in the skin impair calcitriol production. In those with darker skin color (higher melanin content), longer sun exposure time is needed to generate the vitamin than in those with lighter skin color, since melanin blocks some of the UVB rays.

Deficiency: Rickets and Osteomalacia

Vitamin D deficiency is widespread across the United States and world. While deficiency of the vitamin has been linked with several health conditions, as previously discussed, inadequate intakes most notably directly result in the conditions rickets and osteomalacia. In infants and children, vitamin D deficiency causes **rickets**, a condition characterized by seizures as well as growth retardation and failure of bone to mineralize. In vitamin D–deficient infants, the epiphyseal cartilage continues to grow and enlarge without replacement by bone matrix and minerals. These effects are especially visible at the wrists, ankles, and knees, all of which enlarge. In addition, long bones of the legs bow and knees knock as weight-bearing activity such as walking begins. The spine becomes curved, and pelvic and thoracic deformities—such as rachitic rosary, characterized by costochondral beading at the juncture of the ribs and cartilages—occur.

In adults as well as some older children, deprivation of vitamin D leads to bone mineralization defects called **osteomalacia**. The condition results from prolonged elevations in blood PTH (secondary to low serum 25-OH D and calcium concentrations). PTH promotes bone resorption and increased urinary phosphorus excretion, among other changes. Indicators of bone resorption include increased urinary excretion of bone collagen by-products such as hydroxyproline, N-telopeptide, pyridinoline, and deoxypyridinoline. With insufficient serum calcium and phosphorus concentrations, the mineralization of bones cannot occur. Thus, in vitamin D deficiency, as bone turnover occurs, the bone matrix is preserved, but remineralization is impaired. Progressive demineralization results in bone pain (characterized as throbbing or aching) and osteomalacia (soft bone). Muscle weakness and pain also are typically present.

While exposure to sunlight can maintain adequate vitamin D nutrition for most of the world's population, older individuals, people with insufficient sun exposure, and those with certain diseases or conditions may be at risk for vitamin D deficiency. The elderly represent one population group that typically has insufficient vitamin D intake and low sunlight exposure. In addition, aging reduces synthesis of 7-dehydrocholesterol in the skin and reduces the activity of renal 1-hydroxylase in response to PTH. Impaired vitamin D absorption may occur in disorders characterized by fat malabsorption, such as Crohn's disease, pancreatitis, and liver disease. Disorders affecting the parathyroid, liver, or kidneys impair synthesis of the active form of the vitamin. People on anticonvulsant drug therapy may develop an impaired response to vitamin D and exhibit problems with calcium metabolism. Infants may be at risk for deficiency because human milk is low in vitamin D and infants' exposure to sunlight typically is minimal. Thus, it is recommended that vitamin D supplements be given to breast-fed infants.

A number of vitamin D supplements are available for use by those who need them. For example, Rocaltrol (Hoffman-LaRoche) for oral use and Calcijex (Abbott Laboratories) for intravenous use are commonly prescribed brands of calcitriol given to those with kidney disease. Other preparations, such as Calderol (Organon-USA), which provides 25-OH D, and vitamin D_2 and D_3 (i.e., unhydroxylated forms), also are available.

A deficiency of vitamin D for those with normal organ function may be treated with high-dose supplements initially—such as one 50,000 IU (1,250 μg) dose given once per week for 8 weeks followed by lower dosages such as 1,000 IU (25 μg) daily for several months [15,18]. It is estimated that for every 100 IU of vitamin D ingested, serum 25-OH D concentrations increase by 1 ng/mL [24]. Intakes of about 1,000 to 2,000 IU (25–50 μg) daily may be needed to maintain serum 25-OH D concentrations in excess of 75 nmol/L (30 ng/mL) [12].

Toxicity

The Tolerable Upper Intake Level for vitamin D has been set at 4,000 IU (100 μg) for children aged 9 years and older, adolescents, and adults [1]. Although excessive exposure to sunlight may be the primary risk factor in developing skin cancer, it poses no risk of toxicity through overproduction of endogenous vitamin D_3. Cutaneous production of the vitamin reaches a maximum of about 20,000 IU, and extensive whole-body irradiation with ultraviolet light generally raises serum 25-OH D concentrations to about 100 to 200 nmol/L (40–80 ng/mL); levels greater than about 500 nmol/L (200 ng/mL) are associated with toxicity [4,18].

Vitamin D, when ingested in large amounts, is one of the most likely of all vitamins to cause overt toxicity. Toxicity is seen especially in those with vitamin D intakes of 10,000 IU (or more) per day for several months. Manifestations of toxicity include hypercalcemia and calcinosis, the associated calcification of soft tissues including organs such as the kidneys, heart, and lungs, along with blood vessels. In addition, toxicity promotes hyperphosphatemia, hypertension, anorexia, nausea, weakness, headache, renal dysfunction (characterized by polyuria, polydipsia, azotemia, nephrolithiasis, and renal failure), and, in some cases, death. In the 1950s an epidemic of "idiopathic hypercalcemia" among English infants was traced to a daily intake of vitamin D between 2,000 and 3,000 IU. Symptoms of toxicity in the infants included anorexia, nausea, vomiting, hypertension, renal insufficiency, and failure to thrive. Eight people experienced hypervitaminosis from consuming milk (½ to 3 cups daily from a local dairy) that contained up to 232,565 IU of vitamin D_3 per quart; they displayed elevated serum calcium and vitamin D concentrations [25]. Because so many foods are now fortified with vitamin D and many over-the-counter products also contain it, the consumer needs to consider all sources of the vitamin to ensure intake is not excessive.

Assessment of Nutriture

Serum 25-OH D concentrations are most often used to assess vitamin D status. Concentrations less than 25 to 30 nmol/L (10–12 ng/mL) have typically been diagnostic of a vitamin D deficiency; however, newer research suggests serum 25-OH D concentrations less than 50 nmol/L (20 ng/mL) represent deficiency, and concentrations in the range of 50 to 72 nmol/L (20–29 ng/mL) constitute vitamin D insufficiency. Serum 25-OH D concentrations in excess of about 75 or 80 to 100 nmol/L (30 or 32–40 ng/mL) are thought to be needed for bone health [18,26–28]. Toxicity is apparent when serum 25-OH D concentrations exceed about 500 nmol/L (200 ng/mL), although some evidence suggests that concentrations greater than 150 nmol/L (60 ng/mL) may be adverse to health [1,4,18,29].

References Cited for Vitamin D

1. Institute of Medicine, Food and Nutrition Board. Dietary Reference intakes for Calcium and Vitamin D. Washington, DC: National Academy Press. 2011.
2. Omdahl J, Morris H, May B. Hydroxylase enzymes of the vitamin D pathway: expression, function, and regulation. Ann Rev Nutr. 2002; 22:139–66.
3. Heaney RP, Armas LAG, Shary JR, et al. 25-hydroxylation of vitamin D₃: relation to circulating vitamin D₃ under various input conditions. Am J Clin Nutr. 2008; 87:1738–42.
4. Holick M. The use and interpretation of assays for vitamin D and its metabolites. J Nutr. 1990; 120:1464–69.
5. Fleet J. Rapid, membrane-initiated actions of 1,25 dihydroxyvitamin D: what are they and what do they mean? J Nutr. 2004;134:3215–18.
6. MacDonald P, Baudina T, Tokumaru H, et al. Vitamin D receptor and nuclear receptor coactivators. Steroids. 2001; 66:171–76.
7. Haussler MR, Haussler CA, Bartik L, et al. Vitamin D receptor: molecular signaling and actions of nutritional ligands in disease prevention. Nutr Rev. 2008; 66:S98–112.
8. Benn BS, Ajibade D, Porta A, et al. Active intestinal calcium transport in the absence of transient receptor potential vanilloid type 6 and calbindin D9k. Endocrinology. 2008; 149:3196–3205.
9. Fujita H, Sugimoto K, Inatomi S, et al. Tight junction proteins claudin-2 and -12 are critical for vitamin D dependent Ca²⁺ absorption between enterocytes. Molec Biol Cell. 2008; 19:1912–21.
10. Adams JS, Hewison M. Update in vitamin D. J Clin Endocrinol Metab. 2010; 95:471–78.
11. Takasu H. Anti-osteoclastogenic action of active vitamin D. Nutr Rev. 2008; 66 (suppl2):S113–15.
12. Holick MF. The vitamin D deficiency pandemic and consequences of nonskeletal health: mechanisms of action. Molec Aspects Med. 2008; 29:361–68.
13. Samuel S, Sitrin MD. Vitamin D's role in cell proliferation and differentiation. Nutr Rev. 2008; 66(suppl2):S116–24.
14. Martini LA, Wood RJ. Vitamin D and blood pressure connection: update on epidemiologic, clinical and mechanistic evidence. Molec Aspects Med. 2008; 29:291–97.
15. Holick M. Vitamin D: importance in the prevention of cancer, type 1 diabetes, heart disease, and osteoporosis. Am J Clin Nutr. 2004; 79:362–71.
16. Carbone LD, Rosenberg EW, Tolley EA, et al. 25-hydroxyvitamin D, cholesterol, and ultraviolet radiation. Metab Clin Exp. 2008; 57:741–48.
17. Sun Q, Shi L, Rimm EB, et al. Vitamin D intake and risk of cardiovascular disease in US men and women. Am J Clin Nutr. 2011; 94:534–42.
18. Holick M. The vitamin D epidemic and its health consequences. J Nutr. 2005; 135:S2739–48.
19. Whiting S, Calvo M. Dietary recommendations for vitamin D: a critical need for functional end points to establish an estimated average requirement. J Nutr. 2005; 135:304–09.
20. Lips P. Vitamin D physiology. Prog Biophys Molec Biol. 2006; 92:4–8.
21. Holick M. Resurrection of vitamin D deficiency and rickets. J Clin Invest. 2006; 116:2062–72.
22. Mitri J, Dawson-Hughes B, Hu FB, Pittas AG. Effects of vitamin D and calcium supplementation on pancreatic β-cell function, insulin sensitivity, and glycemia in adults at high risk of diabetes: The Calcium and Vitamin D for Diabetes Mellitus (CaDDM) randomized controlled trial. Am J Clin Nutr. 2011; 94:486–94.
23. Collins E, Norman A. Vitamin D. In: Rucker RB, Suttie JW, McCormick DB, Machlin LJ, eds. Handbook of Vitamins. 3rd ed. New York: Marcel Dekker, Inc. 2001 pp. 51–114.
24. Holick MF, Biancuzzo RM, Chen TC, et al. Vitamin D₂ is as effective as vitamin D₃ in maintaining circulating concentrations of 25-hydroxylvitamin D. J Clin Endocrin. 2008; 93:677–81.
25. Jacobus C, Holick M, Shao Q, et al. Hypervitaminosis D associated with drinking milk. N Engl J Med. 1992; 326:1173–77.
26. Bischoff-Ferrari H, Giovannucci E, Willett W, et al. Estimation of optimal serum concentrations of 25-hydroxyvitamin D for multiple health outcomes. Am J Clin Nutr. 2006; 84:18–28.
27. Mullin GE, Dobs A. Vitamin D and its role in cancer and immunity: a prescription for sunlight. Nutr Clin Prac. 2007; 22:305–22.
28. Holick MF. Vitamin D deficiency. New Eng J Med. 2007; 357:266–81.
29. Hathcock JN, Shao A, Vieth R, Heaney R. Risk assessment for vitamin D. Am J Clin Nutr. 2007; 85:6–18.

Suggested Readings

Ceglia L. Vitamin D and skeletal muscle tissue and function. Molec Aspects Med. 2008; 29:407–14.
Norman AW. Minireview: Vvitamin D receptor: new assignments for an already busy receptor. Endocrin. 2006; 147:5542–48.
vanEtten E, Stoeffels K, Gysemans C, et al. Regulation of vitamin D homeostasis: implications for the immune system. Nutr Rev. 2008; 66(suppl2):S125–34.

VITAMIN E

Vitamin E encompasses eight compounds (vitamers). Each of these eight compounds contains a phenolic functional group on a chromanol/chromane ring (sometimes called the head of the molecule) and an attached phytyl side chain (sometimes called the **phytyl tail** of the molecule). The eight compounds (Figure 10.15) are usually divided into two classes:

- the tocopherols, which have saturated side chains with 16 carbons

- the tocotrienols (also called trienols), which have unsaturated side chains with 16 carbons

Each class is composed of four vitamers that differ in the number and location of methyl groups on the chromanol ring. Vitamers in both classes are designated as α, β, γ, or δ. Only α-tocopherol has biologic activity and can meet the body's need (requirement) for the vitamin. Moreover, the body cannot interconvert the vitamers.

All tocopherols and tocotrienols found naturally in foods have an RRR stereochemistry. R and S are used to

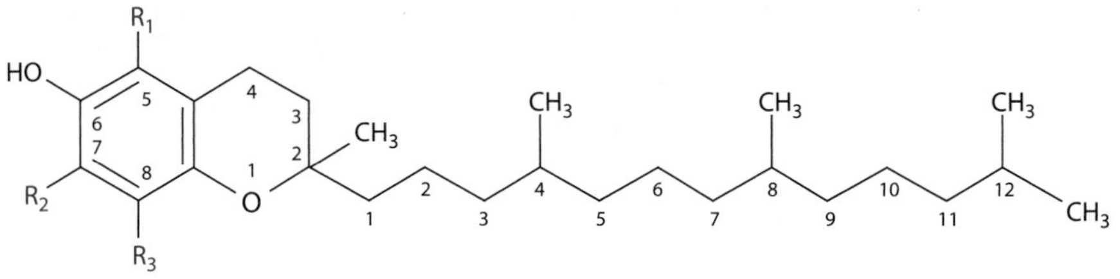

Tocopherols

	R_1	R_2	R_3
α-tocopherol	CH$_3$	CH$_3$	CH$_3$
β-tocopherol	CH$_3$	H	CH$_3$
γ-tocopherol	H	CH$_3$	CH$_3$
δ-tocopherol	H	H	CH$_3$

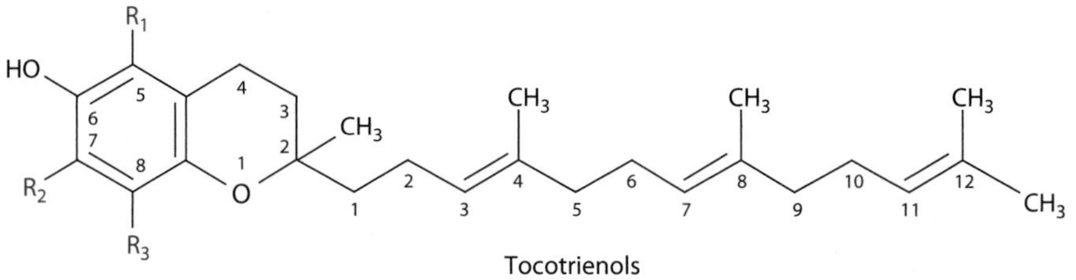

Tocotrienols

	R_1	R_2	R_3
α-tocotrienol	CH$_3$	CH$_3$	CH$_3$
β-tocotrienol	CH$_3$	H	CH$_3$
γ-tocotrienol	H	CH$_3$	CH$_3$
δ-tocotrienol	H	H	CH$_3$

Figure 10.15 The structures of the various forms of the tocopherols and tocotrienols.

designate stereoisomers of asymmetrical molecules such as vitamin E. The most biologically active form is RRR α-tocopherol, which was once called d-α-tocopherol.

Synthetic ester forms of α-tocopherol include all-racemic (all-rac) α-tocopheryl acetate and all-rac α-tocopheryl succinate, which are used in vitamin supplements and fortified foods. These synthetic forms of the vitamin often contain a mixture of eight stereoisomers and thus are not as active as the naturally occurring form, RRR α-tocopherol. Of the eight stereoisomers, four are in the 2R-stereoisomeric form (RRR, RSR, RRS, and RSS) and four are in the 2S-stereoisomeric form (SRR, SSR, SRS, and SSS) [1]. The form of the vitamin should be listed on the food or supplement label. The Food and Nutrition Board recommends that vitamin E activity be limited to naturally occurring RRR α-tocopherol and to three synthetic stereoisomeric forms: RSR-, RRS-, and RSS-α-tocopherol; however, in establishing a Tolerable Upper Intake Level, all supplemental forms of the vitamin were considered [1].

The term *tocopherol* is derived from the Greek word *tokos*, which means "childbirth," and *phero*, which means "to bear or bring forth." This terminology is based upon the vitamin's discovery by H. Evans and K. Bishop in the early 1920s, when they found that rats could not reproduce when given a diet of rancid lard. Wheat germ oil provided the needed vitamin; the oil was later purified, and the vitamin was extracted and named vitamin E (following D, which had been previously discovered).

Sources

Vitamin E, in its various forms, is found primarily in plant foods, especially the oils from plants. Wheat germ (20.3 mg/tablespoon), sunflower (5.6 mg/tablespoon), canola (2.4 mg/tablespoon), and safflower (4.6 mg/tablespoon) oils are especially rich in α-tocopherol, whereas soybean (1.1 mg/tablespoon) and corn (1.9 mg/tablespoon) oils contain less α-tocopherol but considerably higher amounts of γ-tocopherol. Foods (especially full-fat varieties) made from vegetable oils, such as salad dressings, mayonnaise, and margarine, as well as nuts and foods made from them such as peanut butter, represent good sources of vitamin E. Peanuts, cashews, and hazelnuts provide 2.2 mg, 0.3 mg, and 4.3 mg of α-tocopherol, respectively, per ounce, while almonds (especially rich) have about 7.0 mg of α-tocopherol/oz. Margarine has 1.6 mg of α-tocopherol/tablespoon, while mayonnaise has 0.7 mg of α-tocopherol/tablespoon. Unfortunately, people limiting fat intake also limit foods that are high in vitamin E and thus may compromise their ability to meet dietary intake recommendations for the vitamin. Other plant sources of vitamin E include whole-grain cereals and some fruits and vegetables. The green (chloroplast) portions such as the leaves of plants contain mostly α-tocopherol, while the other portions of the plant provide some γ-, δ-, and β-tocopherols. Cooked spinach, broccoli, and collard greens contain 1.9 mg, 1.2 mg, and 0.8 mg of α-tocopherol/½ cup, respectively. Raisin Bran®

and Frosted Mini Wheats® provide 0.45 mg and 0.34 mg of α-tocopherol/cup, respectively.

Tocotrienols, although present in small quantities, are found in legumes, palm oil, and cereal grains, especially the bran and germ fractions of barley, rice, and oats. Palm oil, one of the more saturated oils from a plant source, is also one of the richest natural sources of tocotrienols, with 70% of its vitamin E as tocotrienols and 30% as tocopherols. Rice bran oil is also a good source of γ-tocotrienol.

In foods of animal origin, vitamin E, primarily α-tocopherol, is found concentrated in fatty tissues of the animal. Thus, higher-fat meats, such as ground beef that is 20% fat/80% lean with 0.4 mg of α-tocopherol/3 oz portion, can provide some vitamin E in the diet. Animal products, however, when compared to plants, represent an inferior source of vitamin E.

While the Food and Drug Administration does not require vitamin E to be listed on food labels unless the product has been fortified with the vitamin, the vitamin E content, when present on the label, may be given as a percentage of the Daily Value, which for vitamin E is 30 international units (IU). Two tablespoons of peanut butter, for example, provide 15% of the Daily Value, or 4.5 IU of vitamin E. While the use of IU has been officially discontinued, it is still found on some labels. Conversion factors to calculate intake provided by IU versus mg are given in the section on Recommended Dietary Allowances.

Vitamin E, like other fat-soluble vitamins, is susceptible to destruction during food preparation and storage. The processing of some foods also significantly reduces their vitamin E content; for example, the wheat germ is removed in the milling of wheat to make white flour, and thus substantial amounts of the vitamin are lost. Tocopherols are also oxidized with lengthy exposure to air. In addition, exposure of the vitamin to light and heat also can lead to increased destruction. Thus, the roasting of nuts reduces their vitamin E content.

Digestion and Absorption

Whereas the tocopherols are found free in foods, the tocotrienols are found esterified and must be hydrolyzed before absorption. Similarly, synthetic ester forms of the tocopherols such as tocopheryl acetate must be digested before absorption. Pancreatic esterase and especially duodenal mucosal esterase (also called carboxyl ester hydroxylase) are thought to function in the lumen or at the brush border membrane of enterocytes to hydrolyze tocotrienols and synthetic ester α-tocopherols for absorption.

Vitamin E is absorbed primarily in the jejunum by passive diffusion; bile salts are required for emulsification, solubilization, and micelle formation, thus allowing the vitamin to diffuse across the membrane of the enterocyte. Simultaneous digestion and absorption of dietary lipids with vitamin E improves the vitamin's absorption, which ranges from about 20% to about 50% to 80%. Higher intake of the vitamin appears to reduce its absorption. Little is known about tocotrienol absorption; however, the involvement of a Niemann-Pick C1-like 1 (NPC1L1) transporter in γ-tocotrienol absorption has been suggested.

Transport, Metabolism, and Storage

In the enterocyte, absorbed tocopherols are incorporated into chylomicrons for transport through the lymph and then into circulation. An ATP-binding cassette A1 (ABCA1) membrane transporter is thought to enable secretion of α- and γ-tocopherol across the enterocyte's basolateral membrane for lymphatic transport [2]. During transport in the chylomicrons, tocopherol equilibrates or is transferred among the other lipoproteins, including HDLs and LDLs. LDLs, which possess the highest concentrations of the vitamin, are thought to contain about five to nine α-tocopherol molecules per LDL [3]. Tocotrienols also are found in the same lipoproteins, but in lower concentrations than α-tocopherol. The half-life of RRR α-tocopherol in the plasma is about 48 hours, whereas the stereoisomer SRR α-tocopherol has a half-life of about 13 to 15 hours [4].

Chylomicron remnants deliver vitamin E (absorbed tocopherols and tocotrienols) to the liver. However, only RRR α-tocopherol is incorporated into very-low-density lipoproteins (VLDLs) for resecretion back into the blood and transport to other tissues. It is α-tocopherol transfer protein (αTTP), which is made in the liver (among other tissues), that transfers tocopherol (RRR α-tocopherol preferentially) into VLDLs, which enable distribution of the vitamin to tissues. An ATP-binding cassette protein A1 may also play a role in this process. A deficiency or absence of αTTP caused by gene defects leads to a vitamin E deficiency. It is because of the specificity of αTTP that other forms of the vitamin are not resecreted into the circulation. Thus, α-tocopherol is the primary form of vitamin E found in the blood; normal plasma α-tocopherol (bound within lipoproteins) concentrations range from about 5 to 20 μg/mL.

Tocopherol uptake into cells occurs as lipoproteins are taken up by body tissues. Thus, uptake of the vitamin can occur in several ways: as receptor-mediated uptake of LDLs occurs, through lipoprotein lipase-mediated hydrolysis of chylomicrons and VLDLs, through HDL-mediated nutrient delivery, and possibly by other mechanisms. A phospholipid transfer protein may facilitate vitamin E transfer from the lipoproteins to the cell membranes.

Within the cytosol as well as other parts of the cell, including the nucleus, vitamin E appears to bind to specific proteins (tocopherol-binding proteins) for intracellular transport. ATP–binding cassette (ABC) A1 is thought to be involved in cellular trafficking and efflux of the vitamin from cells. The protein is also known to transport cholesterol and phospholipids.

Within cells, vitamin E is found primarily in cell membranes such as the plasma, mitochondrial, and microsomal membranes. Vitamin E's chromanol group likely is directed toward the membrane surface (near the phosphate region of the phospholipid), and its phytyl tail is directed toward the hydrocarbon region.

There is no single storage organ for vitamin E. The largest amount (over 90%) of the vitamin is concentrated in an unesterified form in fat droplets in adipose tissue. The concentration of vitamin E in adipose tissue increases linearly with the dosage of vitamin E; however, release of vitamin E from adipose tissue is slow even during periods of low vitamin E intake. Other tissues that take up smaller amounts of vitamin E include the liver, lungs, heart, muscle, adrenal glands, spleen, and brain. The vitamin E concentration in these tissues remains constant or increases only at a slow rate with increased ingestion of the vitamin. Yet, during times in which vitamin E intake is low, the liver and plasma provide a readily available source of the vitamin, in addition to skeletal muscle, which, because of its large mass, contains appreciable amounts.

Functions and Mechanisms of Action

The principal function of vitamin E is as an antioxidant. It is in this capacity that the vitamin maintains membrane integrity of body cells. The mechanism by which vitamin E protects the membranes from destruction is through its ability to prevent the oxidation (peroxidation) of unsaturated fatty acids contained in the phospholipids of the membranes. Though the phospholipids of the mitochondrial membrane and endoplasmic reticulum contain more unsaturated fatty acids than the cell's plasma membrane and thus are at greater risk of oxidation, cell membranes are still vulnerable. Tissues with cell membranes especially susceptible to oxidation include the lungs, brain, and erythrocytes. Erythrocyte membranes, for example, are vulnerable because they are high in polyunsaturated fatty acids and they are exposed to high concentrations of oxygen. A discussion of vitamin E's role as an antioxidant follows, with a brief description of the generation of carbon-centered and peroxyl radicals. More information on how free radicals are generated and how they can damage cell membranes may be found in this chapter's Perspective.

Antioxidant Role

As an antioxidant, vitamin E can destroy singlet molecular oxygen and can stop reactions involving free radicals (sometimes called free radical termination or chainbreaking). This section addresses each of these aspects of vitamin E function.

Singlet Molecular Oxygen Destruction Singlet molecular oxygen, $^1O_2$, is a very reactive and destructive compound that may be formed in the body from lipid peroxidation of membranes, transfer of energy from light (photochemical reactions), or the respiratory burst occurring in neutrophils (enzymatic reactions). Singlet molecular oxygen readily reacts with organic molecules such as protein, lipids, and DNA and thus can damage cellular components unless removed. As discussed earlier in this chapter in the section on the antioxidant functions of carotenoids, quenching is a process by which electronically excited molecules, such as singlet molecular oxygen, are inactivated. Specifically, physical quenching occurs when the singlet excited oxygen is deactivated without light emission and generally involves electron energy transfer. Like carotenoids, vitamin E has oxygen-quenching abilities. The ability of vitamin E to physically quench singlet oxygen is related to the free hydroxyl group in position 6 of vitamin E's chromane ring (Figure 10.15). Yet, all tocopherols are not equal in their quenching abilities: α-tocopherol was found to be as or more effective in the quenching of singlet molecular oxygen than β-tocopherol, followed in descending order by γ-tocopherol and then δ-tocopherol [5]. Moreover, the $^1O_2$-quenching ability of the carotenoids lycopene and β-carotene is about two orders of magnitude greater than that of vitamin E; however, given the lower plasma concentrations of the carotenoids, vitamin E's role in quenching singlet oxygen is of greater physiological significance [5].

Free Radical Termination The structure of vitamin E, specifically the phenolic hydroxyl group, provides hydrogen ions to free radicals. Of the different forms of the vitamin, α-tocopherol is more effective than β-, γ-, or δ-tocopherol in its ability to donate hydrogen atoms. The hydrogen ions from α-tocopherol effectively and quickly react with and terminate a variety of free radicals before the free radicals can destroy cell membranes and other cell components.

Free radicals are generated in the course of many body processes involving enzymatic reactions or with exposure to ultraviolet light, among other events. Free radicals can start a series of reactions that can be terminated by vitamin E. The reactions occur in three phases: initiation, propagation (ongoing generation), and termination, with the last involving vitamin E. A description of the three phases, including the reactions occurring in each, is presented next.

Initiation typically begins with an initiator such as a free radical. For example, **hydroxyl radicals** ($^•OH$) are highly reactive, rapidly taking electrons from their surroundings. Often the electron taken by the reactive free hydroxyl radical is from a nearby organic molecule. If the organic molecule is a polyunsaturated fatty acid (PUFA) present in the phospholipid portion of the cell membrane, the membrane is damaged. Membrane lipid peroxidation is thought to represent a primary event in oxidative cellular damage. Specifically, hydrogen atoms from the methylene groups ($-CH_2-$) found between double bonds in polyunsaturated fatty acids ($-CH=CHCH_2CH=CH-$) are primary targets for proton abstraction by radicals. Examples of initiation reactions follow:

- The reaction between lipid compounds (LH) such as PUFA and free hydroxyl radicals ($^{\bullet}OH$) leads to the formation of a lipid carbon-centered or alkyl radical ($L^{\bullet}$) and water, as shown here and in Figure 10.16:

$$LH + {}^{\bullet}OH \longrightarrow L^{\bullet} + H_2O$$

- Alternately, lipid compounds (LH) can react with molecular oxygen (O_2) to generate lipid carbon-centered or alkyl radicals and the **hydroperoxyl radical** $HO_2^{\bullet}$, as follows:

$$LH + O_2 \longrightarrow L^{\bullet} + HO_2^{\bullet}$$

Once lipid carbon-centered or alkyl radicals are formed, they may react to form additional radicals in propagation reactions. Propagation is the second step in the process of lipid peroxidation.

- Lipid carbon-centered or alkyl radicals can react with molecular oxygen in a propagation reaction to form a lipid **peroxyl radical** $LOO^{\bullet}$ and promote peroxidation, as shown here and in Figure 10.16:

$$L^{\bullet} + O_2 \longrightarrow LOO^{\bullet} \text{ (Also written } LO_2^{\bullet})$$

Lipid peroxyl radicals ($LOO^{\bullet}$), once formed, can abstract a hydrogen atom from other organic compounds including more polyunsaturated fatty acids ($L'H$) in membranes or in lipoproteins to generate lipid hydroperoxides (LOOH) and a chain reaction with the $L^{\bullet}$, as shown here and in Figure 10.16:

$$LOO^{\bullet} + L'H \longrightarrow L'^{\bullet} + LOOH$$

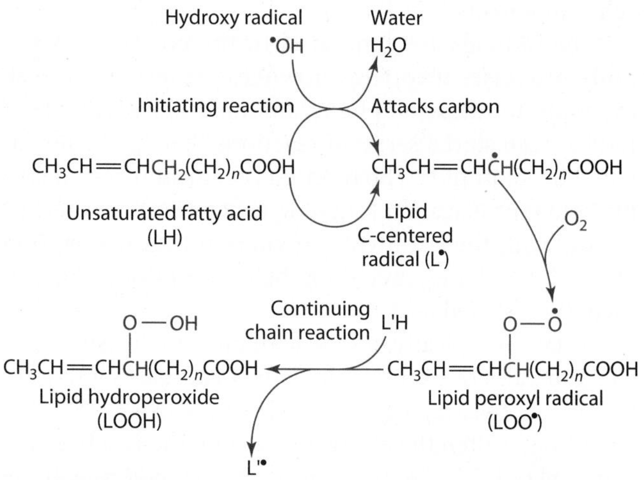

Termination of chain reactions (also referred to as free radical scavenging) is the final step. Without termination, one initiating event could result in the generation of thousands of lipid peroxides and massive cellular damage. Vitamin E located in or near membrane surfaces can react with peroxyl radicals ($LOO^{\bullet}$) before they interact with fatty acids in cell membranes or other cell components. Thus, vitamin E terminates chain-propagation reactions. Vitamin E is less effective, however, in terminating peroxidation that generates free hydroxyl radicals ($^{\bullet}OH$) or **alkoxyl radicals** ($RO^{\bullet}$). Specifically, vitamin E (EH, reduced state), because of the reactivity of the phenolic hydrogen on its carbon 6 hydroxyl group and the ability of the chromanol ring system to stabilize an unpaired electron, provides a hydrogen for the reduction of lipid peroxyl radicals, as shown here:

$$LOO^{\bullet} + EH \longrightarrow LOOH + E^{\bullet}$$

Vitamin E (EH) also provides a hydrogen for the reduction of lipid carbon-centered radicals:

$$L^{\bullet} + EH \longrightarrow LH + E^{\bullet}$$

In these reactions, vitamin E, after hydrogen donation, becomes oxidized. $E^{\bullet}$ represents oxidized vitamin E (also called an α-tocopherol radical or a tocopheroxyl radical). This tocopheroxyl radical can react with another peroxyl radical to form an inactive product such as tocopherylquinone. Alternately, the tocopheroxyl radical that is generated may be reduced; such a reaction is important since it enables the vitamin's reuse. Regeneration of the reduced form of vitamin E (Figure 10.17) requires reducing agents, such as vitamin C (ascorbic acid), reduced glutathione (GSH), NADPH, ubiquinol, or dihydrolipoic acid; see also the Perspective at the end of this chapter. Vitamin E is only one line of defense against oxidative tissue damage, and consequently alone or with other antioxidants may be protective against disease.

Vitamin E and Heart Disease Heart disease is thought to arise, in part, with the oxidation of LDLs, which contributes to plaque formation along with an accumulation of lipid-laden foam cells in the blood vessel walls (arterial intima). The accumulation of lipid-laden foam cells results from monocyte adhesion to endothelial cells lining blood vessels and migration of monocytes into the arterial intima (the innermost layer of blood vessels), where they become macrophages, take up oxidized cholesterol in LDL, develop into foam cells, and over time generate fatty streaks and plaque. The antioxidant properties of vitamin E enable it to inhibit the oxidation of LDLs; it may also help prevent blood clot formation [1]. Thus, it

Figure 10.16 Initiating and chain reactions caused by hydroxy free radical attack on unsaturated fatty acid.

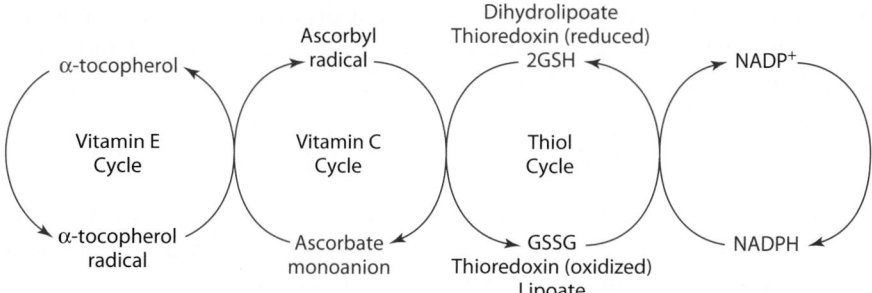

Figure 10.17 The regeneration of vitamin E (α-tocopherol).

is logical that diets rich in vitamin E or supplementation with vitamin E may be associated with a reduced risk of heart disease.

Unfortunately, unlike the results of some studies conducted in the 1990s, more recent randomized clinical trials and other types of studies have not shown beneficial effects of vitamin E supplementation (generally providing 400 IU, 600 IU, or 600 μg of vitamin E) on reducing risk for heart disease in healthy populations and in those with one or more risk factors for heart disease [6–15]. Only a few studies have reported slowed progression of atherosclerosis in those with heart disease, decreased cardiovascular disease mortality, or reduced risk of venous thromboembolism [15–17], while the results of other studies have documented either no beneficial effects or increased health risks in those consuming supplemental vitamin E [18–21]. For example, the Heart Outcomes Prevention Evaluation (HOPE) and HOPE-TOO studies found no difference in rates of death from heart attack, stroke, or heart-related conditions in over 10,000 men and women with heart disease, peripheral vascular disease, a previous stroke, or diabetes who took 400 IU of α-tocopherol for seven years, compared with rates in a placebo group [6,7]. However, in the HOPE-TOO trial, 5.8% of participants taking the vitamin E (400 IU) were hospitalized with heart failure, compared with 4.2% of participants taking the placebo [19]. In a meta-analysis of 19 randomized trials of vitamin E, which included about 136,000 people, a dose-response relationship between vitamin E and all-cause mortality was reported in those who took at least 400 IU of vitamin E per day for at least one year [20]. Postmenopausal women with heart disease ($n = 423$) randomized to receive 400 IU of vitamin E and 500 mg of vitamin C twice daily had significantly higher total mortality and cardiovascular mortality than those receiving a placebo [18]. Similarly, randomly assigned daily supplements of 500 mg of vitamin C, 400 IU of synthetic α-tocopherol, both, or a placebo to a group of over 14,000 male physicians ≥ 50 years of age did not affect the incidence of cardiovascular events [11]. However, the incidence of hemorrhagic stroke significantly increased in those receiving vitamin E [11]. Given the adverse health events documented in many of these recent studies, the risks versus the benefits of vitamin E supplementation

need to be considered carefully, and there is clearly insufficient evidence to support vitamin E supplementation in cardiovascular disease prevention and treatment.

Vitamin E and Cancer   Vitamin E's antioxidant abilities also form the basis for its use to reduce the risk of cancer. Free radical–induced damage is thought to trigger cancer through the activation of certain signaling pathways, alterations in gene expression, disruption of normal repair systems, alterations in enzyme activity, alterations in cell growth or differentiation, and/or direct production of toxic compounds, among other theories [22]. Unfortunately, the results of studies investigating the effects of high dietary vitamin E intakes and the use of vitamin E supplements have revealed no association with lower risk of cancers [8,15,19,23–29], and the findings from two studies suggest that the vitamin may increase mortality [30,31].

Vitamin E and Eye Health   Vitamin E has been suggested in the treatment and prevention of cataracts and age-related macular degeneration, major causes of blindness, especially in older people. Descriptions of these two disorders are provided in the "Eye Health" section in the discussion of vitamin C in Chapter 9. Poor antioxidant status or intake, especially of vitamins E and C, has been shown in many but not all studies to be associated with development of cataracts and age-related macular degeneration. Because radical-induced damage is thought to contribute to the development of these ocular conditions, and because vitamin E functions as an antioxidant, it is logical that vitamin E, like vitamin C and β-carotene, may help in their prevention or treatment. Unfortunately, although several epidemiological and prospective cohort studies suggest a protective effect of vitamin E primarily related to cataract development or progression [32–37], other studies have failed to show such effects [38–40]. Further, because multivitamin preparations are often used in these studies, any observed effects cannot be attributed solely to one vitamin. Thus, at present, evidence in favor of recommending vitamin E in the prevention or treatment of eye disease, especially cataracts, must be considered insufficient [41,42].

Vitamin E and Other Diseases/Conditions   Vitamin E supplementation has also been suggested to diminish oxidation in those individuals with conditions characterized by increased lipid peroxidation such as iron toxicity and diabetes. Vitamin E may also improve plasma membrane structure to enhance cellular glucose uptake (which is important for those with diabetes). In neurodegenerative diseases such as Alzheimer's disease, protein aggregates typically accumulate and are coupled with the loss of specific neuronal cell populations. Because oxidative stress is thought to be linked (at least in part) with the development of some neurodegenerative conditions, provision of antioxidants such as vitamin E is thought to be beneficial. As with other conditions, while a few studies have shown diminished cognitive decline in the elderly and in individuals with Alzheimer's disease with vitamin E supplementation, other studies have failed to support its use [43–45]. Thus, there is no substantial evidence that Alzheimer's disease, other neurodegenerative diseases such as Parkinson's disease, and other forms of dementia can be successfully or partially prevented with vitamin E (or other antioxidant) supplementation [46,47]. Lastly, the effectiveness of topical vitamin E use to prevent scar formation appears to be questionable and requires further study.

Cell Signaling, Gene Expression, and Other Roles

Vitamin E also functions as a cell signaling molecule. In this capacity it interacts with cell receptors and transcription factors, thereby affecting signaling cascades as well as gene expression, enzyme activity, and protein concentrations. One of the most investigated roles is vitamin E's inhibition of protein kinase C, a serine/tyrosine kinase that functions in the transduction of signals from G protein–coupled tyrosine kinase receptors and nonreceptor tyrosine kinases to the nucleus by hydrolysis of phospholipids [48]. Genes transcriptionally regulated by vitamin E are involved in steroidogenesis (including cholesterol synthesis), lipid uptake, antioxidant defense, the cell cycle, inflammation, cell adhesion, and blood coagulation, among other activities, as reviewed by Rimbach and others [49]. Vitamin E also impacts specific micro (mi)RNAs, a group of noncoding RNAs that bind to untranslated regions on mRNA to inhibit translation of the mRNA into protein. One miRNA is suggested to be able to interact with 100 different target mRNAs and thus inhibit multiple genes and silence entire pathways [49,50].

While α-tocopherol is one of the more well-studied of vitamin E's vitamers, research into the functions of tocotrienols is fast emerging. Tocotrienols suppress the activity of the rate-limiting enzyme 3-hydroxy-3-methyl-glutaryl (HMG)-CoA reductase in cholesterol synthesis and have been shown to reduce plasma cholesterol concentrations. Roles of tocotrienols, especially γ-tocotrienol, in cell signaling (involving estrogen and insulin receptors) as well as in anti-inflammatory, antiproliferative, and anti-apoptotic activities have been documented. Such involvement suggests that the tocotrienols may function in neuroprotective, hypocholesterolemic, and anticancer roles in the body [51–53].

Interactions with Other Nutrients

Because the antioxidant functions of vitamin E in the body are closely tied to those of selenium-dependent glutathione peroxidase (an enzyme that converts lipid peroxides into lipid alcohols), an interrelationship exists between vitamin E and selenium. The actions of both nutrients are complementary, and higher concentrations of one nutrient can reduce the effects of lower concentrations of the other nutrient. Similarly, some of vitamin C's functions also complement vitamin E, and vitamin C can regenerate vitamin E following its oxidation.

A relationship between vitamin E and dietary polyunsaturated fatty acids has been suggested because the requirement for the vitamin increases or decreases as the degree of unsaturation of fatty acids in body tissues rises or falls; body tissue lipids, in turn, are influenced by dietary lipid intake [1]. However, foods high in polyunsaturated fatty acids also tend to be relatively good sources of vitamin E.

High intake of vitamin E can interfere with other fat-soluble vitamins. For example, vitamin E inhibits β-carotene absorption and its metabolism in the intestine [54,55]. Vitamin E also impairs vitamin K absorption and its metabolism, including the conversion of phylloquinone (K$_1$) to menoquinone [56]. The effects of vitamin E may increase the risk for bleeding secondary to interference in vitamin K's role in blood clotting.

Metabolism and Excretion

Hepatic metabolism of vitamin E begins with an ω-hydroxylation reaction, requiring cytochrome P-450, to form hydroxychromanol. Next, a series of reactions analogous to β-oxidation of fatty acids follows to effectively truncate vitamin E's phytyl side chain. The end products include a group of carboxyethyl hydroxychromans (abbreviated CEHC). Prior to urinary or fecal excretion, these carboxyethyl hydroxychromans are usually conjugated to glucuronic acid or sulfate. Urinary excretory products of the vitamin also include α-tocopheronic acid and α-tocopheronolactone conjugated to either glucuronic acid or sulfate.

Recommended Dietary Allowance

The RDA for vitamin E for adult men and women (including during pregnancy for women) is 15 mg (22.4 IU) of RRR α-tocopherol [1]. During lactation, recommendations are slightly higher, with an RDA of 19 mg (28.4 IU) of α-tocopherol for women [1]. The RDA for vitamin E for adults is based upon the vitamin E requirement plus twice the coefficient of variation, rounded to the nearest mg [1]. People who smoke may have higher requirements for vitamin E, but specific recommendations for this population have not been made [57].

Recommendations for vitamin E are based upon intake of the natural form (RRR) of α-tocopherol and the synthetic all-rac 2R-stereoisomeric forms (RSR, RRS, and RSS) of α-tocopherol used in fortified foods and vitamin supplements [1]. The equivalent of 1,500 IU of RRR α-tocopherol is 1,000 mg of α-tocopherol. To estimate mg of all-rac (synthetic) 2R α-tocopherol in a supplement, multiply the dose by 0.45 mg/IU, and to estimate mg of RRR (natural) α-tocopherol in a supplement, multiply the dose by 0.67 mg/IU [58]. Conversions from IU to mg are: 1 IU = 0.67 mg α-tocopherol if the vitamin E is from natural sources, whereas 1 IU = 0.45 mg α-tocopherol if a synthetic form of vitamin E is used. Conversely, to convert from mg to IU: 1 mg α-tocopherol = 1.49 IU from natural sources and = 2.22 IU from synthetic sources.

Deficiency

A deficiency of vitamin E in humans is rare. Only a few population groups are at risk for deficiency, including premature infants (who typically exhibit impaired fat utilization secondary to prematurity) and individuals with fat malabsorption disorders such as cystic fibrosis (characterized by pancreatic lipase deficiency) and hepatobiliary system disorders, particularly chronic cholestasis (characterized by decreased bile production). Individuals with genetic defects in either lipoproteins or the α-tocopherol transfer protein are also at risk. For example, individuals with abetalipoproteinemia may develop a vitamin E deficiency because of a lack of microsomal transfer protein needed to assemble or secrete lipoproteins containing apolipoprotein B, while those with an αTTP defect cannot appropriately release α-tocopherol into the blood for distribution to tissues. Treatment of both disorders necessitates the ingestion of large (gram) doses of the vitamin.

Some symptoms of vitamin E deficiency are skeletal muscle pain (myopathy) and weakness, ceroid pigment accumulation, hemolytic anemia, and degenerative neurological problems, including peripheral neuropathy, ataxia, loss of vibratory sense, and loss of coordination of limbs. Plasma α-tocopherol concentrations less than 5 μg/mL are suggestive of deficiency.

Toxicity

Vitamin E appears to be one of the least toxic of the vitamins, although mild gastrointestinal problems may occur with intakes between 200 and 800 mg. However, it is because of an increased tendency for bleeding (due to antiplatelet effects and/or abnormal blood clotting) that a

Tolerable Upper Intake Level of 1,000 mg of α-tocopherol (1,500 IU of natural RRR α-tocopherol or 1100 IU of synthetic all-rac tocopherol)/day for adults has been established by the Food and Nutrition Board [1]. This recommendation for an upper level of intake includes any form of supplemental α-tocopherol [1]. In addition to increased bleeding, higher intakes of the vitamin (1,000 mg or greater) also have been associated with gastrointestinal distress, including nausea, diarrhea, and flatulence; impaired blood coagulation; possible increased severity of respiratory infections; and occasional reports of muscle weakness, fatigue, and double vision. Increased mortality risk also has been shown in some randomized trials providing vitamin E [20,21].

Assessment of Nutriture

Evaluation of vitamin E status relies primarily on blood analyses. Plasma concentrations are responsive to dietary intake under deficiency and toxicity situations. Normal plasma vitamin E concentrations range from about 5 to 20 μg/mL in adults. Plasma concentrations < 5 μg/mL indicate deficiency and reflect dietary intake, while concentrations exceeding about 20 μg/mL reflect toxicity.

A crude estimate of vitamin E status also can be obtained from an erythrocyte hemolysis test that compares the amount of hemoglobin released by red blood cells during incubation with dilute hydrogen peroxide with the amount released during distilled water incubation. The result is expressed as a percentage, with > 20% indicating deficiency and generally associated with plasma α-tocopherol concentrations below 5 μg/mL; however, variables other than vitamin E status influence *in vitro* hemolysis.

References Cited for Vitamin E

1. Food and Nutrition Board, Institute of Medicine. Dietary Reference Intakes. Washington, DC: National Academy Press. 2000 pp. 186–283.
2. Reboul E, Trompier D, Moussa M, et al. ATP-binding cassette transporter A1 is significantly involved in the intestinal absorption of α- and γ-tocopherol but not in that of retinyl palmitate in mice. Am J Clin Nutr. 2009; 89:177–84.
3. Singh U, Devaraj S, Jialal I. Vitamin E, oxidative stress, and inflammation. Ann Rev Nutr. 2005; 25:151–74.
4. Traber MG. Vitamin E regulatory mechanisms. Ann Rev Nutr. 2007; 27:347–62.
5. Kaiser S, Mascio P, Murphy M, Sies H. Physical and chemical scavenging of singlet molecular oxygen by tocopherols. Arch Biochem Biophys. 1990; 277:101–08.
6. HOPE Study Investigators. Vitamin E supplementation and cardiovascular events in high risk patients. N Engl J Med. 2000; 342:154–60.
7. Yusuf S, Dagenais G, Pogue J, et al. Vitamin E supplementation and cardiovascular events in high risk patients: the Heart Outcomes Prevention Study Investigators. N Engl J Med. 2000; 342:154–60.
8. Heart Protection Study Collaborative Group. MRC/BHF heart protection study of antioxidant vitamin supplementation in 20536 high risk individuals: a randomized placebo-controlled trial. Lancet. 2002; 360:23–33.

9. Primary Prevention Project Group. Low-dose aspirin and vitamin E in people at cardiovascular risk: a randomized trial in general practice. Lancet. 2001; 357:89–95.

10. Knekt P, Ritz J, Pereira MA, et al. Antioxidant vitamins and coronary heart disease risk: a pooled analysis of 9 cohorts. Am J Clin Nutr. 2004; 80:1508.

11. Sesso HD, Buring JE, Christen WG, et al. Vitamins E and C in the prevention of cardiovascular disease in men: the Physicians' Health Study II randomized controlled trial. JAMA. 2008; 300:2123–33.

12. Cook NR, Albert CM, Gaziano JM, et al. A randomized factorial trial of vitamins C and E and beta carotene in the secondary prevention of cardiovascular events in women. Arch Intern Med. 2007; 167:1610–18.

13. Jialal I, Devaraj S. Vitamin E supplementation and cardiovascular events in high-risk patients. N Engl J Med. 2000; 342:154–60.

14. Kataja-Tuomola MK, Kontto JP, Mannisto S, et al. Effect of alpha-tocopherol and beta-carotene supplementation on macrovascular complications and total mortality from diabetes: results of the ATBC study. Ann Med. 2010; 42:178–86.

15. Lee I, Cook NR, Gaziano JM, et al. Vitamin E in the primary prevention of cardiovascular disease and cancer: the Women's Health Study: a randomized controlled trial. JAMA. 2005; 294:56–65.

16. Glynn RJ, Ridker PM, Goldhaber SZ, et al. Effects of random allocation to vitamin E supplementation on the occurrence of venous thromboembolism: report from the Women's Health Study. Circulation. 2007; 116:1497–1503.

17. Salonen RM, Nyyssonen K, Kaikkonen J, et al. Six-year effect of combined vitamin C and E supplementation on atherosclerotic progression: the Antioxidant Supplementation in Atherosclerosis Prevention (ASAP) Study. Circulation. 2003; 107:947–53.

18. Waters DD, Alderman EL, Hsia J, et al. Effects of hormone replacement therapy and antioxidant vitamin supplements on coronary atherosclerosis in postmenopausal women: a randomized controlled trial. JAMA. 2002; 288:2432–40.

19. Lonn E, Bosch J, Yusuf S, et al. Effects of long-term vitamin E supplementation on cardiovascular events and cancer: randomized controlled trial. JAMA. 2005; 293:1338–47.

20. Miller E, Pastor-Barriuso R, Dalal D, et al. Meta-analysis: high dosage vitamin E supplementation may increase all-cause mortality. Ann Intern Med. 2005; 142:37–46.

21. Bjelakovic G, Nikolova D, Gluud LL, et al. Mortality in randomized trials of antioxidant supplements for primary and secondary prevention: systematic review and meta-analysis. JAMA. 2007; 297:842–57.

22. Seifried HE, Anderson DE, Fisher EI, Milner JA. A review of the interaction among dietary antioxidants and reactive oxygen species. J Nutr Biochem. 2007; 18:567–79.

23. Bardia A, Tleyjeh IM, Cerhan JR, et al. Efficacy of antioxidant supplementation in reducing primary cancer incidence and mortality: systematic review and meta-analysis. Mayo Clin Proc. 2008; 83:23–34.

24. Bjelakovic G, Nagorni A, Nikolova D, et al. Meta-analysis: antioxidant supplements for primary and secondary prevention of colorectal adenoma. Aliment Pharmacol Ther. 2006; 24:281–91.

25. Bjelakovic G, Nikolova D, Simonetti RG, Gluud C. Systematic review: primary and secondary prevention of gastrointestinal cancers with antioxidant supplements. Aliment Pharmacol Ther. 2008; 28:689–703.

26. Lippman SM, Klein EA, Goodman PJ, et al. Effect of selenium and vitamin E on risk of prostate cancer and other cancers: the selenium and vitamin E cancer prevention trial (SELECT). JAMA. 2009; 301:39–51.

27. Wu K, Willett WC, Chan JM, et al. A prospective study on supplemental vitamin E intake and risk of colon cancer in women and men. Cancer Epidemiol Biomarkers Prev. 2002; 11:1298–1304.

28. Lin J, Cook NR, Albert C, et al. Vitamins C and E and beta carotene supplementation and cancer risk: a randomized controlled trial. J Natl Cancer Inst. 2009; 101:14–23.

29. Coulter ID, Hardy ML, Morton SC, et al. Antioxidants vitamin C and vitamin E for the prevention and treatment of cancer. J Gen Intern Med. 2006; 21:735–44.

30. Bjelakovic G, Nikolova D, Simonetti RG, Gluud C. Antioxidant supplements for prevention of gastrointestinal cancers: a systematic review and meta-analysis. Lancet. 2004; 364:1219–28.

31. Klein EA, Thompson IM, Tangen CM, et al. Vitamin E and the risk of prostate cancer. The Selenium and Vitamin E Cancer Prevention Trial (SELECT). JAMA 2011; 306:1549–56.

32. Jacques PF, Taylor A, Moeller S, et al. Long-term nutrient intake and 5-year change in nuclear lens opacities. Arch Ophthalmol. 2005; 123:517–26.

33. Mares-Perlman JA, Lyle BJ, Klein R, et al. Vitamin supplement use and incident cataracts in a population-based study. Arch Ophthal. 2000; 118:1556–63.

34. Tan AG, Mitchell P, Flood VM, et al. Antioxidant nutrient intake and the long-term incidence of age-related cataract: the Blue Mountains Eye Study. Am J Clin Nutr. 2008; 87:1899–1905.

35. Chylack LT, Brown NP, Bron A, et al. The Roche European American Cataract Trial (REACT): a randomized clinical trial to investigate the efficacy of an oral antioxidant micronutrient mixture to slow progression of age-related cataract. Ophthalmic Epid. 2002; 9:49–80.

36. Fletcher AE, Bentham GC, Agnew M, et al. Sunlight exposure, antioxidants and age-related macular degeneration. Arch Ophthalmol. 2008; 126:1396–1403.

37. Age-related Eye Disease Study Research Group. A randomized placebo-controlled clinical trial of high dose supplementation with vitamins C and E, β carotene, and zinc for age-related macular degeneration and vision loss. Arch Ophthalmol. 2001; 119:1417–36.

38. Christen WG, Glynn RJ, Sesso HD, et al. Age-related cataract in a randomized trial of vitamins E and C in men. Arch Ophthalmol. 2010; 128:1397–1405.

39. Gritz DC, Srinivasan M, Smith SD, et al. The antioxidants in prevention of cataracts study: effects of antioxidant supplements on cataract progression in South India. Br J Ophthalmol. 2006; 90:847–51.

40. Ferrigno L, Aldigeri R, Rosmini F, et al. Associations between plasma levels of vitamins and cataract in the Italian-American clinical trial of nutritional supplements and age-related cataract (CTNS): CTNS report #2. Ophthalmic Epid. 2005; 12:71–80.

41. Chong E, Wong TY, Kreis AJ, et al. Dietary antioxidants and primary prevention of age related macular degeneration: systematic review and meta-analysis. BMJ. 2007; 335:755–62.

42. Chiu C, Taylor A. Nutritional antioxidants and age-related cataract and maculopathy. Exp Eye Res. 2007; 84:229–45.

43. Morris MC, Evand DA, Bienias JL, et al. Vitamin E and cognitive decline in older persons. Arch Neurol. 2002; 59:1125–32.

44. Zandi PP, Anthony JC, Khachaturian AS, et al. Reduced risk of Alzheimer disease in users of vitamin antioxidant supplements: the Cache County Study. Arch Neurol. 2004; 61:82–88.

45. Usoro OB, Mousa SA. Vitamin E forms in Alzheimer's disease: a review of controversial and clinical experiences. Crit Rev Food Sci Nutr. 2010; 50:414–19.

46. Galli F, Azzi A. Present trends in vitamin E research. Biofactors. 2010; 36:33–34.

47. Isaac MG, Quinn R, Tabet N. Vitamin E for Alzheimer's disease and mild cognitive impairment. Cochrane Database Sys Rev. 2008; CD002854.

48. Engin KN. Alpha-tocopherol: looking beyond an antioxidant. Molec Vision. 2009; 15:855–60.

49. Rimbach G, Moehring J, Huebbe P, Lodge JK. Gene-regulatory activity of α-tocopherol. Molecules. 2010; 15:1746–61.

50. Lewis BP, Burge CB, Bartel DP. Conserved seed pairing, often flanked by adenosines, indicates that thousands of human genes are microRNA targets. Cells. 2005; 120:15–20.

51. Sen CK, Khanna S, Rink C, Roy S. Tocotrienols: the emerging face of natural vitamin E. Vit Hormones. 2007; 76:203–61.

52. Colombo ML. An update on vitamin E, tocopherol and tocotrienol: perspectives. Molecules. 2010; 15:2103–13.

53. Devaraj S, Jialal I. Failure of vitamin E in clinical trials: is γ tocopherol the answer? Nutr Rev. 2005; 63:290–93.

54. Food and Nutrition Board, Institute of Medicine. Dietary Reference Intakes. Washington, DC: National Academy Press. 2001 pp. 82–161.
55. Traber MG. The ABCs of vitamin E and β-carotene absorption. Am J Clin Nutr. 2004; 80:3–4.
56. Traber MG. Vitamin E and K interactions: a 50-year-old problem. Nutr Rev. 2008; 66:624–29.
57. Bruno RS, Traber MG. Cigarette smoke alters human vitamin E requirements. J Nutr. 2005; 135:671–74.
58. Traber MG. How much vitamin E?. . . just enough. Am J Clin Nutr. 2006; 84:959–60.

VITAMIN K

Vitamin K was named after the Danish word *koagulation*, which means "coagulation." In the 1920s, H. Dam discovered that chicks fed a low-fat and cholesterol-free diet became hemorrhagic (i.e., they bled excessively) and that their blood took a long time to clot. The missing vitamin called K that corrected the problem was identified in the early 1940s. Dam (along with Doisy) was recognized with a Nobel prize in medicine in 1941 for the discovery.

Compounds with vitamin K activity have a 2-methyl 1, 4-naphthoquinone ring with a substitution at position 3. The naturally occurring forms of vitamin K are phylloquinone (vitamin K_1), which has a phytyl group at position 3 of the ring (2-methyl 3-phytyl 1,4-naphthoquinone), and menaquinone (vitamin K_2), which has an unsaturated multiprenyl group at position 3. Based upon the number of isoprenoid groups, menaquinones (abbreviated MK) are designated with a number (*n*; such as MK-*n*) to indicate the number of isoprenoid units in the side chain. Some menaquinones, such as MK-4, can be synthesized in the body from phylloquinone. Additionally, menadione (2-methyl 1,4-naphthoquinone), a synthetic form of vitamin K sometimes used in animal feeds, can be alkylated by tissue enzymes to generate MK-4, also called menatetrenone. Figure 10.18 depicts menadione, phylloquinone, and menaquinone-7 (MK-7).

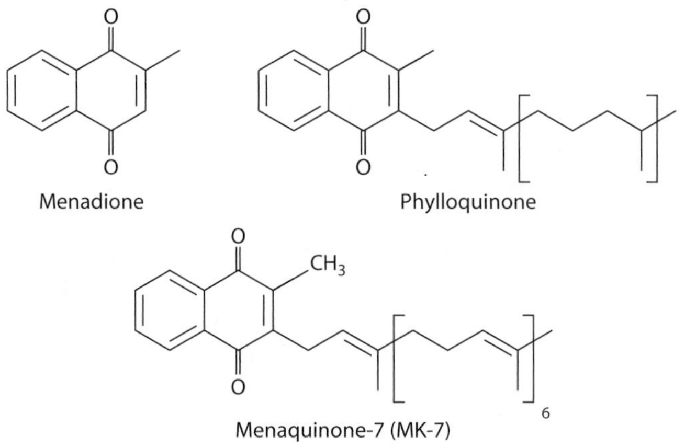

Figure 10.18 Biologically active forms of vitamin K.

Sources

Dietary vitamin K is provided mostly as phylloquinone from ingestion of plant foods. The richest vegetable sources and the main dietary sources of vitamin K include leafy green vegetables, especially collards, spinach, turnip greens, some salad greens, and broccoli. Oils and margarine from plants represent the second major source of the vitamin [1]. Rapeseed and soybean oils are particularly rich (142–200 μg phylloquinone/100 g), while olive oil contains 55 μg of phylloquinone/100 μg of oil. Sunflower, safflower, walnut, and sesame oils provide only 6 to 15 μg of phylloquinone/100 g, and peanut and corn oils contain <3 μg/100 g [2]. Smaller amounts of phylloquinone are found in cereals, fruits, dairy products, and meats. Table 10.2 provides information about selected vitamin K–rich foods. The average adult is thought to consume up to several hundred micrograms of phylloquinone per day [1,3]. Vitamin K's Daily Value, used to express the nutrient's content on food and supplement labels, is 80 μg; however, the vitamin K content of foods is seldom listed on food labels. Exposure of the vitamin to light and heat can result in significant vitamin K destruction.

Menaquinones are synthesized by a variety of facultative and obligate anaerobic bacteria that reside in the body's intestines, although small amounts of menaquinones also may be found in a few foods such as liver, fermented cheeses, and soybean products. Examples of menaquinone-producing obligate anaerobes include *Bacteroides*, *Bacillus fragilis*, *Eubacterium*, *Propionibacterium*, and *Arachnia*; the facultative anaerobe *Escherichia coli* also produces menaquinone [4]. Bacterial synthesis of vitamin K is not sufficient to meet the needs of children or adults [1].

Supplements of vitamin K as phylloquinone (such as Mephyton and Konakion) are available. Water-soluble

Table 10.2 Vitamin K Content of Selected Foods

Phylloquinone (μg/100 g)			
<10	10–50	>100	>200
Milk	Asparagus	Cabbage	Broccoli
Butter	Celery	Lettuce	Kale
Eggs	Green beans	Brussels sprouts	Swiss chard
Cheese	Avocado	Mustard greens	Turnips
Meats	Kiwi		Watercress greens
Fish	Pumpkin (canned)		Collards
Corn	Peas		Spinach
Cauliflower	Peanut butter		Salad greens
Grains	Lentils		
Fruits (most)	Kidney beans		
Tea (brewed)	Pinto beans		
	Soybeans		
	Coffee (brewed)		

Source: Adapted from Booth et al., Vitamin K1 content of foods. Journal of Food Composition and Analysis 1993; 6: 109–20. Reprinted by permission.

forms of the vitamin (such as AquaMephyton, Synkayvite, and Kappadione) are also manufactured for people with fat malabsorptive disorders.

Absorption

Phylloquinone, which requires no digestion, is absorbed from the small intestine, particularly from the jejunum, as part of micelles. Thus, its absorption is enhanced by the presence of dietary fats, bile salts, and pancreatic juice. Some phylloquinone also may be absorbed by active transport from the proximal small intestine (i.e., the duodenum and jejunum).

Menaquinones that are synthesized by some bacteria in the lower digestive tract are absorbed by passive diffusion from the ileum and colon; however, the ability to absorb and use the bacterially produced vitamin varies considerably from human to human and has been difficult to determine accurately [1].

Transport, Metabolism, and Storage

Within the enterocytes, phylloquinone is incorporated into chylomicrons that enter the lymphatic and then the circulatory system for transport to tissues. Chylomicron remnants deliver any vitamin K not taken up by other tissues to the liver. Both phylloquinone and menaquinone can be metabolized by the liver and/or can be incorporated into very-low-density lipoproteins (VLDLs) for secretion back into the blood and transport to extrahepatic tissues. Normal plasma phylloquinone concentrations range from about 0.15 to 1.15 ng/mL (0.3–2.5 nmol/L).

Vitamin K is stored primarily in cell membranes in several tissues, including the lungs, kidneys, bone marrow, and adrenal glands. The liver rapidly metabolizes the vitamin but retains little in storage. Hepatic concentrations of phylloquinone range from about 2 to 20 ng per g of liver, and are about 10 times lower than those of the menaquinones [5]. MK-4 is also found in a variety of tissues, including the pancreas, salivary glands, brain, and bone. Various tissues are able to convert phylloquinone to MK-4; however, the quantity of MK-4 synthesized by the tissues has not been established. The body's pool of vitamin K, estimated at 50 to 100 mg, is low for a fat-soluble vitamin and smaller than that of vitamin B_{12} [6]. Turnover of the body's vitamin K pool is fairly rapid, at about 1.5 days [6].

Functions and Mechanisms of Action

Vitamin K is necessary for the posttranslational carboxylation of specific glutamic acid (glutamyl) residues in proteins to form γ-carboxyglutamic acid (GLA) residues. These interactions are necessary for blood clotting (hemostasis) and bone mineralization, among other processes including apoptosis, growth, and signal transduction. The role of vitamin K in blood clotting and vitamin K's roles in bone and nonosseous tissues are reviewed next.

Vitamin K and Blood Clotting

The vitamin K–dependent posttranslational carboxylation of glutamic acid residues forms γ-carboxyglutamic acid on several major proteins required for the coagulation of blood. The four most well-studied vitamin K–dependent blood-clotting proteins, called *factors,* are factors II (prothrombin), VII, IX, and X. In addition, proteins C, S, Z, and M, also involved in blood clotting, require vitamin K for carboxylation.

Overview of Blood Clotting For blood to clot, fibrinogen, a soluble protein, must be converted to fibrin, an insoluble fiber network. Two pathways, intrinsic and extrinsic, lead to clot formation, as shown in Figure 10.19 and briefly described here.

In the intrinsic pathway, the coagulation process is initiated by the adsorption of factor XII, which circulates in the blood, onto a substance such as collagen, which becomes exposed with tissue injury. Upon contact, factor XII becomes *activated*, as indicated by the letter *a* next to the factor. Through a series of reactions in the intrinsic pathway and via the extrinsic pathway (which is activated by the release of thromboplastin by injured tissue), vitamin K–dependent factor X becomes activated by factors IXa and VIIa, respectively. It is factor Xa that in turn activates another vitamin K–dependent factor, factor II (prothrombin), to produce IIa (thrombin). Thrombin catalyzes the proteolysis of fibrinogen to yield fibrin. Fibrin molecules aggregate to form a mesh-like polymer, which then undergoes cross-linking by fibrin stabilizing factor to form an insoluble fibrin clot and stop bleeding (hemorrhage).

Other blood clotting proteins, designated C, S, Z, and M, also have been identified as vitamin K–dependent carboxylated proteins. The function of protein M is unknown, but the other three proteins inhibit the blood-clotting process and thus exhibit anticoagulant functions. Protein Z inhibits factor Xa. Protein C inactivates factors VIIIa and Va and, along with protein S, enhances fibrinolysis to disrupt the clotting process. Protein S has been also found in bone, suggesting other functions in the body.

The Role of Vitamin K in Carboxylation of Glutamic Acid Residues This section uses prothrombin as a model to describe the carboxylation process; however, remember that in addition to prothrombin (factor II), blood-clotting factors VII, IX, and X; proteins C, S, M, and Z; and proteins presented in the section discussing bone and nonosseous roles of vitamin K depend upon vitamin K for carboxylation.

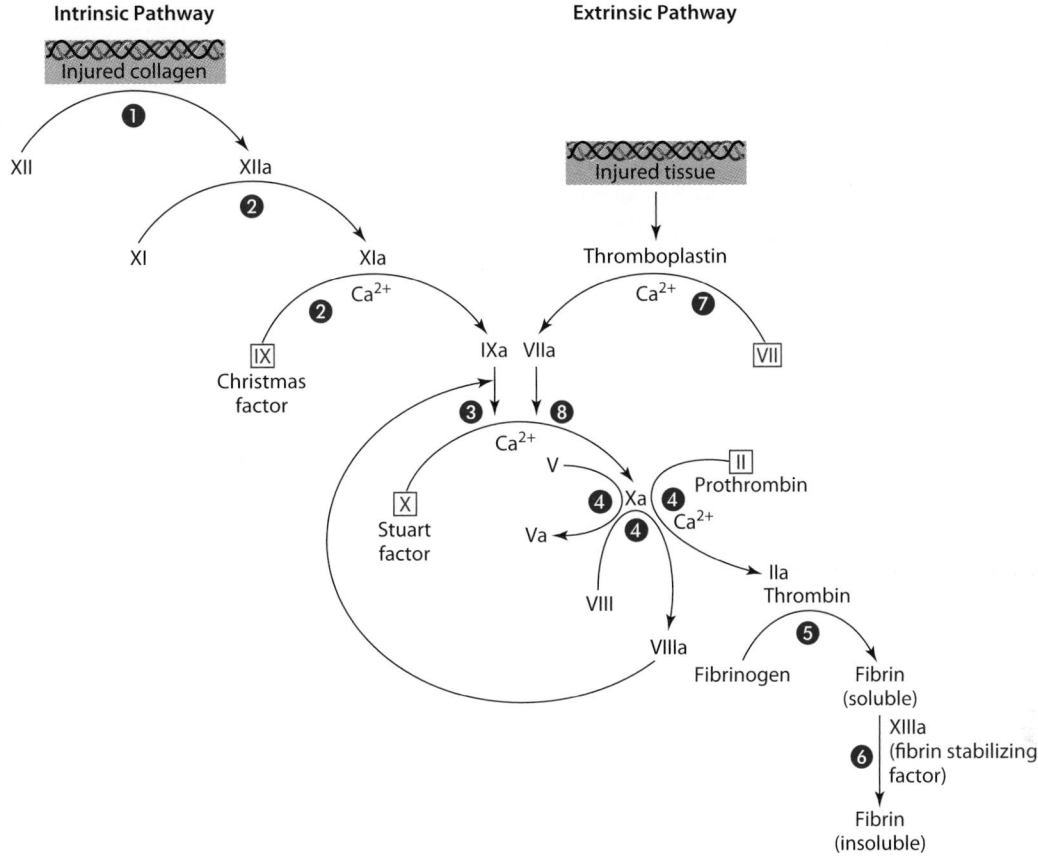

Intrinsic Pathway

Extrinsic Pathway

❶ Initial step: Factor XII adsorbs onto a substance such as collagen, which becomes exposed with injury to a tissue. Upon contact, factor XII becomes activated (denoted by an "a").

❷ Factor XIa, which becomes activated by XIIa, activates factor IX, a vitamin K–dependent protein.

❸ Factor IXa activates factor X, another vitamin K–dependent protein.

❹ Factor Xa converts factor II, prothrombin (vitamin K–dependent) into thrombin.

❺ Thrombin alters fibrinogen to produce fibrin for clot formation.

❻ Factor XIIIa, fibrin stabilizing factor, creates insoluble fibrin for final clot formation.

❼ In the extrinsic pathway, factor VII, a vitamin K–dependent protein, becomes activated in the presence of thromboplastin released by injured tissue.

❽ Factor VIIa works with factor IXa to activate factor X.

Figure 10.19 An overview of blood clotting. Vitamin K–dependent proteins are boxed.

Proteins like prothrombin require a vitamin K–dependent enzyme for the carboxylation of 10 to 13 glutamic acid residues residing in the N-terminal. Once carboxylated, this glutamic acid portion forms γ-carboxyglutamic acid (Gla), as shown in Figure 10.20. The carboxylation is required for the protein to become functional. The enzyme responsible for the γ-carboxylation, called vitamin K–dependent γ-glutamyl carboxylase, is associated with the rough endoplasmic reticulum (where vitamin K–dependent proteins are carboxylated), primarily in the liver. The liver is also where the hemostatic factors are synthesized. The enzyme, however, is found in all human tissues. This widespread occurrence of γ-glutamyl carboxylase suggests that the need for carboxylated proteins that can bind calcium is broad.

Gla residues are synthesized posttranslationally. All glutamic acid residues must be carboxylated for the protein to function. Gla residues on the blood clotting proteins function to bind calcium. The calcium then mediates the binding of Gla proteins to negatively charged phospholipids on membrane surfaces of blood platelets and endothelial cells at the site of injury. This adsorption is essential in hemostasis.

The participation of vitamin K in the carboxylation of proteins is a cyclic process, often called the vitamin K cycle. The γ-glutamyl carboxylase enzyme requires vitamin K in its reduced form, referred to as dihydrovitamin KH_2, dihydroxy, or hydroquinone vitamin K. However, vitamin K is generally present in the body in its oxidized quinone form because of the presence of oxygen in the blood.

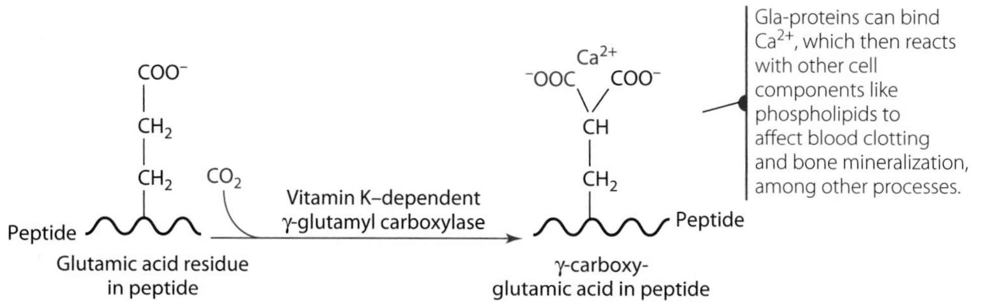

Figure 10.20 Production of γ-carboxylglutamic acid (Gla) via vitamin K–dependent carboxylation.

The steps of the vitamin K cycle, in which vitamin K is converted to its reduced form and functions in the carboxylation process, are shown in Figure 10.21 and briefly reviewed here.

- Reduction of vitamin K quinone to dihydroquinone KH_2 is accomplished by quinone reductases that require either dithiol (RSH-HSR) or NAD(P)H. The dithiol-dependent quinone reductase appears to be the main physiological pathway for generating dihydroquinone KH_2 from the quinone. (See steps 1 and 2 of Figure 10.21.)

- Once dihydroquinone KH_2 is present, along with oxygen and carbon dioxide as the carboxyl precursor, γ-glutamyl carboxylase can carboxylate (add a CO_2 onto) the glutamic acid residues of specific proteins. The carboxylation enables the protein to interact with calcium. (See steps 3 and 4 of Figure 10.21.)

- The carboxylation of glutamic acid is believed to be coupled with the formation of vitamin K 2,3-epoxide (Figure 10.21, step 5). No energy is required for the carboxylation reaction; the reaction is probably accomplished by the free energy produced through the oxidation of dihydroquinone KH_2 to vitamin K 2,3-epoxide, whereby vitamin K provides reducing equivalents [7].

- To complete the cycle (step 6 of Figure 10.21), vitamin K 2,3-epoxide is converted back to vitamin K quinone by an epoxide reductase.

Anticoagulants Coumadin (warfarin) is an anticoagulant that may be prescribed to people at risk for a thrombotic event (e.g., a heart attack). Anticoagulants such as warfarin antagonize the synthesis of vitamin K by interfering with the activity of epoxide reductase (step 6 of Figure 10.21). Ingestion of diets high in vitamin K, as obtained from about a pound of broccoli daily, override the effects of warfarin [8]. Thus, people who are taking anticoagulant medications are instructed to maintain a consistent intake of vitamin K, but also to avoid consumption of large quantities of foods rich (about 700–1,500 μg or more of phylloquinone) in vitamin K at a single meal.

Vitamin K and Bone

Two vitamin K–dependent proteins have been identified in bone, cartilage, and dentine: osteocalcin (also sometimes called bone Gla protein) and matrix Gla protein (MGP). The synthesis of both osteocalcin and MGP appears to be stimulated by calcitriol and by retinoic acid. Osteocalcin is secreted by osteoblasts during bone extracellular matrix (protein) formation, around the onset of hydroxyapatite and mineral deposition. Osteocalcin comprises about 10% to 20% of noncollageneous protein in bone. With vitamin K–dependent carboxylation, the three Gla residues on osteocalcin facilitate the binding of calcium ions to the hydroxyapatite lattice in the extracellular matrix of bone. Although its physiological role remains unclear, osteocalcin appears to be involved in bone remodeling, and it is γ-carboxylation of osteocalcin that is thought to represent the primary mechanism underlying the hypothesized protective influence of vitamin K on bone [9]. Because small amounts of the protein are released into circulation, plasma osteocalcin is often used as an index of bone formation.

MGP is found in bone, dentine, and cartilage and is also associated with bone's extracellular (protein) matrix, where it may promote calcification of bone. A lack of MGP is associated with extensive arterial calcification, suggesting a protective role against soft tissue calcification. However, as with osteocalcin, the exact physiological role of MGP is uncertain. Given that mRNA for MGP has been found in a variety of tissues, including the brain, heart, kidneys, liver, lungs, and spleen, broader roles for the protein are likely.

Vitamin K and Bone Health Associations between serum vitamin K and bone mineral density or fracture risk are numerous in the scientific literature; however, evidence showing a protective influence of dietary intake of vitamin K (ranging from about 45 mg of MK-4 to 500 to 1000 μg of phylloquinone/day) on bone health remains equivocal [9–14]. Some of the reasons for the conflicting results are likely related to differences in the study populations (age and gender), the studied bone site(s), vitamin K forms

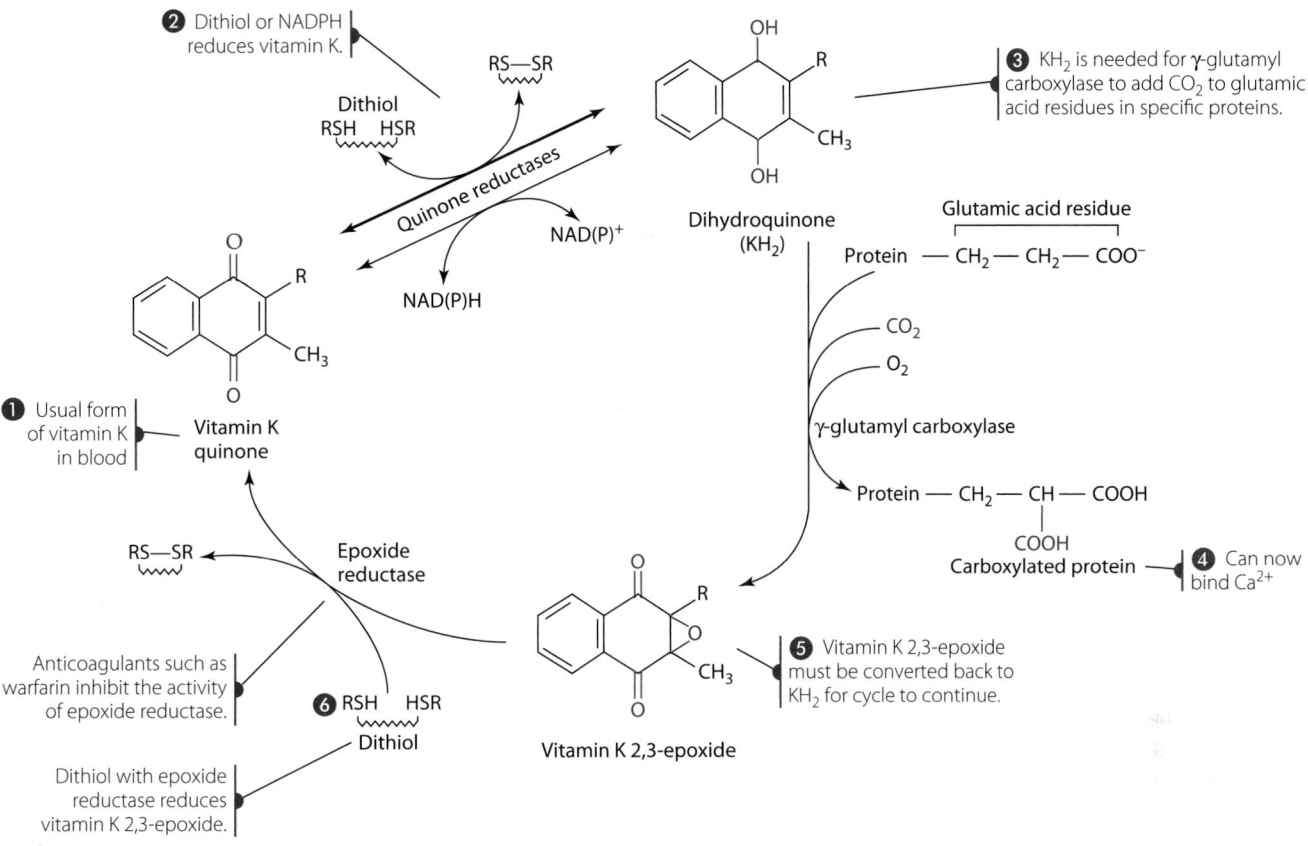

2 Dithiol or NADPH reduces vitamin K.

3 KH₂ is needed for γ-glutamyl carboxylase to add CO₂ to glutamic acid residues in specific proteins.

Dithiol
RSH   HSR

RS—SR

Quinone reductases

NAD(P)⁺

NAD(P)H

Dihydroquinone (KH₂)

Glutamic acid residue

Protein — CH_2 — CH_2 — COO^-

CO_2

O_2

γ-glutamyl carboxylase

Protein — CH_2 — CH — COOH
                        |
                      COOH

Carboxylated protein

4 Can now bind Ca^{2+}

1 Usual form of vitamin K in blood

Vitamin K quinone

RS—SR

Epoxide reductase

Anticoagulants such as warfarin inhibit the activity of epoxide reductase.

6 RSH   HSR
Dithiol

Vitamin K 2,3-epoxide

5 Vitamin K 2,3-epoxide must be converted back to KH₂ for cycle to continue.

Dithiol with epoxide reductase reduces vitamin K 2,3-epoxide.

Figure 10.21 The vitamin K cycle.

and dosages provided, other provided nutrients, and study time frames, among others. Given the high prevalence of osteoporosis, additional studies are clearly warranted.

Vitamin K and Nonosseous Tissue Proteins

In nonosseous tissues, other vitamin K–dependent proteins have been identified, including growth arrest specific gene (Gas) 6 (in smooth muscle, endothelial cells, and natural killer cells), atherocalcin (in atherosclerotic blood vessels), periostin (in the heart and tissues undergoing remodeling), transforming growth factor β-inducible protein (in multiple tissues), transmembrane Gla proteins (in multiple extrahepatic tissues), and renal Gla protein (in the cortex of the kidneys) [15,16]. The functions of these proteins, which are γ-carboxylated primarily in extrahepatic tissues, have not been clearly defined, but their presence indicates that vitamin K performs several different roles in the body.

Interactions with Other Nutrients

Vitamins A and E are known to antagonize vitamin K; excesses of both interfere with vitamin K absorption. Vitamin E's antagonistic effects also include possible interference with vitamin K metabolism. Specifically, vitamin E is thought to inhibit metabolism of MK-4 to phylloquinone and to increase hepatic oxidation and excretion of all forms of vitamin K [17].

Metabolism and Excretion

Phylloquinone is almost completely metabolized to a variety of metabolites (many uncharacterized) before being excreted. The metabolism usually involves step-wise oxidation of the phytyl side chain at position 3 with subsequent conjugation. Most of phylloquinone's metabolites are conjugated with glucuronic acid for excretion primarily in the feces by way of the bile; however, some metabolites are also excreted in the urine.

Relatively little is known about the metabolism and excretion of menaquinone. Metabolism of menadione (the synthetic form of the vitamin) generates menadiol, which then reacts with phosphate, sulfate, or glucuronide. Menadiol phosphate and menadiol sulfate are excreted in both the feces and urine, while menadiol glucuronides are excreted mostly in the feces.

Adequate Intake

Lack of data has hampered the Food and Nutrition Board in its efforts to estimate requirements for vitamin K [1]. Adequate Intake (AI) recommendations of 120 and 90 μg per day for adult males and females (including those who are pregnant or lactating), respectively are recommended. Bacterial-generated menaquinones are generally not sufficiently produced or used to maintain adequate vitamin K status [1]. Metabolic studies suggest that the current vitamin K recommendations, which are based upon the vitamin's need for coagulation function, may be inadequate to maximize carboxylation of proteins needed for bone health [10,18].

Deficiency

A deficiency of vitamin K is unlikely in healthy adults. The population groups that appear to be most at risk for a vitamin K deficiency are newborn infants, people being treated chronically with antibiotics, people with severe gastrointestinal malabsorptive disorders, and the elderly. Newborns are particularly at risk because their food is limited to milk, which is low in vitamin K; their stores of the vitamin are low because inadequate amounts cross the placenta; and their intestinal tract is not yet populated by vitamin K–synthesizing bacteria. Supplementation with vitamin K is considered advisable for all newborns; currently, intramuscular injection of 0.5 to 1 mg of phylloquinone shortly after birth is recommended for all infants [1].

People consuming vitamin K–poor diets and on prolonged sulfonamides and broad-spectrum antibiotic drug therapy are at risk for vitamin K deficiency owing to the coupled effects of low dietary intake and antibiotic-induced destruction of gastrointestinal bacteria that manufacture the vitamin and contribute a source of vitamin K. Individuals with fat malabsorptive disorders such as cystic fibrosis, obstructive jaundice, Crohn's disease, intestinal bypass surgery, chronic pancreatitis, and liver disease are also at risk of deficiency. Because vitamin K is fat soluble, it is absorbed best with dietary fat. Consequently, people who malabsorb fat will also malabsorb fat-soluble vitamins. Lastly, while the elderly tend to consume inadequate amounts of the vitamin, other researchers suggest the problem is more widespread in the United States, where vitamin K intakes are often less than 80 μg daily [1].

Subclinical vitamin K deficiency has been induced in healthy adults fed a diet providing about 10 μg of phylloquinone per day [19]. The 13-day low–vitamin K diet resulted in a significant reduction in plasma vitamin K concentrations. Urinary γ-carboxyglutamic acid excretion significantly decreased in younger subjects but remained unchanged in older adults. Prothrombin time did not change; however, undercarboxylated prothrombin concentrations increased significantly in subjects [19].

Severe vitamin K deficiency is associated with bleeding episodes (hemorrhage). The undercarboxylated blood-clotting factors cannot effectively bind calcium and interact with cell membrane phospholipids exposed on tissue injury, an interaction necessary for thrombin generation and clot formation.

Subclinical vitamin K deficiency may be associated with diminished bone mineral density and increased fracture rates, although the results of studies are not consistent (as previously discussed in the "Vitamin K and Bone Health" section). Additionally, vitamin K deficiency has been linked to cardiovascular disease or arterial calcification, and inflammation, among other conditions, as reviewed by McCann and Ames [15].

Toxicity

Ingestion of large amounts of phylloquinone and menaquinone has not been shown to cause toxicity, and no Tolerable Upper Intake Level for vitamin K has been established [1]. The synthetic form menadione, however, is toxic if consumed in large amounts, causing hemolytic anemia and liver damage (indicated by hyperbilirubinemia and severe jaundice). Menadione is thought to combine with sulfhydryl groups such as those in glutathione, resulting in glutathione oxidation and ultimately membrane damage induced by phospholipid oxidation.

Assessment of Nutriture

Multiple biomarkers are generally used to assess vitamin K status since no single index or biomarker clearly indicates deficiency and adequacy. Plasma or serum concentrations of phylloquinone reflect recent (within about 24 hours) intake of the vitamin; concentrations less than about 0.5 μg/L are associated with deficiency. Whole blood clotting times and prothrombin (or other blood-clotting proteins) time are often used to identify potential deficiency of vitamin K. Prothrombin time, which measures the time required for a fibrin clot to form following the addition of calcium and other substances to citrated plasma, is normally between about 11 and 14 seconds; times greater than 25 seconds are associated with major bleeding and may indicate possible vitamin K deficiency. This test, however, is relatively insensitive because plasma prothrombin concentrations must usually decrease considerably (sometimes 50% or more) before any effects on prothrombin time are observed.

Another fairly sensitive means of assessing vitamin K status is to measure the percentage of under-carboxylated vitamin K–dependent proteins, such as prothrombin or osteocalcin, or the ratio of under- to fully carboxylated proteins. Vitamin K deficiency results in the secretion of under- or partially carboxylated proteins into the blood from either the liver (as with prothrombin) or the bone (as with osteocalcin). However, one protein (such as prothrombin) may be 100% carboxylated while another protein (such as osteocalcin) is only 10% to 40% carboxylated; the physiological significance of these differences is not clear at present [15].

References Cited for Vitamin K

1. Food and Nutrition Board, Institute of Medicine. Dietary Reference Intakes. Washington, DC: National Academy Press. 2001 pp. 162–96.

2. Booth S, Sadowski J, Weihrauch J, Ferland G. Vitamin K1 (phylloquinone) content of foods: a provisional table. J Food Comp Anal. 1993; 6:109–20.

3. Booth S, Golly I, Sacheck J, et al. Effect of vitamin E supplementation on vitamin K status in adults with normal coagulation status. Am J Clin Nutr. 2004; 80:143–48.

4. Suttie J. The importance of menaquinones in human nutrition. Ann Rev Nutr. 1995; 15:399–417.

5. Geleijnse J, Vermeer C, Grobbee D, et al. Dietary intake of menaquinone is associated with a reduced risk of coronary artery disease: The Rotterdam Study. J Nutr. 2004; 134:3100–05.

6. Olson RE, Chao J, Graham D, et al. Total body phylloquinone and its turnover in human subjects at two levels of vitamin K intake. Br J Nutr. 2002; 87:543–53.

7. Berkner KL. The vitamin K-dependent carboxylase. Ann Rev Nutr. 2005; 25:127–49.

8. Kempin S. Warfarin resistance caused by broccoli. N Eng J Med. 1983; 308:1229–30.

9. Shea MK, Booth SL. Uptake on the role of vitamin K in skeletal health. Nutr Rev. 2008; 66:549–57.

10. Cashman KD, O'Connor E. Does high vitamin K_1 intake protect against bone loss in later life? Nutr Rev. 2008; 66:532–38.

11. Bolton-Smith C, McMurdo ME, Paterson CR, et al. Two-year randomized clinical trial of vitamin K_1 (phylloquinone) and vitamin D_3 plus calcium on the bone health of older women. J Bone Mineral Res. 2007; 22:509–19.

12. Booth SL, Dallal G, Shea MK, et al. Effect of vitamin K supplementation on bone loss in elderly men and women. J Clin Endocrinol Metab. 2008; 93:1217–23.

13. Braam LA, Knapen MH, Geusens P, et al. Vitamin K_1 supplementation retards bone loss in postmenopausal women between 50 and 60 years of age. Calcif Tissue Int. 2003; 73:21–26.

14. Rejnmark L, Vestergaard P, Charles P. No effect of vitamin K_1 intake on bone mineral density and fracture risk in perimenopausal women. Osteoporosis Int. 2006; 17:1122–32.

15. McCann JC, Ames BN. Vitamin K, an example of triage theory: is micronutrient inadequacy linked to diseases of aging? Am J Clin Nutr. 2009; 90:889–907.

16. Bellido-Martin L, deFrutos PG. Vitamin K-dependent actions of Gas6. Vitam Horm. 2008; 78:185–209.

17. Traber MG. Vitamin E and K interactions: a 50-year-old problem. Nutr Rev. 2008; 66:624–29.

18. Adams J, Pepping J. Vitamin K and bone health. Am J Heath-Syst Pharm. 2005; 62:1574–81.

19. Ferland G, Sadowski J, O'Brien M. Dietary induced subclinical vitamin K deficiency in normal human subjects. J Clin Invest. 1993; 91:1761–68.

THE ANTIOXIDANT NUTRIENTS, REACTIVE SPECIES, AND DISEASE

Although different sections in several chapters of this book have discussed nutrients with antioxidant functions, nowhere within those chapters is this information brought together to provide a more comprehensive review of how these individual nutrients function together to protect the body from destructive radicals and nonradical species. That is the purpose of this Perspective, which first reviews free radical chemistry; next addresses how selected free radicals and nonradicals are generated in the body, and the damage caused by these species; and finally explains how the antioxidant nutrients function together to eliminate destructive radical and nonradical species.

FREE RADICAL CHEMISTRY

Back in probably one of your first chemistry courses, you learned about atoms. It is here that a brief review of free radical chemistry begins. Atoms contain protons and neutrons, which are found in the nucleus. You may remember that the atomic weight of an element is a function of its number of protons and neutrons, whereas the atomic number represents solely the number of protons. Atoms also have electrons, which revolve in orbitals (also called shells) around the nucleus. An atomic orbital holds a maximum of two electrons, which are generally found in pairs in the orbitals. The term *free radical* represents an atom or molecule that has one or more unpaired electrons. The unpaired electron is found alone in the outer orbital and is usually denoted by a superscript dot, but it may be indicated by a dash or combination. Thus, a superoxide radical can be denoted with a superscript dot ($O_2^{\bullet}$), a superscript dash (O_2^{-}), or both ($O_2^{-\bullet}$). The imbalance in electrons in the orbitals results in most cases in the high reactivity of the free radicals. Free radicals that contain oxygen are called reactive oxygen species (ROS), and free radicals containing nitrogen are called reactive nitrogen species (RNS). The term *reactive* is most appropriately used when comparing different radicals because reactivity with other compounds is relative. The terms *reactive oxygen species* and *reactive nitrogen species*, however, include not only free radicals but also nonradicals, as shown in Table 1.

Table 1 does not include all free radical or reactive species. Oxygen itself is a biradical because it has two unpaired electrons, residing in separate orbitals, that cannot form a pair. An example of a reactive sulfur species radical is thiyl ($RS^{\bullet}$), generated from amino acids and thiols. Trichloromethyl ($CCl_3^{\bullet}$), formed during metabolism of carbon tetrachloride (CCl_4) by cytochrome P-450 enzymes in the liver, is

a chloride-based carbon-centered radical, meaning that the unpaired electron resides on the carbon atom.

GENERATION OF REACTIVE SPECIES

A variety of reactive species are generated daily from multiple sites in the body. In general, the reactive oxygen species are formed on exposure to substances such as smog, ozone, chemicals, drugs, radiation, and high levels of oxygen, among others, and during normal physiological processes, especially in the defense against microbes and other foreign substances. Generally, reactions occurring as part of oxidative phosphorylation in the mitochondria and as part of immune defense in neutrophils, macrophages, monocytes, and eosinophils produce reactive oxygen species. Additionally, the peroxisomes and cytochrome P-450 enzymes generate damaging radicals and nonradicals. Radicals also breed more radicals, as seen in several of the reactions shown in this Perspective. Production of superoxide radicals; hydrogen peroxide; hydroxyl, peroxyl, hydroperoxyl, and carbon-centered (alkyl) radicals; lipid peroxides; and singlet molecular oxygen is reviewed in this section and shown in Figure 1. A few reactive nitrogen species (nitric oxide, **peroxynitrite, nitrogen dioxide**, and **peroxynitrate**) also are discussed.

The Superoxide Radical

The superoxide radical (designated hereafter as $O_2^{\bullet}$) is an oxygen-centered radical; that is, the unpaired electron resides on the oxygen. Remember that molecular oxygen has two unpaired electrons in different orbitals. The addition of an electron to molecular oxygen leaves only one unpaired electron.

$$O_2 \xrightarrow{\ e^- \ } O_2^{\bullet}$$

Superoxide radicals can be made when oxygen molecules (O_2) react with different compounds, such as with the catecholamines epinephrine and dopamine or with the coenzyme form of the vitamin folate, as tetrahydrofolate. The electron transport chain also produces superoxide radicals as a result of autoxidation reactions and the leaking of electrons from the electron transport chain onto oxygen—that is, a one-electron reduction of oxygen to generate the superoxide radical. This leaking of electrons onto oxygen occurs during the passage of electrons from CoQH$^{\bullet}$ (coenzyme Q) as part of the electron transport chain. In the electron transport chain, electrons ultimately are transferred to oxygen (O_2) for ATP production; however, upon interaction between CoQH$^{\bullet}$ and O_2, shown here, the superoxide radical is formed:

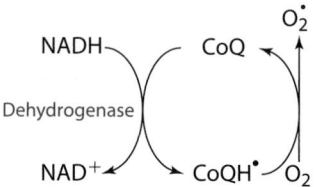

Cytochrome P-450 enzymes also generate superoxide radicals. These heme enzymes found in the endoplasmic reticulum membrane consist of a cytochrome P-450 reductase that transfers electrons from NADPH, and a second cytochrome P-450 that binds molecular oxygen and the substrate being hydroxylated. A variety of substrates, including fatty acids, steroids, and therapeutic drugs, are hydroxylated by this system. The reactions catalyzed by some of the cytochrome P-450 enzymes convert nonpolar compounds to polar compounds. This change in polarity enables elimination (fecal or urinary) of the compound from the body.

Superoxide radicals also are produced in the body in substantial quantities in activated white blood cells, such as macrophages, monocytes, and neutrophils conducting phagocytosis, to assist in destroying foreign substances such

Table 1 Some Reactive Oxygen and Nitrogen Species

Reactive Oxygen Species		Reactive Nitrogen Species	
Oxygen-Containing Radicals	**Oxygen-Containing Nonradicals**	**Nitrogen-Containing Radicals**	**Nitrogen-Containing Nonradicals**
Superoxide $O_2^{\bullet}$	Ozone O_3	Nitric oxide $^{\bullet}NO$	Nitrous acid HNO_2
Hydroxyl $^{\bullet}OH$	Singlet oxygen $^1O_2$	Nitrogen dioxide $^{\bullet}NO_2$	Peroxynitrite $ONOO^{\bullet}$
Hydroperoxyl $HO_2^{\bullet}$	Hypochlorous acid HOCL		Alkyl peroxynitrite LOONO$^{\bullet}$
Alkoxyl $LO^{\bullet}$ or $RO^{\bullet}$	Hydrogen peroxide H_2O_2		
Peroxyl O_2^{2-} or $LO_2^{\bullet}$ or $RO_2^{\bullet}$			

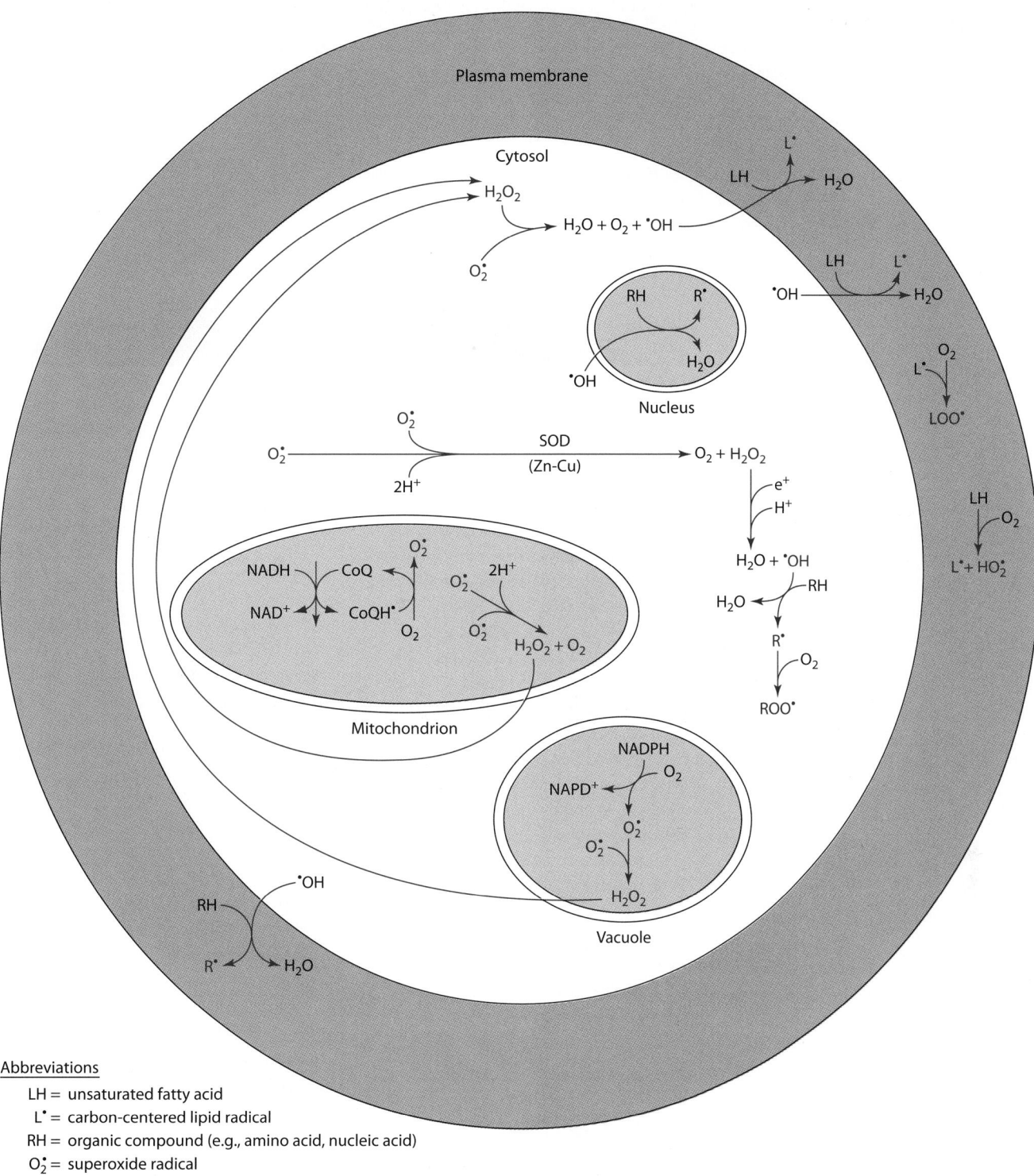

Abbreviations

LH = unsaturated fatty acid
L• = carbon-centered lipid radical
RH = organic compound (e.g., amino acid, nucleic acid)
$O_2^{•}$ = superoxide radical
•OH = hydroxy radical
R• = carbon-centered nonlipid radical
H_2O_2 = hydrogen peroxide
ROO• = nonlipid peroxy radical
LOO• = peroxy radical
$HO_2^{•}$ = hydroperoxyl radical

Figure 1 Generation of reactive species.

as bacteria and viruses. The superoxide radicals in these cells are needed for the subsequent production of other toxic reactive oxygen species, such as hydrogen peroxide (H_2O_2), to further help destroy foreign bacteria and other organisms. In addition, superoxide radicals generated by neutrophils heighten the inflammatory response by acting as chemoattractants for other neutrophils. Production of superoxide radicals in activated white blood cells is thought to begin with the action of NADPH oxidase while a foreign substance is being engulfed by a white blood cell. Specifically, the NADPH oxidase reduces oxygen and produces multiple superoxide radicals. This reaction is shown here:

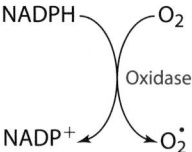

The radicals in turn help kill the bacteria and other foreign substances. The extensive oxygen-requiring process by which white blood cells destroy organisms is sometimes called the *respiratory* or *oxidative burst*.

Although superoxide radicals help to destroy bacteria, viruses, fungi, and the like, in white blood cells, these same radicals, which may reach concentrations of up to 10^{-11} M in cells, can do harm. They are a potent initiator of chain reactions and can lead to the production of other reactive oxygen species, such as hydrogen peroxide and hydroperoxyl radicals ($HO_2^{\bullet}$). The superoxide radical also can react with nitric oxide ($^{\bullet}NO$) to generate several reactive nitrogen species, including peroxynitrite ($ONOO^{\bullet}$). Fortunately, superoxides are not lipid soluble and thus do not diffuse too far away from their site of production.

Hydrogen Peroxide

Hydrogen peroxide (H_2O_2) is not a radical, because it has no unpaired electrons, but it is considered a reactive oxygen species and easily diffuses throughout cells, causing damage. Hydrogen peroxide is generated through the action of several enzymes. A major hydrogen peroxide producer (found extracellularly and intracellularly, in both the cell cytosol and mitochondria) is superoxide dismutase (SOD). Extracellular and cytosolic SOD require both zinc and copper, whereas mitochondrial SOD is manganese dependent. The reaction catalyzed by this enzyme, which removes superoxide radicals, is shown here:

$$O_2^{\bullet} + O_2^{\bullet} + 2H^+$$
$$\downarrow \text{Superoxide dismutase}$$
$$H_2O_2 + O_2$$

Vitamin C (AH_2), like SOD, also can generate hydrogen peroxide while trying to eliminate superoxide radicals. The vitamin, normally present in the body in its reduced ascorbate (also called ascorbate (mono)anion),(AH^-), form, reacts with the radical and generates an ascorbyl radical ($A^{\bullet}$) and hydrogen peroxide as shown:

$$AH^- + O_2^{\bullet} + H^+ \longrightarrow A^{\bullet} + H_2O_2$$

Hydrogen peroxide also is produced in large quantities during the oxidation of compounds in peroxisomes. Peroxisomes are cytoplasmic organelles responsible for the degradation of molecules such as very long-chain (20+ carbons) fatty acids, among others.

Additionally, reactive oxygen species such as hydrogen peroxide are generated with injury or damage, especially if it involves ischemia (inadequate blood flow and, thus, oxygen supply). Possible reasons for the free radical and nonradical production observed in ischemia include (1) neutrophil activation by compounds released by the damaged tissues, (2) disruption of the electron transport chain, and (3) secondary production associated with the generation of xanthine oxidase, especially if the ischemia affects the intestine or endothelial cells of blood vessels. In some tissues during ischemia, xanthine dehydrogenase gets converted into xanthine oxidase by oxidation of sulfhydryl groups, proteolysis, or both. Xanthine oxidase, a molybdenum-, iron-, and riboflavin-dependent enzyme, catalyzes hypoxanthine and xanthine degradation but, unlike xanthine dehydrogenase, it generates hydrogen peroxide. In hypoxic tissue, ADP is degraded (because of lack of oxygen for ATP generation), producing hypoxanthine. During the medical treatment of ischemia, oxygen is administered to the patient. Although this oxygen helps to prevent organ damage, the large quantities of oxygen given with reperfusion provide xanthine oxidase with the oxygen needed to oxidize hypoxanthine and xanthine but also produce large amounts of H_2O_2, which can further damage the already injured tissue.

Other cellular oxidases such as amine oxidase (which is copper dependent) also generate hydrogen peroxide. The reaction catalyzed by amine oxidase, found in the blood and body tissues, is as follows:

$$RCH_2NH_2 \xrightarrow{O_2 \quad H_2O_2} RCH + {}^+NH_4$$

Concentrations of hydrogen peroxide, like superoxide radicals, need to be controlled in the body cells to prevent cellular destruction. Hydrogen peroxide easily diffuses in water and in lipids, within cells and to tissues, to cause damage. It also can react with superoxide radicals to produce a highly reactive and destructive hydroxyl radical.

The Hydroxyl Radical

The hydroxyl radical ($^{\bullet}OH$) is an oxygen-centered radical. It can be produced when the body is exposed to γ rays, low-wavelength electromagnetic radiation. These rays split water in the body to form the hydroxyl radical:

$$H_2O \longrightarrow H^+ + {}^{\bullet}OH$$

Hydroxyl radicals also are produced from a reaction between hydrogen peroxide and a superoxide radical (known as the Haber-Weiss reaction), as shown here,

$$H_2O_2 + O_2^{\bullet} \longrightarrow O_2 + OH^- + {}^{\bullet}OH$$

or from other electrons and protons, as shown here:

$$H_2O_2 \xrightarrow{e^- \quad H^+} H_2O + {}^{\bullet}OH$$

Hydrogen peroxide in contact with free ferrous iron can result in the formation of hydroxyl radicals. However, iron normally is bound to proteins and is not found free in cells. If the iron is freed from the protein, for example, from interaction with a superoxide radical, reduced iron could be generated (protein-bound $Fe^{3+} + O_2^{\bullet} \longrightarrow$ free $Fe^{3+} + O_2^{\bullet} \longrightarrow O_2 + Fe^{2+}$); such events could then trigger what is referred to as the Fenton reaction:

$$H_2O_2 \xrightarrow{Fe^{2+} \quad Fe^{3+}} OH^- + {}^{\bullet}OH$$

In this reaction, the hydrogen peroxide is functioning as an iron-oxidizing agent, and a hydroxyl radical is produced. The iron in the reaction can be substituted with copper, as both are able to react with hydrogen peroxide, but copper, like iron, is bound to proteins *in vivo*.

The hydroxyl radical, thought to be one of the most potent or reactive radicals, rapidly attacks (by taking electrons) virtually all molecules in the body. In fact, the hydroxyl radical is thought to be a major initiator of lipid peroxidation. It also reacts with nucleic acids in DNA, forming 8-hydroxyguanosine (a compound used to estimate DNA damage). Hydroxyl radicals fragment proteins, primarily at proline and histidine residues, triggering damage and premature degradation of the protein. Thus, removing free hydroxyl radicals is important to prevent destruction of cell components.

Peroxyl and Hydroperoxyl Radicals, Carbon-Centered Radicals, and Lipid Peroxides

Peroxyl (O_2^{2-}) and hydroperoxyl ($HO_2^{\bullet}$) radicals (oxygen-centered) can be formed in the body from superoxide radicals reacting with an additional electron and hydrogen, as shown here:

$$O_2^{\bullet} \xrightarrow{e^-} O_2^{2-} \xrightarrow{H^+} HO_2^{\bullet}$$
Superoxide radical   Peroxyl radical   Hydroperoxyl radical

The peroxyl radical, as well as the hydroxyl and alkoxyl ($RO^{\bullet}$ or $LO^{\bullet}$) radicals, is more reactive than the superoxide radical.

Lipid carbon-centered radicals ($L^{\bullet}$) are produced in the body when radicals such as hydroxyl radicals ($^{\bullet}OH$) attack polyunsaturated fatty acids (LH) in the phospholipids of membranes or attack other organic compounds. The initiation reaction in the attack of a polyunsaturated fatty acid may be written as follows:

$$LH + {}^{\bullet}OH \longrightarrow L^{\bullet} + H_2O \text{ (initiation)}$$

Alternately, the reaction may be viewed showing part of the polyunsaturated fatty acid, as shown here:

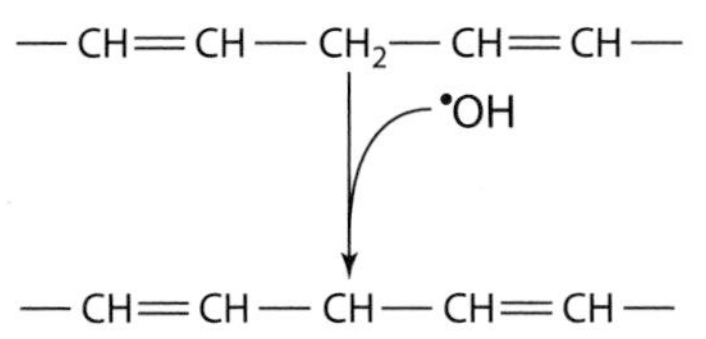

$$
\begin{array}{c}
-CH=CH-CH_2-CH=CH- \\
\downarrow \quad {}^{\bullet}OH \\
-CH=CH-CH-CH=CH-
\end{array}
$$

Propagation follows the initiation step, with products formed in one reaction being used as reactants in another reaction. Oxygen, for example, can react with the lipid carbon-centered radical to generate a lipid peroxyl (LOO$^{\bullet}$) radical as follows:

$$L^{\bullet} + O_2 \longrightarrow LOO^{\bullet}$$

or alternately, this reaction may be expressed as follows:

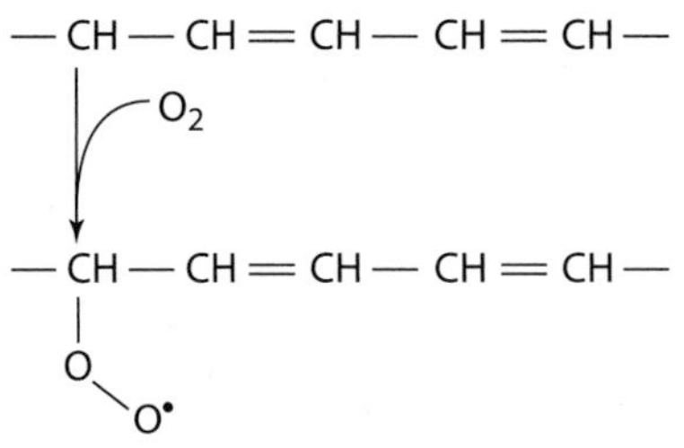

$$
\begin{array}{c}
-CH-CH=CH-CH=CH- \\
\downarrow \quad O_2 \\
-CH-CH=CH-CH=CH- \\
\quad | \\
\quad O \\
\quad \quad O^{\bullet}
\end{array}
$$

Oxygen also can react with polyunsaturated fatty acids to form carbon-centered radicals and hydroperoxyl radicals:

$$LH + O_2 \longrightarrow L^{\bullet} + HO_2^{\bullet}$$

In additional propagation reactions, lipid peroxyl radicals (LOO$^{\bullet}$) may attack (abstract a hydrogen atom or proton from) other polyunsaturated fatty acids (L'H) in cell membranes to generate lipid peroxides (LOOH) and another carbon-centered radical.

$$LOO^{\bullet} + L'H \longrightarrow LOOH + L'^{\bullet}$$

This reaction also may be depicted as follows:

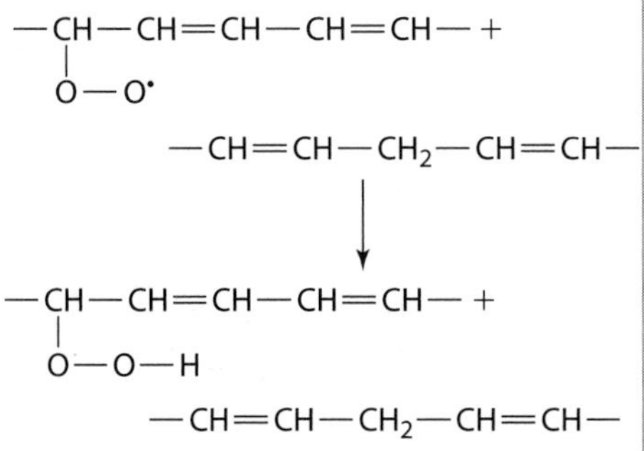

$$
\begin{array}{c}
-CH-CH=CH-CH=CH- \;+ \\
\quad | \\
\quad O-O^{\bullet} \\
\quad \quad -CH=CH-CH_2-CH=CH- \\
\downarrow \\
-CH-CH=CH-CH=CH- \;+ \\
\quad | \\
\quad O-O-H \\
\quad \quad -CH=CH-CH_2-CH=CH-
\end{array}
$$

Should lipid peroxides (LOOH), also known as peroxidized fatty acids, come in contact with free iron, alkoxyl (LO$^{\bullet}$) and

peroxyl (LOO$^{\bullet}$) radicals also can be generated, as shown in these two reactions:

$$LOOH + Fe^{2+} \longrightarrow LO^{\bullet} + OH^- + Fe^{3+}$$
$$LOOH + Fe^{3+} \longrightarrow LOO^{\bullet} + H^+ + Fe^{2+}$$

Like peroxyl radicals, the alkoxyl radical can in turn initiate chain reactions with other polyunsaturated fatty acids in membranes, as follows:

$$LO^{\bullet} + L'H \longrightarrow LOH + L'^{\bullet}$$

However, again it is important to note that *in vivo*, little or no free iron appears to be available to initiate such reactions.

Singlet Molecular Oxygen

Singlet molecular oxygen, also called singlet oxygen ($^1O_2$), possesses higher energy and is more reactive than ground-state oxygen. Specifically, in singlet oxygen, the peripheral electron in the oxygen structure is excited to an orbital above the one it normally occupies. This excited form of oxygen can be generated from lipid peroxidation of membranes by enzymatic reactions, such as occur between hydrogen peroxide and hypochlorous acid in the respiratory burst in white blood cells (i.e., $H_2O_2 + HOCl \longrightarrow {}^1O_2 + H_2O + HCl$), or through photochemical reactions, as shown here:

$$O_2 \xrightarrow{h\nu} {}^1O_2$$

Singlet oxygen, being a reactive oxygen species, can, like free radicals, damage cells and tissues unless it is removed from the body.

Nitric Oxide

Nitric oxide ($^{\bullet}NO$), a widely studied and known vasorelaxant, functions in cells through the activation of guanylate cyclase, increasing cyclic GMP concentrations and thus mediating a cascade of cell signals. Nitric oxide's role as a vasorelaxant is applied in medicine. Nitroglycerin, for example, taken by people experiencing ischemic chest pain (angina), generates nitric oxide in the body, which relaxes coronary blood vessels and increases blood (and thus oxygen) flow to the heart. Nitric oxide also is associated, however, with other beneficial and detrimental effects at the vascular and cellular levels. For example, nitric oxide can react with oxygen to form nitrogen dioxide ($^{\bullet}NO + O_2 \longrightarrow {}^{\bullet}NO_2$), another reactive nitrogen species. Moreover, when nitric oxide reacts with superoxide radicals ($O_2^{\bullet}$), peroxynitrite (ONOO$^{\bullet}$) is generated; peroxynitrite also acts as an oxidizing agent in the body. Thiols (RSH) also can react with nitric oxide, as shown in the general reaction: $^{\bullet}NO + RSH \longrightarrow RSNO + O_2 + H^+$. The **nitrosothiol** (RSNO) that is produced is harmful in that it may attack other compounds unless it is terminated by combining with another thiol (R'SH) to produce RSH + R'SNO or RSSR' + HNO. In contrast to these radical-producing reactions, nitric oxide, by removing superoxide radicals and other radicals, can be viewed as an eliminator or terminator

of free radicals (as discussed further under elimination of lipid peroxides). It also appears to work directly with uric acid to generate nitrosated uric acid; the nitroso group is then transferred to glutathione for transport to other molecules.

Peroxynitrite

Peroxynitrite (ONOO$^{\bullet}$), formed by reactions between nitric oxide and superoxide radicals, is a strong oxidant. It directly attacks amino acids such as cysteine, methionine, and tyrosine in proteins, causing protein **nitrosation** and extensive functional damage to the protein. Peroxynitrite also decomposes to generate more destructive radicals including the hydroxyl radical ($^{\bullet}OH$) and nitrogen dioxide ($^{\bullet}NO_2$). Alternately, and, more likely in human tissues and fluids, peroxynitrite reacts with carbon dioxide (CO_2) to produce carbonate ($CO_3^{-\bullet}$) and nitrogen dioxide ($^{\bullet}NO_2$). Both carbonate and nitrogen dioxide preferentially react with nutrients such as lipids and amino acids within proteins (primarily tyrosine, tryptophan, and cysteine) to form nitrated molecules, which disrupt normal cellular processes.

Nitrogen Dioxide and Peroxynitrate

Nitrogen dioxide ($^{\bullet}NO_2$) is a free radical and a fairly potent oxidant. It is formed when nitric oxide reacts with oxygen ($^{\bullet}NO + O_2 \longrightarrow {}^{\bullet}NO_2$). Nitrogen dioxide, for example, in addition to co-acting with carbonate ($CO_3^{-\bullet}$) radicals to produce nitrated compounds, reacts with unsaturated fatty acids by abstracting a hydrogen atom and induces isomerization of *cis*-double bonds in unsaturated fatty acids by a reversible addition reaction. These actions damage the lipids and, if the lipids are part of a cell membrane, damage the membrane. Peroxynitrate ($O_2NOO^{\bullet}$) is made from the reaction between nitrogen dioxide and a superoxide radical. It typically decomposes to form singlet oxygen and $NO_2^{-\bullet}$.

DAMAGE DUE TO REACTIVE SPECIES

Once formed, free radicals attack, taking electrons from cell constituents (including nucleic acid in DNA in the nucleus of cells). They also take electrons from proteins (especially amino acids such as tyrosine, tryptophan, proline, histidine, or arginine and those with sulfhydryl groups, such as cysteine) and polyunsaturated fatty acids in cell membranes or in the membranes of intracellular organelles, such as the nucleus, mitochondria, or endoplasmic reticulum. Hydroxyl radical–induced changes in purine and pyrimidine bases in DNA may lead to mutations or breakages, which if not repaired may result, for example, in cancer. Attacks on amino acids in proteins by reactive oxygen species may break the peptide bonds in the protein backbone or disrupt the protein structure. Oxidative damage to proteins may cause crosslinking between amino acids, or aggregation, resulting in changes in the secondary or tertiary structures. Such events may even lead to premature degradation of the protein. Free radical attack on polyunsaturated fatty acids present in the phospholipid portion of the cell membranes can lead to degradation of the lipid. Extensive damage in a red blood cell, for example, may cause hemolysis of the membrane and thus the cell. Aqueous peroxyl and peroxy nitrite radicals may induce oxidation of LDLs. Furthermore, radicals give rise to more radicals and thus, more damage.

ANTIOXIDANT NUTRIENT FUNCTIONS

Overproduction of reactive oxygen and nitrogen species and their attack on DNA, proteins, and polyunsaturated fatty acids have been implicated as a cause of or contributor to a variety of conditions and diseases such as cancer, heart disease, cataracts, and complications of diabetes mellitus, among others. Vitamins, along with several other antioxidant compounds, help control or eliminate free radicals. However, the term *antioxidant* is a bit of a misnomer because once it works, the antioxidant itself becomes a radical. Some have suggested that the term *redox agent* be used instead of the term *antioxidant.* Whether or to what extent an overproduction of vitamin radicals may be associated with diseases is unclear; however, the results of many clinical trials providing antioxidant vitamins to treat or prevent various diseases have failed to show beneficial results, and some have even found that supplementation was detrimental to health. The destruction of reactive species by some of the antioxidant nutrients and compounds is reviewed in this section and shown in Figure 2.

Elimination of Superoxide Radicals

Several antioxidant nutrients help dispose of superoxide radicals, including vitamin C and three minerals (zinc, copper, and manganese) that function as cofactors for enzymes involved in oxidant defense. Vitamin C (present under physiological conditions as ascorbate AH^-), being water soluble and hydrophilic, is found in the aqueous parts of the body, such as the blood or the cytosol of the cells. The vitamin provides electrons to reduce the superoxide radical and forms hydrogen peroxide, as shown here:

$$AH^- + O_2^{\bullet} + H^+ \longrightarrow A^{\bullet} + H_2O_2$$

Superoxide radicals also may be eliminated by the action of the enzyme superoxide dismutase (SOD), which works considerably faster than vitamin C in inactivating superoxide radicals. The extracellular form of superoxide dismutase is found in exceptionally high concentrations in arterial blood vessels. Both the extracellular and the cytosolic forms of the enzyme depend upon the presence of two minerals, zinc and copper; the mitochondrial form depends on manganese for activity. Thus, zinc, copper, and manganese are important minerals in the body's oxidant defense system. Superoxide dismutase effectively eliminates superoxide radicals but generates hydrogen peroxide, as shown here:

$$O_2^{\bullet} + O_2^{\bullet} + 2H^+$$
$$\downarrow \text{Superoxide dismutase}$$
$$H_2O_2 + O_2$$

Elimination of Hydrogen Peroxide

Hydrogen peroxide may be disposed of by several mechanisms in cells and tissues. Vitamin C readily reacts with hydrogen peroxide, as do some enzymes. Two enzymes that help to dispose of hydrogen peroxide are glutathione peroxidase and catalase. A third enzyme, myeloperoxidase, uses hydrogen peroxide to generate other radicals needed to help fight bacteria and viruses invading body cells.

In a reaction catalyzed by ascorbate peroxidase, vitamin C (as AH^-), found in the blood and cell cytosol, provides the needed electrons to convert hydrogen peroxide into water and dehydroascorbic acid.

Glutathione peroxidase, found in the plasma as well as the cell's cytosol and mitochondria, is an important enzyme necessary not only for removal of hydrogen peroxide but also for reduction of other peroxides. The enzyme requires the mineral selenium (four atoms) as a cofactor, and its activity is impaired if selenium status is poor. Because of selenium's role in glutathione peroxidase, the mineral is considered an antioxidant nutrient. Additionally, the enzyme requires glutathione (composed of glycine, cysteine, and glutamic acid) in its reduced form (GSH). Glutathione is one of many thiols found in both aqueous and lipophilic parts of the body. Thiols are characterized by the presence of sulfhydryl groups (R-SH) and include glutathione, thioredoxin, and lipoic acid, among others. Glutathione (GSH) serves as a reducing agent; more specifically, each of the two glutathione molecules gives up a hydrogen from its sulfhydryl group (SH). A radical center is formed on the sulfur atom ($GS^{\bullet}$) until two glutathiyl radicals join to form a disulfide bond between the two now oxidized glutathione molecules (designated as GSSG or GS-SG).

$$\begin{array}{ccc} H_2O_2 & & 2\,H_2O \\ & \text{Glutathione} & \\ & \text{peroxidase} & \\ 2\,GSH & \longrightarrow & GSSG \end{array}$$

Catalase is another key enzyme in hydrogen peroxide removal. This heme iron–dependent enzyme is found mostly in cell peroxisomes (cytosolic organelles where lots of hydrogen peroxide is produced during the oxidation of very long-chain fatty acids, among other molecules). Smaller amounts of the enzyme also are found in the cytosol, mitochondria, and microsomes of cells. Neutrophils and other white blood cells contain fairly high quantities of catalase to dispose of hydrogen peroxide no longer needed in the respiratory burst required for the phagocytosis of foreign bacteria, viruses, and fungi. Higher concentrations of hydrogen peroxide are required for catalase activity than for glutathione peroxidase activity. The reaction catalyzed by catalase is shown here:

$$\begin{array}{c} \text{Catalase} \\ 2\,H_2O_2 \longrightarrow 2\,H_2O + O_2 \end{array}$$

The accumulation of H_2O_2 in the body is thought to be prevented primarily by catalase and glutathione peroxidase. Glutathione peroxidase, because of its dual (mitochondrial and cytosolic) locations in the cell and because of its greater activity at lower hydrogen peroxide concentrations, is

thought to be more active than catalase in removing hydrogen peroxide from body cells. Figure 2 shows the complex interaction among components of the oxidant defense system, including the roles of iron-dependent catalase, selenium-dependent glutathione peroxidase, and copper-, zinc-, and manganese-dependent superoxide dismutase.

A final enzyme (found mostly within activated white blood cells) is myeloperoxidase; this enzyme, which is also heme iron dependent, uses hydrogen peroxide for the respiratory burst. Remember that the respiratory burst is required to destroy bacteria, viruses, and other harmful substances. Myeloperoxidase, within activated white blood cells, is released from granules into vacuoles that contain the engulfed foreign substance. In the vacuoles, the hydrogen peroxide, produced from the superoxide radical, is used to generate a potent toxic acid, hypochlorous acid (HOCl).

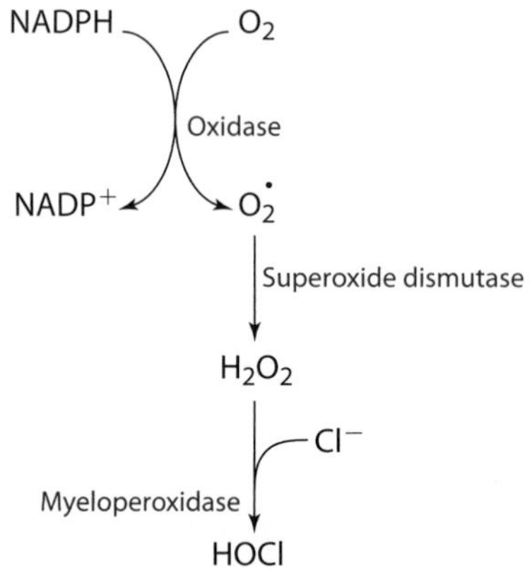

$$\begin{array}{ccc} NADPH & & O_2 \\ & \searrow \quad \nearrow & \\ & \text{Oxidase} & \\ & \nearrow \quad \searrow & \\ NADP^+ & & O_2^{\bullet} \\ & & \downarrow \text{Superoxide dismutase} \\ & & H_2O_2 \\ & & \downarrow \quad \longleftarrow Cl^- \\ & \text{Myeloperoxidase} & \downarrow \\ & & HOCl \end{array}$$

Hypochlorous acid, along with other potent compounds, helps to destroy the foreign bacteria's cell membrane to promote death (lysis) of the foreign substance.

Elimination of Hydroxyl Radicals

Vitamin C and other water-soluble compounds, such as uric acid, thiols including glutathione and dihydrolipoic acid, and possibly other substances such as metallothionein, serve to defend against hydroxyl radicals. Vitamin E, in contrast, is less effective in eliminating hydroxyl radicals.

In aqueous solutions such as blood, vitamin C rapidly and effectively reacts with hydroxyl radicals before they can initiate oxidative damage.

$$\begin{array}{ccc} AH^- & & AH^{\bullet} \\ & \searrow \quad \nearrow & \\ {}^{\bullet}OH & \longrightarrow & H_2O \end{array}$$

Glutathione may also react directly with hydroxyl radicals in aqueous or lipid environments, as shown here:

$$\begin{array}{ccc} GSH & & GSSG \\ & \searrow \quad \nearrow & \\ {}^{\bullet}OH & \longrightarrow & H_2O \end{array}$$

Dihydrolipoic acid (DHLA), the reduced form of lipoic acid (also called thioctic acid), functions in the body as a reducing agent. Dietary or endogenously generated lipoic acid

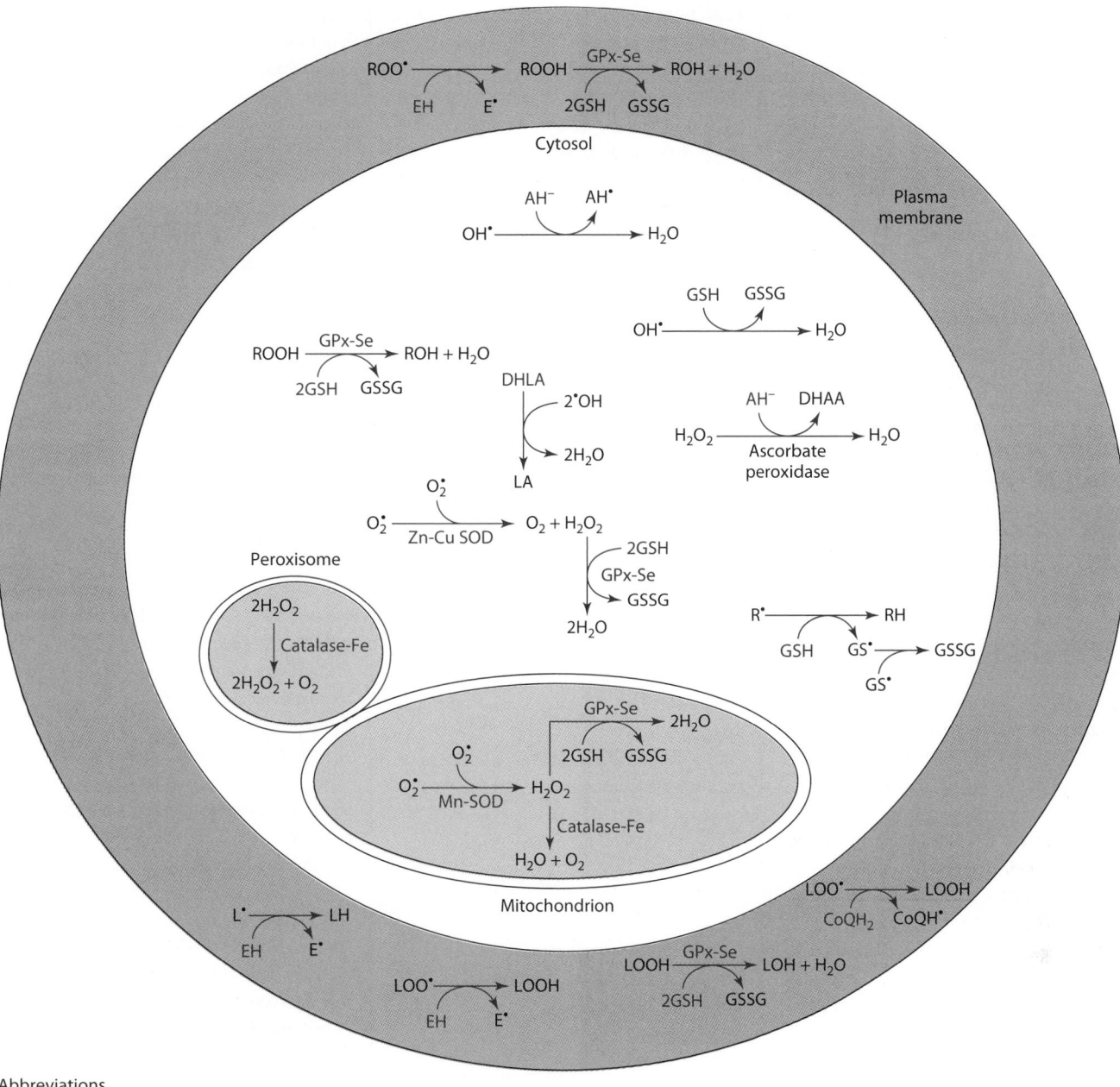

Abbreviations

EH = vitamin E
AH$_2$ = vitamin C
SOD = superoxide dismutase
GSH = reduced glutathione
GSSG = oxidized glutathione
O$_2^{\bullet}$ = superoxide radical
LOO$^{\bullet}$ = peroxy radical
LH = unsaturated fatty acid

L$^{\bullet}$ = carbon-centered lipid radical
RH = organic nonlipid compound
R$^{\bullet}$ = carbon-centered nonlipid radical
H$_2$O$_2$ = hydrogen peroxide
ROO$^{\bullet}$ = nonlipid peroxy radical
ROOH = nonlipid peroxides
LOOH = lipid peroxides
DHLA = dihydrolipoic acid
LA = lipoic acid

Figure 2 The interactions among selected antioxidant nutrients to prevent cell damage.

is reduced in cells to dihydrolipoic acid by dihydrolipamide dehydrogenase, glutathione reductase, or thioredoxin reductase. Dihydrolipoic acid in turn functions in aqueous and lipophilic environments as a reducing agent to diminish oxidative stress under some conditions and to eliminate radicals such as hydroxyl radical (among others) as shown here:

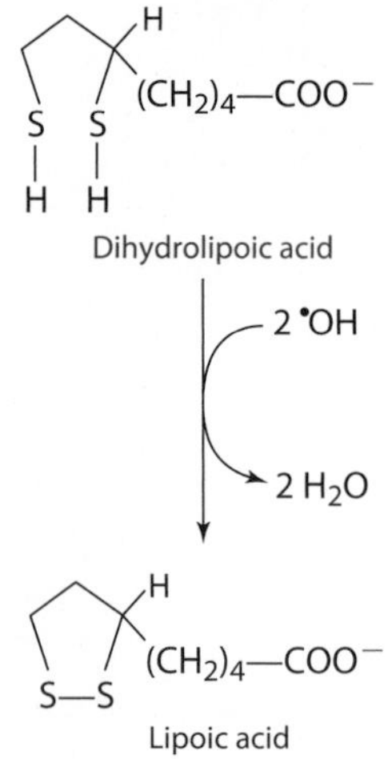

Dihydrolipoic acid

$$2 \, ^{\bullet}OH$$
$$2 \, H_2O$$

Lipoic acid

Ubiquinol (also called coenzyme Q, CoQ_{10}, or Q_{10}; Figure 3) and uric acid (Figure 4) also may act as reducing agents in aqueous solutions. Both ubiquinol and uric acid scavenge various free oxygen radicals, including $^{\bullet}OH$. Metallothionein, a protein rich in cysteine residues and thus sulfhydryl groups, is also thought to scavenge hydroxyl radicals.

Elimination of Peroxyl, Hydroperoxyl, and Carbon-Centered Radicals, Lipid Peroxides, and Some Reactive Nitrogen Species

Several nutrients and compounds, including vitamin E, carotenoids, manganese, ubiquinol, vitamin C, uric acid, and glutathione, along with the selenium-dependent enzyme glutathione peroxidase, actively eliminate carbon-centered, peroxyl, and hydroperoxyl radicals as well as lipid peroxides and some reactive nitrogen species.

Vitamin E, being lipid soluble and located near or in membranes, effectively reacts with many radicals, especially carbon-centered radicals and those that initiate peroxidation, such as peroxyl radicals. Specifically, vitamin E donates its phenolic hydrogen on the carbon 6 hydroxyl group. Vitamin E's chromanol ring then stabilizes the unpaired electron.

● Vitamin E (EH) terminates carbon-centered radicals (as shown below) before they abstract further hydrogens from other polyunsaturated fatty acids:

$$L^{\bullet} + EH \longrightarrow LH + E^{\bullet}$$

● Vitamin E (EH) prevents peroxidation of polyunsaturated fatty acids by reacting with peroxyl radicals ($LOO^{\bullet}$), as illustrated in this reaction:

$$LOO^{\bullet} + EH \longrightarrow LOOH + E^{\bullet}$$

Thus, vitamin E terminates chain-propagation reactions.

Carotenoids such as β-carotene also have the ability to react directly with peroxyl radicals involved in lipid peroxidation. β-carotene is thought to carry out this role to a lesser extent than vitamin E and perhaps to function more in the interior of the cell, whereas vitamin E functions on or at the surface.

Some transition metals, such as manganese, may be able to scavenge peroxyl radicals, as shown here:

$$Mn^{2+} \qquad Mn^{3+}$$
$$LOO^{\bullet} \longrightarrow LOOH$$

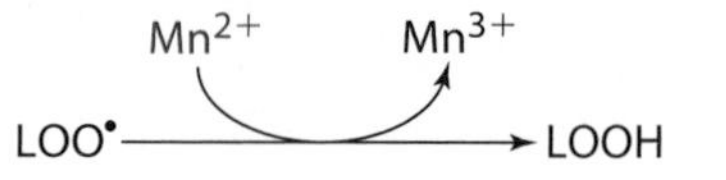

In addition to vitamin E, carotenoids, and manganese, ubiquinol has been shown to provide hydrogens to terminate peroxyl radicals and appears to be a potent antioxidant.

Ubiquinol, the reduced form of coenzyme Q_{10} ($CoQH_2$), is a small fat-soluble molecule that transports electrons and ultimately generates ATP in the electron transport chain in the mitochondria. Ubiquinol has been found in small quantities in lipoproteins, where it is thought to be used before vitamin E in the termination of peroxyl radicals (as shown hereafter) and thus prevent LDL oxidation.

$$CoQH_2 + LOO^{\bullet} \longrightarrow CoQH^{\bullet} + LOOH$$

Vitamin C effectively scavenges alkoxyl ($RO^{\bullet}$) and non-lipid peroxyl ($ROO^{\bullet}$) radicals to produce a hydroxyl acid (ROH) and nonlipid peroxide (ROOH), as shown here:

$$AH^{-} + RO^{\bullet} \longrightarrow A^{\bullet} + ROH$$
$$AH^{-} + ROO^{\bullet} \longrightarrow A^{\bullet} + ROOH$$

Nitric oxide ($^{\bullet}NO$) also can act as an antioxidant to terminate lipid alkoxyl ($LO^{\bullet}$) and peroxyl ($LOO^{\bullet}$) radicals, as shown here:

$$^{\bullet}NO + LO^{\bullet} \longrightarrow LONO$$
$$^{\bullet}NO + LOO^{\bullet} \longrightarrow LOONO$$

Most of the resulting LOONO homolyzes to produce nitrogen dioxide, $^{\bullet}NO_2$, and an alkoxyl radical, $LO^{\bullet}$, and then recombines to produce alkylnitrates ($LONO_2$); however, a small percentage remains as free radicals. Additionally, uric acid removes peroxynitrite ($ONOO^{\bullet}$) before it causes protein nitrosation.

Although eliminating peroxyl radicals ($LOO^{\bullet}$) is helpful, the often simultaneous generation of lipid peroxides/peroxidized fatty acids (LOOH) can cause problems if the peroxidized fatty acids are within hydrophobic regions of cell membranes. The problems occur because peroxidized fatty acids are polar compounds, and the polarized peroxidized fatty acids, once liberated from the phospholipid in the membrane by the actions of phospholipase A_2, destroy the normal architecture of the cell as they migrate from the nonpolar region where they are generated.

Thiols and the selenium-dependent enzyme glutathione peroxidase help to eliminate lipid peroxides. Thiols like glutathione and thioredoxin [$Trx(SH)_2$] act in both aqueous and lipid environments as antioxidants by providing reducing equivalents (hydrogen ions). Glutathione peroxidase uses glutathione in its reduced form (GSH) and catalyzes the conversion of the peroxides (LOOH) to hydroxy acids (LOH) as follows:

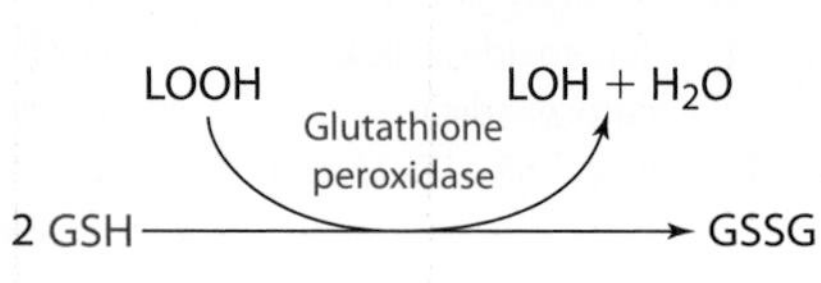

$$LOOH \qquad LOH + H_2O$$
Glutathione peroxidase
$$2 \, GSH \longrightarrow GSSG$$

Elimination of Singlet Molecular Oxygen

Carotenoids as well as vitamin C, uric acid, and thiols (especially lipoic acid) may quench singlet molecular oxygen. Carotenoids such as β-carotene and lycopene have the ability to directly quench hundreds of singlet oxygen molecules either in solution or in membrane systems; lycopene, in fact, appears to be more effective than β-carotene in quenching

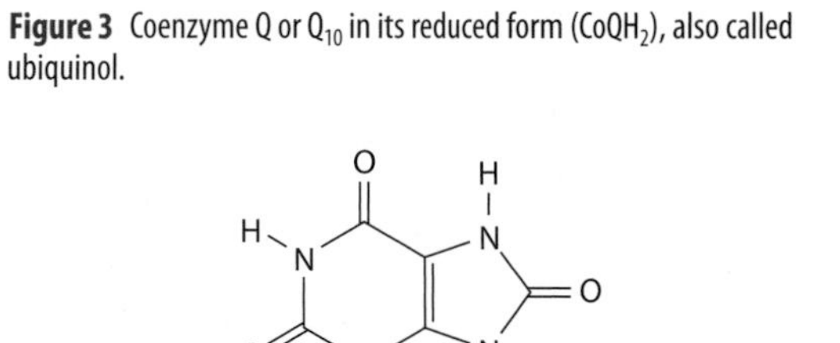

Figure 3 Coenzyme Q or Q_{10} in its reduced form ($CoQH_2$), also called ubiquinol.

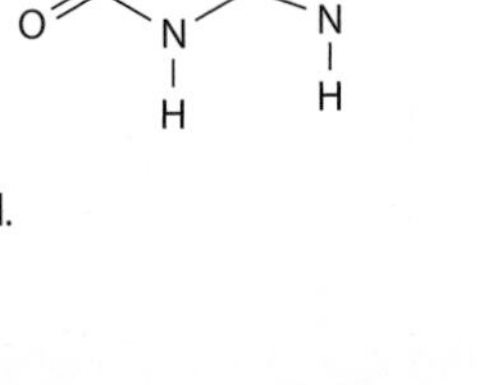

Figure 4 Uric acid.

singlet oxygen [1]. *Quenching* is a process by which electronically excited molecules, such as singlet molecular oxygen, are inactivated. The ability of carotenoids to quench singlet oxygen is attributed to the conjugated double-bond systems within the carotenoid structure. The carotenoids can absorb energy from the singlet oxygen without chemical change to return the "excited" $^1O_2$ to its ground state. Carotenoids then release the energy in the form of heat (as shown hereafter) and thus do not need to be regenerated.

$$^1O_2 + \beta\text{-carotene} \longrightarrow {}^3O_2 + \text{excited}$$
$$\beta\text{-carotene}$$
$$\longrightarrow \beta\text{-carotene} + \text{heat}$$

REGENERATION OF ANTIOXIDANTS

When antioxidants provide reducing equivalents, the antioxidants are oxidized. Regenerating the antioxidants is important for further defense against free radicals. Without the recycling of antioxidants, the body would quickly succumb to oxidative stress. Uric acid, which is thought to account for almost half of the antioxidant capacity of human plasma, depends on vitamin C for its regeneration [2]. It has been estimated that fewer than nine vitamin E molecules exist for every one to two thousand unsaturated fatty acids in cell membrane phospholipids or lipoprotein molecules. Thus, regenerating or recycling oxidized vitamins is critical to prevent massive damage. This next section discusses the recycling of antioxidants.

Vitamin E Regeneration

The regeneration of vitamin E is thought to initially require the migration of the vitamin to the membrane surface. At the cell surface, several compounds regenerate vitamin E. Vitamin C (AH^-) can regenerate α-tocopherol from its radical form ($E^•$), but it too will then need to be regenerated.

$$AH^- \qquad AH^•$$
$$E^• \longrightarrow EH$$

Ubiquinol ($CoQH_2$) also recycles vitamin E, as shown here:

$$E^• \qquad EH$$
$$\text{Ubiquinol} \longrightarrow \text{Ubisemiquinone}$$
$$(CoQH_2) \qquad\qquad (CoQH^•)$$

Glutathione in its reduced form (GSH) may donate its hydrogen atom to re-form vitamin E, as follows:

$$GSH \qquad GS^•$$
$$E^• \longrightarrow EH$$

Ubiquinol (Coenzyme QH$_2$) and Thioredoxin Regeneration

Regeneration of vitamin E by ubiquinol ($CoQH_2$) results in the formation of ubisemiquinone ($CoQH^•$). Ubisemiquinone can be converted back to ubiquinol through the electron transport chain in the mitochondria, by dihydrolipoic acid (DHLA), as shown here:

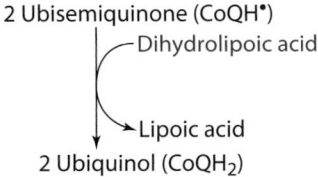

$$\text{2 Ubisemiquinone (CoQH}^•\text{)}$$
$$\text{Dihydrolipoic acid}$$
$$\text{Lipoic acid}$$
$$\text{2 Ubiquinol (CoQH}_2\text{)}$$

or by the thioredoxin-thioredoxin reductase system. This system, ubiquitous in the body, includes thioredoxin (Trx), a small protein with a dithiol (two sulfhydryl groups -$[SH]_2$), and the selenium-dependent flavoenzyme (FAD) thioredoxin reductase with a selenocysteine residue at its active site. The recycling of ubiquinol is shown here:

$$\text{2 Ubisemiquinone (CoQH}^•\text{)}$$
$$\text{Trx-(SH)}_2$$
$$\text{Trx-S}_2$$
$$\text{2 Ubiquinol (CoQH}_2\text{)}$$

Thioredoxin reductase (TrxR) then functions to reduce thioredoxin, using reducing equivalents from NADPH, as shown here:

$$\text{Trx-S}_2$$
$$\text{NADPH + H}^+$$
$$\text{TrxR}$$
$$\text{NADP}^+$$
$$\text{Trx-(SH)}_2$$

Glutathione Regeneration

Glutathione reductase, a flavoprotein that requires FAD as a cofactor, regenerates oxidized glutathione (GSSG) with niacin as NADPH providing the reducing equivalents, as shown next:

$$\text{NADPH + H}^+ \qquad\qquad \text{NADP}^+$$
$$\text{Glutathione reductase}$$
$$\text{GSSG} \longrightarrow \text{2 GSH}$$

Dihydrolipoic acid (DHLA) also is thought to be able to regenerate glutathione, as shown here:

$$\text{DHLA} \qquad \text{Lipoic acid}$$
$$\text{GSSG} \longrightarrow \text{2 GSH}$$

Vitamin C Regeneration

Niacin, dihydrolipoic acid, and thiols such as glutathione and thioredoxin help to regenerate some, but not all, vitamin C. In a reaction catalyzed by semidehydroascorbic acid reductase, niacin in its coenzyme form, NADH, provides for the regeneration of vitamin C, as follows:

$$\text{2 AH}^• + \text{NADH} + \text{H}^+ \longrightarrow \text{2 AH}^-$$
$$+ \text{NAD}^+$$

Dihydrolipoic acid provides hydrogens to the ascorbyl radical form of vitamin C to recycle the vitamin:

$$\text{DHLA} \qquad \text{Lipoic acid}$$
$$\text{A}^• \longrightarrow \text{AH}^-$$

The next few reactions depict some of the recycling efforts contributed by glutathione (GSH) and thioredoxin.

$$\text{2 GSH + 2 A}^• \longrightarrow \text{GSSG + 2 AH}^-$$

$$\text{Trx-(SH)}_2 \qquad \text{Trx-S}_2$$
$$\text{DHAA} \longrightarrow \text{AH}_2$$

An interaction between two vitamin C radicals also permits the regeneration of vitamin C, as follows:

$$\text{2 A}^• \longrightarrow \text{AH}_2 + \text{DHAA}$$

ANTIOXIDANTS AND DISEASE

Overproduction of reactive species, which leads to an imbalance within the body's defense system, is referred to as oxidative or nitrosative stress, and is thought to contribute to aging and the development of several diseases and conditions including some cancers, heart disease, cataracts, diabetes mellitus complications, rheumatoid arthritis, and ischemia-reperfusion injury, among others. Nutrients *in vitro* often demonstrate specific functions or abilities, such as inhibiting lipoprotein cholesterol oxidation or inhibiting cell proliferation or transformation, that are thought to provide protection against the development of disease. Despite the promising results of many *in vitro* studies, the results of supplementation trials *in vivo* to prevent or treat disease are not consistent, and sometimes have shown that vitamin supplementation may be detrimental to health. Similarly, although many studies have shown that people who either consume diets rich in foods (especially fruits and vegetables) that contain antioxidant nutrients or who have high plasma antioxidant nutrient concentrations have a reduced risk of many diseases or conditions, others do not support such associations (see Suggested Readings). New supplementation trials are being conducted, as are *in vitro* and *in vivo* studies, to better elucidate the roles and effects of antioxidants. As these studies continue to clarify the roles of the antioxidant nutrients, scientists and other health professionals will continue to reevaluate current recommendations and perhaps develop new guidelines defining optimal levels of nutrients to prevent diseases. However, enjoying a diet rich in fruits, vegetables, and whole grains is always encouraged to help prevent disease and maintain health.

References Cited

1. Bohm F, Haley J, Truscott T, Schalch W. Cellular bound β-carotene quenches singlet oxygen in man. J Photochem Photobiol B Biol. 1993; 21:219—21.

2. So A, Thorens B. Uric acid transport and disease. J Clin Invest. 2010; 120:1791—99.

Suggested Readings

Age-related Eye Disease Study Research Group. A randomized placebo-controlled clinical trial of high dose supplementation with vitamins C and E, β carotene, and zinc for age-related macular degeneration and vision loss. Arch Ophthalmol. 2001; 119:1417—36.

Agte V, Tarwadi K. The importance of nutrition in the prevention of ocular disease with special reference to cataract. Ophthalmic Res. 2010; 44:166—72.

α-tocopherol, β-carotene (ATBC) Cancer Prevention Study Group. The effect of vitamin E and β carotene on the incidence of lung cancer and other cancers in male smokers. N Engl J Med. 1994; 330:1029—35.

Bardia A, Tleyjeh IM, Cerhan JR, et al. Efficacy of antioxidant supplementation in reducing primary cancer incidence and mortality: systematic review and meta-analysis. Mayo Clin Proc. 2008; 83:23—34.

Bjelakovic G, Nikolova D, Simonetti RG, Gluud C. Systematic review: primary and secondary prevention of gastrointestinal cancers with antioxidant supplements. Aliment Pharmacol Ther. 2008; 28:689—703.

Bjelakovic G, Nikolova D, Gluud LL, et al. Mortality in randomized trials of antioxidant supplements for primary and secondary prevention: systematic review and meta-analysis. JAMA. 2007; 297:842—57.

Christen WG, Liu S, Glynn RJ, et al. Dietary carotenoids, vitamins C and E, and risk of cataract in women: a prospective study. Arch Ophthalmol. 2008; 126:102—09.

Christen WG, Glynn RJ, Sesso HD, et al. Age-related cataract in a randomized trial of vitamins E and C in men. Arch Ophthalmol. 2010; 128:1397—1405.

Chiu C, Taylor A. Nutritional antioxidants and age-related cataract and maculopathy. Exp Eye Res. 2007; 84:229—45.

Cook NR, Albert CM, Gaziano JM, et al. A randomized factorial trial of vitamins C and E and beta carotene in the secondary prevention of cardiovascular events in women. Arch Intern Med. 2007; 167:1610—18.

Farbstein D, Kozak-Blickstein A, Levy AP. Antioxidant vitamins and their use in preventing cardiovascular disease. Molecules. 2010; 15:8098—110.

Fernandez MM, Afshari NA. Nutrition and the prevention of cataracts. Curr Opin Ophthalmol. 2008; 19:66—70.

Fletcher AE, Bentham GC, Agnew M, et al. Sunlight exposure, antioxidants and age-related macular degeneration. Arch Ophthalmol. 2008; 126:1396—1403.

Kataja-Tuomola MK, Kontto JP, Mannisto S, et al. Effect of alpha-tocopherol and beta-carotene supplementation on macrovascular complications and total mortality from diabetes: results of the ATBC study. Ann Med. 2010; 42:178—86.

Levine M, Espey MG, Chen Q. Losing and finding a way at C: new promise for pharmacologic ascorbate in cancer treatment. Free Radic Biol Med. 2009; 47:27—29.

Lin J, Cook NR, Albert C, et al. Vitamins C and E and beta carotene supplementation and cancer risk: a randomized controlled trial. J Natl Cancer Inst. 2009; 101:14—23.

Lippman SM, Klein EA, Goodman PJ, et al. Effect of selenium and vitamin E on risk of prostate cancer and other cancers: the selenium and vitamin E cancer prevention trial (SELECT). JAMA. 2009; 301:39—51.

Omenn G, Goodman G, Thomquist M, et al. Effects of a combination of β carotene and vitamin A on lung cancer and cardiovascular disease. N Engl J Med. 1996; 334:1150—55.

Omenn G, Goodman G, Thornquist M, et al. Risk factors for lung cancer and for intervention effects in CARET, the β-carotene and retinol efficacy trial. J Natl Cancer Inst. 1996; 88:1550—59.

Parisi V, Tedeschi M, Gallinaro G, et al. Carotenoids and antioxidants in age-related maculopathy Italian study: multifocal electroretinogram modifications after 1 year. Ophthalmology. 2008; 115:324—33.

SanGiovanni JP, Chew EY, Clemons TE, et al. The relationship of dietary carotenoid and vitamin A, E, and C intake with age-related macular degeneration in a case-control study: AREDS Report #22. Arch Ophthalmol. 2007; 125:1225—32.

Sesso HD, Buring JE, Christen WG, et al. Vitamins E and C in the prevention of cardiovascular disease in men: the Physicians' Health Study II randomized controlled trial. JAMA. 2008; 300:2123—33.

Tan AG, Mitchell P, Flood VM, et al. Antioxidant nutrient intake and the long-term incidence of age-related cataract: the Blue Mountains Eye Study. Am J Clin Nutr. 2008; 87:1899—1905.

Trumbo PR, Ellwood KC. Lutein and zeaxanthin intakes and risk of age-related macular degeneration and cataracts: an evaluation using the Food and Drug Administration's evidence-based review system for health claims. Am J Clin Nutr. 2006; 84:971—74.

Voutilainen S, Nurmi T, Mursu J, Rissanen T. Carotenoids and cardiovascular health. Am J Clin Nutr. 2006; 83:1265—71.

Wojcik M. A review of natural and synthetic antioxidants important for health and longevity. Curr Med Chem. 2010; 17:3262—88.

Web Sites

National Cancer Institute
http://www.cancer.gov

American Heart Association
www.heart.org

American Cancer Society
www.cancer.org

Prevent Cancer Foundation
www.preventcancer.org

Produce for Better Health Foundation
www.fruitsandveggiesmorematters.org

MAJOR MINERALS

THE IMPORTANCE OF MINERALS IN NORMAL NUTRITION and metabolism cannot be overstated, despite the fact that they constitute only about 4% of total body weight. Their functions are many and varied. They provide the medium essential for normal cellular activity, determine the osmotic properties of body fluids, impart hardness to bones and teeth, and function as obligatory cofactors in metalloenzymes.

Historically, the awareness that minerals are required in normal nutrition evolved from knowledge of the mineral composition of body tissues and fluids. This knowledge has expanded greatly as a result of accumulating improvements in analytical techniques for quantifying minerals.

Major minerals, also called macrominerals, are distinguished from the trace minerals, also called microminerals or microelements, by their abundance in the body. The major minerals are typically required by adults in amounts greater than 100 mg per day. The remaining minerals are sometimes divided into two groups, trace and ultratrace elements/minerals. The trace elements are required by adults in amounts between about 1 mg and 100 mg per day, while the ultratrace minerals are required by adults in amounts less than 1 mg per day.

The major minerals of the human body include calcium, phosphorus, magnesium, sodium, potassium, and chloride, shown on the periodic table in Figure 11.1. Because of their role in maintaining electrolyte balance in body fluids, sodium, chloride, and potassium are discussed in association with water in Chapter 12. Although sulfur is found in the body and is considered a major mineral, the mineral is not discussed as a subsection of this chapter because the body does not use sulfur alone as a nutrient. Sulfur is found in the body associated structurally with vitamins such as thiamin and biotin, and as part of the sulfur-containing amino acids methionine, cysteine, and taurine. Thus, sulfur is commonly found within proteins, especially those found in skin, hair, and nails.

Table 11.1 provides an overview of the major minerals, including information on general functions, approximate body content, some enzyme cofactors, deficiency signs, food sources, and recommended intakes. A similar overview of the trace and ultratrace minerals may be found in Chapters 13 and 14. Note the difference in body content between the major and trace minerals, with the major mineral content of the body ranging from ~35 to 1,400 g, and the trace mineral content ranging from <1 mg to ~4 g. In considering the body's mineral content, keep in mind that a pound is equal to 454 g and an ounce is about 28.4 g.

CALCIUM

Calcium is the most abundant divalent cation in the body, representing about 40% of the body's mineral mass and 1.5% to 2% of total body weight, or between ~1,000 and 1,400 g in the human body. Bones and teeth contain

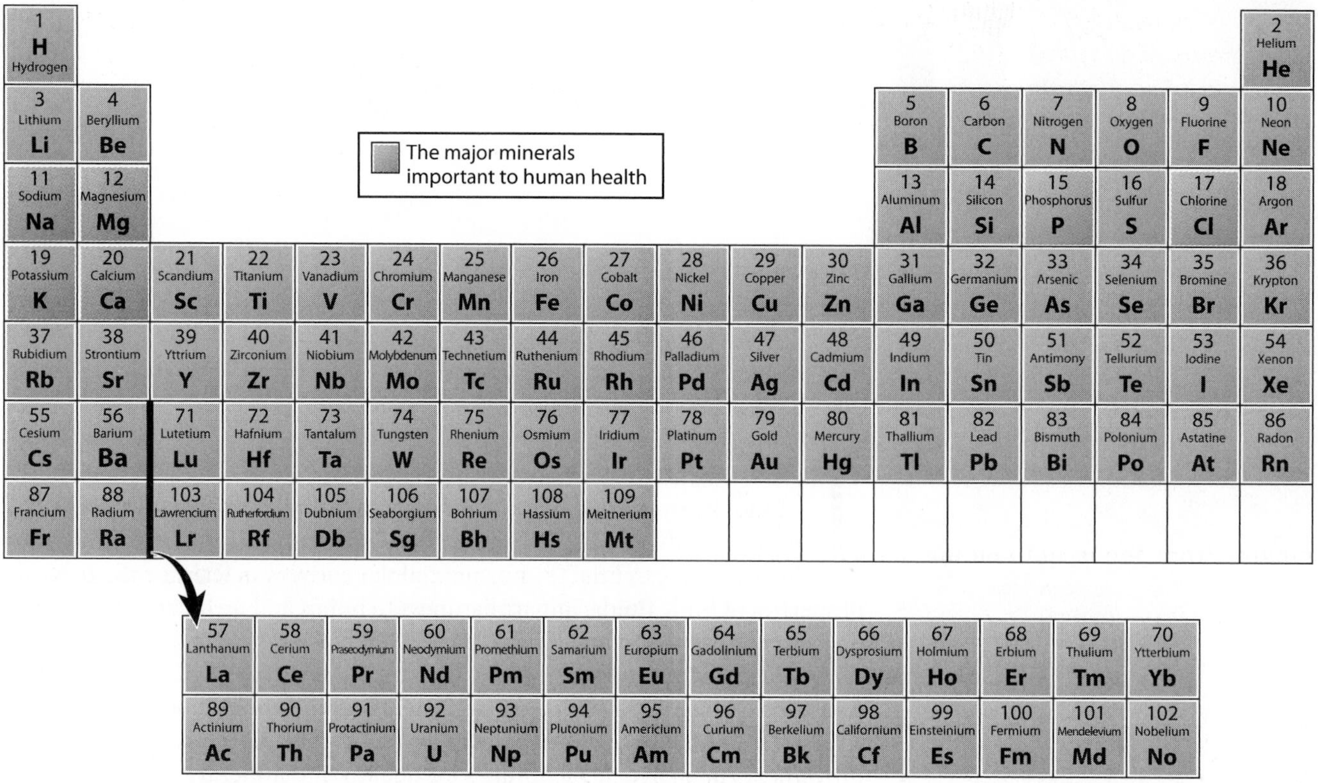

The major minerals important to human health

Figure 11.1 The periodic table highlighting the body's major (macro) minerals.
Source: Derived from Beerman/McGuire, Nutritional Sciences, 1/e. © Cengage Learning.

Table 11.1 Macrominerals[a]: Functions, Body Content, Deficiency Symptoms, and Recommended Dietary Allowances (RDAs)

Mineral	Selected Physiological Functions	Approximate Body Content	Selected Enzyme Cofactors	Deficiency Symptoms	Selected Food Sources	RDA
Calcium	Structural component of bones and teeth; role in cellular processes, muscle contraction, blood clotting, enzyme activation	1,400 g	Adenylate, cyclase, kinases, protein kinase, Ca^{2+}/Mg^{2+}-ATPase (for others, see Table 11.4)	Rickets, osteomalacia, osteoporosis, tetany	Milk, milk products, sardines, clams, oysters, turnip and mustard greens, broccoli, legumes, dried fruits	1,000 mg, 19–50 years
Magnesium	Component of bones; role in nerve impulse transmission, protein synthesis; enzyme cofactor	25 g	Hydrolysis and transfer of phosphate groups by phosphokinase; important in numerous ATP-dependent enzyme reactions	Neuromuscular hyperexcitability, muscle weakness, tetany	Nuts, legumes, whole-grain cereals, leafy green vegetables	400 mg males; 310 mg females; 19–30 years
Phosphorus	Structural component of bone, teeth, cell membranes, phospholipids, nucleic acids, nucleotide coenzymes, ATP-ADP phosphate transferring system in cells, pH regulation	850 g	Activates many enzymes in phosphorylation and dephosphorylation	Neuromuscular, skeletal, hematologic, and cardiac manifestations; rickets, osteomalacia	Meat, poultry, fish, eggs, milk, milk products, nuts, legumes, grains, cereals	700 mg, 19+ years
Sulfur	Component of sulfur-containing amino acids, lipoic acid, and two vitamins (thiamin, biotin)	175 g		Unknown	Protein foods: meat, poultry, fish, eggs, milk, cheese, legumes, nuts	Not established

Note: Abbreviations: ATP, adenosine triphosphate; ADP, adenosine diphosphate.
[a]The electrolyte macrominerals (sodium, chloride, and potassium) are discussed in Chapter 12.

about 99% of the body's calcium. The other 1% is distributed in intra- and extracellular fluids. Within body fluids, calcium is found in its ionic form, Ca^{2+}.

Sources

The best food sources of calcium include dairy products, especially milk, cheese, and yogurt, and selected seafood, such as salmon and sardines (with bones), clams, and oysters. Milk and yogurt, depending on type, typically provide between 200 and 400 mg of calcium/cup, and cheeses generally provide 100 to 200 mg of calcium/oz. Seafoods such as sardines (with bones) contain up to 400 mg of calcium per 3-oz portion. Selected vegetables, such as turnip and mustard greens, broccoli, cauliflower, and kale also provide relatively large amounts of calcium, ranging from about 30 to 80 mg per half-cup cooked serving. Legumes and legume products, especially tofu (soybean curd), and nuts provide some calcium. One cup of cooked kidney, pinto, or navy beans contains 64, 79, or 126 mg of calcium, respectively. Almonds provide about 75 mg of calcium per ounce, while walnuts contain 28 mg, pecans 20 mg, and peanuts 15 mg of calcium/ounce. The calcium content of tofu ranges from about 125 to 227 mg per half cup depending on type of tofu and brand. Other excellent food sources of calcium include those fortified with it, such as fruit juices (especially orange juice, which provides up to about 350 mg of calcium/8 fl oz) and breads. The Daily Value for calcium, which is used on food and supplement labels, is 1,000 mg. Thus, one-half cup of low-fat cottage cheese providing 10% of the Daily Value contains 100 mg of calcium.

In contrast to the aforementioned foods, meats and grains (not fortified) are relatively poor sources of calcium. Some vegetables such as spinach, rhubarb, and Swiss chard also are poor sources because they contain large amounts of oxalic acid, which binds calcium and inhibits its absorption, as discussed in the "Factors Influencing Absorption" section.

Several different calcium supplements are available, including calcium carbonate, calcium citrate, calcium acetate, calcium lactate, calcium gluconate, and calcium monophosphate. The two most widely available supplements contain calcium citrate and calcium carbonate. Calcium citrate is beneficial for those with limited gastric acid production (as may occur in older individuals) and, unlike most other supplements, can be ingested without food. Calcium carbonate is a relatively inexpensive form, but its use is often associated with gastrointestinal side effects such as constipation, gas, and/or bloating. Calcium carbonate contains about 40% calcium by weight. Because the percentage of calcium by weight in different supplements varies, different amounts of supplements must be consumed to obtain a specific amount of calcium. For example, to obtain 500 mg of calcium from calcium carbonate, 1.26 g would need to be ingested, whereas a person would need to ingest 5.49 g of calcium gluconate, 3.53 g of calcium lactate, 2.37 g of calcium citrate, or 2.16 g of calcium acetate. Sources of calcium used for supplements, however, also should be considered. For example, calcium carbonate from fossilized oyster shell or dolomite may be contaminated with aluminum and lead and should not be used. Bone meal preparations may also contain lead and should be avoided.

Digestion, Absorption, and Transport

Digestion

Calcium is present in foods and dietary supplements as relatively insoluble salts. Calcium can be solubilized (to exist as free Ca^{2+}) from most calcium salts in about 1 hour at an acidic pH (as occurs in the stomach). Solubilization does not necessarily ensure better absorption, however, because free calcium can bind to other dietary constituents, limiting its bioavailability, as discussed in the "Factors Influencing Absorption" section.

Absorption

Calcium absorption in the small intestine is thought to involve two main transport systems:

- saturable, carrier-mediated, active transport
- diffusion

Two other modes of absorption in the small intestine have been proposed but are not fully elucidated and accepted at this time.

The main transport system for calcium operates primarily in the duodenum and proximal jejunum, is saturable (at low to moderate calcium intakes), requires energy, and is regulated by calcitriol (the active form of vitamin D). At a calcium intake of about 400 to 500 mg/meal, this system accounts for more than 60% of total calcium absorption in the small intestine [1]. Absorption of calcium from the lumen of the gastrointestinal tract across the enterocyte's brush border membrane, then across the cytosol of the enterocyte and into the plasma using this system requires: a vitamin D–dependent membrane channel protein called transient receptor potential (TRP) vanilloid (V)6 (abbreviated TRPV6 but also called calcium transporter 1 or CaT1); a vitamin D–dependent cytosolic binding protein called calbindin D9k that shuttles the calcium across the cell cytosol; and a vitamin D–dependent calcium-ATPase pump on the luminal side (basolateral membrane) of the enterocyte to release the calcium into the plasma. (The expression of both TRPV6 and calbindin decline with age; this decline accounts in part for the higher calcium intake recommendations for older individuals.)

The second major route for calcium absorption is paracellular diffusion, a passive, nonsaturable, nonregulated process (no carriers or energy needed) that is concentration dependent and occurs throughout the small intestine but mostly in the jejunum and ileum. Paracellular absorption is absorption that occurs between cells, rather than through them. The paracellular process allows the movement of calcium through normally very tight junctions between the intestinal cells. This transport occurs typically when high calcium concentrations are present in the lumen, and thus a gradient of calcium concentrations exists between the lumen and the basolateral side of the enterocyte. Increases in the concentration of intracellular calcium ions are thought to mediate the process through a series of reactions to ultimately "open" the junctions between cells to facilitate calcium absorption. Additionally, vitamin D has been shown to enhance the expression of genes that code for selected transmembrane proteins, called claudins, which have been shown to be essential for paracellular intestinal calcium absorption [2]. Fructose oligosaccharides, inulin, and other nondigestible saccharides also have been shown to enhance paracellular calcium absorption [3].

Two other systems thought to perhaps contribute in a minor capacity to calcium absorption in the small intestine are vesicular transport and transcaltachia. Vesicular transport involves endocytosis of calcium across the intestinal cell's brush border membrane, after which the calcium is sequestered in vesicles. These vesicles merge with lysosomes to facilitate the release of calcium into the cell cytosol. Further details of this mechanism are not clear at this time. Transcaltachia occurs within minutes of calcitriol binding to receptors on an enterocyte's basolateral membrane. While this mechanism has not been fully elucidated, a vitamin D–binding protein receptor called membrane-associated rapid response steroid-binding protein (MARRS) is thought to be involved in transcaltachia [1].

A final minor contributor to calcium absorption occurs in the large intestine, where bacteria may release calcium that is bound to some fermentable fibers such as pectins. About 4% to 10% (or ~8 mg) of dietary calcium is absorbed by the colon each day. This amount, however, may be higher in people who absorb less calcium in the small intestine.

Overall, calcium absorption in adults averages about 25% to 30%. Calcium absorption from calcium supplements (providing 250 mg of calcium) varies from about 27% to 39%, depending upon the specific calcium salt used in the supplement, the amount of calcium ingested, and whether it is consumed under fasting conditions or with food; ingestion with food generally enhances absorption. Absorption also tends to be higher when calcium is consumed in amounts less than 500 mg. Relative to calcium absorption from milk as a reference and under fasting conditions, calcium absorption from calcium lactate exceeded that from milk, while absorption

from calcium carbonate, citrate, and succinate was similar to milk [4]. Relative to calcium absorption from milk as a reference and testing with coingestion of a meal, calcium absorption from calcium carbonate, lactate, citrate malate, and gluconate was similar to milk; in contrast, calcium absorption from tricalcium phosphate was well below that from milk [4]. In a food/supplement matrix, calcium absorption from calcium citrate malate and calcium sulfate appears to be best [4].

Factors Influencing Absorption While adequate vitamin D status is important to promote calcium absorption, several situations or conditions within the gastrointestinal tract may directly enhance or inhibit intestinal calcium absorption (Table 11.2). Diets that are low in calcium (<400 mg) lead to enhanced calcium absorption because of the resulting drop (below the lower limit of normal) in plasma calcium concentrations and increase in parathyroid hormone (PTH) secretion. The increased serum PTH in turn stimulates calcitriol synthesis and can increase calcium absorption by about 10%. Growth, pregnancy, and lactation also improve absorption. (Note that requirements are also increased in these situations.) Infants and young children, for example, absorb up to about 60% of dietary calcium, in contrast to adults, who absorb up to about 30%. With aging and with estrogen deficiency in females, calcium absorption diminishes to about 15% to 20% because of decreased calcitriol production and its diminished effects on TRPV6 channels.

Dietary components also can enhance calcium absorption. Ingesting food or lactose along with the calcium source appears to improve overall calcium absorption, possibly by improving solubility. The effects of lactose on calcium diffusion, especially in the ileum, are thought to be more pronounced in infants than in adults. Other sugars, sugar alcohols (such as xylitol), and protein also may enhance calcium absorption and decrease its secretion into the gastrointestinal tract.

Several dietary components diminish calcium absorption or promote its secretion from the blood back

Table 11.2 Interactions between Calcium and Selected Nutrients/Substances

Nutrients/Substances Enhancing Calcium Absorption	Nutrients/Substances Inhibiting Calcium Absorption
Vitamin D	Fiber
Sugars and sugar alcohols	Phytic acid
Protein	Oxalic acid
	Excessive divalent cations (Zn, Mg)
	Unabsorbed fatty acids

Nutrients Enhancing Urinary Calcium Excretion	Nutrients Whose Absorption May Be Inhibited by Excessive Calcium
Sodium	Phosphorus
Protein	Iron
Caffeine	Fatty acids

into the gastrointestinal tract. Ingestion of caffeine, for example, increases the secretion of calcium into the gut, thereby leading to increased endogenous fecal calcium losses.

Phytic acid (also called phytate or inositol hexaphosphate; shown later in Figure 11.7), found in whole-grain breads, seeds, and legumes, inhibits calcium absorption. Specifically, phytic acid binds calcium and decreases its availability, especially when present in a phytic acid:calcium molar ratio > 0.2. Some fibers, such as wheat bran, also may bind to calcium and decrease its absorption. However, most individuals in the United States do not consume enough phytic acid and fiber to profoundly affect calcium absorption.

Calcium absorption in the intestine is also inhibited by the presence of oxalic acid (Figure 11.2), which chelates the ionized calcium, has a very low solubility (<0.1 mmol/L; optimal solubility is thought to range from about 0.1 to 10.0 mmol/L), and increases fecal calcium excretion. Oxalic acid (oxalate) is found in a variety of vegetables (e.g., spinach, rhubarb, Swiss chard, beets, celery, eggplant, greens, okra, squash), fruits (e.g., currants, strawberries, blackberries, blueberries, gooseberries), nuts (pecans, peanuts), and beverages (tea, Ovaltine, cocoa), among other foods.

Divalent cations such as magnesium and zinc can interact with calcium to inhibit calcium absorption. For example, magnesium and calcium compete with each other for intestinal absorption whenever an excess of either is present in the gastrointestinal tract. Similarly, zinc and calcium may interact to diminish calcium absorption, especially when the diet is low in calcium and contains an excess of zinc in the form of a supplement.

Unabsorbed dietary fatty acids found in significant quantities in the gastrointestinal tract associated with steatorrhea (>7 g of fecal fat per day) can interfere with calcium absorption by forming insoluble calcium "soaps" (calcium–fatty acid complexes) in the lumen of the small intestine. These calcium soaps cannot be absorbed and are excreted in the feces. Steatorrhea is a problem associated with some gastrointestinal tract disorders, such as inflammatory bowel diseases, as well as with disorders affecting the pancreas, such as pancreatitis and cystic fibrosis.

Finally, individuals taking medications known as proton pump inhibitors (e.g., Prilosec [omeprazole], Prevacid [lansoprazole], Nexium [esomeprazole]; often used to treat gastroesophageal reflux disease or ulcers) may exhibit diminished calcium absorption due to insufficient production of gastric acid needed to solubilize the calcium in the stomach.

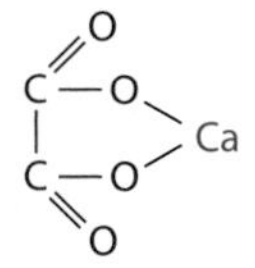

Transport

Calcium is transported in the blood in three forms. Some calcium (~40%) is bound to proteins, mainly albumin and prealbumin. Some calcium (up to ~10%) is complexed with sulfate, phosphate, or citrate. About 50% of calcium is found free (ionized) in the blood. From the blood, most calcium is deposited in bone, which serves as a reservoir should blood calcium concentrations decrease below the lower limit of normal. Figure 11.3 provides an overview of calcium digestion, absorption, and transport.

Regulation of Calcium Concentrations Calcium concentrations are tightly controlled both intracellularly and extracellularly. In the blood plasma/serum (i.e., extracellular), calcium concentrations between about 8.5 and 10.5 mg/dL (2.12–2.63 mmol/L) are maintained.

Extracellular Calcium Concentration Regulation The three main hormones involved in calcium homeostasis in the blood serum/plasma are PTH, calcitriol, and calcitonin. This section describes each of these hormones and their actions involving calcium; calcitriol and PTH are discussed primarily together. An overview of calcium regulation is shown in Figure 11.4.

- PTH is secreted from the chief cells of the parathyroid gland in response to low plasma concentrations of calcium (i.e., <8.5 mg/dL) or, to a lesser extent, magnesium. Calcium-sensing receptors (CaR) found on the parathyroid gland (as well as the kidney tubular cells) monitor calcium and magnesium concentrations in the blood. Increased concentrations of calcium and magnesium appear to initiate a conformational change in an exterior portion of the receptor that, through a second messenger, signals the parathyroid gland to diminish PTH release. When serum calcium concentrations drop below the lower limit of normal (~8.5 mg/dL), the parathyroid gland releases PTH into the blood.

- PTH increases extracellular fluid (blood plasma/serum) calcium concentrations through interactions with the kidney and bone. In the kidney, PTH increases the synthesis of calcitriol from 25-OH vitamin D. Calcitriol production results in increased renal tubular reabsorption of calcium by promoting the synthesis of calbindin D28k, a vitamin D–dependent calcium transporter found in the kidneys. In bone, PTH interacts with receptors on osteoblasts (bone-building cells). Calcitriol also may be involved in this process. The osteoblasts produce two proteins, macrophage colony stimulating factor and receptor activator of nuclear

Figure 11.2 The binding of calcium by oxalic acid.

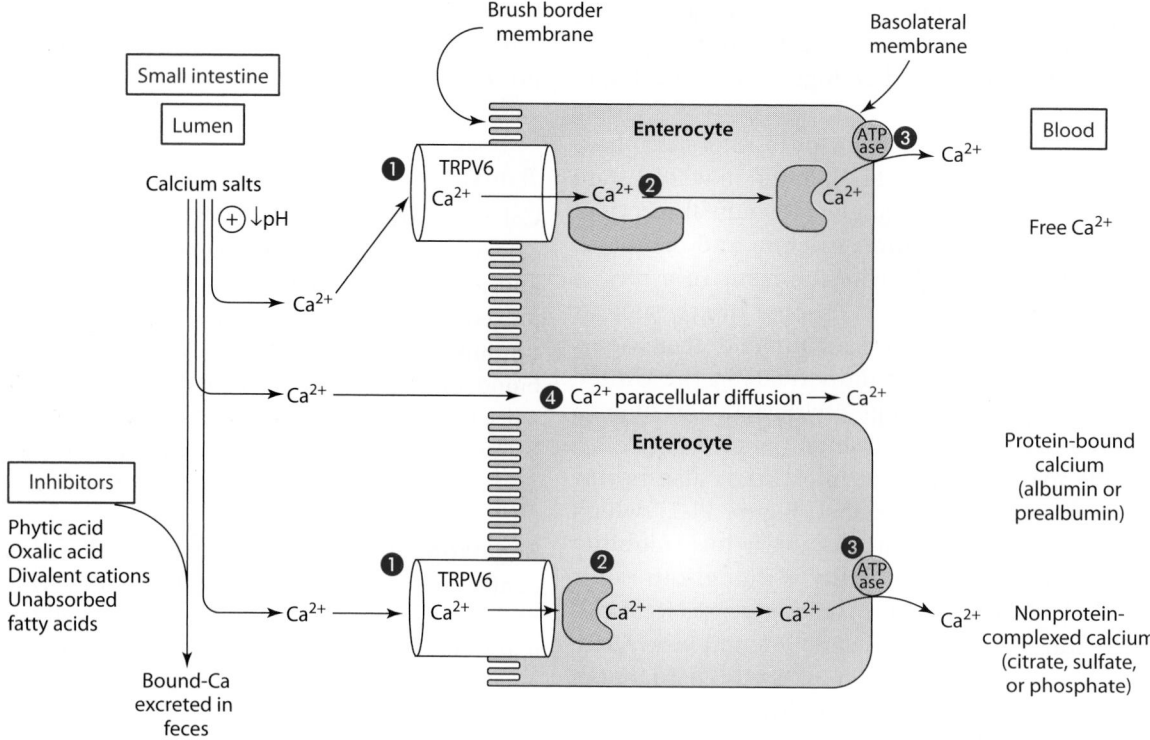

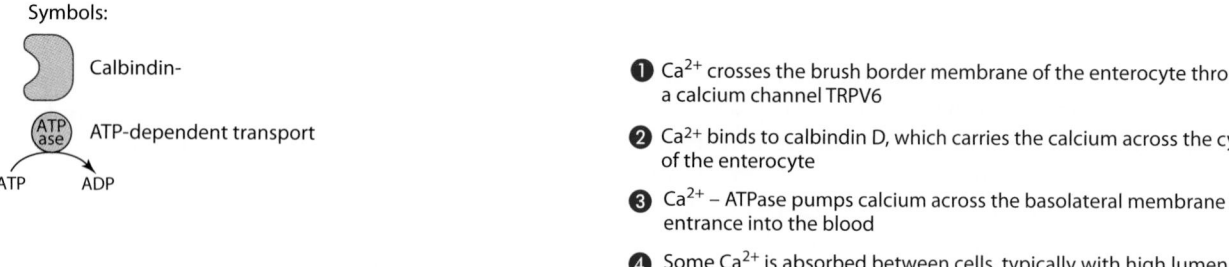

Figure 11.3 Calcium digestion, absorption, and transport.

factor κ B ligand (RANKL), which bind to RANK receptors on osteoclast precursor cells to stimulate their proliferation and differentiation into osteoclasts (bone-breaking cells). Osteoclasts release proteases and acids that degrade (resorb) bone, and promote the release of calcium from the bone into the blood.

● Calcitriol acts in the intestine in multiple ways to improve calcium absorption. Calcitriol interacts with nuclear vitamin D receptors to induce the transcription of the gene that codes for calbindin D9k, which functions as a calcium-binding protein to promote calcium transport through the cytosol of the enterocyte. Calcitriol also enhances calcium absorption at the brush border membrane by increasing TRPV6 channels and at the basolateral membrane by increasing calcium-ATPase pumps. The vitamin also appears to facilitate paracellular absorption by promoting the synthesis of specific claudin proteins. Thus, the net effect of these actions by PTH and calcitriol is to increase serum calcium concentrations into the normal range.

● Calcitonin, synthesized in the parafollicular (also called C) cells of the thyroid gland, functions in opposition to PTH and calcitriol to lower serum calcium concentrations should they rise above the upper end of the normal range (>10.5 mg/dL). Calcitonin suppresses PTH production and release, and inhibits the activity of osteoclasts to prevent mobilization of Ca^{2+} from bone. Table 11.3 summarizes the actions of parathyroid hormone, vitamin D, and calcitonin.

Intracellular Calcium Concentration Regulation Low free Ca^{2+} concentrations (100 nmol/L, or approximately 0.0001 times the concentration in the extracellular fluid) are maintained within the cytosol of cells. In response to cell activation by depolarization, neurotransmitters, or hormones, calcium enters the cytosol of cells either directly from extracellular sites through channels (such as voltage-dependent slow channels, ligand-gated channels, or stretch-activated channels) or by release from intracellular sites such as the endoplasmic (or sarcoplasmic)

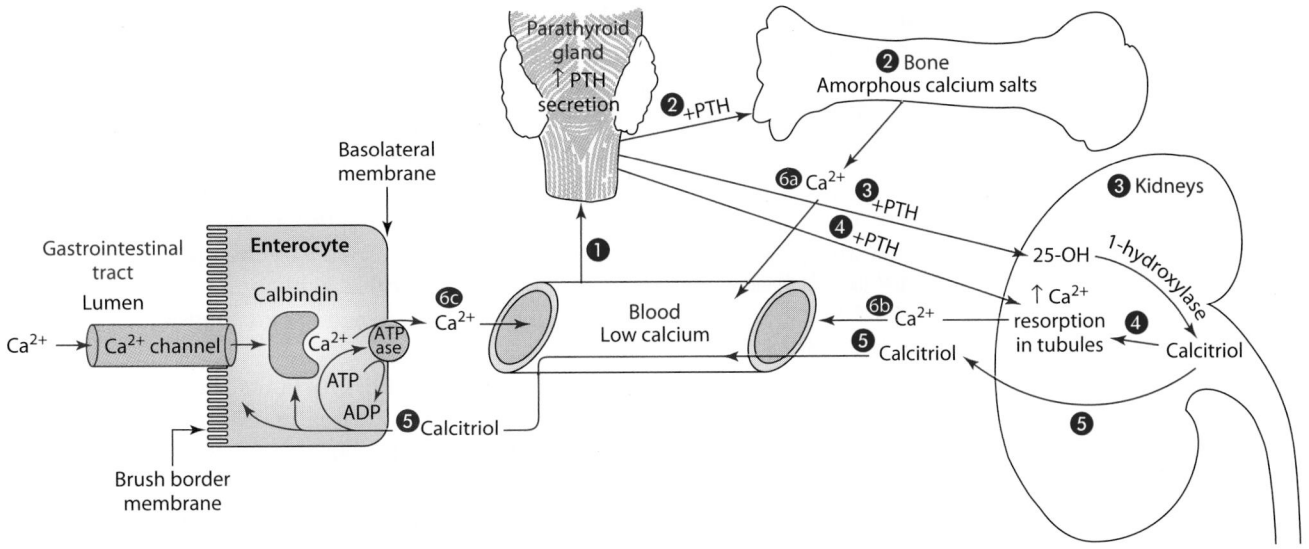

① Low blood calcium signals the parathyroid gland to release parathyroid hormone (PTH) into the blood.

② PTH binds to bone cell receptors and triggers the resorption or breakdown of bone mineral for the release of calcium into the blood.

③ PTH acts on the kidneys to synthesize the active form of vitamin D, calcitriol.

④ PTH and calcitriol promote the reabsorption of calcium from the kidney and into the blood.

⑤ Calcitriol leaves the kidney and travels to the intestine, where it promotes calcium absorption across the brush border membrane, its transport in the cell cytosol, and egress into the blood.

⑥ Calcium enters the blood **ⓐ** after release from bone, **ⓑ** after release from kidneys, and **ⓒ** after absorption from intestinal cells.

Figure 11.4 An overview of blood calcium regulation by parathyroid hormone (PTH) and calcitriol (also called 1,25(OH)$_2$ vitamin D) in response to low blood calcium concentrations.

Table 11.3 A Summary of the Effects of Parathyroid Hormone (PTH), Calcitriol, and Calcitonin on Calcium Balance

	PTH	Calcitriol	Calcitonin
Serum calcium	↑	↑	↓
Bone calcium	↓	*	↑
Renal calcium reabsorption	↑	↑	↓
Intestinal calcium absorption	↑	↑	No effect

*Works with PTH

reticulum and the mitochondria, among other organelles. This efflux of organelle-sequestered calcium into the cytosol typically requires a Ca^{2+}-ATPase pump or release channel (such as the ryanodine receptor of the sarcoplasmic reticulum in skeletal muscle).

Raising the concentration of cytosolic Ca^{2+} allows Ca^{2+} to carry out its cellular functions. Yet, following the release of Ca^{2+} into the cytosol, the concentration of calcium is returned within a short time period to its normal level. To achieve its resting concentration, calcium is exported from cells by ATP-dependent pumps. The main system responsible for releasing calcium from cells is the $Ca^{2+}/3Na^+$ exchanger, which has low affinity but exhibits a high capacity for calcium. In contrast, the $Ca^{2+}/2H^+$ (proton)-ATPase pump, which exhibits high affinity but

a low capacity for calcium, extrudes calcium in exchange for two hydrogen ions (protons); it is thought to account for minor adjustments needed in cellular calcium concentrations. In addition to being pumped out of the cell, calcium can be sequestered (stored/re-stored) in cellular organelles such as the mitochondria, endoplasmic (or sarcoplasmic) reticulum, nucleus, and vesicles. This function is performed by Ca^{2+}-ATPases, which pump Ca^{2+} from the cytosol into the organelles for storage until needed by the cell. Within organelles, calcium binds to proteins (such as calsequestrin in the sarcoplasmic reticulum) or complexes with phosphate (as in the mitochondrion). Some of the ATPases responsible for maintaining calcium concentrations are shown later in Figure 11.6.

Functions and Mechanisms of Action

Calcium plays several vital roles in the body, including skeleton (bone) formation, nerve transmission, muscle contraction, blood clot formation, and signal transduction/serving as a messenger. Of these roles, calcium's most widely known function is in the mineralization of bone, of which there are two main types: cortical and trabecular. Most bones possess an outer layer of cortical bone that surrounds trabecular bone. Some bones also contain a cavity for bone marrow. Some characteristics of cortical and trabecular bone are listed hereafter:

Cortical Bone	Trabecular Bone
• is compact or dense	• has a spongy appearance
• represents about 75–80% of total bone in the body	• represents about 20% to 25% of total bone in the body
• consists of layers of mineralized protein (mostly type I collagen)	• consists of an interconnected system of mineralized proteins (mostly type I collagen)
• is found mainly on the surfaces of all bones and the shaft of long bones of the limbs	• is found in relatively high concentrations in the axial skeleton (vertebrae and pelvic region) and the ends of long bones

Trabecular bone is more active metabolically, with a high turnover rate, and thus can be more rapidly depleted of calcium with poor calcium intake than is cortical bone; consequently, it is more susceptible to osteoporosis, as discussed in the Perspective at the end of this chapter.

Bone Mineralization

Approximately 99% of total body calcium is found in teeth and bones, both cortical and trabecular. About 50% to 66% of the weight of bones is minerals, with the remaining 34% to 50% being water, ground substance (described later in this chapter), and protein. Minerals, or the mostly inorganic portion of bone, consist largely of calcium and phosphorus but also include fluoride, magnesium, potassium, sodium, and strontium. Some of these minerals along with hydroxyl groups make up **hydroxyapatite,** a crystal latticelike substance found bound to proteins and ground substance. Carbonate is also found in bone, usually associated with calcium, potassium, and sodium.

The organic parts of the bone contain several proteins and ground substance, which together form the bone matrix or scaffolding (also called the extracellular matrix). Proteins in bone include primarily type I collagen (about 85–90% of proteins), with smaller amounts of several other proteins including osteonectin, osteopontin, bone sialoprotein, osteocalcin (also called bone Gla protein), and matrix Gla protein. Of these noncollagenous proteins, osteonectin, a phosphoprotein, is the most abundant and binds both calcium and collagen. Osteopontin binds to both hydroxyapatite and bone cells. Osteocalcin and matrix Gla protein, which are dependent on vitamin K for carboxylation of their glutamic acid residues, function in calcium and hydroxyapatite binding and mineral deposition. The synthesis of these two proteins is enhanced by calcitriol. Bone sialoprotein promotes hydroxyapatite crystal nucleation. Calcium generally facilitates interactions between proteins and between proteins and phospholipids in bone cell membranes to strengthen bone.

In addition to protein, the bone matrix is made up of ground substance, which consists mostly of glycoproteins and proteoglycans. Glycoproteins are composed of proteins covalently bound to typically short chains of carbohydrate. Proteoglycans are similar to glycoproteins but typically are larger, consisting of a core protein covalently conjugated to one or more glycosaminoglycans (made up of long chains of repeating disaccharides). It is the glycosaminoglycan portion of the proteoglycan that interacts with matrix proteins to enhance bone strength and resilience. Hyaluronic acid and chondroitin sulfate are two glycosaminoglycans associated with bone and cartilage.

Proteins and ground substance are synthesized by bone cells. Among the three main types of bone cells (osteoblasts, osteocytes, and osteoclasts), osteoblasts, which originate from the bone marrow, are the bone-building cells. Under the influence of PTH, calcitriol, and estrogen, among other hormones, osteoblasts secrete collagen and other proteins as well as ground substance—that is, the bone matrix/extracellular matrix surrounding the bone cells that becomes mineralized over time. As the osteoblasts secrete the proteins and ground substance and mineralization occurs, the osteoblasts become embedded in the protein and ground substance matrix. With further embedding in the matrix, some osteoblasts undergo apoptosis and others undergo differentiation and morphological changes to become osteocytes. Osteocytes—that is, osteoblasts that have been incorporated into bone matrix—are important to maintaining the integrity of the surrounding bone. Other osteoblasts differentiate into another cell type called lining cells. Lining cells, which have a relatively flat shape, form a membrane (called the periosteum) that covers the bone surface and regulate the flux of minerals into and out of bone.

During mineralization, calcium, phosphorus, magnesium, and other minerals enter bone fluid from blood and then attach to bone proteins and ground substance. Phosphorus is thought to be laid down first; calcium is thought to then bind to the phosphorus. Calcium is initially present as Ca^{2+} and then as amorphous (noncrystal or poorly crystalline) calcium forms, such as $Ca_3(PO_4)_2$, that are deposited between collagen and noncollagen proteins and ground substance. Other amorphous forms of minerals in bone include carbonate bound to calcium, phosphorus, or magnesium, and, for example, $Ca_3(PO_4)_2$ (tricalcium phosphate), $Mg_3(PO_4)_2$ (trimagnesium phosphate), and $CaHPO_4 \cdot 2H_2O$ (brushite). These salts ultimately are converted to more crystalline compounds such as $Ca_8H_2(PO_4)_6 \cdot 5H_2O$ (octacalcium phosphate) and hydroxyapatite crystals, $Ca_{10}(PO_4)_6(OH)_2$. Osteoblasts are thought to secrete onto the bone surface substances that enhance the precipitation or deposition of calcium and other minerals. These substances also break down substances released by osteoclasts that prevent bone mineralization. Whether osteoblasts facilitate the movement of calcium and other minerals from the blood to the bone surface is unclear. The process of calcification and mineralization of the bone matrix has yet to be clearly delineated.

Osteoclasts, another type of bone cell, are large, multinucleated (with about 2 to 10 nuclei) cells that resorb (break down) previously made bone. These cells attach onto a selected area on the bone surface and start the degradation process. Resorption is thought to begin when two proteins, macrophage colony stimulating factor (M-CSF) and receptor activator of nuclear factor κ B ligand (RANKL), are produced by osteoblasts. These proteins in turn bind to RANK receptors on osteoclast precursor cells to stimulate their proliferation, differentiation, and fusion to produce mature osteoclasts. To regulate the process, osteoblasts also produce osteoprotegerin, a protein that binds to RANKL to prevent it from binding to receptors on osteoclastic cells. Thus, osteoprotegerin inhibits osteoclast differentiation and activity. Osteoclasts contain lysosomes that release acids (such as citric and lactic acids); bone resorption, in fact, is initiated by the release of hydrochloric acid. The acids function to dissolve amorphous mineral complexes. Lysosomes also release enzymes such as cathepsin K, matrix metalloproteinases, and hydrolases that break down the bone protein matrix. Osteoclasts respond to PTH, calcitriol, and calcitonin, among other hormones and signaling compounds. Osteoclasts play an important role in increasing blood calcium concentrations to a normal level in times of inadequate calcium intake and contribute to bone fragility and osteoporosis if not balanced by adequate bone formation.

In children and adolescents, skeletal turnover occurs such that formation of bone exceeds resorption of bone. Skeletal turnover continues into adulthood, with peak bone mass occurring in early adulthood. During the fifth decade, bone mass begins to decline. Although the need for calcium in bone modeling is continuous, its greatest benefits in promoting the formation of a sturdy skeletal mass occur during linear bone growth and the years immediately following.

Other Roles

The small amount (1%) of body calcium that is nonosseous (not associated with bone) is found both intracellularly within organelles such as the mitochondria, endoplasmic reticulum (sarcoplasmic reticulum in muscle), nucleus, and vesicles and extracellularly in the blood, lymph, and body fluids. Of the calcium in the blood plasma, about 50% is ionized. This ionized calcium is active, which means that the numerous regulatory functions of calcium are performed by < 0.5% of the total body calcium.

Free ionized calcium is essential for a number of processes, a few of which will be briefly reviewed. Calcium is required for blood clotting. Specifically, calcium is needed for clot formation, which involves the binding of

cell membrane phospholipids with Gla residues of specific blood clotting proteins (see Chapter 10).

Skeletal muscle contraction necessitates increased intracellular calcium concentrations, which are typically achieved by calcium secretion through calcium release channels in the membranes of intracellular storage sites such as the sarcoplasmic reticulum. The released calcium then binds to troponin C, which has four calcium binding sites. The binding of Ca^{2+} to troponin C results in a conformational change in the protein and alters interactions with other proteins to enable an interaction between actin and myosin, resulting in muscle contraction. Once the plasma membrane repolarizes, calcium is pumped back into cisternae of the sarcoplasmic reticulum via a Ca^{2+}-ATPase and bound to calsequestrin, and myosin and actin no longer interact to sustain muscle contraction. Visceral smooth muscle contraction also requires increased intracellular calcium concentrations; however, the calcium influx into the visceral smooth muscle cell's cytosol comes from the extracellular fluid through gated channels rather than from intracellular organelles.

Membrane permeability is affected by calcium, which may bind to both membrane proteins and phospholipids. Changes in membrane fluidity occur with calcium-protein interactions that affect protein cross-linking. Enhanced membrane rigidity and electrical resistance may result from calcium's interaction with membrane phospholipids.

Ion channels (porelike protein structures in membranes) are involved in the generation of action potentials in nerve cells. Various neurotransmitters interact with receptors on nerve cells to open ion channels, especially calcium and sodium channels. Calcium, for example, can enter the nerve ending and trigger the release of acetylcholine. The acetylcholine in turn diffuses to and binds to receptors to trigger another serious of events, ultimately including depolarization to generate an action potential.

In many body cells, calcium carries out its functions in association with various binding proteins. Calmodulin, a cytosolic calcium-binding protein operative in most body cells, consists of two similar globular lobes (each with two Ca^{2+}-binding sites) joined by a long helix. The binding of Ca^{2+} activates calmodulin by changing its conformation (Figure 11.5); this conformational change allows the protein to stimulate or interact with a variety of enzymes, such as:

- calcineurin, a phosphatase that dephosphorylates and inactivates calcium channels
- myosin light-chain kinase, which phosphorylates the light chain of myosin and, following a sequence of events, causes smooth muscle contraction
- phosphorylase kinase, which activates phosphorylase (the enzyme responsible for glycogenolysis, i.e., degrading glycogen to glucose-1-PO_4)
- calcium calmodulin kinases, of which there are several, with several functions

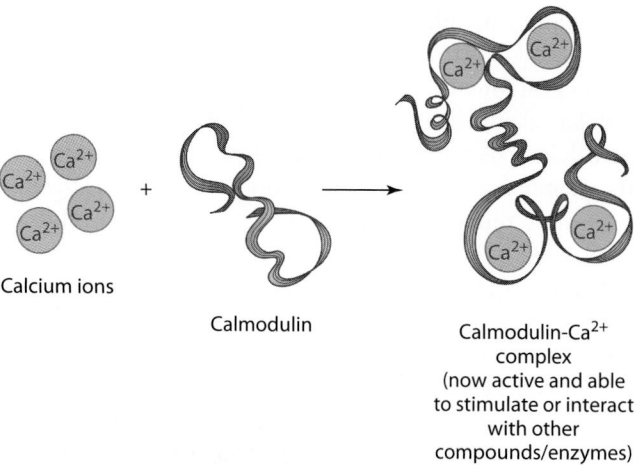

Figure 11.5 Schematic representation of the structural change that occurs in calmodulin following the binding to calcium (Ca^{2+}) ions.

Calcium, either alone or as part of calmodulin or other calcium-binding proteins, acts as an important messenger within many cells. For example, increased intracellular concentrations of Ca^{2+} can activate phospholipase A_2, which hydrolyzes fatty acids like arachidonic acid from phospholipids in cell membranes. The newly released arachidonic acid can in turn be metabolized to form thromboxanes, prostaglandins, or leukotrienes. Phosphodiesterase, which hydrolyzes cyclic AMP (cAMP) to 5′ AMP, is also dependent on Ca^{2+}. Cyclic AMP, formed from ATP by adenylate cyclase, activates protein kinases, thereby influencing intermediary metabolism. Calcium also activates protein kinase C, which is involved in a number of cellular processes such as phosphorylating enzymes to activate or inactivate metabolic pathways. Some other enzymes that may be affected either directly by increased free cytosolic Ca^{2+} or through increases in protein-bound Ca^{2+} are listed in Table 11.4. Figure 11.6 shows some of calcium's intracellular actions and mechanisms by which cytosolic calcium concentrations are maintained. Clearly, calcium affects a wide range of enzymes and cellular processes in the body.

Interactions with Other Nutrients

Nutrients or substances that inhibit or enhance calcium absorption were discussed in the section on calcium

Table 11.4 Selected Enzymes Regulated by Calcium and/or Calmodulin

Adenylate cyclase	Myosin kinase
Ca-dependent protein kinase	NAD kinase
Ca/Mg-ATPase	Nitric oxide synthase
Ca/phospholipid-dependent protein kinase	Phospholipase A_2
Cyclic nucleotide phosphodiesterase	Phosphorylase kinase
Glycerol-3-phosphate dehydrogenase	Pyruvate carboxylase
Glycogen synthase	Pyruvate dehydrogenase
Guanylate cyclase	Pyruvate kinase

absorption. Additional interactions (Table 11.2) related to the effects of calcium on phosphorus, iron, and fatty acids are addressed here.

Ingestion of large amounts of calcium with a phosphorus-containing meal inhibits phosphorus absorption. The use of calcium supplements (2–3 g per day, or in a calcium to phosphorus ratio >3:1) to inhibit intestinal phosphorus absorption has thus often been employed in the medical management of kidney failure, which is associated with elevated plasma phosphorus concentrations. This strategy, however, is used less often than in the past due to possible calcium phosphate deposition in soft tissues.

Calcium from dietary sources as well as from various supplements (especially in doses of 800 mg or more) has been shown in several studies to decrease primarily nonheme (but also heme) iron absorption [5]. The inhibitory effect, however, appears to be of short duration, and adaptation results such that iron status is not negatively impacted [6]. Calcium is thought to transiently inhibit iron absorption by causing the iron transporter ferroportin to relocate temporarily from the enterocyte's basolateral membrane to the cytosol, although effects on DMT1 (which transports iron across the brush border membrane) availability and changes in membrane fluidity also may play roles [6].

Calcium also diminishes the absorption of fatty acids and thus influences serum lipid concentrations and bile's fatty acid profile. Calcium (especially when consumed in gram amounts with a meal) may inhibit bile acid reabsorption in the ileum and promote increased fecal bile acid excretion. This situation necessitates the use of body cholesterol for the synthesis of new bile to replace what was excreted in the feces. Calcium also may directly bind the fatty acids in the small intestine to form insoluble soaps that are excreted in the feces. These interactions between calcium (observed with daily intakes of about 1.2 to 3 g) and fatty acids can reduce serum concentrations of total and low-density lipoprotein cholesterol and thus may decrease the risk for heart disease. Calcium supplementation of 2 or 3 g daily also may decrease chenodeoxycholate concentrations in bile and the lithocholate:deoxycholate ratio in the feces. Such changes are favorable to the colonic environment and may help prevent colon cancer.

Excretion

Calcium is excreted in the urine and feces, although up to about 182 mg (average, 60 mg) may be lost daily from the skin, especially with extreme sweating [7]. Of the calcium that is filtered, most is reabsorbed by the kidneys such that urinary calcium losses range from about 100 to 240 mg (2.5–6 mmol) per day, with an average of about 170 mg. Most of the filtered calcium is reabsorbed passively in

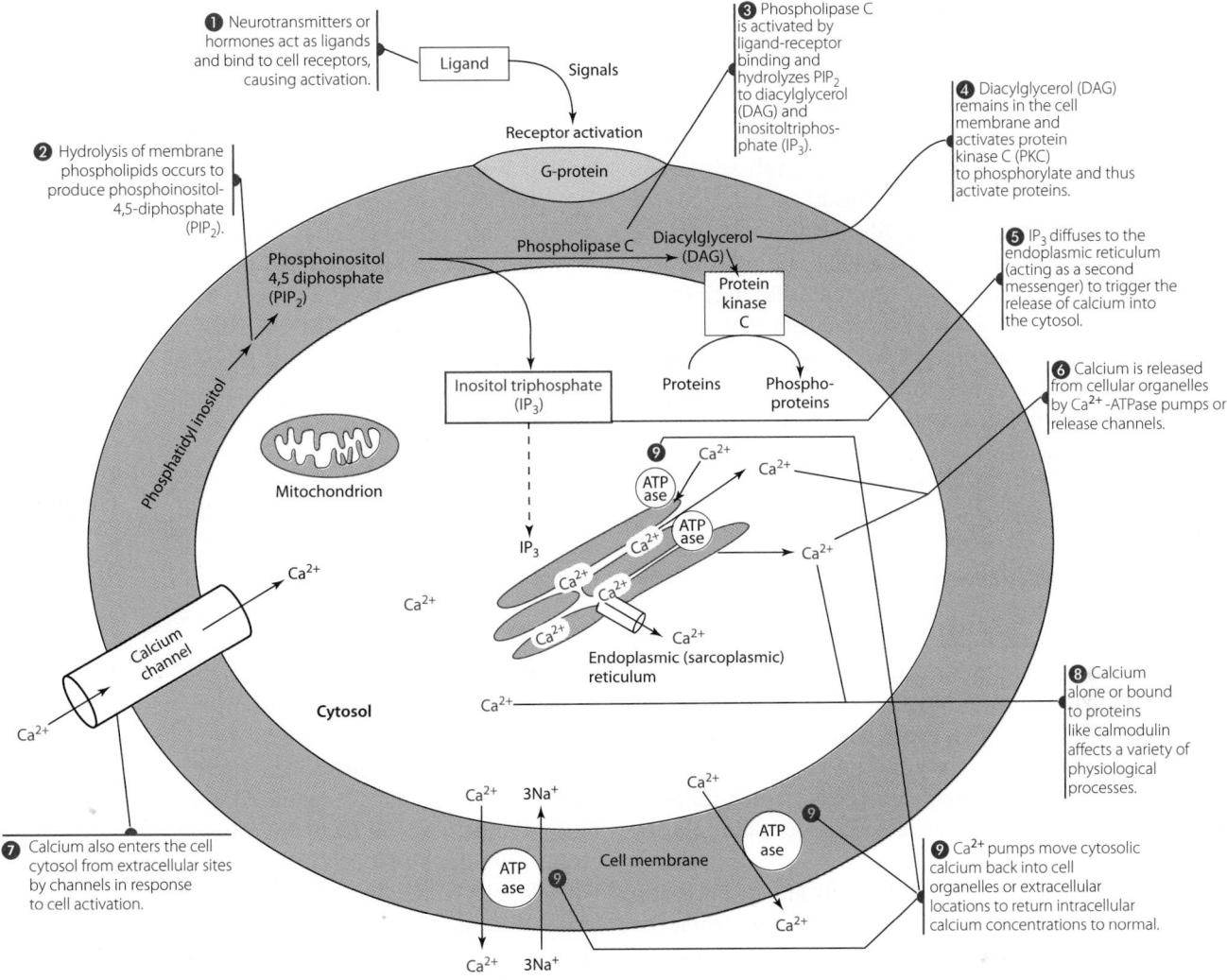

Figure 11.6 Some of calcium's intracellular actions and mechanisms by which cytosolic calcium concentrations are maintained.

the proximal tubule. In the ascending loop of Henle, calcium-sensing receptors respond to serum calcium concentrations and adjust active reabsorption accordingly. Transient receptor potential calcium channel vanilloid (TRPV) 5 and calbindin D28k (which are under the influence of calcitriol) regulate active calcium absorption in the distal tubule.

Protein, caffeine, and sodium have been shown to increase urinary calcium excretion. (The effect of phosphorus on calcium excretion appears to be negligible, although it once was thought to be of significance.) Yet, while high intakes of protein may increase urinary calcium excretion, it is thought that protein's ability to enhance calcium absorption and inhibit calcium secretion into the gastrointestinal tract cancel out its promotion of urinary calcium losses. Urinary calcium losses associated with caffeine consumption are small, about 2 to 3 mg calcium loss in the urine per cup of ingested coffee (providing <100 mg of caffeine). Thus, caffeine intake in moderation is not thought to compromise calcium balance as long as

calcium intake is adequate. Urinary sodium and calcium excretion are linked in the proximal renal tubule, as they share a common resorption mechanism. Sodium consumption of 500 mg per day, for example, can increase urinary calcium excretion by about 10 mg per day [8].

Fecal losses of calcium from endogenous sources (the sloughing of mucosal cells and calcium that is not reabsorbed from digestive juices—saliva, gastric juice, pancreatic juice, and bile) range from about 45 to 100 mg (1.12–2.5 mmol) per day.

Recommended Dietary Allowance

In 2010, the Recommended Dietary Allowance (RDA) for calcium was set at 1,000 mg daily for adult men age 19 to 70 years and women age 19 to 50 years, including pregnant and lactating women [9]. For females age 51 years and older and males age 71 years and older, the recommendations for calcium intake are slightly higher at 1,200 mg per day. The inside covers of this book provide additional recommendations for calcium for other age groups.

The U.S. Food and Drug Administration (FDA) has approved some health claims related to calcium. One example claim is "Regular exercise and a healthy diet with enough calcium help teen and young adult white and Asian women maintain good bone health and may reduce the risk of osteoporosis later in life" [10]. Another claim added to the aforementioned statement on foods providing 40% or more of the Daily Value (1,000 mg) states, "Adequate calcium intake is important, but daily intakes above about 2,000 mg are not likely to provide any additional benefit" [10]. Foods citing these claims should not provide more phosphorus than calcium on a weight-for-weight basis [10].

Deficiency

Inadequate calcium intake, poor calcium absorption, excessive calcium losses, or some combination of these factors contribute to calcium deficiency. Individuals with fat malabsorption (which diminishes vitamin D absorption and thus status), immobilization (which promotes calcium loss from bone), decreased gastrointestinal transit time (which diminishes intestinal calcium absorption), and long-term use of thiazide diuretics (which increase urinary calcium excretion) are at risk of developing a calcium deficiency.

Calcium deficiency most profoundly affects bone and muscle. Rickets occurs in infants and children when the amount of calcium accretion per unit of bone matrix (i.e., bone mineralization) is deficient; the condition, however, is more commonly associated with a codeficiency of vitamin D. Low levels of free ionized Ca^{2+} in the blood (hypocalcemia) may result in **tetany**, a condition characterized by intermittent muscle contractions that fail to relax; muscles of the arms and legs (extremities) are usually most affected. Muscle pain, muscle cramps or spasms, and paresthesia (numbness or tingling in the hands and feet) also are common signs of tetany. Convulsions also may occur. A prolonged period of calcium deficiency increases the risk for developing osteoporosis—the loss of bone mass (protein matrix and bone minerals), which causes increased bone fragility and fracture risk. Unfortunately, much of the U.S. population, particularly females over 12 years of age, fails to consume the recommended amount of calcium. Osteoporosis and diet are discussed further in the Perspective at the end of the chapter.

In addition to increasing the risk for osteoporosis, inadequate calcium intake has been associated with hypertension, colon cancer, type 2 diabetes mellitus, and obesity. The Perspective "Macrominerals and Hypertension" at the end of Chapter 12 addresses this first relationship. A protective effect of calcium, alone and in combination with vitamin D, and/or of dairy products,

in reducing the risk for colorectal cancers and/or for the formation of its precursor colorectal adenomas has been reported in a few studies and meta-analyses [11–14]. In most of these studies the amount of calcium provided has ranged from about 800 to 1,200 mg. The mechanism(s) by which calcium reduces colon cancerogenesis is not clear, but calcium is thought to reduce proliferation and promote normal differentiation of colonic cells. Calcium may also bind and precipitate bile acids to prevent their negative impact on colonic cells. At present, data demonstrating a positive association are deemed promising but inconsistent [9,15,16]. Thus, the evidence is considered insufficient to recommend the routine use of a calcium supplement to reduce or prevent colon cancer [9,16].

An inverse association has been reported between the risk for type 2 diabetes and dietary calcium intake and/or dairy production consumption [17–21]. The mechanism(s) by which increased calcium/dairy product intake decreases the risk of type 2 diabetes is not clear. Some proposed theories suggest the effects are related to an increased circulating concentration of insulin-like growth factor-1, which promotes glucose uptake, and/or to reductions in insulin resistance and inflammation, among other possible factors [20–23].

Low intakes of calcium and/or dairy products have also been associated with an increased risk of obesity and/or body weight. These effects are thought to be due to increased circulating serum concentrations of vitamin D and PTH (which occur secondary to low calcium intake and low blood calcium concentrations). In this situation, calcium entry into adipocytes is theorized to be greater than normal; the elevation in intracellular calcium affects gene expression, increasing de novo lipogenesis and inhibiting lipolysis. Conversely, increases in dietary calcium reduce plasma PTH and vitamin D concentrations, reduce calcium uptake into adipocytes, and reduce intracellular calcium concentrations. This "lower-calcium environment" in the cell promotes lipolysis and inhibits expression of genes that enhance lipogenesis. While the modulation of body weight by calcium and/or dairy remains under investigation (and has been shown to be beneficial in some trials) [24–27], meta-evaluations of randomized clinical trials along with additional studies report no consistent effect from the ingestion of calcium and/or dairy products on weight and/or alterations in fat metabolism [28–32].

Toxicity

A Tolerable Upper Intake Level of 2,500 mg of calcium has been recommended for adults 19 to 50 years of age. The recommendation decreases to 2,000 mg of calcium for those age 51 years and older [9]. However, the use of calcium supplements, even in amounts less than the Tolerable Upper Intake Level, may cause gastrointestinal side effects, especially constipation, bloating, and/or gas.

Milk- (or calcium-) alkali syndrome has been documented in those consuming excessive quantities of calcium in the form of milk, but more commonly from calcium-containing antacids, as may be used in the treatment of ulcers, heartburn, and sometimes renal failure. With these large intakes of calcium (especially in excess of 3 g per day), hypercalcemia (serum calcium concentrations in excess of 10.5 mg/dL or 2.63 mmol/L) occurs as well as deposition of calcium in soft tissues (which over time may lead to hardening of blood vessels, among other problems). Hypercalcemia and systemic alkalosis may be associated with lethargy, anorexia, nausea, vomiting, and heart arrhythmias. Serum calcium concentrations in excess of about 12 mg/dL may cause **hypercalciuria** (urinary calcium excretion greater than about 250–300 mg/day). Individuals with idiopathic hypercalciuria (urinary calcium levels > 4 mg/kg body weight per day) who consume excessive amounts of calcium may increase their risk of developing calcium-containing kidney stones.

Assessment of Nutriture

No routine biochemical method appears to assess calcium status accurately. Serum calcium is so exquisitely regulated that it usually indicates little about calcium status. However, serum ionized calcium, Ca^{2+}, can reflect alterations in calcium metabolism, and use of serum calcium concentrations may require corrections based on an individual's protein status. In the presence of normal serum albumin concentrations, the ratio between bound calcium and ionized calcium remains constant. However, when serum albumin concentrations are depressed, corrections are needed to adjust for the corresponding decrease that occurs in the protein-bound fraction of calcium. For each 1 g/dL decrease in serum albumin, serum calcium decreases 0.8 mg/dL. The following equations can be used for estimating protein-bound calcium: Protein-bound calcium (mg/dL) = 0.44 + [0.76 × albumin (g/dL)] or [0.8 × (normal albumin – actual albumin)] + measured calcium (mg/dL).

Because the majority of calcium is found in bone, it is common to assess bone mineral density, especially in those at risk for osteoporosis. Assessment of bone minerals is accomplished by several methods. Measurement by dual-energy X-ray absorptiometry (abbreviated DEXA or DXA) is thought to be one of the best tools. The method involves scanning specific sites at two different energy levels using an X-ray tube. Radiation exposure is low, and the procedure is relatively quick. Bone density also can be assessed through computerized tomography (CT) scans, which measure variances in tissue density. X-rays are taken as the person is held in a scanner. Radiation pulses are emitted, collected, and processed to reconstruct the image and calculate bone density. This method, however, is less precise and accurate than DEXA. Neutron activation, in

which γ rays are counted following administration of ^{48}Ca into the body and exposure of the body to a low neutron flux, enables assessment of total body calcium content. Results of neutron activation correlate with single-photon absorptiometry, which measures total bone mineral content. Single-photon absorptiometry exposes a portion of a limb, usually the radius (forearm) or os calcis (heel), to radiation. The quantity of bone mineral is inversely proportional to the amount of photon energy transmitted from the bone, as measured by a scintillation counter.

References Cited for Calcium

1. Fleet JC, Schoch RD. Molecular mechanism for regulation of intestinal calcium absorption by vitamin D and other factors. Crit Rev Clin Lab Sci. 2010; 47:181–95.
2. Fujita H, Sugimoto K, Inatomi S, et al. Tight junction proteins claudin-2 and -12 are critical for vitamin D dependent Ca^{2+} absorption between enterocytes. Molec Biol Cell. 2008; 19:1912–21.
3. Suzuki T, Hana H. Various nondigestible saccharides open a paracellular calcium transport pathway with the induction of intracellular calcium signalling in human intestinal caco-2 cells. J Nutr. 2004; 134:1935–41.
4. Rafferty K, Walters G, Heaney RP. Calcium fortificants: overview and strategies for improving calcium nutriture of the US population. J Food Sci. 2007; 72:R152–58.
5. Gaitan D, Flores S, Saavedra P, et al. Calcium does not inhibit the absorption of 5 milligrams of nonheme or heme iron at doses less than 800 milligrams in nonpregnant women. J Nutr. 2011; 141:1652–56.
6. Lonnerdal B. Calcium and iron absorption: mechanisms and public health relevance. Interntl J Vit Nutr Res. 2010; 80:293–99.
7. Charles P, Eriksen EF, Hasling C, et al. Dermal, intestinal, and renal obligatory losses of calcium: Relation to skeletal calcium loss. Am J Clin Nutr. 1991; 54:S266–73.
8. Devine A, Criddle R, Dick I, et al. A longitudinal study of the effect of sodium and calcium intake on regional bone density in postmenopausal women. Am J Clin Nutr. 1995; 62:740–45.
9. Institute of Medicine, Food and Nutrition Board. Dietary Reference intakes for Calcium and Vitamin D. Washington DC: National Academy Press. 2011.
10. FDA Food Guidance, Compliance and Regulatory Information. www.fda.gov/food/LabelingNutrition/default.htm
11. Bonithon-Kopp C, Kronborg O, Giacosa A, et al. Calcium and fibre supplementation in prevention of colorectal adenoma recurrence: a randomized intervention trial. Lancet. 2000; 356:1300–06.
12. Barron JA, Beach M, Mandel JS, et al. Calcium supplements for the prevention of colorectal adenomas. N Engl J Med. 1999; 340:101–07.
13. Grau MV, Baron JA, Sandler RS, et al. Vitamin D, calcium supplementation, and colorectal adenomas: results of a randomized trial. J Natl Cancer Inst. 2003; 95:1765–71.
14. Cho E, Smith-Warner SA, Spiegelman D, et al. Dairy foods, calcium, and colorectal cancer: a pooled analysis of 10 cohort studies. J Natl Cancer Inst. 2004; 96:1015–22.
15. Kushi LH, Byers T, Doyle C, et al. The American Cancer Society 2006 Guidelines on nutrition and physical activity for cancer prevention: reducing the risk of cancer with healthy food choices and physical activity. Cancer J Clin. 2006; 56:254–81.
16. Weingarten MA, Zalmanovici A, Yaphe J. Dietary calcium supplementation for preventing colorectal cancer and adenomatous polyps. Cochrane Database Syst Rev 2008; CD003548.
17. Malik VS, Sun Q, van Dam RM, et al. Adolescent dairy product consumption and risk of type 2 diabetes in middle-aged women. Am J Clin Nutr. 2011; 94:854–61.
18. Villegas R, Gao Y, Dai Q, et al. Dietary calcium and magnesium intakes and the risk of type 2 diabetes: the Shanghai Women's health Study. Am J Clin Nutr. 2009; 89:1059–67.

19. Van Dam RM, Hu FB, Rosenberg L, et al. Dietary calcium and magnesium, major food sources, and risk of type 2 diabetes in U.S. black women. Diabetes Care. 2006; 29:2238–43.

20. Pittas AG, Lau J, Hu FB, Dawson-Hughes B. The role of vitamin D and calcium in type 2 diabetes: a systematic review and meta-analysis. J Clin Endocrinol Metab. 2007; 92:2017–29.

21. Tremblay A, Gilbert JA. Milk products, insulin resistance syndrome, and type 2 diabetes. J Am Coll Nutr. 2009; 28(suppl 1):S91–102.

22. Holmes MD, Pollak MN, Willett WC, Hankinson SE. Dietary correlates of plasma insulin-like growth factor 1 and insulin like growth factor binding protein 3 concentrations. Cancer Epid Biomarkers Prev. 2002; 11:852–61.

23. Larrson SC, Wolk A. Magnesium intake and risk of type 2 diabetes: a meta-analysis. J Intern Med. 2007; 262:208–14.

24. Major GC, Chaput JP, Ledoux M, et al. Recent developments in calcium-related obesity research. Obes Rev. 2008; 9:428–45.

25. Zemel MB, Miller SL. Dietary calcium and dairy modulation of adiposity and obesity risk. Nutr Rev. 2004; 62:125–31.

26. Shahar DR, Schwarzfuchs D, Fraser D, et al. Dairy calcium intake, serum vitamin D, and successful weight loss. Am J Clin Nutr. 2010; 92:1017–22.

27. Onakpoya IJ, Perry R, Zhang J, Ernst E. Efficacy of calcium supplementation for management of overweight and obesity: systematic review of randomized clinical trials. Nutr Rev. 2011; 69:335–43.

28. Lanou AJ, Barnard ND. Dairy and weight loss hypothesis: an evaluation of the clinical trials. Nutr Rev. 2008; 66:272–79.

29. Trowman R, Dumville JC, Hahn S, Torgerson DJ. A systematic review of the effects of calcium supplementation on body weight. Br J Nutr. 2006; 95:1033–38.

30. Bortolotti M, Rudelle S, Schneiter P, et al. Dairy calcium supplementation in overweight or obese persons: its effect on markers of fat metabolism. Am J Clin Nutr. 2008; 88:877–85.

31. Yanovski JA, Parikh SJ, Yanoff LB, et al. Effects of calcium supplementation on body weight and adiposity in overweight and obese adults. Ann Intern Med. 2009; 150:821–29.

32. Weaver CM, Campbell WW, Teegarden D, et al. Calcium, dairy products, and energy balance in overweight adolescents: a controlled trial. Am J Clin Nutr. 2011; 94:1163–70.

Suggested Readings

Bronner F. Recent developments in intestinal calcium absorption. Nutr Rev. 2009; 67:109–13.

Patel AM, Goldfarb S. Got calcium? welcome to the calcium-alkali syndrome. J Am Soc Nephrology. 2010; 21:1440–43.

Straub DA. Calcium supplementation in clinical practice; a review of forms, doses, and indications. Nutr Clin Pract. 2007; 22:286–96.

PHOSPHORUS

Among the minerals, phosphorus is second only to calcium in abundance in the body. The human body contains about 560 to 850 g of phosphorus, representing about 0.8% to 1.2% of body weight. Of total body phosphorus, about 85% is in the skeleton, 1% is in the blood and body fluids, and the remaining 14% is associated with soft tissue such as muscle.

Sources

Phosphorus is widely distributed in foods. The best food sources include protein-rich foods like meat, poultry, fish, eggs, milk, and milk products. Dairy products, for example, contain about 200 to 350 mg of phosphorus per serving. An egg has about 100 mg of phosphorus. Meats, fish, and poultry provide about 150 to 250 mg of phosphorus per 3-oz serving. Nuts, legumes, cereals, and grains also represent good sources of phosphorus. For example, an ounce of peanuts provides about 101 mg of phosphorus and an ounce each of walnuts and pecans contains 98 mg and 79 mg, respectively. Peanut butter has 57 mg of phosphorus per tablespoon. Cooked black, kidney, and pinto beans (1 cup) provide 241 mg, 233 mg, and 251 mg of phosphorus, respectively. A slice of whole-wheat bread has about 57 mg, and one cup of wheat bran cereal with raisins provides 20% of the Daily Value (which is 1,000 mg), or 200 mg of phosphorus. Cola-type soft drinks contain phosphoric acid and, depending upon consumption habits, can contribute substantially to dietary intake. A 12-oz soft drink provides about 25 to 40 mg of phosphorus. Coffee and tea contain fairly little phosphorus, less than 10 mg/cup. In addition to dietary sources, phosphate-containing supplements, including K-Phos and Neutra-Phos K, are available commercially and also provide potassium. Such supplements are usually needed only for people whose phosphorus stores have been depleted by malnutrition.

Dietary phosphorus occurs as inorganic phosphates as well as organic forms. In its organic form, phosphorus is bound to proteins, sugars, and lipids. The relative amounts of inorganic and organic phosphorus vary within foods and the diet. For example, about one-third of the phosphorus in milk is as inorganic phosphates, and the remaining two-thirds are bound to organic nutrients. Similarly, meats contain phosphorus that is largely bound to organic compounds and thus require hydrolysis for absorption to occur. Over 80% of the phosphorus in grains such as wheat, rice, and corn is found as phytic acid (Figure 11.7). Phosphorus in the form of phytic acid is also found in beans, legumes, and nuts. The bioavailability of phosphorus from phytic acid is limited to about 50%, as discussed in the "Factors Influencing Absorption" section.

Digestion, Absorption, and Transport

Digestion

Regardless of its dietary form, most phosphorus is absorbed from the gastrointestinal tract as inorganic phosphate ions. Thus, organically bound phosphorus must be digested enzymatically to release inorganic

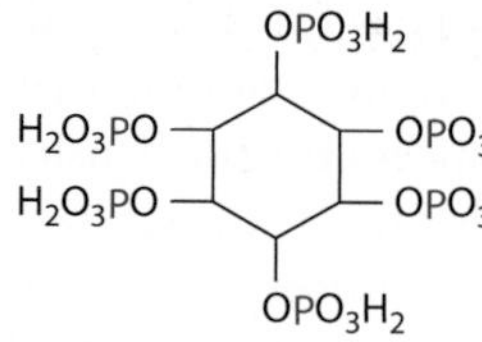

Figure 11.7 Phytic acid (phytate).

phosphate (P_i) for absorption. Phospholipase C, a zinc-dependent enzyme, for example, hydrolyzes the glycerophosphate bond in phospholipids. Alkaline phosphatase, another zinc-dependent enzyme whose activity is stimulated by calcitriol, functions at the brush border membrane of the enterocyte to free phosphate from some, but not all, bound forms. For example, it cannot free phytic acid-bound phosphorus.

Absorption

Phosphorus absorption occurs throughout the small intestine, but primarily in the duodenum and jejunum. About 50% to 70% of dietary phosphorus is absorbed, with absorption from animal products at the upper end of the range, and that from phytic acid–containing foods at the lower end.

Phosphorus absorption occurs by two processes:

- saturable, carrier-medicated, active transport
- diffusion

Due to typically high inorganic phosphate concentrations, the absorption of phosphate is thought to occur primarily by passive diffusion. Specifically, passive diffusion is thought to be possible in the slightly acidic pH of the proximal duodenum [1]. In this region, the concentration of the mineral would be high (after eating), and the valence of the phosphate ions would shift toward $H_2PO_4^-$ to enable passive transport along the electrochemical gradient [1]. The intercellular junctions of the small intestine are thought to exhibit low permeability to phosphate ions ($H_2PO_4^-$ and HPO_4^{2-}), thus minimizing the likelihood of much paracellular diffusion [1].

Active transport of the mineral is thought to be more widely used when phosphate intake is low. The active transport of phosphorus involves a sodium-phosphate cotransporter, which carries two sodiums for each phosphate, as either $H_2PO_4^-$ or HPO_4^{2-}. Calcitriol and low-phosphorus diets have been shown to increase the number of cotransporters in the intestinal brush border membrane; however, calcitriol is not essential for this up-regulation [2].

Factors Influencing Absorption A number of factors either positively or negatively influence phosphorus absorption, as noted in Table 11.5. The main enhancer of phosphorus absorption is calcitriol, which stimulates carrier-mediate absorption in both the duodenum and the jejunum.

Several substances inhibit phosphorus absorption. Phytic acid, with its six phosphate groups (see Figure 11.7), is the major form of phosphate in grains and legumes. The bioavailability of phosphorus from phytic acid is poor, however, because humans do not produce phytase, a phosphate esterase that liberates phosphate from phytic acid. Yeasts in breads possess phytase that can hydrolyze some phytates to yield some phosphorus available for absorption. However, when phytic acid–containing foods are consumed with foods rich in Ca^{2+} or Zn^{2+}, phytic acid forms cation-phytic acid complexes and prevents these nutrients from being absorbed.

Several minerals, including magnesium, aluminum, and calcium, also impair phosphorus absorption. Phosphorus and magnesium are thought to form a complex, $Mg_3(PO_4)_2$, within the gastrointestinal tract to render each other unavailable for absorption. Aluminum hydroxide (3 g) given with a meal has been shown to reduce phosphorus absorption from 70% to 35%. Aluminum, magnesium (as hydroxides), and calcium (as carbonate or acetate) are common components of antacids and for years were given in pharmacological doses to bind dietary phosphate in people with **hyperphosphatemia** (high blood phosphorus concentrations) caused by kidney disease.

Transport

Phosphorus is quickly absorbed from the intestine and into the blood, appearing in the blood within about an hour after ingestion in animal studies. Transport across the enterocyte's basolateral membrane for entrance into the blood is thought to occur by facilitated diffusion. Phosphorus is found in the blood in both organic and inorganic forms. About 70% of phosphorus is present as organic phosphate, such as that found as phospholipids in lipoproteins. Of the remaining 30% of phosphorus, most ($\sim$85%) is present as HPO_4^{2-} due to its greater solubility in blood than $H_2PO_4^-$ and the trivalent anion PO_4^{3-} (which is present in trace amounts). A small percentage of inorganic phosphates, mainly HPO_4^{2-}, are found complexed with calcium, magnesium, or sodium as salts in the blood. Figure 11.8 provides an overview of phosphorus digestion, absorption, and transport.

Plasma inorganic phosphate concentrations usually range from about 2.5 to 4.5 mg/dL (0.81–1.45 mmol/L). Dietary phosphate, age, time of day, various hormones such as parathyroid hormone (PTH) and fibroblast growth factor (FGF) 23, and renal function contribute to the variability of the serum phosphate concentration. Circulating plasma phosphate is in equilibrium with skeletal and cellular inorganic phosphate as well as with organic phosphates formed in intermediary metabolism. Uptake of phosphorus into cells is thought

Table 11.5 Factors Enhancing and Inhibiting Intestinal Phosphorus Absorption

Substances Enhancing Absorption	Substances Inhibiting Absorption
Vitamin D	Phytic acid
	Excessive intakes of:
	• Magnesium
	• Aluminum
	• Calcium

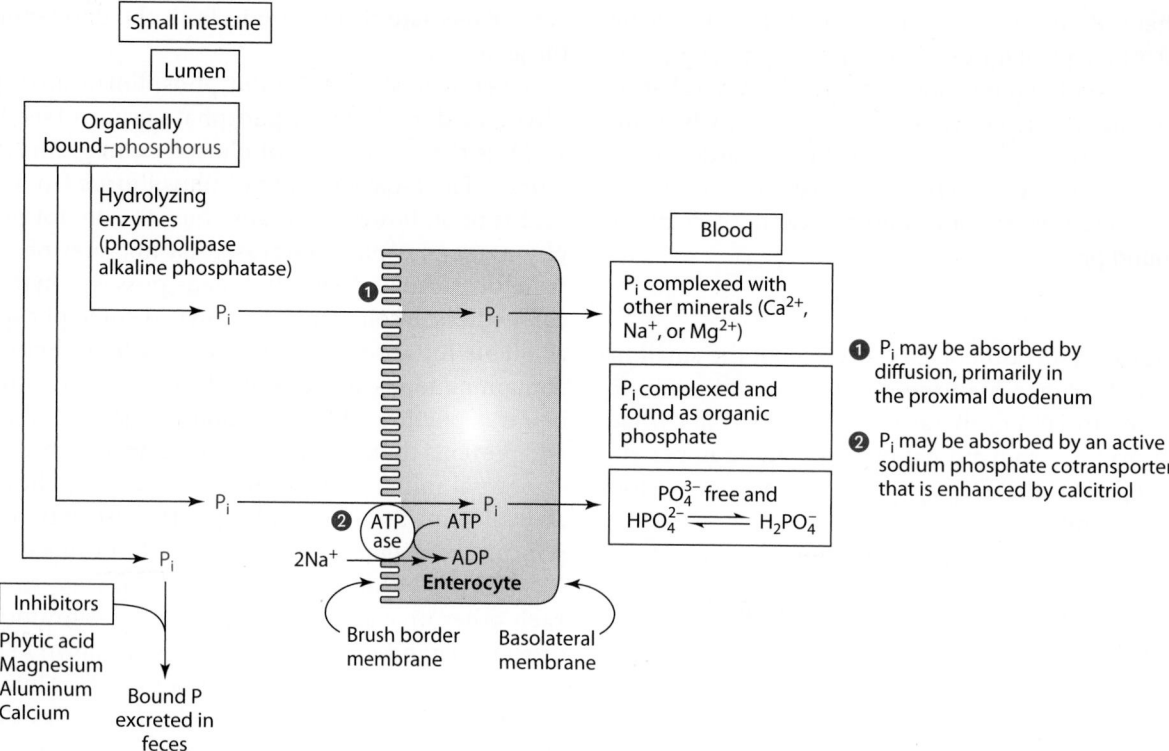

Figure 11.8 Digestion, absorption, and transport of phosphorus.

to occur passively (driven by the chemical gradient), but the mechanism has not been thoroughly examined. Phosphorus is found in all cells of the body, especially those of bone and muscle.

Functions and Mechanisms of Action

Phosphorus has many functions in the body, with involvement in several biologically important compounds. Examples include roles in bone mineralization, energy transfer and storage, nucleic acid formation, cell membrane structure, and acid-base balance. This section briefly discusses each of these roles.

Bone Mineralization

Phosphate is of prime importance in the development of skeletal tissue, which in itself accounts for 85% of body phosphorus. In bone, phosphorus is found in amorphous calcium phosphate forms, including, for example, $Ca_3(PO_4)_2$, $CaHPO_4 \cdot 2H_2O$, and $Ca_3(PO_4)_2 \cdot 3H_2O$, and in more crystalline forms such as hydroxyapatite, $Ca_{10}(PO_4)_6(OH)_2$, which is laid down on collagen in the ossification process of bone formation. In amorphous bone, the ratio of calcium to phosphorus is about 1.3:1, similar to extracellular fluid; however, in crystalline bone,

the ratio is about 1.5 to 2.0:1. Phosphorus that is not part of bone is found either in extracellular fluids, such as blood, or in soft tissues. Within cells, phosphorus is the major anion and is involved in a host of processes.

PTH, calcitriol, and calcitonin influence phosphorus balance in the body. Calcitonin promotes the use of phosphorus in bone mineralization. Thus, calcitonin decreases serum phosphorus concentrations (as it does serum calcium). PTH has the opposite effect of calcitonin; PTH (along with calcitriol) stimulates resorption of phosphate from bone, possibly through enhanced alkaline phosphatase activity. This action increases serum phosphorus levels; however, PTH also stimulates the excretion of phosphorus in urine. The PTH-induced urinary excretion of phosphorus typically is sufficient to override bone resorption of phosphorus so as to effect a net decrease in plasma phosphate. The actions of calcitriol in the intestine stimulate phosphate absorption. The net effect of these hormones is to regulate phosphorus and ensure that the mineral is available to perform its numerous functions in the body.

In addition to its role in bone, phosphorus is a structural component of many other important compounds, some of which are shown in Figure 11.9 and described hereafter.

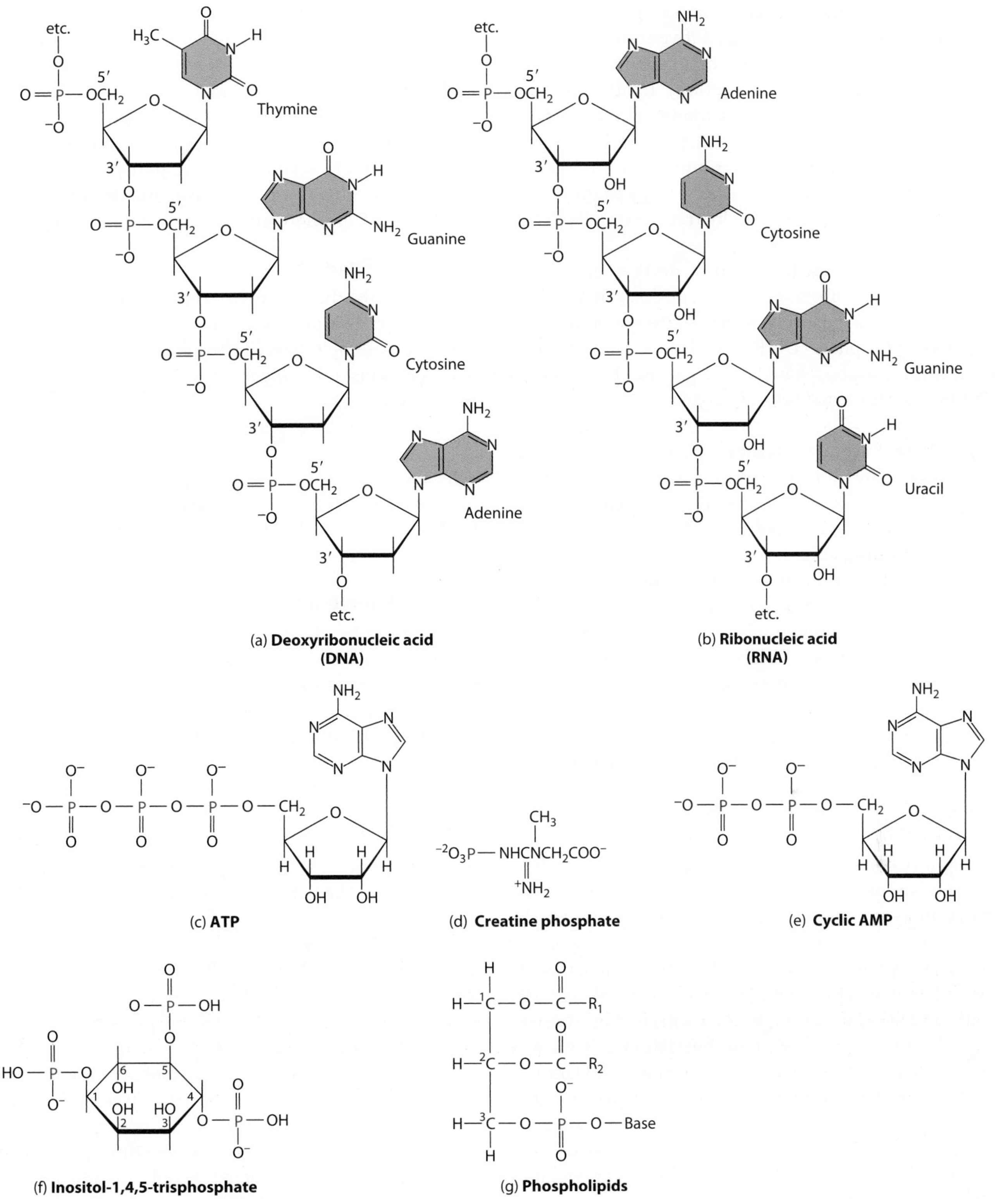

Figure 11.9 Some examples of important phosphorus-containing compounds in the body.

Nucleotide/Nucleoside Phosphates

Structural Roles Phosphate is an important component of the nucleic acids DNA and RNA (Figure 11.9a and b), alternating with pentose sugars to form the linear backbone of these molecules.

Energy Storage and Transfer Phosphorus is of vital importance in the intermediary metabolism of the energy nutrients in the form of high-energy phosphate bonds, such as those in the nucleoside triphosphate adenosine triphosphate (ATP) (Figure 11.9c). The energy released as the phosphate bond of ATP is broken provides for numerous cellular functions (e.g., active transport pumps for nutrient absorption and for maintenance of ion concentrations, muscle cell contraction). In addition to its presence in ATP, phosphorus is found in creatine phosphate (also called phosphocreatine; Figure 11.9d). Creatine phosphate, synthesized in muscle from ATP and creatine, provides and replenishes energy to muscles as needed (e.g., during exercise) by transferring its PO_4 to ADP using creatine kinase.

Another nucleoside triphosphate, uridine triphosphate (UTP), activates substances in intermediary metabolism. For example, UTP hydrolysis enables the coupling of uridine monophosphate (UMP) and glucose-1-phosphate to form uridine diphosphate (UDP)-glucose. UDP-glucose is critical for the synthesis of glycogen.

Intracellular Second Messenger Phosphorus as part of cyclic adenosine monophosphate (cAMP) (Figure 11.9e), which is derived from ATP, functions as a second messenger to affect cellular metabolism. cAMP, which acts within cells by activating certain protein kinases, is generated in response to the binding of certain hormones to cell receptors. Another phosphorus-containing second messenger is cyclic guanosine monophosphate (cGMP), which activates protein kinases. Inositol triphosphate (IP_3; Figure 11.9f) also functions as a second messenger to trigger intracellular calcium release from cellular organelles. Its actions are mediated by protein kinases. The role of protein kinases as they function in enzyme activation is discussed next.

Phosphoproteins and Phosphorylated Forms of Vitamins

Phosphorus also is of vital importance in intermediary metabolism of the energy nutrients through the phosphorylation of different substrates in the body. Protein kinases activated by cAMP, a phosphate-containing second messenger, phosphorylate specific target proteins within the cell, thereby changing cellular activities. Many enzymatic activities, for example, are controlled by alternating phosphorylation or dephosphorylation. An example of the role of phosphorylation and dephosphorylation of enzymes can be found in the discussion of glycogen degradation (see Chapter 3). In addition to phosphorylating proteins, phosphorus is needed for the actions of some vitamins, including thiamin and vitamin B_6 (pyridoxine). The active coenzyme forms of both of these vitamins—thiamin as thiamin pyro-/diphosphate and vitamin B_6 as pyridoxal phosphate, pyridoxamine phosphate, and pyridoxine phosphate—require phosphorus.

Phospholipids

Cell membranes are made up, in part, of lipids, including phospholipids, which (as their name implies) contain phosphorus. Phospholipids, with their polar and nonpolar regions, are important to the bilayer structure of cell membranes. Each phospholipid contains a glycerol backbone with two fatty acyl chains attached at carbons 1 and 2; the phosphate group is attached to glycerol carbon 3 and to a base (Figure 11.9g). The bases include choline (forming phosphatidylcholine), inositol (forming phosphatidylinositol), serine (forming phosphatidylserine), and ethanolamine (forming phosphatidylethanolamine). See Chapter 5 for more information on phospholipids.

Acid–Base Balance

Phosphate also functions in acid–base balance. Within cells, phosphate is the main intracellular buffer. Within the kidney, for example, filtered phosphate reacts with secreted hydrogen ions, releasing sodium ions in the process, as shown here:

$$Na_2HPO_4 + H^+ \longrightarrow NaH_2PO_4 + Na^+$$

This action removes free hydrogen ions and therefore increases pH. The following reaction also increases pH: $HPO^{2-} + H^+ \longrightarrow H_2PO_4^-$. These reactions may be reversed to lower pH.

Oxygen Availability

Phosphate is involved indirectly in oxygen delivery. In red blood cells, the synthesis of 2,3-diphosphoglycerate, which influences oxygen release from hemoglobin, requires phosphorus. Decreased 2,3-diphosphoglycerate associated with phosphorus deficiency can diminish release of oxygen to tissues.

Excretion

About 67% to 90% of phosphorus in inorganic form is excreted in the urine. The remaining 10% to 33% of phosphorus is excreted in the feces. The proximal tubule reabsorbs about three-quarters of filtered phosphorus, and the distal tubule reabsorbs about 10%; about 15% is typically excreted. A sodium phosphate cotransporter $[2Na^+ - H_2PO_4^-$ or $HPO_4^{2-}]$ is responsible for most phosphorus reabsorption in the proximal tubule.

Unlike calcium, high dietary phosphorus leads to high serum phosphorus, which leads to increased urinary phosphorus excretion. In other words, maintenance of the phosphate balance is achieved largely through renal excretion. The amount of dietary phosphorus and absorbed phosphorus has approximately a linear relationship with urinary phosphorus if the amount of phosphorus filtered is greater than the tubular maximum for phosphorus. The tubular maximum for phosphorus (TmP) is the amount (mmol) of phosphorus reabsorbed per unit time. However, if phosphorus intake and plasma phosphorus concentrations are low, then most filtered phosphorus is reabsorbed. This reabsorption helps maintain the plasma phosphorus concentration.

Urinary phosphorus excretion is typically promoted (i.e., tubular reabsorption of phosphorus is inhibited) by increased dietary phosphorus intake, parathyroid hormone, acidosis, and phosphatonins (also called phosphotonins, such as fibroblast growth factor [FGF]-23). FGF23, secreted by osteoblasts and osteocytes, reduces the renal synthesis of calcitriol and the expression of the sodium-phosphate co-transporter in the kidney. Phosphate excretion in the urine is typically inhibited by phosphorus deficiency, calcitriol, alkalosis, estrogen, and thyroid and growth hormones.

Recommended Dietary Allowance

The RDA for phosphorus is 700 mg/day for males and females (including those who are pregnant or lactating) age 19 years and older [3]. An estimated requirement (580 mg/day) for phosphorus was determined based upon the relationship between dietary phosphorus intake and plasma phosphorus concentrations as well as a known efficiency of intestinal absorption [3]. A coefficient of variation of 10% was added to the requirement and rounded to establish this recommended intake. The inside covers of the book provide the RDAs for phosphorus for other age groups.

Deficiency

Phosphorus deficiency is rare. It is typically confined to people (e.g., those with renal disease) who are receiving large amounts of antacids containing calcium, magnesium, aluminum, or some combination (which bind phosphorus in the gastrointestinal tract and inhibit its absorption). In addition, people who are malnourished and are being refed enterally through a tube or parenterally (intravenously) without being given additional phosphorus have been known to exhibit phosphate deficiency, also called refeeding syndrome. Premature infants can be at risk for deficiency because of their higher needs for the mineral and the insufficient amount found in human milk. Genetic deficiency disorders involving phosphorus include X-linked hypophosphatemia and hypophosphatemic rickets (also called Dent's syndrome). These disorders result from defects in phosphorus reabsorption in the kidneys, and thus cause excessive phosphorus loss. Deficiency of phosphorus, manifested biochemically by low serum phosphorus concentrations (<1.5 mg/dL), usually results in anorexia, leukocyte dysfunction, reduced cardiac output, decreased diaphragmatic contractility, arrhythmias, skeletal muscle and cardiac myopathy, weakness, and neurological problems (ataxia and paresthesia), as well as possible death.

Toxicity

While toxicity from phosphorus is rare, a Tolerable Upper Intake Level of 4 g of phosphorus has been recommended for those age 9 to 70 years to minimize the likelihood of hyperphosphatemia (high blood phosphate concentrations). After age 70 years, the tolerable level drops to 3 g of phosphorus daily; this decrease is associated with an increased likelihood of impaired renal function that often occurs with aging [3]. For pregnant and lactating women, the Tolerable Upper Intake Levels are 3.5 g and 4 g, respectively [3]. Hyperphosphatemia (plasma phosphorus concentrations greater than the upper limit of normal or about 4.5 mg/dL [1.45 mmol/L]) as well as plasma phosphorus concentrations at the upper end of the normal range has been linked with heart disease.

Assessment of Nutriture

The assessment of phosphorus nutriture is not a major consideration because deficiency is so rare. Serum phosphorus concentrations and urinary excretion are most often assessed; however, their specificity and sensitivity are low. Serum phosphate concentrations, for example, can be maintained at the expense of tissues.

References Cited for Phosphorus

1. Cross HS, Debiec H, Peterlik M. Mechanism and regulation of intestinal phosphate absorption. Miner Electrolyte Metab. 1990; 16:115–24.
2. Segawa H, Kaneko I, Yamanaka S, et al. Intestinal Na-Pi cotransporter adaption to dietary Pi content in vitamin D receptor null mice. Am J Physiol Renal Physiol. 2004; 287; F39–47.
3. Food and Nutrition Board, Institute of Medicine. Dietary Reference Intakes. Washington, DC: National Academy Press. 1997, pp. 146–89.

Suggested Readings

Bergwitz C, Juppner H. Regulation of phosphate homeostasis by PTH, vitamin D, and FGF23. Ann Rev Nutr. 2010; 61:91–104.
Ellam TJ, Chico TJA. Phosphate: the new cholesterol? The role of the phosphate axis in non-uremic vascular disease. Atherosclerosis 2012; 220:310-18.

MAGNESIUM

Of the major minerals, magnesium ranks sixth ($Ca^{2+} > P > K^+ > Na^+$ and $Cl^- > Mg^{2+}$) in overall abundance in the body, but intracellularly the cation is second only to potassium. The human body contains about 25 g of magnesium (close to 1% of body weight), of which approximately 50% to 60% is located in bone, another 39% to 49% in soft tissues, and about 1% in extracellular fluids.

Sources

Magnesium is found in a wide variety of foods. Foods particularly high in magnesium include nuts, legumes, and whole-grain cereals (especially oats and barley). Beans (such as navy, pinto, kidney, and garbanzo) and black-eyed peas, for example, provide about 40 to 50 mg/ ½-cup cooked serving. Peanut butter contains about

50 mg of magnesium/2 tablespoons, and sunflower seeds have about 40 mg of magnesium/¼ cup. Whole-grain bread (1 slice) and oatmeal (½ cup) each contain about 25 mg of magnesium. Spices, seafood, and green leafy vegetables also provide good amounts of magnesium. Chlorophyll found in the green leafy vegetables contains magnesium. Spinach, for example, contains about 150 mg of magnesium/cup. Seafood such as halibut is rich in magnesium, with about 100 mg/3-oz serving. Milk and yogurt provide about 25 to 40 mg of magnesium per cup. Other particularly good food sources of magnesium are chocolate (36–51 mg/2 oz) depending on the type, blackstrap molasses (43 mg/tablespoon), corn (48 mg/cup), peas (23 mg/½ cup), and brown rice (40 mg/½ cup). Some magnesium is also found in coffee (about 48 mg/2 oz espresso) and cocoa (about 25 mg/6-oz cup of hot chocolate). Tap water also may represent a source of the mineral. Water can be high in magnesium (hard water) or high in sodium (soft water). The Daily Value for magnesium, used on food and supplement labels, is 400 mg.

Magnesium salts—such as magnesium sulfate ($MgSO_4$, or Epsom salts), magnesium oxide (MgO), magnesium chloride ($MgCl_2$), magnesium lactate, magnesium acetate, magnesium gluconate, and magnesium citrate—are commonly available supplemental forms of the mineral. Absorption of magnesium from magnesium oxide tends to be less than that from other magnesium salts. Absorption also may be better from effervescent tablets than from capsules. To maximize absorption, magnesium supplements should not be taken at the same time as other mineral supplements, such as iron. Supplements of magnesium are sometimes needed for people with diseases associated with fat malabsorption, such as inflammatory bowel and pancreatic diseases, because the malabsorption of fat leads to increased loss of magnesium in the feces.

Food processing and preparation may substantially reduce the magnesium content of some foods. For example, refining whole wheat, which removes the germ and outer layers, can substantially reduce its magnesium content (by over 75%).

Digestion, Absorption, and Transport

Digestion and Absorption

Unlike calcium and phosphorus, dietary magnesium does not require digestion prior to absorption. Magnesium (as Mg^{2+}) absorption occurs throughout the small intestine, mainly in the jejunum and ileum. However, the colon also may play a role in absorbing magnesium, especially if disease has interfered with magnesium absorption in the small intestine. Two transport systems are thought to be responsible for magnesium absorption in the small intestine:

• saturable, carrier-mediated active transport
• diffusion

The active magnesium transporter is a transient receptor potential (TRP) melastatin divalent cation-permeable channel protein called TRPM6. This channel protein is found on the brush border membrane of enterocytes (mostly in the duodenum). The channel is inhibited by high cytosolic magnesium concentrations. Thus, absorption decreases with increased intracellular magnesium concentrations. This carrier system operates mostly with low magnesium intakes.

Paracellular absorption of magnesium increases as intraluminal magnesium concentrations increase. Much of magnesium is thought to be absorbed by this passive, concentration-dependent route when magnesium intakes are high.

About 30% to 60% of dietary magnesium is absorbed from the intestine. Absorption declines to less than 30% as magnesium intake increases above about 550 mg. Conversely, magnesium absorption increases above 60% (up to ~75%) when magnesium intake is low (less than 40 mg). Efflux of magnesium from cells is thought to occur by a Na^+/Mg^{2+} antiport system that depends on a Na^+/K^+-ATPase to sustain the sodium gradient. Figure 11.10 illustrates magnesium absorption and transport.

Factors Influencing Absorption Magnesium absorption is influenced by several dietary factors, as listed in Table 11.6. For example, unabsorbed fatty acids present in high quantities, as with steatorrhea, in the gastrointestinal tract may bind to magnesium to form soaps. These magnesium–fatty acid soaps are excreted in the feces. Minerals such as phosphorus also inhibit magnesium absorption. Magnesium and phosphorus form a complex, $Mg_3(PO_4)_2$, within the gastrointestinal tract to render each other unavailable for absorption. The inhibition is most apparent when magnesium consumption is low and intake of phosphorus is high. Additionally, phytic acid and nonfermentable fiber (such as cellulose) have been shown to impair magnesium absorption, but only to a small extent [1].

Magnesium absorption may be improved by vitamin D, protein, and selected carbohydrates. Vitamin D, in pharmacological doses, and protein, in some but not all studies, have been shown to increase magnesium absorption and/or its retention [2]. Carbohydrates, such as fructose and oligosaccharides, also may increase magnesium absorption [3].

Table 11.6 Substances/Nutrients Affecting Intestinal Absorption of or Interacting with Magnesium at an Extraintestinal Site

Substances Enhancing Absorption	Substances Inhibiting Absorption	Nutrient Interactions
Vitamin D	Phytic acid	Calcium
Protein	Fiber	Phosphorus
Carbohydrates	Excessive unabsorbed fatty acids	Potassium
Fructose		
Oligosaccharides		

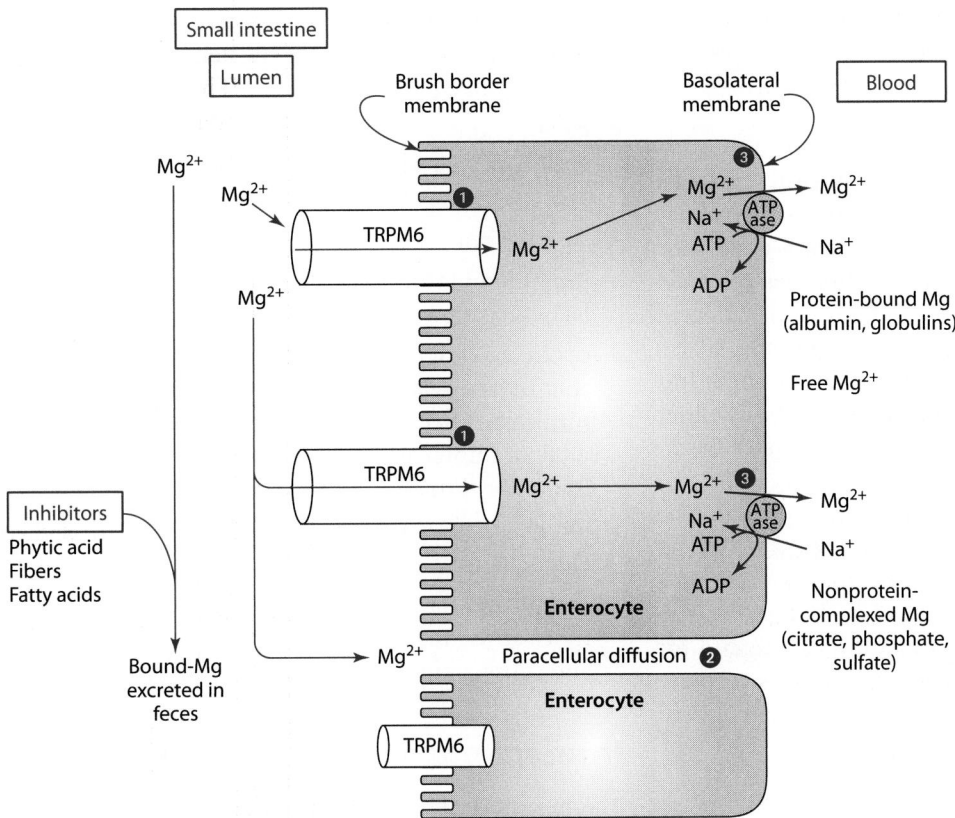

① Mg^{2+} crosses the brush border membrane of the enterocyte through a magnesium channel, TRPM6

② Mg^{2+} also may be absorbed between cells; this transport is influenced by the electron chemical gradient and solvent drag

③ Mg^{2+} is pumped out of the cell across the basolateral membrane by a sodium- dependent ATPase

Figure 11.10 Magnesium absorption and transport.

Transport

In the plasma, most magnesium (50–55%) is found free in its ionic form as Mg^{2+}, about 33% is bound to protein, and 13% is complexed with citrate, phosphate, sulfate, or other negatively charged anions or compounds. Of the 33% of magnesium that is protein bound, most is bound to albumin, with the remainder usually bound to globulins. Plasma magnesium concentrations are maintained between about 1.7 and 2.2 mg/dL (0.75–1.0 mmol/L); however, the homeostatic mechanism of control is unclear. Maintenance of these constant serum values appears to depend upon gastrointestinal absorption, renal excretion, and cellular flux of magnesium rather than on hormonal regulation. However, several hormones appear to affect, but not regulate, magnesium metabolism. Parathyroid hormone, for example, increases intestinal magnesium absorption, diminishes renal magnesium excretion, and enhances bone magnesium resorption, thereby raising plasma magnesium concentrations.

Free intracellular concentrations of magnesium are also rigidly maintained—at about 0.2 to 1.0 mmol/L—by altering membrane uptake, intracellular storage in organelles, and cellular flux. Most intracellular magnesium is bound to nucleic acids, ATP, proteins, and negatively charged phospholipids. Several plasma membrane magnesium transporters have been identified, including TRPM7 (in the heart, adipose tissue, and bone), MagT1 (in epithelial cells), NIPA Mg^{2+} transporter, and SLC41 Mg^{2+} transporter; the latter system may mediate cellular magnesium efflux [4]. Additionally, MMgT1 and 2 appear to control magnesium metabolism within the Golgi complex and post-Golgi vesicles [4].

Functions and Mechanisms of Action

About 50% to 60% of magnesium in the body is found associated with bone. Bone magnesium is divided between that found associated with phosphorus and calcium as part of the crystal lattice (~70%) and that found on the surface in an amorphous form (~30%). Bone surface magnesium is thought to represent an exchangeable magnesium pool that is able to maintain serum concentrations. In contrast, the magnesium in the crystal lattice is probably deposited at the time of bone formation. Magnesium may be present in bone as $Mg(OH)_2$ or $Mg_3(PO_4)_2$, for example.

Magnesium that does not function as part of bone is found in extracellular fluids (1%); in soft tissues, primarily skeletal muscle (about 25%); and in organs such as the liver and kidneys. Within cells, magnesium is associated with phospholipids as part of cell membranes (plasma, endoplasmic reticulum, and mitochondrial), where it may help in membrane stabilization. Magnesium is also associated with proteins (enzymes). Magnesium is important for over 300 different enzymatic reactions either as a structural cofactor or as an allosteric activator of enzyme activity.

Up to about 90% of intracellular magnesium may be associated with ATP or ADP. In ATP, magnesium is linked to the oxygen atoms of the phosphate groups, forming a complex that assists in the transfer of an ATP phosphate group. Figure 11.11 depicts magnesium as a ligand for the phosphate groups of ATP. Protein kinases transfer the γ-phosphate of magnesium ATP to a substrate. Listed here are some of magnesium's roles in the body:

- glycolysis: hexokinase, glucokinase, and phosphofructokinase
- TCA cycle: oxidative decarboxylation
- pentose phosphate pathway (hexose monophosphate shunt): transketolase reaction
- creatine phosphate formation: creatine kinase
- β-oxidation: initiation by thiokinase (acyl-CoA synthetase)
- activities of alkaline phosphatase and pyrophosphatase
- nucleic acid synthesis
- DNA synthesis and degradation, as well as the physical integrity of the DNA helix
- DNA replication and RNA transcription

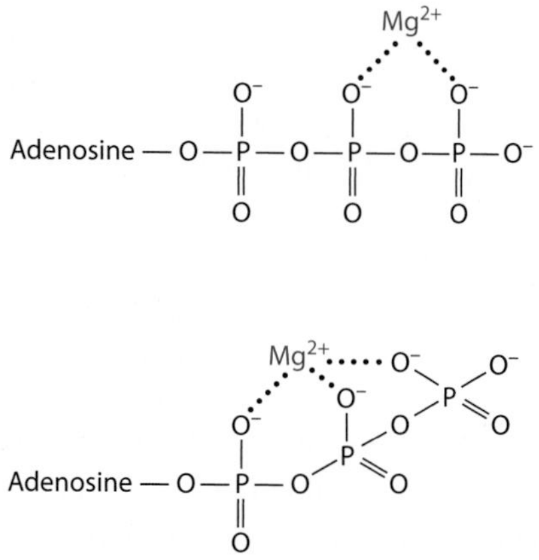

- amino acid activation
- protein synthesis (e.g., with ribosomal aggregation and binding messenger RNA to ribosome subunits)
- cardiac and smooth muscle contractibility (direct action as well as influence on calcium ion transport and use)
- vascular reactivity
- inhibition of thrombosis formation and reduced platelet aggregation
- cyclic adenosine monophosphate (cAMP) formation by adenylate cyclase; because of its function in forming cAMP, magnesium mediates, in part, the effects of numerous hormones, including parathyroid hormone
- ion channel regulation, especially potassium and calcium channels
- insulin and insulin action (such as tyrosine kinase activity at the insulin receptor, postreceptor signaling, and subsequent cellular glucose uptake)

Interactions with Other Nutrients

Magnesium interacts with a number of nutrients, most notably vitamin D, calcium, phosphorus, and potassium. For example, the hydroxylation of vitamin D in the 25-position requires magnesium. Several interrelationships link calcium and magnesium. Calcium and magnesium use overlapping transport systems in the kidney and thus compete in part with each other for reabsorption. Magnesium also may mimic or displace calcium from calcium-binding sites, decrease the flux of calcium across the cell membrane, further inhibit the release of calcium from the sarcoplasmic reticulum in response to increased influx from extracellular sites, and activate the Ca^{2+}-ATPase pump to decrease intracellular Ca^{2+} concentrations. Magnesium may compete with calcium for nonspecific binding sites on troponin C and myosin to alter muscle contraction. Additionally, in smooth muscle, magnesium, if bound to sites that are normally occupied by calcium, can inhibit contraction. The magnesium-calcium relationship has implications for people with respiratory disease because increased intracellular calcium promotes bronchial smooth muscle contraction [5].

Magnesium inhibits phosphorus absorption. As magnesium intake increases, phosphorus absorption decreases. The two minerals are thought to precipitate as $Mg_3(PO_4)_2$. Magnesium acetate (600 mg), for example, has been shown to reduce phosphorus absorption from about 77% to 34% [6].

A close interrelationship also exists between magnesium and potassium. Magnesium influences the balance between extracellular and intracellular potassium, but its

Figure 11.11 Modes by which Mg^{2+} provides stability to ATP.

mechanism of action is unclear. Magnesium depletion is associated with increased potassium efflux from cells (i.e., cellular potassium depletion) and subsequent renal potassium excretion. When magnesium and potassium deficiencies coexist, as may occur with some diuretic drug therapies, magnesium infusions—but not potassium infusions—normalize muscle potassium.

Excretion

Excess magnesium is excreted from the body through the kidneys, which help to maintain magnesium homeostasis along with the small intestine. Of the filtered magnesium (that which is not bound to protein), about 65% to 75% is reabsorbed in the ascending limb of the loop of Henle, another 10% to 15% is reabsorbed in the proximal convoluted tubule, and the remainder is reabsorbed in the distal convoluted tubule. Paracellin, an intercellular magnesium transporter found in the ascending limb of the loop of Henle, and TRPM6, an active magnesium transporter found in the distal convoluted tubule, are involved in urinary magnesium excretion. About 3% to 5% of the filtered magnesium is excreted in the urine. Increased plasma magnesium concentrations, which are monitored by renal divalent cation sensors, inhibit magnesium reabsorption from the distal convoluted tubule. Activation of these sensors also reduces the kidney's response to hormones such as parathyroid hormone, which normally reduces magnesium excretion [7]. Diuretic loop medications, as well as protein, alcohol, and caffeine consumption, increase urinary magnesium excretion.

Fecal magnesium concentrations represent unabsorbed magnesium and a small amount of endogenous magnesium. About 25 to 50 mg of magnesium from endogenous sources is usually excreted daily in the feces [8]. Magnesium also may be lost in sweat, in amounts estimated at approximately 15 mg/day [7,8].

Recommended Dietary Allowance

The RDAs for magnesium vary with age. Among those 19 to 30 years of age, males need 400 mg and females need 310 mg magnesium per day, and among those 31 years and older, males need 420 mg and females need 320 mg magnesium daily [8]. Requirements used to establish these recommendations, however, are thought to be high by some researchers [9]. Pregnant women age 19 to 30 years should ingest 350 mg daily, and those age 31 to 50 years should consume 360 mg of magnesium [8]. During lactation, women age 19 to 30 years should ingest 310 mg daily, and those age 31 to 50 years should consume 320 mg of magnesium [8]. The inside covers of the book provide the RDAs for magnesium for other age groups.

Deficiency

Pure magnesium deficiency from inadequate dietary intake has not been reported, but deficiency has been induced under research protocols and demonstrated in individuals with a rare genetic disorder, Gitelman-Bartter 104 syndrome. Individuals at an increased risk of developing a deficiency include those with malabsorptive disorders (associated with excessive losses of magnesium through vomiting or diarrhea), excessive alcohol use (which is usually coupled with poor intake), chronic diuretic use (which increases urinary magnesium losses), parathyroid disease (which alters magnesium excretion), and burns (which cause excessive dermal loss of magnesium).

With deficiency, hypomagnesemia (plasma magnesium concentrations less than ~1.7 mg/dL) occurs within a relatively short time. Other biochemical changes include low blood concentrations of calcitriol, potassium, and calcium. Effects on PTH concentrations vary, but concentrations are usually low because PTH secretion is diminished; low PTH levels typically result in hypocalcemia (low blood calcium). **Hypokalemia** (low blood potassium) also results from alterations in cellular transport systems that maintain the potassium gradient. Calcitriol synthesis may be altered by decreases in PTH secretion or renal resistance to PTH. Bone is also typically affected [10].

Symptoms associated with magnesium deficiency or disturbances in balance (which may not occur until serum concentrations are < ~1 mg/dL) include nausea, vomiting, headache, anorexia, muscle weakness, spasms and tremors, mental confusion, personality changes, and hallucinations. Changes in cardiovascular and neuromuscular function follow, including, for example, ataxia, paresthesias, neuromuscular hyperexcitability, seizures, and cardiac dysrhythmias—either rapid heart rate (tachycardia), or skipped heartbeats, or irregular heart beat (fibrillation), which may lead to death.

Poor magnesium status and/or low magnesium intakes have been associated with hypertension and cardiovascular disease, as well as diabetes mellitus. A discussion of magnesium as it relates to hypertension is found in the Perspective at the end of Chapter 12. Heart disease appears to develop more quickly in the presence of magnesium deficiency; this accelerated development may result from increased oxidative stress, increased blood cholesterol concentrations, increased thrombosis, and/or inflammation, among other possible mechanisms [11–14]. However, studies reporting an inverse association between magnesium and heart disease are inconsistent [15–17]. Further, while magnesium supplements have been shown to improve brachial artery endothelial function and to inhibit platelet-dependent thrombosis, other supplementation trials have not demonstrated significant benefits [18–21].

Inconsistent findings also have been documented for an association between dietary magnesium intake and/or serum magnesium concentrations and the risk of diabetes [11,22–27]. Links between diabetes and magnesium are plausible given the many roles that magnesium plays in glucose metabolism including, for example, involvement in tyrosine kinase activity at the insulin receptor, intracellular calcium concentrations, ATP-dependent reactions, and interactions between insulin and the insulin receptor [14,23,24]. While some supplementation trials providing magnesium (in amounts up to ~325 mg/day) have shown beneficial effects (e.g., on glucose metabolism, reducing fasting plasma glucose), others have not [17,28–31]. Consequently, given the insufficient evidence of clear beneficial effect(s), magnesium supplementation in the absence of deficiency is not currently recommended for those with diabetes [14,32].

Toxicity

An excessive intake of magnesium is not likely to cause toxicity except in those with impaired renal function, since healthy kidneys can normally excrete magnesium fairly rapidly (thus preventing significant increases in serum concentrations). Excessive intake of magnesium salts (3–5 g), such as from $MgSO_4$, may, however, have a cathartic effect, leading to diarrhea and possible dehydration. Signs of magnesium toxicity include nausea, flushing, double vision, slurred speech, and muscle weakness, which usually appears at plasma magnesium concentrations of about 9 to 12 mg/dL (3.7–4.9 mmol/L). Deep tendon reflexes may disappear with plasma magnesium concentrations of about 4.9 to 7.3 mg/dL (2–3 mmol/L). Acute magnesium toxicity from excessive intravenous administration of magnesium may cause nausea, depression, and paralysis [8]. Muscular paralysis and cardiac and/or respiratory failure may occur if plasma magnesium concentrations exceed about 15 mg/dL (6 mmol/L). A Tolerable Upper Intake Level of 350 mg magnesium from nonfood sources has been recommended for people age 9 years and older (including during pregnancy and lactation) [8]. However, grams doses (>1 g) of magnesium (given intravenously) are often used in the treatment of preeclampsia and eclampsia [33–35].

Assessment of Nutriture

Assessment of magnesium status is difficult because extracellular magnesium represents only about 1% of total body magnesium and appears to be homeostatically regulated. Despite low sensitivity and specificity (e.g., normal serum levels may persist despite severe intracellular deficits), serum magnesium concentrations are routinely measured to assess magnesium status and, when the serum magnesium concentration is below normal (<~1.7 mg/dL or 0.7 mmol/L), an inadequate amount of intracellular magnesium is a certainty. Erythrocyte magnesium concentrations decrease more slowly than plasma or serum concentrations with magnesium deficiency and may reflect longer-term magnesium status because of the life span of the red blood cell.

Determining magnesium status more definitively usually involves measurement of renal magnesium excretion. Normally, 80% of an intravenous magnesium load is excreted within 24 hours; however, with deficiency, excretion decreases. Renal magnesium excretion should be measured before and after the administration of the magnesium load.

References Cited for Magnesium

1. Coudray C, Demigne C, Rayssiguier Y. Effects of dietary fibers on magnesium absorption in animals and humans. J Nutr. 2003; 133:1–4.
2. Brink EJ, Beynen AC. Nutrition and magnesium absorption: a review. Prog Food Nutr Sci. 1992; 16:125–62.
3. Milne DB, Nielsen FH. The interaction between dietary fructose and magnesium adversely affects macromineral homeostasis. J Am Coll Nutr. 2000; 19:31–37.
4. Quamme GA. Molecular identification of ancient and modern mammalian magnesium transporters. Am J Physiol Cell Physiol. 2010; 298:C407–29.
5. Landon R, Yound E. Role of magnesium in regulation of lung function. J Am Diet Assoc. 1993; 93:674–77.
6. Fine K, Santa Ana C, Porter J, Fordtran J. Intestinal absorption of magnesium from food and supplements. J Clin Invest. 1991; 88:396–402.
7. Vormann J. Magnesium: nutrition and metabolism. Mol Aspects Med. 2003; 24:27–37.
8. Food and Nutrition Board, Institute of Medicine. Dietary Reference Intakes. Washington, DC: National Academy Press. 1997, pp. 190–249.
9. Hunt CD, Johnson LK. Magnesium requirements: new estimations for men and women by cross-sectional statistical analyses of metabolic magnesium balance data. Am J Clin Nutr. 2006; 84:843–52.
10. Rude R, Gruber H, Norton H, et al. Bone loss induced by dietary magnesium reduction to 10% of the nutrient requirement in rats is associated with increased release of substance P and tumor necrosis factor alpha. J Nutr. 2004; 134:79–85.
11. Barbagallo M, Dominguez LJ, Galioto A. Role of magnesium in insulin action, diabetes, and cardio-metabolic syndrome X. Mol Aspects Med. 2003; 24:39–52.
12. Mazur A, Maier JAM, Rock E. Magnesium and the inflammatory response: potential physiopathological implications. Arch Biochem Biophys. 2007; 458:48–56.
13. Rosanoff A, Seelig MS. Comparison of mechanism and functional effects of magnesium and statin pharmaceuticals. J Am Coll Nutr. 2004; 23:S501–05.
14. Bo S, Pisu E. Role of dietary magnesium in cardiovascular disease prevention, insulin sensitivity and diabetes. Curr Opin Lipidol. 2008; 19:50–56.
15. Al-Delaimy WK, Rimm EB, Willett WC. Magnesium intake and risk of coronary heart disease among men. J Am Coll Nutr. 2004; 23:63–70.
16. Abbott RD, Ando F, Masaki KH, Dietary magnesium intake and the future risk of coronary heart disease (The Honolulu Heart Program). Am J Cardiol. 2003; 92:665–69.
17. Song Y, Manson J, Buring J, Liu S. Dietary magnesium intake in relation to plasma insulin and risk of type 2 diabetes in women. Diab Care. 2004; 27:59–65.

18. Karaszewski B, Kozera G, Dorosz A. High magnesium or potassium hair accumulation is not associated with ischemic stroke risk reduction: a pilot study. Clin Neurol Neurosurg. 2007; 109:676–79.

19. Shechter M, Sharir M, Paul Labrador MJ. Oral magnesium therapy improves endothelial function in patients with coronary artery disease. Circulation. 2000; 102; 2353–58.

20. Shechter M, Bairey Merz CN, Paul Labrador M. Oral magnesium supplementation inhibits platelet-dependent thrombosis in patients with coronary artery disease. Am J Cardiol. 1999; 84:152–56.

21. Shechter M. Does magnesium have a role in the treatment of patients with coronary artery disease? Am J Cardiovasc Drugs. 2003; 3:231–39.

22. Bo S, Durazzo M, Guidi S. Dietary magnesium and fiber intake, inflammatory and metabolic parameters in middle-aged subjects from a population-based cohort. Am J Clin Nutr. 2006; 84:1062–69.

23. Larsson SC, Wolk A. Magnesium intake and risk of type 2 diabetes: a meta-analysis. J Intern Med. 2007; 262:208–14.

24. Martini LA, Catania AS, Ferreira SRG. Role of vitamins and minerals in prevention and management of type 2 diabetes mellitus. Nutr Rev. 2010; 68:341–54.

25. Schulze MB, Schulz M, Schienkiewitz A, et al. Fiber and magnesium intake and incidence of type 2 diabetes: a prospective study and meta-analysis. Arch Intern Med. 2007; 167:956–65.

26. Hopping BN, Erber E, Grandinetti A, et al. Dietary fiber, magnesium, and glycemic load alter risk of type 2 diabetes in a multiethnic cohort in Hawaii. J Nutr. 2010; 140:68–74.

27. Sales C, Pedrosa L. Magnesium and diabetes mellitus: their relation. Clin Nutr. 2006; 25:554–62.

28. Ma B, Lawson AB, Liese AD. Dairy, magnesium, and calcium intake in relation to insulin sensitivity: approaches to modeling a dose-dependent association. Am J Epidemiol. 2006; 164:449–58.

29. Psaltopoulou T, Ilias I, Alevizaki M. The role of diet and lifestyle in the primary, secondary, and tertiary prevention: a review of meta-analyses. Rev Diab Studies. 2010; 7:26–35.

30. Lopez-Riadura R, Willett WC, Rimm EB. Magnesium intake and risk of type 2 diabetes in men and women. Diabetes Care. 2004; 27:134–40.

31. Rodriguez-Moran M, Guerrero-Romero P. Oral magnesium supplementation improves insulin sensitivity and metabolic control in type 2 diabetic subjects: a randomized double-blind controlled trial. Diabetes Care. 2003; 26:1147–52.

32. American Diabetes Association. Nutrition recommendations and interventions for diabetes. Diabetes Care. 2008; 31(suppl):S61–78.

33. Euser AG, Cipolla MJ. Magnesium sulfate for the treatment of eclampsia. Stroke. 2009; 40:1169–75.

34. Guerrera MP, Volpe SL, Mao JJ. Therapeutic uses of magnesium. Am Fam Physician. 2009; 80:157–62.

35. Duley L, Matar HE, Almerie MQ, Hall DR. Alternative magnesium sulphate regimens for women with pre-eclampsia and eclampsia. Cochrane Database Syst Rev 2010; 8:CD007388.

Suggested Readings

Musso CG. Magnesium metabolism in health and disease. Nephrol Rev 2009; 41:357–62.

San-Cristobal P, Dimke H, Hoenderop JGJ, Bindels RJM. Novel molecular pathways in renal Mg^{2+} transport: a guided tour along the nephron. Curr Opin Nephrol Hypertens. 2010; 19:456–62.

OSTEOPOROSIS AND DIET

One in every 2 women and 1 in every 4 men over the age of 50 years will suffer a fracture because of osteoporosis sometime during their lives [1,2]. Treating the fracture, however, does not necessarily restore health. About 20% of people with hip fractures attributable to osteoporosis die within 1 year of sustaining the fracture [3]. About 33% of people who have had an osteoporosis-induced hip fracture are no longer able to care for themselves and move into nursing homes within the year following the fracture, and another 17% (although they do not require nursing home care) are not able to return to their previous, prefracture lifestyle [4,5].

In the United States, osteoporosis affects approximately 30 to 50 million people, 80% of whom are women. The condition results in about 1.5 million fractures per year; this number is expected to double to 3 million fractures by 2025. Fractures affecting the spine occur most frequently, followed by fractures of the hip and wrist. The cost of treating osteoporotic fractures exceeds $14 billion per year.

Osteoporosis is a systemic skeletal disease characterized by the deterioration of the microarchitecture of bone tissue and low bone mineral density, as shown in Figure 1 [4]. The condition results in fragile bones at increased risk for fracture. Although bone turnover occurs throughout life, after about age 30 to 35 years bone resorption (breakdown) exceeds

bone formation. This bone resorption, including mineral loss, occurs at a rate of up to ~10% per decade in both men and women. However, during the first 5 to 8 years after menopause, the rate of loss accelerates considerably in women. The decline in estrogen production that occurs with menopause, coupled with the generally smaller body and bone mass of women, contributes to the higher prevalence of osteoporosis in women than in men.

Osteoporosis affects both cortical and trabecular bone, although trabecular bone has a higher turnover rate (~25%/year) and is affected to a greater extent than is cortical bone, with a turnover rate of about 4%/year. Cortical or compact bone is found mostly in the shaft of long bones of the limbs but also on the outer walls of all bones. Trabecular (or cancellous) bone is the honeycomb or lattice-type bone found in the vertebrae of the spine, the pelvis (hip area), and the ends of long bones (such as the wrist). Thus, sites containing trabecular bone—the vertebral

bodies (~95% trabecular bone), the femoral neck in the pelvis (~45% trabecular bone), and the radius (~5% trabecular bone)—are the principal sites affected with osteoporosis, especially in women (Figure 2). In addition, teeth

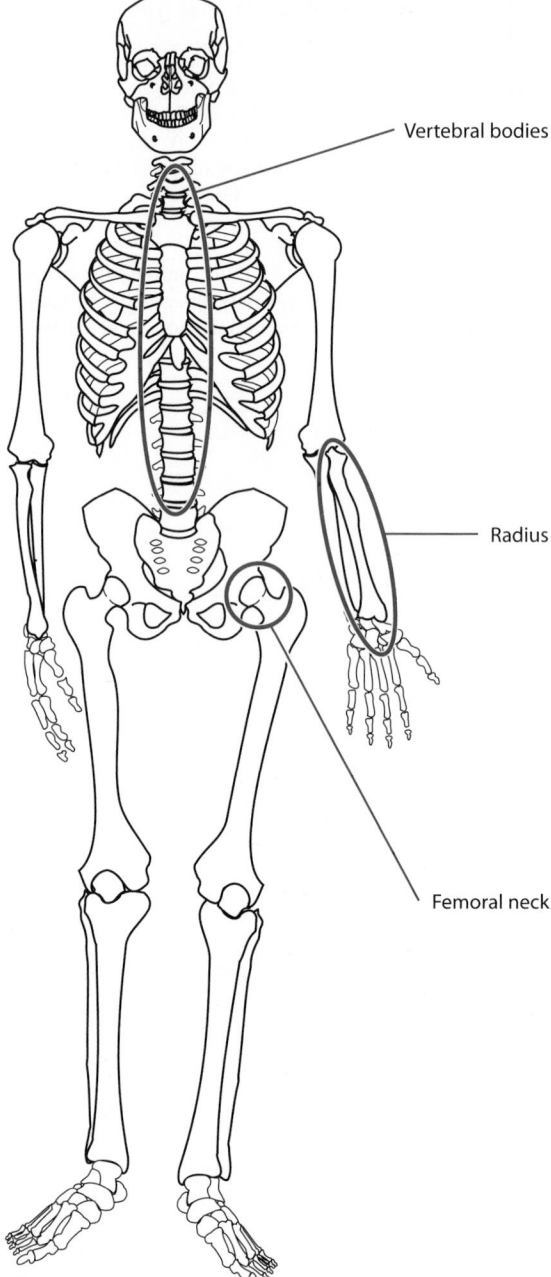

Figure 2 Major sites affected by osteoporosis.

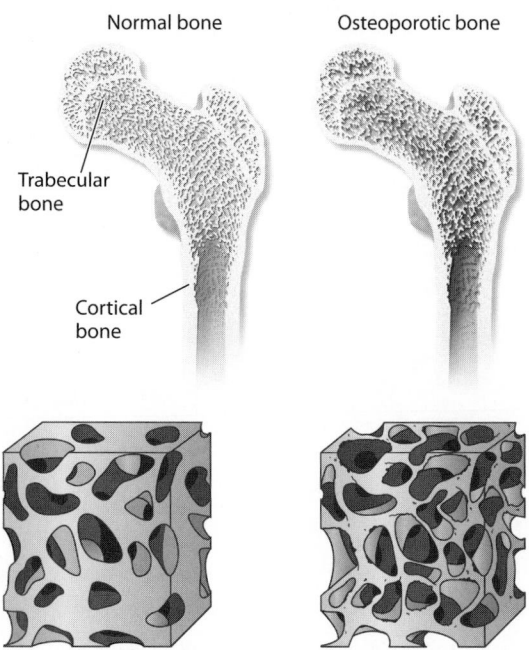

Figure 1 Normal bone/osteoporotic bone.

also may become loose or fall out because some trabecular bone in the jaw is lost. Osteoporosis that affects the vertebrae is associated with loss in height, vertebral pain, and rounding of the shoulders (**kyphosis,** a hunchback-type curvature of the spine, also called **dowager's hump**). The kyphosis in turn reduces the space in the chest and abdominal cavity, resulting in decreased lung capacity and thus shortness of breath, abdominal pain, reduced appetite, and premature satiety. Osteoporosis-induced vertebral fractures also typically limit mobility. The limited mobility causes excessive bed rest, which further weakens muscles and bones, and predisposes the person to falling and suffering further fractures. The excessive bed rest also increases the person's risk for pressure sores, also called decubitus ulcers.

Diagnosis of osteoporosis is based on measurements of bone mineral density, primarily by dual-energy X-ray absorptiometry (DEXA). DEXA scans use X-rays at two energy levels to assess bone mineral content. Peripheral DEXA scans typically measure the extremities including the heel, wrist, or finger. Axial (central) DEXA scans focus on the spine/vertebrae and hip. Software used with the DEXA scan calculates bone mineral density of various regions of interest. Bone mineral density represents the average concentration of minerals per unit area, or how tightly the bone mineral tissue is compressed in a given area. Bone density is reported for comparison purposes as a T score or Z score. T scores represent the number of standard deviations away from the mean bone density of gender- and race-matched young (usually 25- to 45-year-old) adults. A T score equal to 0 means that the person's bone mineral density is at the mean for young adults (considered to represent peak bone mass) of the same gender and race. Osteoporosis is diagnosed if bone mineral density is greater than 2.5 standard deviations below the bone mineral density of young adults [4]. Alternately, osteoporosis may be diagnosed if a fracture involving no or minimal trauma occurs. A T score of −1 to −2.49 is classified as osteopenia, while a T score of 0 to −0.99 is normal [4]. For every 1 standard deviation below the mean, the risk of fracture doubles. Thus, those with osteoporosis are at considerable risk for fracture, and those with osteopenia are at risk for fracture as well as for the development of osteoporosis. Z scores are similar to T scores but represent the number of standard deviations from the mean bone density of age-matched as well as gender- and race-matched people. Thus, for older people, T scores will likely be lower than Z scores.

Individuals most at risk for osteoporosis are those with a family history of the disorder, those who are Caucasian or Asian, and those with a small frame size or low body mass index (especially $< 19 \text{ kg/m}^2$). People using medications such as glucocorticoids, thyroid hormones (taken in excess), and antiepileptic drugs also are at increased risk for bone loss and thus osteoporosis. Although the effects of aging and genetic factors (and sometimes drug therapies) cannot be eliminated, other factors contributing to the development of osteoporosis may be modified. Factors interfering with the attainment of peak bone mass as well as factors accelerating the rate of bone loss are influential in the development of osteoporosis. Some of these factors, including estrogen, physical activity, and intakes of calcium, vitamin D, sodium, protein, acid load, potassium, and magnesium, and a few other nutrients thought to play lesser roles, are addressed in this Perspective.

ESTROGEN

Estrogen, which is produced mainly by the ovaries, has positive effects on bone formation and mineralization, and its influence is especially evident at puberty. Estrogen deficiency promotes bone resorption in all age groups, but in adolescence estrogen deficiency also prevents attainment of peak bone mass. Although estrogen's effects are thought to be mediated by changes in the activities of osteoblasts (bone-forming cells) and osteoclasts (bone-destroying cells), the exact mechanisms by which estrogen affects bone formation and resorption have not been elucidated.

Estrogen concentrations decrease in women around the time of menopause (perimenopause). Estrogen concentrations also are low in women who undergo a surgical ovariectomy (removal of the ovaries) and may be low in young women who are athletes or have eating disorders, especially anorexia nervosa. This estrogen deficit, whether it occurs in older women at menopause or with an ovariectomy, in adolescent girls, or in young women, increases the risk for development of osteoporosis unless estrogen levels can be quickly restored.

Because of estrogen's protective effect on bone, many health care providers believe that estrogen replacement should be recommended on an individual basis, but especially for women who are going through menopause, are immediately postmenopausal, or have had an ovariectomy. Estrogen replacement in the form of oral contraceptive agents also is important for young women who have low estrogen concentrations because of an eating disorder or considerable physical activity. Moreover, use of oral contraceptive agents in women over the age of 40 years decreases subsequent risk of hip fractures after menopause and improves bone mineral density [6]. Estrogen or estrogen replacement therapy (ERT) for peri- or postmenopausal women attenuates bone loss to slow turnover rates and decreases vertebral and nonvertebral fracture rates. It also may increase vertebral and hip bone density [7]. ERT and recovery from amenorrhea, however, have not been associated with normalization of bone density [8]. In addition, use of ERT is not without risk; major side effects include increased risk of breast and uterine cancers and cardiovascular events [7].

PHYSICAL ACTIVITY

The effects of the absence of physical activity (i.e., a sedentary lifestyle) on bone are apparent in people on complete bed rest, because of injury, for example. Similarly, the negative influence of weightlessness, as occurs with space travel, on mineral balance has long been recognized. It follows, therefore, that weight-bearing exercises, including carrying one's own body weight by walking, running, dancing, or weight training (among other activities), on a regular basis should have a protective effect on bone. Indeed, many studies have demonstrated beneficial effects of exercise including improved bone mineral density (primarily the spine and hip), and/or decreased bone loss [9–12]. Perhaps equally beneficial are the improvements in muscle strength and balance associated with exercise (even walking 4 hours per week), which diminish the likelihood of falling and thus of fracturing bones [7,9–12]. Extreme physical activity, however, when associated with amenorrhea (lack of menstruation and thus low blood estrogen), is counterproductive to maintaining bone mass.

CALCIUM AND VITAMIN D

Adequate intakes of calcium and vitamin D are important throughout life. Both nutrients are critical for the attainment of the full genetic expression of peak skeletal mass that occurs sometime in early adulthood. Attainment of dense bones during the early years offers the best protection against weakened, osteoporotic bones in later years.

Adequate intakes of calcium and vitamin D (whether obtained through dietary sources and/or through food plus supplements) in children and adolescents improve bone mass and bone mineral density and thus help achievement of peak bone mass [13–15]. Although peak bone mass is achieved by early adulthood, adequate calcium and vitamin D are needed throughout life for function in bone as well as in other body tissues. While calcium is directly needed to mineralize bone, vitamin D helps to decrease serum parathyroid hormone concentrations (which if elevated promote bone resorption), increase bone mass, and decrease risk of falling. Many studies have found that supplementation with calcium alone (1,000–1,200 mg or more) or in combination with vitamin D (400–1,000 IU or more) prevents the loss of bone mineral density, especially in the spine and sometimes in the hip, in postmenopausal women; however, significant reductions in fracture risk have not consistently been demonstrated [4,16–28]. Consequently, calcium (together with vitamin D) is generally deemed beneficial to prevent bone loss, mainly from the hip and spine, but is considered to have questionable long-term effectiveness in reducing fracture risk [16,25–28].

SODIUM

High sodium intake can be detrimental to body calcium and thus interfere with the attainment of peak bone mass. A direct relationship exists between sodium and calcium: The two nutrients are co-excreted in the urine. Further, because dietary sodium intake in the United States greatly exceeds needs, most ingested sodium is excreted in the urine. A sodium load of 100 mmol (2.3 g) per day increases urinary calcium excretion by 0.5 to 1.5 mmol (20–60 mg) per day [29]. Thus, if the amount of calcium absorbed is not adequate to compensate quantitatively for the increased urinary calcium loss, then bone mass may be compromised [29]. However, other studies and analyses have found that high dietary sodium intake does not significantly affect biomarkers of bone resorption or formation, especially in young adults, and that an adequate potassium intake can reduce or prevent the salt- or sodium-induced increase in urinary calcium excretion [26,29–32].

PROTEIN

An adequate protein intake is necessary for bone health, yet concerns have been raised that high protein intakes may be detrimental to bone (and thus a risk factor for osteoporosis). While it has been demonstrated that doubling protein intake without changing intake of other nutrients results in about a 50% increase in urinary calcium, this rise in urinary calcium is associated with increased calcium absorption and is not associated with increased bone resorption [33–35]. More-over, in natural foods, proteins are usually present with sub-stances that counteract protein's effect on calcium excretion. Large, prospective, epidemiological observations together with intervention studies suggest that diets relatively high in protein are associated with increased bone mineral mass and reduced incidence of osteoporotic bone fractures, and such diets attenuate the decrease in bone mineral density associated with fractures [33,36]. Inadequate protein intake negatively affects bone health and healing from fractures, while protein supplementation or a high-protein diet ap-pears to enhance production of bone growth factor (insulin-like growth factor [IGF]-1), which promotes bone formation [33,35,36].

ACID LOAD, POTASSIUM, AND MAGNESIUM

The pH of body cells and fluids, especially the blood, is tightly regulated. A more acidic blood pH is thought to contribute to osteoporosis because it promotes the demineralization of bone to provide buffers to neutralize the blood. The blood is thought to become mildly acidic when the diet contains an abundance of foods that generate acids (referred to as acid ash) and insufficient foods that provide buffers to neutral-ize the acids. Acid ash is produced in the body in varying amounts based upon the foods consumed; ingesting meat, fish, eggs, and cheese (and to a lesser extent, most grain products) generates more acid ash in the body than inges-tion of other food groups. Most of the acids generated from these foods are thought to arise from the oxidation of the sulfur-containing amino acids. Consuming soft drinks also provides considerable amounts of acids (especially phos-phoric acid) that are absorbed into the body. The blood pH is normally maintained between about 7.35 and 7.45. As the acid concentration of the blood increases, the pH of the blood drops, causing a mild or low-grade metabolic acidosis.

Excess acids in the blood can be buffered by various compounds and can be excreted in the urine by the kidneys; however, the pH of the urine can go only so low—usually not less than about 4.5. Thus, while some of the acids may be excreted in the urine, the kidneys cannot always completely eliminate the acid load at a fast enough rate to prevent low-grade acidosis [26]. To fully correct the acidosis (in the blood), consumption of foods that provide buffers or precur-sors of buffers, such as bicarbonate, to neutralize the acids is

needed. Diets rich in potassium and magnesium and organic anions like citrate, especially available from fruits and veg-etables, have been shown to favorably affect acid-base bal-ance, bone mineral density, and bone metabolism [37–39]. Citrate and alkaline salts, like potassium citrate and potas-sium bicarbonate, neutralize the endogenous acids, and thus ingestion of fruits and vegetables, which provide potassium and bicarbonate, helps to negate an acid load. Potassium and magnesium intakes have been positively associated with bone mineral density in men and women [38,39].

Insufficient intakes of fruits and vegetables coupled with the ingestion of diets that are high in acid ash increase bone resorption and renal calcium loss, and/or decrease bone formation [40]. Daily cola (diet and regular) consumption has been associated with reduced hip (but not spine) bone mineral density in women [41]. Yet urinary calcium excretion was not excessive following the consumption of noncaf-feinated carbonated phosphoric acid–containing beverages [42]. The urinary loss of calcium associated with excretion in acidic urine has been estimated at 66 mg calcium/day [43]. Over time this daily loss of 66 mg of calcium has been calcu-lated as a 24 g loss per year, or a 480 g loss of calcium over 20 years; this 480 g loss is almost half of the skeleton's ~1,150 g calcium content and is consistent with severe osteoporosis [43]. Studies supplementing the diet with buffers, usually as potassium bicarbonate, and/or supplemental fruits and vegetables, have generally shown significant reductions in urinary calcium excretion and in markers of bone resorption [31,44,45].

VITAMINS C AND K

Vitamins C and K are important for the synthesis and func-tion of various proteins found in bone. Remember that vitamin C is needed for the synthesis of hydroxylysine and hydroxyproline, which contribute to triple helix formation of collagen, one of the main proteins in bone. Positive cor-relations between vitamin C intake and bone mineral den-sity have been shown in adolescents and in adult women [45,46]. In older men, lower bone (femoral neck) loss has been associated with higher vitamin C intake [47]. Further, significant reductions in hip and nonvertebral fractures have been demonstrated in men and women with high vitamin C intakes [48]. Yet, the results from other studies are mixed, and because some significant findings have been reported in only certain subpopulations, a more complex interaction between vitamin C and bone health has been suggested and requires further research [28].

In addition to collagen, bone also contains many other proteins, including osteocalcin and matrix Gla protein. Osteo-calcin and matrix Gla protein require vitamin K to function. With inadequate vitamin K status, these two proteins are not fully carboxylated and have limited ability to bind calcium and facilitate bone mineralization. Serum undercarboxylated osteocalcin concentrations (a sign of poor vitamin K status) have been found to be inversely correlated with bone min-eral density in the **Ward's triangle** (a region within the hip) and femoral neck in women during the first decade

of menopause [51]. In addition, low vitamin K intake has been associated with lower bone mineral density and in-creased incidence of hip fractures in elderly men and women [52–54]. However, supplemental vitamin K has not consis-tently improved bone mineral density [55,56].

OTHER LIFESTYLE FACTORS

Smoking negatively affects bone health. Smoking is associ-ated with lower bone density and, in women, with earlier menopause, increased postmenopausal bone loss, and increased risk of fracture, especially of the hip and spine [57–59].

Caffeine minimally affects calcium balance and therefore is thought to be weakly associated with the development of osteoporosis. Caffeine reduces the renal reabsorption of cal-cium, which leads to a temporary (~1- to 3-hour) increase in urinary calcium losses. The loss is typically followed by a period of reduced urinary calcium excretion with no net ef-fect [60,61]. It has been estimated that 1 cup of caffeinated coffee promotes the loss of about 6 mg calcium in the urine [62,63]. Caffeine in amounts of 300 to 400 mg increased urinary calcium by 10 mg/day [64]. However, caffeine may also promote increased secretion of calcium into the gut to enhance calcium loss from the body; whether the secreted calcium is reabsorbed, and the extent of the secretion, have not been determined. Caffeine intake has been positively associated with risk of hip fracture in middle-aged women, especially those whose calcium intake is low [62]. However, no association was reported between current caffeine intake and bone density in postmenopausal women [65].

SUMMARY

Maintenance of desirable skeletal status clearly is multifacto-rial. A person's genetic makeup cannot be changed, nor can the physiological changes accompanying aging be reversed. People usually do have the option, however, of choosing a lifestyle in which good nutrition (i.e., eating a variety of foods—especially fruits and vegetables—and getting recommended intakes of all nutrients) and weight-bearing exercise are practiced regularly [66]. Clearly, consuming recommended intakes of calcium and vitamin D is critical throughout life, as the ability of these two nutrients to reverse bone loss and completely prevent osteoporosis-associated fractures after menopause remains doubtful. To prevent os-teoporosis, reductions in dietary sodium consumption are worthwhile, and efforts should be made to increase the in-gestion of potassium- and magnesium-rich foods, especially fruits and vegetables, which are also rich in buffers. Ingesting foods to meet the recommended intakes of vitamins, espe-cially C and K (and likely others), should also be promoted to contribute to good bone health. Consumption of soft drinks and caffeinated beverages is probably best done in moderation. In addition to a good diet and exercise, atten-tion to the hormonal environment is also critical to attenuat-ing bone loss during periods of low estrogen concentration such as may occur with eating disorders or excessive exercise, or during the peri- and postmenopausal stages of life for women. With bone density monitoring and early diagnosis of problems, drug therapies may be started to slow or halt the progression of osteoporosis; however, prevention of osteoporosis is better. See the "Suggested Readings" section for articles providing reviews of drug therapies available for the treatment of osteoporosis.

References Cited

1. Brewer L, Williams D, Moore A. Current and future treatment options in osteoporosis. Eur J Clin Pharmacol. 2011; 67:321–31.

2. Bone Health and Osteoporosis: A report of the Surgeon General. Rockville, MD: U.S. Dept of Health and Human Services. 2004.

3. Rotella D. Osteoporosis: challenges and new opportunities for therapy. Curr Opin Drug Disc Devel. 2002; 5:477–86.

4. NIH Consensus Development Panel on Osteoporosis: osteoporosis prevention, diagnosis, and therapy. JAMA. 2001; 285:785–95.

5. Sayegh R, Stubblefield P. Bone metabolism and the perimenopause. Obstet Gynecol Clin N Am. 2002; 29:495–510.

6. Kuohung W, Borgatta L, Stubblefield P. Low dose oral contraceptive and bone mineral density: an evidence-based analysis. Contraception. 2000; 61:77–82.

7. Nelson H. Postmenopausal osteoporosis and estrogen. Am Fam Physic. 2003; 68:606–12.

8. Kaufman B, Warren M, Dominguez J, et al. Bone density and amenorrhea in ballet dancers are related to a decreased resting metabolic rate and lower leptin levels. J Clin Endo Metab. 2002; 87:2777–83.

9. Feskanich D, Willett W, Colditz G. Walking and leisure-time activity and risk of hip fracture in postmenopausal women. JAMA. 2002; 288:2300–06.

10. Martyn-St. JM, Carroll S. Meta-analysis of walking for preservation of bone mineral density in postmenopausal women. Bone. 2008; 43:521–31.

11. Bonaiuti D, Shea B, Iovine R, et al. Exercise for preventing and treating osteoporosis in postmenopausal women. Cochrane Database Syst Rev 2002; CD000333.

12. Lau EM, Suriwongpaisal P, Lee JK, et al. Risk factors for hip fracture in Asian men and women: the Asian osteoporosis study. J Bone Miner Res. 2001; 16:572–80.

13. Nowson CA, Green RM, Hopper JL, et al. A co-twin study of the effect of calcium supplementation on bone density during adolescence. Osteoporosis Int. 1997; 7:219–25.

14. Cheng S, Lyytikainen A, Kroger H, et al. Effects of calcium, dairy product, and vitamin D supplementation on bone mass accrual and body composition in 10–12-y-old girls: a 2-y randomized trial. Am J Clin Nutr. 2005; 82:1115–26.

15. Merrilees MJ, Smart EJ, Gilchrist NL, et al. Effect of dairy food supplements on bone mineral density in teenage girls. Eur J Nutr. 2000; 39:256–62.

16. Jackson RD, LaCroix AZ, Gass M, et al. Calcium plus vitamin D supplementation and the risk of fractures. N Engl J Med. 2006; 354:669–83.

17. Tang BM, Eslick GD, Nowson C, et al. Use of calcium or calcium in combination with vitamin D supplementation to prevent fractures and bone loss in people aged 50 years and older: a meta-analysis. Lancet. 2007; 370:657–66.

18. Avenell A, Gillespie WJ, Gillespie LD, O'Connell D. Vitamin D and vitamin D analogues for preventing fractures associated with involutional and postmenopausal osteoporosis. Cochrane Database Syst Rev 2009; CD000227.

19. Boonen S, Lips P, Bouillon R, et al. Need for additional calcium to reduce the risk of hip fracture with vitamin D supplementation: evidence from a comparative meta-analysis of randomized controlled trials. J Clin Endocrinol Metab. 2007; 92:1415–23.

20. Shea B, Wells G, Cranney A. Meta-analyses of therapies for postmenopausal osteoporosis. Endocrin Rev. 2002; 23:552–59.

21. Shea B, Wells G, Cranney A, et al. Osteoporosis Methodology Group. Calcium supplementation on bone loss in postmenopausal women. Cochrane Database Syst Rev 2004; 1(1):CD004526.

22. Chapuy M, Arlot M, Delmas P, Meunier P. Effect of calcium and cholecalciferol treatment for three years on hip fractures in elderly women. BMJ. 1994; 308:1081–82.

23. Tuck S, Francis R. Osteoporosis. Postgrad Med J. 2002; 78:526–32.

24. Bischoff-Ferrari HA, Rees JR, Grau MV, et al. Effect of calcium supplementation on fracture risk: a double-blind randomized controlled trial. Am J Clin Nutr. 2008; 87:1945–51.

25. Bischoff-Ferrari HA, Dawson-Hughes B, Baron JA, et al. Calcium intake and hip fracture risk in men and women: a meta-analysis of prospective cohort studies and randomized controlled trials. Am J Clin Nutr. 2007; 86:1780–90.

26. Institute of Medicine, Food and Nutrition Board. Dietary Reference intakes for Calcium and Vitamin D. Washington DC: National Academy Press. 2011.

27. Spangler M, Phillips BB, Ross MB, Moores KG. Calcium supplementation in postmenopausal women to reduce the risk of osteoporotic fractures. Am J Health-Syst Pharm. 2011; 68:309–18.

28. Tucker KL. Osteoporosis prevention and nutrition. Curr Osteoporosis Rep. 2009; 7:111–17.

29. Heaney RP. Role of dietary sodium in osteoporosis. J Am Coll Nutr. 2006; 25:S271–76.

30. Cohen A, Roe F. Review of risk factors for osteoporosis with particular reference to a possible etiological role of dietary salt. Food Chem Toxicology. 2000; 38:237–53.

31. Sellmeyer D, Schlotter M, Sebastian A. Potassium citrate prevents increased urine calcium excretion and bone resorption induced by high sodium chloride diet. J Clin Endocrinol Metab. 2002; 87:2008–12.

32. Lin P-H, Ginty F, Appel L, et al. The DASH diet and sodium reduction improve markers of bone turnover and calcium metabolism in adults. J Nutr. 2003; 133:3130–36.

33. Heaney RP. Bone health. Am J Clin Nutr. 2007; 85:S300–03.

34. Kerstetter JE, O'Brien KO, Caseria DM, et al. The impact of dietary protein on calcium absorption and kinetic measures of bone turnover in women. J Clin Endocrinol Metab. 2005; 90:26–31.

35. Bonjour J. Dietary protein: an essential nutrient for bone health. J Am Coll Nutr. 2005; 24:S526–36.

36. Schurch M, Rizzoli R, Slosman D, et al. Protein supplements increase serum insulin-like growth factor 1 levels and attenuate proximal femur bone loss in patients with recent hip fracture: a randomized, double-blind, placebo-controlled trial. Ann Intern Med. 1998; 128:801–09.

37. New SA, Robins SP, Campbell MK, et al. Dietary influences on bone mass and bone metabolism: further evidence of a positive link between fruit and vegetable consumption and bone health. Am J Clin Nutr. 2000; 71:142–51.

38. Tucker KL, Hannan MT, Chen H, et al. Potassium, magnesium, and fruit and vegetable intakes are associated with greater bone mineral density in elderly men and women. Am J Clin Nutr. 1999; 69:727–36.

39. Zhu K, Devine A, Prince RL. The effects of high potassium consumption on bone mineral density in a prospective cohort study of elderly postmenopausal women. Osteoporo Int. 2009; 20:335–40.

40. Lemann J, Bushinsky D, Hamm L. Bone buffering of acid and base in humans. Am J Physiol Renal Physiol. 2003; 285:F811–32.

41. Tucker KL, Morita K, Qiao N, et al. Colas, but not other carbonated beverages, are associated with low bone mineral density in older women: the Framingham Osteoporosis Study. Am J Clin Nutr. 2006; 84:936–42.

42. Heaney RP, Rafferty K. Carbonated beverages and urinary calcium excretion. Am J Clin Nutr. 2001; 74:343–47.

43. Fenton TR, Eliasziw M, Lyon AW, et al. Meta-analysis of the quantity of calcium excretion associated with the net acid excretion of the modern diet under the acid-ash diet hypothesis. Am J Clin Nutr. 2008; 88:1159–66.

44. Lanham-New SA. The balance of bone health: tipping the scales in favor of potassium-rich bicarbonate-rice foods. J Nutr. 2008; 138:S172–77.

45. Freudenheim J, Johnson N, Smith E. Relationships between usual nutrient intake and bone mineral content of women 35–65 years of age: longitudinal and cross sectional analysis. Am J Clin Nutr. 1986; 44:863–76.

46. Gunnes M, Lehmann E. Dietary calcium, saturated fat, fiber, and vitamin C as predictors of forearm cortical and trabecular bone mineral density in healthy children and adolescents. Acta Paediatr. 1995; 84:388–92.

47. Sahni S, Hannan MT, Gagnon D, et al. High vitamin C intake is associated with lower 4-year bone loss in elderly men. J Nutr. 2008; 138:1931–38.

48. Sahni S, Hannan MT, Gagnon D, et al. Protective effect of total and supplemental vitamin C intake on the risk of hip fracture: a 17-year follow-up from the Framingham Osteoporosis Study. Osteoporosis Int. 2009; 20:1853–61.

49. Wolf RL, Cauley JA, Pettinger M. Lack of a relationship between vitamin and mineral antioxidants and bone mineral density: results from the Women's Health Initiative. Am J Clin Nutr. 2005; 82:581–88.

50. Simon JA, Hudes ER. Relation of ascorbic acid to bone mineral density and self-reported fractures among US adults. Am J Epidemiol. 2001; 154:427–33.

51. Knapen M, Kruseman A, Wouters R, Vermeer C. Correlation of serum osteocalcin fractions with bone mineral density in women during the first 10 years after menopause. Calcif Tiss Int. 1998; 63:375–79.

52. Szulc P, Arlot M, Chapuy M, et al. Serum undercarboxylated osteocalcin correlates with hip bone mineral density in elderly women. J Bone Miner Res. 1994; 9:1591–95.

53. Booth S, Tucker K, Chen H, et al. Dietary vitamin K intakes are associated with hip fracture but not with bone mineral density in elderly men and women. Am J Clin Nutr. 2000; 71:1201–08.

54. Macdonald HM, McGuigan FE, Lanham-New SA, et al. Vitamin K1 intake is associated with higher bone mineral density and reduced bone resorption in early postmenopausal Scottish women: no evidence of gene-nutrient interactions with apolipoprotein E polymorphism. Am J Clin Nutr. 2008; 87:1513–20.

55. Bolton-Smith C, McMurdo ME, Paterson CR, et al. Two-year randomized controlled trial of vitamin K1 (phylloquinone) and vitamin D3 plus calcium on the bone health of older women. J Bone Miner Res. 2007; 22:509–19.

56. Booth SL, Dallal G, Shea MK, et al. Effect of vitamin K supplementation on bone loss in elderly men and women. J Clin Endocrinol Metab. 2008; 93:1217–23.

57. Ward KD, Klesges RC. A meta-analysis of the effects of cigarette smoking on bone mineral density. Calcif Tissue Int. 2001; 68:259–70.

58. Vestergaard P, Mosekilde L. Fracture risk associated with smoking: a meta-analysis. J Intern Med. 2003; 254:572–83.

59. Kanis JA, Johnell O, Oden A, et al. Smoking and fracture risk: a meta-analysis. Osteoporos Int. 2005; 16:155–62.

60. Fitzpatrick L, Heaney RP. Got soda? J Bone Mineral Res. 2003; 18:1570–72.

61. Barger-Lux MJ, Heaney RP, Stegman MR. Effects of moderate caffeine intake on the calcium economy of premenopausal women. Am J Clin Nutr. 1990; 52:722–25.

62. Hernandez-Avila M, Colditz G, Stampfer M, Rosner B. Caffeine, moderate alcohol intake, and risk of fractures of the hip and forearm in middle-aged women. Am J Clin Nutr. 1991; 54:157–63.

63. Heaney R, Recker R. Effects of nitrogen, phosphorus and caffeine on calcium balance in women. J Lab Clin Med. 1982; 99:46–55.

64. Massey LK, Whiting SJ. Caffeine, urinary calcium, calcium metabolism and bone. J Nutr. 1993; 123: 1611–14.

65. Lloyd T, Rollings N, Eggli D, et al. Dietary caffeine intake and bone status of postmenopausal women. Am J Clin Nutr. 1997; 65:1826–30.

66. Nieves JW. Osteoporosis: the role of micronutrients. Am J Clin Nutr. 2005; 81(suppl):S1232–39.

Suggested Reading

Grossman JM. Osteoporosis prevention. Curr Opin Rheumatol. 2011; 23:203–10.

Henriksen K, Bollerslev J, Everts V, Karsdal MA. Osteoclast activity and subtypes as a function of physiology and pathology: implications for future treatments of osteoporosis. Endoc Rev. 2011; 32:31–63.

Mayes S. Review of postmenopausal osteoporosis pharmacotherapy. Nutr Clin Prac. 2007; 22:276–85.

Neve A, Corrado A, Cantatore FP. Osteoblast physiology in normal and pathological conditions. Cell Tissue Res. 2011; 343; 280–302.

Riek AE, Towler DDA. The pharmacological management of osteoporosis. Missouri Med. 2011; 108:118–23.

Rude RK, Singer FR, Gruber HE. Skeletal and hormonal effects of magnesium deficiency. J Am Coll Nutr. 2009; 28:131–41.

Sharif PS, Abdollahi M, Larijani B. Current, new and future treatments of osteoporosis. Rheumatol Int. 2011; 31:289–300.

Thorpe MP, Evans EM. Dietary protein and bone health: harmonizing conflicting theories. Nutr Rev. 2011; 69:215–30.

Vermeer C, Theuwissen E. Vitamin K, osteoporosis, and degenerative diseases of ageing. Menopause Int. 2011; 17:19–23.

12 WATER AND ELECTROLYTES

CHAPTER 1, IN PARTICULAR, and the subsequent chapters dealing with nutrient metabolism emphasize the specialized nature of the cells comprising the organ systems of the body. Despite the great diversity of specialized cellular functions, the composition of the body fluids (the internal environment) enveloping the cells remains relatively constant under normal conditions. This constant composition, or **homeostasis,** of the internal environment is necessary for optimal activity of the cells. It is maintained by homeostatic mechanisms involving most of the body's organ systems, especially the circulatory, respiratory, and renal systems as well as the central nervous system (CNS) and the endocrine regulation system. Many minor disturbances inevitably occur in water distribution, electrolyte balance, and pH of the body fluids during metabolism. As disturbances arise, compensatory mechanisms of the regulatory organs make appropriate corrections to maintain homeostasis.

WATER DISTRIBUTION IN THE BODY

Water accounts for about 60% of the total body weight in a normal adult, making it the most abundant constituent of the human body. In terms of volume, the total body water in a man of average weight (70 kg) is roughly 42 L. Water provides the medium for the solubilization and passage of a multitude of nutrients, both organic and inorganic, from the blood to the cells and for the return of metabolic products to the blood. It also serves as the medium in which the vast number of intracellular metabolic reactions take place.

Total body water can theoretically be compartmentalized into two major reservoirs: the intracellular compartment, which includes all water enclosed within cell membranes, and the extracellular compartment, which includes all water external to cell membranes. Of the 42 L of total body water, the intracellular and extracellular compartments account for about 28 L and 14 L, respectively. The anatomic extracellular water is functionally subdivided into the plasma (the cell-free, intravascular water compartment) and the interstitial fluid (ISF). The ISF directly bathes the extravascular cells and provides the medium for the passage of nutrients and metabolic products back and forth between the blood and cells. In addition, the pericardial, pleural, peritoneal, and synovial spaces or cavities that are normally empty except for a small volume of viscous lubricating fluid are considered part of the ISF compartment. The body water compartment volumes for a 70-kg man are summarized in Table 12.1.

The fraction of total body weight that is water and the percentage of total body water that is extracellular or intracellular do not remain constant during growth. Expressed as a percentage of body weight, total body water

Table 12.1 Fluid Compartment Values

	Percentage of Body Weight	Percentage of Total Body Water	Volume (L) in 70-kg Man
Total body water	60	—	42
Extracellular water	20	33	14
Plasma	5	8	3.5
Interstitial fluid	15	25	10.5
Intracellular water	40	67	28

decreases during gestation and early childhood, reaching adult values by about 3 years of age. During this time, the extracellular water (as percentage of body weight) decreases while the intracellular water (as percentage of body weight) increases.

MAINTENANCE OF FLUID BALANCE

Most available body water enters by the oral route as beverages (water and water-based beverages) or as liquids contained in foods. A relatively small amount of water is formed within the body as a product of metabolic reactions (metabolic water). These two sources together account for a daily intake of about 2,500 mL of fluid, of which the oral route contributes about 2,300 mL, or >90%.

The routes by which water is lost from the body can vary according to environmental and physiological conditions, such as ambient temperature and extent of physical exercise. At an ambient temperature of 68°F (20°C), about 1,400 mL of the 2,300 mL taken in is normally lost in the urine, 100 mL in the sweat, and 200 mL in the feces. The remaining 600 mL leaves the body as insensible water loss, so called because the subject is not aware of the water loss as it is occurring. Evaporation from the respiratory tract and diffusion through the skin are examples of insensible water loss.

Osmotic Pressure

One of the more important factors determining the distribution of water among the water compartments of the body is **osmotic pressure.** When a membrane permeable to water but impermeable to solute particles separates two fluid compartments of unequal solute concentrations, a net movement of water takes place through the membrane from the solution with higher water (lower solute) concentration toward the solution with lower water (higher solute) concentration. In other words, water moves from the more dilute solution to the more concentrated solution. The movement of water across a

semipermeable membrane is called **osmosis.** Osmosis can be blocked by applying an external pressure across the membrane in the opposite direction to the water flow. The amount of pressure required to exactly oppose osmosis (i.e., water movement) into a solution across a semipermeable membrane separating the solution from pure water is the osmotic pressure of the solution. The direction of osmosis across a membrane is dependent upon the number of independent particles on each side of the membrane.

There are several ways to characterize the concentration of a solution (and thus its osmotic pressure). Osmolality is a measure of the individual particles of the solute that contribute to the osmotic pressure of a solution, expressed as osmoles of solute per a certain *weight* (1 kg) of *solvent* (osm/kg). *Osmoles* refers to the number of moles of each *particle* in the solution. Molarity, in contrast, denotes the molar concentration (i.e., number of moles) of solute in a designated *volume* of *solution* (1 L). A third measure, osmolarity, denotes the osmoles of solute particles in a designated *volume* (1 L) of *solution* (osm/L). Note that 1 mole of a compound may dissociate into 2 or more osmoles of particles in solution. For example, whereas in a solution containing glucose or urea, which does not disassociate, moles and osmoles of the solute are equal; in a solution of NaCl, which disassociates into 2 ions, there are twice as many osmoles as moles of the solute. Thus, a NaCl solution that has a molarity of 1 mole/L has an osmolarity of 2 osm/L. The use of osmolality—osmoles per kg of solvent—provides a constant ratio of solute particles to molecules of solvent that is independent of temperature (aqueous solutions expand as they are heated). In dilute aqueous solutions, as found in the human body, only a small numerical difference exists between osmolarity and osmolality, and both the terms and values are often used interchangeably. Because osmolality is less convenient to use and calculate than osmolarity, osmolarity is often preferred in clinical practice.

The theoretic osmotic pressure presupposes that the solute particles are unable to pass freely through the membrane. When the membrane is permeable to a solute, it does not contribute to the actual, or *effective,* osmotic pressure. The higher the permeability of a membrane is to a solute, the lower the effective osmotic pressure of a solution of that solute at a given osmolality. As an example, cell membranes are much more permeable to a nonionic substance such as urea than to sodium and chloride ions. Therefore, the effective osmotic pressure of a solution of urea across the cell membrane would be much less than that of a solution of sodium chloride of the same osmolality.

The effective osmotic pressure of plasma and interstitial fluid across the capillary endothelium that separates them is caused mainly by macromolecules, such as proteins, that cannot pass through the endothelium. Protein concentration is much higher in the plasma than in the interstitial fluid, conferring on the plasma a relatively high osmotic pressure, or water-attracting property. Proteins and other macromolecules too large to traverse the capillary endothelium are sometimes called **colloids,** and the osmotic pressure attributed to them is appropriately termed the *colloid osmotic pressure.*

Filtration Forces

Water distribution across the capillary endothelial surface is controlled by the balance of forces that tend to move water from the plasma to the interstitial fluid (filtration forces) and forces that move water from the interstitial fluid into the plasma (reabsorption forces). The major filtration force in the capillaries is hydrostatic pressure (P_{pl}) caused by the pumping of the heart. A much weaker filtration force is the ISF colloid osmotic pressure (II_{isf}); this force is weak because of the negligible concentration of protein in the ISF. Another weak filtration force is a small, negative ISF hydrostatic pressure (P_{isf}). The major reabsorption force countering the filtration forces is the plasma osmotic pressure (II_{pl}), which is approximately 28 mm Hg.

At the arteriolar end of the capillaries, the average values of these forces are P_{pl} (hydrostatic pressure): 25 mm Hg; II_{isf} (colloid osmotic pressure): 5 mm Hg; P_{isf} (interstitial hydrostatic pressure): −6 mm Hg; and II_{pl} (plasma osmotic pressure): 28 mm Hg. The net result of these four forces can be described by Starling's equation:

$$\text{Filtration pressure} = (P_{pl} + II_{isf}) - (II_{pl} + P_{isf})$$

Substituting the average values, we have

$$\begin{aligned}\text{Filtration pressure} &= (25 + 5) - (28 + [-6]) \\ &= (25 + 5) - (28 - 6) \\ &= (30) - (22) \\ &= 8 \text{ mm Hg}\end{aligned}$$

This positive filtration pressure indicates that a net filtration of water from the plasma to the ISF occurs at the arteriolar end of the capillaries. When filtration pressure is negative, a net reabsorption of water from the ISF to the plasma occurs. This situation exists at the venule end of the capillaries, where P_{pl} is substantially reduced while the concentration of plasma protein, and therefore II_{pl}, correspondingly increases. The net effect of these forces on the water distribution between plasma and ISF along the course of the capillary is shown in Figure 12.1.

From what you have read to this point, you should understand that osmotic pressure, together with proper intake of water and its output by body mechanisms, is a very important factor in maintaining fluid balance and compartmentalization. The body's extracellular water volume, for example, is determined mainly by its osmolarity. The osmolarity, in turn, acts as the signal to the regulatory

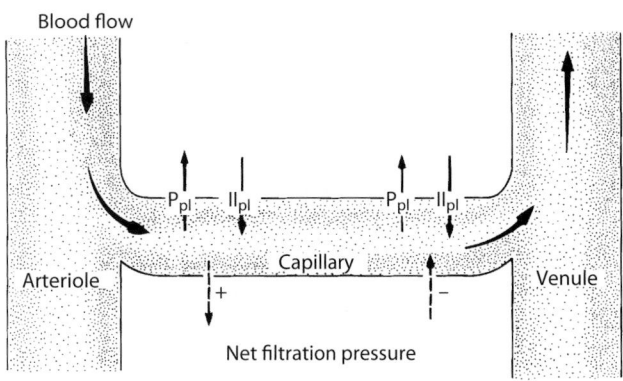

Figure 12.1 Starling's hypothesis of water distribution between plasma and interstitial fluid compartments. The relative magnitudes of the pressures, Ppl (plasma hydrostatic pressure) and IIpl (plasma osmotic pressure), are represented by the thickness of their respective arrows. There is a positive net filtration pressure at the arteriolar end of the capillary and a negative net filtration pressure at the venule end.
Source: Clinical Chemistry: Theory, Analysis, and Correlation, 2nd ed., Kleinman, L.I., Lorenz, J.M., 'Physiology and pathophysiology of body water and electrolytes,' p. 373. Copyright © Elsevier 1989.

factors responsible for maintaining fluid homeostasis. The regulation of extracellular water osmolarity and volume is largely the responsibility of the hypothalamus, the renin-angiotensin-aldosterone system, and the kidneys.

THE KIDNEY'S ROLE

The functional unit of the kidney is the nephron. Each kidney contains about 1 to 1.5 million nephrons. The five components of the nephron are the Bowman's capsule, proximal convoluted tubule, loop of Henle, distal convoluted tubule, and collecting duct. The excretion process starts in the Bowman's capsule, the proximal (nearest the Bowman's capsule) end of the renal tubule, which encapsulates a tuft of about 50 capillaries linking the afferent (flowing into the capsule) and efferent (flowing from the capsule) arterioles that surround the tubule segments after they leave the capsule. The capillary network in the Bowman's capsule is called the glomerulus, and it accounts for the particularly rich blood supply that the kidney enjoys. An estimated 25% of the volume of blood pumped by the heart into the systemic circulation is circulated through the kidneys, a particularly significant situation in view of the fact that the kidneys constitute only about 0.5% of total body weight. The major components of the nephron are shown schematically in Figure 12.2.

The capillaries in the glomerular network have large pores and act as a filter in removing water and other substances, including electrolytes, glucose, amino acids, and metabolic waste products, from plasma. The capillaries of the glomerulus are 100 to 400 times more permeable to water and dissolved solutes than are the capillaries of skeletal muscle. The filtered substances make up what is known as the glomerular filtrate. In the absence of disease, no blood cells (or proteins that exceed a molecular weight of about 50,000 daltons) normally enter the glomerular

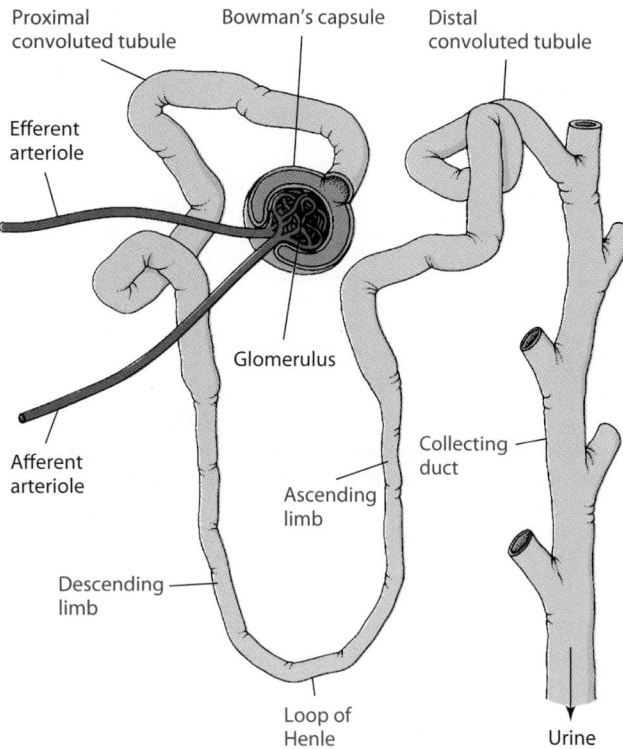

Figure 12.2 A schematic representation of the major components of the nephron.

filtrate because their larger size prevents them from passing through the pores of the capillary endothelium.

Each segment of the tubules is functionally distinct in its permeability to water and the solutes of the glomerular filtrate. The tubular segments are surrounded by a network of capillaries into which glomerular filtrate materials can be selectively reabsorbed into the bloodstream as a salvage mechanism. These capillaries surrounding the nephron may also secrete certain substances from the blood into the renal tubule.

The removal of potentially toxic waste products, a major function of the kidneys, is accomplished through the formation of urine. Urine formation involves three basic processes:

- *filtration*, through which the glomerular filtrate is formed
- *reabsorption* of selected filtrate substances into the bloodstream
- *secretion* of materials into the tubules from the surrounding capillaries

Through these same processes, the kidneys are able to regulate fluid and electrolyte homeostasis for the proper functioning of the body's cells. In healthy people, the kidneys are highly sensitive to fluctuations in fluid and electrolyte intake, and compensate for these fluctuations by varying the volume and constituents of the urine. The glomerular capillaries differ from other capillaries in the body in that the hydrostatic pressure within them

is approximately three times greater than in other capillaries. As a result of this high pressure, substances are filtered through the semipermeable membrane into the Bowman's capsule at a rate of about 130 mL/minute. This glomerular filtration rate (GFR) amounts to over 187 L of filtrate formed per day, yet only about 1,400 mL of urine is produced during this time. This difference in the volumes of filtrate and urine means that < 1% of the filtrate is excreted as urine, and the remaining 99% is reabsorbed into the blood. An overview of urine formation is provided here, with emphasis on its hormonal and enzymatic regulation. For more detail, consult a textbook on human physiology such as [1].

Vasopressin

You have read that the hypothalamus, renin-angiotensin-aldosterone system, and kidneys are responsible for maintaining extracellular fluid volume and osmolarity. Actually, the three work in concert because the hypothalamic hormone, vasopressin (also called arginine vasopressin [AVP] or antidiuretic hormone [ADH]), and aldosterone, produced in the adrenal cortex, exert their effects through the kidneys.

Vasopressin is a nine–amino acid peptide that is produced in the supraoptic nucleus of the hypothalamus but stored in and secreted by the posterior pituitary gland. Arginine vasopressin contains the amino acid arginine and is the hormone found in humans. (Animals such as pigs produce other forms of vasopressin that contain lysine in place of arginine.) The secretion of vasopressin into the circulation is triggered by increased extracellular water osmolarity or by decreased intravascular volume. The hypothalamic response to high extracellular fluid osmolarity is attributed to shrinkage of neurons within the gland, caused by the movement of water out of the neurons into the higher-osmolarity interstitial fluid. This shrinkage then acts as the signal to the posterior pituitary to release the hormone. The induction of the thirst sensation by vasopressin in response to plasma osmolarity is illustrated graphically in Figure 12.3.

Vasopressin has two primary functions in the kidney. First, it is a potent water-conserving hormone. In the absence of vasopressin, the distal portion of the ascending loop of Henle and the collecting ducts (see Figure 12.2) are impermeable to water. Vasopressin increases the water permeability of the distal convoluted tubule and the collecting duct by binding with specific hormone-binding sites called V_2 receptors, which stimulate the production of cAMP and movement of aquaporins from intracellular vesicles to the cell surface by exocytosis. The aquaporins are water channels that increase water permeability in proportion to the level of vasopressin present. The osmolarity gradient between the glomerular filtrate in the tubule and the surrounding interstitial fluid causes water to

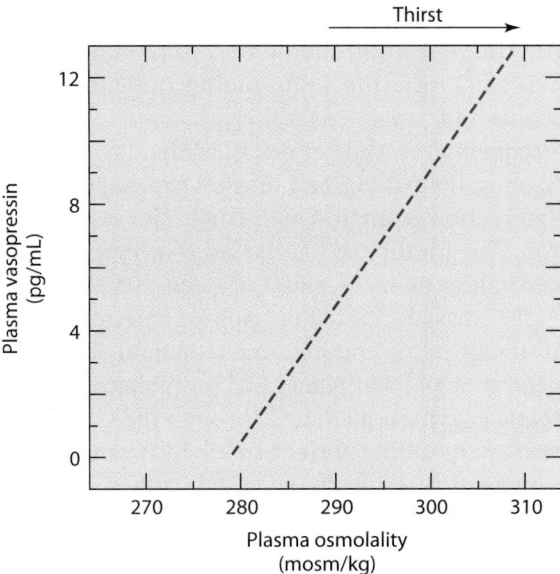

Figure 12.3 Relationship of plasma vasopressin to plasma osmolality. The arrow indicates the plasma osmolality at which the sensation of thirst is stimulated.
Source: Vokes T., Water homeostasis. Annual Review of Nutrition, 1987; 7:386. Reprinted by permission.

move across the cell lining of the tubule into the capillaries [1]. The second function of vasopressin is to regulate, via the same V_2 receptors, the discretionary reabsorption of sodium through Na^+ channels (NaC) that increase the reabsorption of Na^+. NaC are present in aldosterone-sensitive cells in the distal portion of the nephron [2]. Vasopressin also binds to the hormone-binding V_1 receptors, which are abundant in the smooth muscle of the thick portion of the distal part of the glomerulus, causing contraction. This contraction increases blood pressure and the glomerular filtration rate, resulting in the increased excretion of Na^+ [3].

About 80% of the water has been removed from the filtrate before it reaches the distal portion of the loop of Henle, the distal convoluted tubule, and the collecting ducts where vasopressin acts. When vasopressin is present, additional water is reabsorbed. Under conditions of hyper- or overhydration, vasopressin is not released, and in its absence the distal portion of the glomerulus and the collecting duct are impermeable to water. Thus, in this situation the 20% of the water that has not been reabsorbed at this point is excreted as urine. Because this portion of the nephron remains permeable to electrolytes, the kidney can excrete urine of different osmolarities. Vasopressin promotes a limited amount of Na^+ retention and K^+ excretion.

Renin-Angiotensin-Aldosterone System

The major regulatory factor controlling sodium ion retention and potassium ion excretion is the renin-angiotensin-aldosterone system (RAAS). The RAAS is the most potent system involved in the regulation of Na^+ and K^+. The sequence of events that make up the RAAS is illustrated in

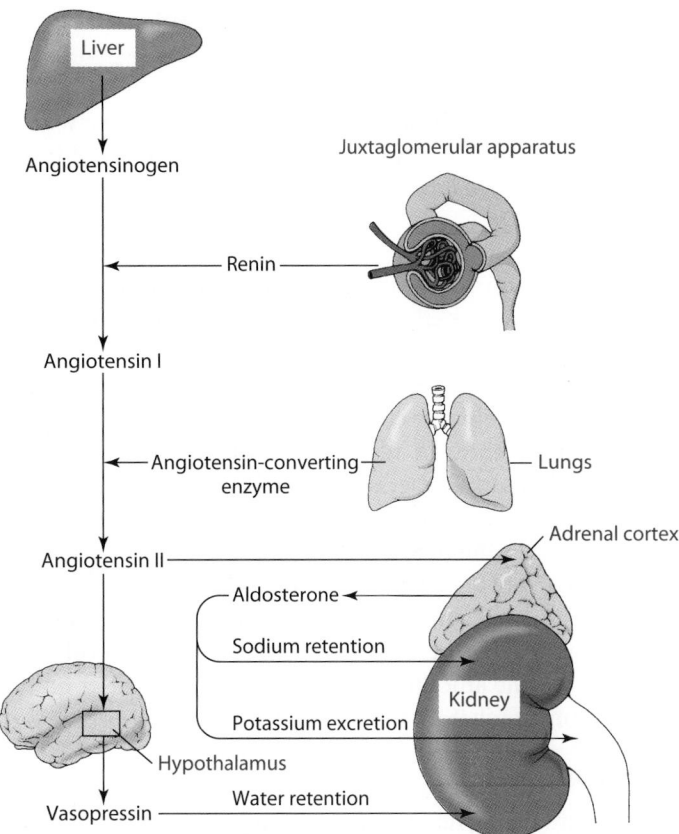

Figure 12.4 The renin-angiotensin-aldosterone system, illustrating the cooperation of kidneys, liver, lungs, adrenals, and hypothalamus in this mechanism of fluid homeostasis.

Figure 12.4. Renin is secreted by cells of the afferent arteriole of the glomerulus in response to a fall in plasma Na^+, Cl^-, ECF volume, or blood pressure. This starts a series of reactions, discussed later, that ultimately result in the release of aldosterone from the adrenal cortex. The kidneys and aldosterone are involved in most of the regulation of excretion and retention of Na^+, K^+, and Cl^-.

The plasma concentrations of several different substances influence the release of aldosterone from the adrenal cortex. Listed in decreasing order of their potency in stimulating aldosterone release, they are:

❶ The increased angiotensin II. This potent polypeptide hormone participates in the renin-angiotensin-aldosterone system. It reacts with receptors on cell membranes of the adrenal cortex, stimulating the synthesis and release of aldosterone.

❷ Decreased atrial natriuretic peptide (ANP) and brain natriuretic peptide (BNP). ANP is a peptide hormone synthesized in atrial cells of the heart and released in response to increased arteriolar stretch, which indicates elevated blood pressure. BNP is synthesized in the ventricles of the heart. ANP is more potent than BNP. Both function in opposition to aldosterone in that they inhibit sodium reabsorption in the kidney and thereby promote sodium excretion [1].

❸ Increased plasma potassium concentration.

❹ Decreased plasma sodium.

Each of these stimulants of aldosterone release will be discussed briefly. A physiology text [1] can provide additional information on renal physiology.

Renin

Renin is a hormone and proteolytic enzyme synthesized in a variety of cells as an inactive preprorenin that is cleaved to form prorenin, which is also inactive, in the endoplasmic reticulum of these cells [4]. The enzymatically active renin is secreted by granular cells in the juxtaglomerular (near or adjoining the glomerulus) apparatus of the kidney. The granular cells are innervated by the sympathetic nervous system and are stimulated to release renin when the blood pressure falls below normal. Specifically, renin secretion is stimulated by decreased renal perfusion pressure, which is sensed by the distention receptors and baroreceptors within the juxtaglomerular apparatus. The amount of renin released is based upon the level of stimulation of the granular cells.

Angiotensin

The circulating renin hydrolyzes angiotensinogen—a large, freely circulating protein constantly synthesized by the liver and present in high concentrations—to angiotensin I, another inactive decapeptide. Angiotensin I is then acted on by a second proteolytic enzyme, angiotensin-converting enzyme (ACE), synthesized in vascular endothelial cells in the blood vessels of the lung, producing the active octapeptide angiotensin II. Angiotensin II then interacts with specific receptors on adrenal cortical cells, leading to the synthesis and release of aldosterone. Angiotensin II is also a potent vasoconstrictor that increases blood pressure. Note that ACE inhibitors, one of the family of drugs used to control blood pressure in hypertensive individuals, function by reducing the conversion of angiotensin I to angiotensin II [1].

A sequential cascade of reactions that involves G proteins, phospholipase C, and inositol triphosphate follows the interaction of angiotensin II with its membrane receptor. Phospholipase C raises the intracellular Ca^{2+} concentration by increasing Ca^{2+} conductance through Ca^{2+} channels, and inositol triphosphate releases Ca^{2+} from storage in the endoplasmic reticulum. The elevated concentration of intracellular Ca^{2+} stimulates appropriate synthetic enzymes, mediated through the Ca^{2+}-binding protein calmodulin, present in all eukaryotic cells [1]. This interaction results in increased synthesis and release of aldosterone. Figure 11.6 illustrates this type of hormonal mechanism.

Angiotensin II can be hydrolyzed further to angiotensin III (a process that is not shown in Figure 12.4) by the hydrolytic removal of an aspartic acid residue by a plasma aminopeptidase. Angiotensin III is also physiologically active. In fact, it has been observed to be more potent than angiotensin II in its aldosterone-stimulating ability. However, the plasma concentration of angiotensin III is considerably less than that of angiotensin II, and therefore its contribution to maintaining fluid balance is less dramatic.

In addition to its role in conserving body water through aldosterone action, angiotensin II is a potent vasoconstrictor, reducing the glomerular filtration rate and therefore the filtered load of sodium. Also, angiotensin II stimulates the hypothalamic thirst center and the release of vasopressin, both of which increase body water volume. Figure 12.5 illustrates the central role of the hypothalamus and the action of angiotensin II in the hormonal regulation of fluid homeostasis.

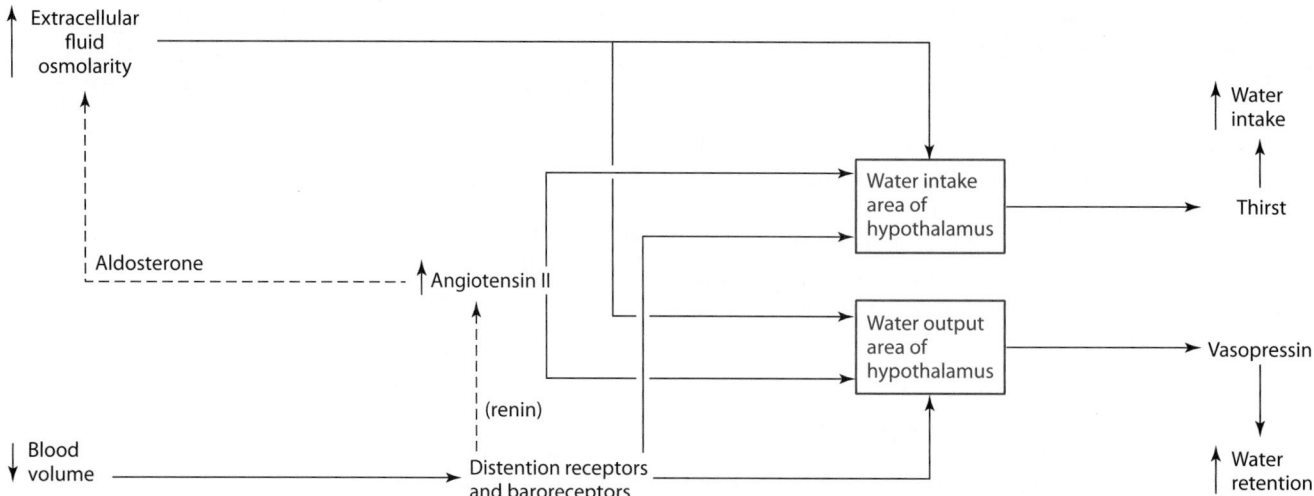

Figure 12.5 A summary of the mechanisms by which fluid homeostasis is maintained. Water depletion stimuli such as increased extracellular fluid osmolarity or decreased blood volume can stimulate the hypothalamus either directly or through the production of angiotensin II, formed by the action of the renal protease renin. The renin-angiotensin-aldosterone system (shown by dashed arrows) increases extracellular fluid osmolarity by promoting renal tubular reabsorption of sodium.

Aldosterone

Aldosterone works on the cells of the distal ascending loop of Henle and collecting ducts by inserting additional Na^+ channels into the luminal membrane and additional Na^+–K^+ pumps into the basolateral membrane [1]. The result is an influx of Na^+ into the cells lining the distal ascending loop of Henle and collecting tubules from the lumen and the active pumping of Na^+ out of the lumen into the plasma. The Cl^- follows the Na^+. This promotes retention of both salt and water and hence reverses the conditions that triggered the release of renin—that is, the salt depletion, reduced plasma volume, and decreased arterial blood pressure. Angiotensin II also increases blood pressure by constricting systemic arterioles, stimulating thirst (which increases water intake), and stimulating vasopressin release (which increases water reabsorption by the kidneys). Together, the actions of aldosterone and angiotensin II contribute to expanded plasma volume and increased blood pressure.

If the Na^+ load, ECF (including the plasma volume), and blood pressure are elevated, renin secretion is inhibited. If renin is not released, the RAAS does not function and aldosterone is not released. In the absence of aldosterone, Na^+ is lost in the urine. Although aldosterone regulates only about 8% of the filtered Na^+, the reduction in reabsorption with low aldosterone levels can account for a large loss of Na^+ in the course of a day because of the large amount of fluid filtered by the glomerulus. The mechanisms of fluid homeostasis are illustrated in Figure 12.5.

Natriuretic Peptides

Opposing the RAAS are the atrial natriuretic peptide (ANP) and the brain natriuretic peptide (BNP). ANP, the more potent of the two peptides, is produced and stored in granules in cardiac myocytes of the atrium. BNP was first discovered in the brain (which gave it its name) but is mostly produced and stored by cardiac myocytes of the ventricles of the heart. ANP and BNP are released into circulation when the heart muscle is stretched by an expansion of ECF that results from the retention of Na^+ and H_2O, and increased arterial blood pressure. The natriuretic peptides promote Na^+ and water excretion, which decreases the plasma volume and lowers blood pressure. Their action inhibits the RAAS by inhibiting renin secretion, which in turn inhibits aldosterone secretion. The peptides also promote dilation of the afferent arterioles and constriction of the efferent arterioles. The result is an increase in glomerular pressure, which increases the glomerular filtration rate, making more Na^+ and H_2O available for excretion. ANP and BNP directly lower blood pressure by lowering cardiac output and reducing peripheral vascular resistance [5,6].

MAINTENANCE OF ELECTROLYTE BALANCE

Electrolytes are the anions and cations that are distributed throughout the fluid compartments of the body. They are distributed in such a way that within a given compartment—the blood plasma, for example—electrical neutrality is always maintained, with the anion concentration exactly balanced by the cation concentration. The cationic electrolytes of the extracellular fluid include sodium, potassium, calcium, and magnesium (Ca^{+2} and Mg^{+2} are covered in Chapter 11). These cations are electrically balanced by the anions chloride, bicarbonate, and negatively charged proteins, along with relatively low concentrations of organic acids, phosphate, and sulfate. The major electrolytes, most of which are categorized nutritionally as macrominerals, are listed in Table 12.2. The maintenance of pH and electrolyte balance is a responsibility that rests almost exclusively with the kidney.

All filterable substances in plasma—that is, all the plasma solutes except the larger proteins—freely enter the glomerular filtrate from the blood. Some of these substances (such as urea and detoxified drugs) are metabolic waste products and are excreted in the urine with little or no reabsorption in the tubules. However, most of the materials in the glomerular filtrate (such as Na^+, amino acids, glucose) are needed by the body and must be salvaged. This salvage operation is accomplished through their tubular reabsorption by either active or passive mechanisms. Active transport (transport requiring energy) allows substances to pass across membranes against concentration gradients by the action of ATP-dependent membrane transport systems (Chapter 1). Glucose is a

Table 12.2 Electrolyte Composition of Body Fluids

	Plasma (mEq/L)	Interstitial Fluid (mEq/L H_2O)	Intracellular Water (mEq/L H_2O)
Cations	153	153	195
Na^+	142	145	10
K^+	4	4	156
Ca^{2+}	5	2–3	3.2
Mg^{2+}	2	1–2	26
Anions	153	153	195
Cl^-	103	116	2
HCO_3^-	28	31	8
Protein	17	—	55
Others	5	6	130
Osmolality (mosm/kg H_2O)	285–293*	~300	~300

* Normal range

prime example of a solute that can be actively transported across the tubular cells from the urine into the blood, even though the blood concentration of glucose normally is 20 times that of urine. Another group of solutes, including ammonium, potassium, and phosphate ions, occurs in relatively high concentration in urine compared to blood. These substances are transported from blood into the tubular cells, also against a concentration gradient. Passive transport, the simple diffusion of a material across a membrane from a compartment of higher concentration of the material to a compartment of lower concentration, is not energy demanding. This process, too, functions within the renal tubular cells.

Alterations in food intake can profoundly affect water and electrolyte balance. During the initial days of a period of fasting, for example, renal excretion of Na^+ increases markedly, whereas prolonged fasting tends to conserve sodium ions. Refeeding causes a marked retention of Na^+, probably caused by the ingestion of carbohydrate. Consequently, a rapid regain of body weight follows, caused by an increase in total body water secondary to the stimulation of vasopressin and thirst by the rise in plasma osmolality. These alterations in sodium and water balance as a result of early-phase fasting and refeeding account for weight loss and weight regain of a greater magnitude than would be predicted from the changes in energy balance.

Clinically, the concentration of electrolytes is generally expressed in terms of milliequivalents (mEq). Milliequivalents are determined by dividing the number of millimoles of the ion by its valence (electrical charge). For Na^+, K^+, and Cl^- the valence is one, so the mmol and mEq are the same. For an ion like Mg^{+2} or Ca^{+2} the number of mmol must be divided by 2 (the ion's valence). A solution that contains 1 mmol of Mg^{+2} thus contains 0.5 mEq of Mg^{+2}. Stating electrolyte concentrations in terms of mEq accounts for cations and anions of different valences (such as Mg^{+2}, Ca^{+2}, HPO_4^{+2}, or SO_4^{+2}) since they must balance out.

Table 12.2 shows that, in terms of electrolyte balance, the contribution of sodium to the body's total cation mEq is clearly quite large compared to that of potassium, calcium, and magnesium, and a correspondingly high percentage of anion mEq is contributed by chloride and bicarbonate together. The concentration of these three major ions is used to calculate the so-called anion gap, a clinically useful parameter for establishing metabolic disorders that can alter electrolyte balance. The value is calculated by subtracting the measured anion (chloride + bicarbonate) concentration from the measured cation (sodium) concentration: Measured cations (Na^+) − measured anions (Cl^- + HCO_3^-) = anion gap. Under normal conditions, the anion gap value is about 12 mEq/L, but it may range from 8 to 18 mEq/L. Deviation from a normal anion gap is most commonly associated with increases

or decreases in the concentration of certain unmeasured anions such as proteins, organic acids, phosphate, or sulfate. For example, the production of excessive amounts of organic acids, such as would occur in lactic acidosis or ketoacidosis, increases the unmeasured anion concentration at the expense of the measured anion bicarbonate that is neutralized by the acids. Such a condition would therefore cause a greater anion gap.

Considering the effect of plasma osmolality on water intake and retention, it is logical that, should sodium ions accumulate in the body water for any reason, a concomitant rise in blood pressure (essential hypertension) would result. Clinical evidence for this correlation is provided by the hypertension experienced by patients with adrenal adenomas, whose high levels of aldosterone cause excessive retention of sodium. An apparent causal relationship also exists between dietary intake of sodium (as sodium chloride) and the etiology of hypertension, as suggested by studies conducted through one or more of the following designs:

- relating salt consumption to the prevalence of hypertension
- tracking development of hypertension in animals fed high-salt diets
- measuring response of hypertensive patients fed low-salt diets

Electrolytes, particularly salt (NaCl), exert a profound impact on hypertension. The Perspective on macrominerals and hypertension at the end of this chapter explores this topic further. Here, we will discuss the food sources, absorption, transport, functions, and excretion of as well as the Adequate Intakes (AIs) for the electrolytes sodium, potassium, and chloride.

SODIUM

About 30% of the approximately 105 g of sodium in the body (of a 70-kg human) is located on the surface of bone crystals. From that site, it can be released into the bloodstream should **hyponatremia** (low serum sodium) develop. The remainder of the body's sodium is found in the extracellular fluid, primarily plasma; in the interstitial fluid; and, in lower levels, intracellularly in nerve and muscle tissue. Sodium constitutes about 93% of the cations in the body, making it by far the most abundant member of this family (Table 12.2).

Sources

The major source of sodium in the diet is added salt in the form of sodium chloride. Sodium comprises 40% by weight of sodium chloride. One teaspoon of salt provides 2,300 mg (2.3 g) of sodium. Because salt is so extensively used in food processing and manufacturing, processed foods account for an estimated 75% of total sodium consumed. Canned meats and soups, condiments, pickled foods, and traditional snacks (chips, pretzels, crackers, etc.) are particularly high in added salt. For example, 400 to 500 mg of sodium are typically provided by a half-cup of soup or stew or a tablespoon of condiments such as ketchup and mustard. Smoked, processed, or cured meats (such as luncheon meats, ham, corned beef, hot dogs), processed cheeses, and canned fish provide about 400 to 800 mg of sodium in a 2- to 3-oz serving. Moreover, some condiments, like soy sauce, contain >1,000 mg of sodium/tablespoon. Naturally occurring sources of sodium such as milk, meat, eggs, and most vegetables furnish only about 10% of consumed sodium. Milk, for example, provides about 120 mg of sodium per cup. Meats, poultry, and fish (not processed) provide only about 25 mg of sodium per ounce. Breads provide about 160 mg of sodium/slice, although quick breads (muffins, biscuits) contain >300 mg sodium in a biscuit or a 2-oz muffin. Fresh vegetables provide typically less than 40 mg of sodium per half-cup, although celery is an exception, containing about 100 mg of sodium per cup. In contrast, canned vegetables contain >200 mg of sodium per half-cup. Instant pasta and rice dishes are exceptionally high in sodium, often providing over 700 mg of sodium per half-cup, as prepared. Salt added during cooking and at the table provides roughly 15% of total sodium, and water supplies <10%. Depending upon the method of assessment, estimates of sodium ingested by Americans range from approximately 3,000 to 5,000 mg/day.

Terms such as *free*, *very low*, *low*, *reduced*, or *light* in conjunction with sodium on food labels are associated with specific amounts of sodium per serving. For example, "free" means <5 mg of sodium per serving, "very low" means <35 mg per serving, and "low" means <140 mg of sodium per serving. The term *reduced* or *less* indicates at least 25% less sodium per serving than the appropriate reference food. The term *light* may be used if the food is low in calories and fat, and the sodium content has been reduced by at least 50%. The Daily Value for sodium used on food labels is 2,400 mg.

Sodium intake has been linked with high blood pressure (hypertension) in some people, as discussed in the Perspective "Macrominerals and Hypertension" at the end of this chapter. The U.S. Food and Drug Administration has approved health claims stating "Diets low in sodium may reduce the risk of high blood pressure, a disease associated with many factors" as well as "Development of hypertension or high blood pressure depends on many factors. [This product] can be part of a low-sodium and low-salt diet that might reduce the risk of hypertension or high blood pressure" [7].

Absorption, Transport, and Function

About 95% to 100% of ingested sodium is absorbed, with the remaining 0% to 5% excreted in the feces. Three basic pathways operate in absorption of sodium across the enterocyte brush border membrane. One of these pathways (the Na^+/glucose cotransport system) functions throughout the small intestine. Another pathway (an electroneutral Na^+ and Cl^- cotransport system) is active in both the small intestine and the proximal portion of the colon. The third pathway (an electrogenic sodium absorption mechanism) operates principally in the colon.

The Na^+/glucose cotransport system involves a carrier on the brush border (apical) membrane of the small intestine. Na^+ and glucose bind to the carrier, which shuttles them from the outer surface to the inner surface of the cell membrane. There both are released before the carrier returns to the outer surface. Absorbed Na^+ is then pumped out across the enterocyte's basolateral (serosal) membrane by the Na^+/K^+-ATPase pump, while the glucose diffuses across the membrane by a facilitated transport pathway. The Na^+ gradient created by the Na^+/K^+-ATPase pump provides the energy needed to maintain the absorptive direction of the ion. Cotransport of Na^+ by this mechanism also can occur with solutes other than glucose, including amino acids, di- and tripeptides, and many B vitamins.

The existence of an electroneutral Na^+ and Cl^- cotransport mechanism has been proposed because of the observation that a significant portion of sodium uptake requires the presence of chloride, and vice versa [8]. Precisely how this system functions has not yet been established. However, the cotransport is believed to involve Na^+/H^+ exchange working in concert with a Cl^-/HCO_3^- mechanism [1]. The mechanism allows the entrance of both Na^+ and Cl^- into the cell, where they are exchanged for H^+ and HCO_3^-. Protons (H^+) and HCO_3^- are produced within the cell by the action of carbonic anhydrase on CO_2. Absorbed Na^+ is pumped across the basolateral membrane by the Na^+/K^+-ATPase pump, and followed by Cl^-, which crosses by diffusion.

The colonic mechanism is called an electrogenic sodium absorption mechanism because the absorbed sodium ion is the only ion moving transcellularly, allowing its transport to be monitored. It enters the luminal membrane of the colonic mucosal cell through Na^+-conducting pathways called Na^+ channels, diffusing inwardly by the downhill concentration gradient of the ion. The absorbed sodium is accompanied by water and anions, resulting in net water and electrolyte movement from the luminal side to the bloodstream side of the colonic cells. It is pumped out across the basolateral membrane on the bloodstream side of the cell by the Na^+/K^+-ATPase pump.

All three of these mechanisms are depicted schematically in Figure 12.6. Note that the common driving force for sodium absorption in all these processes is the inwardly directed gradient maintained by the basolateral Na^+ pump, which maintains a low intercellular Na^+ concentration.

Once absorbed into the body, sodium is transported freely in the blood. Serum sodium concentrations are maintained within a fairly narrow range (~135–145 mEq/L) by several hormones, including vasopressin, aldosterone, and atrial natriuretic hormone.

Within the body, sodium plays important roles in the maintenance of fluid balance, nerve transmission/impulse conduction, and muscle contraction (Table 12.3). Although proteins play a role in fluid balance, they normally remain within either the cell or extracellular fluid. Sodium, potassium, and chloride therefore display the most movement of charged particles (ions) across cell membranes to maintain osmotic pressure and thus fluid balance. Sodium's roles in nerve transmission and muscle contraction involve sodium as part of the Na^+/K^+-ATPase pump found in the plasma membrane of cells. With the exchange of sodium for potassium and the hydrolysis of ATP, an electrochemical potential gradient generates nerve or impulse conduction.

Interactions with Other Nutrients

It has long been recognized (since before 1940) that dietary sodium intake increases urinary calcium excretion. Studies have shown that accompanying the calciuria are decreased fecal calcium excretion and increased calcium absorption. Such calcium-elevating effects partially offset the urinary calcium losses. The sodium-calcium interaction and its possible association with osteoporosis are presented in more detail in the Perspective "Osteoporosis and Diet" at the end of Chapter 11.

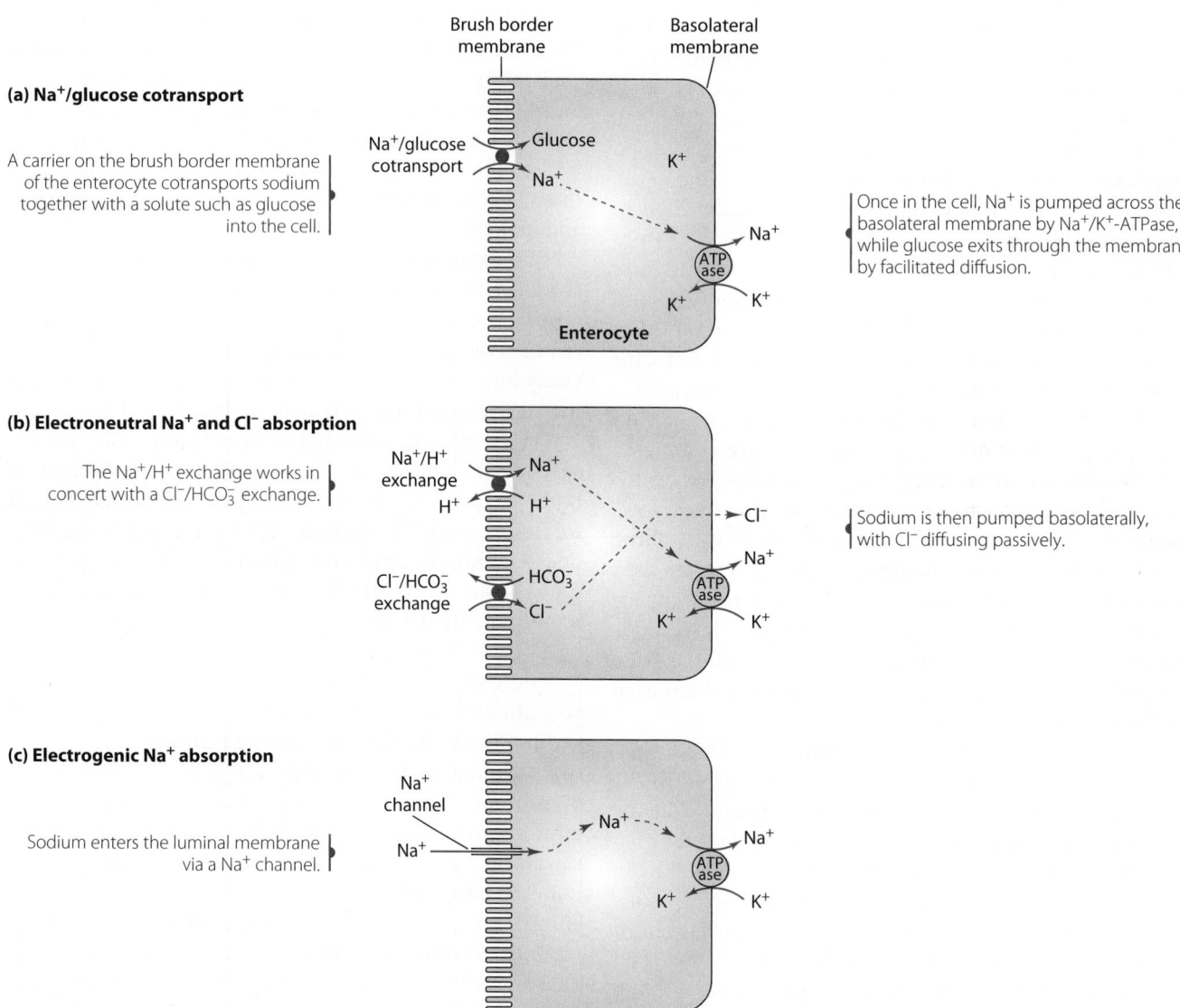

Figure 12.6 Absorption mechanisms for sodium in the intestine (a–c).

Table 12.3 Electrolytes: Functions, Body Content, Deficiency Symptoms, and Adequate Intakes (AIs)

Mineral	Selected Physiological Functions	Approximate Body Content	Selected Enzyme Cofactors	Deficiency Symptoms	Selected Food Sources	AI
Sodium	Water, pH, and electrolyte regulation; nerve transmission, muscle contraction	105 g	Na^+/K^+-ATPase	Anorexia, nausea, muscle atrophy, poor growth, weight loss	Table salt, meat, seafood, cheese, milk, bread, vegetables (abundant in most foods except fruits)	1,500 mg, 19–50 years
Potassium	Water, electrolyte, and pH balances; cell membrane transfer	245 g	Pyruvate kinase, Na^+/K^+-ATPase	Muscular weakness, mental apathy, cardiac arrhythmias, paralysis, bone fragility	Avocados, bananas, dried fruits, oranges, peaches, potatoes, dried beans, tomatoes, wheat bran, dairy products, eggs	4,700 mg, 19+ years
Chloride	Primary anion; maintains pH balance, enzyme activation, component of gastric hydrochloric acid	105 g		In infants: loss of appetite, failure to thrive, weakness, lethargy, severe hypokalemia, metabolic acidosis	Table salt, seafood, milk, meat, eggs	2,300 mg, 19–50 years

Excretion

Because nearly all ingested sodium is absorbed, much larger amounts are absorbed than are required by the body. Sodium in excess of that needed by the body is excreted, primarily by the kidneys, but also through the skin by sweating. Under conditions of moderate temperature and level of exercise, sodium losses in sweat are small. However, because the sodium content of sweat is about 50 mEq/L, it can be reasoned that conditions of high temperature or sustained vigorous exercise can account for significant losses.

The maintenance of the body's sodium load is an important component of homeostasis. An increased sodium load increases ECF volume and blood pressure. Multiple mechanisms help to maintain physiological levels of sodium. As stated previously, vasopressin is released into circulation in response to an increase in extracellular fluid osmolarity or decreased plasma volume (indicators of insufficient body water and dehydration). Vasopressin enhances the reabsorption of water by the ascending loop of Henle and the collecting ducts, stimulates the thirst centers of the brain to increase the consumption of water, and causes the reabsorption of Na^+ through Na^+ channels on the epithelial cell membrane that are aldosterone sensitive.

Aldosterone, however, is the major hormone that controls sodium excretion. Released in the presence of increased angiotensin II levels, decreased levels of the natriuretic peptides ANP and BNP, increased plasma K^+, or decreased Na^+, aldosterone causes increased Na^+ (along with Cl^-) and water reabsorption. It also stimulates the release of vasopressin, which further increases the reabsorption of both water and Na^+. When the body's load of Na^+ is elevated, renin is not secreted, the RAAS is not activated, and Na^+ is excreted in the urine rather than reabsorbed. The RAAS is opposed by the natriuretic peptides, which promote Na^+ and water excretion, thus decreasing the plasma volume and lowering blood pressure.

Deficiency

Dietary deficiencies of sodium do not normally occur because of the abundance of the mineral across a broad spectrum of foods. However, with excessive sweating involving a loss of more than about 3% of total body weight, deficiencies of sodium have been reported. Symptoms include muscle cramps, nausea, vomiting, dizziness, shock, and coma.

Adequate Intake and Assessment of Nutriture

The National Research Council has suggested an Adequate Intake of 1,500 mg (65 mmol) of sodium (or 3.8 g of salt) for adults per day [9]. The minimum amount of sodium needed to replace losses (with no sweat and maximal adaptation) is estimated at about 180 mg (8 mmol); however, this amount is not thought to represent the requirement [9]. A Tolerable Upper Intake Level of 2,300 mg (100 mmol) of sodium for adults per day has been established [9]. Given that the average person consumes between 3 and 5 g of sodium per day, most people greatly exceed these intake recommendations. Interestingly, patients with various health conditions such as hypertension or kidney disease are put on sodium-restricted diets providing 2 g/day (more than the current Adequate Intake). Such diets typically restrict intake of foods high in sodium (i.e., canned soups; canned and brined vegetables; smoked, cured, and processed meats, fish, and cheeses; quick breads; salted snack foods; prepared, frozen foods; instant rice, pasta, and potato dishes; and condiments). Additional recommendations for sodium for other age groups are provided on the inside front cover of the book. The Perspectives at the end of this chapter provide further information on sodium as it relates to hypertension and prolonged exertion.

Sodium is measured routinely in clinical laboratories, especially to determine electrolyte balance. Sodium in the serum and other biological fluids is usually quantified by the technique of ion-selective electrode **potentiometry**. This method measures Na^+ in the same way a pH meter measures protons. A 24-hour urinary sodium excretion level is most often used as a reflection of sodium intake.

POTASSIUM

Potassium is the major intracellular cation. In fact, in contrast to sodium, about 95% to 98% of the body's potassium is found within cells. Potassium constitutes up to about 0.35% of total body weight, or up to about 245 g in a 70-kg human.

Sources

Potassium is widespread in the diet and is especially abundant in unprocessed foods, which provide potassium along with anions like phosphate and citrate (note that citrate is thought to be important for acid–base balance because it can serve as a precursor to bicarbonate as it is decarboxylated via the TCA cycle; see Chapter 3). Foods exceptionally rich in potassium (usually greater than 300 mg per cup) include some fruits like prune juice, avocados, bananas, cantaloupe, honeydew melon, mango, and papaya, and some vegetables (winter squash, leafy green vegetables, and yams). Other good sources of potassium, containing between about 200 and 300 mg of potassium per cup, are legumes, nuts and seeds, peanut butter, selected vegetables (such as potatoes, asparagus, mushrooms, and okra), and fruits (like oranges, grapefruits, peaches, pears, kiwi, and nectarines). Milk and yogurt also provide potassium—about 300 mg per cup. In addition to unprocessed sources, salt substitutes often contain potassium in place of sodium.

Diets high in potassium are associated with lower blood pressure; this topic is discussed further in the Perspective "Macrominerals and Hypertension" at the end of this chapter. The Food and Drug Administration has approved the health claim: "Diets containing foods that are good sources of potassium and low in sodium may reduce the risk of high blood pressure and stroke" [7]. To use this claim, a food must contain at least 350 mg (10% Daily Value) of potassium; must contain ≤140 mg of sodium, ≤3 g of total fat, ≤1 g of saturated fat, and ≤20 mg of cholesterol; and must provide ≤15% of energy (kcal) from saturated fat [7]. For food labeling purposes, to be considered a "rich," "excellent," or "high" source of potassium (or any other nutrient), a food must contain 20% or more of the Daily Value; to be a "good" source of potassium, the food must contain 10% to 19% of the Daily Value [7].

Absorption, Transport, and Function

The mechanisms by which potassium is absorbed from the gastrointestinal tract are not as clearly understood as the mechanisms of sodium absorption. Over 85% of ingested potassium is absorbed, although the exact sites along the small intestine where absorption takes place have not been precisely identified. In addition to being absorbed in the small intestine, K^+ may be absorbed across the colonic mucosal cells. Depending upon concentration, potassium is thought to be absorbed by passive diffusion or by a K^+/H^+-ATPase pump. This pump exchanges intracellular H^+ for luminal K^+. Alternatively, K^+ may enter the enterocyte through brush border membrane channels that also serve as secretory pathways.

To enter the blood, the K^+ accumulated in the enterocyte diffuses across the basolateral membrane through the K^+ channel. Uptake of potassium from blood into nonintestinal cells occurs by active transport. High intracellular potassium concentrations are maintained by Na^+/K^+-ATPase pumps, which are stimulated by hormones, especially insulin and some catecholamines. This cellular uptake of the ion helps to maintain the serum K^+ concentration within its normal range of about 3.5 to 5.0 mEq or mmol/L after K^+ ingestion. **Hypokalemia** (low serum potassium) reduces insulin secretion from the pancreas following a meal, which impacts the metabolism of carbohydrate from the meal.

Potassium influences the contractility of smooth, skeletal, and cardiac muscle and profoundly affects the excitability of nerve tissue. It is also important in maintaining electrolyte and pH balance.

Interactions with Other Nutrients

Like sodium, potassium affects the urinary excretion of calcium. However, its effect is opposite to that of sodium: whereas sodium increases calcium excretion, potassium decreases it. Replacement of some of the NaCl in the diet with KCl to reduce the amount of NaCl consumed has been shown to reduce urinary calcium excretion [10]. The addition of potassium citrate (90 mmol/day) to a diet high in salt (225 mmol or about 8 g of salt/day) can prevent the normal increase in urinary calcium associated with a high-salt diet [11]. Moreover, this addition of potassium citrate significantly decreases markers of bone resorption that have been associated with a high salt intake in postmenopausal women [11]. A discussion of potassium and bone is found in the Perspective at the end of Chapter 11.

Excretion

Most potassium (up to ~90%) is excreted from the body via the kidneys, with only small amounts excreted in the feces. Eighty percent of the K^+ in the glomerular filtrate is reabsorbed in the proximal tubule unregulated. In general, the regulation of K^+ excretion is controlled by the same hormones as Na^+ excretion, but in the opposite direction. For example, as Na^+ is being reabsorbed in the ascending loop of Henle and the collecting duct in response to vasopressin, K^+ is being excreted in the urine. Likewise, aldosterone also enhances the excretion of K^+ as Na^+ is being reabsorbed from the distal tubule and the collecting ducts.

Recall that one of the conditions that stimulates aldosterone release from the adrenal glands independently from the RAAS is increased K^+ plasma concentration. Potassium is primarily an intracellular cation; plasma concentrations of K^+ are low, and small changes can have a pronounced effect on its urinary excretion. In addition to prompting the excretion of K^+ as Na^+ is being reabsorbed, aldosterone causes the secretion of K^+ from the capillaries into the tubular cells and then into the lumen of the collecting duct. The mechanism for this secretion is a Na^+/K^+ pump that moves Na^+ out of the cell and K^+ into it. The high concentration of the intracellular K^+ causes it to move passively through K^+ channels located on the lumen side of the tubule cell into the tubule lumen. In other segments of the tubule, the K^+ channels are located on the basolateral membrane, causing the K^+ to be excreted. If K^+ plasma concentration is low, less aldosterone is released and less K^+ is excreted [1].

Recent research has suggested another mechanism for the tight control of serum K^+ that functions as a high-K^+ meal is being consumed. This mechanism involves insulin, glucagon, and an unidentified protein that causes K^+ to be removed from serum prior to any changes in K^+ concentration in ECF [12,13]. The molecular events comprising this mechanism are still unclear.

Deficiency and Toxicity

Deficiency of potassium does not occur through dietary inadequacies, primarily because of the abundance of potassium in commonly eaten foods. The condition most often results from situations causing profound fluid loss, such as severe vomiting and diarrhea. Additionally, the use of some medications such as thiazide and loop diuretics, which are used to treat high blood pressure, increase urinary potassium excretion and may cause deficiency. Severe potassium deficiency causes hypokalemia (serum potassium concentrations $< {\sim}3.5$ mEq or mmol/L), which in turn may result in cardiac arrhythmias, muscular weakness, nervous irritability, hypercalciuria, glucose intolerance, and mental disorientation. Hypokalemia also may occur as part of refeeding syndrome, which develops when malnourished people are being refed (usually intravenously or through a tube) a diet lacking enough supplemental potassium to replace that lost from the cells during the starvation period and needed by the body as it synthesizes new lean body mass. A moderate deficiency of potassium (without hypokalemia) may be associated with elevations in blood pressure, increased urinary calcium excretion, and abnormal bone turnover (increased bone resorption and decreased bone formation). The Perspectives at the end of this chapter and Chapter 11 provide further information on these topics. Too much potassium in the blood/serum is referred to as **hyperkalemia** (an abnormally high serum potassium concentration). Hyperkalemia, which most often results from impaired renal function, can cause cardiac arrhythmias and even cardiac arrest.

Adequate Intake and Assessment of Nutriture

The National Research Council has suggested an Adequate Intake of 4,700 mg (120 mmol) of potassium per day for adults [9]. Recommendations for potassium for other population groups are provided on the inside front cover of the book. The potassium intake of most Americans (about 3,300 mg) does not meet recommendations, and even consuming a diet rich in fruits and vegetables, such as the DASH (Dietary Approaches to Stop Hypertension) diet used to treat hypertension, can still leave a person just short of meeting recommendations. Thus, it takes careful diet planning to achieve the Adequate Intake. No Tolerable Upper Intake Level has been established for potassium from foods; however, note that potassium supplements should be used only with the recommendations and supervision of medical personnel because too much (or too little) potassium in the blood can be lethal.

Potassium status is typically assessed based upon plasma potassium concentrations, which normally range from approximately 3.5 to 5.0 mEq or mmol/L. Serum potassium levels, like those of sodium, are determined primarily by ion-selective electrode potentiometry.

CHLORIDE

Chloride is the most abundant anion in the ECF, with approximately 88% of chloride found in the ECF and just 12% intracellularly. Its negative charge neutralizes the positive charge of the Na^+ with which it is usually associated. In this respect, it is of great importance in maintaining electrolyte balance. Total body chloride content is similar to that of sodium, representing about 0.15% of body weight, or about 105 g in a 70-kg human.

Sources

Nearly all the chloride consumed in the diet is associated with sodium in the form of sodium chloride, or salt. Salt, which is about 60% chloride, is abundant in a large number of foods, particularly in snack items and processed foods. Chloride also is found in eggs, fresh meats, and seafood. The average adult consumes an estimated 50 to 200 mmol, or 2,000 to 8,000 mg, of chloride/day.

Absorption, Transport, and Secretion

Chloride is almost completely absorbed in the small intestine. Its absorption closely follows that of sodium in the establishment and maintenance of electrical neutrality and osmotic balance. The absorptive mechanisms, however, generally are different. For example, in the Na^+-glucose cotransport system (described in the section on sodium), chloride follows the actively absorbed Na^+ passively through a so-called paracellular pathway. The absorbed Na^+ creates an electrical gradient that provides the drive for the accompanying inward diffusion of Cl^- between cells. The electroneutral Na^+/Cl^- cotransport absorption system also contributes to the movement of chloride into the enterocytes, although the relative contribution of this system to total chloride absorption is not well established. Sodium absorbed by the electrogenic Na^+ absorption mechanism also is accompanied by chloride, which follows the absorbed sodium passively (paracellularly) to maintain electrical neutrality and osmotic pressure. Clearly, regardless of which absorptive mechanism is functioning, wherever sodium goes, chloride cannot be far behind!

Secretory mechanisms for the electrolytes throughout the gastrointestinal tract center on chloride, which is the major secretory product of the stomach and the rest of the gastrointestinal tract. The well-defined mechanism is an electrogenic Cl^- secretion. Cl^- is the only ion actively secreted by the gastrointestinal tract cells, and its movement can be monitored by changes in electrical potentials. Cells take up chloride from the blood across the basolateral membrane by way of a $Na^+/K^+/Cl^-$ cotransport pathway. An appropriate gradient is set up by the Na^+/K^+-ATPase pump, which maintains a low concentration of intracellular sodium. Potassium channels on the basolateral membrane allow potassium recycling out of the cell. Chloride accumulating in the enterocyte exits through the brush border membrane into the lumen through the Cl^- channels. Figure 12.7 illustrates the chloride secretory mechanism.

Recent evidence shows that Cl^- can be actively transported, through Cl^- channels, into and out of cells lining the colon and the distal portion of the ascending loop of Henle. These cells express genes coding for transporters such as a Na-independent Cl^--HCO_3^- cotransporter that pumps Cl^- into the cell. This research suggests that Cl^- moves into some cells by active as well as passive means. This active transport of Cl^- results in a high cellular concentration, which in turn results in fluid secretion when Cl^- passively exits the cell through Cl^- channels, and Na^+ and water accompany it [14].

Dysfunction of chloride transport is experienced by people with cystic fibrosis, a genetic disorder that results from a mutation in a protein called the cystic fibrosis transmembrane conductance regulator. Defects in the protein result in the production of extremely thick mucus that obstructs many of the body's glands and causes many organs, especially the lungs and pancreas, to malfunction.

Functions

Chloride has important functions in addition to its role as a major electrolyte. The formation of gastric hydrochloric acid requires chloride, which is secreted along with protons from the parietal cells of the stomach. Chloride is released by white blood cells during phagocytosis to assist in the destruction of foreign substances. Also, chloride acts as the exchange anion for HCO_3^- in red blood cells, in a process sometimes called the chloride shift. The purpose is to allow the transport of tissue-derived CO_2 back to the lungs in the form of plasma HCO_3. Waste CO_2 from tissues enters the red blood cell, where it is converted to HCO_3^- by carbonic anhydrase. A transporter protein (chloride bicarbonate exchanger) then transports the HCO_3^- out of the cell into the plasma as it simultaneously transports plasma Cl^- into the cell. In the absence of chloride, bicarbonate transport ceases.

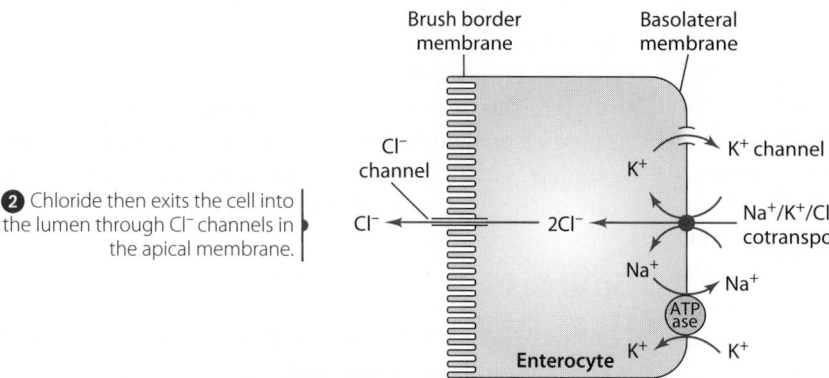

❷ Chloride then exits the cell into the lumen through Cl^- channels in the apical membrane.

❶ Chloride is cotransported along with Na^+ and K^+ from the circulation across the basolateral membrane and into the mucosal cell.

❸ The driving force is provided by active removal of Na^+ by the Na^+/K^+-ATPase pump and the recycling of potassium through K^+ channels on the basolateral membrane.

Figure 12.7 Intestinal chloride secretory mechanism.

Excretion

Chloride excretion occurs through three primary routes: the gastrointestinal tract, the skin, and the kidneys, with losses through each route closely reflecting those of sodium. Excretion of chloride through the gastrointestinal tract normally is minimal, approximately 1 to 2 mEq/day for the average adult. Losses through the skin are similar quantitatively to sodium losses, that is, normally quite small except in cases of high temperature and vigorous exercise. The major route of chloride excretion is through the kidney, where it is primarily regulated indirectly through sodium regulation.

Deficiency

Dietary deficiency of chloride does not occur under normal conditions. As is the case for the other electrolytes, deficiency arises chiefly through gastrointestinal tract disturbances such as severe diarrhea and vomiting. Convulsions typically occur with chloride deficiency.

Adequate Intake and Assessment of Nutriture

The National Research Council recommends an Adequate Intake of 2,300 mg (65 mmol) of chloride per day [9]. A Tolerable Upper Intake Level for chloride is 3.6 g (100 mmol) [9]. The chloride and sodium AIs and ULs are the same when expressed as mmoles.

Chloride status is assessed through evaluation of its concentration in the serum, which usually ranges from about 101 to 111 mEq or mmol/L. However, like that of all serum solutes, chloride concentration depends upon the body water status. It is possible, for example, for the total body store of chloride to be diminished and fluid concentrations of chloride to appear normal and even be elevated if body water accompanies the losses. Two widely used methods for determining chloride concentration in serum are ion-selective electrode potentiometry and a **coulometric titration** (a method of measuring the volume of reagent required for a reaction) with silver ions.

ACID–BASE BALANCE: THE CONTROL OF HYDROGEN ION CONCENTRATION

The maintenance of the hydrogen ion concentration in body fluids within a narrow range, which is vital to normal physiological function, is achieved via the lungs and kidneys. In fact, acid–base regulation is one of the most important aspects of homeostasis because even slight deviations from normal acidity can cause marked alterations in enzyme-catalyzed reaction rates in the cells.

Hydrogen ion concentration can also affect both the cellular uptake and regulation of metabolites and minerals and the uptake and release of oxygen from hemoglobin. Because the body regulates acid–base balance in conjunction with fluid-electrolyte balance, we will address it here.

The degree of acidity or alkalinity of any fluid is determined by its concentration of protons (H^+). The hydrogen ion concentration in body fluids is generally quite low: it is regulated at approximately 4×10^{-8} mol/L. Concentrations can vary from as low as 1.0×10^{-8} mol/L to as high as 1.0×10^{-7} mol/L, but values outside this range are not compatible with life. From these values, it is apparent that expressing H^+ in terms of its actual concentration is awkward. The concept of pH, which is the negative logarithm of the H^+ concentration, was devised to simplify the expression. It enables concentrations to be expressed as whole numbers rather than as negative exponential values:

$$pH = -\log [H^+]$$

Bracketed values symbolize concentrations. Throughout this discussion, this designation is used to signify concentrations of substances other than protons. The pH of extracellular fluid, in which the H^+ concentration may be assumed to be approximately 4×10^{-8} mol/L, can therefore be calculated as follows:

$$pH = -\log (4 \times 10^{-8})$$
or
$$pH = \log (1/(4 \times 10^{-8}))$$
(dividing)
$$pH = \log (0.25 \times 10^{8})$$
$$pH = \log 0.25 + \log 10^{8}$$
(taking logs)
$$pH = -0.602 + 8$$
$$pH = 7.4$$

As the molar concentration of H^+ becomes smaller and the value of the negative exponent of 10 becomes larger, the pH correspondingly increases. Low acidity therefore denotes low H^+ concentration and high pH, whereas high acidity is associated with high H^+ concentration and low pH.

An acid, as it relates to fluid acid–base regulation, may be defined as a substance capable of releasing protons (H^+). The metabolism of the major nutrients continuously generates organic acids, which must be neutralized. Chapter 3 explains how lactic acid and pyruvic acid can accumulate in periods of oxygen deprivation, and Chapter 5 describes how fatty acids are released from triacylglycerols during lipolysis. Also, the acidic ketone bodies, acetoacetic acid and β-hydroxybutyric acid, can increase substantially during periods of prolonged starvation or low carbohydrate intake. Carbon dioxide, the product of the complete oxidation of energy nutrients, is itself indirectly acidic because it forms carbonic acid (H_2CO_3) on combination with H_2O. Acidic salts of sulfuric and phosphoric acids are also generated metabolically from sulfur- or phosphorus-containing substances.

The term *acidosis* refers to a rise in extracellular (principally plasma) H^+ concentration (a lower pH) beyond the normal range. Abnormally low H^+ concentration (i.e., high plasma pH), in contrast, results in **alkalosis.** To guard against such fluctuations in pH, three principal regulatory systems are available:

- buffer systems within the fluids that immediately neutralize acidic or basic compounds
- the respiratory center, which regulates breathing and the rate of exhalation of CO_2
- renal regulation, by which either acidic or alkaline urine can be formed to adjust body fluid acidity

Acid–Base Buffers

A buffer is anything that can reversibly bind protons. In the body, a buffer is a chemical solution designed to resist changes in pH despite the addition of acids or bases. A buffer usually consists of a weak acid, which can be represented as HA, and its conjugate base (A^-). The conjugate base, therefore, is the residual portion of the acid following the release of the proton. The conjugate base of a weak acid is basic because it tends to attract a proton and to regenerate the acid. Therefore, the dissociation of a weak acid and the reunion of its conjugate base and proton comprise an equilibrium system:

$$HA \longleftrightarrow H^+ + A^-$$

The equilibrium expression for this reaction, called the acid dissociation constant (K_a), is represented as

$$K_a = \frac{[H^+]\,[A^-]}{[HA]}$$

The equation can be rearranged to

$$[H^+] = \frac{K_a\,[HA]}{[A^-]}$$

Taking the negative logarithm of both sides of the equation gives

$$-\log\,[H^+] = -\log K_a - \log \frac{[HA]}{[A^-]}$$

These values become

$$pH = pK_a + \log \frac{[A^-]}{[HA]}$$

This equation, referred to as the Henderson-Hasselbalch equation, shows how a buffer system composed of a weak acid and its conjugate base resists changes in pH if a strong acid or base is added to the system. For example, if the molar concentrations of the conjugate base and the acid are equal, then the ratio of $[A^-]$ to $[HA]$ is 1.0, and the logarithm of this ratio is 0, making the pH of the system equal to the pK_a of the acid.

The pK_a, which is the negative logarithm of the acid dissociation constant (K_a), of any weak acid is a constant for that particular acid and simply reflects its strength (i.e., its tendency to release a proton). If a strong acid or a strong base is added to this system, the ratio of $[A^-]$ to $[HA]$ changes and therefore the pH changes, but only slightly. Suppose, for example, that both the conjugate base and the free acid are present at 0.1 mol/L concentrations, and suppose also that the pK_a of the acid is 7.0. As shown previously, if the ratio is 0.1:0.1, the pH is 7.0. The addition of enough hydrochloric acid (a strong acid) to the buffer in the example to make its final concentration 0.05 mol/L shifts the equilibrium to the left (to make HA). The 0.05 mol/L of H^+ (from the fully dissociated HCl) will combine with an equal molar amount of A^- to form HA. The new $[A^-]$ concentration therefore becomes 0.05 mol/L ($0.1 - 0.05$), and $[HA]$ is 0.15 mol/L ($0.1 + 0.05$). The logarithm of this new ratio (0.05:0.15, or 0.33) is -0.48. Inserting this value into the Henderson-Hasselbalch equation, we can see that the pH decreases by only 0.48. In other words, the pH decreased from 7.0 to 6.52 by making the system 0.05 mol/L hydrochloric acid. In contrast, this same concentration of HCl in an unbuffered, aqueous solution would produce an acid pH between 1.0 and 2.0.

The physiologically important buffers that maintain the narrow pH range of extracellular fluid at approximately 7.35 to 7.45 are proteins and the bicarbonate (HCO_3^-)–carbonic acid (H_2CO_3) system. Proteins have the most potent buffering capacity among the physiological buffers, and, because of its high concentration in whole blood, hemoglobin is most important in this respect. The binding of oxygen to hemoglobin is influenced by the pH of the blood. For the proper uptake and release of oxygen in the erythrocyte to occur, it is crucial for the pH regulation to be operating. As **amphoteric** substances (substances that possess both acidic and basic groups on their amino acid side chains), proteins are capable of neutralizing either acids or bases. For instance, the two major buffering groups on a protein are carboxylic acid (R—COOH) and amino (R—NH_3^+) functions, which dissociate as shown:

1. $R—COOH \longleftrightarrow R—COO^- + H^+$
2. $R—NH_3^+ \longleftrightarrow R—NH_2 + H^+$

At physiological pH, the carboxylic acid is largely dissociated into its conjugate base and a proton, so the equilibrium as shown is shifted strongly to the right. At that same pH, however, the amino group, being much weaker as an acid (a stronger base), is only weakly dissociated, and its equilibrium greatly favors the right-to-left direction. If protons, in the form of a strong acid, are added to a protein solution, they are neutralized by reaction 1 because their presence will cause a shift in the equilibrium toward the undissociated acid (right to left). Strong bases, as contributors of hydroxide (OH^-) ions, will likewise be neutralized because, as they react with the protons to form water, the equilibrium of reaction 2 (as illustrated) shifts to the right to restore the protons that were neutralized.

The bicarbonate–carbonic acid buffer system is of particular importance because it is through this system that respiratory and renal pH regulation is exerted. This buffer system is composed of the weak acid carbonic acid (H_2CO_3) and its salt or conjugate base, bicarbonate ion (HCO_3^-). The carbonic acid dissociates reversibly into H^+ and HCO_3^-:

$$H_2CO_3 \leftrightarrow H^+ + HCO_3^-$$

The buffering capacity of this reaction arises from the fact that either added protons or added hydroxide ions will be neutralized by corresponding shifts in the equilibrium, similar to the carboxy-amino group buffering by proteins described earlier. The H_2CO_3 can be formed not only from the acidification of HCO_3^-, as shown in the previous right-to-left reaction, but also from the reaction of dissolved CO_2 with water. Recall that CO_2 is formed as a result of total oxidation of the energy nutrients as well as various decarboxylation reactions. The gas diffuses from tissue cells into the extracellular fluids and then into erythrocytes, where its reaction with water to form H_2CO_3 is accelerated by the zinc metalloenzyme carbonic anhydrase. The overall reaction involving carbon dioxide, carbonic acid, and bicarbonate ion is as follows:

3. $\underset{\text{(gas)}}{CO_2} \leftrightarrow \underset{\text{(dissolved)}}{CO_2} \leftrightarrow H_2CO_3 \leftrightarrow H^+ + HCO_3^-$

In the lungs, these equilibrium reactions are shifted strongly to the left in the circulating erythrocytes because of the release of protons from hemoglobin as hemoglobin acquires oxygen to become oxyhemoglobin. This shift allows the exhalation of carbon dioxide.

Normally, the ratio of the concentration of HCO_3^- to H_2CO_3 in plasma is 20:1, and the apparent pK_a value for H_2CO_3 is 6.1. Using the Henderson-Hasselbalch equation, we can show how a normal plasma pH of 7.4 results from these values:

$$pH = pK_a + \log \frac{[HCO_3^-]}{[H_2CO_3]}$$
$$= 6.1 + \log \frac{20}{1}$$
$$= 6.1 + 1.3$$
$$pH = 7.4$$

Alterations in the 20:1 ratio of $[HCO_3^-]$ to $[H_2CO_3]$ clearly change the pH. The next section shows how respiratory and renal regulatory systems function to keep this ratio, and therefore the pH, relatively constant.

Respiratory Regulation of pH

If plasma levels of CO_2 rise, perhaps because of accelerated metabolism, more H_2CO_3 is formed. This reaction, in turn, causes a fall in pH as the acid dissociates to release protons (reaction 3). The elevated CO_2 itself, as well as the resulting increase in hydrogen ion concentration, is detected by the respiratory center of the brain, resulting in an increase in the respiratory rate. This hyperventilation increases CO_2 loss through the lungs substantially and therefore decreases the amount of H_2CO_3. This mechanism increases the ratio of HCO_3^- to H_2CO_3 by reducing H_2CO_3, thus elevating the pH to a normal value. Conversely, if plasma pH rises for any reason (because of either an increase in HCO_3^- or a decrease in H_2CO_3), the respiratory center is signaled accordingly and causes a slowing of the respiration rate. As CO_2 then accumulates, the H_2CO_3 concentration rises and the pH decreases.

Renal Regulation of pH

Although the respiratory system acts as an immediate (in minutes) regulator of the HCO_3^-/H_2CO_3 system, long-term control (hours or days) is exerted by renal mechanisms. The kidneys regulate pH by controlling the secretion of H^+, by conserving or producing HCO_3^-, and by synthesizing ammonium ions. The secretion of H^+ occurs in conjunction with the tubular reabsorption of Na^+ ions through the mechanism of countertransport, an active process involving a common Na^+/H^+ carrier protein and energy sufficient to move the protons from the tubular cells into the tubule lumen against a concentration gradient of protons. With consumption of a normal diet, about 50 to 100 mEq of H^+ are generated daily. Renal secretion of the protons is necessary to prevent a progressive metabolic acidosis. The renal tubules are not very permeable to HCO_3^- because of the charge and the relatively large size of the ions. Bicarbonate ions therefore are reabsorbed by a special indirect process. The hydrogen ions in the glomerular filtrate convert filtered HCO_3^- to H_2CO_3, which dissociates into CO_2 and H_2O. The CO_2 diffuses into the tubular cell, where it combines with water, in a reaction catalyzed by carbonic anhydrase, to form H_2CO_3. The relatively high tubular-cell pH allows the dissociation of the H_2CO_3 into HCO_3^- and H^+, after which the bicarbonate reenters the extracellular fluid and the proton is actively returned to the lumen by the Na^+/H^+ carrier. The net result is to excrete an H^+ and to reabsorb a bicarbonate ion, even though it is not the same bicarbonate ion. These events, by which hydrogen ions are secreted against a concentration gradient in exchange for Na^+, and bicarbonate is returned to the plasma from the glomerular filtrate, are summarized in Figure 12.8.

The pH of the urine normally falls within the range of 5.5 to 6.5, despite the active secretion of hydrogen ions throughout the tubules. This pH is largely achieved by partial neutralization of the hydrogen ions by ammonia, which is secreted into the lumen by the tubular cells. Ammonia is produced in large amounts from the metabolic

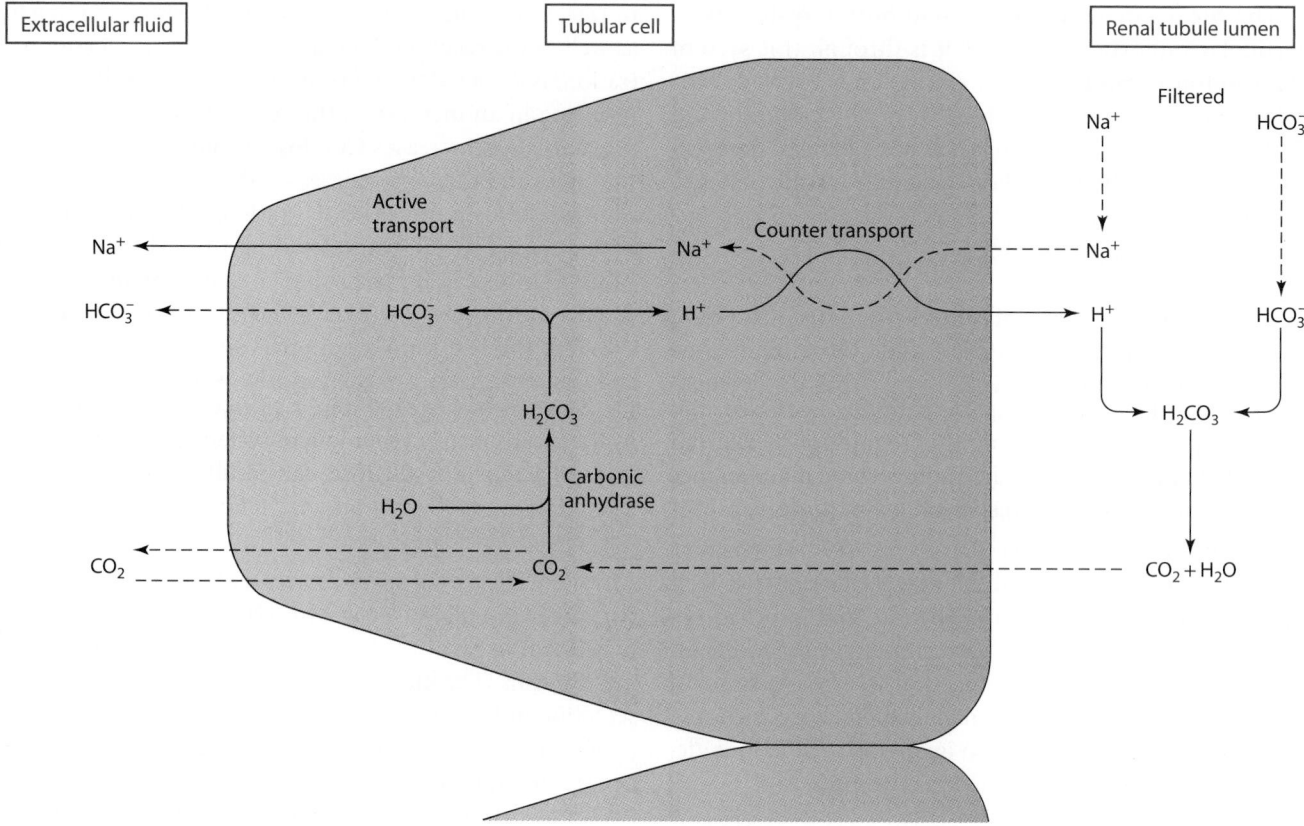

Figure 12.8 Renal tubular cell reactions illustrating the origin of and the active secretion of hydrogen ions in exchange for sodium ions, as well as the mechanism for tubular reabsorption of bicarbonate. Solid arrows indicate reactions or active transport, while dashed arrows signify diffusion.

breakdown of amino acids. In the renal tubule cells, ammonia is hydrolytically released from glutamine by glutaminase and is secreted into the urine (Chapter 6). Because it is a basic substance, ammonia immediately combines with protons in the collecting ducts to form ammonium ions (NH_4^+), which are excreted in the urine primarily as their chloride salts.

Should metabolic acidosis occur, such as in starvation or diabetes, urinary excretion of ammonia increases concomitantly to compensate. This increase occurs because the diminished intake and use of carbohydrate stimulate gluconeogenesis and therefore enhance excretion of ammonia, which is formed from the higher rate of amino acid catabolism.

Like respiratory regulation, renal regulation of pH is directed at maintaining a normal ratio of $[HCO_3^-]$ to $[H_2CO_3]$. In alkalosis, for example, in which the plasma ratio of $[HCO_3^-]$ to $[H_2CO_3]$ increases as the pH rises above 7.4, a net increase occurs in the excretion of bicarbonate ions. This increase occurs because the high extracellular HCO_3^- concentration increases its filtration, while the relatively low concentration of H_2CO_3 decreases the secretion of H^+. Therefore, the fine balance between

HCO_3^- and H^+ that normally exists in the tubules no longer is in effect. Also, because no HCO_3^- ions can be reabsorbed without first reacting with H^+ (Figure 12.8), all the excess HCO_3^- passes into the urine, neutralized by sodium ions or other cations. In effect, therefore, HCO_3^- is removed from the extracellular fluid, restoring the normal ratio of HCO_3^- to H_2CO_3 and pH.

In acidosis, the ratio of plasma $[HCO_3^-]$ to $[H_2CO_3]$ decreases, meaning that the rate of H^+ secretion rises to a level far greater than the rate of HCO_3^- filtration into the tubules. As a result, most of the filtered HCO_3^- is converted to H_2CO_3 and reabsorbed as CO_2 (Figure 12.8), while the excess H^+ is excreted in the urine. As a consequence, the extracellular fluid ratio of $[HCO_3^-]$ to $[H_2CO_3]$ increases, as does the pH. The importance of the kidney in the homeostatic control of body water, as well as in electrolyte and acid–base balance, is emphasized in this chapter. The material is presented as a review of the principles involved in such control and of the effect of diet on fluid and electrolyte homeostasis. Although a detailed account of renal physiology is beyond the scope of this text, excellent sources that deal specifically with this subject are available [15].

SUMMARY

Maintaining body fluids and electrolytes is vitally important for sound health and nutrition. Intracellular fluid provides the environment for the myriad of metabolic reactions that take place in cells. The interstitial fluid compartment of the extracellular fluid mass allows nutrients to migrate into cells from the bloodstream and metabolic waste products from the cells to return to the bloodstream. These fluids contain the electrolytes, dissolved minerals that have important physiological functions. Their concentrations and their intracellular and extracellular distribution must be precisely regulated, and the mechanism for achieving this regulation is exerted largely through the kidney. The homeostatic maintenance of fluid volume is also the responsibility of this organ.

Fluid volume control by the kidney is mostly hormone mediated. Vasopressin, produced in the hypothalamus, stimulates the tubular reabsorption of water from the glomerular filtrate. Aldosterone, a product of the adrenal cortex, increases the reabsorption of sodium ions, which indirectly stimulate vasopressin release through the resulting rise in extracellular fluid osmotic pressure. Thirst centers in the brain, which respond to fluctuations in blood volume or extracellular fluid osmolality, are also important regulators of fluid balance by their influence on the amount of fluid intake.

The macrominerals sodium, potassium, and chloride along with other ions of nutritional importance such as calcium and magnesium are freely filtered by the renal glomerulus but are selectively conserved by tubular reabsorption through active transport systems. Potassium is an example of a mineral that is regulated in part by tubular secretion into the filtrate. Secretion of the ion from the distal tubular cells increases as its concentration in those cells rises because of increased dietary intake. Potassium, like sodium, is regulated by aldosterone. Elevated plasma potassium stimulates the release of aldosterone, which exerts opposing renal effects on the two minerals—enhanced reabsorption of sodium and an increase in potassium excretion. Normal physiological function depends upon proper control of the body fluid acid–base balance.

Many metabolic enzymes have a narrow range of pH at which they function adequately, and these catalysts are intolerant of pH swings of more than several tenths of a unit from the average normal value of 7.4 for extracellular fluids. The plasma is well buffered, primarily by proteins and by the bicarbonate–carbonic acid system. However, conditions of acidosis or alkalosis can result in situations such as an overproduction of organic acids, as would occur in diabetes or starvation, or respiratory aberrations that may cause abnormal carbon dioxide ventilation. Therefore, restoration of normal pH may be necessary and is accomplished through compensatory mechanisms of the kidneys and lungs. These organs function to maintain a normal ratio of bicarbonate to carbonic acid. The bicarbonate concentration is under the control of the kidneys, which can either conserve the ion by reabsorbing it to a greater extent or increase its excretion, depending upon whether the ratio needs to be decreased or increased to compensate for a pH disturbance. The carbonic acid value is controlled by the respiratory center. Its concentration can be increased or decreased by changes in the respiratory rate. Hyperventilation, for example, lowers the value by "blowing off" carbon dioxide, whereas a slowing of respiration retains carbon dioxide and therefore raises the carbonic acid level. From their effects on the bicarbonate: carbonic acid ratio, one can reason that hyperventilation can raise the pH and suppression of the respiratory rate can lower the pH in a compensatory manner.

References Cited

1. Sherwood L. Human Physiology: From Cells to Systems. 7th ed. Belmont, CA: Cengage Learning. 2010.
2. Rossier BC, Stutts MJ. Activation of the epithelial sodium channel (ENaC) by serine proteases. Ann Rev Physiol. 2008; 71:361–79.
3. Stockand JD. Vasopressin regulation of renal sodium excretion. Kid Internat. 2010; 78:849–56.
4. Kurtz A. Renin release: sites, mechanism, and control. Ann Rev Physiol. 2011; 73:377–99.
5. Potter LR. Matriuretic peptide metabolism, clearance and degradation. FEBS J 2011; 278:1808–17.
6. Clerico A, Giannoni A, Vittorini S, Passino C. Thirty years of the heart as an endocrine organ: physiological role and clinical utility of cardiac natriuretic hormones. Am J Physiol Heart Circ Physiol. 2011; 301:H12–20.
7. Guidance for Industry: A Food Labeling Guide. Appendix C: Health Claims. 2009. http://www.fda.gov/Food/GuidanceComplianceRegulatoryInformation/GuidanceDocuments/FoodLabelingNutrition/FoodLabelingGuide/ucm064919.htm
8. Frizzell RA, et al. Sodium-coupled chloride transport by epithelial tissues. Am J Physiol. 1979; 236:F1–8.
9. Food and Nutrition Board, Institute of Medicine. Dietary Reference Intakes. Washington, DC: National Academy Press, 2004.
10. Bell RR, Eldrid MM, Watson FR. The influence of NaCl and KCl on urinary calcium excretion in healthy young women. Nutr Res. 1992; 12:17–26.
11. Sellmeyer D, Schlotter M, Sebastian A. Potassium citrate prevents increased urine calcium excretion and bone resorption induced by high sodium chloride diet. J Clin Endocrinol Metab. 2002; 87:2008–12.
12. Young JH, McDonough AA. Recent advances in understanding integrative control of potassium homeostasis. Annu Rev Physiol. 2009; 71:381–401.
13. Giebish GH, Wang WH. Potassium transport-an update. J Nephroh. 2010; 23:S97–S104.
14. Duran C, Thompson CH, Xiao Q, Hartzell HC. Chloride channels: often enigmatic, rarely predictable. Annu Rev Physiol. 2010; 72:95–121.
15. Eaton DC, Pooler JP. Vander's Renal Physiology. 7th ed. McGraw Hill Medical. New York. 2009.

Suggested Readings

Klaplan L, Pesce A. Clinical Chemistry: Theory, Analysis, and Correlation. St. Louis: Mosby. 2009. Chap. 28. Physiology and pathophysiology of body water and electrolytes.

A clearly written clinical approach to fluid and electrolyte homeostasis, with diagrammatic illustrations of the regulatory mechanisms of fluid and electrolyte control.

Eaton DC, Pooler JP. Vander's Renal Physiology. 7th ed. New York: McGraw Hill Medical. 2009. Chapter 6. Basic renal process for sodium, chloride and water and Chapter 7 Control of sodium and water excretion: Regulation of plasma volume.

A brief basic physiology textbook that provides good illustrations of the role of the kidney in water, sodium, and potassium homeostasis.

Web Sites

http://nkdep.nih.gov/patients/kidney_disease_information.htm
National Institutes of Health Web site on kidney function and disease
www.kidney.org/atoz
National Kidney Foundation Web site, which provides information on kidney disease including nutritional aspects.

MACROMINERALS AND HYPERTENSION

Hypertension (high blood pressure) affects over 33% of Americans [1], and in 2005, the condition accounted for about 395,000 preventable deaths in the United States [2]. Hypertension, which is diagnosed when systolic and/or diastolic blood pressure values are ≧ 140/90 mm Hg, respectively, typically results from increased cardiac output and/or increased peripheral vascular resistance. Increased peripheral vascular resistance occurs when the luminal diameter of the arteries, arterioles, or both decreases (such as from plaque accumulation on blood vessel walls and with thickening of the media layer of blood vessels, which is also associated with plaque accumulation). The condition may be classified as primary (also called essential) or secondary. Causes of essential hypertension are generally unknown and thought to be multifactorial, perhaps related to a malfunction in sodium excretion and/or of the renin-angiotensin, aldosterone, catecholamine, and/or sympathetic nervous systems, among other factors. Essential hypertension accounts for greater than 90% of hypertension cases. The remaining cases of hypertension occur secondary to other conditions, such as kidney, endocrine, or neurological diseases. Whether it is essential or secondary, hypertension is a risk factor for stroke, renal disease, and heart disease. In fact, the risk for heart disease increases progressively as blood pressure increases above 115/75 mm Hg [3,4].

Although some risk factors for hypertension are not controllable (e.g., genetic predisposition, race, aging), others can be modified by a person's commitment to lifestyle changes that include diet modifications. Yet, because hypertension is a heterogeneous disease with a variety of precipitating factors, dietary modifications work for some but not all hypertensive individuals. This Perspective focuses on four of the major minerals (sodium, potassium, calcium, and magnesium) and blood pressure, and briefly addresses some other dietary factors that may also be associated with the condition.

SODIUM

Sodium, as salt—sodium chloride—was one of the first nutrients directly linked to hypertension. Dozens of studies (epidemiological and observational) and meta-analyses of studies have been conducted over several decades examining salt and/or sodium and blood pressure across and within population groups. Study designs, time periods, and subjects included and excluded have varied, as have the means used to assess sodium intake (analysis of diet or urinary sodium excretion), often leading to conflicting results. However, overall evidence now shows relatively consistently that reductions in sodium intake are associated with small reductions in blood pressure. The Dietary Approaches to Stop Hypertension (DASH) trials provided some of the most convincing evidence [4–9]. In these trials (as well as others), decreasing sodium intake resulted in significant reductions in blood pressure in those with and without hypertension [5–10]. Meta-analyses of studies also have provided useful information. For example, a meta-analysis of 17 trials including hypertensive individuals and 11 trials including normotensive individuals showed that modest reductions in sodium intake, of at least 4 weeks duration, resulted in significant reductions in blood pressure [10]. Urinary sodium excretion decreased by 78 mmol (equivalent to 4.6 g of salt) and 74 mmol (equivalent to 4.3 g of salt) in hypertensive and normotensive individuals, respectively. A dose response between blood pressure and change in urinary sodium excretion was observed; decreasing sodium intake by 100 mmol (6 g of salt) per day predicted a reduction in blood pressure of 7.11/3.88 mm Hg in hypertensive individuals and of 3.57/1.66 mm Hg in normotensive individuals [11]. Similar results were found in another meta-analysis of randomized controlled trials whereby salt restriction was associated with reductions of 27 to 39 mmol/day in urinary sodium excretion and reductions of 1 to 4 mm Hg in systolic blood pressure [12]. Additionally, clinical trials show that reduction in sodium intake by normotensive individuals decreases the risk of developing hypertension [13,14]. A progressive and direct dose-response effect exists between sodium intake and blood pressure in both hypertensive individuals and normotensive individuals [13]; however, reductions in sodium intake generally produce greater reductions in blood pressure in those with hypertension than in those without hypertension [11,15].

No one mechanism is thought to be responsible for salt-induced elevations in blood pressure. In some people, salt ingestion is thought to cause sodium and water retention and extracellular volume expansion, with the resulting release of a substance or substances that increase heart and blood vessel contractile activity and affect the renin-angiotensin-aldosterone system [16,17]. Elevations (even in the normal range) in plasma sodium concentrations appear to be associated with arterial thickening and narrowing and impaired endothelial cell elasticity, factors that increase blood pressure [15,18]. Alternatively, sodium may cause abnormal handling of other ions into and out of plasma and vascular smooth muscle, causing elevations in blood pressure [16,19]. Sodium retention decreases nitric oxide production; nitric oxide promotes vasodilation of blood vessels [16]. Sodium promotes urinary calcium excretion, also associated with elevations in blood pressure. Sensitivity to sodium correlates with low plasma renin activity (reflecting volume overload), a decreased capacity of the renin-angiotensin system to respond to physiological stimuli, and insulin resistance [20]. Further, in such people, sodium restriction appears to increase plasma renin activity and sympathetic nervous system activity to improve blood pressure [20].

Policy recommendations for sodium intake continue to be controversial. Some experts are passionate in their promotion of reductions in salt intake for the general population, while others believe such recommendations go beyond available data [21]. The Institute of Medicine set 1.5 g of sodium (65 mmol) per day (which corresponds to 3.8 g of salt) as the Adequate Intake recommendation for adults, and 2.3 g of sodium (100 mmol) per day (which corresponds to 5.8 g of salt) as the Tolerable Upper Intake Level [13]. Meeting such recommendations requires careful attention to the sodium content of processed foods as well as limiting both the amount of salt directly added to foods and the consumption of foods with visible salt (e.g. pretzels, some crackers, among other foods).

POTASSIUM

High potassium intake is also known to affect blood pressure—but inversely. Epidemiological, observational studies as well as clinical trials show an association between higher potassium intake (alone or relative to sodium intake) and lower blood pressure. Systolic and diastolic blood pressure reductions of 4.4 mm Hg and 2.5 mm Hg, respectively, have been reported in those with hypertension excreting at least 2 g (50 mmol) of potassium/day in the urine, and systolic and diastolic blood pressure reductions of 1.8 mm Hg and 1.0 mm Hg, respectively, have been reported in normotensive individuals excreting at least 2 g of potassium/day in the urine [22]. Meta-analyses of controlled potassium supplementation trials also report significant reductions in both systolic and diastolic blood pressure [22,23]. However, the effects of potassium supplementation on blood pressure are typically greater in African Americans and in those with hypertension than in whites and those who are normotensive [22–27]. Furthermore, the effects of potassium supplementation are typically greater in people ingesting large amounts of sodium and in those who are salt sensitive [13,16,24].

The mechanisms by which potassium affects blood pressure are multiple. Potassium promotes urinary sodium excretion (**natriuresis**) and thus diminishes body sodium.

Increased potassium intake also is associated with reduced urinary excretion of calcium and magnesium (which can in turn affect blood pressure) [13,27]. Potassium may induce vascular smooth muscle relaxation and thus reduce peripheral resistance [16]. It can inhibit platelet aggregation, arterial thrombosis, and proliferation of smooth vascular muscle cells to decrease peripheral vascular resistance [20].

While most studies support the inverse relationship between potassium intake and blood pressure, the results of other meta-analyses do not concur, suggesting that the evidence is inconclusive [28]. The Institute of Medicine recommends 4.7 g of potassium (120 mmol) per day as an Adequate Intake [13]; this is about the same amount of potassium as was provided in the DASH trials. Unfortunately, most Americans do not meet this recommendation. Recommendations to increase potassium intake to 4.7 g suggest the inclusion of additional fruits and vegetables into the diet plan, but not the use of potassium supplements for healthy, hypertensive, or at-risk individuals.

CALCIUM

A possible relationship between calcium and hypertension was first recognized with the discovery in the early 1970s that communities supplied with hard water (high calcium content) had a lower death rate from cardiovascular disease. A number of individual studies and meta-analyses of studies conducted in the 1990s [29–32] also supported a relationship between calcium and blood pressure. In most of the meta-analyses examining calcium supplementation (400 mg to 2 g), only small (less than 4 mm Hg and often less than 2 mm Hg) reductions in systolic, and typically not diastolic, blood pressure were found [30–33]. Findings from the Women's Health Initiative, which followed over 36,000 postmenopausal women, found that calcium (1,000 mg) along with vitamin D (400 IU) had no significant effects on blood pressure [34]. While studies continue to show associations between calcium and blood pressure [35], evidence in favor of a causal association between calcium supplementation and blood pressure reductions has been considered weak and insufficient to recommend calcium supplementation as an approach to lower blood pressure [4,31,33].

How calcium exhibits antihypertensive effects is uncertain. Calcium has a membrane-stabilizing and vasorelaxing effect on the smooth muscle cells [20,36]. It also affects the central and peripheral sympathetic nervous systems and modifies calcium homeostasis through effects on the actions of PTH and calcitriol. For example, calcium may suppress PTH-induced elevations in serum calcium concentrations to in turn reduce vascular resistance [36]. Increased intracellular calcium concentrations correlate directly with increased blood pressure. Calcium may also exert its effects through interactions with other nutrients. For example, increased calcium intake causes natriuresis and minimizes sodium-induced calciuria, which in turn can lower blood pressure.

The Institute of Medicine has established a Recommended Dietary Allowance of 1,200 mg per day of calcium for adults older than 50 years [37]. Given the evidence, individuals should strive to meet these recommendations; however, additional calcium consumption beyond the Recommended Dietary Allowance for those with hypertension or for those trying to prevent hypertension is not suggested at this time [4,31,33].

MAGNESIUM

While epidemiological data as well as animal and human studies suggest an inverse relationship between blood pressure and magnesium (intake and/or serum) [38–41], the effects of magnesium supplementation on blood pressure in clinical trials are inconsistent and less convincing [4,42–44]. Dickinson and associates [43], in analysis of 12 randomized controlled trials providing magnesium supplements, reported that diastolic blood pressure dropped by 2.2 mm Hg, but no significant reduction was observed in systolic blood pressure. Yet, despite the small, significant drop in diastolic blood pressure, because of few well-controlled trials, differences in treatment protocols, variations in forms of magnesium salts used, and the heterogeneity of the population, these authors concluded that the association between magnesium supplementation and blood pressure reduction is weak [43]. An additional meta-analysis examining trials providing combinations of magnesium, calcium, and potassium also found a lack of robust evidence in favor of supplementation of any combination of these three major minerals [45].

How magnesium directly impacts blood pressure is not clear (see [44] for an excellent review on the subject). Magnesium is known to promote relaxation of vascular smooth muscle as well as to interact with calcium [36,44]. In fact, low serum magnesium (indicative of low magnesium status) is associated with increased smooth muscle tension, vasospasms, and higher blood pressure [17,44]. Increased blood pressure also is associated with low intracellular calcium and with increased calcium and magnesium excretion [44]. Magnesium is a required cofactor for enzymes involved in fatty acid metabolism and the synthesis of prostaglandins, which are known to influence blood pressure.

The Institute of Medicine has established a Recommended Dietary Allowance for those ≥ 31 years of age of 420 mg of magnesium for males and 320 mg of magnesium for females per day [45]. The use of magnesium supplements in the prevention and treatment of hypertension is not recommended at this time. Supplementation of magnesium above the Recommended Dietary Allowance is suggested only for those with magnesium deficiency or those with increased urinary magnesium losses secondary to diuretic use [46].

OTHER DIETARY FACTORS

A direct, dose-dependent relationship exists between alcohol consumption (especially ingesting three or more drinks per day) and blood pressure [4]. Stimulation of the sympathetic nervous system, changes in hormones (such as renin, angiotensin, aldosterone, insulin, and cortisol), changes in vascular tone (e.g., inhibition of vascular relaxing substances, such as nitric oxide, or increased intracellular concentrations of calcium or electrolytes in vascular smooth muscle), as well as changes in baroreflex sensitivity have been suggested as mechanisms by which alcohol may influence blood pressure [19,47]. Recommendations to lower blood pressure suggest moderation of alcohol intake (among those who drink); moderation is defined as ≤ 1 drink per day for women and ≤ 2 drinks per day for men [4]. A drink is defined as 12 oz beer, 5 oz wine (12% alcohol), or 1.5 oz of 80-proof distilled spirits.

The effectiveness of fish oil supplements, rich in the omega-3 fatty acids eicosapentaenoic acid (EPA) and decosahexanoic acid (DHA), on blood pressure has been examined in several clinical trials and meta-analyses of studies. Small, but significant, reductions in systolic and diastolic blood pressure (about 3–5 mm Hg systolic and 2–4 mm Hg diastolic) have been typically observed in those with hypertension (but not in those who are normotensive) with the daily consumption of at least 3 g of omega-3 fatty acids [48–51]. The blood pressure–lowering effects of fish oil have been attributed, in part, to enhanced production of prostaglandins that promote vasodilation and inhibit platelet aggregation, and to decreased formation of thromboxane A_2, which promotes vasoconstriction and platelet aggregation [52]. In spite of studies showing omega-3 fatty acid–associated reductions in blood pressure, the American Heart Association suggests omega-3 fatty acids have a limited role in the treatment of hypertension [52]. Others also suggest that fish oil supplements should not be routinely recommended to lower blood pressure [4]. For those who choose to ingest supplements, the Food and Drug Administration recommends the use of no more than 3 g of eicosapentaenoic acid and decosahexanoic acid per day, with not more than 2 of the 3 g derived from dietary supplements [53].

Lifestyle approaches also have been investigated in the prevention and treatment of hypertension. The randomized trial Dietary Approaches to Stop Hypertension (DASH) reported that low-fat diets rich in fruits, vegetables, and low-fat dairy products were more effective in reducing blood pressure than a control diet low in fruits and vegetables and average in fat (~36% of kcal) [4–9]. The DASH diet provides 3 g of sodium, about 4,500 mg of potassium, 8 to 10 servings of fruits and vegetables, and 2 to 3 servings of low-fat dairy products daily; limits red meat, fats, and sugar-sweetened foods and beverages; and emphasizes nuts, seeds, and legumes. The DASH-sodium study, which compared the effects of the DASH diet with three levels of sodium intake (3.3 g, 2.4 g, and 1.5 g) with those of a control diet, further showed that additional blood pressure reduction could be achieved through reduction in dietary sodium to 1.5 g/day [6,9].

Other lifestyle modification approaches have been investigated. The PREMIER Trial, which included weight loss, increased physical activity, sodium reduction, and the DASH diet, was found to be beneficial to those with hypertension not on medications (−14.2 mm Hg systolic and −7.4 mm Hg diastolic) and to those without hypertension (−9.2 mm Hg systolic and −5.8 mm Hg diastolic) [54]. The effectiveness of lifestyle interventions for hypertension, investigated in a meta-analysis, also showed that weight reduction, regular exercise, alcohol restriction, and salt restriction were associated with significant reductions in systolic and diastolic blood pressure; however, evidence did not support the use of relaxation therapies or potassium, calcium, or magnesium supplements to reduce blood pressure [55].

In summary, several dietary modifications can be made to help to lower blood pressure, including reducing sodium intake; increasing potassium, calcium, and magnesium intakes to meet recommendations; consuming alcohol in moderation (for those who drink); and following a healthy diet plan such as DASH. These findings are consistent with recommendations by the Joint National Committee on Prevention, Detection, Evaluation, and Treatment of High Blood Pressure, which promote the consumption of diets that supply adequate dietary intakes of calcium, potassium, and magnesium and not the use of supplements [56].

References Cited

1. High blood pressure facts. http://www.cdc.gov/bloodpressure/facts.htm

2. Denaei G, Ding EL, Mozaffarian D, et al. The preventable causes of death in the United States: comparing risk assessment of dietary, lifestyle, and metabolic risk factors. PLos Med. 2009; 6:e1000058.

3. Lewington S, Clarke R, Qizibash N, et al. Age-specific relevance of usual blood pressure to vascular mortality: a meta-analysis of individual data for one million adults in 61 prospective studies. Lancet. 2002; 360:1903–13.

4. Appel LJ, Brands MW, Daniels SR, et al. Dietary approaches to prevent and treat hypertension. Hypertens. 2006; 47:296–308.

5. Vollmer WM, Sacks FM, Ard J, et al. Effects of diet and sodium intake on blood pressure: subgroup analysis of the DASH-sodium trial. Ann Intern Med. 2001; 135:1019–28.

6. Bray GA, Vollmer WM, Sacks FM, et al. A further subgroup analysis of the effects of the DASH diet and three dietary sodium levels on blood pressure: results of the DASH-sodium Trial. Am J Cardiol. 2004; 94:222–27.

7. Appel LJ, Moore TJ, Obarzanek E, et al. A clinical trial of the effects of dietary patterns on blood pressure: DASH Collaborative Research Group. N Engl J Med. 1997; 336:1117–24.

8. Svetkey LP, Simmons-Morton D, Vollmer WM, et al. Effects of dietary patterns on blood pressure: subgroup analysis of Dietary Approaches to Stop Hypertension (DASH) randomized clinical trial. Arch Intern Med. 1999; 159:285–93.

9. Sacks FM, Svetkey LP, Vollmer WM, et al. for the DASH-sodium Collaborative Research Group. Effects on blood pressure of reduced dietary sodium and the Dietary Approaches to Stop Hypertension (DASH) diet: DASH-Sodium Collaborative Research Group. N Engl J Med. 2001; 344:3–10.

10. Kumanyika SK, Cook NR, Cutler JA, et al. for the Trials of Hypertension Prevention Collaborative Research Group. Sodium reduction for hypertension prevention in overweight adults: further results from the Trials of Hypertension Prevention Phase II. J Hum Hypertens. 2005; 19:33–45.

11. He FJ, MacGregor GA. Effect of modest salt reduction on blood pressure: a meta-analysis of randomized trials. Implications for public health. J Hum Hypertension. 2002; 16:761–70.

12. Taylor RS, Ashton KE, Moxham T, et al. Reduced dietary salt for the prevention of cardiovascular disease: a meta-analysis of randomized controlled trials (Cochrane Review). Am J Hypertens. 2011; 24:843–53.

13. Institute of Medicine. Dietary Reference Intakes: Water, Potassium Sodium Chloride, and Sulfate. Washington, DC: National Academy Press, 2004.

14. Stevens VJ, Obarzanek E, Cook NR, et al. Long-term weight loss and changes in blood pressure: results of the Trials of Hypertension Prevention Phase II. Ann Intern Med. 2001; 134:1–11.

15. Intersalt Cooperative Research Group: Intersalt: An international study of electrolyte excretion and blood pressure. Results for 24 hour urinary sodium and potassium excretion. Br Med J. 1998; 297:319–28.

16. Bussemaker E, Hillebrand U, Hausberg M, et al. Pathogenesis of hypertension: interactions among sodium, potassium, and aldosterone. Am J Kidney Dis. 2010; 55:1111–20.

17. Das UN. Nutritional factors in the pathobiology of human essential hypertension. Nutrition. 2001; 17:337–46.

18. Reuter S, Bussemaker E, Hausberg M, et al. Effect of excessive salt intake: role of plasma sodium. Curr Hypertens Rep. 2009; 11:91–97.

19. Suter PM, Sierro C, Vetter W. Nutritional factors in the control of blood pressure and hypertension. Nutr Clin Care. 2002; 5:9–19.

20. Buemi M, Senatore M, Corica F, et al. Diet and arterial hypertension: is the sodium ion alone important? Med Res Rev. 2002; 22:419–28.

21. Hollenberg NK. The influence of dietary sodium on blood pressure. J Am Coll Nutr. 2006; 25:S240–46.

22. Whelton P, He J, Culter J, et al. Effects of oral potassium on blood pressure: meta-analysis of randomized controlled clinical trials. JAMA. 1997; 277:1624–32.

23. Geleijnse J, Kok F, Grobbee D. Blood pressure response to changes in sodium and potassium intake: a metaregression analysis of randomized trials. J Hum Hypertens. 2003; 17:471–80.

24. Morris R, Sebastian A, Forman A, et al. Normotensive salt-sensitivity: effects of race and dietary potassium. Hypertension. 1999; 33:18–23.

25. Barri Y, Wingo C. The effects of potassium depletion and supplementation on blood pressure: a clinical review. Am J Med Sci. 1997; 314:37–40.

26. Kotchen T, Kotchen J. Dietary sodium and blood pressure: interactions with other nutrients. Am J Clin Nutr. 1997; 65:S708–11.

27. Sellmeyer D, Schlotter M, Sebastian A. Potassium citrate prevents increased urine calcium excretion and bone resorption induced by high sodium chloride diet. J Clin Endocrinol Metab. 2002; 87:2008–12.

28. Dickinson HO, Nicolson DJ, Campbell F, et al. Potassium supplementation for the management of primary hypertension in adults. Cochrane Database Sys Rev. 2006; 3:CD004641.

29. Cappuccio F, Elliott P, Allender P, et al. Epidemiologic association between dietary calcium intake and blood pressure: a meta-analysis of published data. Am J Epidemiol. 1995; 142:935–45.

30. Bucher H, Cook R, Guyatt G, et al. Effects of dietary calcium supplementation on blood pressure: a meta-analysis of randomized controlled trials. JAMA. 1996; 275:1016–22.

31. Allender P, Cutler J, Follmann D, et al. Dietary calcium and blood pressure: a metaanalysis of randomized clinical trials. Ann Intern Med. 1996; 124:825–31.

32. Griffith LE, Guyatt GH, Cook RJ, et al. The influence of dietary and nondietary calcium supplementation on blood pressure: a meta-analysis of randomized controlled trials. Am J Hypertens. 1999; 12:84–92.

33. Dickinson HO, Nicolson DJ, Campbell F, et al. Calcium supplementation for the management of primary hypertension in adults. Cochrane Database Sys Rev. 2006; 3:CD004639.

34. Margolis KL, Ray RM, Horn LV, et al. for the Women's Health Initiative Investigators. Effect of calcium and vitamin D supplementation on blood pressure: the Women's Health Initiative randomized trial. Hypertension. 2008; 52:847–55.

35. Sabanayagam C, Shankar A. Serum calcium levels and hypertension among US adults. J Clin Hypertens. 2011; 13:716–21.

36. Hatton D, Yue Q, McCarron D. Mechanisms of calcium's effects on blood pressure. Semin Nephrol. 1995; 15:593–602.

37. Institute of Medicine, Food and Nutrition Board. Dietary Reference intakes for Calcium and Vitamin D. Washington, DC: National Academy Press, 2011.

38. Joffres MR, Reed DM, Yano K. Relation of magnesium intake and other dietary factors to blood pressure: the Honolulu heart study. Am J Clin Nutr. 1987; 45:469–75.

39. Paolisso G, Barbagallo M. Hypertension, diabetes mellitus, and insulin resistance: the role of intracellular magnesium. Am J Hypertens. 1997; 10:346–55.

40. Ma J, Folsom AR, Melnick SL. Associations of serum and dietary magnesium with cardiovascular disease, hypertension, diabetes, insulin and carotid arterial wall thickness: the ARIC study. J Clin Epidemiol. 1995; 48:927–40.

41. Song Y, Sesso HD, Manson JAE. Dietary magnesium intake and risk of incident hypertension among middle-aged and older US women in a 10-year follow-up study. Am J Cardiol. 2006; 98:1616–21.

42. Jee SH, Miller E, Guallar E, et al. The effect of magnesium supplementation on blood pressure: a meta-analysis of randomized clinical trials. Am J Hypertens. 2002; 15:691–96.

43. Dickinson HO, Nicolson DJ, Campbell F, et al. Magnesium supplementation for the management of essential hypertension in adults. Cochrane Database Sys Rev. 2006; 3:CD004640.

44. Touyz RM. Role of magnesium in the pathogenesis of hypertension. Molec Aspects Med. 2003; 24:107–36.

45. Food and Nutrition Board, Institute of Medicine. Dietary Reference Intakes. Washington, DC: National Academy Press, 1997.

46. Beyer FR, Dickinson HO, Nicolson DJ, et al. Combined calcium, magnesium, and potassium supplementation for the management of primary hypertension in adults. Cochrane Database Sys Rev. 2006; 3:CD004805.

47. Cushman WC. Alcohol consumption and hypertension. J Clin Hyperten. 2001; 3:166–70.

48. Howe PR. Dietary fats and hypertension: focus on fish oil. Ann NY Acad Sci. 1997; 827:339–52.

49. Morris MC, Sacks F, Rosner B. Does fish oil lower blood pressure? a meta-analysis of controlled trials. Circulation. 1993; 88:523–33.

50. Appel LJ, Miller ER, Seidler AJ, Whelton PK. Does supplementation of diet with fish oil reduce blood pressure? a meta-analysis of controlled trials. Arch Intern Med. 1993; 153:1429–38.

51. Geleijnse JM, Giltay EJ, Grobbee DE, et al. Blood pressure response to fish oil supplementation: metaregression analysis of randomized trials. J Hypertens. 2005; 20:1493–99.

52. Kris-Etherton PM, Harris WS, Appel LJ. for the Nutrition Committee. AHA scientific statement: fish consumption, fish oil, omega-3 fatty acids, and cardiovascular disease. Circulation. 2002; 106:2747–57.

53. FDA announces qualified health claims for omega-3 fatty acids. http://www.fda.gov/SiteIndex/ucm108351.htm

54. Appel LJ, Champagne CM, Harsha DW, et al. for the PREMIER Collaborative Research Group. Effect of comprehensive lifestyle modification on blood pressure control: main results of the PREMIER clinical trial. JAMA. 2003; 289:2083–93.

55. Dickinson HO, Mason JM, Nicolson DJ, et al. Lifestyle interventions to reduce raised blood pressure: a systematic review of randomized controlled trials. J Hypertens. 2006; 24:215–33.

56. The seventh report of the Joint National Committee on Prevention, Detection, Evaluation, and Treatment of High Blood Pressure (JNC 7). 2003. www.nhlbi.nih.gov/guidelines/hypertension.

Web Sites

www.americanheart.org
www.nlm.nih.gov/medlineplus/highbloodpressure.html
www.cdc.gov/nchs/fastats/hyprtens.htm

Suggested Readings

Appel LJ, Frohlich ED, Hall JE, et al. The importance of population-wide sodium reduction as a means to prevent cardiovascular disease and stroke. Circulation. 2011; 123:1138–43.

Carey RM. Overview of endocrine systems in primary hypertension. Endocrinol Metab Clin N Am. 2011; 40:265–77.

Rosendorff C, Black HR, Cannon CP, et al. Treatment of hypertension in the prevention and management of ischemic heart disease. Circulation. 2007; 115:2761–88.

FLUID BALANCE AND THE THERMAL STRESS OF EXERCISE

An important dimension of the demands of sport and exercise is **thermoregulation,** the control of body temperature within a narrow range. Strenuous exercise challenges this control because it increases the metabolic rate and therefore is markedly thermogenic. (Recall that the energy-producing systems are <40% efficient and the remainder of the energy is given off as heat.) A drop in deep body (core) temperature of 10°F (5.5°C) or an increase of just 5°F (3.0°C) above normal is tolerated, but fluctuation beyond this range can result in death. Heat stress mortality and morbidity are particularly a problem in the young, ages 15 to 19. The Centers for Disease Control and Prevention (CDC) estimates that between 2005 and 2009, an average of 9,237 time-loss heat-related illnesses per year were reported by high school athletes [1]. The team sport with the highest incidence of heat-related deaths is football. A total of 39 heat-related deaths of football players were reported in the United States between 1995 and 2008; 29 of these individuals were of high school age and 2 were professional players [2]. These heat-related deaths and illnesses are preventable with a few precautions.

Various mechanisms of thermoregulation maintain thermal balance in the body. Muscular activity is one of the most influential factors contributing to increases in body core temperature; others include hormonal effects, the thermic effect of food, postural changes, and environmental changes. Countering the heat gain factors are mechanisms that protect against hyperthermia by removing heat from the body, such as radiation, conduction, and convection, mechanisms for dry heat exchange that are facilitated by augmented blood flow to the skin. In an otherwise normal adult engaged in strenuous exercise, evaporation (of sweat), a wet mechanism for heat exchange, provides the most important physiological defense against overheating. Dry heat exchange is more important in children because they have a higher relative skin surface area–to–body mass ratio, and the adult capacity for sweating and its regulation do not fully develop until several years following puberty [3].

Evaporation of 1.0 mL of sweat is equivalent to about 0.6 kcal of body heat loss. Therefore, even at maximal exercise—at which 4.0 L of O_2/minute are consumed, equivalent to about 20 kcal/minute of heat produced—core temperature would be expected to rise just 1°F every 5 to 7 minutes. This gradual rise occurs because sweating, assumed to be maximal at 30 mL/minute, would cool the body only to the extent of about 18 kcal/minute.

Approximately 60% of the energy released during exercise is in the form of heat. If this heat is not removed from the body, the combined heat load from metabolic activity and the environment could lead to a dramatic increase in body temperature during strenuous activity. Hyperthermia can result in lethal heat injury. As stated previously, the major mechanism for heat loss for an adult is the evaporation of sweat. Nearly 600 kcal are eliminated by the cooling effect of the evaporation of 1 L of sweat. (Note that cooling results from the *evaporation* rather than the *formation* of sweat.) Among the remaining mechanisms for heat removal, radiation is the next most important for the adult. In radiation, heat generated in the working muscles is transported by blood flow to the skin, from which it can subsequently be exchanged with the environment. For both of these thermoregulatory mechanisms, body water is clearly the major participant; therefore, much research focuses on strategies for replacing lost fluids during strenuous exercise.

Firm evidence indicates that depletion of body water (dehydration) from loss of more than 2% of body weight as sweat can impair performance of endurance activities but does not decrease the strength of strength athletes. The most likely explanations for the impairment in endurance athletes are:

- A reduced plasma volume and therefore reduced hemodynamic capacity to achieve maximal cardiac output and peripheral circulation. As plasma volume declines, reduced skin blood flow and a fall in stroke volume follow. Heart rate increases to compensate but cannot offset the stroke volume deficit [4].

- Altered sweat gland function, whereby sweating ceases in an autonomic control attempt to conserve body water.

As a result of these reactions, body temperature rises quickly, drastically increasing the chance of cramps, exhaustion, and even heatstroke, a condition that has a mortality rate of 80%. Sweat losses of 1.5 L/hour are commonly encountered in endurance sports, and under particularly hot or warm-humid conditions, sweat rates exceeding 2.5 L/hour have been measured in fit individuals. Marathon runners can lose 6% to 8% of body weight in water during the 26.2-mile (42.2 km) event, and plasma volume may fall 13% to 18%. It is common, therefore, for a 150-lb (68-kg) runner to lose 0.5 lb (1.1 kg) of water (equivalent to an 8-oz glass of water) per mile in a hot environment.

Dehydration results when fluid loss exceeds intake, and the degree of dehydration is directly proportional to the fluid disparity. The primary goal of fluid replacement is to maintain plasma volume so that circulation and sweating can proceed at maximal levels. The maximum rate of sweating is greater than the maximum rate for absorbing water from the intestinal tract, so at maximum exercise effort, some dehydration is bound to occur. The endurance athlete has difficulty avoiding a negative water balance because attempting to replenish the copious amount lost in the course of a marathon or other long-duration event is impractical. Moreover, it is distasteful because the necessary intake far exceeds the thirst desire, a stimulus that is delayed behind rapid dehydration. Athletes allowed to drink in response to their thirst desire replace only about half the water lost during exercise [3]. Force-feeding of fluids to exactly balance fluids lost is ideal from the standpoint of athletic performance, although the dramatic effects of lesser amounts of fluid replenishment during exercise are also well documented. The experimental design on which such conclusions are generally based is comparison of the extent of fluid intake with performance and certain physiological parameters, such as heart rate and body temperature. Study groups are commonly composed of subjects who, in the course of prolonged exercise, are (1) force-fed fluids beyond the thirst desire, (2) allowed to drink fluid ad libitum (as desired), or (3) deprived of fluid intake. Force-fed subjects display superior performance, lower heart rate, and lower body core temperature than the other groups, and the ad libitum group outperforms the deprived group in these circumstances [5].

A controversial issue in sports nutrition is whether electrolyte replacement is necessary during prolonged exercise. Based upon the knowledge that sweat contains electrolytes (sodium, potassium, chloride, and magnesium), it was once reasoned that because substantial amounts of electrolytes were lost during endurance athletics, replacing them was necessary to optimize performance. Sports drinks supplemented with electrolytes and sometimes glucose (glucose-electrolyte solutions [GES drinks]) began to appear on the market in the 1970s and are currently sold under names such as Gatorade, PowerAde, and All Sport. Whether such supplementation is necessary depends upon the length and level of intensity of the exercise and therefore on the quantity of sweat lost. GES drinks containing about 8% or less of carbohydrate have been shown not to decrease stomach emptying time, and they facilitate rapid absorption of water. Along with the quantity, the nature of the carbohydrate, which may include glucose, sucrose, fructose, high-fructose corn syrup, and/or maltodextrins, is important. Polyglucose (maltodextrin, a water-soluble polymer of glucose units connected by

Table 1 Average Electrolyte Concentrations in Sweat and Blood Serum (mEq/L)

	Na$^+$	K$^+$	Cl$^-$	Mg^{2+}
Sweat	40–45	3.9	39	3.3
Blood serum	140	4	110	1.5–2.1

α[1–4] linkages) increases the amount of glucose absorbed from a GES drink and has a small effect on osmolality.

The typical electrolyte content of sweat is very low compared with that of body fluids, with the exception of Mg^{+2}, as shown in Table 1. Dehydration through sweating has the effect of concentrating sodium and chloride ions in extracellular and intracellular water because of their relatively low concentration in sweat. Therefore, in marathon-level exertion, in which a total sweat loss of 5 to 6 L or less is incurred, rehydration with water alone is adequate, because only about 200 mEq of sodium and chloride would be lost from a relatively large body store. Some research suggests, however, that flavored water or pleasant-tasting electrolyte-glucose solutions encourage the athlete to consume more fluid than he or she would if using plain water for hydration [5]. This enhanced fluid intake is probably beneficial, even though the electrolytes might not be needed. In addition, drinking plain water lowers the osmolality of the blood, which reduces the thirst reflex.

The American Academy of Pediatrics makes recommendations for active children, including the use of flavored beverages that contain electrolytes, for the reasons stated previously [6].

Although some researchers regard potassium losses during exercise in the heat as constituting a potential health problem, this view too is controversial given the relatively small amount of the ion lost. Assuming a typical sweat potassium concentration (Table 1), a sweat loss of 5 L would induce an estimated potassium deficit of <20 mEq, or well under 1% of the estimated total body store of 3,000 mEq for a 70-kg man.

Only under severe conditions of prolonged, high-intensity exercise (during events such as the ultra-marathon or Ironman competition) in the heat would electrolyte replacement be indicated. In such a case, electrolyte loss may exceed the amount provided in the daily diet, and some sodium supplementation may be necessary. Whether potassium supplementation is called for under similar conditions is doubtful, for the reasons discussed.

References Cited

1. Heat illness among high school athletes: United States, 2005–2009. Morbidity and Mortality Weekly. 2010; 59:1009–13.

2. Marshall SW. Heat injury in youth sport. Br J Sorts Med. 2010; 44:8–12.

3. Falk B, Dotan R. Temperature regulation and elite young athletes. Med Sport Sci. 2011; 56:126–49.

4. Becker JA, Stweart LK. Heat-related illness. Am J Fam Physician. 2011; 83:1325–30.

5. Montain SJ. Hydration recommendations for sport: 2008. Curr Sports Med Rep. 2008; 7:187–92.

6. McArdle W, Katch F, Katch V. Exercise Physiology. 7th ed. Baltimore, MD: Williams & Wilkins. 2010; Chap. 25.

Web Sites

www.umass.edu/cnshp/index.html
Center for Nutrition in Sport and Human Performance at the University of Massachusetts

www.gssiweb.org
A Web site of the Gatorade Sports Science Institute. It contains many summary articles on exercise science, sports nutrition, and sports medicine.

www.beverageinstitute.org
A Web site sponsored by the Coca-Cola Company that contains articles at the consumer and professional level on fluid and beverage intake.

13 ESSENTIAL TRACE AND ULTRATRACE MINERALS

THE TRACE MINERALS OR TRACE ELEMENTS (also called microminerals) initially gained the description "trace" because their concentrations in tissue were not easily quantified by early analytical methods. Today, however, trace minerals can be analyzed by a variety of techniques. Trace minerals or elements are now typically defined as minerals that are needed by the body in small amounts, that is, less than 100 mg per day. However, some of the trace elements may be categorized as ultratrace if required in amounts of less than 1 mg per day.

Figure 13.1 shows the periodic table, highlighting some of the essential trace and ultratrace elements. This chapter describes the sources, digestion, absorption, transport, storage, functions, interactions with other nutrients, excretion, recommended intakes, deficiency, toxicity, and assessment of nutriture for the trace minerals iron, zinc, and copper, and the ultratrace minerals selenium, iodine, and molybdenum, for which Recommended Dietary Allowances have been established by the Food and Nutrition Board. In addition, these same topics are covered for the trace mineral manganese and the ultratrace mineral chromium, for which Adequate Intakes have been established by the Food and Nutrition Board.

Very little is known about the need for many other trace and ultratrace elements, including nickel, silicon, vanadium, arsenic, and boron; therefore, no recommendations for intake exist. Chapter 14 addresses these elements, as well as fluoride, a nonessential element with established Adequate Intakes.

Table 13.1 provides an overview of the minerals addressed in the chapter, including information on the approximate quantities in the body of these trace minerals, which range from <1 mg to about 4 g. Keeping in mind that an ounce weighs about 28.4 g, contrast these amounts with the body concentrations of the major minerals, which range from about 35 to 1,400 g.

IRON

The human body contains about 2 to 4 g of iron, or ~38 mg iron/kg body weight for women and ~50 mg iron/kg body weight for men. Over 65% (~1.3–2.6 g) of body iron is found in hemoglobin, up to about 10% (~0.2–0.4 g) is found as myoglobin, about 1% to 5% (up to 0.1–0.2 g) is found as part of enzymes, and the remaining body iron (about 20% or 0.4–0.8 g) is found in the blood or in storage. While the metal exists in several oxidation states varying from Fe^{6+} to Fe^{2-} depending on its chemical environment, the only states that are stable in the aqueous environment of the body and in food are the ferric (Fe^{3+}) and the ferrous (Fe^{2+}) forms.

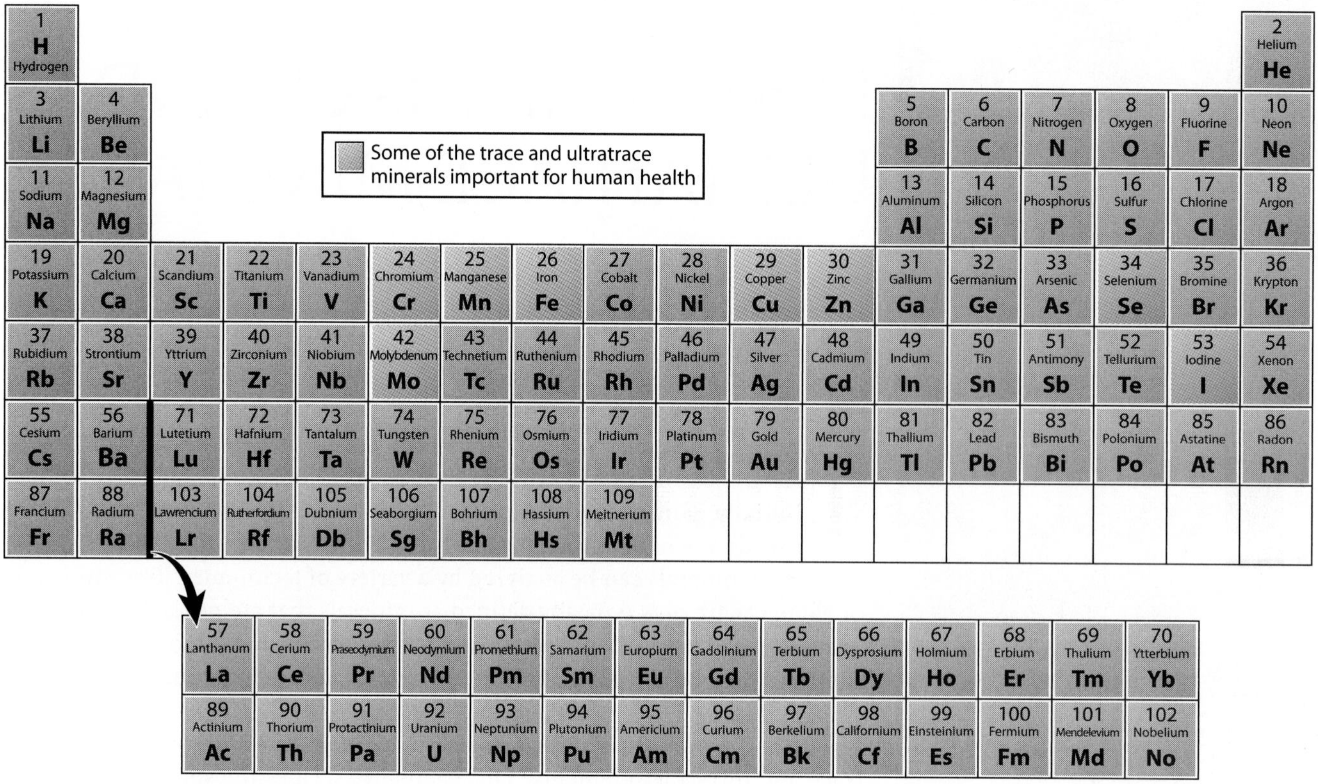

1 Hydrogen **H**																	2 Helium **He**
3 Lithium **Li**	4 Beryllium **Be**											5 Boron **B**	6 Carbon **C**	7 Nitrogen **N**	8 Oxygen **O**	9 Fluorine **F**	10 Neon **Ne**
11 Sodium **Na**	12 Magnesium **Mg**											13 Aluminum **Al**	14 Silicon **Si**	15 Phosphorus **P**	16 Sulfur **S**	17 Chlorine **Cl**	18 Argon **Ar**
19 Potassium **K**	20 Calcium **Ca**	21 Scandium **Sc**	22 Titanium **Ti**	23 Vanadium **V**	24 Chromium **Cr**	25 Manganese **Mn**	26 Iron **Fe**	27 Cobalt **Co**	28 Nickel **Ni**	29 Copper **Cu**	30 Zinc **Zn**	31 Gallium **Ga**	32 Germanium **Ge**	33 Arsenic **As**	34 Selenium **Se**	35 Bromine **Br**	36 Krypton **Kr**
37 Rubidium **Rb**	38 Strontium **Sr**	39 Yttrium **Y**	40 Zirconium **Zr**	41 Niobium **Nb**	42 Molybdenum **Mo**	43 Technetium **Tc**	44 Ruthenium **Ru**	45 Rhodium **Rh**	46 Palladium **Pd**	47 Silver **Ag**	48 Cadmium **Cd**	49 Indium **In**	50 Tin **Sn**	51 Antimony **Sb**	52 Tellurium **Te**	53 Iodine **I**	54 Xenon **Xe**
55 Cesium **Cs**	56 Barium **Ba**	71 Lutetium **Lu**	72 Hafnium **Hf**	73 Tantalum **Ta**	74 Tungsten **W**	75 Rhenium **Re**	76 Osmium **Os**	77 Iridium **Ir**	78 Platinum **Pt**	79 Gold **Au**	80 Mercury **Hg**	81 Thallium **Tl**	82 Lead **Pb**	83 Bismuth **Bi**	84 Polonium **Po**	85 Astatine **At**	86 Radon **Rn**
87 Francium **Fr**	88 Radium **Ra**	103 Lawrencium **Lr**	104 Rutherfordium **Rf**	105 Dubnium **Db**	106 Seaborgium **Sg**	107 Bohrium **Bh**	108 Hassium **Hs**	109 Meitnerium **Mt**									

Some of the trace and ultratrace minerals important for human health

57 Lanthanum **La**	58 Cerium **Ce**	59 Praseodymium **Pr**	60 Neodymium **Nd**	61 Promethium **Pm**	62 Samarium **Sm**	63 Europium **Eu**	64 Gadolinium **Gd**	65 Terbium **Tb**	66 Dysprosium **Dy**	67 Holmium **Ho**	68 Erbium **Er**	69 Thulium **Tm**	70 Ytterbium **Yb**
89 Actinium **Ac**	90 Thorium **Th**	91 Protactinium **Pa**	92 Uranium **U**	93 Neptunium **Np**	94 Plutonium **Pu**	95 Americium **Am**	96 Curium **Cm**	97 Berkelium **Bk**	98 Californium **Cf**	99 Einsteinium **Es**	100 Fermium **Fm**	101 Mendelevium **Md**	102 Nobelium **No**

Figure 13.1 The periodic table highlighting some of the essential trace and ultratrace elements.
Source: Derived from Beerman/McGuire, Nutritional Sciences, 1/e. © Cengage Learning.

Sources

Dietary iron is found in one of two forms in foods, heme and nonheme. Heme iron represents iron that is contained within the porphyrin ring structure shown in Figure 13.2. Heme iron is derived mainly from hemoglobin and myoglobin and thus is found in animal products, especially meat, fish, and poultry. About 50% to 60% of the iron in meat, fish, and poultry is heme iron; the rest is nonheme iron. Nonheme iron is found primarily in plant foods (nuts, fruits, vegetables, grains, tofu) and dairy products (milk, cheese, eggs), although dairy products contain very little iron and represent a very poor iron source.

Foods particularly high in iron include liver, with about 5 mg of iron/3 oz, and other organ meats; however, these foods are not popular items in most American diets. More popular foods that are relatively good sources of iron

include meats, especially red meats, and seafoods such as oysters and clams. For example, two typical forms of beef, eye of the round roast and hamburger, both provide about 2 mg of iron/3 oz. A 3-oz chicken breast contains about 1 mg of iron, and a similar serving of dark meat turkey has about 2 mg of iron. Clams and oysters are quite rich in iron, providing about 12 mg and 8 mg, respectively, per 3-oz serving. Beans (such as navy, lima, and black) provide about 1.8 to 2.2 mg of iron per half cup. The dark green leafy vegetables spinach (cooked) and collard greens (cooked) provide about 3.7 mg and 2.2 mg of iron per half cup, respectively. Raisins, a dried fruit, contain about 0.68 mg of iron per quarter cup. Other good sources of iron are listed in Table 13.1. Although iron is widely distributed in food, its content in an average American diet is estimated at 5 to 7 mg iron per 1,000 kcal.

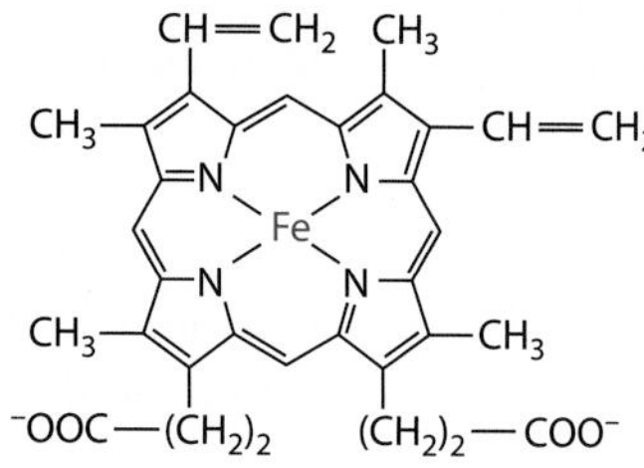

In addition to the amount of iron found naturally in foods, foods such as breads, rolls, pasta, cereals, grits, and flour are often fortified with iron. Fortified flour, for example, contains 20 mg of iron per lb, and corn grits, corn meal, and rice contain from 13 to 26 mg per lb. Pasta has 13 to 16.5 mg per lb, and bread, rolls, and buns contain 12.5 mg iron per lb. A breakfast cereal such as wheat bran with raisins, for example, provides 25% of the Daily Value for iron (which is 18 mg) or 4.5 mg iron per 1 cup. Cooked, enriched spaghetti (1 cup) has about 2 mg of iron. One whole-grain English muffin has 8% of the Daily Value, or about 1.44 mg of iron. Elemental iron,

Figure 13.2 Heme iron, a metalloporphyrin.

Table 13.1 Approximate Body Content, Selected Functions, Deficiency Symptoms, Food Sources, and Recommended Dietary Allowance (RDA) or Adequate Intake (AI) for the Essential Trace and Ultratrace Minerals

Mineral	Approximate Body Content	Selected Physiological Roles	Selected Enzyme Cofactor Roles	Selected Deficiency Symptoms	Selected Food Sources	RDA or AI* (Adults)
Chromium	4–6 mg	Possibly potentiates insulin signaling		Glucose intolerance, glucose and lipid metabolism abnormalities	Mushrooms, green peppers, organ meats, whole grains, Brewer's yeast	35 μg* male; 25 μg* female
Copper	50–150 mg	Iron use; synthesis of collagen, pigment, neurotransmitters	Superoxide dismutase, lysyl oxidase, cytochrome c oxidase, dopamine monooxygenase, amine oxidase, peptidylglycine α-amidating monooxygenase	Anemia, neutropenia, bone and blood vessel abnormalities, impaired immune function	Liver, shellfish, whole grains, legumes, eggs, meat, fish	900 μg
Iodine	15–20 mg	Thyroid hormones synthesis		Enlarged thyroid gland (goiter)	Iodized salt, salt-water seafood, milk, liver, eggs, yogurt, legumes	150 μg
Iron	2–4 g	O₂ transport and use; amino acid metabolism; antioxidant; carnitine, collagen, and thyroid hormone synthesis	Catalase, cytochromes, myeloperoxidase, thyroperoxidase, lysine and proline dioxygenases, phosphoenolpyruvate (PEP) carboxykinase	Anemia, fatigue, impaired work performance, decreased resistance to infection	Organ meats (liver), meat, molasses, clams, oysters, nuts, legumes, green leafy vegetables, dried fruits, enriched/whole grains	8 mg male; 18 mg female
Manganese	10–20 mg	Brain function, collagen, bone, growth, urea synthesis, glucose and lipid metabolism, CNS function	Glucosyltransferase, arginase, pyruvate carboxylase, PEP carboxykinase, superoxide dismutase, glutamine synthetase	In animals, possibly humans: impaired growth, skeletal abnormalities, impaired CNS function	Wheat bran, legumes, hazelnuts, blueberries, pineapple, seafood, poultry, meat	2.3 mg* male; 1.8 mg* female
Molybdenum	2 mg	Metabolism of purines, pyrimidines, pteridines, aldehydes; oxidation	Xanthine dehydrogenase/oxidase, aldehyde oxidase, sulfite oxidase	Hypermethioninemia, ↑ urinary xanthine, sulfite excretion, ↓ urinary sulfate and urate excretion	Legumes, meat, poultry, fish, grains	45 μg
Selenium	20 mg	Protection against hydrogen peroxide and free radicals, thyroid hormone production	Glutathione peroxidase, 5'-deiodinase, thioredoxin reductase, selenoprotein P, selenophosphate synthesis	Myalgia, cardiac myopathy, poor growth, abnormal sulfur metabolism	Oysters, tuna, meat, poultry, fish, whole grains, Brazil nuts	55 μg
Zinc	1.5–3.0 g	Nutrient metabolism, collagen formation, alcohol detoxification, carbon dioxide elimination, sexual maturation, cell replication and growth	DNA-RNA polymerase, carbonic anhydrase, alcohol dehydrogenase, carboxypeptidase, alkaline phosphatase, deoxythymidine kinase, superoxide dismutase	Poor wound healing, subnormal growth, anorexia, abnormal taste/smell; impaired reproductive system development	Oysters, wheat germ, beef, liver, poultry, whole grains	11 mg male; 8 mg female

* Indicates Adequate Intake values

ferrous ascorbate, ferrous carbonate, ferrous citrate, ferrous fumarate, ferrous gluconate, ferrous lactate, ferric ammonium citrate, ferric chloride, ferric citrate, ferric pyrophosphate, and ferric sulfate are approved and used for food fortification.

Oral supplements of ferrous iron are available in complexes with sulfate, succinate, citrate, lactate, tartrate, fumarate, and gluconate. These oral iron supplements provide nonheme iron and are used typically to treat iron deficiency. Amino acid-iron chelates, such as iron glycine, are also marketed; however, iron administered as a chelate has not been shown to be absorbed better than iron given as ferrous sulfate or ferrous ascorbate. Iron dextrans can be administered intravenously if oral supplements are not correcting the iron deficiency.

Digestion, Absorption, Transport, and Storage

Figure 13.3 provides an overview of iron digestion, absorption, and transport, as well as some of iron's fates in the enterocyte.

Heme Iron Digestion and Absorption

Heme iron must be hydrolyzed from the globin portion of hemoglobin and myoglobin before absorption. This digestion is accomplished by proteases in both the stomach and the small intestine and results in the release of heme from the globin. Heme, containing the iron bound to the porphyrin ring (also called a metalloporphyrin), remains soluble, especially in the presence of the degradation products (amino acids and peptides) of globin, and

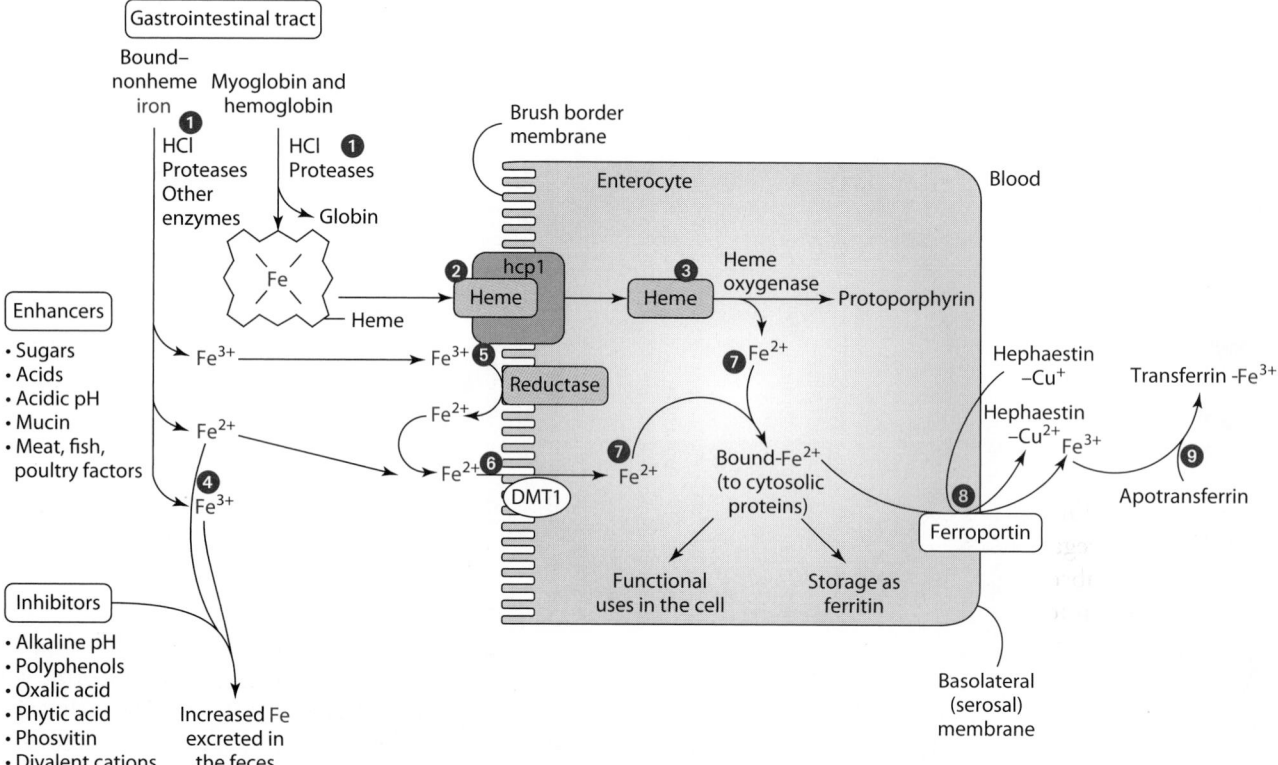

① Iron is released from bound food components. Some HCl in the stomach may reduce Fe^{3+} to Fe^{2+}.

② Free heme is absorbed intact by heme carrier protein (hcp) 1, located primarily in the proximal small intestine.

③ Within the enterocyte, heme is catabolized by heme oxygenase to protoporphyrin and Fe^{2+}.

④ Nonheme iron in the small intestine may react with one or more inhibitors, which promote the fecal excretion of iron.

⑤ Any of three reductases, cytochrome b reductase 1, cytochrome b (558) ferric cupric reductase, and six trans-membrane epithelial antigen of the prostate (steap) 2, may reduce Fe^{3+} to Fe^{2+}.

⑥ Divalent metal transporter (DMT) 1 carries Fe^{2+} across the brush border membrane into the cytosol of the enterocyte, although endocytosis of DMT1 as part of transcytosis may also enable iron absorption.

⑦ Fe^{2+} may bind to poly rC binding protein or a yet unidentified protein for transport in the cytosol; iron may also be used within the cell or stored as part of ferritin.

⑧ Ferroportin transports iron across the basolateral membrane. Iron transport is coupled with its oxidation to Fe^{3+} by hephaestin.

⑨ Fe^{3+} attaches to transferrin for transport in the blood.

Figure 13.3 Iron digestion, absorption, enterocyte use, and transport.

is readily absorbed intact across the brush border of the enterocyte by heme carrier protein 1 (hcp1). A proton-coupled folate transporter (PCFT) also has been identified as a heme carrier but is not thought to contribute substantially to heme absorption. Heme carrier protein 1 is found mainly in the proximal small intestine. While iron absorption occurs throughout the small intestine, it is most efficient in the proximal portion, particularly the duodenum. Within the enterocyte, the absorbed heme porphyrin ring is hydrolyzed by heme oxygenase into ferrous iron and protoporphyrin. This released iron is thought to associate with cytosolic proteins and can be used by the enterocyte, stored as ferritin, excreted with the sloughing of the enterocytes, or, following transport out of the enterocyte, used by other body tissues.

Nonheme Iron Digestion and Absorption

Nonheme iron, which is typically bound to components of foods, must be enzymatically freed (hydrolyzed) in the gastrointestinal tract to be absorbed. Gastric secretions, including hydrochloric acid and proteases in the stomach and small intestine, aid in the release of nonheme iron, mostly as Fe^{3+}, from some food components. The acidic environment of the stomach results in the reduction of some, but not all, ferric iron (Fe^{3+}) to the ferrous state (Fe^{2+}). Ferrous iron remains fairly soluble in both the acidic environment of the stomach and the more alkaline environment of the small intestine.

Once ferric iron passes from the stomach into the small intestine, it mixes with alkaline juices secreted into the intestine from the pancreas. In this more alkaline environment, some ferric iron may complex to produce ferric hydroxide ($Fe(OH)_3$), a relatively insoluble compound that tends to aggregate and precipitate, making the iron less available for absorption. Alternately, ferric iron may undergo reduction to a ferrous state by one or more reductases found primarily on the enterocyte's (duodenum's) brush border membrane, including cytochrome b reductase 1, cytochrome b (558) ferric cupric reductase, and six-transmembrane epithelial antigen of the prostate (steap) 2. Vitamin C may be needed for the activity of ferric cupric reductase, which also has the ability to reduce copper from the cupric (Cu^{2+}) to the cuprous state (Cu^{1+}) [1].

The main transporter for ferrous iron in the intestine is divalent cation (also called mineral) transporter 1 (abbreviated DCT or DMT); hereafter, the transporter is abbreviated DMT1. In the gastrointestinal tract, the DMT1 transporters are found primarily in the duodenum and transport not only iron but also, to a lesser extent, other minerals such as zinc, manganese, copper, nickel, and lead. Mineral transport using DMT1 may be coupled with H^+ transport (symport) into the enterocyte. DMT1 operates at acidic pH (about 5.5). Synthesis of DMT1 is affected by iron status, with increased transporter synthesis associated with the presence of low iron stores, and decreased expression of DMT1 associated with increased enterocyte iron concentrations.

The mechanism(s) by which ferric iron is absorbed is not clearly delineated and likely plays only a minor role in iron uptake for body use. A membrane protein called integrin may facilitate ferric iron absorption across the brush border membrane of the enterocyte. Integrin is thought to exist as part of the paraferritin complex, which includes an intracellular iron transport protein, mobilferrin, and a flavin-dependent ferrireductase.

Factors Influencing Iron Absorption

Several chelators/ligands may bind with nonheme iron to either inhibit or enhance its absorption. **Chelators** are small organic compounds that form a complex with a metal ion. Ligands are compounds that also bind or complex with minerals. Whether chelated iron or iron attached to a ligand is absorbed or not absorbed depends in part on the nature of the iron chelate ligand complex. If the iron chelate ligand complex maintains solubility and the iron is loosely bonded, the iron typically can be released at the enterocyte and absorption is enhanced. However, if the iron chelate ligand is strongly bonded and insoluble, iron is not absorbed; this iron is then excreted in the feces as part of the chelate ligand.

Enhancers of Nonheme Iron Absorption Some dietary factors that have been found to enhance nonheme iron absorption include:

- sugars, especially fructose and sorbitol
- acids, such as ascorbic, citric, lactic, and tartaric
- meat, poultry, and fish or their digestion products
- mucin

Sugars, such as fructose and sorbitol, are thought to form chelates or serve as ligands for iron. Ascorbic acid (vitamin C), along with citric, lactic, and tartaric acids, for example, acts as a reducing agent as well as forms a chelate with nonheme ferric iron at an acidic pH. Meat, poultry, and fish factors that enhance nonheme iron absorption have not been clearly identified, although digestion products from animal tissues high in the contractile proteins actin and myosin and the amino acids cysteine and histidine have been shown to promote iron absorption [2].

The amount of iron available for absorption can be estimated from the quantity of vitamin C and meat, fish, or poultry that is ingested with the nonheme iron source, assuming ~500 mg body iron stores. Seventy-five units of ascorbic acid or meat, fish, or poultry (MFP) factor (one unit = 1.3 g of raw or 1 g of cooked meat, fish, or poultry or 1 mg of ascorbic acid) has been shown to maximize iron absorption when consumed with the iron source [3].

Units in excess of 75 seem to have no further benefit. The absence of enhancing factors predicts a nonheme iron absorption of only 2% to 3%, but 75 units of these factors can increase absorption of nonheme iron to 8% (some suggest up to 20% if the person is also iron deficient) [4].

Mucin, an endogenously synthesized chelator, is a small protein made in both gastric and intestinal cells. Gastric mucin (sometimes called gastroferrin) is released into the lumen of the gastrointestinal tract, although some mucin is also found on the brush border membrane of intestinal cells. Mucin binds multiple ferric iron atoms (as well as possibly zinc and chromium) at an acid pH and maintains ferric iron solubility in the alkaline pH of the small intestine to enhance iron absorption. Histidine, ascorbic acid, and fructose, other chelators of iron, are thought to donate the iron to mucin in the small intestine. In addition to the aforementioned compounds, a more acidic environmental pH such as that found in the upper duodenum favors iron absorption.

Inhibitors of Nonheme Iron Absorption Many dietary factors inhibit iron absorption, including:

- polyphenols such as tannin derivatives of gallic acid, chlorogenic acids, monomeric flavinoids, and polyphenolic polymerization products (found in tea and coffee)

- oxalic acid (found in spinach, chard, berries, chocolate, and tea, among other sources)

- phytic acid, also referred to as phytate, inositol hexaphosphate, or polyphosphate (found in maize, whole grains, legumes)

- phosvitin, a protein containing phosphorylated serine residues (found in egg yolks)

- divalent cations such as calcium, zinc, and manganese

Polyphenols or polyphenolic compounds, when consumed with a source of nonheme iron, can reduce iron absorption by over 50%. Coffee consumption, with or just after a meal, may reduce iron absorption by 40%.

Phytic and oxalic acids complex with iron, as well as a few other minerals, including zinc and copper. The phytic acid–mineral and oxalic acid–mineral complexes are insoluble and poorly absorbed. Fermentation of bread dough reduces the phytic acid content and improves the absorption of some minerals, but, in general, mineral absorption is better without the presence of phytic or oxalic acids. (Figure 13.10, in the section on zinc, shows the structures of both phytic acid and oxalic acid.) Most individuals in the United States, however, do not consume enough phytic acid and oxalic acid to profoundly inhibit iron absorption.

Several other minerals can reduce the absorption of iron, especially nonheme iron. Calcium in amounts of 300 to 600 mg and in many forms (such as calcium phosphate, calcium citrate, calcium carbonate, and calcium chloride and in milk), when given with up to 18 mg of iron as ferrous sulfate or when incorporated into food, substantially decreases iron absorption. The inhibitory effect, however, appears to be of short duration, and adaptation results such that iron status is not negatively impacted [5]. Specifically, calcium is thought to transiently inhibit iron absorption by causing the iron transporter ferroportin to relocate temporarily from the enterocyte's basolateral membrane to the cytosol, although effects on DMT1 availability and changes in membrane fluidity also may play roles [5]. (See the next section for a discussion on the role of ferroportin.) In addition to calcium, zinc and manganese also interact with iron and may negatively affect each other's absorption by an undefined mechanism [6–8]. Inhibition of absorption (often by greater than 50%) of iron (usually as ferrous sulfate) has been demonstrated with the coingestion of zinc, usually as zinc sulfate, in solution, and in amounts greater than those of iron. However, lesser amounts of the nutrients in other forms also may reduce iron absorption [7].

Other intraluminal factors inhibitory to iron absorption include rapid transit time, malabsorption syndromes, achylia (absence of digestive juices), and excess alkalinization (i.e., increased pH) of the gastrointestinal tract. The alkalinization of the gastrointestinal tract is frequently associated with the use of medications (antacids, H_2 receptor blockers [such as Zantac (ranitidine), Tagamet (cimetidine), or Pepcid (famotidine)], and proton pump blockers [such as Prevacid (lansoprazole) or Prilosec (omeprazole)]) that are commonly taken to treat heartburn, gastroesophageal reflux disease (GERD), and ulcers. A more alkaline environment in the gastrointestinal tract may also occur with aging due to age-related reductions in gastric acid production.

Overall absorption of iron from the U.S. diet is estimated at about 10% to 18%, but a person's iron status also affects iron absorption. Absorption, for example, may range from about 10% (for persons with normal iron status) up to about 35% (for persons who are iron deficient). In other words, iron absorption can rise to 3 to 6 mg daily when the body has low iron stores and can fall to 0.5 mg or less daily when iron stores are high. Additional information on the regulation of iron absorption follows the section about intestinal cell iron use. A review of algorithms used to predict iron availability reports that the effects of iron status on iron absorption can be estimated based on selected biochemical indicators of iron status [9].

Intestinal Cell Iron Use

The preceding sections have reviewed digestion and absorption, including factors inhibiting and enhancing iron absorption into the enterocyte. Following absorption across the enterocyte's brush border membrane, iron enters the cytosol of the cell. Because of the potential for free iron to initiate oxidative damage, little iron is thought to exist unbound within the enterocyte (or any cell). However, at present, it is not clear what substance(s) iron attaches to within cells. Possible carriers include amino acids, such as cysteine and histidine, as well as protein(s). One identified protein, poly (rC) binding protein 1 (PCBP1), has been shown to bind up to three iron atoms with high affinity. Another possibility for iron transport within cells is transcytosis, whereby DMT1-bound ferrous iron is endocytosed into the cell and carried through the cytosol. Additionally, ferric iron has been reported to interact with a membrane receptor, integrin, and then bind to a cytosolic protein, mobilferrin. However, studies using DMT1 knock-out mice suggest that DMT1 mediates most iron absorption into enterocytes.

As depicted in Figure 13.3, once in the enterocyte, iron is either:

- used by the intestinal cell in a functional capacity, or
- stored in ferritin, or
- transported across the enterocyte's basolateral membrane to enter circulation for transport to body tissues

Iron is used functionally within enterocytes. These functions are presented in the "Functions and Mechanisms of Action" section.

Iron that is not needed for functional uses may be incorporated into (apo)ferritin in the intestinal cell for short-term storage. As iron is incorporated into ferritin, it is oxidized to its ferric state for deposition and storage. The stored ferric iron can be released from ferritin and reduced back to the ferrous state should the iron be needed by the enterocyte or other (nonintestinal) cells. If not needed, the iron remains attached as part of ferritin and is excreted when the short-lived (2–3 days) enterocytes are sloughed off into the lumen of the gastrointestinal tract. Ferritin synthesis in the intestine and other tissues is directly affected by cellular iron concentrations, with increased ferritin synthesis associated with increased iron absorption and decreased synthesis associated with low iron absorption. Ferritin is described in further detail in the section on storage. The mechanism by which iron affects the synthesis of ferritin is described in the "Regulation of Iron Absorption" section.

Iron transport across the enterocyte's basolateral membrane for entrance into the blood requires the iron to bind to the membrane transport protein ferroportin (fp or fpn). This transport of iron is also coupled with iron's oxidation to Fe^{3+} by a copper-containing protein called hephaestin (or, in the absence of hephaestin, by the copper-containing protein ceruloplasmin). Hephaestin is found on the enterocyte's basolateral membrane near ferroportin. This role of copper as part of hephaestin and ceruloplasmin in the oxidation of iron is crucial to iron metabolism. In fact, copper deficiency results in decreased ceruloplasmin and hephaestin, iron accumulation in the intestine and liver, and reduced iron transport to tissues. The copper-dependent oxidation of iron to the ferric state allows the transport of iron in the blood as part of the protein transferrin. Specifically, transferrin carries one or two ferric iron atoms (becoming monoferric transferrin or diferric transferrin, respectively) for delivery to body tissues.

Regulation of Iron Absorption

The main regulator of iron absorption is the protein hepcidin, which is released from the liver when body iron stores are adequate or high. The liver is thought to recognize the body's iron status, at least in part, by the binding of diferric transferrin to transferrin receptors 1 (TfR1) found on liver cells. This binding in turn releases a high-iron (HFe) protein from TfR1; this released HFe protein then binds to hepatic TfR2, another type of transferrin receptor. The HFe-TfR2 complex is thought to serve as a "sensor" of the body's iron status and in turn stimulates hepcidin synthesis through an intracellular signaling pathway. Several other proteins also influence hepcidin synthesis and may be involved in iron sensing, including β2-microglobulin, hemojuvelin (HJV), bone morphogenic protein 6 (BMP6), and transmembrane serine protease s6 (TMPRSS6; also called matripase 2), among others.

Hepcidin, upon release from the liver, travels in the blood, targeting ferroportin on the basolateral cell membranes of enterocytes and cell membranes of macrophages. Specifically, hepcidin binds ferroportin, resulting in internalization and degradation (via ubiquitin and lysosomes) of both the hepcidin and the ferroportin. With the hepcidin-induced loss of ferroportin from the cell membranes, iron cannot be transported out of the enterocyte or out of the macrophage and thus cannot get into the blood for use by other tissues. Consequently, increased hepcidin concentrations result in increased enterocyte and macrophage iron concentrations. In the case of the enterocyte, the availability of newly absorbed iron to the body is decreased.

With low iron status, little hepcidin is released from the liver, and ferroportin concentrations on enterocyte and macrophage cell membranes remain sufficient for iron export out of the cells. This situation enables iron to get into the blood for distribution and use by body tissues.

Defects in any of the genes coding for proteins known to modulate hepcidin synthesis impact iron status. For example, individuals with a genetic mutation in the matripase 2 gene have been found to overproduce hepcidin; the result is a condition known as iron-refractory iron-deficiency anemia. In contrast, an absence of hepcidin (e.g., due to a genetic defect) causes iron to continue to be absorbed into the body and can result in the accumulation of iron in the body (see the "Toxicity" section).

In addition to hepcidin's role in the regulation of iron absorption and thus iron status, a cell's iron content affects iron absorption. In cells, iron is incorporated into binding proteins (called iron regulatory/response element binding proteins [IRE-BP] or iron response proteins [IRP]), which affect the translation of mRNA for proteins involved in intestinal iron absorption, cellular iron uptake, and storage (Figure 13.4). With little available cellular iron, the IRE-BP exists as a 3Fe-4S cluster and functions as a binding protein. As a binding protein, the IRE-BP binds to iron response elements (IREs), which are stem loop structures of about 30 nucleotides located in specific 3' and 5' untranslated regions of mRNA. IREs are present in the mRNA for several proteins involved in iron utilization, such as transferrin receptors, ferritin, cytochrome b reductase, and DMT1. In the case of ferritin in low-iron situations, the IRE-BP binds to an IRE in the 5' untranslated region of ferritin mRNA and acts as a repressor to inhibit the translation of the ferritin protein. Thus, less ferritin is made in cells when the cellular iron content is low. From a physiological standpoint, this inhibition makes sense because ferritin stores iron, and not much ferritin would be needed if the cell's iron content were low. Under the opposite conditions, in which the cell has a relatively high iron content, the IRE-BP contains a 4Fe-4S cluster, exhibits aconitase (a TCA cycle enzyme) activity, and does not bind to the IRE on the ferritin mRNA. Consequently, the ferritin mRNA undergoes translation. Thus, more ferritin protein is made in cells when cellular iron concentrations are high.

Transport

Iron in its oxidized ferric state is transported in the blood attached to the protein transferrin. Transferrin's role in iron transport and the importance of protein in iron binding in the body are reviewed next.

Transferrin, a glycoprotein made primarily in the liver, has two binding sites for minerals, one near its carboxy (C)-terminal end and the other near its amino (N)-terminal end. Both binding sites have a high affinity for ferric iron, but the one near the amino (N)-terminal end also binds other minerals, such as chromium, followed in descending order by copper, manganese, cadmium, zinc, and nickel. The binding of ferric iron to transferrin requires the presence of an anion, usually bicarbonate, at each binding site. The plasma iron pool typically contains about 4 mg of iron bound to transferrin. Transferrin in the plasma is typically about one-third (33%) saturated with ferric iron. (Note: If all of transferrin's binding sites were occupied [e.g., as in a toxicity situation], then the transferrin would be fully [100%] saturated.)

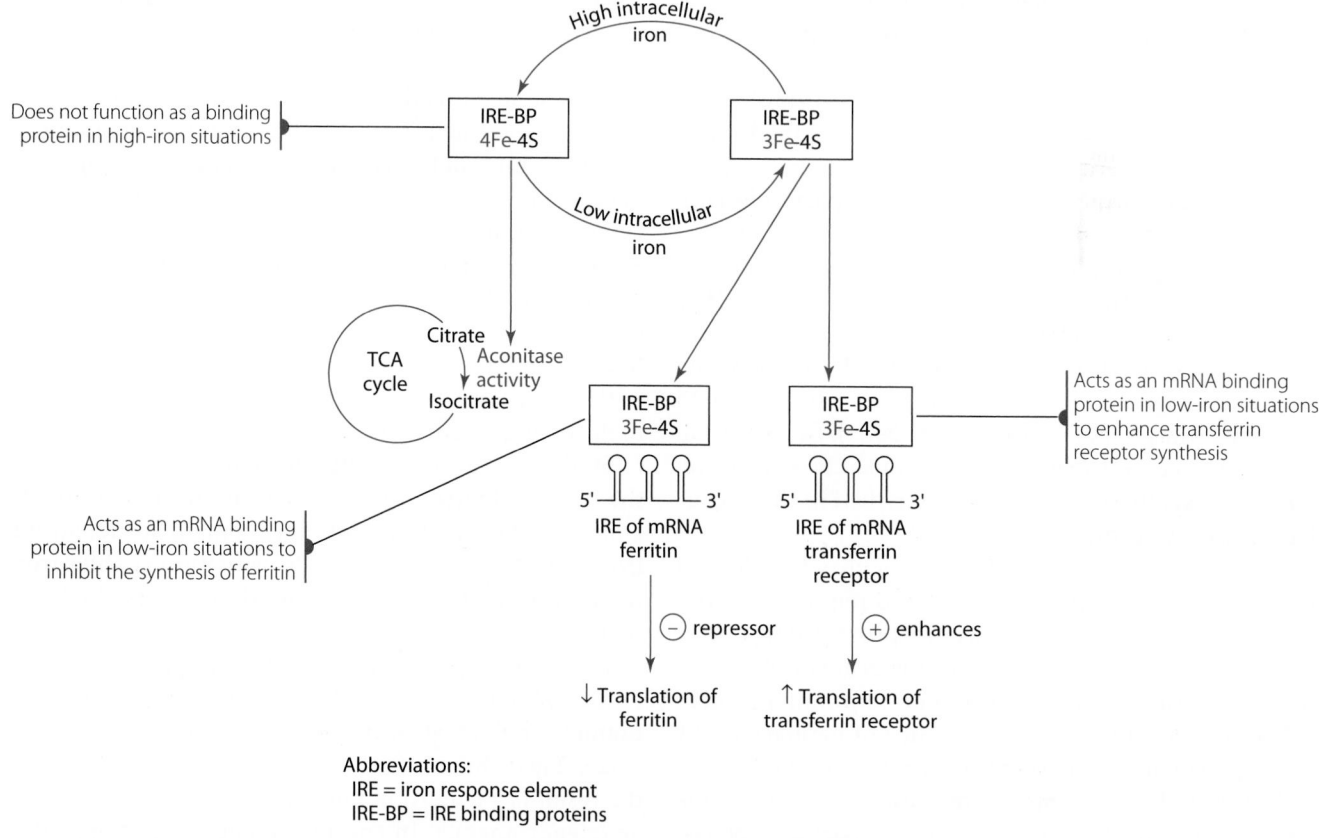

Figure 13.4 The influence of intracellular iron on the translation of ferritin mRNA and transferrin receptor mRNA.

The role of proteins in the transport as well as storage of iron is important because of iron's redox activity. The binding of iron by proteins serves as a protective mechanism. When iron is left unbound, its redox activity can lead to the generation of harmful free radicals. Free ferrous iron (Fe^{2+}), for example, readily reacts with hydrogen peroxide (H_2O_2) in what is known as the Fenton reaction: $Fe^{2+} + H_2O_2 \longrightarrow Fe^{3+} + OH^- + \cdot OH$. This reaction generates a hydroxyl anion and a free hydroxyl radical ($\cdot OH$), which is extremely reactive and damaging to cells. In addition, the binding of iron by protein is important to ensure that bacteria that may be present in the body, as with an infection, are unable to use the iron for their own (bacterial) growth. Free iron—but not protein-bound iron—is readily used by bacteria for proliferation and growth. Bacteria cannot multiply without nutrients, such as iron, acquired from the host. Thus, keeping iron attached to proteins in the body diminishes bacterial replication.

Transferrin binds and transports not only newly absorbed dietary iron that has crossed the basolateral membrane of the enterocyte, but also iron that has been released following the degradation of iron-containing compounds in the body. In fact, most of the iron entering the plasma for distribution by transferrin is contributed from hemoglobin destruction. Thus, transferrin ferries iron throughout the body, delivering both new and recycled iron to tissues. Transferrin has a half-life of about 7 to 10 days.

Cellular Iron Uptake The amount of iron taken up by the tissues depends in part upon transferrin's saturation level and the presence of transferrin receptors on cell membranes. For example, iron delivery is greater from diferric transferrin (transferrin containing two bound iron atoms) than from monoferric transferrin (transferrin containing only one bound iron atom). The mono- and diferric transferrin bind to transferrin receptors (TfRs) on cell membranes (Figure 13.5). Most cell membranes contain a form of transferrin receptors abbreviated TfR1; liver and intestinal cells, however, contain an isoform known as TfR2, which preferentially binds diferric transferrin. Transferrin receptors consist of two subunits that each bind one transferrin molecule.

Once the transferrin molecule with its bound iron attaches to the transferrin receptor, a complex is formed.

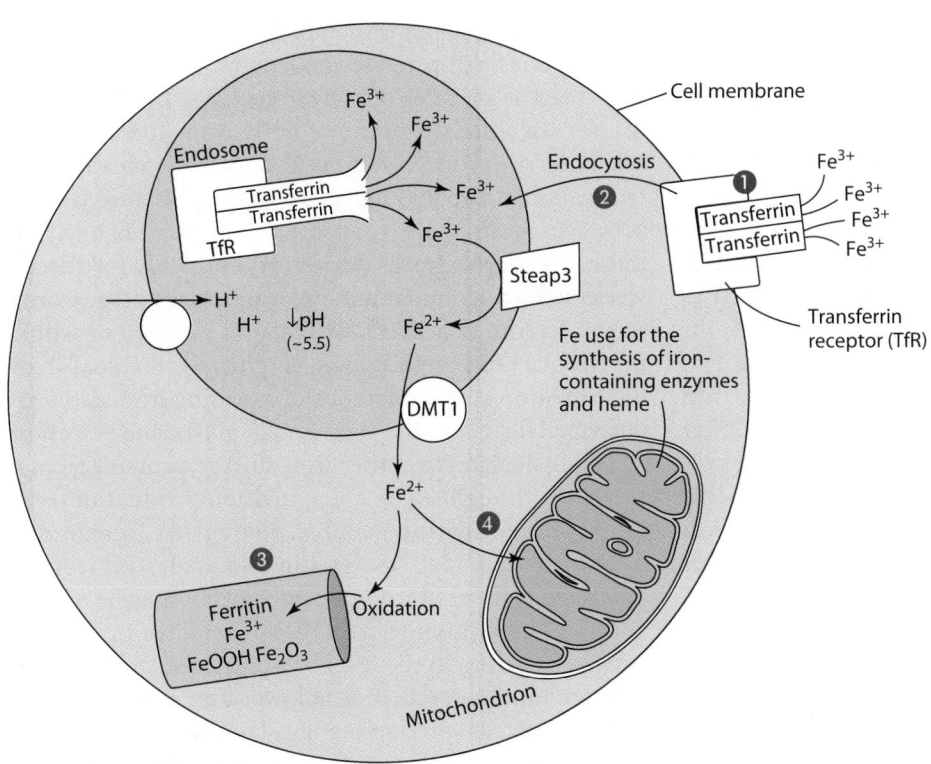

① Transferrin with its bound Fe^{3+} atoms attaches to transferrin receptors on the cell membranes. Following attachment, the complex is endocytosed into the cell cytosol where it forms an endosome.

② A drop in pH in the endosome helps initiate the release of Fe^{3+}, which is then reduced by steap3 and transported out of the endosome by a transporter such as DMT1.

③ Fe^{2+} released from the endosome may be oxidized and stored as part of ferritin.

④ Fe^{2+} may be used within the cell functionally.

Figure 13.5 Overview of iron uptake and storage.

The transferrin receptor–transferrin complex is next internalized by endocytosis and forms a vesicle (also called an endosome) within the cell's cytosol. Next, in an ATP-dependent process, protons are pumped into the endosome and reduce the pH from about 7.4 to about 5.5. In the presence of the acidic pH and possibly other factors, ferric iron atoms are released from the transferrin molecule. The apotransferrin is then thought to return to the cell surface and plasma. Use of the released ferric iron requires reduction and transport across the endosomal membrane. Reduction of ferric iron to a ferrous state is thought to be accomplished by the ferrireductase activity of steap3. DMT1 is thought to transport the ferrous iron out of the endosome. Iron released from the endosome is typically transported to other sites for use.

The number of transferrin receptors on cell membranes increases or decreases depending on intracellular iron concentrations. In other words, intracellular iron affects the genetic expression of transferrin receptors. The mRNA for the transferrin receptor contains IREs in the 3' untranslated region; remember: IREs are stem loop structures found in the mRNA. In a low–cellular-iron situation, IRE-BPs contain 3Fe-4S clusters and readily bind to the IRE and stabilize the transferrin receptor mRNA. This stabilized transferrin receptor mRNA exhibits a longer half-life, and consequently more transferrin receptors are synthesized (Figure 13.4). Once made, these transferrin receptors become embedded in the cell's plasma membrane to promote cellular iron uptake. Thus, in conditions of low cellular iron, transferrin receptor synthesis is increased. If the intracellular iron concentration is adequate or relatively high, fewer transferrin receptors are translated. In this situation, IRE-BPs exist as 4Fe-4S clusters and exhibit aconitase activity in the mitochondria, and thus do not act as binding proteins. Without the IRE-BPs bound to the IREs of transferrin receptor mRNA, the mRNA is not as stable and is more quickly degraded. This decreased stability and increased degradation in turn diminish translation of the mRNA and result in fewer transferrin receptor proteins being produced. The synthesis of fewer transferrin receptor proteins means that fewer receptors are available on the cell surface, and less iron is brought into the cell. Thus, transferrin receptor expression indicates the cell's need for iron uptake.

Storage

Iron not needed in a functional capacity is stored in three main sites: the liver, bone marrow, and spleen. Transferrin delivers iron to these sites, especially the liver, which is thought to store about 60% of the body's iron in both reticuloendothelial (RE) cells and hepatocytes. The remaining 40% is found in reticuloendothelial cells within the spleen and bone marrow (and possibly between muscle fibers). Most of the iron stored in reticuloendothelial cells is derived from phagocytosis of red blood cells and subsequent degradation of the hemoglobin within those cells.

Ferritin is the primary storage form of iron in cells; the role of iron in the control of ferritin synthesis was previously described in the "Regulation of Iron Absorption" section. The protein is initially synthesized as apoferritin, containing no iron atoms; it has a hollow spherelike shape and is composed of 24 protein subunits. Once iron enters apoferritin, the protein is referred to as ferritin. Ferritin's subunits are classified based upon molecular mass as H or L, and the proportions of H and L subunits within ferritin vary between tissues. The L form, for example, predominates in the liver and spleen and takes up iron rather slowly, compared with the H form, which is found in higher amounts in the heart and red blood cells. Iron enters apoferritin through channels or pores. The pores serve as the site of the oxidation of the ferrous iron and generate ferric oxyhydroxide crystals ($4Fe^{2+} + O_2 + 6H_2O \longrightarrow 4FeOOH + 8H^+$) and ferrihydrite ($5Fe_2O_3 + 9H_2O$); molecular oxygen functions as the electron acceptor. Ferric oxyhydroxide and ferrihydrite are deposited in the interior of the protein shell. As many as 4,500 iron atoms can be stored in ferritin; however, the protein more commonly stores about 800 to 1,500 atoms.

Ferritin is not a stable compound but rather is constantly being degraded and resynthesized, providing an available intracellular iron pool. Equilibration occurs between tissue ferritin and serum ferritin. Thus, serum ferritin is used as an index of body iron stores: 1 ng of ferritin/mL serum equals ~10 mg of body iron stores. Normal serum ferritin concentrations (for adults) typically range from about 18 to 250 ng/mL; however, because ferritin acts as an acute-phase (reactant) protein, it is not a reliable indicator of iron stores during, and possibly for several weeks following, inflammation or illness. In other words, serum ferritin concentrations may be elevated or within the normal range in the blood, despite an individual's having little iron stores. Methods of assessing iron status are described further in the "Assessment of Nurture" section.

Hemosiderin is another iron storage protein. Hemosiderin is thought to be a degradation product of ferritin, representing, for example, aggregated ferritin or a deposit of degraded apoferritin and coalesced iron atoms. The content of iron in hemosiderin may be as high as 50%. The ratio of ferritin to hemosiderin in the liver varies according to the level of iron stored in the organ, with ferritin predominating at lower iron concentrations, and hemosiderin predominating at higher concentrations (iron overload). Although iron in hemosiderin can be labilized to supply free iron, iron is released at a slower rate from hemosiderin than from ferritin.

The release of iron from ferritin stores requires mobilization and reduction of Fe^{3+}. Reductases and/or reducing substances such as riboflavin ($FMNH_2$), niacin (NADH), or vitamin C may play roles in the reduction of the iron.

While the superoxide radical ($O_2 \cdot$) has been found to initiate iron release from ferritin *in vitro*, only one or two iron atoms from ferritin are freed, even with extended exposure to superoxide radicals [10].

Following this reduction of iron to release it from storage, Fe^{2+} is transported to the cell's plasma membrane, where it must bind to ferroportin and be reoxidized. This reoxidation of iron requires ceruloplasmin and enables it to bind to transferrin for transport in the blood to other tissues.

$$Fe^{2+} \longrightarrow Fe^{3+}(\text{which can now bind to transferrin})$$
$$\text{Ceruloplasmin-Cu}^{2+} \quad \text{Ceruloplasmin-Cu}^{1+}$$

Functions and Mechanisms of Action

Iron functions in the body as part of several proteins, including the dozens of enzymes for which it serves as a cofactor. These iron-dependent proteins are involved in diverse body processes (Table 13.2), as described in this section. Moreover, the iron in the proteins is found in different forms. For example, in many body proteins, iron is present as part of heme, while in others, iron is found in a cluster with sulfur (2Fe-2S, 4Fe-4S, or 3Fe-4S), by itself as a single atom, or as part of a bridge with oxygen. Heme proteins represent the largest group and include hemoglobin, myoglobin, and cytochromes, as well as some enzymes. Iron-sulfur proteins also include several enzymes with diverse roles that participate in electron transport, the TCA cycle, and heme synthesis. Proteins that contain single iron atoms are mostly mono- and dioxygenase enzymes, and the one iron-oxygen bridge protein is found in the enzyme ribonucleotide reductase.

Heme: Hemoglobin and Myoglobin

The essentiality of iron is due in part to its presence in heme, which functions as a prosthetic group for some

Table 13.2 Selected Functions of Iron

Hemoglobin and myoglobin
Electron transport: ATP production
Amino acid metabolism: phenylalanine, tyrosine, tryptophan, arginine
Niacin synthesis
Carnitine synthesis
Procollagen synthesis
Nitric oxide synthesis
Antioxidant: protection
Destruction of bacteria, viruses, and microbes
Thyroid hormone synthesis
Sulfite oxidation
DNA purine base catabolism
Carbohydrate metabolism
DNA synthesis

proteins. The atom of iron in the center of the heme molecule enables oxygen transport to tissues (hemoglobin); transitional storage of oxygen in tissues, particularly muscle (myoglobin); and transport of electrons through the respiratory chain (cytochromes).

Hemoglobin is synthesized in red blood cells and carries about 98.5% of the total oxygen found in the blood. Hemoglobin, a conjugated tetrameric protein, consists of four heme groups and globin, which is made up of four polypeptide chains (see Figure 6.20). Each polypeptide chain is associated with one of the heme molecules. Heme is an iron-containing derivative of porphyrin. Porphyrins, in turn, are cyclic compounds made up of four pyrrole rings joined together by methenyl bridges. Nitrogen atoms in each of the four pyrrole rings bind to the iron atom, and these bonds hold the iron atom in the plane of the porphyrin ring. The iron atom in the center of the heme has two remaining coordinate bonds available for binding. One is with an amino acid (often the nitrogen atom of histidine) of the protein to which the heme is attached. For example, in hemoglobin, the iron in the heme binds to the nitrogen of an amino acid in the protein globin; heme is found in a hydrophobic pocket of the protein. The sixth and last coordinate bond in heme proteins that bind oxygen—namely, hemoglobin and myoglobin—is positioned between the iron and oxygen. The oxygen is held quite loosely so that transfer to tissues can be rapid. In heme proteins that do not bind oxygen, the sixth coordinate bond is with atoms of amino acid groups in the protein (such as an enzyme) with which the heme group is associated. Heme synthesis accounts for the largest use of functional iron in the body. In fact, each red blood cell is thought to contain millions of hemoglobin molecules, and all the red blood cells in the body together contain about two-thirds of total body iron. Any one red blood cell may carry up to a billion oxygen atoms.

To synthesize heme for hemoglobin, iron is needed in the erythropoietic cells in the bone marrow. These cells possess transferrin receptors on their plasma membranes; thus, transferrin delivers the iron for heme synthesis to the erythropoietic cells. Mitoferrin transports the iron, following its release from the endosome, into the mitochondrial matrix, and a chaperone, frataxin, is thought to further transport the iron to the site of heme synthesis. Alternately, degradation of old red blood cells within the bone marrow can directly provide the necessary iron for hemoglobin synthesis without the use of transferrin (see the "Turnover" section).

Briefly, the synthesis of heme (shown in Figure 13.6) occurs as follows:

• Glycine and succinyl-CoA combine to form Δ-aminolevulinic acid (ALA) in the cell's mitochondria. The reaction is catalyzed by Δ-aminolevulinic acid synthase, a vitamin B_6–dependent enzyme that is inhibited by

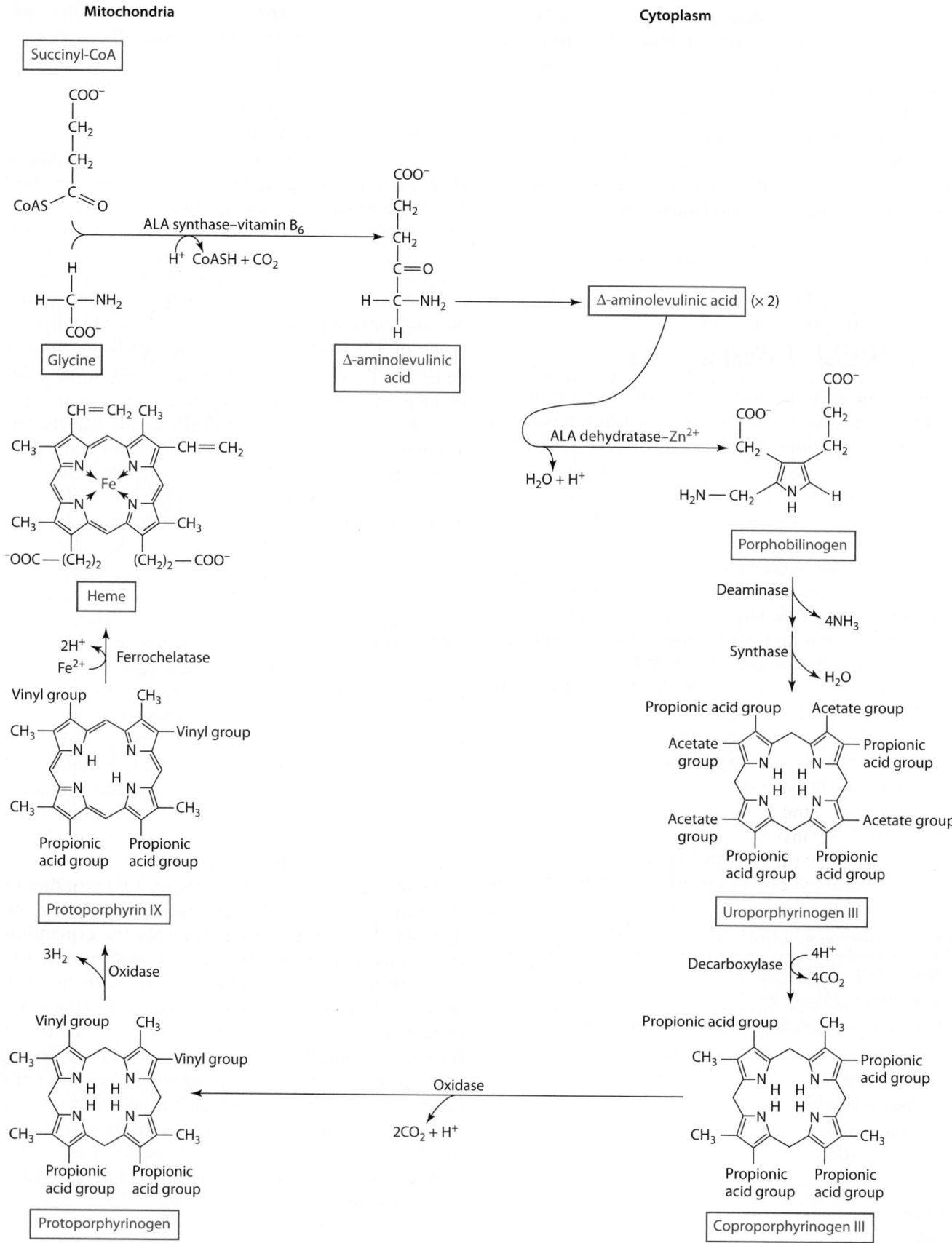

Figure 13.6 Heme biosynthesis. Vinyl group: $CH=CH_2$; propionic acid group: $(CH_2)_2COO^-$; acetate group: CH_2COO^-.

the final end product (heme) and whose synthesis is also thought to be regulated by iron.

- Next, ALA enters the cytosol, where a zinc-dependent dehydratase catalyzes the condensation of two ALA molecules to form porphobilinogen. This enzyme is sensitive to lead, which binds to its sulfhydryl groups to inactivate the enzyme.

- Next, in a series of cytosolic reactions involving a de-aminase, a synthase, and a decarboxylase, four porphobilinogens condense to form a tetrapyrrole that cyclizes. Side chains are modified, and coproporphyrinogen III is formed and enters the mitochondria.

- Coproporphyrinogen is converted in the mitochondria to protoporphyrinogen.

- Protoporphyrinogen is oxidized to form protoporphyrin IX.

- Last, an iron (Fe^{2+}) atom is inserted into protoporphyrin IX to yield heme. The insertion of iron into the heme is catalyzed by ferrochelatase, a 2Fe-2S cluster protein. The transcription of the ferrochelatase enzyme appears to be regulated by iron.

Unlike the tetrameric hemoglobin, myoglobin consists of a single hemoprotein chain. Myoglobin, which is found in the cytosol of the muscle cells, facilitates the diffusion rate of dioxygen from hemoglobin in capillary red blood cells to the cytosol and mitochondria of muscle cells.

Cytochromes and Other Enzymes Involved in Electron Transport: Energy Production

Heme-containing cytochromes in the electron transport chain, such as cytochromes b and c, pass along single electrons. The transfer of electrons along the chain is made possible by the change in the oxidation state of iron. In the reduced cytochromes, the iron atom is in the ferrous state. The iron atom of the reduced cytochrome becomes oxidized to the ferric state when a single electron is transferred to the next cytochrome. The iron atom of the cytochrome receiving the electron then becomes reduced. Nonheme iron–sulfur enzymes involved in electron transport include NADH dehydrogenase, succinate dehydrogenase, and ubiquinone–cytochrome c reductase. See Chapter 3 for a more thorough discussion of electron transport. Whether iron is carrying oxygen or transporting electrons, its essentiality in energy transformation is without question.

Monooxygenases and Dioxygenases: Amino Acid Metabolism, Carnitine Synthesis, and Procollagen Synthesis

Many additional enzymes involved in a variety of processes besides energy production also require iron. Some monooxygenases, which insert one of two oxygen atoms into a substrate, require a single iron atom to function; examples (all needed for amino acid metabolism) include:

- phenylalanine monooxygenase
- tyrosine monooxygenase
- tryptophan monooxygenase

Specifically, these enzymes insert an oxygen atom into the aromatic amino acids phenylalanine, tyrosine, and tryptophan, respectively and use cosubstrates to furnish the hydrogen atoms that reduce the second oxygen atom to water. Tetrahydrobiopterin is frequently used as a co-substrate in reactions involving amino acids, and during the reactions tetrahydrobiopterin is oxidized to dihydro-biopterin. The reactions catalyzed by these three enzymes are shown in Figures 6.10 and 6.11, and are important for amino acid metabolism. In other words, the use of these three amino acids for functions other than protein synthesis (including catecholamine, serotonin, and melatonin synthesis) depends on iron-dependent enzymes.

Many dioxygenases, which catalyze the insertion of two oxygen atoms into a substrate, also need iron. These include:

- tryptophan dioxygenase (needed for amino acid metabolism)
- homogentisate dioxygenase (needed for amino acid metabolism)
- trimethyllysine dioxygenase and 4-butyrobetaine dioxygenase (needed for carnitine synthesis)
- lysine dioxygenase and proline dioxygenase (needed for procollagen synthesis)
- nitric oxide synthase (needed for amino acid metabolism)

Heme-containing tryptophan dioxygenase (also called a pyrrolase) converts the amino acid tryptophan to N-formylkynurenine (Figure 6.11), representing the first step of tryptophan catabolism for the generation of energy and the B vitamin niacin. Iron deficiency has been shown to reduce the efficacy of tryptophan as a precursor of niacin [11].

Homogentisate dioxygenase is also involved in amino acid metabolism, specifically that of tyrosine. During tyrosine catabolism to generate energy, tyrosine is transaminated to produce hydroxyphenylpyruvate, which is then converted to homogentisate (homogentisic acid). Homogentisate in turn is converted to (4-)maleylacetoacetate by homogentisate dioxygenase, a single atom iron-dependent enzyme (Figure 6.10). Defects in this enzyme result in the genetic disorder alkaptonuria, which is characterized by high concentrations of homogentisic acid in the urine. When this urine is excreted and the homogentisic acid is exposed to air, the compound turns a very dark color, causing the urine to appear almost black. In those with alkaptonuria, the homogentisic acid also accumulates in joints, causing arthritis.

Two of the four steps required for carnitine synthesis involve iron-dependent dioxygenases. Recall that carnitine is an important nitrogen-containing compound necessary for the transport of long-chain fatty acids into the mitochondria for oxidation. The first step in carnitine synthesis (Figure 6.23), in which trimethyl lysine is converted to 3-OH trimethyl lysine, requires a single iron-containing trimethyl lysine dioxygenase, and the final step, in which 4-butyrobetaine is converted to carnitine, requires 4-butyrobetaine dioxygenase, another single iron–containing enzyme.

Hydroxylation reactions for procollagen synthesis are shown in Figure 9.4. Both lysine and proline dioxygenases contain single iron atoms. These reactions are important for the synthesis of the protein collagen, a component of bone, cartilage, skin, and blood vessels, among other body structures.

Two isoforms of nitric oxide synthase, a dioxygenase needed for the synthesis of nitric oxide from the amino acid arginine, contain heme iron. Nitric oxide is a potent biological effector molecule that is involved in a variety of physiological processes including regulation of blood pressure (relaxation of vascular smooth muscle) and intestinal motility, inhibition of platelet aggregation, and macrophage function, to name a few.

Peroxidases: Antioxidant Roles and Thyroid Hormone Synthesis

Other important reactions required to protect the body also involve iron-containing enzymes.

• Catalase, with four heme groups, converts hydrogen peroxide to water and molecular oxygen: $2H_2O_2 \longrightarrow 2H_2O + O_2$. Catalase is one of the major antioxidant enzymes of the body and thus helps prevent cellular damage that can be induced by hydrogen peroxide (see the Perspective in Chapter 10).

• Myeloperoxidase (also called chloroperoxidase), another heme-containing enzyme, is found in the plasma as well as in neutrophils (white blood cells). During phagocytosis, myeloperoxidase is released into the phagocytic vesicle within the neutrophil. The phagocytic vesicle contains a variety of destructive compounds, including hydrogen peroxide (H_2O_2), free hydroxyl radicals (•OH), and other ions such as chloride (Cl⁻). Myeloperoxidase catalyzes the following reaction: $H_2O_2 + Cl^- \longrightarrow H_2O + OCl^-$. The OCl⁻ (hypochlorite) formed in the reaction is a strong cytotoxic oxidant responsible for the destruction of foreign substances, such as bacteria. The activity of myeloperoxidase may be impaired with iron deficiency, resulting in increased susceptibility to or severity of infection.

Peroxidases also are important in producing the thyroid hormones, T_3 and T_4.

• Thyroperoxidase (also called thyroid peroxidase), a heme-dependent enzyme, is necessary for organification of iodide (a process in which two iodides are added to tyrosine residues on thyroglobulin). This same enzyme also conjugates the thyroglobulins to form the thyroid hormones (see the "Functions and Mechanisms of Action" section in the "Iodine" portion of this chapter). Iron deficiency, in fact, is associated with decreased thyroperoxidase activity resulting in decreased T_3 and T_4 synthesis [12]. See Figure 13.18.

Oxidoreductases

Some oxidoreductases that are iron (and also molybdenum) dependent include:

• aldehyde oxidase, which converts aldehydes (RCOH) to alcohols (RCOOH)

• sulfite oxidase, an iron- and sulfur-containing enzyme, converts sulfite (SO_3) to sulfate (SO_4)

• xanthine oxidase and dehydrogenase, iron-sulfur cluster enzymes, metabolize hypoxanthine generated from DNA purine base catabolism to uric acid

These reactions are discussed in detail in the "Functions and Mechanisms of Action" section for molybdenum.

Other Iron-Containing Enzymes: Carbohydrate Metabolism, DNA Synthesis, and Lipid, Steroid, and Drug Metabolism

Two enzymes involved in carbohydrate oxidation require iron as a cofactor. In glycolysis, the flavoenzyme glycerol phosphate dehydrogenase has a nonheme iron component. In addition, phosphoenolpyruvate (PEP) carboxykinase, important in gluconeogenesis, also requires iron for its functioning.

Another iron-dependent enzyme involved in DNA synthesis, and thus cell replication, is ribonucleotide reductase, which converts adenosine diphosphate (ADP) into deoxy ADP. This enzyme contains nonheme iron as part of a bridge with oxygen ($Fe^{3+} - O_2 - Fe^{3+}$).

A few additional heme iron-containing cytochromes include cytochrome b5 involved in lipid metabolism, and the cytochrome P450 family involved in drug metabolism and steroid hormone synthesis.

Iron as a Pro-oxidant

As a pro-oxidant, free ferrous iron may catalyze the nonenzymatic Fenton reaction: $Fe^{2+} + H_2O_2 \longrightarrow Fe^{3+} + OH^- + •OH$. In this reaction, ferrous iron reacts with hydrogen peroxide to generate ferric iron and the free hydroxyl radical (•OH). In a reaction known as the Haber-Weiss reaction, the superoxide radical, $O_2^{•-}$, reacts with hydrogen peroxide to generate molecular oxygen and free hydroxyl radicals (•OH): $O_2^{\bullet} + H_2O_2 \longrightarrow O_2 + {}^{\bullet}OH + OH^-$. Hydroxyl radicals ($OH^-$) are dangerous membrane oxidants.

Turnover

Although dietary iron is important in maintaining the long-term adequacy of body iron for its various roles, the amount of iron absorbed (about 0.06% of the total body iron content) cannot meet the daily iron needs of the body. Rather, avid conservation and constant recycling (turnover) of body iron ensure an adequate supply.

Most of the iron entering the plasma for distribution or redistribution by transferrin results from hemoglobin, ferritin, and hemosiderin degradation (Figure 13.7). Hemoglobin is degraded primarily by phagocytes of the reticuloendothelial system (found in the liver, spleen, and bone marrow). Ferritin and hemosiderin are also degraded primarily in the liver, spleen, and bone marrow. Ferritin degradation is covered in the section on iron storage. Briefly, hemoglobin degradation occurs in this way. Most old (senescent) red blood cells, which live for about 120 days, are taken up and degraded (phagocytosed) by macrophages and reticuloendothelial cells in the spleen; however, reticuloendothelial cells and macrophages in bone marrow and Kupffer cells (macrophages) in the liver also may degrade the red blood cells. During red blood cell degradation, the heme portion of the hemoglobin molecule in the red blood cell is catabolized by heme oxygenase to release iron and protoporphyrin.

Protoporphyrin is subsequently degraded to biliverdin, which is then converted into bilirubin; the bilirubin is secreted into the bile for excretion from the body. With this heme degradation, reticuloendothelial cells and macrophages release about 20 to 25 mg of iron per day for reuse. Ferroportin, the same protein responsible for iron efflux from intestinal cells, enables the transport of iron out of the macrophages and reticuloendothelial cells. Specifically, ferroportin facilitates the transport of iron into vesicles, from which it is subsequently secreted into the blood. Oxidation of the iron by ceruloplasmin is also required as the iron is transported out of the cell by ferroportin; as stated previously, this oxidation of iron enables iron transport in the blood by transferrin.

The release of iron from the reticuloendothelial cells and macrophages is facilitated by low hepcidin concentrations. Iron released from these cells may be reused, for example, for erythropoiesis, or for incorporation into iron-dependent enzymes, or the iron may be deposited for storage. In situations with increased hepcidin (as would occur with increased body iron), ferroportin is degraded, and iron is retained within the macrophages and reticuloendothelial cells. Hepcidin concentrations are also elevated, however, with inflammatory conditions and infections, because many cytokines, released by macrophages and other white blood cells, induce hepcidin synthesis.

Although most red blood cells are degraded in the reticuloendothelial system, some (up to ~10%) red blood cell lysis occurs within the blood. Two proteins synthesized in the liver, haptoglobin and hemopexin, remove the released hemoglobin and any free heme, respectively, from the blood. Haptoglobin forms complexes with

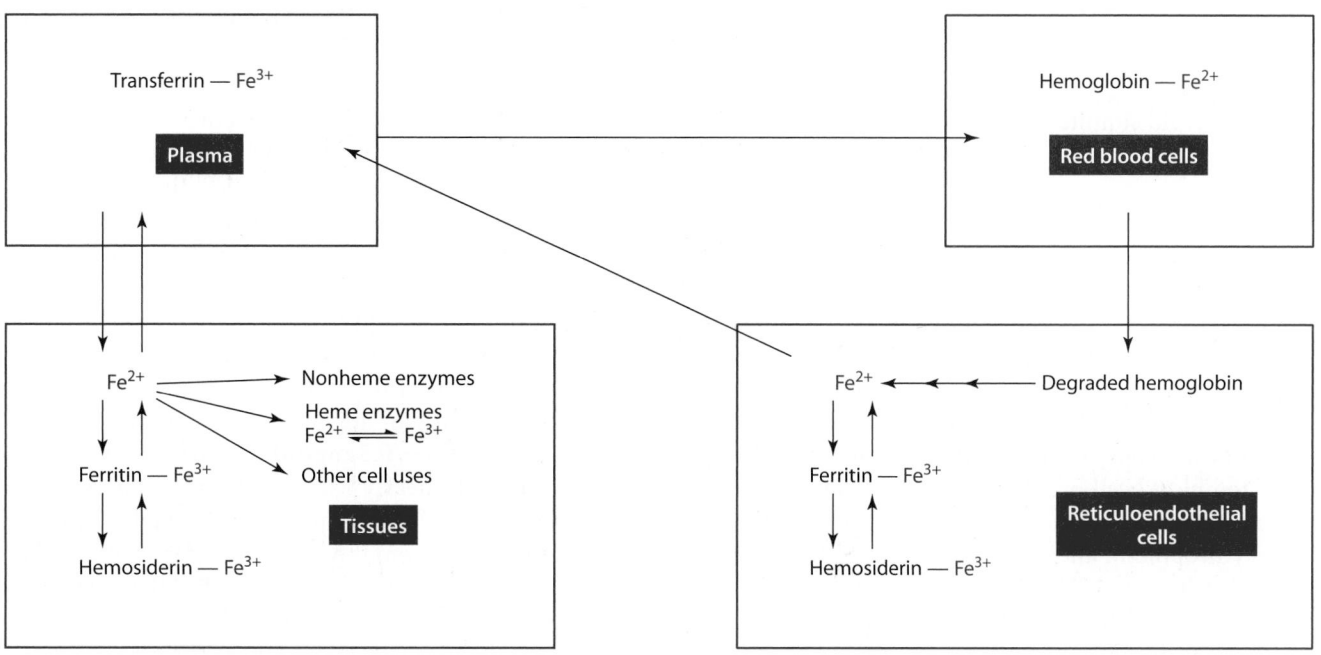

Figure 13.7 Internal iron exchange.

free hemoglobin, and hemopexin forms a complex with free heme in the blood. The proteins then deliver the iron-containing compounds to the liver, where further degradation occurs to enable reuse of the iron. With significant hemolysis, the quantity of iron passing through the plasma can expand to six to eight times the normal amount. In contrast, should erythropoiesis decline dramatically, as occurs on descent from high altitudes, the quantity of iron in the plasma pool may decrease to as little as one-third of normal. Figure 13.7 represents schematically the internal iron exchange in the body.

Interactions with Other Nutrients

You have read that iron and ascorbic acid interact, enhancing iron absorption and maintaining iron in the appropriate valence state for enzyme function. The potential also may exist for vitamin C–induced release of ferric iron from ferritin, with subsequent reduction of iron to the ferrous form [13]. Whether such reactions result in Fenton reactions and occur *in vivo* is unclear.

An interaction also occurs between iron and copper whereby a copper deficiency causes iron-deficiency anemia. In the 1920s, studies revealed that iron supplements were unable to cure anemia in rats; however, ashed foodstuffs containing copper replenished blood hemoglobin concentrations [14]. Specifically, the copper was needed for the ferroxidase activity of hephaestin and ceruloplasmin, which in turn enabled iron to be mobilized and used for hemoglobin synthesis.

Another interaction involves iron and zinc. Just as zinc inhibits iron absorption (see the "Inhibitors of Iron Absorption" section), iron inhibits zinc absorption. The inhibition occurs primarily if the two minerals are ingested together in the absence of food and if iron is present as nonheme iron in a ratio with zinc of 2 (or higher):1 [15–18]. Consequently, care should be taken to avoid simultaneous coingestion of these minerals in supplement forms if trying to treat an iron or zinc deficiency.

Vitamin A and iron also interact. Reduced vitamin A status causes iron accumulation in organs such as the spleen and liver. Inadequate vitamin A status also is associated with altered red blood cell morphology and decreased plasma iron and blood hemoglobin and hematocrit. The interaction between the nutrients appears to be mediated at least in part through erythropoietin, a hormone made in the kidneys that stimulates erythropoiesis (red blood cell production). Specifically, vitamin A as retinoic acid binds to a response element on the gene for erythropoietin and stimulates transcription of erythropoietin. Thus, with insufficient vitamin A, the erythropoietin gene is not transcribed adequately, red blood cell synthesis is diminished, and iron remains in stores. Supplementation of vitamin A in people with poor vitamin A and iron status increases erythropoietin synthesis and increases iron release from stores to provide the iron that is needed for erythropoiesis [19]. Another possible means by which vitamin A may influence iron is through interactions between retinoic acid and the transferrin receptor gene.

Iron and lead also interact. Lead inhibits the activity of Δ-aminolevulinic acid dehydratase, which is required for heme synthesis. Lead also inhibits the activity of ferrochelatase, the enzyme that incorporates iron into heme. Thus, lead poisoning is associated with iron-deficiency anemia secondary to decreased hemoglobin production. In addition, increased absorption of lead occurs with iron deficiency and could be problematic for children, who are often iron deficient and may have increased exposure to lead. The mechanism by which lead absorption is enhanced in situations of iron deficiency is unknown, but it may involve increased lead uptake through the enterocyte transporter DMT1.

Excretion

Total daily iron losses for an adult male are ~0.9 to 1.2 mg/day. Iron losses for women (postmenopausal) are a bit lower, ~0.7 to 0.9 mg/day because of women's smaller surface area [20]. Losses of iron occur from three main sites:

- the gastrointestinal tract
- the skin
- the kidneys

Of these sites, most (0.6 mg) iron losses occur through the gastrointestinal tract. Of this 0.6 mg, about 0.45 mg is lost through minute (~1 mL) blood loss (which occurs even in healthy people), and another 0.15 mg through losses in bile and desquamated mucosal cells. The skin losses of ~0.2 to 0.3 mg of iron occur with desquamation of surface cells from the skin. Finally, a very small amount, about 0.08 mg, is lost in the urine via the kidneys. Losses of iron, however, may be greater in people with gastrointestinal ulcers or intestinal parasites, or with hemorrhage induced by surgery or injury.

Total iron losses in premenopausal women are estimated to be ~1.3 to 1.4 mg/day because of iron loss in menses. The average loss of blood during a menstrual cycle is ~35 mL, with an upper limit of ~80 mL. The iron content of blood is ~0.5 mg/mL of blood, which translates into a loss of nearly 17.5 mg of iron per period. Averaged out over a month, iron loss attributable to menses is ~0.5 mg/day; in some women, however, iron loss during menses alone may exceed 1.4 mg/day. Balancing iron losses from the body with iron absorption is important to health. Iron deficiency remains one of the most common nutritional deficiencies worldwide.

Recommended Dietary Allowance

For adult men, the requirement and Recommended Dietary Allowance (RDA) for iron are 6 mg/day and 8 mg/day, respectively. For postmenopausal women, the requirement and RDA for iron are 5 mg/day and 8 mg/day, respectively [20]. Because of the greater losses associated with menses, premenopausal women require 8.1 mg iron/day; the recommended intake is 18 mg/day [20]. During pregnancy, though no menstrual losses occur, iron is needed for the fetus, for expanding blood volume, and for tissue and storage such that the RDA for iron is 27 mg/day. The RDA for iron is 9 mg/day during lactation [20]. The inside front cover of the book provides additional RDAs for iron for other age groups.

Deficiency

Iron deficiency occurs most often due to inadequate iron intake. Iron intake is frequently inadequate in four population groups:

- infants and young children (6 months to about 4 years) because of the low iron content of milk and other preferred foods, rapid growth rate, and insufficient body reserves of iron to meet needs beyond about 6 months

- adolescents in their early growth spurt because of rapid growth and the needs of expanding red blood cell mass

- females during childbearing years because of menstrual iron losses

- pregnant women because of their expanding blood volume, the demands of the fetus and placenta, and blood losses that are incurred in childbirth

In addition, many nonpregnant females in their childbearing years fall short of the RDA for iron because of restricted energy (caloric) intake and inadequate consumption of iron-rich foods. Further, individuals with renal disease develop iron deficiency because of an impaired ability to synthesize red blood cells due to reductions in erythropoietin synthesis by the diseased kidney.

The need for iron also may be increased secondary to greater iron losses or impaired iron absorption. Conditions associated with increased iron losses include hemorrhage, renal replacement therapy (also called dialysis), decreased (faster than normal) gastrointestinal transit time associated with diarrhea, and infection with parasites. Impaired iron absorption may occur with parasites, protein-energy malnutrition, renal disease, achlorhydria (the absence of hydrochloric acid in gastric juice), and prolonged use of medications such as antacids and proton pump inhibitors used in the treatment of heartburn, gastroesophageal reflux disease, and ulcers. Individuals that rely on a plant-based diet, in which the iron is typically less bioavailable, also are more likely to develop iron deficiency.

Figure 13.8 depicts the gradual depletion of the body's iron content. Iron deficiency is associated with suboptimal health, and, if not treated, usually progresses to iron-deficiency anemia. Iron-deficiency anemia is diagnosed typically when blood hemoglobin concentrations (and hematocrit) drop to less than the lower limit of normal (see the "Assessment of Nutriture" section); however, these two changes typically do not occur until the iron content of the body is quite low.

Iron-deficiency anemia impairs the oxygen carrying capacity of the blood. Signs and symptoms of iron deficiency, mostly demonstrated in children, include pallor, listlessness, behavioral disturbances, impaired performance in some cognitive tasks, some irreversible impairment of learning ability, and short attention span. In adults, work performance and productivity are most commonly impaired with iron deficiency. Further details about iron deficiency with and without anemia as it relates to changes that occur in indices of iron status are covered in the "Assessment of Nutriture" section.

The treatment of iron deficiency usually requires supplements. The initial effects of oral iron supplements, given in amounts up to about 120 mg/day, on improvements in red blood cell counts and hemoglobin concentrations take about 2 weeks. The use of iron supplements is frequently associated with constipation, dark stools, nausea, and/or stomach pain. Iron therapy to increase body stores of iron may be needed for 3 months to 1 year. Parenteral (intravenous) iron therapy also is available as iron dextran, sodium ferric gluconate, and iron sucrose should oral supplements not adequately improve iron status.

Toxicity

The Tolerable Upper Intake Level for iron for adults is 45 mg. Acute iron toxicity is mostly observed with accidental iron overload, as may occur with the ingestion of excessive numbers of iron pills or iron-containing vitamin/mineral pills. With acute toxicity, the excessive presence of an overload of iron atoms is thought to exceed the transport carrying capacity of transferrin. The unbound iron in turn behaves in a free radical manor to damage both the gastrointestinal tract and other tissues.

Chronic iron toxicity is generally associated with the genetic disorder hemochromatosis, which is most often seen in Caucasian males and becomes evident around 20 years of age. An estimated 50 per 10,000 people in the United States are homozygous for the disorder. Hemochromatosis is characterized by increased (at least two times normal) iron absorption. Mutations in one of several genes that result in diminished hepcidin synthesis cause the condition and result in the inability of the body to accurately sense iron stores and down-regulate

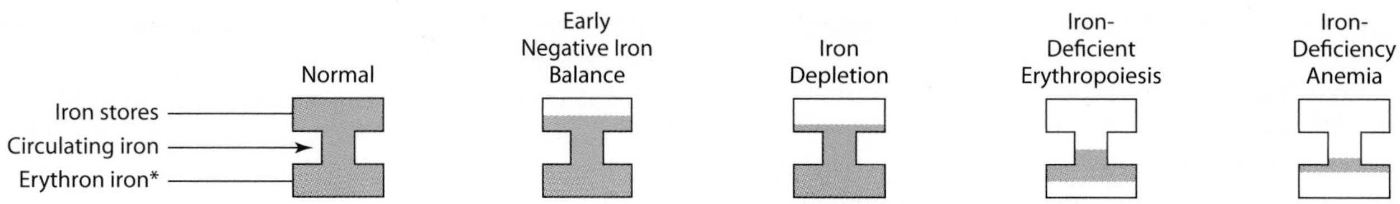

	Normal	Early Negative Iron Balance	Iron Depletion	Iron-Deficient Erythropoiesis	Iron-Deficiency Anemia
Iron stores → Circulating iron → Erythron iron* →					
Reticuloendothelial marrow iron	2–3$^+$	1$^+$	0–1$^+$	0	0
Transferrin iron-binding capacity (µg/dL)	330±30	330–360	360	390	410
Plasma ferritin (µg/L)	100±60	<25	20	10	<10
Iron absorption (%)	5–10	10–15	10–15	10–20	10–20
Plasma iron (µg/dL)	115±50	<120	115	<60	<40
Transferrin saturation (%)	35±15	30	30	<15	<15
Sideroblasts (%)	40–60	40–60	40–60	<10	<10
Erythrocyte protoporphyrin (µg/dL)	30	30	30	100	200
Erythrocytes	Normal	Normal	Normal	Normal	Microcytic Hypochromic
Serum transferrin receptors	Normal	Normal–high	High	Very high	Very high
Ferritin iron	Normal	Normal–low	Low	Very low	Very low

* Iron within circulating erythrocytes and their precursors.

Figure 13.8 Sequential changes in iron status associated with iron depletion.

Source: Adapted from Victor Herbert, 'Recommended dietary intakes (RDI) of iron in humans', American Journal of Clinical Nutrition, 1987; 45:679–686. Copyright © American Society for Clinical Nutrition. Reprinted by permission.

intestinal iron absorption. For example, in the C282Y mutation in the HFE protein, tyrosine is substituted for cysteine because of a single base change; this alteration inhibits HFE's ability to stimulate the synthesis of hepcidin, which tells the intestinal cells to down-regulate iron absorption. Similarly, the H63D mutation also reduces hepcidin synthesis, whereas a mutation (Q248H) in ferroportin promotes hemochromatosis due to continued ferroportin expression.

Although several mutations can cause hemochromatosis, in most people with the condition, iron absorption generally continues despite high iron stores. The absorbed iron is progressively deposited throughout the body, including within joints and tissues, especially the liver, heart, and pancreas, causing extensive organ damage and ultimately organ failure. Iron deposition in the liver, for example, leads to cirrhosis, usually by about 50 years of age. Heterozygotes for the condition do not develop severe organ dysfunction but exhibit abnormal iron status. For example, if untreated, serum ferritin concentrations continue to rise in the blood and may exceed 1,000 µg/L (normal: <250 µg/L). Treatment of hemochromatosis requires frequent phlebotomy (removal of blood), usually the weekly removal of about 1 unit (~400–500 mL) of blood, which contains about 200 to 250 mg of iron.

In addition, deferoxamine may be given. Deferoxamine works by chelating (binding to) iron in the body and increasing urinary iron excretion. Treatment of hemochromatosis usually continues as described until serum ferritin concentrations are less than about 20 to 50 µg/L, and transferrin saturation is less than about 30% [21]. Once these levels are achieved, the frequency with which the person undergoes phlebotomy can be diminished.

Other people at particularly high risk for iron overload are those with iron-loading anemias, thalassemia, and sideroblastic anemia. The elevated erythropoiesis in the bone marrow in people so affected causes increased iron absorption.

Iron toxicity has been linked with an increased risk of hepatic cancer. On the other hand, although studies once linked high body iron (serum ferritin >200 µg/L) to a higher risk of heart attack and heart disease, a larger and more recent group of studies has shown no such association.

Assessment of Nurture

Numerous measurements are used to assess iron nurture. The most common indices are hemoglobin (amount of iron-containing protein found in red blood cells per unit, usually deciliter or liter, of blood) and hematocrit (that proportion of the total blood volume that is red blood cells). However, although these indices indicate the presence of anemia, they are among the last to change as iron deficiency develops.

In the first stages of iron deficiency, iron stores in the liver, spleen, and bone marrow are diminished. Although iron stores can be aspirated and measured from bone marrow, the routine test involves measurement of plasma (or serum) ferritin. Decreases in plasma ferritin concentration are thought to parallel the decrease in the amount of iron found in stores. Plasma ferritin concentrations less than about 12 ng/mL are associated with iron deficiency. However, if inflammation or infection is present, the plasma ferritin concentration rises, an occurrence unrelated to iron stores. Thus, plasma ferritin may appear within normal range or high while the body's iron status is quite low; measurement of the levels of C-reactive protein or alpha1 acid glycoprotein in the blood can be used to detect the presence of inflammation or infection. Once iron stores are depleted, the plasma ferritin concentration no longer reflects the tissue iron pool.

As iron deficiency progresses into the second stage, iron stores typically remain low, and transport iron decreases. Thus, plasma ferritin concentrations continue to be diminished, and circulating iron begins to decrease. Iron circulates in the blood bound to transferrin. With deficiency, transferrin saturation decreases to less than 16% (from its normal saturation of about 33%). Transferrin saturation can be calculated by multiplying the serum iron concentration by 100 and then dividing by the total iron-binding capacity (TIBC). TIBC represents the amount of iron that plasma transferrin can bind and normally ranges from ~250 to 400 μg/dL. Levels greater than 400 μg/dL suggest iron deficiency. Serum iron concentrations, which represent the amount of iron bound to transferrin and other blood proteins, also are affected with iron deficiency, decreasing to <~50 μg/dL (normal values range from ~50 to 165 μg/dL).

As circulating iron diminishes, functional or cellular iron also becomes limited. With diminished iron, free protoporphyrin concentrations in erythrocytes rise. Protoporphyrin is a precursor of heme (for hemoglobin) and accumulates within red blood cells when iron is not available. Erythrocyte protoporphyrin levels greater than 70 μg/dL red blood cells are associated with iron deficiency. In iron deficiency, the number of transferrin receptors on the cell surface, especially of immature red cells, also increases. The increased receptor number represents an up-regulation to enable cells to better compete for transferrin-bound iron. With iron deficiency, concentrations of serum transferrin receptors (sTfR), truncated forms of the membrane receptor protein, increase to greater than 8.0 mg/L and are thought to be directly proportional to the functional tissue (i.e., cellular) iron deficit after depletion of iron stores.

In the final stages of iron deficiency, anemia occurs. With anemia, blood hemoglobin concentrations drop below the lower limit of normal, which is typically 12 g/dL and 13 g/dL for females and males, respectively. Hematocrit concentrations with anemia also decrease below the lower limit of normal, less than about 37% and 40% for women and men, respectively. Characterization of red blood cells with respect to size (mean corpuscular volume, or MCV) and amount of hemoglobin they contain (mean corpuscular hemoglobin, or MCH, and mean corpuscular hemoglobin concentration, or MCHC) typically shows that they are smaller and lower in hemoglobin than normal in the final stages of iron-deficiency anemia. Descriptions of these assessments follow.

- MCV (fL) represents the size of the red blood cell. It is calculated by dividing hematocrit by red blood cells and then multiplying by 10.

- MCH (pg/rbc) represents the average hemoglobin content of each individual red blood cell. It is calculated by dividing hemoglobin by number of red blood cells and then multiplying by 10.

- MCHC represents the amount of hemoglobin in grams per deciliter (%) of red blood cells. It is calculated by dividing hemoglobin by hematocrit and then multiplying by 100.

Thus, red blood cells are pale (hypochromic) and small (microcytic) with iron-deficiency anemia. Figure 13.8 illustrates the changes that occur in the various measurements.

References Cited for Iron

1. Atanasova B, Mudway I, Laftah A, et al. Duodenal ascorbate levels are changed in mice with altered iron metabolism. J Nutr. 2004; 134:501–05.
2. Hurrell R, Lynch S, Trinidad T, et al. Iron absorption in humans: bovine serum albumin compared with beef muscle and egg white. Am J Clin Nutr. 1988; 47:102–07.
3. Monsen E, Balintfy J. Calculating dietary iron bioavailability: refinement and computerization. J Am Diet Assoc. 1982; 80:307–11.
4. Monsen, E. Iron nutrition and absorption: Dietary factors which impact iron bioavailability. J Am Diet Assoc. 1988; 88:786–90.
5. Lonnerdal B. Calcium and iron absorption: mechanisms and public health relevance. Interntl J Vit Nutr Res. 2010; 80:293–99.
6. Whittaker P. Iron and zinc interactions in humans. Am J Clin Nutr. 1998; 68:S442–46.
7. Herman S, Griffin IJ, Suwarti S, et al. Cofortification of iron-fortified flour with zinc sulfate, but not zinc oxide, decreases iron absorption in Indonesian children. Am J Clin Nutr. 2002; 76:813–17.
8. Kelleher SL. Lonnerdal B. Zinc supplementation reduces iron absorption through age-dependent changes in small intestine iron transporter expression in suckling rat pups. J Nutr. 2006; 136:1185–91.
9. Hunt JR. Algorithms for iron and zinc bioavailability: are they accurate? Int J Vitam Nutr Res. 2010; 80:257–62.
10. Bolann B, Ulvik R. On the limited ability of superoxide to release iron from ferritin. Eur J Biochem. 1990; 193:899–904.
11. Oduho G, Han Y, Baker D. Iron deficiency reduces the efficacy of tryptophan as a niacin precursor. J Nutr. 1994; 124:444–50.

12. Zimmermann M. The influence of iron status on iodine utilization and thyroid function. Ann Rev Nutr. 2006; 26:367–89.

13. Herbert V, Shaw S, Jayatilleke E. Vitamin C–driven free radical generation from iron. J Nutr. 1996; 126:S1213–20.

14. Waddell J, Steenbock H, Elvehjem C, Hart E. Iron salts and iron containing ash extracts in the correction of anemia. J Biol Chem. 1927; 77:777–95.

15. Sandstrom B, Davidsson L, Cederblad A, Lonnerdal B. Oral iron, dietary ligands and zinc absorption. J Nutr. 1985; 115:411–14.

16. Solomons N, Jacob R. Studies on the bioavailability of zinc in humans: effects of heme and nonheme iron on the absorption of zinc. Am J Clin Nutr. 1981; 34:475–82.

17. Kordas K, Stoltzfus RJ. New evidence of iron and zinc interplay at the enterocyte and neural tissues. J Nutr. 2004; 134:1295–98.

18. O'Brien KO, Zaveleta N, Caulfield LE, et al. Prenatal iron supplementation impairs zinc absorption in pregnant Peruvian women. J Nutr. 2000; 130:2251–55.

19. Zimmermann M, Biebinger R, Rohner F, et al. Vitamin A supplementation in children with poor vitamin A and iron status increases erythropoietin and hemoglobin concentrations without changing total body iron. Am J Clin Nutr. 2006; 84:580–86.

20. Food and Nutrition Board, Institute of Medicine. Dietary Reference Intakes. Washington, DC: National Academy Press. 2001 pp. 290–393.

21. Pietrangelo A. Hereditary hemochromatosis. Ann Rev Nutr. 2006; 26:251–70.

Suggested Readings

Collins JF, Wessling-Resnick M, Knutson MD. Hepcidin regulation of iron transport. J Nutr. 2008; 138:2284–88.

Collins JF, Prohaska JR, Knutson MD. Metabolic crossroads of iron and copper. Nutr Rev. 2010; 68:133–47.

Fleming R, Britton R. HFE and regulation of intestinal iron absorption. Am J Physiol Gastrointest Liver Physiol. 2006; 290:590–94.

Garrick MD, Garrick LM. Cellular iron transport. Biochim Biophys Acta. 2009; 1790:309–25.

Ma Y, Yeh M, Yeh K, Glass J. Transport of iron through the intestinal epithelium. Am J Physiol Gastrointest Liver Physiol. 2006; 290:G417–22.

Nemeth E. Iron regulation and erythropoiesis. Curr Opin Hematol. 2008; 15:169–75.

Nemeth E, Ganz T. Regulation of iron metabolism by hepcidin. Ann Rev Nutr. 2006; 26:323–42.

Piperno A, Mariani R, Thrombini P, Girelli P. Hepcidin modulation in human diseases: from research to clinic. World J Gastroenterol. 2009; 15:538–51.

Web Site for Nutrient Composition Information

http://www.ars.usda.gov/Services/docs.htm?docid=18877

ZINC

The human body contains about 1.5 to 3.0 g of zinc. Zinc is found in all organs, tissues, and body fluids. Zinc, a metal, can exist in several different valence states, but it is almost universally found as the divalent ion (Zn^{2+}) in the human body.

Sources

Zinc is found in foods complexed with nucleic acids and with amino acids that are part of peptides and proteins. The zinc content of foods varies widely (Table 13.3).

Very good sources of zinc are red meats (especially organ meats) and seafood (especially oysters and mollusks). Other good animal sources of zinc include poultry, pork, and dairy products. Animal products are thought to provide between 40% and 70% of zinc consumed by most people in the United States. Whole grains (especially bran and germ) and vegetables (leafy and root) represent good plant sources of zinc. Cereals are thought to provide about 30% of the zinc in the U.S. diet. Fruits contain little zinc. Plant sources not only have a lower zinc content, but zinc from plants is also absorbed to a lesser extent than zinc from animal sources (e.g., meat). The Daily Value for zinc (used on food and supplement labels) is 15 mg.

Processing of certain foods may affect zinc availability. Heat treatment can cause zinc in food to form complexes that resist hydrolysis, thereby making zinc unavailable for absorption. Maillard reaction products—that is, amino acid–carbohydrate complexes resulting from browning, for example—are particularly notable for inhibiting zinc's availability for absorption.

Zinc supplements are available in several forms including oral tablets and lozenges, throat or nasal sprays, and nasal gels. Zinc is typically found in supplements as zinc oxide, zinc sulfate, zinc acetate, zinc chloride, and zinc gluconate. These various forms provide differing

Table 13.3 Zinc Content of Selected Foods

Food/Food Group	Zinc (mg)
Seafood	
Oyster (1)	12.8
Crabmeat (3 oz)	3.8
Shrimp (3 oz)	1.8
Flounder/sole (3 oz)	0.5
Meat and poultry	
Liver (beef) (3 oz)	4.3
Chicken (dark meat) (3 oz)	2.4
Beef, ground (3 oz)	3.8
Veal (3 oz)	3.5
Pork (3 oz)	1.8
Eggs and dairy products	
Egg (1)	0.5
Milk (1 cup)	1.0
Cheeses (1 oz)	0.5–1.2
Legumes (cooked, 1/2 cup)	1.0–2.7
Nuts (1 oz)	0.9–1.5
Grains and cereals	
Rice and pasta (cooked, 1 cup)	0.7–1.2
Bread (whole-wheat, 1 slice)	0.3
Bread (white, 1 slice)	0.1
Vegetables (cooked, 1 cup)	0.1–0.7
Fruits	<0.1

Source: USDA.

amounts of zinc. Zinc gluconate, for example, is approximately 14.3% zinc, whereas zinc sulfate is 23% zinc, and zinc chloride is 48% zinc. Zinc chloride and zinc sulfate are very soluble, as is zinc acetate. In contrast, zinc carbonate and zinc oxide are fairly insoluble. Zinc supplements for oral consumption should be consumed on an empty stomach, without simultaneously ingesting other mineral supplements such as iron or calcium. Abdominal pain (e.g., gastric irritation), dyspepsia, nausea, vomiting, and diarrhea are commonly reported side effects of zinc supplements.

Topical zinc products, which usually provide zinc as zinc oxide or zinc chloride, may be used in wound management and include paste bandages, occlusive adhesive dressings, alginates, stockings, and zinc-saline dressings. The percutaneous absorption of the zinc depends on the skin's integrity and requires (in the case of zinc oxide or chloride) the acidic moisture on the skin's surface to release the zinc. If skin is not intact (as may occur with burns or other injury), much more zinc is absorbed. In the presence of an intact skin barrier, zinc binds to the sulfhydryl groups in epidermal keratin upon release from the zinc oxide or chloride salt in the acidic environment. A small amount of the zinc will then penetrate beyond the superficial keratinocytes and enter circulation in a process that takes about 60 minutes from the time of topical application. The rest of the zinc (not making it into circulation) binds to metallothionein (which is induced with topical zinc application) in epidermal keratinocytes and will eventually be sloughed off with skin cell turnover.

Endogenous sources of zinc, especially pancreatic and biliary secretions that are released daily into the gastrointestinal tract, augment the amounts absorbed from dietary food sources and supplements. Carboxypeptidase, for example, is a zinc metalloenzyme, and with its hydrolysis zinc is released. The released zinc is then available for absorption and reuse in the body. This reuse of endogenous zinc, especially from pancreatic secretions, is important for the body's zinc homeostasis.

Digestion, Absorption, Transport, and Storage

Figure 13.9 provides an overview of zinc digestion, absorption, and transport as well as some of zinc's fates in the enterocyte.

Digestion

Zinc, like iron, needs to be hydrolyzed from amino acids and nucleic acids before it can be absorbed. Zinc is believed to be liberated from food during the digestive process, most likely by the acidic environment of the stomach and upper duodenum and by proteases and nucleases in the stomach and small intestine.

Absorption

Zinc absorption in the gastrointestinal tract occurs primarily in the proximal small intestine, that is, the duodenum and upper jejunum. However, the relative contribution of each segment of the small intestine (duodenum, jejunum, and ileum) toward overall zinc absorption has not been demonstrated.

Two mechanisms (carrier-medicated transport and diffusion) are responsible for intestinal zinc absorption (Figure 13.9). The primary means of zinc absorption into the enterocyte with intakes up to about 7 to 9 mg of zinc per day is saturable and carrier-mediated [1]. The protein carrier Zrt- and Irt-like protein (ZIP) 4 is the major transporter of zinc across the brush border membrane and into the cytosol of the enterocyte; this transporter is expressed throughout the gastrointestinal tract. Zinc intake influences ZIP4. With high zinc intakes, ZIP4 is degraded more rapidly to down-regulate absorption, whereas zinc restriction enhances ZIP4 mRNA stability, rapidly induces ZIP4 synthesis, and shifts ZIP4 proteins to the brush border membrane. The enhanced ZIP4 synthesis is mediated by up-regulation of the transcription factor Kruppel-like factor 4 (KLF4), which binds to the promoter region on the ZIP4 gene.

A mutation in ZIP4 causes the disorder acrodermatitis enteropathica. The condition is characterized by poor zinc absorption and is clinically manifested by skin lesions (which often become infected), especially on the face, knees, and buttocks; impaired growth; and low plasma zinc concentrations, representing signs and symptoms of zinc deficiency. If untreated, the condition can be fatal. The provision of high doses of zinc that can be absorbed by diffusion typically helps compensate for the impaired ZIP4 transporters.

Although other carrier proteins present in the gastrointestinal tract bind zinc, they are not thought to contribute except in a minor capacity to zinc absorption. For example, DMT1 (divalent mineral transporter 1) was once thought to be highly involved in brush border zinc uptake. However, although zinc appears to up-regulate DMT1 mRNA expression, the DMT1 transporter does not appear to transport significant quantities of zinc into intestinal cells. Similarly, some zinc may bind to amino acids such as histidine and perhaps enter the enterocyte using amino acid transporters; however, this contribution to zinc absorption is minor. ZIP11 is also found on the brush border membrane, and its synthesis is up-regulated with zinc restriction; however, at this time, its role in zinc absorption is thought to be small, if any [1].

In addition to carrier-mediated transport, paracellular (meaning between cells) diffusion of zinc through the tight junctions of the enterocytes enables absorption. This process is thought to contribute to the absorption of zinc when zinc intakes (typically 20 mg or more) exceed the capacity of the ZIP4 carriers. Zinc (given in dosages

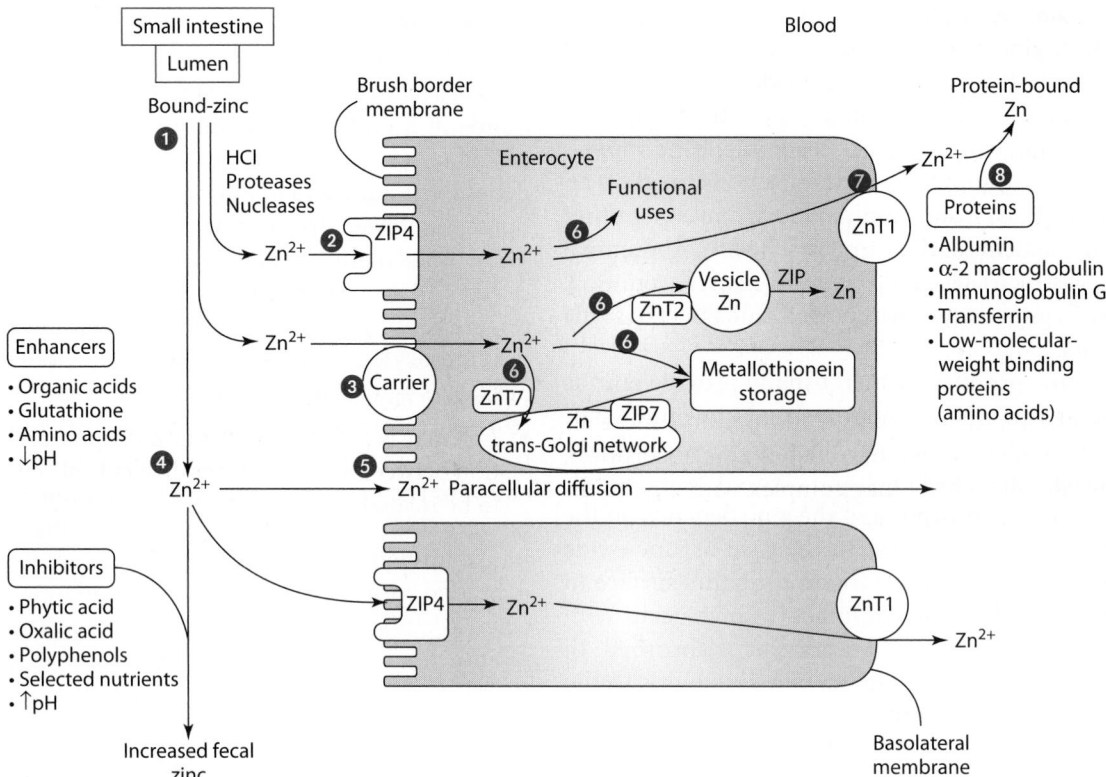

Figure 13.9 Digestion, absorption, enterocyte use, and transport of zinc.

1 Bound zinc is released from food components, primarily proteins and nucleic acids.

2 Most zinc is absorbed by Zrt- and Irt-like protein (ZIP) 4 across the brush border membrane.

3 Divalent mineral transporter (DMT) 1 and amino acids may play a minor role in zinc absorption across the brush border membrane.

4 Some zinc may be directed into the feces if bound to inhibitors, or absorption may be enhanced by organic acids, ↓pH, or chelators.

5 With high zinc intakes, zinc may be absorbed between cells (i.e., paracellularly).

6 Within cells, zinc may be used functionally or stored in vesicles, in the trans-Golgi network, or as part of metallothionein.

7 Zinc may be transported across the basolateral membrane by ZnT1.

8 Zinc binds any of several proteins for transport in the blood.

of 30–150 mg) used in the treatment of acrodermitis enteropathica is likely absorbed paracellularly.

Overall, about 20% to 30% of zinc is absorbed from the typical U.S. diet. However, fractional zinc absorption varies from approximately 10% to 80%; at higher intakes (such as 20 mg or more) absorption diminishes, whereas at lower intakes absorption increases. For example, 100% of zinc may be absorbed at an intake less than 1 mg, whereas about 40% may be absorbed with a zinc intake of 12 mg [1]. This up- and down-regulation of absorption and the ability to increase and decrease zinc excretion are important for maintaining zinc homeostasis in the body.

Factors Influencing Zinc Absorption

As is the case with iron, chelators or ligands bind to zinc. Whether these substances are enhancers or inhibitors of zinc absorption depends on the digestibility and absorbability of the zinc chelates or ligands formed.

Enhancers of Zinc Absorption Ligands or chelators including organic acids (like citric acid and picolinic acid) and prostaglandins may bind and promote zinc absorption. Pancreatic secretions are thought to contain an unidentified constituent that enhances zinc absorption. In addition, glutathione (a tripeptide composed of cysteine, glutamate, and glycine) and products of protein digestion, such as tripeptides and amino acids, are purported to serve as ligands. Zinc typically binds to sulfur (e.g., cysteine alone, or as part of glutathione) and nitrogen (e.g., histidine) within these ligands. Amino acids serving as ligands help maintain zinc's solubility in the gastrointestinal tract; whether zinc bound to amino acid ligands can be absorbed using amino acid transporters is unclear.

Absorption of zinc also is enhanced by an acidic environment. Thus, the use of medication such as antacids, H_2 receptor blockers (such as Zantac [ranitidine], Tagamet [cimetidine], or Pepcid [famotidine]), and proton pump blockers (such as Prevacid [lansoprazole] or Prilosec [omeprazole]), which are commonly taken to treat heartburn, gastroesophageal reflux disease, and ulcers, increases gastric and proximal intestinal pH and results in decreased zinc absorption.

Inhibitors of Zinc Absorption In addition to a more alkaline environment, which diminishes zinc absorption, many compounds in food may complex with zinc to inhibit its absorption. Some examples of inhibitors include:

- *Phytic acid* is found in plant foods, particularly legumes, seeds, and cereals such as maize and bran. It binds to zinc (as well as other minerals) via oxygen within the compound's phosphate groups. The zinc-phytic acid complex is large, insoluble, and poorly absorbed. However, fermentation of bread reduces the phytic acid content and improves zinc absorption. Figure 13.10 depicts the binding of zinc by phytic acid. Most individuals in the United States, however, do not consume enough phytic acid or oxalic acid (discussed later in this chapter) to significantly inhibit zinc absorption.

- *Oxalic acid* (oxalate), another inhibitor of zinc absorption, is found in a variety of foods, most notably spinach, chard, berries, chocolate, and tea. The binding of zinc by oxalic acid is shown in Figure 13.10. The typical U.S. diet is not high in oxalic acid, and it is thus unlikely to negatively impact zinc absorption.

- *Polyphenols* (such as tannins and gallic acid) in tea and coffee and certain *fibers* found in whole grains, fruits, and vegetables also bind zinc and inhibit its absorption.

Most individuals in the United States, however, consume well under the recommended amount of dietary fiber and are thus unlikely to experience fiber-induced inhibition of zinc absorption.

- *Folate* (a B vitamin) supplements may negatively impact zinc absorption. The results of studies examining folate's inhibition of zinc absorption (with folic acid given in amounts of 350–800 μg and zinc in amounts of 3.5–50 mg) are equivocal. However, given the use of folic acid supplements to prevent neural tube defects in women during childbearing years, additional studies are warranted.

- *Iron* may negatively affect zinc absorption. The interaction between zinc and other divalent cations is thought to be related to competition between cations for binding ligands in the intestinal lumen or within the cell as well as possibly for transporters on the brush border of the enterocytes. Nonheme iron and zinc interact to inhibit zinc absorption primarily when coingested in solution and when iron is ingested in amounts of 20 mg or more; the effects are not always apparent when given with a meal and seem to vary depending on the population being studied and the form of the nutrients provided [2,3]. Given the possibility of an interaction between the two nutrients, to maximize zinc absorption, a zinc supplement should not be consumed at the same time as a nonheme iron supplement.

- *Calcium* may inhibit zinc absorption. The effects of calcium on zinc absorption and balance are also equivocal. Some studies have shown that ingestion of calcium (500 mg to ~2 g) as calcium carbonate, hydroxyapatite, or calcium citrate malate has no effect on zinc absorption, whereas other studies providing similar amounts of calcium as milk, calcium phosphate, and calcium carbonate found reductions in net zinc absorption and zinc balance [4–6]. Results appear to vary with the forms and amounts of the nutrients provided and the study populations. To minimize the likelihood of interactions, it is prudent to not take mineral supplements at the same time, to avoid the ingestion of calcium supplements at meals providing significant amounts of zinc, and to ensure adequate dietary intake of zinc.

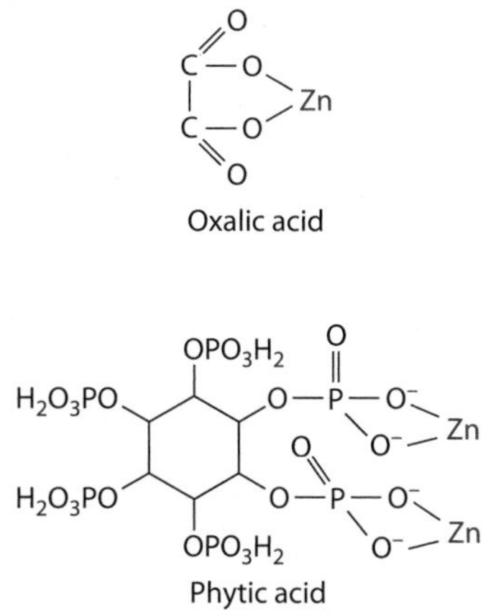

Intestinal Cell Zinc Use

Zinc entering the enterocyte has several possible fates. The zinc may be:

- used functionally within the enterocyte, or
- stored or sequestered in the enterocyte, or
- transported through the cytosol and across the basolateral membrane for entry into the blood and thus use by other tissues

Oxalic acid

Phytic acid

Figure 13.10 The binding of zinc by oxalic acid and phytic acid.

The functional use of zinc within the enterocyte is similar to its use in other body cells and is described further in the "Functions and Mechanisms of Action" section.

If not used functionally within cells such as enterocytes, zinc is largely sequestered or bound to proteins; in other words, little zinc is found free. Zinc transporters function to remove zinc from the environment; that is, they lower intracellular (cytosolic) zinc concentrations, mediating both zinc efflux from cells and movement of zinc into intracellular compartments. Intracellularly, zinc is sequestered in vesicles, secretory granules, endosomes, or the trans-Golgi network (complex). The intracellular trafficking protein ZnT7 in the enterocyte is thought to be involved in zinc movement into the trans-Golgi network, while ZIP7 may transport the mineral out of the trans-Golgi network; however, the exact roles of these two transporters have not been clearly established. ZnT2 appears to sequester zinc in endosome-like vesicles within enterocytes. Overall, however, how zinc is transported within the cytosol (i.e., intracellular trafficking) is not well delineated.

The protein metallothionein (sometimes called thionein if free of metals) serves as zinc's main storage protein and as an intracellular binding ligand. Metallothionein contains an unusually high content (30%) of cysteine, which functions in metal binding. Metallothionein is thought to both transport zinc to zinc-requiring enzymes and store zinc. The metallothionein-bound zinc can be released for cellular use, but if not used, it will be lost into the feces with the sloughing of enterocytes that is part of normal intestinal cell turnover. Metallothionein is covered in further detail in the "Storage" section.

Zinc needed for extraintestinal use will be carried across the basolateral membrane of the enterocyte for release into the blood. Zinc transporter (ZnT) 1, which does not require sodium or ATP, preferentially transports zinc out of duodenal and jejunal cells, likely in exchange for H^+ or K^+; ZnT1 is also found on several other cell membranes. The synthesis of ZnT1 is increased with high dietary zinc intake but does not appear to be affected with decreased zinc intake. Specifically, ZnT1 synthesis is regulated by the zinc-responsive metal transcription factor (MTF) 1, which binds to metal response elements in the promoter region of the ZnT1 gene; (MTF1 is discussed more thoroughly in the "Gene Expression" section). In addition to ZnT1, a sodium-zinc exchanger has been identified that appears to direct sodium-dependent active extrusion of zinc from some cells. DMT1, found on the basolateral membrane of enterocytes, also may play a minor role in intestinal cell zinc efflux into the blood.

Transport

Zinc passing into portal blood from the intestinal cell is mainly transported loosely bound to albumin. Most zinc is then taken to the liver, where the mineral is initially concentrated. Zinc leaving the liver for transport in the blood may again be bound to albumin but also may be attached to other proteins including transferrin, α-2 macroglobulin, and immunoglobulin (Ig) G (Figure 13.9). Albumin is thought to transport up to ~60% of zinc in the blood. Transferrin, α-2 macroglobulin, and IgG are thought to transport ~15% to 40% of the zinc in the blood. Two amino acids, histidine and cysteine, loosely bind and transport up to about 8% of the zinc; these amino acids form a ternary (histidine-zinc-cysteine) complex in the blood. A tiny amount (<0.01%) of zinc also may travel free in the blood. Normal plasma zinc concentrations range from about 70 to 120 μg/dL (10–18 μmol/L).

Multiple transporters, including at least 14 ZIPs and 10 ZnTs, facilitate cellular zinc uptake and release, yet many of the mechanisms remain unclear. ZIP carriers 1, 2, 4, 5, 6, 7, 8, and 14 appear to be involved in cellular zinc uptake from extracellular locations and the release of zinc from intracellular stores, both to effect increased cytosolic zinc concentrations. ZIP14, for example, transports zinc into hepatocytes, and its activity appears to be increased as part of the acute-phase (reactant) response (as occurs with infections and trauma). The transporter ZIP5 is expressed in the intestinal cell as well as the pancreas, liver, and kidneys. In the intestine, ZIP5 is found on the basolateral membrane, where it is thought to facilitate serosal to mucosal zinc transport. In other words, ZIP5 moves zinc out of the circulation, that is, from the blood into the intestinal cell. The zinc transporter ZnT6, found on the enterocyte's brush border membrane, is thought to mediate the exocytosis of zinc from the intestinal cell back into the lumen for ultimate excretion in the feces. Not all ZIP carriers, however, solely transport zinc; many, such as ZIP14, which transports both Fe^{2+} and Zn^{2+}, carry other minerals as well.

Storage

Zinc is found in all body organs, most notably the liver, kidneys, muscle, skin, and bones. Within cells, about 30% to 40% of zinc is bound to proteins in the nucleus, about 50% is in the cytosol, and the remaining zinc is found in cell membranes. The zinc content of most soft tissues (including muscle, brain, heart, and lungs) is relatively stable. This soft-tissue zinc does not respond to or equilibrate with other zinc pools to release zinc when dietary zinc intake is low. Similarly, although zinc is found in bones as part of apatite, bones release the mineral very slowly and cannot be depended on to supply zinc during dietary deprivation. Instead, when dietary zinc intake is insufficient, catabolism of selected "less essential" zinc-containing metalloproteins (enzymes) and liver metallothionein occurs to enable the release and redistribution of zinc to meet particularly crucial needs for the mineral.

Zinc is thought to be stored in the body attached to metallothionein, which contains a high proportion of cysteine residues that bind metals including not only zinc (7 atoms/molecule), but also copper, cadmium, and mercury. Metallothionein is found in most body tissues, including the liver, pancreas, kidneys, intestine, keratinocytes, and red blood cells. Various forms of the protein exist and are designated by number as metallothionein (MT)-1 through MT-4. MT-1 and MT-2 appear to be the most common tissue forms. Although metallothionein is thought to serve as a storage form of zinc, other roles also have been attributed to the protein. Metallothionein may regulate the distribution (serving like a transporter or chaperone) and transfer of zinc to enzymes, gene-regulatory molecules, or other acceptor proteins. Metallothionein also exhibits antioxidant-type functions. For example, the protein is known to scavenge free hydroxyl radicals. In times of cell injury/stress, metallothionein synthesis increases and helps control free radical concentrations. This response is part of the body's acute-phase response, and the enhanced thionein gene expression results in part from the increased release of glucagon and the cytokine interleukin 1 (which is synthesized and secreted by monocytes and activated macrophages). The induction in thionein gene transcription during infection promotes zinc storage and prevents bacterial use of the mineral. Should zinc be needed within cells, it may be released from metallothionein by the action of lysosomal proteases. At an acidic pH, these proteases degrade metallothionein to release the zinc for use by cells.

Zinc regulates the gene expression of thionein. Specifically, metal regulatory (also called response) elements (MREs), consisting of specific nucleotide sequences, are found in the promoter region of the thionein gene. A metal transcription factor dependent on zinc interacts with the MRE to induce thionein synthesis. See the "Gene Expression" section for a more complete description of how zinc affects gene transcription.

Functions and Mechanisms of Action

Zinc has many seemingly divergent functions, probably because it is a component of numerous metalloenzymes. As a component of metalloenzymes, zinc (1) provides structural integrity to the enzyme by binding directly to amino acid residues and thereby stabilizing the enzyme's tertiary structure and/or (2) participates in the reaction at the catalytic site. Zinc affects many fundamental life processes. Zinc appears to be part of more enzyme systems than all the rest of the trace minerals combined. Enzymes (at least 70 and perhaps over 200) from every enzyme class (oxidoreductases, hydrolases, lyases, isomerases, transferases, and ligases) require zinc. A few of these zinc-dependent enzymes are listed in Table 13.4 and are described in the next section.

Table 13.4 Selected Functions of Zinc

Metalloenzyme component
Carbonic anhydrase
Alkaline phosphatase
Alcohol dehydrogenase
Carboxypeptidases
Aminopeptidases
Delta aminolevulinic acid dehydratase
Superoxide dismutase
Phospholipase C
Polyglutamate hydrolase
Matrix metalloproteinases
Polymerases
Kinases
Nucleases
Transcriptases
Gene expression: zinc fingers
Membrane/cytoskeletal stabilization
Immune function
Sexual maturation
Fertility and reproduction

Zinc-Dependent Enzymes

Carbonic Anhydrase: Acid–Base Balance Carbonic anhydrase has a very high affinity for zinc, which plays a catalytic role. The enzyme, found primarily in erythrocytes and in renal tubule cells, is essential for acid–base balance/buffering and respiration. More zinc (about eight to nine times) is found associated with this enzyme in red blood cells than is found in the plasma. The enzyme catalyzes the following reaction, thereby allowing the rapid disposal of carbon dioxide: $CO_2 + H_2O \longrightarrow H_2CO_3 \longrightarrow H^+ + HCO_3^-$. The H^+ dissociated from carbonic acid reduces oxyhemoglobin as oxygen is released to the tissues; the bicarbonate passes into the plasma to participate in buffering reactions. Concentrations of the enzyme are not significantly affected by zinc deprivation, but activity in red blood cells diminishes with low-zinc (3.8 mg/day for several weeks) diets [7].

Alkaline Phosphatase: Phosphate Digestion Alkaline phosphatase contains four zinc atoms per enzyme molecule. Two of the four atoms are required for enzyme activity. The other two are needed for structural purposes. The enzyme, found mainly in bones and in the liver (with small amounts in the plasma), lacks substrate specificity, hydrolyzing monoesters of phosphates from various compounds. Enzyme activity decreases with zinc deficiency.

Alcohol Dehydrogenase: Nonspecific Aldehyde Synthesis Alcohol dehydrogenase also contains four zinc atoms per enzyme molecule, with two of the four required for catalytic activity and two required for structural purposes (protein conformation). This enzyme, which generally lacks specificity, is important in the NADH-dependent conversion of alcohols to aldehydes. For example, the enzyme converts a form of vitamin A, retinol, to retinal; retinal is needed for the visual cycle and night vision. In addition, the enzyme converts ethanol to acetyl-aldehyde, a reaction important in alcohol metabolism.

Carboxypeptidases A and B and Aminopeptidases: Protein Digestion Carboxypeptidases A and B, exopeptidases secreted by the pancreas into the duodenum, are necessary for protein digestion. Zinc is bound tightly to carboxypeptidases and is essential for enzymatic activity; in fact, enzyme activity decreases with zinc deficiency. Figure 13.11 shows the zinc-containing portion of the carboxypeptidase A enzyme.

Aminopeptidases consist of a group of enzymes also involved in protein digestion. Aminopeptidases typically contain one or two zinc atoms, needed for catalytic activity. The enzymes cleave amino acids from the amino (N)-terminal end of proteins or polypeptides that are being digested in the intestinal tract.

Delta (Δ)-Aminolevulinic Acid Dehydratase: Heme Synthesis Δ-aminolevulinic acid dehydratase, involved in heme synthesis, is also zinc dependent. This enzyme is made up of eight subunits, each of which binds one zinc atom. Zinc is essential for the maintenance of free thiols (-SH) in the enzyme because zinc prevents the oxidation of thiol groups and consequently disulfide bond formation within the enzyme. The enzyme catalyzes the condensation of two Δ-aminolevulinic acids to form porphobilinogen (Figure 13.6). Lead, if present in the body in high concentrations (as occurs with lead poisoning), replaces zinc in the dehydratase and diminishes heme synthesis.

Superoxide Dismutase: Antioxidant Superoxide dismutase (SOD) found in the cell cytosol requires two atoms each of zinc and copper for function; zinc appears to have a structural role in the enzyme. An extracellular form of the enzyme that is also zinc and copper dependent has been characterized and appears to be more sensitive to zinc than is the cytosolic form of the enzyme. The extracellular form is found in the plasma, lymph, synovial fluid, and lungs; it exists in equilibrium between cell surfaces and the plasma. Both the cytosolic and extracellular forms of superoxide dismutase serve important antioxidant defense roles in the body by catalyzing the removal of superoxide radicals, $O_2^{\bullet-}$.

$$2O_2^{\bullet-} + 2H^+ \xrightarrow{\text{Superoxide dismutase}} H_2O_2 + O_2$$

Further information on this enzyme is found in the section on copper, in the "Functions and Mechanisms of Action" subsection.

Phospholipase C: Phospholipid Metabolism Phospholipase C requires three zinc atoms for catalytic activity. This enzyme hydrolyzes the glycerophosphate bond in phospholipids.

Polyglutamate Hydrolase: Folate Digestion Polyglutamate hydrolase, also called γ-glutamylhydrolase or pteroylglutamate hydrolase, is a zinc-dependent enzyme necessary to digest the vitamin folate in the gastrointestinal tract. Folate is found in foods bound to several (poly) glutamic acid residues. For folate to be absorbed, all but

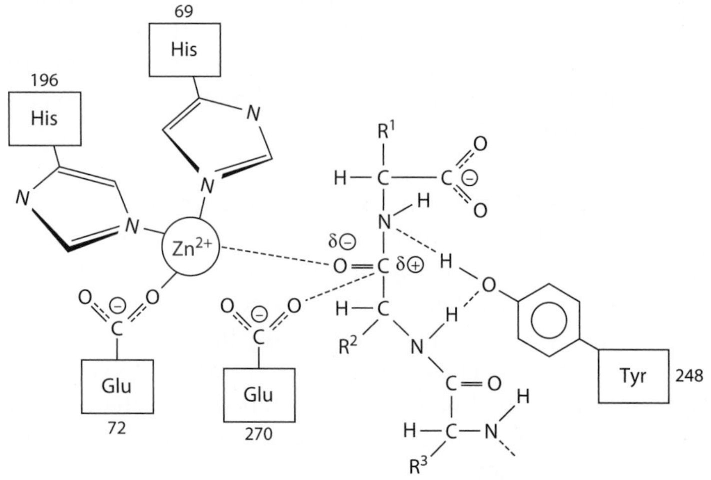

Figure 13.11 Partial structure of carboxypeptidase A.

one of the glutamic acids must be removed. The enzyme polyglutamate hydrolase removes all but one of the glutamic acids from folate.

$$\text{Polyglutamate folate} \xrightarrow{\text{Polyglutamate hydrolase}} \text{Monoglutamate folate}$$
$$\searrow$$
$$\text{Glutamic acids}$$

The monoglutamate folate can then be actively transported into intestinal cells. Poor zinc status can diminish folate absorption.

Matrix Metalloproteinases: Wound Repair Matrix metalloproteinases include a group of zinc-containing endopeptidases (with zinc located at the catalytic site where the substrate binds) that are found in keratinocytes, macrophages, fibroblasts, and endothelial cells. The enzymes are synthesized as inactive zymogens and become active in the presence of several soluble mediators and extracellular matrix compounds that are generated with cell injury. The matrix metalloproteinases generally function in wound healing, degrading components of the extracellular matrix (among other roles) to allow for remodeling of extracellular matrix proteins and tissue repair. Based on structural elements, the enzymes may be categorized, for example, as: collagenases (important for wound debriding), gelatinases, matrilysins, or stromelysins (needed for wound contraction).

Polymerases, Kinases, Nucleases, Transferases, Phosphorylases, and Transcriptases: Nucleic Acid Synthesis and Cell Replication and Growth Polymerases, kinases, nucleases, transferases, phosphorylases, and transcriptases all require zinc. Paramount in nucleic acid synthesis are the zinc metalloenzymes DNA and RNA polymerase and deoxythymidine kinase. Deoxythymidine kinase is necessary for the conservation or salvaging of thymine, the pyrimidine unique to DNA. Additionally, catabolism of RNA appears to be regulated by zinc because of zinc's influence on ribonuclease activity. Enzymes such as deoxynucleotidyl transferase, nucleoside phosphorylase, and reverse transcriptase also depend on zinc.

Gene Expression

Zinc plays a major role in regulating gene transcription. To perform this function, zinc binds to transcription factors (proteins). The binding of zinc to transcription factors results in a conformational change in the shape of the transcription factor protein such that it resembles a "finger." *Zinc fingers* is the term used to indicate the secondary shape (configuration) of the transcription factor proteins when bound to zinc. About 30 amino acids held together by one zinc atom are thought to make up a zinc finger; the zinc, attached to four of the amino acids through cysteine residues or a combination of cysteine and histidine

residues, stabilizes the structure. These zinc fingers, once formed, interact with specific DNA sequences, called metal response or regulatory elements (MREs), located in the promoter region of selected genes to either enhance or repress transcription (Figure 13.12). About 2,000 transcription factors have been identified and nearly half appear to require zinc. In addition, some zinc finger proteins may interact with mRNA to repress translation.

Other Roles

Physiological functions of zinc include tissue or cell growth, cell membrane integrity, cell replication, bone formation, skin integrity, cell-mediated immunity, and generalized host defense. The role of zinc in tissue growth is related primarily to its function in regulating protein synthesis, which includes its influence on polysome conformation as well as the synthesis and catabolism of the nucleic acids.

The effect of zinc on cell membranes may occur through direct effects on the membrane proteins' conformation or on protein-to-protein interactions. Zinc may affect the activity of several enzymes attached to plasma membranes, including alkaline phosphatase, carbonic anhydrase, and superoxide dismutase, among others. Zinc itself also is believed to stabilize membrane structure by stabilizing phospholipids and thiol (SH) groups that need to be maintained in a reduced state. Zinc may also stabilize membranes by quenching free radicals as part of metallothionein and by promoting associations between membrane skeletal and cytoskeletal proteins. Zinc in cells is found bound to tubulin, a protein that makes up the microtubules. Microtubules are thought to act as a framework for structural support of the cell as well as enable movement. Because of zinc's roles in maintaining

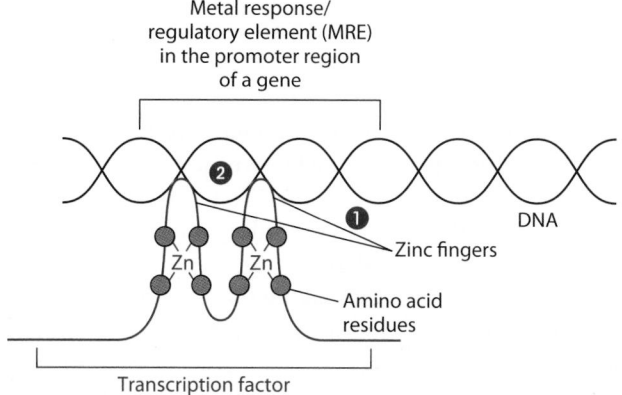

Figure 13.12 The role of zinc in gene expression.

❶ Zinc fingers are proteins with a secondary structure or shape like a finger due, in part, to the presence of a zinc atom linked through cysteinyl or histidyl residues in the protein.

❷ Zinc fingers are found within many transcription factors, which bind to the metal response/regulatory elements in the promoter regions of genes to enhance or inhibit transcription.

cell membranes, the use of zinc, either alone or with anti-oxidants such as vitamins C and E and beta-carotene, has been thought to be beneficial in the treatment of the eye disorder macular degeneration. Unfortunately, data regarding the benefits of zinc in delaying the progression of age-related macular degeneration have been inconclusive.

Zinc is involved with insulin and thus influences carbohydrate metabolism. Zinc is transported into pancreatic beta-cells by zinc transporters ZnT5 and ZnT8. Pancreatic beta-cells are responsible for insulin production and secretion. Once synthesized, insulin is stored with zinc in granules in the pancreatic beta-cells until it is released into the blood. Zinc deficiency decreases the insulin response, resulting in impaired glucose tolerance. Zinc also appears to regulate the protein kinase mammalian target of rapamycin (mTor), thereby affecting insulin-signaling and protein-synthesis pathways that occur when insulin binds to cell receptors.

Zinc has several other diverse roles. For example, basal metabolic rate may be influenced by zinc; a decrease in thyroid hormones and basal metabolic rate has been observed in individuals receiving a zinc-restricted diet. Zinc is also important for taste; it is a component of gustin, a protein involved in taste acuity.

Finally, zinc is important for cell survival and immune function. Zinc deficiency affects both cell-mediated and humoral immunity. The literature in this area is extensive, but an example of one of the effects of zinc is illustrated through its actions on thymulin, a zinc-dependent hormone peptide that binds to T-cells and promotes their differentiation and functions (including cytokine release). T-cells are critical to immune system function and with zinc deficiency, thymulin activity diminishes and profoundly affects T-cell numbers and functions, and pre-T-cell apoptosis (programmed cell death) [8]. The relationship between immunity and zinc has led many to use zinc to self-treat colds. However, a meta-analysis of the use of zinc supplements (taken orally as a lozenge, or as a nasal spray or gel) for the treatment of colds suggested study findings were inconclusive [9–13]. Given these equivocal findings, the known side effects of excessive zinc consumption (see the "Toxicity" section), and the increased likelihood of exceeding recommended zinc intake when taking cold-remedy zinc supplements, caution should be exercised if taking these products.

Although many functions of zinc are known, many others are not. The effects of zinc deficiency on the body fail to explain fully the manifestations of zinc deprivation.

Interactions with Other Nutrients

Substances that interact with zinc in the gastrointestinal tract to inhibit its absorption have been addressed in the section on absorption. Other types of interactions between zinc and selected nutrients are presented here.

Zinc and vitamin A interact in a couple of ways. From the discussion on zinc functions, you may remember that zinc is required for alcohol dehydrogenase structure and activity. Retinol (the alcohol form of vitamin A) serves as a substrate for this enzyme, which converts retinol to retinal (retinaldehyde), the aldehyde form of vitamin A. This metabolism of the vitamin is necessary for its function in the body. In addition, zinc is necessary for the hepatic synthesis of retinol-binding protein, which transports vitamin A in the blood. Zinc deficiency is associated with both decreased mobilization of retinol from the liver (even with adequate liver vitamin A stores) as well as decreased plasma retinol-binding protein concentrations.

The detrimental effect of excessive zinc intake on copper absorption is thought to be attributable to zinc's stimulation of the synthesis of metallothionein, which has a higher affinity for copper than for zinc. With increased intestinal concentrations of metallothionein induced by high zinc levels, copper ingested in foods readily binds to the metallothionein within the enterocyte and becomes "trapped," preventing its passage into the plasma. The danger of copper deficiency precipitated by zinc supplementation has led to the recommendation of a Tolerable Upper Intake Level for elemental zinc of 40 mg daily [14].

Diminished calcium absorption has been observed with the ingestion of zinc supplements when calcium intake is low (<300 mg/day of calcium) [15]. However, calcium absorption appears to be unaffected by zinc when calcium intake is at adequate (recommended) levels.

Cadmium, if present in high concentrations in the body, appears to bind to sites to which zinc would normally bind and thus disrupts normal zinc functions. For example, cadmium can replace zinc in zinc fingers, preventing the fingers from functioning as they would with zinc present.

Excretion

There are three routes of zinc loss from the body including the:

- gastrointestinal tract
- kidneys
- skin

Most zinc (up to 80%) is lost from the body through the gastrointestinal tract in the feces; the amount lost in the feces may be increased or decreased depending on body zinc concentrations, although absorption is also regulated to control the body's overall zinc content. Zinc in the feces comes from unabsorbed dietary zinc, sloughed intestinal cells, and endogenous sources (such as zinc-containing metalloproteins secreted by the salivary glands, intestinal mucosa, pancreas [main source], and liver into the gastrointestinal tract), which may be adjusted depending upon how much zinc has been absorbed. The purposeful intestinal excretion of zinc, for example, can be accomplished by ZIP5, which facilitates the movement of zinc from the blood across the basolateral membrane and into the enterocyte, followed by the action of ZnT6 on the enterocyte's brush border membrane, which mediates the exocytosis of zinc from the intestinal cell into the lumen for excretion in the feces.

In contrast to intestinal zinc losses, renal and skin (dermal) losses of zinc, as well as zinc losses in semen and menses, are relatively constant and small. Most zinc filtered by the kidneys is reabsorbed by the tubules. ZnT1 is thought to control renal zinc resorption. About 0.3 to 0.7 mg of zinc/day is typically excreted in the urine. The zinc appearing in the urine is believed to be derived from the small percentage of plasma zinc that is complexed with histidine and cysteine. Zinc losses of ~0.4 to 0.6 mg/day occur with exfoliation of skin and with sweating. Other minor routes of zinc loss include (for men) semen (0.1 mg/day) and (for women) menses (0.1 mg/day). Hair contains ~0.1 to 0.2 mg zinc/g of hair [14].

Recommended Dietary Allowance

Zinc recommendations are based on the intake needed to maintain balance as well as on estimates of zinc absorption and body losses. Total daily zinc losses for adult men and women were calculated at 3.84 mg and 3.3 mg, respectively [14]. Zinc losses for men consisted of 0.63 mg urinary zinc, 0.54 mg integuemental and sweat zinc, 0.1 mg semen zinc, and 2.57 mg endogenous intestinal zinc; for women, urinary zinc losses were 0.44 mg, integuemental and sweat zinc losses were 0.46 mg, menses zinc losses were 0.1 mg, and endogenous intestinal zinc losses were 2.3 mg [14]. To account for absorption, the daily requirements for zinc for adult men and women were set at 9.4 mg and 6.8 mg, respectively, and the RDAs were set at 11 mg and 8 mg, respectively. The RDA for zinc during pregnancy is 11 mg/day to cover the calculated need for growth of the fetus and placenta [14]. The zinc recommendation for lactating women is 12 mg/day [14]. The inside front cover of the book provides additional RDAs for zinc for other age groups.

Deficiency

Signs and symptoms of zinc deficiency observed in children are growth retardation (caused by inadequate cell division needed for growth), skeletal abnormalities (from impaired development of epiphyseal cartilage, or defective collagen synthesis or cross-linking), poor wound healing, diarrhea, skin rash/lesions/dermatitis (especially around body orifices), and delayed sexual maturation. Some signs and symptoms of deficiency in adults include anorexia, diarrhea, lethargy, depression, skin rash/lesions/dermatits, hypogeusia (blunting of sense of taste), alopecia (hair loss), and impaired immune function, protein synthesis, and wound healing.

Some population groups—especially the elderly, children of low income, vegetarians, and those with alcoholism—have been found to consume less than adequate amounts of zinc. Conditions associated with an increased need for intake include trauma, sickle cell anemia, and malabsorption.

Toxicity

Excessive intakes of zinc cause toxicity. An acute zinc toxicity (such as from 4 g of zinc gluconate, which provides 570 mg of elemental zinc) produces some of the following symptoms: metallic taste, headache, nausea, vomiting, epigastric pain, abdominal cramps, and bloody diarrhea. In addition, reduced immune function and alterations in copper and iron status may occur. Chronic ingestion of zinc in amounts of about 40 mg (lower for some people) results in a copper deficiency (see the "Interactions with Other Nutrients" section) as well as neurologic problems such as numbness, weakness, ataxia, and spastic gait [14]. Zinc used intranasally (spray or gel) has been reported to cause anosmia (permanent loss of smell) in some individuals. The Tolerable Upper Intake Level for zinc has been set at 40 mg daily based on its interaction with copper [14].

Assessment of Nutriture

Evaluating zinc nutriture is difficult, owing to homeostatic control of body zinc. A variety of indices have been used to assess zinc status, including measurements of zinc in red blood cells, leukocytes, neutrophils, and plasma or serum. The most common basis for assessment is serum or plasma zinc, with fasting concentrations less than about 70 µg/dL (10 µmol/L) suggesting deficiency. Low fasting plasma zinc concentrations indicate that little zinc is present in the exchangeable zinc pool and may reflect a loss of tissue zinc (especially from the liver). Plasma zinc concentrations, however, must be interpreted with caution because concentrations are influenced by many factors unrelated to zinc depletion, including meals, time of day (diurnal variation), stress, infection, and medications such as steroid therapy. In fact, postprandial (after eating) plasma zinc concentrations have been found to be more sensitive to low dietary zinc intake than fasting plasma zinc concentrations.

Metallothionein also has been used to assess zinc status. Concentrations of metallothionein respond to changes in dietary zinc. For example, liver and red blood cell metallothionein concentrations diminish as dietary zinc intake decreases and are thought to reflect zinc status or stores. Serum zinc and serum metallothionein concentrations can be used to indicate poor zinc status if both are low. Elevations in serum metallothionein coupled with low serum zinc, however, usually suggest an acute-phase response, and in such conditions these indices are not reliable.

Urinary zinc excretion remains fairly constant over a range of intakes and is thought to be a useful marker of status in those with moderate to severe zinc deficiency [15]. Low hair zinc may be associated with chronic intake of dietary zinc in suboptimal amounts; however, the concentration of zinc in hair depends not only upon delivery of zinc to the root but also on the rate of hair growth, which is affected by other conditions (including protein status).

Measurement of the activity of zinc-dependent enzymes also has been employed as an index of zinc status. Studies using enzymes as indicators typically have measured carbonic anhydrase or alkaline phosphatase, which "hold" zinc less securely than other zinc metalloenzymes. Ideally, measurements of activity should be taken before and after zinc supplementation.

References Cited for Zinc

1. King JC. Does zinc absorption reflect status? Int J Vitam Nutr Res. 2010; 80:300–06.
2. Walker CF, Kordas K, Stoltzfus RJ, Black RE. Interactive effects of iron and zinc on biochemical and functional outcomes in supplementation trials. Am J Clin Nutr. 2005; 82:5–12.
3. Kordas K, Stoltzfus RJ. New evidence of iron and zinc interplay at the enterocyte and neural tissues. J Nutr. 2004; 134:1295–98.
4. McKenna A, Ilich J, Andon M, et al. Zinc balance in adolescent females consuming a low- or high-calcium diet. Am J Clin Nutr. 1997; 65:1460–64.
5. Dawson-Hughes B, Seligson FH, Hughes VA. Effects of calcium carbonate and hydroxyapatite on zinc and iron retention in postmenopausal women. Am J Clin Nutr. 1986; 44:83–88.
6. Wood R, Zheng J. High dietary calcium intakes reduce zinc absorption and balance in humans. Am J Clin Nutr. 1997; 65:1803–09.
7. Lukaski H. Low dietary zinc decreases erythrocyte carbonic anhydrase activities and impairs cardiorespiratory function in men during exercise. Am J Clin Nutr. 2005; 81:1045–51.
8. Fraker P. Roles for cell death in zinc deficiency. J Nutr. 2005; 135:359–62.
9. Marshall I. Zinc for the common cold. Cochrane Database Systematic Review. 1999; (2); CD001364.
10. Turner RB. Ineffectiveness of intranasal zinc gluconate for prevention of experimental rhinovirus colds. Clin Infect Dis. 2001; 33:1865–70.
11. Turner RB, Cetnarowski W. Effect of treatment with zinc gluconate or zinc acetate on experimental and natural colds. Clin Infect Dis. 2000; 31:1202–08.
12. Prasad AS, Fitzgerald J, Bao B, et al. Duration of symptoms and plasma cytokine levels in patients with common cold treated with zinc acetate: a randomized double-blind, placebo- controlled trial. Ann Intern Med. 2000; 133:245–52.
13. Hirt M, Nobel S, Barron E. Zinc nasal gel for treatment of common cold symptoms: a double-blind, placebo-controlled trial. Ear Nose Throat J. 2000; 79:778–80.
14. Food and Nutrition Board, Institute of Medicine. Dietary Reference Intakes. Washington, DC: National Academy Press. 2001 pp. 442–501.
15. Spencer H. Mineral and mineral interactions in human beings. J Am Diet Assoc. 1986; 86:864–67.
16. Lowe NM, Fekete K, Decsi T. Methods of assessment of zinc status in humans: a systemic review. Am J Clin Nutr. 2009; 89(suppl):S2040–51.

Suggested Readings

Bellayr IH, Mu X, Li Y. Biochemical insights into the role of matrix metalloproteinases in regeneration: challenges and recent developments. Future Med Chem. 2009; 1:1095–1111.
Cousins RJ. Gastrointestinal factors influencing zinc absorption and homeostasis. Int J Vitam Nutr Res. 2010; 80:243–48.
Landsdown ABG, Mirastschijski U, Stubbs N, et al. Zinc in wound healing: theoretical, experimental, and clinical aspects. Wound Rep Reg. 2007; 15:2–16.
Klug A. The discovery of zinc fingers and their development for practical applications in gene regulation and genome manipulation. Quart Rev Biophys. 2010; 43:1–21.
Maret W, Sandstead HH. Zinc requirements and the risks and benefits of zinc supplementation. J Trace Elem Med Biol. 2006; 20:3–18.
Toth K. Zinc in neutrotransmission. Ann Rev Nutr. 2011; 31:139–53.
Wang X, Zhou B. Dietary zinc absorption: a play of Zips and ZnTs in the gut. Life 2010; 62:176–82.

Web Site for Nutrient Composition Information

http://www.ars.usda.gov/Services/docs.htm?docid=18877

COPPER

The copper content of the human body ranges from about 50 to 150 mg. Copper is found in all body tissues and most secretions. In the aqueous environment of the body, copper is found in either of two valence states, the cuprous state (Cu^{1+}) or cupric state (Cu^{2+}).

Sources

The copper content of food varies widely, reflecting the origin of the food and the conditions under which the food was produced, handled, and prepared for use. The richest sources of copper are meats (especially organ meats like liver) and shellfish (especially oysters and lobster), as shown in Table 13.5. Plant food sources rich in copper include nuts (especially cashews), seeds, legumes, and dried fruits. Potatoes, whole grains, and cocoa also are good sources. In contrast, milk and dairy products are poor sources of the mineral. In the United States, the median copper intake from foods by adults ranges from about 1,000 to 1,600 μg/day [1]. The Daily Value for copper (used on food and supplement labels) is 2 mg (over twice the recommended intake of the mineral).

The main form of copper found in mineral-fortified food products and supplements is copper sulfate; however, cupric oxide is also found in some supplements. The use of cupric oxide as a source of copper is discouraged because the copper has been shown to be unavailable for absorption from the gastrointestinal tract of animals; in fact, it is no longer used as a copper supplement in animal nutrition [2]. In addition to copper sulfate (~25% copper), other bioavailable forms of copper include cupric chloride (~47% copper), cupric acetate (~35% copper), and copper carbonate (~57% copper) [2].

Table 13.5 Copper Content of Selected Foods

Food/Food Group	Copper (mg)	Food/Food Group	Copper (mg)
Seafood		Meat and poultry	
Oysters (3 oz)	6.4	Liver, beef (3 oz)	12.4
Crabmeat (3 oz)	1.0	Chicken (3 oz)	0.04 – 0.07
Lobster (3 oz)	1.6	Beef, ground (3 oz)	0.07
Salmon (3 oz)	0.05	Pork (3 oz)	0.06 – 0.14
Eggs and dairy products		Legumes (cooked, 1 cup)	0.35 – 0.61
Egg (1)	0.007	Nuts (1 oz)	0.11 – 0.45
Milk (1 cup)	0.02–0.06	Fruits	0.02 – 0.09
Cheeses (1 oz)	0.007–0.12	Vegetables (cooked, 1 cup)	0.02 – 0.06
Grains and cereals		Potato (1 baked)	0.335
Rice and pasta (cooked, 1 cup)	0.14–0.20	Other, cocoa powder (1 Tbsp)	0.2
Bread white/whole-wheat (1 slice)	0.06/0.11		

Source: USDA.

Copper from endogenous sources is also found in and absorbed from the gastrointestinal tract. Relatively large amounts of copper are secreted daily into the gastrointestinal tract in digestive juices. For example, the copper contents of saliva and gastric juice are ~400 μg and 1,000 μg, respectively; pancreatic and duodenal juices may contain up to 1,300 μg and 2,200 μg, respectively [3]. This re-use of copper is important to the body's copper homeostasis.

Digestion, Absorption, Transport, and Storage

Figure 13.13 provides an overview of copper digestion, absorption, and transport as well as some of copper's fates in the enterocyte.

Digestion

Most copper in foods is found as Cu^{2+} and is bound to organic components, especially amino acids that make up food proteins. Thus, digestion is needed to free the bound copper before absorption can occur. Gastric hydrochloric acid and pepsin facilitate the release of bound copper in the stomach. Additional proteolytic enzymes in the small intestine hydrolyze proteins further to release copper.

Absorption

Copper is absorbed primarily in its reduced (cuprous/Cu^{1+}) state from the proximal small intestine, especially the duodenum. While a small amount may be absorbed from the stomach, gastric copper absorption is thought to contribute relatively little to the overall absorption of the mineral.

The reduction of copper (from Cu^{2+} to Cu^{1+}) may occur in the acidic environment of the stomach, but more likely results from the action of one or more reductases, including cytochrome b ferric/cupric reductase, six-transmembrane epithelial antigen of the prostate (steap) 2, and/or cytochrome b reductase 1 found on

intestinal cell membranes. Vitamin C also may facilitate the reduction.

Copper absorption across the enterocyte's brush border membrane is accomplished by one or more carrier proteins. One such carrier is copper transporter (Ctr) 1 (also designated hCtr1), which transports copper in its Cu^{1+} state. Ctr1 is found not only on the enterocyte's brush border membrane, but also associated with vesicles in the cytosol of intestinal cells; it is also found on most extra-intestinal cell membranes to facilitate copper uptake. Synthesis of Ctr1 appears to be regulated by the transcription factor Sp1 and is responsive to the body's copper status. However, the mechanism by which body copper influences Sp1 and Ctr1 synthesis is not clear at present.

In addition to Ctr1, divalent mineral (cation) transporter 1 (DMT1 or DCT1) also serves as a copper transporter, specifically cotransporting (symporting) Cu^{1+} and H^+ across the enterocyte's brush border membrane. Competition between iron and copper for enterocyte brush border membrane absorption using DMT1 has been suggested [4,5]. Additional, but as of yet unidentified, copper transporters may also facilitate intestinal copper absorption.

Typically, the gastrointestinal tract absorbs about 50% to 80% of ingested copper. Fractional absorption of copper increases as copper intake decreases, and vice versa. Absorption, for example, may average about 20% when copper intake is high, such as >5 mg/day, but increases to over 50% when intake is <1 mg/day [3–6]. Copper absorption was calculated at 75% with an intake of 350 μg of copper, an amount that is about one-half of an adult's requirement for the mineral [1].

Factors Influencing Copper Absorption

Copper transport across the enterocyte's brush border membrane may be influenced by a variety of dietary components, with some having a positive effect and others exerting a negative influence on absorption.

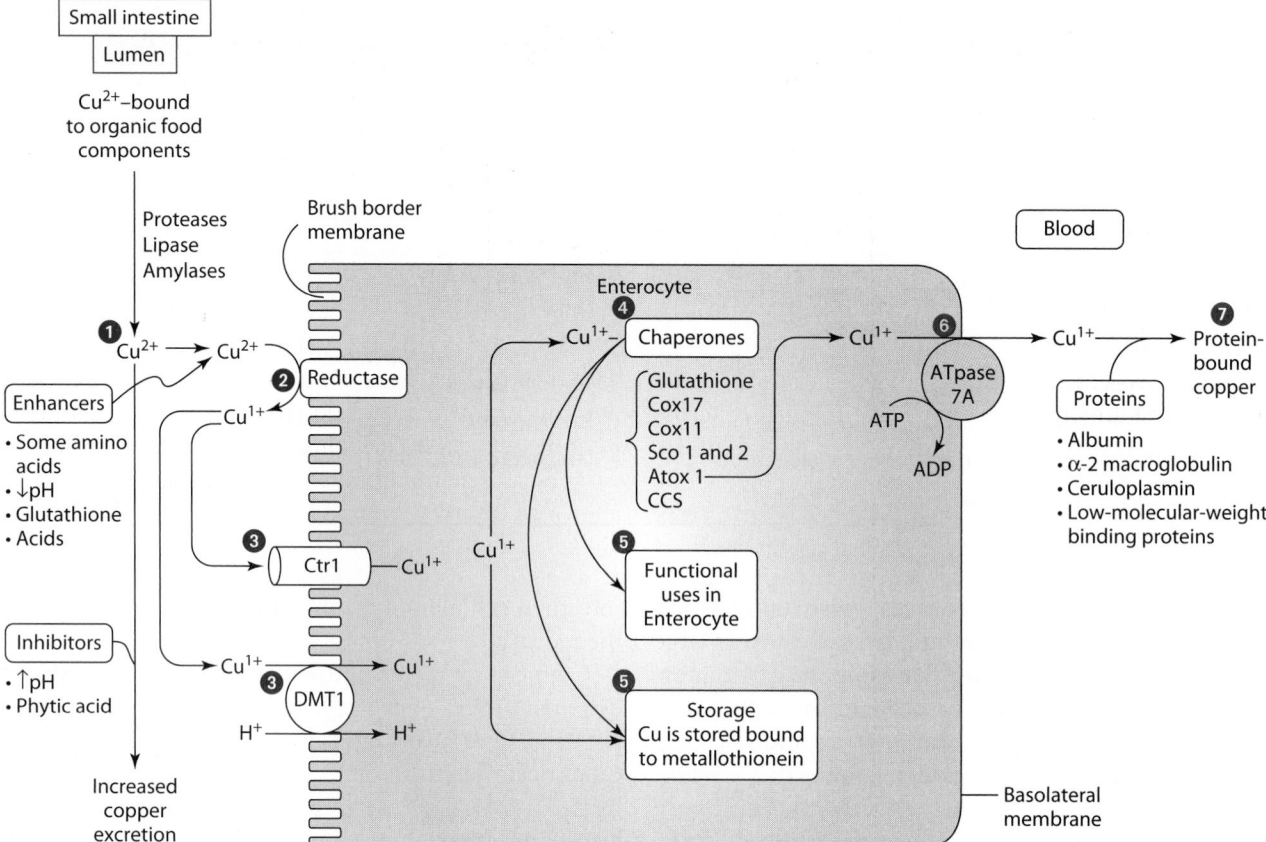

Figure 13.13 Overview of copper digestion, absorption, enterocyte use, and transport.

❶ Cu^{2+} is released from food components.

❷ Copper is reduced to Cu^{1+}, most likely by cytochrome b ferric/cupric reductase, cytochrome b reductase 1, and/or steap2.

❸ Cu^{1+} crosses the brush border membrane by a high-affinity Ctr1 transporter, and to a lesser extent by DMT1. Amino acid transporters (not shown) may play a minor role.

❹ Within the cytosol, copper binds to one of several chaperones for transport and delivery to target enzymes. Atox1 transports Cu^{1+} to the basolateral membrane.

❺ Copper is delivered to enzymes by chaperones to enable its use in the cells, or it binds to metallothionein for storage.

❻ ATP7A transports Cu^{1+} across the basolateral membrane. A defect in this ATPase causes Menkes' disease.

❼ Copper attaches to proteins for transport in the blood.

Enhancers of Copper Absorption Examples of ligands or chelators that facilitate copper absorption include amino acids, especially histidine and cysteine. Whether copper bound to these amino acids can be absorbed through amino acid carrier systems is not clear. Copper also forms ligands with sulfhydryl groups in cysteine residues that are found within the tripeptide glutathione. Glutathione is found both within the lumen of the gastrointestinal tract and intracellularly.

The presence of organic acids in foods also improves copper absorption. Citric, gluconic, lactic, acetic, and malic acids act as binding ligands to improve solubilization and thus absorption of copper. Citric acid, for example, forms a stable complex with copper and improves its absorption. A more acidic environment, as found in the proximal intestine versus the distal intestine, also favors copper absorption.

Inhibitors of Copper Absorption Just as an acidic environment facilitates copper absorption, the opposite is true of an alkaline environment. Excessive antacid ingestion or the use of medications such as H_2 receptor blockers (such as Zantac [ranitidine], Tagamet [cimetidine], or Pepcid [famotidine]), and proton pump blockers (such as Prevacid [lansoprazole] or Prilosec [omeprazole]), which are commonly taken to treat heartburn, gastroesophageal reflux disease, and ulcers, results in a high-pH (more alkaline) environment and can diminish copper absorption. Copper atoms in an alkaline medium often bind to hydroxides (OH), forming insoluble compounds that are not readily absorbable. In addition to these pH effects, substances found in foods may bind to copper to diminish its absorption.

Phytic acid (Figure 13.10), found mainly in plant foods (cereals, legumes), is a known inhibitor of the absorption of copper (among other minerals, including iron, zinc, and calcium). Most individuals in the United States, however, do not consume enough phytic acid to negatively affect copper status.

Zinc can also impede copper absorption. The use of zinc supplements, typically in amounts of about 40 mg or more, has been shown to impair copper absorption and diminish copper status. The detrimental effect of excessive zinc intake on copper absorption is thought to result from zinc's stimulation of metallothionein synthesis in intestinal cells. Although its synthesis is stimulated by zinc, metallothionein more avidly binds copper than zinc, and thus reduces copper's luminal-to-serosal flux (i.e., from the lumen of the gastrointestinal tract across the basolateral membrane) and entry into the blood. Copper deficiency induced by high zinc intake can be difficult to correct. For example, when zinc (110–165 mg) supplements were taken for 10 months, discontinuation of the zinc and 2 months of oral copper supplementation failed to correct the copper deficiency. Intravenous administration of cupric chloride for 5 days (total dose of 10 mg) was needed to bypass the intestinal cells and correct the deficiency, suggesting that the correction of a zinc-induced copper deficiency is a slow process [7].

The effects of supplemental iron and/or iron fortification on copper absorption remain unclear, with conflicting reports depending on the forms and amounts of the nutrients provided, and the populations being studied.

Intestinal Cell Copper Use

Once within the enterocyte, copper is bound to amino acids (especially histidine and cysteine), glutathione (a tripeptide composed of glycine, cysteine, and glutamate, which transports Cu^{1+}), and/or proteins/chaperones. Like iron, free copper ions may damage cells through nonenzymatic reactions (see the "Other Roles" section). Consequently, copper is usually found attached to compounds within the body.

Copper entering the enterocyte has several possible fates. The copper may be:

- stored or sequestered in the enterocyte, or
- used functionally within the enterocyte, or
- transported through the cytosol and across the basolateral membrane for entry into the blood and thus use by other tissues

Copper can be stored temporarily within enterocytes (and other cells) in cytosolic vesicles; the protein Ctr2 serves to transport copper out of the cell cytosol and into cytosolic vesicles for temporary storage. Storage of copper also occurs as part of the protein metallothionein (discussed further in the "Storage" section). While metallothionein may in some cases only temporarily hold onto the copper, the copper, if not released from metallothionein, will be lost into the feces with intestinal cell turnover, approximately every 2 to 3 days. Copper's uses in the intestinal cell are similar to its uses in the body and are discussed in the "Functions and Mechanisms of Action" section.

Copper transport across the intestinal cell's basolateral membrane occurs primarily via active transport as Cu^{1+} by the ATPase ATP7A. ATP7A is expressed in most body cells with the exception of hepatocytes, which express a similar transporter, ATP7B. Mutations in the ATP7A gene result in Menkes' disease, an X-linked disorder characterized by defective copper efflux from cells. People with Menkes' disease have increased intestinal cell copper concentrations and impaired delivery of copper to peripheral tissues. The condition is also characterized by vascular and neurological problems that are only partially alleviated by intravenous administration of copper. Individuals with Menkes' disease typically die within the first few years of life.

Transport

From the intestinal cells, copper is transported in portal blood to the liver bound loosely to the proteins albumin (specifically the amino [N]-terminus of albumin) and α-2 macroglobulin (which binds two copper atoms and may have a higher affinity for the mineral than albumin) [8]. Amino acids are not thought to contribute to copper transport in the blood [8].

The uptake of copper into the liver (and other tissues) occurs by multiple carrier proteins, including Ctr1; however, Ctr2 (which has been identified on the plasma membrane of some cells), DMT1, and likely unidentified carriers also may be involved in cellular copper uptake [8]. Reduction of copper from the Cu^{2+} to the Cu^{1+} state, which is needed for carrier transport, is likely facilitated by reductases on cellular membranes. Ascorbic acid, once thought to facilitate copper uptake, did not enhance cellular copper uptake from α-2 macroglobulin [8].

Once within the cytosol of hepatocytes, copper first appears to bind to glutathione and/or metallothionein and then is thought to be transferred to chaperones, which carry the copper to copper-requiring enzymes; however, copper may directly bind to the chaperones. Copper chaperones are soluble intracellular proteins that bind intracellular copper and deliver it to various, but specific, locations following cellular copper uptake. The chaperone atox1 transports Cu^{1+} to the trans-Golgi network, where ATP7B directs the copper for insertion into ceruloplasmin (as well as other cuproenzymes). Six copper ions (as Cu^{1+} and Cu^{2+}) are attached posttranslationally to form ceruloplasmin. Three of the six copper atoms are involved in electron transfer, and the other three function at ceruloplamin's catalytic site (and give the protein a blue color). Although copper does not appear to influence ceruloplasmin synthesis, ceruloplasmin activity is diminished without sufficient copper, and ceruloplasmin's half-life is shortened.

Ceruloplasmin is released into the blood from the liver and constitutes about 60% to 70% of circulating copper in the blood; the remainder circulates loosely bound to albumin and α-2 macroglobulin for delivery to tissues. Plasma ceruloplasmin concentrations typically range from about 20 to 50 mg/dL; serum copper concentrations normally range from about 70 to 150 μg/dL (10–24 μmol/L).

Ceruloplasmin delivers copper (but not the copper found at its active oxidase site) to tissues after binding to specific membrane receptors. Reduction of Cu^{2+} to Cu^{1+} is likely accomplished by reductases present on cell membranes and enables cellular copper uptake using Ctr1 or other plasma cell membrane carriers [9].

Storage

The liver is the main organ that stores copper and that controls copper homeostasis in the body. However, compared to other trace minerals, relatively little copper (up to about 150 mg) is found in the body. On a percentage basis, the skeleton followed by muscles and then the liver contains the most copper; on an absolute basis, the organs with the most copper per gram are the kidneys, liver, brain, and skeleton. Within cells, copper is stored bound to the protein metallothionein. Metallothionein stores 12 copper atoms (as well as zinc atoms) per molecule; it is also thought to regulate cellular zinc distribution and to scavenge free hydroxyl radicals, thereby acting in an antioxidant capacity. Copper positively influences hepatic and renal, but not intestinal, metallothionein synthesis. The mechanism by which copper influences metallothionein synthesis is not well defined.

Functions and Mechanisms of Action

The essentiality of copper is due, in part, to its participation as an enzyme cofactor, either at the enzyme's active site (perhaps as an intermediate in electron transfer) or at the enzyme's allosteric regulatory site. Before addressing the coenzyme roles of copper, a brief discussion of copper chaperones is needed because it is the chaperones that function within cells to transport the copper to the specific enzymes in need of copper for their function. In other words, these chaperones direct intracellular trafficking of the mineral. Some of the identified chaperones for copper include:

- Cyclooxygenase (cox) 17 and cox 11
- Sco1 and Sco2
- CCS (copper chaperone for superoxide dismutase)
- Atox1 (also called hAtx or Hah1)

Cox17, found in the cytosol, and cox 11, Sco1, and Sco2, found in the mitochondria, are thought to transport Cu^{1+} for cytochrome c oxidase synthesis. CCS, which is found in the mitochondria and cytosol, appears to deliver Cu^{1+} for the synthesis of superoxide dismutase. Atox1 ferries Cu^{1+} to ATPases ATP7A and ATP7B, which are necessary for cellular export of copper. For example, atox1 transports Cu^{1+} to the trans-Golgi network, where ATP7B then directs it for insertion into cuproenzymes such as ceruloplasmin. Another possible chaperone is murr1, which is also associated with ATP7B in the liver; murr1 is thought to facilitate copper excretion in the bile. This section addresses a few of the body's cuproenzymes (copper-requiring metalloenzymes) and the reactions they catalyze (Table 13.6).

Ceruloplasmin: Ferroxidase and Antioxidant

Ceruloplasmin, a glycoprotein, is not simply a transporter of copper in the blood. It is also a multifaceted oxidative enzyme (oxidase) that is found in the blood and bound to cell surface receptors on the plasma membranes of cells. Ceruloplasmin, also known as ferroxidase I, oxidizes minerals, most notably ferrous (Fe^{2+}) iron but also manganese (Mn^{2+}). Its role in the oxidation of iron (Fe^{2+} to Fe^{3+}) is critical to enable iron to bind to transferrin for transport to the body's tissues.

$$Fe^{2+} \longrightarrow Fe^{3+}$$
$$Ceruloplasmin\text{-}Cu^{2+} \qquad Ceruloplasmin\text{-}Cu^{1+}$$

Another proposed function of ceruloplasmin is as an antioxidant or modulator of the inflammatory process. As modulators of the inflammatory process, acute-phase (also called reactant) proteins like ceruloplasmin increase in the blood in response to severe infections and other inflammatory events (such as injury). This rise in blood levels is important because during infections, for

Table 13.6 Selected Functions of Copper

Ceruloplasmin: iron oxidation and antioxidant
Superoxide dismutase: antioxidant
Cytochrome c oxidase: ATP production
Amine oxidases: oxidation of biogenic amines
Lysyl oxidase: collagen and elastin cross-linking
Dopamine monooxygenase/hydroxylase: norepinephrine (catecholamine) synthesis
Tyrosinase: melanin pigment production
p-hydroxyphenylpyruvate hydroxylase: tyrosine degradation
Peptidylglycine α-amidating monooxygenase: activation of selected hormones
Factors V and VIII: blood clotting
Immune function
Gene expression

example, phagocytosis of invading organisms by white blood cells generates superoxide radicals, among other damaging compounds. These compounds, while normally produced by cells, are generated in larger amounts with infections and inflammation and must be eliminated (by ceruloplasmin, superoxide dismutase, or other enzymes) to prevent excessive damage to body cells.

Superoxide Dismutase: Antioxidant

Superoxide dismutase (SOD) is a copper- and zinc-dependent enzyme (although another form in the mitochondria is manganese dependent). In the enzyme, copper and zinc are linked to the enzyme by an imidiazole group, and histidine and aspartate residues. Copper (Cu^{2+}) is found at the enzyme's active site, where the superoxide substrate binds to the enzyme. Removal of copper, but not zinc, results in reduced cytosolic superoxide dismutase activity. Specifically, superoxide dismutase catalyzes the removal (dismutation) of the superoxide radicals ($O_2^{\bullet}$). During the reaction, copper is reduced along with the oxygen radical to initially generate molecular oxygen (O_2) and then, by reoxidation, hydrogen peroxide (H_2O_2).

$$2O_2^{\bullet} + 2H^+ \xrightarrow{\text{Superoxide dismutase}} O_2 + H_2O_2$$

Superoxide radicals along with other free radicals can cause peroxidative damage to the phospholipid component of cell membranes, especially disrupting unsaturated double bonds in fatty acids, as well as damaging other cellular components. Superoxide dismutase therefore assumes an important protective function. The enzyme is found in the cytosol of most cells of the body and in extracellular locations. Extracellular superoxide dismutase is found in the blood and other body fluids (e.g., lymph, synovial fluid, lungs); it is also secreted and bound to heparan sulfate on the surface of cells and is found in relatively large concentrations in the arterial wall. Increased peroxidation of cell membranes is observed with copper deficiency.

Cytochrome c Oxidase: Energy Production

Cytochrome c oxidase contains three copper atoms per molecule. One subunit of the enzyme contains two copper atoms and functions to receive electrons from cytochrome c and then transfer the electrons to the second subunit. The second subunit contains another copper atom and is involved in reducing molecular oxygen and ultimately in energy production. Cytochrome c oxidase functions in the terminal oxidative step in mitochondrial electron transport (Figure 3.25). It is when the enzyme transfers an electron so that molecular oxygen (O_2) is reduced to form water molecules that enough free energy is generated to permit ATP production. Severe copper deficiency impairs the activity of this enzyme.

Amine Oxidases (Monoamine and Diamine Oxidases): Biogenic Amine Oxidation

Amine oxidases are also copper dependent. Copper appears to function as an allosteric structural component of these enzymes. Histidine residues in the enzyme serve as ligands for the copper; TOPA quinone (6-hydroxydopa) serves as the enzyme's cofactor. Amine oxidases, including monoamine and diamine oxidases, are found both in the blood and in body tissues. The enzymes catalyze the oxidation of biogenic amines, such as tyramine, histamine, and dopamine, as well as serotonin (5-hydroxytryptamine), norepinephrine, and polyamines, to form aldehydes and ammonium ions (NH_4 is generated from the cleaved amine group). In the reaction, oxygen (O_2) is reduced to form hydrogen peroxide (H_2O_2). Because of the wide range of biogenic amines oxidized by copper-dependent amine oxidases, suboptimal copper status can result in a broad range of neurological and physiological manifestations.

$$RCH_2NH_2 \xrightarrow[\text{Amine oxidase}]{O_2 \quad H_2O_2} RCH{=}O + {}^+NH_4$$

Lysyl Oxidase: Collagen Synthesis

Lysyl oxidase, secreted by connective tissue cells (bone, blood vessels, etc.), generates cross-links between connective tissue proteins, including collagen and elastin. Specifically, lysyl oxidase catalyzes the removal (oxidative deamination) of the epsilon (ε) amino group of lysyl and hydroxylysyl residues of a collagen and elastin polypeptide and the oxidation of the terminal carbon atom of an aldehyde to form cross-links. The cross-linking is needed to stabilize the extracellular matrix. Lysyl oxidase activity decreases with inadequate copper intake, negatively affecting the strength of connective tissues [10]. While lysyl oxidase is an amine oxidase, it is listed separately from the previous section because of its different physiological role in the body.

Dopamine Monooxygenase/Hydroxylase, Tyrosinase, and p-hydroxyphenylpyruvate Hydroxylase: Tyrosine Metabolism and Pigment Synthesis

In tyrosine metabolism (Figure 6.10), norepinephrine, melanin pigments, and homogentisic acid production are all copper dependent. Norepinephrine synthesis, which occurs mainly in the adrenal medulla and neurons, begins with tyrosine, which is converted in an iron-dependent reaction to 3,4-dihydroxyphenylalanine (also called L-dopa). The L-dopa is then decarboxylated to form dopamine. To synthesize norepinephrine from dopamine, the enzyme dopamine monooxygenase/hydroxylase, which contains up to eight copper atoms per molecule, is required for the hydroxylation reaction as shown. Norepinephrine functions in the body as both a hormone and neurotransmitter, affecting a wide range of physiological processes.

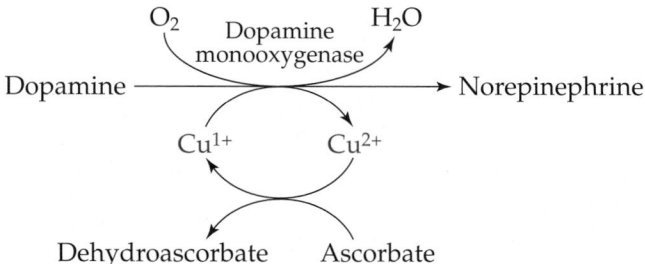

While in some cells L-dopa is used to form dopamine, in melanocytes, which are found in the epidermal layer of skin and in the eyes and hair, L-dopa can be oxidized by the copper-dependent enzyme tyrosinase (also called catechol oxidase) to produce dopaquinones. The dopaquinones then polymerize to form pigments called melanin. Melanin provides color to the iris of the eye, skin, and hair. A mutation in the tyrosinase enzyme causes the condition called albinism, which is characterized by lighter than normal skin color, white hair, and light-colored eyes.

In tyrosine catabolism for energy production (Figure 6.10), the conversion of p-hydroxyphenylpyruvate to homogentisate (homogentisic acid) requires the copper-dependent enzyme p-hydroxyphenylpyruvate hydroxylase and vitamin C, as shown.

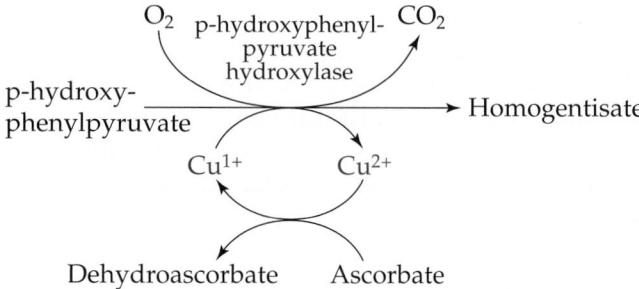

Peptidylglycine α-amidating Monooxygenase: Hormone Activation

Amidation of peptide hormones, such as bombesin, calcitonin, gastrin, and cholecystokinin, is necessary for hormone function. The amidation requires the copper-dependent enzyme peptidylglycine α-amidating monooxygenase, which is found mostly in the brain. This enzyme cleaves a carboxy terminal glycine residue off peptides that have a C-terminal glycine. The amino group of glycine is retained by the peptide as a terminal amide. The oxidized residue is released as glyoxylate. Peptidylglycine α-amidating monooxygenase also requires vitamin C to reduce Cu^{2+} back to Cu^{1+}, and is shown in Figure 9.5.

Because of the divergent roles that these hormones play in the body once activated by amidation, copper indirectly has wide-ranging effects on multiple body processes.

Other Roles

Copper also plays a variety of other roles in the body, some of which are not well characterized. The blood clotting proteins (factors) V and VIII both contain copper atoms. Copper is also involved in angiogenesis, immune system function, nerve myelination, and endorphin action. Copper influences gene expression by binding to specific transcription factors, which in turn bind to promoter sequences on DNA. Once the copper-bound transcription factors interact with DNA, transcription may be enhanced or suppressed. These interactions are not well characterized.

Pro-Oxidant Role

As a pro-oxidant, copper (if free) behaves similarly to iron. Copper reacts with superoxide radicals and catalyzes the formation of hydroxyl radicals through the Fenton reaction: $Cu^{1+} + H_2O_2 \longrightarrow Cu^{2+} + OH^- + {}^\bullet OH$. Associated with the generation of reactive oxygen species is increased oxidative damage to DNA (base oxidation and strand breaks), proteins, and lipids (peroxidation), especially membrane lipids.

Interactions with Other Nutrients

Copper is known to interact with a number of dietary constituents. Those that affect copper absorption have been described previously. Additional interactions with iron and molybdenum that are unrelated to intestinal copper absorption are discussed here.

The importance of copper in normal iron metabolism is evidenced by the anemia that results from prolonged copper deficiency. This anemia is caused by impaired mobilization and use of iron, stemming from the reduced ferroxidase activity of hephaestin in enterocytes and of ceruloplasmin, which is largely responsible for oxidation of iron to its trivalent (Fe^{3+}) state. Remember that iron must be in this oxidized state to bind to its transport protein transferrin for delivery to tissues. With copper deficiency, the activity of ceruloplasmin and the expression of hephaestin are reduced, and iron remains mostly trapped within cells. Thus, copper deficiency results in a secondary iron-deficiency anemia, and treatment with copper (and not iron) is required to correct the problem.

Another nutrient that interacts with copper is molybdenum, which can enhance copper excretion. Urinary copper excretion has been shown to rise as molybdenum intake increases. For example, urinary copper excretion rose from 24 to 77 μg/day as molybdenum intake increased from 160 to 1,540 μg/day [11]. No changes in fecal copper excretion were noted, suggesting that molybdenum may have increased copper mobilization from tissues and promoted excretion [11]. Molybdenum's effect on copper is exploited in the treatment of Wilson's disease (see the "Toxicity" section).

Excretion

Copper is excreted primarily (>95%) through the bile into the feces. In fact, biliary copper excretion is regulated by the liver to maintain copper balance (homeostasis). Thus, with high dietary copper intake, biliary copper excretion via the feces increases, and with low dietary copper intake, fecal copper excretion decreases. At a copper intake of about 1.4 mg/day, fecal copper excretion is about 2.4 mg/day [12].

The ATPase ATP7B plays a major role in copper excretion. With high (excess) concentrations of copper in hepatocytes, copper is directed into cytosolic compartments (vesicles), and ATP7B is translocated from the trans-Golgi network to the hepatocyte's canalicular membrane. The movement of ATP7B is associated with its kinase-dependent phosphorylation, which increases in response to elevations in cellular copper. ATP7B facilitates the exocytosis of the copper-containing vesicles (in a process that involves the chaperone murr1) across the

hepatic canalicular membrane for excretion into the bile (Figure 13.14). Wilson's disease, an inherited disorder of copper metabolism, is characterized by defective biliary copper excretion and thus copper toxicity. The disorder results from a mutation(s) in ATP7B and is discussed further in the "Toxicity" section.

Other minor routes of copper excretion/losses include the urine, sweat and skin cell desquamation, menses (for women), semen (for men), hair, and nails. Copper loss via the urine is small (<60 μg). Urinary copper excretion does not typically change with changes in copper intake except under extreme conditions such as with Wilson's disease [13]. Similarly, only small amounts (<50 μg) of copper are lost in sweat and with desquamation of skin cells. Women experience trace losses of copper in normal menstrual flow; however, a woman's copper status, unlike her iron status, is not compromised by menstruation. Together, losses from menses or semen, along with losses from hair and nails, are not thought to exceed surface losses [1].

Recommended Dietary Allowance

The results of depletion and repletion studies, along with other studies permitting factorial analysis of obligatory losses over a range of intakes, have enabled estimates of

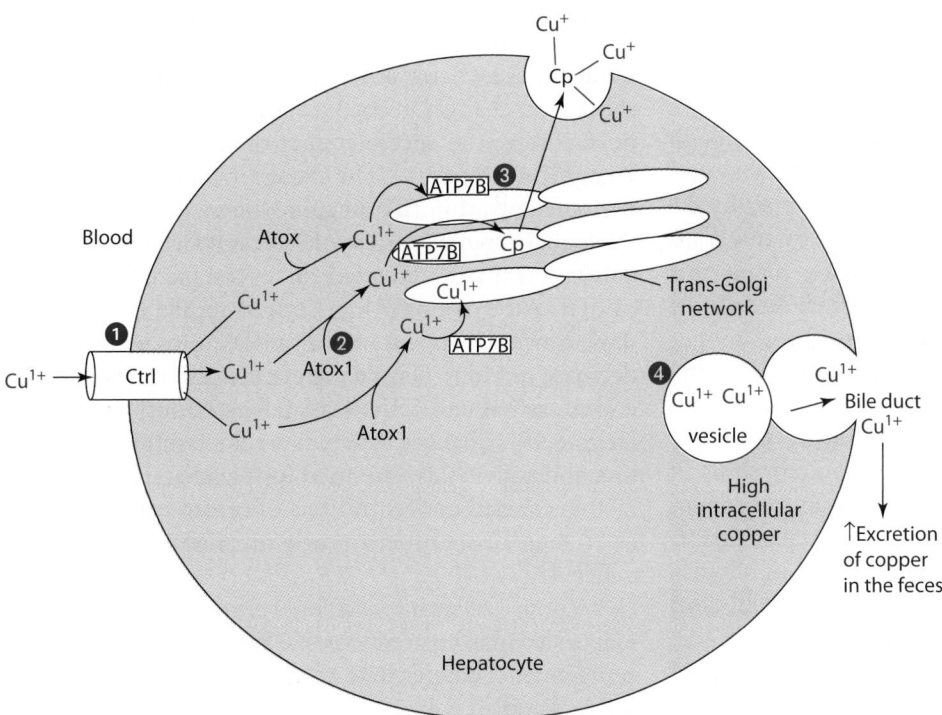

❶ Ctrl transports copper into the hepatocytes from the blood.

❷ Atox1 functions as a chaperone to take Cu^{1+} to the trans-Golgi network.

❸ ATP7B transports Cu^{1+} across the trans-Golgi network membrane and into the Golgi network, where it is incorporated into ceruloplasmin (Cp) and other cuproenzymes.

❹ In the presence of excess copper, ATP7B moves to the canalicular membrane to mediate the secretion of copper from vesicles into the bile duct.

Figure 13.14 The role of ATP7B in copper use and excretion in the liver.

copper requirements. Based on a copper requirement for adults of 700 μg, a 30% coefficient of variation of the requirement, and rounding to the nearest 100 μg, an RDA for copper was set at 900 μg/day [1]. Recommendations during pregnancy and lactation are 1,000 μg and 1,300 μg, respectively [1]. RDAs for copper for other age groups are found on the inside front cover of the book.

Deficiency

Various clinical manifestations are associated with copper deficiency. Most commonly recognized signs and symptoms include anemia, leukopenia (specifically neutropenia, a lower-than-normal number of neutrophils), hypopigmentation or depigmentation of skin and hair, impaired immune function, bone abnormalities, altered cholesterol metabolism, and cardiovascular and pulmonary dysfunction [14]. The likelihood of copper deficiency increases in persons consuming excessive amounts of zinc (40 mg/day). In addition, deficiency is more likely with prolonged use of medications (such as proton pump inhibitors) that diminish copper absorption. Additionally, persons with conditions that promote increased loss of copper from the body, such as the renal disorder nephrosis or gastrointestinal malabsorptive disorders such as celiac disease, Crohn's disease, and ulcerative colitis, are at greater risk of deficiency.

Toxicity

Copper toxicity is fairly rare in the United States, although acute poisonings have occurred because of water contamination and accidental ingestion. A Tolerable Upper Intake Level for copper was set at 10 mg per day by the Food and Nutrition Board [1], although intakes below this level, such as 5 mg, may cause gastrointestinal discomfort in some individuals. Ingestion of a large dose of copper (such as 64 mg elemental copper provided by 250 mg copper sulfate) may cause acute toxicity characterized typically by epigastric pain, nausea, vomiting, diarrhea, weakness, lethargy, and anorexia. Other symptoms of toxicity with prolonged intake of high amounts of copper include hematuria (blood in urine), liver damage resulting in jaundice, and kidney damage resulting in oliguria (little urine production) or anuria (no urine production) [15]. Copper is lethal in amounts about 1,000 times normal dietary intake [16]. Chronic copper ingestion of 30 mg daily for 2 years followed by 60 mg daily for a year resulted in liver failure in a young man who self-prescribed copper supplements [17].

Wilson's disease, a genetic disorder resulting from a mutation(s) in the gene coding for ATP7B, is characterized by copper toxicity. The incidence of the condition is about 1 in 30,000 live births. The most common mutation in Caucasians is C3207A, which disrupts the binding of ATP to the transporter. The absence or dysfunction of ATP7B in turn disrupts copper excretion into the bile and into the secretory pathway for incorporation into cuproenzymes such as ceruloplasmin. Thus, in Wilson's disease, copper accumulates in the liver but also leaks out (unbound, i.e., not as part of ceruloplasmin) into the blood and is deposited in other organs, especially the brain, kidneys, and eyes (cornea). Symptoms usually are not apparent until at least 7 years of age. The copper deposition in the corneas results in Kayser-Fleischer (greenish gold) rings visible in the eyes. Neurologic or psychiatric problems also may occur secondary to copper deposition in the brain. At present, the condition is treated primarily with chelation medications, such as D-penicillamine therapy, to bind body copper and increase its urinary excretion. Avoidance of high-copper foods is recommended. Additionally, zinc supplements (such as 50 mg zinc as zinc acetate or zinc sulfate given three times a day) along with molybdenum supplements (such as thiomolybdate given in six doses of 20 mg each) also may be recommended to decrease intestinal copper absorption and to enhance urinary copper excretion, respectively [18].

Assessment of Nutriture

Copper status is best assessed using multiple indicators. Serum, plasma, or red blood cell copper is frequently used, but these indicators are likely inadequate to assess short-term changes in copper status. The lower end of the normal range for serum copper concentrations is about 70 μg/dL (10 μmol/L). The change in plasma/serum copper concentration that occurs when subjects consume inadequate copper varies considerably between individuals and is further affected by several factors unrelated to diet. An extremely low copper intake (~0.38 mg/day), however, appears to be sufficient to significantly decrease not only plasma copper but also ceruloplasmin concentration and activity as well as urinary copper excretion [19]. Changes in serum ceruloplasmin concentration and activity also are used to assess copper status. In fact, decreased concentrations of serum ceruloplasmin (<20 mg/dL) are often an early manifestation of copper deficiency.

Response of serum ceruloplasmin to copper supplements also may be used to assess copper status. Typically, supplemental copper first normalizes serum copper and the neutrophil count, then serum ceruloplasmin [20]. Ceruloplasmin concentration increases following supplementation only in copper-deficient subjects. Another useful indicator of copper status is measurement of the activity of copper-dependent enzymes such as superoxide dismutase in the red blood cell. Superoxide dismutase activity is sensitive to longer-term copper deficiency [21].

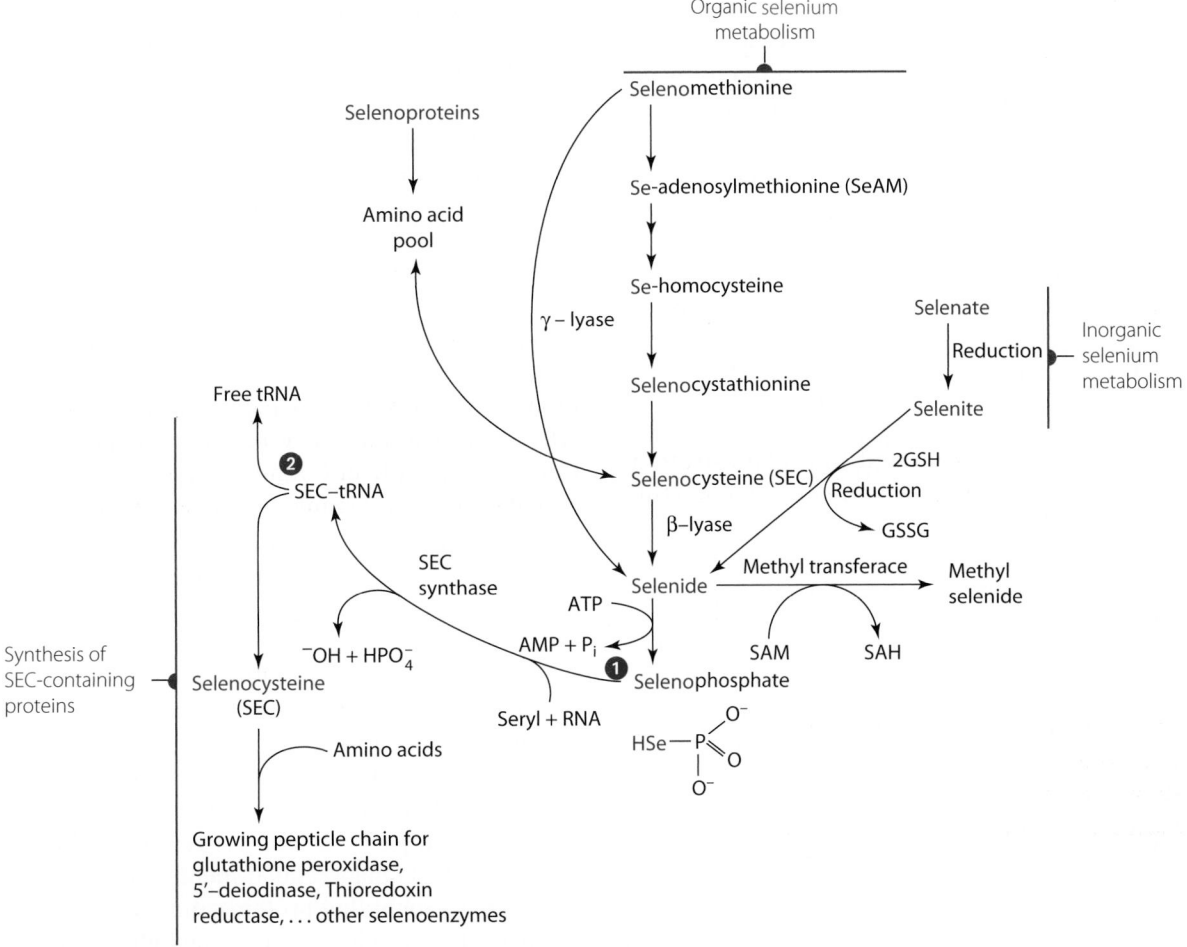

1 Synthesis of selenocysteine-containing proteins begins with selenophosphate and the amino acid serine, which is esterified to a specific transfer (t) RNA to form seryl tRNA^{SEC}. Selenocysteine synthase replaces the hydroxy group of serine with a HSe$^-$ from selenophosphate to form SEC-tRNA^{SEC} (or SEC-tRNA for short).

2 SEC-tRNA delivers selenocysteine to the growing peptide chains of the various SEC-containing proteins like glutathione peroxidase, iodothyronine 5′deiodinase, and thioredoxin reductase, among others.

Figure 13.16 Selenium metabolism.

selenite remains unclear [4]. Selenide may be methylated for excretion or may be utilized to form selenophosphate, which is subsequently used in the synthesis of selenoenzymes, discussed in the "Functions and Mechanisms of Action" section.

Selenomethionine, which is derived from the diet, may be either stored as selenomethionine in an amino acid pool, used for protein synthesis just as the amino acid methionine is used, catabolized in multiple reactions (referred to as trans-selenation) to yield selenocysteine, or directly lysed at the γ-position to generate selenide. This latter reaction is thought to be induced with excessive selenium intakes [1].

Selenocysteine, which is derived either from selenomethionine metabolism or from the diet, is degraded primarily by selenocysteine β-lyase to yield free selenide. Selenide, in turn, can be methylated and excreted in the urine or can be converted by selenophosphate synthase into selenophosphate, an important intermediate in the synthesis of the body's selenium-dependent enzymes, as shown in Figure 13.16.

Interestingly, although selenocysteine is required for selenium-dependent enzyme function, selenocysteine obtained directly from the diet or selenomethionine degradation cannot be utilized. Instead, the selenocysteine must be synthesized in the body from the amino acid serine, while the serine is attached to transfer (t) RNA, and from selenophosphate (Figure 13.16). It is through the activity of the selenocysteine-containing enzyme selenophosphate synthetase 2 that selenophosphate is made. Thus, while attached to tRNA, serine is converted, through a series of reactions involving selenophosphate, into selenocysteine (abbreviated tRNA^{SEC}). Should selenophosphate not be produced in sufficient quantities, the subsequent generation of all selenoproteins becomes diminished. A total abolishment of selenoprotein synthesis is lethal. But diminished activity of even some selenoproteins results in massive cellular damage associated with oxidative stress due to the reduction of the antioxidant/cell redox services normally provided by the selenoproteins.

The incorporation of selenocysteine that is made while attached to the tRNA also involves a novel process whereby the UGA stop codon is reprogrammed to be read as a sense codon. This reprogramming requires (1) tRNA^{SEC}, (2) a selenocysteine insertion sequence (SECIS) in the 3' untranslated section of the mRNA of selenoproteins, (3) SEC insertion sequence binding protein 2 (SBP2), and (4) elongation factor (EF) selenocysteine. The selenocysteine insertion sequence is found in the 3' untranslated part of the mRNA of selenoproteins. The attachment of the SEC insertion sequence binding protein 2 to the insertion sequence on the mRNA enables interaction with a specific elongation factor and with the tRNA^{SEC}. In the presence of these elements, selenocysteine is incorporated at the UGA codon, and UGA is not read as a stop codon.

Functions and Mechanisms of Action

Various incompletely understood roles have been postulated for selenium. Some of the less defined roles include its involvement in maintaining or inducing the cytochrome P450 system, in DNA repair and enzyme activation, and in immune system function. The better-characterized roles of selenium are related to its functions as an integral part of specific enzymes (e.g., selenoproteins) in the body. Over 25 selenoproteins have been identified in humans. These proteins primarily function in antioxidant capacities, and thus regulate cell redox status. The next sections and Table 13.7 describe some of the selenium-dependent enzymes and their metabolic roles.

Glutathione Peroxidase (GPX): Antioxidant

One of the most clearly established functions of selenium is as an integral part of the enzyme glutathione peroxidase. Several glutathione peroxidase enzymes (designated GPX followed by a number) have been characterized, and each catalyzes the same basic reaction but in different tissues. Most GPXs (of which seven have been identified) are selenium dependent, containing selenium as selenocysteine.

Within cells, glutathione peroxidase is found mainly (~70%) in the cytosol and to a lesser extent (~30%) in

the mitochondrial matrix; however, GPX4 is found predominantly associated with cell membranes. GPX1 is found in most body tissues but most notably in the liver, kidneys, and red blood cells. GPX2 is found mainly in the gastrointestinal tract and liver. GPX3 originates in the kidney but is released into the plasma (extracellular); GPX3 accounts for 10% to 30% of selenium in the plasma. Other cells in other organs, including the brain, also express other forms of the enzyme.

Glutathione peroxidase catalyzes the removal of hydrogen peroxides (H_2O_2) and organic hydroperoxides (designated ROOH). GPX4 functions mainly to remove phospholipid hydroperoxides (designated LOOH) associated with membranes. Organic peroxides are derived from nucleic acids and other molecules, including unsaturated fatty acids; however, a peroxide derived from fatty acids is usually designated as a lipid (rather than organic) peroxide. Hydrogen peroxides are generated in many cells throughout the body as part of normal metabolism and may be generated in large amounts by activated white blood cells as they phagocytize foreign substances. The reaction catalyzed by glutathione peroxidase neutralizes or eliminates hydrogen peroxide and organic (including lipid) peroxides. In fact, glutathione peroxidase is more active than catalase in reducing organic peroxides and hydrogen peroxides. If not removed, these peroxides typically damage cellular membranes and other cell components including proteins and DNA. Glutathione, a tripeptide of glycine, cysteine, and glutamate found in most body cells, is needed in its reduced form (GSH) for the glutathione peroxidase-catalyzed reaction and furnishes the reducing equivalents, as shown in the following reactions.

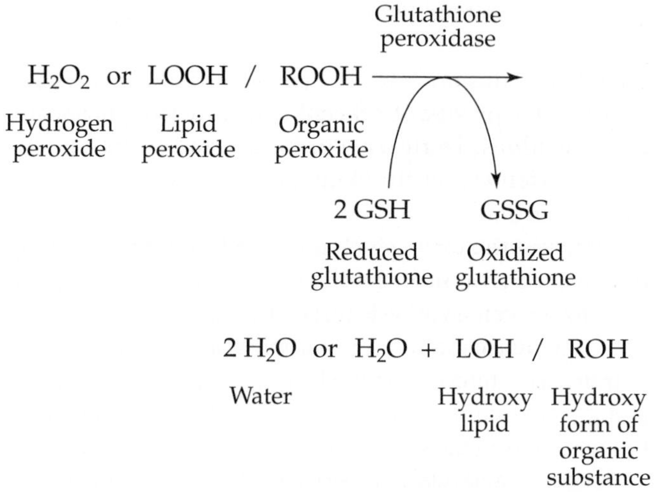

$$\text{H}_2\text{O}_2 \text{ or LOOH / ROOH} \xrightarrow{\text{Glutathione peroxidase}}$$

Hydrogen peroxide   Lipid peroxide   Organic peroxide

2 GSH   GSSG

Reduced glutathione   Oxidized glutathione

$$2\,\text{H}_2\text{O} \text{ or } \text{H}_2\text{O} + \text{LOH / ROH}$$

Water   Hydroxy lipid   Hydroxy form of organic substance

The oxidized glutathione (GSSG) that is formed as a result of glutathione peroxidase activity must be regenerated back to its reduced form (GSH). Reduced glutathione is thought to be the most abundant antioxidant found in cells. This regeneration of reduced glutathione

Table 13.7 Selected Functions of Selenium

Glutathione peroxidase: antioxidant

Selenoprotein P: antioxidant

Selenophosphate synthetase 2: selenoprotein synthesis

Thioredoxin reductase: cellular redox state maintenance

Iodothyronine 5'-deiodinases: thyroid hormone synthesis and metabolism

Methionine sulfoxide reductases: oxidative damage repair

Other selenoproteins: antioxidant, intracellular protein processing and folding, calcium regulation is imperative for cells to maintain appropriate redox states. Glutathione reductase, a flavoenzyme, catalyzes this reduction in a reaction dependent on $NADPH + H^+$, which is derived from the pentose phosphate pathway (hexose monophosphate shunt). The regeneration of reduced glutathione is shown here:

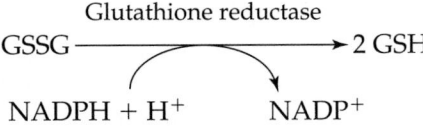

Selenium availability affects glutathione peroxidase activity and mRNA levels, especially that of GPX1. With selenium deficiency, the incorporation of selenocysteine into glutathione peroxidase during translation is decreased and thus causes increased degradation of the glutathione peroxidase mRNA. With inadequate selenium, any available selenium is shifted to other, more critical selenoproteins, such as selenoprotein P. With selenium supplementation, glutathione peroxidase mRNA increases rapidly to control levels, and enzyme activity gradually increases.

Selenoprotein P: Antioxidant

Selenoprotein P, a glycoprotein, is synthesized mostly in the liver but also the brain and is found throughout the body, including in association with capillary endothelial cells. It is the major selenium-containing protein in the blood, accounting for up to about 80% of plasma selenium. Selenoprotein P transports selenium to tissues for use. The protein appears to be taken up into cells to deliver selenium by receptor-mediated endocytosis.

Selenoprotein P, unlike most selenoenzymes (which contain one to four selenium atoms as selenocysteine), contains up to 10 selenocysteine residues. However, under conditions in which selenium is limited, selenoprotein P may be synthesized with fewer selenocysteine residues. In other words, instead of having 10 selenocysteines, selenoprotein P may only have two or three or so selenocysteines if sufficient selenium is not available in the cells. Moreover, when selenium is limited, selenoprotein P appears to preferentially receive selenium over other selenoenzymes such as glutathione peroxidases [5].

Selenoprotein P is thought to function in the body as an antioxidant, especially in removing the damaging peroxynitrite ($ONOO^\bullet$) radical. Peroxynitrite is synthesized by activated white blood cells from superoxide radicals ($O_2^{\bullet-}$) and nitrogen monooxide ($NO^\bullet$). If not inactivated, peroxynitrite, for example, can cause DNA single-strand breaks and lipid peroxidation. Selenoprotein P may also catalyze the reduction of membrane phospholipid hydroperoxides to alcohols, similar to the function of GPX4.

Selenophosphate Synthetase 2: Selenoprotein Synthesis

At least two forms of selenophosphate synthetase have been identified. One form (designated SPS1) does not contain selenocysteine and is thought to recycle selenium from selenocysteine. The selenophosphate synthetase 2 isoform, which contains selenocysteine, catalyzes the synthesis of selenophosphate from selenide, as shown here:

$$H_2Se \xrightarrow[\text{ATP} \quad \text{AMP} + P_i]{\text{Selenophosphate synthetase}} HSePO_3^{2-}$$

Selenide ATP AMP + P_i Selenophosphate

Selenophosphate is a key compound needed in the body to synthesize other selenocysteine-containing proteins/enzymes (Figure 13.16) such as glutathione peroxidase, deiodinase, thioredoxin reductase, selenoprotein P, and others. Mutations in selenophosphate synthetase 2 or defective selenophosphate synthetase 2 activity significantly reduces selenoprotein synthesis. This in turn leads to increased reactive oxygen species generation and cellular apoptosis.

Thioredoxin Reductase: Antioxidant

Thioredoxin reductase is a flavoenzyme (containing FAD) that, like glutathione peroxidase, selenoprotein P, and selenophosphate synthetase 2, contains selenocysteine at its active site. The enzyme is found in three forms designated by numbers; forms 1 and 2 are found in the blood and most body tissues, while form 3 is found in the testes. Within cells (in the cytosol, mitochondria, and nucleus), thioredoxin reductase helps maintain the redox state by reducing oxidized thioredoxin (TrxS-SxrT) and oxidized glutaredoxin, as well as other substrates that have become oxidized, including transcription factors, receptors, and enzymes. An example of an enzyme substrate is ribonucleotide reductase, important in the conversion of ribonucleotides to deoxyribonucleotides in DNA synthesis.

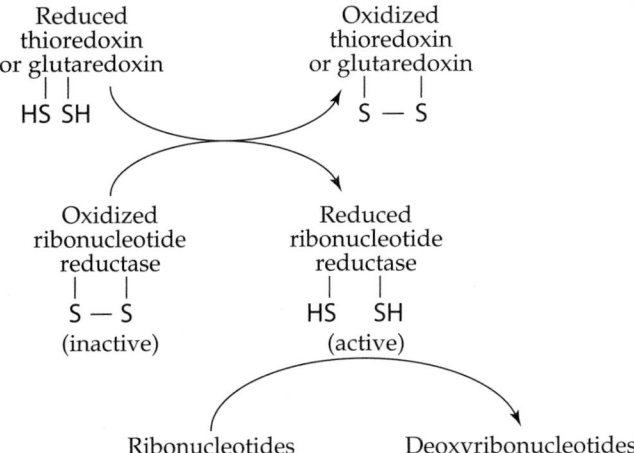

Specifically, thioredoxin reductase transfers reducing equivalents from NADPH through its bound FAD to reduce disulfide bonds (S-S) within the oxidized substrate, as shown next.

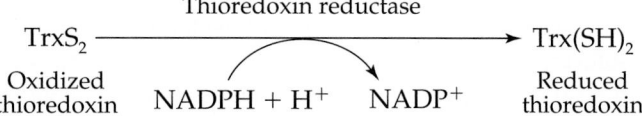

Because of the oxidation-reduction roles of thioredoxin, the thioredoxin system regulates cell growth, inhibits apoptosis by inhibiting apoptosis signal-regulating kinase (ASK) 1, and modulates intracellular signaling cascades. The modulation of intracellular signaling, for example, is accomplished by regenerating oxidized transcription factors such as activator protein (AP) 1 and nuclear factor κB.

Iodothyronine 5'-Deiodinases (IDI or DI): Thyroid Hormone Synthesis

Selenium is also necessary for iodine metabolism and may regulate thyroid hormone production [6]. The thyroid gland contains several selenoproteins including selenoprotein P, glutathione peroxidase, thioredoxin reductase, and iodothyronine 5' deiodinase [7,8]. Iodothyronine 5'-deiodinases are selenocysteine-containing enzymes with the selenocysteine present at the active site. Three types of 5'-deiodinases have been characterized. Type 1 is found mainly in the thyroid gland and the liver, kidneys, and pituitary gland, and types 2 and 3 are found in tissues such as skin, pituitary, adipose, skeletal muscle, and brain.

5'-deiodinases catalyze the deiodination (removal of iodine) from the 5 or 5' positions of thyroid hormones and some of their metabolites. For example, deiodinases types 1 and 2 convert the thyroid hormone thyroxine (T_4) to 3,5,3'-triiodothyronine (T_3). T_3 is the body's primary hormonal regulator of metabolism as well as of normal growth and development; a selenium deficiency results in decreased T_3 concentrations and increased T_4 concentrations. In addition to T_3 generation for release into the blood and use by extrahepatic cells, type 1 5'-deiodinase facilitates the degradation of surplus T_3. Type 2 deiodinase provides for the production and use of T_3 within specific tissues.

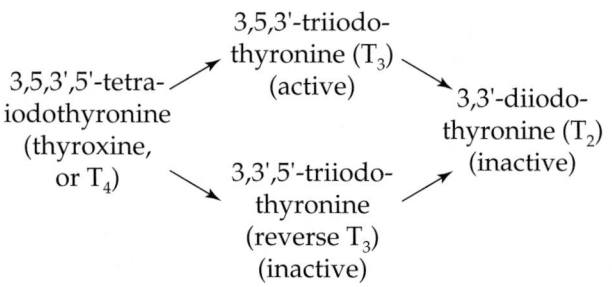

Type 3 deiodinase deiodinates T_3 to T_2 (also called 3,3'-diiodothyronine). Other reactions also can occur. If T_3 is not needed, then, for example, T_4 may be converted by type 3 deiodinase into reverse T_3, an inactive metabolite. For further information regarding thyroid hormone metabolism, see the "Iodine" section.

Methionine Sulfoxide Reductase (Selenoprotein R): Antioxidant

Selenoprotein R is part of a group of methionine sulfoxide reductases (also called methionine R or S sulfoxide reductases); these enzymes contain selenocysteine and are found in both the cytosol and nucleus of cells. The enzymes reduce methionine sulfoxides (oxidized methionines) using reduced thioredoxin. Methionine (met) sulfoxides (met-R-O or met-S-O, representing both R- and S-epimers) are generated in proteins when free radicals cause oxidation of methionine residues. The reaction catalyzed by methionine sulfoxide reductase is as follows:

$$\text{Protein} - \text{met-R-O} + \text{Trx(SH)}_2 \longrightarrow \text{protein} - \text{met} + \text{Trx-S}_2 + H_2O$$

The presence of the sulfoxide within the protein damages the protein so that it is unable to perform its normal function; however, methionine repair and thus return of normal protein function occurs with the action of methionine sulfoxide reductase.

Other Selenoproteins

Several other selenoproteins containing at least one selenocysteine have been identified, but little is known about their functions [9]. Selenoprotein W, a small selenocysteine-containing protein, is found mostly in the cytosol of cells within a number of tissues, but especially those of the heart and skeletal muscle. In these tissues, selenoprotein W may be found bound to reduced glutathione through a cysteine residue. The function of this protein is unclear, but it is speculated to have antioxidant roles and may be important in muscle growth.

Several selenoproteins, including selenoproteins S and K, are found in the endoplasmic reticulum and appear to have roles in the processing and/or folding of proteins. Selenoprotein S is thought to remove misfolded proteins as well as to protect against oxidative damage. Proteins typically must be folded before they are secreted from a cell and into the blood; misfolded proteins must be targeted and degraded. Selenoprotein H, found in the nucleus, may act as a transcription factor to upregulate the expression of other selenoproteins; it may also remove superoxide radicals from neuronal cells. Selenoprotein M, found in neuronal cells, is thought to protect against hydrogen peroxide damage and may also be involved in calcium release. Selenoprotein M, along with selenoprotein 15, also appears to play roles in protein folding. Selenoprotein N may also be involved in calcium regulation and protection against protein oxidation in muscle cells. Selenoprotein T also appears to play a role in calcium mobilization. Other selenoproteins, such as O, I, and V, have been identified, but their functions remain largely unknown.

Disease Prevention

Because of selenium's numerous antioxidant roles in the body, associations between selenium and risk and prevention of disease, primarily cancer and cardiovascular disease, have been examined. Serum selenium concentrations, for example, have been inversely associated with both heart disease risk and the incidence of some cancers [10–12]. Yet, selenium supplementation studies for the prevention of disease report inconsistent findings. For example, the Nutritional Prevention of Cancer (NPC) trial showed that selenium supplementation (200 mg) significantly decreased prostate cancer risk, especially among those with the lowest plasma selenium concentrations [13]. A review and meta-analysis of antioxidant supplementation in reducing primary cancer incidence and mortality showed that selenium supplementation may exhibit anticarcinogenic effects in men but not women [14]. A meta-analysis of antioxidant supplement trials for the prevention of gastrointestinal cancers found that selenium (up to 228 mg) showed significant beneficial effects; however, many of the trials analyzed in the meta-analysis were considered low quality [15,16]. A larger randomized, placebo-controlled study (Selenium and Vitamin E Cancer Prevention Trial, referred to as SELECT) of over 35,000 men found that selenium supplementation (200 mg) for 7 years was not beneficial in preventing prostate, lung, colorectal, or overall primary cancer [17]. Similarly, an antioxidant trial that included selenium supplementation (100–228 mg) showed no beneficial effects in primary or secondary prevention of colorectal adenomas [18]. Despite the lack of consistent demonstrated benefits, a daily selenium intake of 200 μg for at least 6 months has been recommended by some to potentially diminish the risk of these diseases [11].

Interactions with Other Nutrients

A selenium deficiency may develop if the mineral is present in the body only as selenomethionine because, in this situation, the selenium becomes available only as proteins are degraded in the course of normal turnover. However, the risk for such a problem is fairly low if dietary selenium and protein intakes are adequate.

Excretion

Urinary excretion (representing 50–60% or more of losses) is thought to be the means by which selenium homeostasis is maintained in the body; urinary excretion is directly proportional to selenium intake. The major urinary metabolites of selenium are methylated forms of the mineral. The most prevalent urinary metabolite in humans is the selenosugar methylseleno-N-acetylgalactosamine (CH_3Se-GalN) [19]. Other urinary metabolites, especially with higher intakes of the mineral, include methylselenol (CH_3SeH), dimethylselenide [$(CH_3)_2Se$], and trimethylselenonium [$(CH_3)_3Se^+$] [3,19]. Fecal losses of selenium represent up to about 50%. Selenium losses through the lungs and skin also contribute to selenium excretion to a small extent. Pulmonary elimination (i.e., exhalation in the breath) of selenium is usually associated with ingestion of large amounts of the mineral. The main form of selenium that is exhaled is dimethylselenide, which is quite volatile and has a garlicky odor.

Recommended Dietary Allowance

The Food and Nutrition Board set a Recommended Dietary Allowance for selenium for adults of 55 μg/day [20]. Based mostly on balance studies as well as on repletion studies of men with selenium deficiency in regions of China, the adult requirement for selenium was determined to be 45 μg. The requirement was based on calculation of the amount of selenium necessary to plateau concentrations of selected selenoproteins in the plasma. To set the RDA, a 20% coefficient of variation was added, and the final number was rounded to the nearest five. RDAs for selenium for pregnancy and lactation were set at 60 μg and 70 μg, respectively [20]. The inside front cover of the book provides RDAs for selenium for other age groups. Studies, however, suggest that the RDA for selenium for adults may be suboptimal [21].

Deficiency

Selenium deficiency occurs primarily in selected regions of the world such as China, central Africa, and parts of Europe. The deficiency is linked to Keshan disease and Kashin-Beck disease. Keshan disease is characterized by cardiomyopathy involving cardiogenic shock, congestive heart failure, or both, along with multifocal necrosis of heart tissue, which becomes replaced with fibrous tissue. Infection by coxsackie virus appears to be a cofactor in the development of Keshan disease. In the absence of sufficient selenium, mutations occur in benign strains of the virus. These mutations cause the virus to become virulent; the presence of the virus is thought to account for some of the symptoms of Keshan disease [22]. Kashin-Beck disease is characterized by osteoarthropathy involving degeneration and necrosis of the joints and of epiphyseal-plate cartilages of the legs (primarily knees and ankles) and arms (mostly fingers, hands, and elbows). Several factors, including selenium deficiency, are thought to contribute to the development of Kashin-Beck disease.

Selenium deficiency also has been observed in people receiving total parenteral nutrition. Major symptoms of deficiency included poor growth, muscle pain and weakness, loss of pigmentation of hair and skin, and whitening of nail beds. Poor growth may be associated with the role of selenium in thyroid hormone metabolism. Selenium supplementation corrects the deficiency.

Toxicity

Selenium toxicity, also called selenosis, has been observed both in miners and in people who consume excess selenium from supplements. Signs and symptoms of toxicity include nausea, vomiting, fatigue, diarrhea, hair and nail brittleness and loss, paresthesia, interference in sulfur metabolism (primarily oxidation of sulfhydryl groups), and inhibition of protein synthesis [23]. Acute poisoning from gram amounts of selenium is lethal, with damage occurring to most organ systems [23]. A Tolerable Upper Intake Level of 400 μg/day has been set by the Food and Nutrition Board [20].

Assessment of Nutriture

The concentration of selenium in the blood is thought to be a reflection or function of dietary intake within a specific range. For plasma selenium concentrations, a value of 70 ng/mL (0.8 μmol/L) appears to be the cutoff [20]. If a person's plasma selenium concentration is <70 ng/mL, dietary selenium affects the plasma selenium concentration.

The activities and concentrations of selenoproteins have been used to assess selenium status. Selenoprotein P and glutathione peroxidase in tissues (GPX1) and in the plasma (GPX3) are commonly used. Selenoprotein P and glutathione peroxidase concentrations decrease in the plasma as selenium deficiency worsens, thus serving as an index of selenium status in populations with low intake [20,23,24]. Optimization of both selenoprotein P and glutathione peroxidase occurs when plasma selenium concentrations are about 80 to 90 ng/mL [24]. Whole blood glutathione peroxidase activity also can be measured and is thought to reflect longer-term selenium status due to the typical 120-day life span of red blood cells. Urinary selenium concentration may reflect status, especially toxicity [25].

References Cited for Selenium

1. Wastney ME, Combs GF, Canfield WK, et al. A human model of selenium that integrates metabolism from selenite and selenomethionine. J Nutr. 2011; 141:708–11.
2. Finley JW. Selenium accumulation in plant foods. Nutr Rev. 2005; 63:196–202.
3. Thomson CD, Chisholm A, McLachlan SK, Campbell JM. Brazil nuts: an effective way to improve selenium status. Am J Clin Nutr. 2008; 87:379–84.
4. Suzuki KT. Metabolomics of selenium: Se metabolites based on speciation studies. J Hlth Sci. 2005; 51:107–14.
5. Mostert V. Selenoprotein P: properties, functions, and regulation. Arch Biochem Biophys. 2000; 376:433–38.
6. Beckett GJ, Arthur J. Selenium and endocrine systems. J Endocrinol. 2005; 184:455–65.
7. Hess SY. The impact of common micronutrient deficiencies on iodine and thyroid metabolism: the evidence from human studies. Clin Endocrin Metab. 2010; 24:117–32.
8. Combs GF, Midthune DN, Patterson KY, et al. Effects of selenomethionine supplementation on selenium status and thyroid hormone concentrations in healthy adults. Am J Clin Nutr. 2009; 89:1808–14.
9. Reeves MA, Hoffmann PR. The human selenoproteome: recent insights into functions and regulation. Cell Mol Life Sci. 2009; 66:2457–78.
10. Flores-Mateo G, Navas-Acien A, Pastor-Barriuso R, Guallar E. Selenium and coronary heart disease. Am J Clin Nutr. 2006; 84:762–73.
11. Wei W, Abnet C, Qiao Y, et al. Prospective study of serum selenium concentrations and esophageal and gastric cardia cancer, heart disease, stroke and total death. Am J Clin Nutr. 2004; 79:80–85.
12. Brenneisen P, Steinbrenner H, Sies H. Selenium, oxidative stress, and health aspects. Trace Elem Hum Hlth. 2005; 26:256–67.
13. Duffield-Lillico AJ, Dalkin BL, Reid ME, et al. Selenium supplementation, baseline plasma selenium status and incidence of prostate cancer: an analysis of the complete treatment period of the Nutritional Prevention of Cancer Trial. BJU Int. 2003; 91:608–12.
14. Bardia A, Tleyjeh IM, Cerhan JR, et al. Efficacy of antioxidant supplementation in reducing primary cancer incidence and mortality: systematic review and meta-analysis. Mayo Clin Proc. 2008; 83:23–34.
15. Bjelakovic G, Nikolova D, Simonetti RG, Gluud C. Antioxidant supplements for prevention of gastrointestinal cancers: a systematic review and meta-analysis. Lancet. 2004; 364:1219–28.
16. Bjelakovic G, Nikolova D, Simonetti RG, Gluud C. Systematic review: primary and secondary prevention of gastrointestinal cancers with antioxidant supplements. Aliment Pharmacol Ther. 2008; 28:689–703.
17. Lippman SM, Klein EA, Goodman PJ, et al. Effect of selenium and vitamin E on risk of prostate cancer and other cancers: the selenium and vitamin E cancer prevention trial (SELECT). JAMA. 2009; 301:39–51.
18. Bjelakovic G, Nagorni A, Nikolova D, et al. Meta-analysis: antioxidant supplements for primary and secondary prevention of colorectal adenoma. Aliment Pharmacol Ther. 2006; 24:281–91.
19. Francesconi KA, Pannier F. Selenium metabolites in urine: a critical overview of past work and current status. Clin Chem. 2004; 50:2240–53.
20. Food and Nutrition Board, Institute of Medicine. Dietary Reference Intakes. Washington, DC: National Academy Press. 2000 pp. 284–324.
21. Broome C, McArdle F, Kyle J, et al. An increase in selenium intake improves immune function and poliovirus handling in adults with marginal selenium status. Am J Clin Nutr. 2004; 80:154–62.
22. Moghadaszadeh B, Beggs AH. Selenoproteins and their impact on human health through diverse physiological pathways. Physiol. 2006; 21:307–15.
23. Clark RF, Strukle E, Williams SR, Manoguerra AS. Selenium poisoning from a nutritional supplement. JAMA. 1996; 275:1087–88.
24. Xia Y, Hill KE, Li P, et al. Optimization of selenoprotein P and other plasma selenium biomarkers for the assessment of the selenium nutritional requirement: a placebo-controlled, double-blind study of selenomethionine supplementation in selenium-deficient Chinese subjects. Am J Clin Nutr. 2010; 95:525–31.
25. Longnecker M, Stampfer M, Morris J. A 1-year trial of the effect of high selenium bread on selenium concentrations in blood and toenails. Am J Clin Nutr. 1993; 57:408–13.

Suggested Readings

Antioxidants and Redox Signaling 2010 volume 12, issue 7 provides a forum on selenium.

Burk RF, Hill KE. Selenoprotein P: expression, functions, and roles in mammals. Biochim Biophys Acta. 2009; 1790:1441–07.

Germain DLS, Galton VA, Hernandez A. Minireview: defining the roles of the iodothyronine deiodinases: current concepts and challenges. Endocrinology. 2009; 150:1097–107.

Kohrle J, Jakob F, Contempre B, Dumont J. Selenium, the thyroid, and the endocrine system. Endocrine Rev. 2005; 26:944–84.

Lei XG, Cheng W, McClung JP. Metabolic regulation and function of glutathione peroxidase-1. Ann Rev Nutr. 2007; 27:41–61.

Zeng H. Selenium as an essential micronutrient: roles in cell cycle and apoptosis. Molecules. 2009; 14:1263–78.

Web Site for Nutrient Composition Information

http://www.ars.usda.gov/Services/docs.htm?docid=18877

CHROMIUM

Chromium, a metal with a ubiquitous presence in air, water, and soil, exists in several oxidation states from Cr^{2-} to Cr^{6+}. Trivalent chromium, Cr^{3+}, is the stablest of the oxidation states and is often found attached to ligands containing nitrogen, oxygen, or sulfur to form hexacoordinate or octahedral complexes. This trivalent form of chromium is thought to be the most important form in humans. The human body contains about 4 to 6 mg of chromium.

Sources

In foods, chromium exists in the trivalent form. Good sources of dietary chromium include meats, fish, and poultry (especially organ meats) and grains (especially whole grains). Beef (100 g) contains, for example, about 55 μg of chromium; a slice of whole-wheat bread, about 1 μg of chromium. Relatively large amounts of chromium are also found in cheese (e.g., American cheese contains about 40 μg of chromium/oz), peanuts (about 45 μg/ounce), dark chocolate and selected vegetables such as raw mushrooms (about 29 μg/half-cup), green peppers, broccoli (about 5.5 μg/cup), green beans, and spinach. Additionally, chromium is found in some fruits such as apples (about 1.4 μg each), bananas, and orange and grape juices (2–7 μg/cup); in selected spices (such as cinnamon, cloves, bay leaves, turmeric); and in tea, beer, and wine. Brewer's yeast (100 g) provides about 112 mg chromium. The Daily Value for chromium is 120 μg.

Food processing and refining can affect the chromium content of foods. Refining of sugar, for example, diminishes chromium. Thus, molasses and brown sugar are higher in chromium than white sugar. In contrast, chromium is easily solubilized from stainless steel cookware or cans into acidic foods. Thus, the use of stainless steel cookware may increase the amount of chromium in food.

Chromium is available in supplement form as inorganic salts, such as with chloride, or as an organic complex, such as with acetate, nicotinic acid alone or with amino acids, or picolinic acid. Although all forms appear to be absorbed and used, the different forms of the supplement appear to affect tissue concentrations differently. For example, chromium picolinate has been touted as superior to other forms of chromium; however, urinary chromium excretion from chromium picolinate also is higher than other supplemental forms, suggesting poor tissue uptake [1–3].

Digestion, Absorption, Transport, and Storage

Digestion and Absorption

Chromium, Cr^{3+}, may be released from food components in acidic solutions, as would be found in the stomach. Chromium is absorbed throughout the small intestine, especially in the jejunum. Although the mode of absorption in humans is not known, chromium is thought to be absorbed by passive diffusion (as shown in rats), by a carrier-mediated transporter, and/or perhaps by endocytosis [1]. About 0.4% to 2.5% of dietary chromium (with intakes of 40 μg and 10 μg, respectively) is absorbed from the gastrointestinal tract [4–6]. If, for example, absorption averaged 0.5%, a chromium intake of 30 μg would provide 0.15 μg of absorbed chromium.

Factors Influencing Chromium Absorption

Like that of other trace minerals, the absorption of chromium may be influenced by dietary factors.

Enhancers of Chromium Absorption Within the stomach, amino acids or other ligands may chelate chromium. Amino acids such as phenylalanine, methionine, and histidine as well as picolinic acid (picolinate) act as ligands to improve chromium absorption [7]. These chelations typically help chromium remain soluble and prevent olation (see next paragraph) once it reaches the alkaline pH of the small intestine. Lipophilic compounds such as picolinate may enhance Cr^{3+} absorption through the cell's lipid membranes. Vitamin C may also enhance chromium absorption.

Inhibitors of Chromium Absorption Chromium in a neutral or alkaline environment may react with hydroxyl ions (OH^-), which readily polymerize to form high-molecular-weight compounds in a process called olation. This reaction, which occurs more readily with antacid use (e.g., to relieve heartburn), results in chromium precipitation and thus reduced absorption. Phytic acid, found mostly in grains and legumes, also diminishes chromium absorption; however, the quantity of phytic acid provided in most U.S. diets is not thought to substantially inhibit the absorption of dietary chromium.

Transport

In the blood, Cr^{3+}, like Fe^{3+}, binds to transferrin. If transferrin sites are unavailable (due to occupation by iron, for example), albumin is thought to transport chromium. Globulins and possibly lipoproteins also may transport the mineral if present in very high concentrations. Some chromium also may circulate unbound in the blood. The uptake of transferrin-bound chromium into cells is thought to occur like that of iron (see Figures 13.5 and 13.17).

Storage

Chromium is thought to be stored in tissues with ferric iron because of its transport by transferrin. The body contains ~4 to 6 mg of chromium. Tissues especially high in chromium include the kidneys, liver, muscle, spleen, heart, pancreas, and bones. Tissue chromium concentrations appear to decline with age.

Functions and Mechanisms of Action

Chromium is thought to potentiate the action of insulin; however, the mechanism by which potentiation occurs is still under investigation. For decades, this biological action of chromium was believed to be attributable to its complexing with nicotinic acid and amino acids to form the organic compound **glucose tolerance factor** (GTF). GTF was first identified in brewer's yeast, but this factor has never been purified, nor has its exact structure been characterized.

While it is still thought to potentiate the action of insulin, more recent studies have suggested that the biologically active form of chromium is a low-molecular-weight chromium-binding substance called chromodulin. Chromodulin is thought to be produced in response to insulin secretion, which stimulates chromium uptake by cells. Once within the cell, chromium atoms (four) bind to apochromodulin, an oligopeptide that is thought to be composed of glycine, cysteine, aspartate, and one or more glutamates. Once the four chromium atoms bind to the apochromodulin, the complex is called holochromodulin (Cr^4-chromodulin) or chromodulin. This proposed process is shown in Figure 13.17.

Insulin signaling within cells is regulated (in part) by the phosphorylation of tyrosine residues on selected proteins. More specifically, insulin initially binds to the alpha subunit of an insulin receptor; this binding leads to autophosphorylation of specific tyrosine residues on the beta subunit of the insulin receptor and stimulates tyrosine kinase activity of the receptor and of other intracellular (cytosolic) protein substrates (such as insulin receptor substrate 1) involved in signal transduction. For example, the activation of phosphatidylinositol-3-kinase results from the binding of insulin receptor substrates to the enzyme's regulatory subunit; this in turn enables a variety

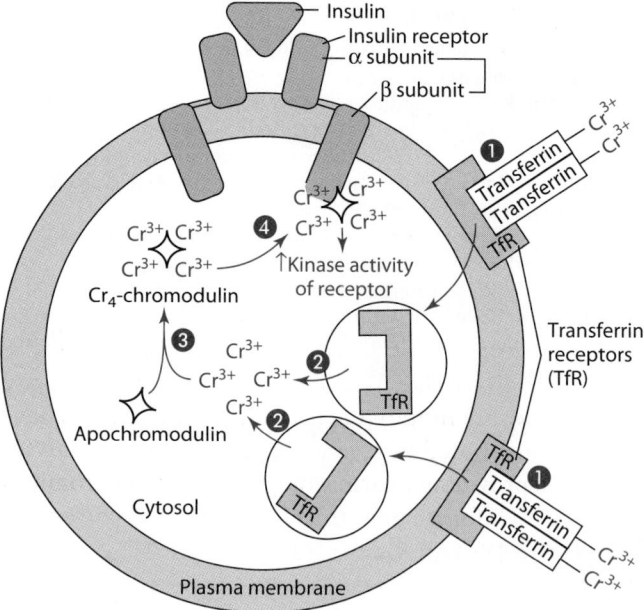

❶ Transferrin delivers Cr^{3+} to transferrin receptors (TfR) on cell membranes.

❷ Cr^{3+} is released inside the cell.

❸ Four Cr^{3+} atoms complex with chromodulin to form holo chromodulin or Cr_4-chromodulin.

❹ Cr_4-chromodulin functions to increase the kinase activity of the beta subunit of the insulin receptor and other cytosolic tyrosine kinases.

Figure 13.17 Proposed role of chromium (Cr^{3+}) as part of chromodulin in potentiating insulin's reactions.

of insulin-dependent cellular activities such as GLUT4 translocation for cellular glucose uptake and protein synthesis, among others. Chromodulin is thought to bind to the cytosolic beta subunit of the insulin receptor, where it stimulates (or amplifies) the kinase activity of the beta subunit of the insulin receptor. Chromodulin also may stimulate the tyrosine kinase activity of other enzymes involved in insulin signaling to effect GLUT4 translocation and improved cellular glucose uptake [8–11]. Cells treated with selected forms of chromium also have been shown to exhibit increased insulin receptor gene expression, improved protein anabolism, decreased protein degradation, and improved insulin sensitivity, although the results of studies on the effects of chromium supplementation on insulin sensitivity have been conflicting [12,13].

Another possibly biologically active form of chromium in the body is chromate. Chromate or chromic acid (CrO_3), which contains the hexavalent form of chromium, can be produced within the body from oxidation of Cr^{3+} by oxidants such as hydrogen peroxide and free radicals. Chromate, similarly to vanadate, may inhibit the activity of phosphotyrosine phosphatase to prolong or enhance insulin signaling; however, the methodological approaches used in chromate studies as well as in some of the studies examining chromodulin's mechanism(s) of action have been questioned [14–16].

In addition to its proposed association with insulin, Cr^{3+} also may affect gene expression and/or maintain the structural integrity of nuclear strands [17]. The expression of a handful of genes in adipose tissue of diabetic mice has shown to be altered in response to niacin-bound Cr^{3+} [17].

Chromium and Health

Diabetes Improvements in measures of glucose control (primarily glycosylated hemoglobin and fasting glucose concentrations) in individuals with type 2 diabetes have been demonstrated in several studies and meta-analyses of studies providing pharmacological doses of chromium [2,18–23]. Unfortunately, the effectiveness of chromium supplementation in the treatment of type 2 diabetes remains controversial, as consistent effects have not been observed. Future studies focusing on selected study populations, such as those with insulin resistance and more extreme elevations in fasting glucose and hemoglobin A1c concentrations, are thought to be needed; it is those with these manifestations who are thought to benefit most from chromium supplementation [20].

Weight Loss/Body Composition Changes Chromium as a supplement also has been purported to effect changes in body composition, weight, and strength performance. However, most well-controlled studies providing chromium supplementation have shown no significant effects on strength gains, muscle accretion, or fat loss; in fact, the Federal Trade Commission ordered the discontinuation of such claims [24]. Effects of chromium on weight loss have been conflicting.

Interactions with Other Nutrients

Because chromium is transported in the blood bound to transferrin, the blood's primary iron-binding protein, one might surmise that chromium, if given in large amounts, might displace iron from transferrin and impair iron status. Indeed, ingesting chromium, as chromium chloride and chromium picolinate, has been associated with impaired iron status in some, but not all, studies.

Excretion

Most chromium (~95%) is excreted from the body in the urine. In absolute terms, urinary chromium excretion ranges from ~0.2 to 0.4 µg per day [6]. In addition to urinary losses, small amounts of chromium are lost with desquamation of skin cells. Fecal chromium represents mostly unabsorbed dietary chromium, not endogenous chromium excreted via the bile into the feces.

Adequate Intake

The Adequate Intakes (AIs) for chromium for adult men and women through age 50 years are 35 µg and 25 µg, respectively; these values drop to 30 µg and 20 µg for men and women, respectively, over 50 years of age [6]. During pregnancy and lactation, intakes of 30 µg and 45 µg of chromium, respectively, are recommended [6]. AIs for chromium for other age groups are provided on the inside front cover of the book.

Deficiency

Chromium deficiency was originally described in individuals receiving intravenous nutrition (total parenteral nutrition). Signs and symptoms of deficiency included weight loss, peripheral neuropathy, elevated plasma glucose concentrations or impaired glucose use (also called insulin resistance, which may be characterized by hyperinsulinemia), and high plasma free fatty acid concentrations. While the reversal of these symptoms with chromium supplementation was viewed as evidence of chromium's essentiality, it is now apparent that the parenteral nutrition solution given to correct the deficiency provided pharmacological amounts of chromium, 2 to 6 µg per day (i.e., more than would typically be absorbed from the diet) [14,25].

Toxicity

Oral supplementation of up to about 1,000 µg of chromium as Cr^{3+} appears to be safe [6]. However, the use of chromium (Cr^{3+}) picolinate has been associated with chromosomal and organ damage [26–30]. Documented chromium-induced DNA damage includes adducts, single- and double-strand DNA breaks, and inter- and intrastrand crosslinks, among other types of destruction [26]. Organ damage, specifically renal failure and hepatic dysfunction, has been reported in those ingesting chromium picolinate supplements providing between 600 and 2,400 µg of chromium [27,28]. Renal problems also were documented in some individuals with higher than normal concentrations of chromium in their blood and urine due to long-term receipt of parenteral nutrition contaminated with high amounts of chromium [25].

Toxicity is also associated with exposure to the hexavalent form (Cr^{6+}) of chromium. Inhalation of or direct contact with hexavalent chromium may result in respiratory disease or in dermatitis and skin ulcerations, respectively. Liver damage may also occur. Cr^{6+} ingested orally is about 10 to 100 times more toxic than Cr^{3+}. Ingesting chromic acid (CrO_3), which contains hexavalent chromium, has resulted in severe acidosis, gastrointestinal hemorrhage, hepatic injury, renal failure, and death [29].

The intracellular reduction of the hexavalent form of chromium results in the production of multiple reactive oxygen species (free radicals) and is likely responsible for many of these observed effects. No Tolerable Upper Intake Level for chromium has been established by the Food and Nutrition Board to date.

Assessment of Nutriture

No specific tests are currently available to determine chromium status. Although a plasma chromium level of ~0.5 ng/mL is considered normal, the chromium content of physiological fluids is not indicative of status [31]. Fasting plasma chromium is not in equilibrium with tissue chromium. Responses of plasma chromium to an oral glucose load are inconsistent. Urinary chromium appears to reflect only recent intake, not status [31].

References Cited for Chromium

1. Kottwitz K, Laschinsky N, Fischer R, Nielsen P. Absorption, excretion and retention of ^{51}Cr from labeled Cr-(III)-picolinate in rats. Biometals. 2009; 22:289–95.
2. Hummel M, Standl E, Schnellet O. Chromium in metabolic and cardiovascular disease. Horm Metab Res. 2007; 39:743–51.
3. DiSilvestro RA, Dy E. Comparison of acute absorption of commercially available chromium supplements in humans. J Trace Elem Exp Med. 2007; 21:274–75.
4. Anderson RA, Kozlovsky AS. Chromium intake, absorption and excretion of subjects consuming self-selected diets. Am J Clin Nutr. 1985; 41:1177–83.
5. Anderson R, Polasky M, Bryden N, Canary J. Supplemental chromium effects on glucose, insulin, glucagon, and urinary chromium losses in subjects consuming controlled low chromium diets. Am J Clin Nutr. 1991; 54:909–16.
6. Food and Nutrition Board, Institute of Medicine. Dietary Reference Intakes. Washington, DC: National Academy Press. 2001 pp. 197–223.
7. Dong F, Kandadi MR, Ren J, Sreejayan N. Chromium (D-phenylalanine)$_3$ supplementation alters glucose disposal, insulin signaling, and glucose transporter-4 membrane translocation in insulin-resistant mice. J Nutr. 2008; 138:1846–51.
8. Vincent JB. Elucidating a biological role for chromium at a molecular level. Acct Chem Res. 2000; 33:503–10.
9. Wang H, Kruszewski A, Brautigan D. Cellular chromium enhances activation of insulin receptor kinase. Biochem. 2005; 44:8167–75.
10. Vincent J. Recent advances in the nutritional biochemistry of trivalent chromium. Proc Nutr Soc. 2004; 63:41–47.
11. Yang X, Palanichamy K, Ontko A, et al. A newly synthetic chromium complex – chromium (phenylalanine)$_3$ improves insulin responsiveness and reduces whole body glucose tolerance. FEBS Letters. 2005; 579:1458–64.
12. Qiao W, Peng Z, Wang Z, et al. Chromium improves glucose uptake and metabolism through upregulating the mRNA levels of IR, GLUT4, GS, and UCP3 in skeletal mucle cells. Biol Trace Elem Res. 2009; 131:133–42.
13. Peng Z, Qiao W, Wang Z, et al. Chromium improves protein deposition through regulating the mRNA levels of IGF-1, IGF-1R, and Ub in rat skeletal muscle cells. Biol Trace Elem Res. 2010; 137:226–34.
14. Vincent JB. Chromium: celebrating 50 years as an essential element? Dalton Trans. 2010; 39:3787–94.
15. Mulyani I, Levina A, Lay PA. Biomimetic oxidation of chromium (III): does the antidiabetic activity of chromium (III) involve carcinogenic chromium (VI)? Angew Chem Int Ed. 2004; 43:4504–07.
16. Levina A, Lay PA. Mechanistic studies of relevance to the biological activities of chromium. Coord Chem Rev. 2005; 249:281–98.
17. Levina A, Lay PA. Chemical properties and toxicity of chromium (III) nutritional supplements. Chem Res Toxicol. 2008; 21:563–71.
18. Lau FC, Bagchi M, Sen CK, Bagchi D. Nutrigenomic basis of beneficial effects of chromium (III) on obesity and diabetes. Mol Cell Biochem. 2008; 317:1–10.
19. Balk EM, Tatsioni A, Lichtenstein AH. Effect of chromium supplementation on glucose metabolism and lipids: a systematic review of randomized controlled trials. Diabetes Care. 2007; 30:2154–63.
20. Cefalu WT, Rood J, Pinsonat P, et al. Characterization of the metabolic and physiologic response to chromium supplementation in subjects with type 2 diabetes mellitus. Metab Clin Exp. 2010; 59:755–62.
21. Jain SK, Croad JL, Velusamy T, et al. Chromium dinicocysteinate supplementation can lower blood glucose, CRP, MCP-1, ICAM-1, creatinine, apparently mediated by elevated blood glucose and adiponectin and inhibition of NFkB, Akt, and Glut-2 in livers of zucker diabetic fatty rats. Mol Nutr Food Res. 2010; 54:1371–80.
22. Krzysik M, Grajeta H, Prescha A, Weber R. Effect os cellulose, pectin, and chromium (III) on lipid and carbohydrate metabolism in rats. J Trace Elem Med Biol. 2011; 25:97–102.
23. Broadhurst CL, Domenico P. Clinical studies on chromium picolinate supplementation in diabetes mellitus: a review. Diabetes Technol Ther. 2006; 8:677–87.
24. Federal Trade Commission Docket #C-3758 Decision and Order. Available at www.ftc.gov/os/1997/07/nutritid.pdf. Accessed 10/12/2010.
25. Moukarzel A. Chromium in parenteral nutrition: too little or too much? Gastroenterol. 2009; 137:S18–28.
26. Thompson CM, Haws LC, Harris MA, et al. Application of the U.S. EPA mode of action framework for purposes of guiding future research: a case study involving the oral carcinogenicity of hexavalent chromium. Toxicol Sci. 2011; 119:20–40.
27. Wasser WG, Feldman NS, D'Agati VD. Chronic renal failure after ingestion of over-the-counter chromium picolinate. Ann Intern Med. 1997; 126:410–11.
28. Cerulli J, Grabe DW, Gauthier I, et al. Chromium picolinate toxicity. Ann Pharmacotherapy. 1998; 32:428–31.
29. Loubieres Y, de Lassence A, Bernier M, et al. Acute, fatal, oral chromic acid poisoning. Clin Toxicol. 1999; 37:333–36.
30. Anderson R. Chromium as an essential nutrient for humans. Regulatory Toxicol and Pharmacol. 1997; 26:S35–41.
31. Anderson R, Polansky M, Bryden N, et al. Effects of chromium supplementation on urinary chromium excretion of human subjects and correlation of chromium excretion with selected clinical parameters. J Nutr. 1983; 113:276–81.

IODINE

Iodine, a nonmetal, typically is found and functions in its ionic form, iodide (I^-). Hence, the term *iodide* is used throughout this section. The human body contains about 15 to 20 mg of iodide, most (70–80%) of which is found in the thyroid gland.

Sources

The iodide concentration in foods is extremely variable because, as is so often the case, it reflects the regionally variable soil concentrations of the element and the amount and nature of fertilizer used in plant cultivation. Thus, the iodide content of grains, vegetables, and fruits varies with the iodide content of the soil, and the iodide content of meats depends upon the iodide of the soil and plants that the animals ate. The amount of iodide in drinking water is an indication of the iodide content of the rocks and soils of a region and closely parallels the incidence of iodine deficiency among the inhabitants of that region. For example, the iodide content of water from goitrous areas in India, Nepal, and Ceylon ranged from 0.1 to 1.2 mg/L, compared to 9.0 mg/L found in nongoitrous Delhi [1]. In the United States, before salt was fortified with iodine in the 1920s, people living in the Great Lakes and Rocky Mountain areas had iodine-poor diets. Iodized salt was introduced in 1924 in the state of Michigan [2]. Yet, in 2007, 29% to 50% of the world's population was thought to be iodine deficient, especially those living in mountainous regions (e.g., the Himalayas, European Alps, and the Andes) and lowland noncoastal regions (such as central Africa and Eastern Europe) [3].

Iodide is found in seafoods; however, large differences in iodide content exist between marine fish and freshwater fish. Edible marine (sea) fish contain about 30 to 300 μg of iodide/100 g, in contrast to only 2 to 4 μg of iodide/100 g in freshwater fish. Cod and shrimp (3 oz) provide about 99 μg and 35 μg of iodide, respectively. Kelp, which is especially rich in iodide, has about 415 μg of iodide per quarter cup. Other protein-rich foods also supply iodide. Milk and yogurt, for example, provide about 55 to 85 μg of iodide/cup, and an ounce of cheddar cheese, about 12 μg. An egg provides about 28 μg of iodide, and meats generally provide about 25 to 35 μg/100 g. Liver, for example, contains 36 μg of iodide/3 oz, and 3 oz of turkey (white meat) provides 34 μg. Beans, such as navy beans, contain about 35 μg of iodide/one-half cup. An additional source of iodide is breads and grain products made from bread dough. Dough oxidizers or conditioners contain iodates (IO_3^-) as food additives to improve cross-linking of the gluten. White bread (1 slice) contains about 23 μg of iodide, and cooked macaroni (enriched), about 27 μg per cup.

Iodized salt (¼ teaspoon or 1.5 g) supplies about 70 μg of iodide. Iodine is usually added to salt as potassium iodate or iodide. About 90% of households in North and South America use iodized salt; in contrast, less than half of households in Europe do. In the United States, processed foods are typically manufactured with noniodized salt. Restricting salt intake (as may be necessary for people being treated for hypertension) may negatively affect iodine status [4]. Iodine in vitamin/mineral supplements is provided as potassium or sodium iodide. The Daily Value for iodine is 150 μg.

Digestion, Absorption, Transport, and Storage

Dietary iodine (I) is either bound to amino acids (sometimes termed organified) or found free, primarily as iodate (IO_3^-) or iodide (I^-). During digestion,

organic bound iodine may be freed and converted to iodide within the gastrointestinal tract. Iodate, for example from breads or iodized salt, is usually reduced to iodide by glutathione within the gastrointestinal tract. Small quantities of iodinated amino acids and other organic forms of iodide that escape digestion may be absorbed, but not as efficiently as the iodide ion. The thyroid hormones thyroxine (T_4) and triiodothyronine (T_3) also are absorbed unchanged, with a bioavailability of about 70%, which allows T_4 medication to be administered orally.

Iodide is absorbed rapidly, mostly from the stomach and to a lesser extent from the duodenum. Overall, absorption of iodide is greater than 90%. Following absorption, free iodide appears in the blood, from which it is capable of permeating all tissues. The mineral selectively concentrates, however, in the thyroid gland, with lesser amounts found in the ovaries, placenta, skin, and salivary, gastric, and mammary glands.

The thyroid gland traps iodide most aggressively, by way of an active transport system against an iodide gradient that is often 20 to 50 times the plasma concentration. Specifically, iodide is taken up into the thyroid gland by a Na^+/I^- symporter located in the basolateral membrane of the thyroid gland; the transporter carries two sodiums and one iodide, with the sodium gradient generated by the Na^+/K^+ ATPase serving as the driving force. The thyroid gland contains 70% to 80% of the total body iodide and takes up about 120 μg of iodide per day. Because the thyroid gland and its synthesis of the thyroid hormones are the focal points of iodide metabolism, information on the transport of iodide into nonthyroidal tissue is sparse. However, iodide uptake by other tissues, such as salivary glands, likely occurs by an active transport mechanism.

Functions and Mechanisms of Action

The main function of iodide is in the synthesis of the thyroid hormones, thyroxine (T_4) and triiodothyronine (T_3). As long as the daily iodide intake is above about 50 μg, uptake of iodide by the thyroid gland is usually sufficient for hormone production [5]. Thyroid-stimulating hormone (also called thyrotropin), released from the pituitary gland, helps to regulate thyroid hormone production and secretion. Four atoms of iodide are needed for each T_4, and three atoms of iodide for each T_3. Amino acids are also needed for the synthesis of the thyroid hormones.

Thyroid Hormone Synthesis

The thyroid gland is made of multiple acini, also called follicles. The follicles are spherical in shape and are surrounded by a single layer of thyroid cells. The follicles are filled with colloid, a proteinaceous material. The events in thyroid hormone synthesis are shown in Figure 13.18 and described here:

- The thyroid cells actively (through an Na^+/K^+-ATPase pump) take up iodide from the blood.
- Once within the cell, iodide (I^-) is oxidized to iodine (I), which is then bound to the number 3 position

of tyrosyl residues of the glycoprotein thyroglobulin (a process called organification of the iodine). This binding of iodine to the tyrosyl residues is catalyzed by the heme iron-dependent enzyme thyroperoxidase and generates thyroglobulin-3-monoiodotyrosine (Thg-MIT). Hydrogen peroxide acts as the electron acceptor.

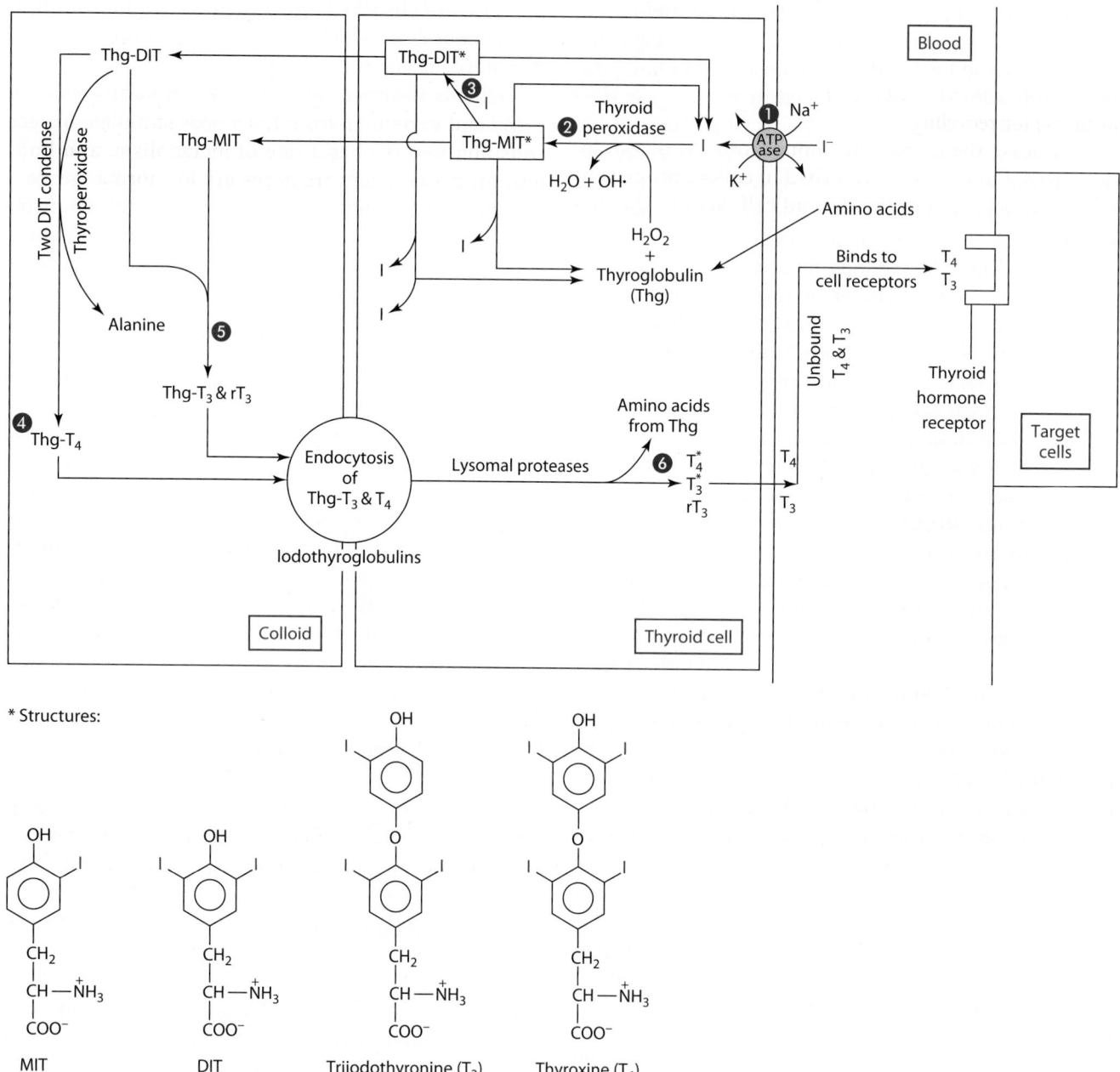

* Structures:

MIT   DIT   Triiodothyronine (T_3)   Thyroxine (T_4)

❶ I^- is actively transported into the thyroid cell.

❷ I is bound to a tyrosine residue on thyroglobulin to form thyroglobulin-3-monoiodotyrosine (Thg-MIT).

❸ Thg-MIT is iodinated to form Thg-DIT, thyroglobulin-3, 5-diodotyrosine, which ❹ condenses with another Thg-DIT in the colloid to form Thg-T_4.

❺ Thg-DIT also can condense with Thg-MIT to form Thg-T_3 and reverse (r)T_3.

❻ T_4 and T_3, active thyroid hormones, are released into the blood following endocytosis of Thg-T_3 and Thg-T_4 back into the thyroid cell and hydrolysis of the Thg by proteases.

Figure 13.18 Overview of iodine intrathyroidal metabolism and hormonogenesis.

- Next, MIT is iodinated in the number 5 position by thyroperoxidase to form thyroglobulin-3,5-diiodotyrosine (Thg-DIT).

- In the colloid, two DITs condense or couple to form Thg-3,5,3′,5′-tetraiodothyronine (Thg-T_4), with the elimination of an alanine side chain. Thyroperoxidase also catalyzes this coupling reaction. DIT also condenses or couples with MIT to form 3,5,3′-triiodothyronine (T_3) and reverse T_3 (rT_3).

DIT and MIT not used for thyroid hormone synthesis in the thyroid cells are deiodinated, and the iodine is made available for recycling.

To release the thyroid hormones into the blood, iodothyroglobulin must be resorbed in colloid droplets by endocytosis back into the thyroid cell. Within the thyroid cell, the iodothyroglobulin (Thg-T_4 and Thg-T_3) is hydrolyzed by lysosomal proteases, and T_4 and T_3 are released into the blood.

Transport of Thyroid Hormones in the Blood

Three transport proteins bind and transport T_4 and T_3 in the blood. The protein thyroxine-binding globulin has the smallest capacity but the greatest affinity for T_4 and T_3. Albumin and transthyretin (also called prealbumin) also transport the thyroid hormones. A very small fraction (<0.1%) of T_4 and T_3 in the blood is not bound to transport proteins; it is in this free form that the hormones are available to the cell receptors and affect physiological processes. The plasma concentration of T_4 is nearly 50 times that of T_3, but T_3 is many times (~20–100) more potent on an equal molar basis. Several tissues—the liver, kidneys, brain, pituitary, and brown adipose, to name a few—deiodinate T_4 to generate T_3, although most T_3 in the blood has been synthesized in the liver from T_4. The conversion of T_4 to T_3 is catalyzed by the selenium-dependent enzyme 5′-deiodinase; this conversion is impaired with selenium deficiency.

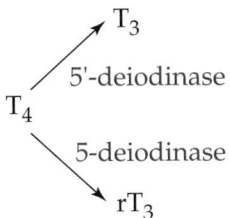

For a more in-depth description of thyroid hormone synthesis, see the reviews by Visser [6] and Vanderpas [7].

Thyroid Hormone Functions

The multiple effects of the thyroid hormones result from the hormones' occupancy of nuclear receptors, with subsequent effects on gene expression. The receptors appear to be the same in all tissues, binding T_3 more avidly than

T_4 and requiring fivefold to sevenfold higher concentrations of T_4 to achieve comparable physiological effects. Thyroid hormones bind to DNA as monomers, homodimers, and heterodimers, such as with retinoid X receptors (discussed under vitamin A in Chapter 10). Additionally, the hormone receptor complex may interact with the DNA through zinc fingers. Although the mechanisms of action of the thyroid hormones are unclear, biological effects occur in response to increased mRNA and protein synthesis triggered by the thyroid hormone receptor complex interactions with DNA.

The effects of thyroid hormones on metabolism are many and varied. Thyroid hormones stimulate oxygen consumption, the basal rate of metabolism, and body heat production, and are necessary for normal nervous system development and linear growth. Directly or indirectly, most organ systems are under the influence of these hormones (Table 13.8).

Interactions with Other Nutrients

The metabolism of the thyroid hormones is largely dependent upon a group of three selenium-dependent iodothyronine 5′-deiodinases. Impaired selenium status results in altered thyroid hormone metabolism and function. The roles of these deiodinases are described further under the section of this chapter addressing selenium, specifically "Iodothyronine 5′-Deiodinases (IDI or DI)."

Like selenium deficiency, iron and vitamin A deficiencies may magnify the effects of inadequate iodine. Heme iron is a component of the enzyme thyroperoxidase, which attaches iodine to tyrosine residues on thyroglobulin, and which then conjugates the thyroglobulins for the production of the thyroid hormones. Iron also may be involved in the binding of T_3 to nuclear receptors. Thus, iron deficiency impairs thyroid hormone synthesis and functions. Similarly, vitamin A deficiency reduces iodine uptake by the thyroid gland and decreases the synthesis of thyroglobulin and the coupling of iodotyrosine residues to form T_4 [8].

Another well-established interaction is that between iodide and goitrogens. Substances that interfere with iodide metabolism to inhibit thyroid hormonogenesis are called goitrogens because their effect is to secondarily

Table 13.8 Selected Physiological Effects of Thyroid Hormones

Adipose tissue: enhances lipolysis

Muscle: enhances contraction

Bone: promotes anabolism (growth and development)

Cardiovascular system: increases heart rate

Gastrointestinal tract: stimulates nutrient digestion and absorption

Metabolism: stimulates metabolic rate and cellular oxygen consumption in metabolically active tissues augment thyroid-stimulating hormone release and consequently thyroid gland enlargement. Goitrogens may affect iodide uptake by the gland, organification of the iodide, or hormone release from the thyroid cells. That some natural foods are goitrogenic was evidenced many years ago when it was discovered that rabbits fed a fresh cabbage diet developed goiters that could be reversed by iodine supplementation. It was later shown that cruciferous vegetables, including cabbage, kale, cauliflower, broccoli, rutabaga, turnips, Brussels sprouts, and mustard greens, contain glucosinolates, which compete with iodide for uptake into the thyroid gland. Perhaps the only food to be identified directly with goiter etiology is cassava, which is consumed in large quantities in many developing countries. Cassava contains the cyanogenic glucoside linamarin that later became known as goitrin (Figure 13.19). The linamarin, once hydrolyzed within the gastrointestinal tract, releases cyanide, which is then metabolized to thiocyanate (SCN^-). Thiocyanate competes with iodide for uptake into the thyroid gland. Cyanogenic glucosides are also found in lima beans, flaxseed, linseed, sorghum, and sweet potatoes.

Other goitrogenic compounds that compete with iodide's active transport into the thyroid cells include halide ions such as bromide (Br^-) and astatide (At^-). Perchlorate (ClO_4^-), along with perrhenate (ReO_4^-) and pertechnetate (Tc_4^-), interferes with organification as well as iodide uptake; perchlorate is a known contaminant in drinking water. Lithium (Li^-), used to treat some psychiatric disorders, inhibits thyroid hormone release from the gland. Some other classes of goitrogens that interfere with iodide metabolism include polycyclic hydrocarbons and phenol compounds derived from coal.

Excretion

The kidneys have no mechanism to conserve iodide, and they therefore provide the major route (~80–$90+\%$) for iodide excretion. Usual urinary iodine excretion exceeds 100 µg/L if intake is adequate [9]. Fecal excretion of iodide (up to 20% of the total excreted) is relatively low, ranging from 6.7 to 42.1 µg/day [10]. Some iodide is also lost in sweat, a loss that can be of consequence in hot, tropical regions where iodide intake may be only marginally adequate.

Recommended Dietary Allowance

Because of its important link to thyroid function, iodide nutriture has been investigated thoroughly for over half a century. Dating as far back as the 1930s, intake

requirements have been published based upon results of balance studies and upon calculations of average daily urinary losses. Adult daily requirements established by those early studies ranged from 100 to 200 µg. The minimum amount (requirement) of iodide to prevent goiter is estimated at 50 to 75 µg/day or ~1 µg/kg of body weight, and has not changed significantly over the years. The RDA for iodine is 150 µg/day for adults [9]. Although the recommendations apply equally to both sexes, iodide needs are higher during pregnancy and lactation: 220 µg and 290 µg, respectively [9]. The inside front cover of the book provides additional RDAs for iodine for other age groups.

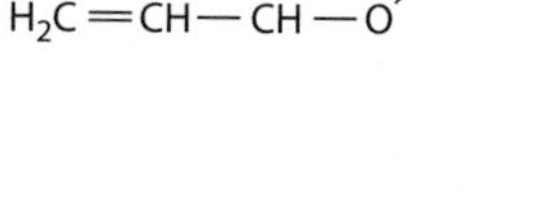

Deficiency

Thyroid Hormone Release as Related to Iodide Deficiency

The release of thyroid hormones by the thyroid gland is controlled. Thyrotropin-releasing hormone secreted by the hypothalamus acts on the pituitary gland to stimulate thyroid-stimulating hormone (TSH). TSH, in response to thyrotropin-releasing hormone, is secreted from the anterior pituitary and increases the activity of the thyroid gland to generate T_4. TSH output is regulated by T_4 through negative feedback to the pituitary. A decline in the blood level of T_4 triggers the release of TSH, resulting in hyperplasia of the thyroid. Elevated T_4 inhibits release of TSH and thyrotropin-releasing hormone.

Iodine Deficiency and Iodine Deficiency Disorders

Iodine deficiency prevails in many areas of the world and is associated most often with dietary insufficiency of iodine (typically less than about 10–20 µg of iodine/day). About 200 to 300 million people worldwide are iodine deficient [11]. Inadequate iodide intake is the main cause of goiter (although other factors, such as ingestion of goitrogens, may cause the disorder), which is characterized by enlargement (hyperplasia) of the thyroid gland. This enlargement is caused by overstimulation by TSH. Iodide deficiency depletes the thyroid gland's iodide stores and therefore reduces the output of T_4 and T_3. This decline in the blood level of T_4 triggers release of TSH, resulting in hyperplasia of the thyroid gland. The growth of the gland is self-restricting, however, because in its enlarged state it traps and processes available iodide more efficiently. The gland can return to normal size over time (months to years) as dietary iodine is increased to adequate amounts.

Because iodide deficiency also affects growth, development, and other health factors, the term *iodide deficiency disorders (IDDs)* has been coined. Iodine deficiency in a fetus results from iodide deficiency of the mother; two types of cretinism can result. Neurological cretinism in the infant is characterized by mental deficiency, hearing loss or deaf mutism, and motor disorders such as

Figure 13.19 Goitrin.

spasticity and muscular rigidity [5]. Hypothyroid cretinism results in thyroid failure. Early treatment of cretinism with iodine can often correct the condition.

Defects in the Na^+/I^- symporter have been characterized and result in the absence of thyroid hormone production [12]. Consequently, hypothyroidism, goiter, and mental retardation, among other signs and symptoms of iodide deficiency, develop if the condition goes untreated.

The addition of iodide to table salt and the administration of iodized oil, potassium iodide or iodine, and iron salts have done much to alleviate the problem of endemic goiter in some goitrous regions of the world. Yet iodide deficiency continues to be a major health problem in many underdeveloped countries, and, in many countries, may be coupled with selenium and iron deficiencies. In the United States, the restriction of salt intake (as may be necessary for people being treated for hypertension) may increase a person's risk for developing iodine deficiency [4]. See Carpenter [13] and Patrick [14] for a review of the history of iodine deficiency.

Toxicity

Poor monitoring and over-supplementation of iodine in several countries with supplementation programs are reportedly resulting in excessive intakes. In addition, in some countries, excessive intake results from overconsumption of foods naturally high in iodine. Some signs of acute iodide toxicity include burning of the mouth, throat, and stomach; nausea; vomiting; diarrhea; and fever. A Tolerable Upper Intake Level for iodine has been set at 1,100 μg (1.1 mg)/day [9]. High iodine intake may cause problems with the thyroid gland, including both hyper- and hypothyroidism and inflammation of the thyroid (thyroiditis).

Assessment of Nutriture

Assessment of iodide status is generally directed at populations living in areas suspected of being iodide deficient, although individuals may be assessed if thyroid problems are suspected. Several methods are used for iodine assessment. Urinary iodine excretion represents an indicator of recent iodine intake; in fact, daily urinary iodine can be used to calculate iodine intake using the following formula: Daily iodine intake = urinary iodine × 0.0235 × body weight, with urinary iodine measured in μg/L and weight measured in kg [9]. Usual urinary iodine excretion exceeds 100 μg/L if intake is adequate. Urinary iodide excretion equal to 100 μg/L is thought to correspond to an iodide intake of about 150 μg [5]. Median urinary iodine concentrations of <100 μg/L suggest inadequate iodine intake and iodine insufficiency or mild iodine deficiency in a population. Urinary iodine concentrations less than 50 μg/L are usually associated with insufficient thyroid

hormone secretion and are indicative of moderate iodine deficiency, while concentrations less than 20 μg/L are considered severe [5]. As dietary iodine intake increases, urinary iodine concentrations also rise. Urinary iodine concentrations equal to or in excess of 500 μg/L have been associated with increasing thyroid volume, which in turn indicates thyroid dysfunction [15].

Thyroid size, measured by ultrasonography or by palpation, is also used to assess goiter, and indirectly iodine status. Enlargement of the gland is associated with suboptimal iodide status; however, the size of the gland may take months to years to return to normal in response to treatment (iodine supplementation) [5]. Thus, this indicator is typically used along with urinary iodine excretion.

In addition to urinary iodide excretion and measurement of the thyroid gland, serum TSH concentrations are an especially sensitive indicator of iodine status in newborn infants from at-risk populations. Serum TSH concentrations greater than about 5 μUnits/L in a population suggest deficiency. Finally, serum concentrations of thyroglobulin, which rise with iodide deficiency as the size of the thyroid gland enlarges, may be used to assess iodine status. Serum thyroglobulin concentrations greater than 10 μg/L suggest inadequate iodine intake.

References Cited for Iodine

1. Karmarkar M, Deo M, Kochupillai N, Ramalingaswami V. Pathophysiology of Himalayan endemic goiter. Am J Clin Nutr. 1974; 27:96–103.
2. Zimmermann MB. Research on iodine deficiency and goiter in the 19th and early 20th centuries. J Nutr. 2008; 138:2060–63.
3. Mithen R. Effect of genotype on micronutrient absorption and metabolism: a review of iron, copper, iodine, and selenium, and folates. Int J Vitam Nutr Res. 2007; 77:205–16.
4. Cann S. Salt in food. Lancet. 2005; 365:845–46.
5. Zimmermann MB. Iodine deficiency. Endocrin Rev. 2009; 30:376–408.
6. Visser TJ. The elemental importance of sufficient iodine intake: a trace is not enough. Endocrinology. 2006; 147:2095–97.
7. Vanderpas J. Nutritional epidemiology and thyroid hormone metabolism. Ann Rev Nutr. 2006; 26:293–322.
8. Hess SY. The impact of common micronutrient deficiencies on iodine and thyroid metabolism: the evidence from human studies. Clin Endocrin Metab. 2010; 24:117–32.
9. Food and Nutrition Board, Institute of Medicine. Dietary Reference Intakes. Washington, DC: National Academy Press, 2001.
10. Vought R, London W, Lutwak L, Dublin T. Reliability of estimates of serum inorganic iodine and daily fecal and urinary iodine excretion from single casual specimens. J Clin Endocr Metab. 1963; 23:1218–28.
11. Ristic-Medic D, Piskackova Z, Hooper L, et al. Methods of assessment of iodine status in humans: a systemic review. Am J Clin Nutr. 2009; 89(suppl):S2052–69.
12. Reed-Tsur MD, De la Vieja A, Ginter CS, Carrasco N. Molecular characterization of V59E NIS, a Na^+/I^- symporter mutant that causes congenital I^- transport defect. Endocrinology. 2008; 149:3077–84.
13. Carpenter K. David Marine and the problem of goiter. J Nutr. 2005; 135:675–80.
14. Patrick L. Iodine: deficiency and therapeutic considerations. Altern Med Rev. 2008; 13:116–27.
15. Zimmermann M, Ito Y, Hess S, et al. High thyroid volume in children with excess dietary iodine intakes. Am J Clin Nutr. 2005; 81:840–44.

Suggested Readings

Molecular and Cellular Endocrinology 2010 volume 322 is devoted to disorders involving iodine utilization.

Burgi H. Iodine excess. Clin Endocrin Metab. 2010; 24:107–15.

Zimmermann MB. The influence of iron status on iodine utilization and thyroid function. Ann Rev Nutr. 2006; 26:367–89.

Web Site for Nutrient Composition Information

http://www.ars.usda.gov/Services/docs.htm?docid=18877

MANGANESE

Although widely distributed in nature, manganese exists primarily as Mn^{2+} or Mn^{3+} in only trace amounts (about 10–20 mg) in the body.

Sources

Whole-grain cereals, dried fruits, nuts, and leafy vegetables are among the common manganese-rich foods. Wheat bran–based breakfast cereals provide about 1.7 mg of manganese/cup. Wheat germ contains about 2.0 mg of manganese/quarter cup, and 1 cup of oatmeal provides about 1.3 mg. Nuts (almonds, pecans, cashews, hazelnuts) provide about 0.5 to 1.8 mg of manganese/oz, while beans (black, kidney, pinto, and navy) have about 0.76 to 0.96 mg/cup. Leafy green vegetables (cooked), such as spinach, collard greens, and turnip greens, contain about 0.8 to 1.7 mg of manganese/half cup. Pineapple is particularly rich in manganese, with 2.3 mg per cup. Blueberries also provide about 0.9 mg per cup. Tea contains relatively large amounts of manganese (about 0.4–1.6 mg/cup). The manganese content of grains varies widely, due partly to plant species differences and partly to the efficiency with which the milling process separates the manganese-rich and manganese-poor parts of the grain. White flour, for example, has a much lower manganese concentration than the wheat grain from which it was produced. A slice of whole-wheat bread provides 0.30 mg of manganese, whereas a slice of white bread contains only 0.15 mg. The usual intake of manganese among Americans ranges from about 3 to 9 mg/day. The Daily Value for manganese is 2 mg. Supplements provide managanese as manganese gluconate, manganese sulfate, manganese ascorbate, and amino acid chelates of manganese.

Digestion, Absorption, Transport, and Storage

Digestion and Absorption

Whether manganese is bound to food components that need to undergo digestion to release manganese prior to its absorption is not clear. Manganese absorption, likely as Mn^{2+}, is typically less than about 5%, with absorption decreasing as intake increases and increasing as intake decreases. Females may absorb greater amounts than males for unclear reasons. Manganese absorption appears to be quickly saturable and is thought to involve a low-capacity, high-affinity, active carrier protein such as divalent mineral transporter (DMT) 1 and/or Zrt- and Irt-like protein (ZIP) 14. Absorption likely occurs throughout the length of the small intestine. Both regulation of intestinal absorption and control of excretion enable manganese homeostasis in the body.

Factors Influencing Absorption Relative to many of the other trace minerals, little information is available on factors influencing manganese absorption. Low-molecular-weight ligands, such as histidine and citrate, enhance manganese absorption. In contrast, but as with other divalent cations, fiber, phytic acid, and oxalic acid may precipitate manganese in the gastrointestinal tract, making the manganese unavailable for absorption. Iron also appears to compete with manganese for absorption, likely using DMT1. Copper also decreases manganese absorption and retention.

Transport and Storage

Manganese entering into the portal circulation from the gastrointestinal tract may either remain free or become bound as Mn^{2+} to α-2 macroglobulin before traversing the liver, where it is almost totally removed. Upon release from the liver, some manganese in the blood may (1) remain free (as Mn^{2+}); (2) be bound (as Mn^{2+}) to albumin, α-2 macroglobulin, β-globulin, or γ-globulin; or (3) be oxidized by ceruloplasmin to Mn^{3+} and complexed with transferrin. Serum manganese concentrations normally range from about 0.6 to 4.3 ng/mL. The mineral has a half-life in the blood of about 10 to 42 days.

Manganese is cleared rapidly from the blood. Zrt- and Irt-like protein (ZIP) 8 (expressed on the cell membranes of cells of the liver, kidneys, lungs, and testes), along with ZIP14 (expressed primarily in the intestine and liver), and DMT1 (ubiquitiously expressed) are thought to transport manganese into cells. In addition, uptake of manganese bound to transferrin occurs through transferrin receptors (see the "Cellular Iron Uptake" section).

Within cells, manganese is found primarily as Mn^{2+} in the mitochondria; unlike iron and copper, manganese is not readily oxidized within tissues. Manganese is found in most organs and tissues (including hair) and does not tend to concentrate significantly in any particular one, although its concentration is highest in the bones, liver, pancreas, and kidneys. In bones (which may contain 25–40% of total body stores), manganese is found as part of the apatite.

Functions and Mechanisms of Action

At the molecular level, manganese, like other trace elements, can function both as an enzyme activator and as a constituent of metalloenzymes. In the activation of enzyme-catalyzed reactions, manganese may bind to the substrate, to ATP, or to the enzyme directly, inducing conformational changes. Enzymes from nearly every class (including transferases, kinases, hydrolases, oxido-reductases, ligases, and lyases) can be activated by manganese in this manner and are numerous and diverse in function. However, largely because the activation of many enzymes is not manganese specific, a manganese deficiency does not impair the activity of most of these enzymes. The metal is typically replaced by other divalent cations like magnesium. One exception to this apparent lack of specificity is the manganese-specific activation of the glycosyl transferases. Examples of roles that manganese-dependent enzymes perform in the body are described in the next section.

Bone, Cartilage, and Connective Tissue Synthesis

Two manganese-dependent transferases important for connective tissue synthesis are xylosyl transferase and glycosyl (also called galactosyl or galacto) transferase. Glycosyl transferase is especially important for the synthesis of glycosaminoglycans, such as chondroitin sulfate, which attach to proteins to form proteoglycans. Remember that proteoglycans are important structural components of connective tissues such as cartilage and bone. Specifically, glycosyl transferase catalyzes the transfer of a sugar moiety (galactose) from uridine diphosphate (UDP) to an acceptor molecule, as shown by the general reaction:

$$\text{UDP-sugar} + \text{acceptor} \xrightarrow{\text{Glycosyl transferase}} \text{UDP} + \text{acceptor-sugar}$$

Manganese deficiency is associated with impaired glycosyl transferase activity.

Manganese also activates the hydrolase prolidase, a dipeptidase with specificity for dipeptides. Prolidase is found in dermal fibroblasts and is important for collagen formation.

Urea Synthesis

Arginase, a hydrolase that requires four manganese atoms per molecule, is a cytosolic enzyme responsible for urea formation. The enzyme is found in high concentrations in the liver, the site of the urea cycle. The enzyme cleaves arginine to generate urea and ornithine. Low-manganese diets in animals have been shown to decrease arginase activity.

Carbohydrate/Nutrient Metabolism

Pyruvate carboxylase, a ligase/synthetase that contains four manganese atoms, converts pyruvate to the TCA cycle intermediate oxaloacetate. Because magnesium can replace manganese in pyruvate carboxylase, minimal changes in pyruvate carboxylase activity occur with manganese deficiency.

Phosphoenolpyruvate carboxykinase (PEPCK), a lyase activated by manganese, converts oxaloacetate to phosphoenolpyruvate and carbon dioxide. This reaction is important in gluconeogenesis. The activity of phosphoenolpyruvate carboxykinase decreases in animals with manganese deficiency.

The enzyme isocitrate dehydrogenase requires either manganese or magnesium. This enzyme catalyzes the conversion of isocitrate to alpha-ketoglutarate in the TCA cycle; $NADP^+$ is needed for the reaction.

Amino Acid Metabolism

Glutamine synthetase, activated by manganese or magnesium, is important in the synthesis of glutamine from glutamate.

Antioxidant Roles

Superoxide dismutase, a manganese-dependent (Mn^{3+}-SOD) oxido-reductase metalloenzyme (not manganese activated), functions in a manner similar to copper- and zinc-dependent superoxide dismutase to prevent lipid peroxidation by superoxide radicals. However, manganese-SOD is found in the mitochondria, whereas copper-zinc-SOD is found extracellularly and in the cell cytosol. Thus, Mn-SOD likely eliminates superoxides before they damage mitochondrial function. The activity of the electron transport/respiratory chain generates large amounts of superoxide radicals, necessitating substantial Mn-SOD activity. Cellular ultrastructural abnormalities associated with manganese deficiency are likely caused by uncontrolled lipid peroxidation in the membranes because of reduced Mn-SOD activity or simply by reduced availability of manganese to directly scavenge free radicals. Manganese, one of a few minerals able to scavenge free radicals, quenches peroxyl radicals as shown in this equation: $Mn^{2+} + ROO^{\bullet} \longrightarrow Mn^{3+} + ROOH$. Low-manganese diets in animals have been shown to decrease Mn-SOD activity. Moreover, Mn-SOD knockout mice die shortly after birth, an indication of Mn-SOD's essential protective role in the body.

Other Roles

Manganese also may act as a modulator of second messenger pathways in tissues. For example, manganese increases cAMP accumulation through binding to ATP and ADP. Manganese can activate guanylate cyclase, and manganese may affect cytosolic calcium levels and thus regulate calcium-dependent processes [14].

Interactions with Other Nutrients

Only a few interactions between manganese and other trace elements are thought to be of significance nutritionally. One such relationship—that between manganese and iron—is detailed in the section on absorption. However, the interaction is reciprocal; that is, iron in excess inhibits manganese absorption, and manganese, when ingested in amounts about four to eight times the recommended intake, decreases iron absorption up to about 40%. Interactions also may occur between manganese and calcium and between manganese and zinc; however, because of the paucity of information and the divergent results from various studies, the nature of such interactions remains undefined.

Excretion

Manganese is excreted primarily (>90%) via the bile in the feces. Excess absorbed manganese from the diet is quickly excreted by the liver into the bile to maintain homeostasis. Very little manganese is excreted in the urine, less than 1 μg/L. Small losses also occur through sweat and skin desquamation [3].

Adequate Intake

The latest recommendation for manganese intake, like previous recommendations, is based on median intake because data are insufficient to calculate requirements for the mineral. Recommended Adequate Intakes of manganese are 2.3 mg for adult men and 1.8 mg for adult women daily [4]. With pregnancy and lactation, recommendations increase to 2 mg and 2.6 mg, respectively [4]. The inside front cover of the book gives additional recommendations for manganese for other age groups.

Deficiency

Manganese deficiency is associated with diverse physiological malfunctions. In humans, manganese deficiency generally does not develop unless the mineral is deliberately eliminated from the diet. Studies in which men received either 0.11 mg manganese per day for 39 days (the diet was also devoid of vitamin K, making it difficult to separate the effects of the manganese and vitamin K deficiencies) or 0.35 mg manganese per day resulted in negative manganese balance [3]. Symptoms and signs of deficiency include nausea; vomiting; dermatitis; decreased serum manganese; decreased fecal manganese excretion; increased serum calcium, phosphorus, and alkaline phosphatase (thought to be associated with skeletal bone changes); decreased growth of hair and nails; changes in hair and beard color; poor bone formation and skeletal defects; decreased clotting proteins; and altered carbohydrate and lipid metabolism [3,4].

Other problems associated with deficiency include the occurrence of ataxia, loss of equilibrium, cell ultrastructure abnormalities, compromised reproductive function, abnormal glucose tolerance, and impaired lipid metabolism [3,4].

Toxicity

Exposure to high levels of oral, parenteral, and air manganese may result in toxicity. Additionally, individuals with liver failure are at greater risk for toxicity because manganese homeostasis is maintained largely by the liver through excretion in the bile. Manganese toxicity secondary to liver failure is characterized by manganese accumulation within the liver and other organs such as the brain; accumulation in the brain results in neurologic abnormalities [5,6]. Motor and cognitive dysfunction also occurs with manganese toxicity. Neonates receiving total parenteral nutrition are thought to be at higher risk for manganese toxicity because of their lack of absorptive control and diminished biliary manganese excretion [7–9]. Symptoms of manganese toxicity with chronic exposure to airborne manganese include cough, bronchitis, pneumonitis, reduced lung function, prolonged reaction time, tremors, diminished memory capacity, and loss of coordination resembling Parkinson's disease [5,6]. Other signs and symptoms of toxicity include insomnia, headache, increased forgetfulness, anxiety, mood changes, compulsive behaviors, reduced response speed, rapid hand movements, and gait disturbance [7–9]. The Tolerable Upper Intake Level for manganese has been set at 11 mg/day [4].

Assessment of Nutriture

Assessment of manganese status typically is based on concentrations of manganese in the plasma/serum and whole blood. Serum concentrations have been found to be somewhat sensitive to large variations in intake but do not necessarily correlate with intake or status [2,9]. Enzyme activity, primarily Mn-SOD and arginase, also has been used but has not been shown to be a good indicator of manganese status [9].

References Cited for Manganese

1. Davis C, Greger J. Longitudinal changes of manganese dependent superoxide dismutase and other indexes of manganese and iron status in women. Am J Clin Nutr. 1992; 55:747–52.
2. Greger JL, Davis CD, Suttie JW, Lyle BJ. Intake, serum concentrations, and urinary excretion of manganese by adult males. Am J Clin Nutr. 1990; 51:457–61.
3. Friedman B, Freeland-Graves J, Bales C, et al. Manganese balance and clinical observations in young men fed a manganese-deficient diet. J Nutr. 1987; 117:133–43.
4. Food and Nutrition Board, Institute of Medicine. Dietary Reference Intakes. Washington, DC: National Academy Press. 2001 pp. 394–419.
5. Santamaria AB. Manganese exposure, essentiality, & toxicity. Ind J Med Res. 2008; 128:484–500.

6. Santamaria AB, Sulsky SI. Risk assessment of an essential element: manganese. J Tox Environ Health. 2010; 73:128–55.

7. Erikson K, Thompson K, Aschner J, Aschner M. Manganese neurotoxicity: a focus on the neonate. Pharmac & Ther. 2007; 113:369–77.

8. Aschner J, Aschner M. Nutritional aspects of manganese homeostasis. Trace Elem Human Hlth. 2005; 26:353–62.

9. Hardy G. Manganese in parenteral nutrition: who, when, and why should we supplement? Gastroenterol. 2009; 137:S29–35.

Suggested Reading

Roth JA. Homeostatic and toxic mechanisms regulating manganese uptake, retention, and elimination. Biol Res. 2006; 39:45–57.

Web Site for Nutrient Composition Information

http://www.ars.usda.gov/Services/docs.htm?docid=18877

MOLYBDENUM

The need for molybdenum was established in humans through the observation that a genetic deficiency of specific enzymes that require molybdenum as a cofactor resulted in severe pathology. In the body, which contains about 2 mg of the mineral, molybdenum, a metal, is found primarily in either of two valence states, Mo^{4+} or Mo^{6+}.

Sources

Molybdenum is widespread among foods, but as with many other minerals, the molybdenum content of a given plant food may vary greatly depending upon the concentration of molybdenum in the soil. Better sources of molybdenum in the diet are legumes, which can provide up to 184 µg/100 g; meat, fish, and poultry, which contain up to ~129 µg/100 g; and grains and grain products, which provide up to ~117 µg/100 g [1,2]. Nuts and vegetables usually contain less than 50 µg/100 g, but fruits and dairy products are especially low in molybdenum, providing less than 12 µg/100 g [1,2]. The Daily Value for molybdenum is 75 µg.

Digestion, Absorption, Transport, and Storage

Molybdenum, which is found in foods primarily as molybdate (MoO_4^{2-}), does not appear to require digestion prior to its absorption from the small intestine, mostly the proximal region. The mechanism by which molybdenum is absorbed is thought to be passive, although some studies suggest the possible involvement of a carrier. Molybdenum absorption increases with increasing dietary intake over a range of 22 to 1,490 µg/day [3]. Molybdenum absorption from foods ranges from ~50% to 85% and, from the supplement ammonium molybdate, absorption is over 90% [3–6]. Sulfates (SO_4^{2-}), if present in large quantities, may compete with molybdate for absorption. Transport of molybdenum in the blood is thought to occur as molybdate, which binds to albumin and α-2 macroglobulin.

The molybdenum content of human tissues is quite low, averaging 0.1 to 1.0 µg/g of wet weight; the human body contains about 2 mg of the mineral. Molybdate uptake by tissues is thought to occur by a high-affinity carrier that perhaps also transports sulfate. The liver, kidneys, and bones contain the most molybdenum in terms of both absolute amount and concentration. Other tissues, such as small intestine, the lungs, spleen, brain, thyroid and adrenal glands, and muscle, also contain the element. In tissues, molybdenum is found in any of three forms: molybdate, free molybdopterin, or molybdopterin that is bound to enzymes.

Functions and Mechanisms of Action

The biochemical role of molybdenum centers around the redox function of the element and its necessity as a cofactor in the form of molybdopterin for four metalloenzymes (sulfite oxidase, aldehyde oxidase, xanthine dehydrogenase/oxidase, and amidoxime reductase), all of which catalyze oxidation-reduction reactions. Molybdopterin is an alkylphosphate-substituted pterin, to which molybdenum is coordinated through two sulfur atoms. Molybdopterin anchors the molybdenum to the apoenzyme at its catalytic site. The molybdenum is further bonded either to two oxygen molecules (called dioxomolybdopterin) or to one oxygen and one sulfur (called oxosulfidomolybdopterin), as shown in Figure 13.20. The inability to synthesize molybdopterin because of genetic defects is usually lethal.

Sulfite Oxidase: Sulfur Metabolism

Sulfite oxidase, a mitochondrial intermembrane enzyme found in many body tissues, especially the liver, heart, and kidneys, has iron-sulfur clusters, two molybdopterins (dioxo cofactor form), and two cytochrome residues. The enzyme catalyzes the terminal step in the metabolism of the sulfur-containing amino acids (methionine and cysteine), in which sulfite (SO_3^{2-}) is converted to sulfate (SO_4^{2-}), as shown here:

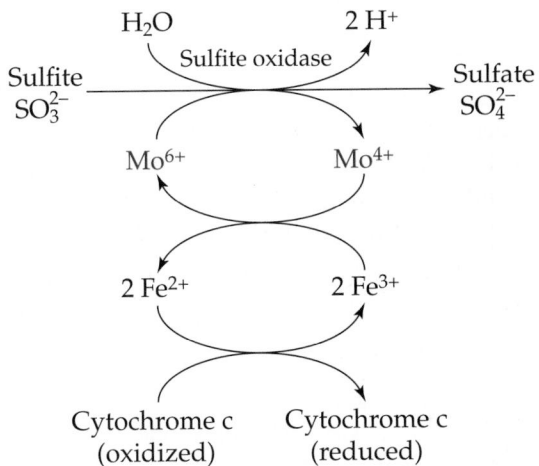

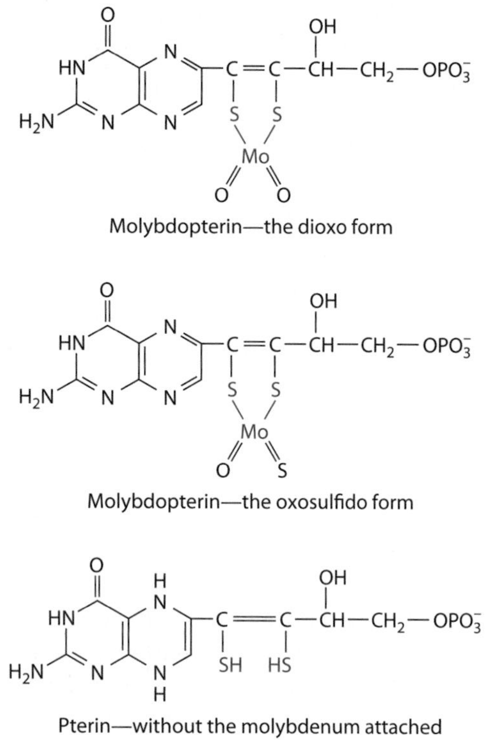

Molybdopterin—the dioxo form

Molybdopterin—the oxosulfido form

Pterin—without the molybdenum attached

Figure 13.20 Molybdopterin structures.

Cytochrome c is the physiological electron acceptor for the reaction.

In addition to originating from the catabolism of methionine and cysteine, sulfites are found in the diet. Sulfites are added to some foods as an antimicrobial agent. Sulfate generated from this reaction typically is excreted in the urine or reused for the synthesis of sulfoproteins, sulfolipids, and mucopolysaccharides (a component of mucus).

Aldehyde Oxidase: Various Roles

Aldehyde oxidase is a molybdoenzyme (using the oxosulfido form) that is similar to xanthine oxidase (see the next section) in size, cofactor composition, and substrate specificity. It presumably functions in the cytosol of liver cells as a true oxidase, using exclusively molecular oxygen as its physiological electron acceptor. The enzyme's primary substrates are thought to include a variety of aldehydes, including, for example, the retinal form of vitamin A and the pyridoxal form of vitamin B_6, as well as acetyladehyde and other drugs. Other enzymes, however, such as an NADH-dependent aldehyde dehydrogenase also found in the liver, are thought to catalyze reactions similar to those catalyzed by this aldehyde oxidase.

Xanthine Dehydrogenase and Xanthine Oxidase: Hydroxylation of Purines, Pteridines, and Pyrimidines, among Other Compounds

Xanthine dehydrogenase and xanthine oxidase (also called oxidoreductases) are interconvertible, iron-dependent (containing 2 iron-2 sulfur centers) enzymes that exist as a homodimer of two identical subunits and that also require FAD and molybdopterin in the oxosulfido cofactor form. The molybdenum is necessary for the oxidative capacity of the enzyme; inactivation of the enzyme results if the mineral is not present. Xanthine dehydrogenase is found in a variety of tissues, including the liver, lungs, kidneys, and intestine. Xanthine oxidase is found in the intestine, thyroid cells, and possibly other tissues. Healthy tissues may contain about 10% of their total xanthine enzymes in the oxidase form [7]. Conversion of xanthine dehydrogenase to xanthine oxidase may occur following the oxidation of sulfhydryl groups or by proteolysis of the dehydrogenase form.

The xanthine dehydrogenase and oxidase enzymes are capable of hydroxylating various purines, pteridines, pyrimidines, and other heterocyclic nitrogen-containing compounds. Hypoxanthine, derived from purine catabolism, is oxidized in most tissues by xanthine dehydrogenase to generate xanthine and then uric acid (Figure 13.21). Xanthine dehydrogenase transfers electrons from the substrate onto NAD^+ to form $NADH + H^+$. Oxidation of hypoxanthine and xanthine by xanthine oxidase also results in uric acid, but in these reactions O_2 accepts the electrons from $FADH_2$ and hydrogen peroxide (H_2O_2) or a superoxide radical is formed.

Unlike sulfite oxidase, reduced xanthine oxidase activity causes no apparent clinical effects. The human inheritable disorder xanthinuria, in which large amounts of xanthine are excreted in the urine, provides evidence of the body's ability to tolerate low xanthine dehydrogenase or oxidase activity. The condition is essentially free of clinical manifestations, except for the possible development of kidney calculi (stones) caused by the high urinary xanthine concentration.

The effects of xanthine oxidase activity, however, are quite damaging in people being treated for ischemia (local or temporary deficiency of blood supply and thus relative oxygen deprivation). Degradation of ATP in hypoxic tissue yields hypoxanthine. Reperfusion of the tissue with oxygen (as occurs with medical treatment of ischemia, for example) helps prevent total destruction of the tissue from lack of oxygen and nutrients, but it also provides xanthine oxidase with the oxygen needed to oxidize the relatively large concentrations of hypoxanthine. Oxidation of hypoxanthine generates large amounts of hydrogen peroxide, which further induces tissue damage (called reperfusion injury). However, the injury also is thought to be mediated partly by neutrophil accumulation and activation, and the reactive oxygen species formed may be involved in signal transduction pathways [8].

Amidoxime Reductase: Drug Metabolism

Amidoxime reductase is found attached to the outer mitochondrial membrane, where it complexes with cytochrome b5 and molybdopterin [9]. The enzyme

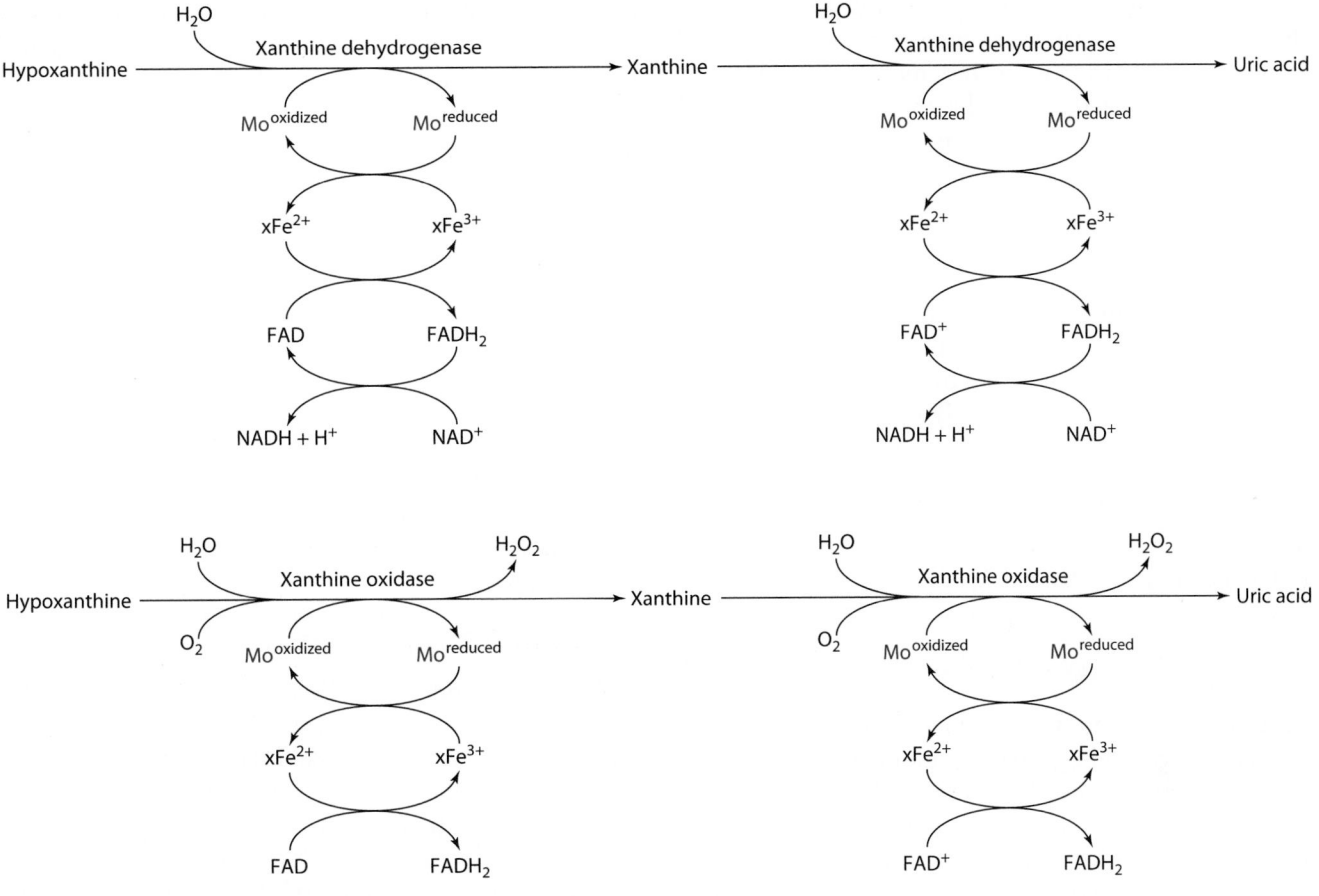

Figure 13.21 The actions of xanthine dehydrogenase and xanthine oxidase on the substrates hypoxanthine and xanthine.

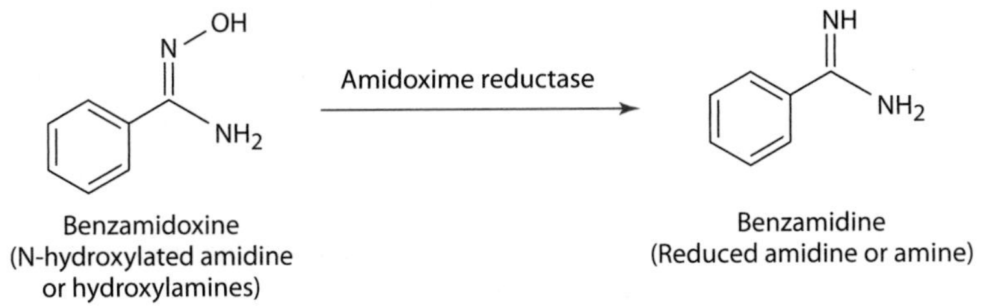

Figure 13.22 The reduction of N-hydroxylated compounds such as benzamidoxine by the molybdenum-dependent enzyme amidoxime reductase.

complex reduces N-hydroxylated amidines and hydroxyamines. N-hydroxylated drugs, for example, are synthesized by drug companies to improve the solubility and absorption of drugs into intestinal cells. Within the body, however, the drug must be reduced to exert its desired effects. Amidoxime reductase enables such a reaction (Figure 13.22).

Interactions with Other Nutrients

The most notable interaction in humans involving molybdenum is with copper. Ingestion of molybdenum as tetrathiomolybdate compromises copper absorption; the compound directly binds to copper in the gastrointestinal tract to inhibit its absorption. Because of this

property, tetrathiomolybdate is used in the treatment of Wilson's disease, a disorder of copper toxicity, as well as some cancers [10–13]. It is molybdenum's direct anti-tumor activity and the ability of molybdenum as tetrathiomolybdate to induce a copper deficiency that is beneficial in cancer treatment [11–13]. Copper is required for the formation of new blood vessels, referred to as angiogenesis. Because angiogenesis provides blood to tumors and enables their growth, substances like molybdenum that can prevent copper-induced angiogenesis have exhibited promising results such as inhibition of tumor growth in some animal studies [12,13]. A relationship between molybdenum intake and copper excretion may also exist. Urinary copper excretion in humans has been shown to rise from 24 μg to 77 μg/day as molybdenum intake increases from 160 μg to 1,540 μg/day [14]. No changes in fecal copper excretion were noted, suggesting perhaps that molybdenum increased copper mobilization from tissues and promoted excretion [14]. These effects were not confirmed, however, in a later study by Turnlund and Keys [15].

Excretion

Most molybdenum is excreted as molybdate in the urine. Urinary excretion of molybdenum increases as dietary molybdenum intake increases. In other words, little molybdenum is retained in the body when dietary intake is high, and the kidneys are thought to play a role in molybdenum homeostasis. Small amounts of molybdenum are excreted from the body in the feces by way of the bile. Small amounts of molybdenum also can be lost in sweat (20 μg) and in hair (0.01 μg/g of hair).

Recommended Dietary Allowance

Based on balance studies as well as depletion and repletion studies providing varying amounts of dietary molybdenum, an Estimated Average Requirement for molybdenum for adults was set at 34 μg [16]. The RDA for molybdenum for adults (men and women) is 45 μg (130% of the requirement), with 50 μg suggested during pregnancy and lactation [16]. The inside front cover of the book provides additional RDAs for molybdenum for other age groups.

Deficiency

Molybdenum deficiency is rarely encountered, although molybdenum deficiency has been documented in a patient maintained for 18 months on total parenteral (intravenous) nutrition. Molybdenum deficiency was associated with high blood concentrations of methionine, hypoxanthine, and xanthine, as well as low blood concentrations of uric acid. Additionally, urinary concentrations of sulfate were low, and those of sulfite were high. Treatment with 300 μg of ammonium molybdate (providing 163 μg of molybdenum) resulted in clinical improvement and normalized sulfur amino acid metabolism and uric acid production.

The importance of sulfite oxidase, and therefore molybdenum, in human nutrition is evidenced in those with sulfite oxidase deficiency, an inherited recessive disorder of metabolism. The genetic disorder is characterized by poor feeding, hypoactivity, dyspnea, dislocation of the ocular lenses, attenuated brain growth, seizures, severe neurological damage, and death in childhood. Elevated levels of urinary sulfite

and thiosulfate, along with biochemical manifestations reflecting aberrant sulfur amino acid metabolism and sulfite oxidation, also are present.

Toxicity

Molybdenum appears to be relatively nontoxic with intakes up to about 1,500 μg/day [5]. However, symptoms such as gout (inflammation of the joints caused by the accumulation of uric acid) have appeared in some people living in regions that contain high soil molybdenum levels and in those with occupational exposure to molybdenum [17]. Gout results from high amounts of uric acid (which likely arise from increased xanthine dehydrogenase activity) that have accumulated in and around joints. A Tolerable Upper Intake Level for molybdenum has been set at 2 mg [16].

Assessment of Nutriture

Molybdenum appears to distribute itself fairly equally between the plasma and red blood cells. Although studies have typically assessed the molybdenum concentrations of plasma/blood, the use of these as indicators of molybdenum status has not been validated. Similarly, while urinary molybdenum concentrations increase with increased molybdenum intake, urinary molybdenum is not necessarily reflective of molybdenum status.

References Cited for Molybdenum

1. Pennington J, Jones J. Molybdenum, nickel, cobalt, vanadium, and strontium in total diets. J Am Diet Assoc. 1987; 87:1646–50.
2. Tsongas TA, Meglen RR, Walravens PA, Chappell WR. Molybdenum in the diet: an estimate of the average daily intake in the United States. Am J Clin Nutr. 1980; 33:1103–07.
3. Novotny JA, Turnlund JR. Molybdenum intake influences molybdenum kinetics. J Nutr. 2007; 137:37–42.
4. Turnlund JR, Weaver CM, Kim SK, et al. Molybdenum absorption and utilization in humans from soy and kale intrinsically labeled with stable isotopes of molybdenum. Am J Clin Nutr. 1999; 69:1217–23.
5. Turnlund JR, Keyes WR, Peiffer GL. Molybdenum absorption, excretion, and retention studied with stable isotopes in young men at five intakes of dietary molybdenum. Am J Clin Nutr. 1995; 62:790–96.
6. Turnlund J, Keyes W, Peiffer G, Chiang G. Molybdenum absorption, excretion, and retention studied with stable isotopes in young men during depletion and repletion. Am J Clin Nutr. 1995; 61:1102–09.
7. McCord J. Free radicals and myocardial ischemia: overview and outlook. Free Rad & Med. 1988; 4:9–14.
8. Meneshian A, Bulkley G. The physiology of endothelial xanthine oxidase: from urate catabolism to reperfusion injury to inflammatory signal transduction. Microcirculation. 2002; 9:161–73.
9. Havemeyer A, Bittner F, Wollers S, et al. Identification of the missing component in the mitochondrial benzamidoxime prodrug-converting system as a novel molybdenum enzyme. J Biol Chem. 2006; 281:34796–802.

10. Brewer GJ. The use of copper-lowering therapy with tetrathiomolybdate in medicine. Expert Opin Investig Drug. 2009; 18:89–97.

11. Bandarra D, Lopes M, Lopes T, et al. Mo(II) complexes: a new family of cytotoxic agents? J Inorganic Biochem. 2010; 104:1171–77.

12. Gartner E. A pilot trial of the antiangiogenic copper lowering agent tetrathiomolybdate in combination with irinotecan, 5-flurouracil, and leucovorin for metastatic colorectal cancer. Invest New Drugs 2009; 27:159–65.

13. Kumar P, Yadav A, Patel SN, et al. Tetrathiomolybdate inhibits head and neck cancer metastasis by decreasing tumor cell motility, invasiveness, and by promoting tumor cell anoikis. Mol Cancer 2010; 9:206–17.

14. Turnlund J. Copper nutriture, bioavailability, and the influence of dietary factors. J Am Diet Assoc. 1988; 88:303–08.

15. Turnlund JR, Keyes WR. Dietary molybdenum: effect on copper absorption, excretion, and status in young men. In: Roussel AM, Anderson RA, Favier A, eds. Trace Elements in Man and Animals, 10th ed. New York: Kluwer Academic. 2000.

16. Food and Nutrition Board, Institute of Medicine. Dietary Reference Intakes. Washington, DC: National Academy Press. 2001 pp. 420–41.

17. Selden AI, Berg N, Soderbergh A, Bergstrom B. Occupational molybdenum exposure and a gouty electrician. Occupational Med. 2005; 55:145–48.

Suggested Readings

Mendel RR. Cell biology of molybdenum. Biofactors. 2009; 35:429–34.

Schwarz G, Mendel RR, Ribbe MW. Molybdenum cofactors, enzymes and pathways. Nature. 2009; 460:839–47.

Web Site for Nutrient Composition Information

http://www.ars.usda.gov/Services/docs.htm?docid=18877

NUTRIENT–DRUG INTERACTIONS

Nutrient–drug interactions represent nutrient-induced changes in the kinetics of a drug or drug-induced changes in nutrient metabolism or nutritional status. Such interactions can be extremely detrimental. Some nutrient interactions can lead to failure of the drug to perform its desired actions or to drug toxicity. Alternately, some drug interactions can promote nutrient deficiencies or toxicities. In addition to these direct interactions, drugs also may influence nutrition status indirectly by, for instance, diminishing appetite, altering taste, or promoting nausea, vomiting, or diarrhea. This Perspective reviews some examples of foods and nutrients that affect the absorption, distribution, metabolism, actions (functions), or excretion of drugs, as well as some examples of drugs that affect the absorption, metabolism, or excretion of nutrients. Table 1 provides an overview of some of the interactions presented in this Perspective.

EFFECTS OF FOODS AND NUTRIENTS ON DRUG ABSORPTION

Foods or nutrients in foods can alter drug absorption by serving as a physical barrier or through effects on transit time (i.e., motility of the gastrointestinal tract), secretions, drug dissolution, chelation, or carrier uptake, among other effects. Many drugs should be taken without food or beverage to prevent interference with drug absorption. For example, the absorption of Fosamax (alendronate), used to treat osteoporosis, is greatly diminished with concurrent ingestion of food or beverages (other than water). Similarly, the antibiotics erythromycin and penicillin (ampicillin), along with the antihypertensive drugs Capoten (captopril) and Univasc or Uniretic (moexipril), should be ingested only with water; food should not be consumed for at least 1 hour. On the other hand, the absorption of many other drugs is enhanced with co-ingestion of food or even specific dietary nutrients such as those provided by a high-fat meal.

Foods or antacids that contain relatively large amounts of magnesium, calcium, zinc, iron, and aluminum need to be avoided or should be ingested separately (by several hours) from antibiotics such as Achromycin and Sumycin (tetracycline antibiotics), Cipro (ciprofloxacin), Maxaquin (lomefloxacin), and Levaquin (levofloxacin), and from other groups of antibiotics and antifungals such as Nizoral (ketoconazole). The divalent and trivalent minerals in the antacids or from the foods chelate (bind to) and decrease the absorption of the drugs.

An appropriate gastrointestinal tract pH is important for dissolving or absorbing some drugs. Thus, ingesting foods or antacids that can promote gastrointestinal secretions or alter pH may be detrimental.

EFFECTS OF FOODS ON DRUG METABOLISM

Many drugs that undergo substantial first-pass metabolism in the gastrointestinal tract are affected by coingestion of grapefruit juice. Some of these medications include the immunosuppressants Neoral and Sandimmune (cyclosporine); some HMG-CoA reductase inhibitors (used to treat high blood cholesterol) such as Zocor (simvastatin), Mevacor (lovastatin), and Lipitor (atorvastatin); Pletal (cilostazol), which is used to treat intermittent claudication and peripheral vascular disease; VePesid (etoposide), which is used to treat some cancers; and Relpax (eletriptan), which is used to treat migraines. The exact compound or compounds in grapefruit juice that cause the interaction are not clear. Grapefruit juice is rich in many phytochemicals, especially flavonoids such as the flavanone naringenin and its glycoside naringin and the flavonol kaempferol. Ingesting grapefruit juice is thought to decrease (down-regulate) the isozyme of cytochrome P450 known as CYP 3A4, which is found in the intestine [1,2]. This enzyme normally begins intestinal cell metabolism of many drugs. Consequently, the down-regulation of this enzyme by ingestion of grapefruit juice causes the drugs to be absorbed without any metabolism and causes blood concentrations of the drugs to be much higher than desired. The high blood concentrations of the drug, in turn, can result in undesirable side effects, including toxicity. Similarly, inhibition of intestinal non-CYP3A enzymes as well as enterocyte transport proteins has been demonstrated *in vitro* and may alter drug metabolism [3,4].

Table 1 An Overview of Some Selected Drug–Nutrient/Food Interactions

Drug(s)	Nutrient(s)/Food(s)
Antibiotics: tetracycline, Achromycin, Sumycin, Cipro, Maxaquin, and Levaquin; **Antifungal:** Nizoral	**Calcium, magnesium, zinc, iron, and aluminum**
Immunosupressant: Neoral; some **HMG-CoA reductase inhibitors:** Zocor, Mevacor, and Lipitor; **Anti-intermittent claudication:** Pletal; **Antimigraine:** Relpax	**Grapefruit juice**
Anti-Parkinson's: Dopar, Larodopa, Sinemet, Parcopa	**Protein and vitamin B$_6$**
Monoamine oxidase inhibitors: Parnate and Nardil; **Antituberculosis:** Isoniazid	**Amine-containing foods:** aged cheeses; smoked, salted, and pickled fish; sausage; salami; pepperoni; corned beef; bologna; meat extracts; wines; and chocolate, among others
Anticoagulants: Coumadin	**Vitamin K**
Bronchodilators: Theo-24, Theolair, Uniphyl, and Elixophyllin	**Caffeine and vitamin B$_6$**
Antimanic: Eskalith, Lithobid, Lithotabs	**Sodium**
Bile-acid sequestrants: Questran	**Fat-soluble vitamins A, D, E, and K; folate; iron; magnesium; calcium; and zinc**
Antituberculosis: Isoniazid	**Vitamin B$_6$**
Anticonvulsants: Phenobarbital, Dilantin, and Phenytek	**Vitamin D and folate**
H$_2$ receptors blockers: Tagament and Zantac; **Proton pump inhibitors:** Prilosec and Prevacid	**Iron, zinc, calcium, magnesium, and vitamin B$_{12}$**
Loop diuretics: Lasix and Bumex	**Potassium, chloride, magnesium, and sodium**

In addition to alterations in drug distribution caused by grapefruit juice, a high protein intake (two to three times recommendations) alters the distribution of the anti-Parkinson drugs Dopar and Larodopa (levodopa), and Sinemet and Parcopa (levodopa and carbidopa). The effects are thought to result from competition for carriers at the blood-brain barrier between the drug and large neutral amino acids (such as phenylalanine, tyrosine, and tryptophan). These large neutral amino acids appear in the blood following consumption of large amounts of protein. Vitamin B_6 also can increase the metabolism of levodopa by enhancing its conversion to dopamine before the drug crosses the blood-brain barrier. Vitamin B_6 is found in liver and other protein-rich foods, such as meats and legumes, as well as seeds and whole grains. Thus, ingesting levodopa with large amounts of protein or vitamin B_6, or regularly consuming a diet high in protein or vitamin B_6 while taking levodopa, is contraindicated.

EFFECTS OF FOODS AND NUTRIENTS ON THE ACTIONS OF DRUGS

Some foods or nutrients can enhance or oppose the actions of drugs. Foods that contain amines, especially tyramine, dopamine, or histamine, are known to interact with a group of drugs known as monoamine oxidase inhibitors (MAOIs), which are used mostly to treat some forms of depression. MAOIs such as Parnate (tranylcypromine sulfate) and Nardil (phenelzine sulfate) prevent the enzyme monoamine oxidase from catabolizing amines in the diet as well as amines made endogenously. Amines consist of vasoactive or pressor amines (e.g., tyramine, serotonin, and histamine) and neurotransmitters or psychoactive amines (e.g., dopamine and norepinephrine). The antituberculosis drug INH (isoniazid) exhibits MAOI-like activity. The problem arises when people on MAOIs or INH eat foods high in amines, especially tyramine or histamine, which may be found in fairly large quantities in some foods. Consuming these foods ordinarily presents no problem because the amines can quickly be inactivated by monoamine oxidase (MAO). However, in people taking MAOIs or isoniazid, these reactions do not occur. Consequently, high dietary amine intake coupled with high endogenous norepinephrine may result in excessive vasoconstriction, manifested as severe headache, acute hypertension or a hypertensive crisis, and cardiac dysrhythmia. People taking MAOIs are counseled against ingesting foods high in amines, such as aged cheeses (cheddar, Camembert, Stilton, Boursault), yeast extracts (e.g., Marmite), and brewer's yeast. Smoked, salted, or pickled fish such as herring or cod, as well as sausage, salami, pepperoni, corned beef, and bologna, also are high in tyramine. Foods moderately high to high in tyramine include meat extracts; tenderizers; red wines, including Chianti, vermouth, sherry, and burgundy; and cheeses such as blue, natural brick, Brie, Gruyère, mozzarella, Parmesan, Romano, and Roquefort. Broad beans (fava, Chinese pea pods), chocolate, large amounts of caffeine, liver (chicken or beef), and selected fruits may also contain large amounts of tyramine. Histamine is not typically found in large quantities in foods, with the exception of improperly stored or spoiled fish. Dopamine is found in fava and broad beans and snow peas.

A nutrient known to antagonize the action of the anticoagulant Coumadin (warfarin) is vitamin K. Coumadin works by inhibiting reactions in the vitamin K cycle that generate the active form of vitamin K needed for blood clotting. By inhibiting production of active vitamin K, the drug prolongs the clotting time of blood. Large amounts of vitamin K oppose the actions of the drug, promoting blood clotting and leading to drug resistance. Ingesting large quantities of foods rich in vitamin K, including green vegetables, some legumes (soybeans, garbanzo beans), and liver should be avoided.

Caffeine, a component of coffee, tea, many soft drinks, and chocolate, counters the actions of tranquilizers and may exacerbate some adverse effects of the bronchodilators: Theo-24, Theolair, Uniphyl, and Elixophyllin (theophylline). Specifically, large amounts of caffeine coupled with use of theophylline promote increased nervousness, insomnia, and tremors. (These drugs also interfere with vitamin B_6 metabolism.)

EFFECTS OF FOODS AND NUTRIENTS ON DRUG EXCRETION

Sodium and the mineral lithium in the antimanic drugs Eskalith, Lithobid, and Lithotabs (lithium carbonate) are known to interact in the kidneys. Specifically, the sodium and lithium compete with each other for reabsorption into the tubules of the kidneys. Thus, a high intake of sodium promotes lithium excretion and thereby diminishes the effects of the drug, whereas a low intake of sodium promotes reabsorption of lithium and thereby enhances the likelihood of drug toxicity.

EFFECTS OF DRUGS ON NUTRIENT ABSORPTION

Drugs may alter the absorption of nutrients through several mechanisms. For example, drugs may alter the transit time of nutrients through the gastrointestinal tract, speeding up or slowing down the passage of its contents. Typically, when contents move quickly through the gastrointestinal tract, fewer nutrients are absorbed; when contents move slowly, more nutrients are absorbed. Changes in the pH of the gastrointestinal tract also may alter nutrient absorption. For example, H_2 receptor blockers such as Tagamet (cimetidine) and Zantac (ranitidine) and proton pump inhibitors such as Prilosec (omeprazole) and Prevacid (lansoprazole), which decrease hydrochloric acid secretion into the stomach and thus increase gastric pH, diminish the absorption of several nutrients, especially iron. H_2 receptor blockers and proton pump inhibitors are used to treat ulcers and gastroesophageal reflux disease (GERD).

The ability of some drugs to chelate or adsorb nutrients or gastrointestinal secretions also diminishes nutrient absorption. For example, bile acid sequestrants such as Questran (cholestyramine) adsorb bile and thus decrease the absorption of the fat-soluble vitamins A, D, E, and K and the carotenoids. In addition, the drug chelates other nutrients (including folate) and some divalent minerals (including iron, magnesium, calcium, and zinc). Bile acid sequestrant drugs are used to treat high blood cholesterol concentrations, a risk factor for heart disease.

EFFECTS OF DRUGS ON NUTRIENT METABOLISM

In addition to altering nutrient absorption, drugs may alter the metabolism of nutrients in body tissues. Isoniazid, used in the treatment of tuberculosis, for example, diminishes the conversion of pyridoxine (vitamin B_6) to its functional coenzyme form in the liver and thus can cause a vitamin B_6 deficiency. Another group of drugs known to alter vitamin metabolism includes the anticonvulsants phenobarbital and phenytoin (Dilantin, Phenytek). These drugs alter the metabolism of vitamin D, leading to (in severe cases) the deficiency conditions rickets and osteomalacia if vitamin supplements (as 25-OH cholecalciferol) are not taken. Specifically, the anticonvulsants are thought to diminish the hepatic conversion of vitamin D as cholecalciferol to 25-OH cholecalciferol. Interestingly, these anticonvulsants also affect the vitamin folate by diminishing its absorption in the intestine.

EFFECTS OF DRUGS ON NUTRIENT EXCRETION

Drugs may increase or decrease the excretion of nutrients from the body. Loop diuretics used to treat high blood pressure such as Lasix (furosemide) and Bumex (bumetanide) promote the urinary excretion of sodium and water (important in lowering blood pressure); however, the drugs also increase losses of potassium, chloride, and magnesium from the ascending portion of the loop of Henle. Dietary replacement of the minerals, especially potassium, is important to prevent low blood potassium concentrations.

SUMMARY

Nutrient–drug interactions can severely affect both nutritional status and the effectiveness of pharmacological treatment. Although accredited health-care facilities are mandated to educate patients about interactions between foods and drugs, many individuals remain unaware of such interactions and their consequences.

References

1. Hanley MJ, Cancalon P, Widmer WW, Greenblatt DJ. The effect of grapefruit juice on drug disposition. Expert Opin Drug Metab Toxicol. 2011; 7:267–86.

2. Seden K, Dickinson L, Khoo S, Back D. Grapefruit-interactions. Drugs. 2010; 70:2373–407.

3. Won CS, Oberlies NH , Paine MF. Influence of dietary substances on intestinal drug metabolism and transport. Curr Drug Metab. 2010; 11:778–92.

4. Bailey DG. Fruit juice inhibition of uptake transport: a new type of food-drug interaction. Br J Clin Pharmacol. 2010; 70:645–55.

Selected Readings

Felipez L, Sentongo TA. Drug-induced nutrient deficiencies. Pediatr Clin N Am. 2009; 56:1211–24.

Genser D. Food and drug interactions: consequences for the nutrition/health status. Ann Nutr Metab. 2008; 52(suppl1):29–32.

Ruggiero A, Cefalo MG, Coccia P, et al. The role of diet on the clinical pharmacology of oral antineoplastic agents. Eur J Clin Pharmacol. 2012; 68:115–122.

14

NONESSENTIAL TRACE AND ULTRATRACE MINERALS

PERSPECTIVE

AS CHAPTER 13 EXPLAINED, TRACE ELEMENTS are those minerals that are needed by the body in amounts less than 100 mg/day, and ultratrace elements are those elements with estimated, established, or suspected requirements of less than 1 mg/day. Based on these definitions, at least 18 elements may be classified as ultratrace elements: aluminum, arsenic, boron, bromine, cadmium, chromium, copper, germanium, iodine, lead, lithium, molybdenum, nickel, rubidium, selenium, silicon, tin, and vanadium. However, while copper, chromium, iodine, molybdenum, and selenium are considered ultratrace elements by the preceding definition, they have been included in Chapter 13 based on their established essentiality and Adequate Intake or Recommended Dietary Allowance set by the Food and Nutrition Board. The elements that are addressed in this chapter—fluoride, arsenic, boron, nickel, silicon, and vanadium—are not, at present, considered essential, although for each, some evidence suggests a possible need. Figure 14.1 shows the location of these elements in the periodic table. Table 14.1 provides an overview of selected functions, food sources, and deficiency symptoms for these nutrients. A brief discussion also is provided for the element cobalt, which is needed but only as part of vitamin B_{12} (cobalamin).

FLUORIDE

Though present in the body in trace amounts, fluoride is not considered an essential nutrient since the element has not been shown to be essential for life and no biochemical role has been identified for it. Fluoride has, however, been shown to exert beneficial effects, especially on teeth, as discussed in the "Functions and Deficiency" section.

Sources

Whereas fluorine (F) is a gaseous chemical element, fluoride (F^-) is typically found bound to a metal, nonmetal, or organic compound. The term *fluoride* is used throughout this section (analogous to the use of the terms *iodide* and *chloride* previously). Community drinking water has been fluoridated (with about 1 ppm or 1 mg of fluoride in a liter of drinking water) for over 60 years in the United States, due to the discovery of the inverse relationship between fluoride intake and the incidence of dental caries. Several beverages, including ready-to-use infant formulas, are made with fluoridated water, but others vary greatly in their fluoride content depending upon the use or nonuse of fluoridated water in their processing.

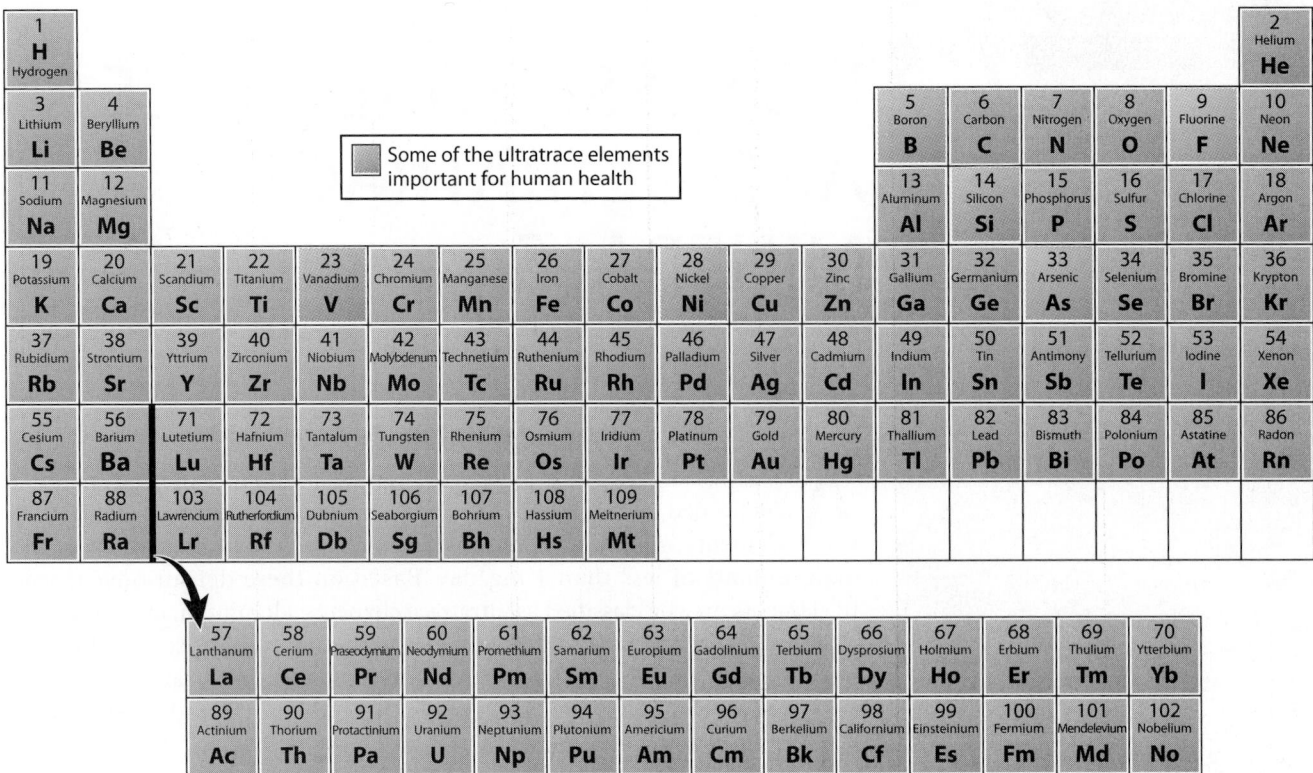

Figure 14.1 The periodic table highlighting important nonessential trace and ultratrace elements.

Table 14.1 Nonessential Trace and Ultratrace Elements: Selected Functions, Deficiency Symptoms, and Food Sources

Mineral	Selected Possible Physiological Roles	Selected Deficiency Symptoms in Animals	Food Sources
Fluoride	Maintenance of teeth and bone structure	Dental caries, bone problems (in humans)	Fish, meat, legumes, grains, drinking water (variable)
Arsenic	Methyl group use, signal transduction	Impaired growth and reproduction	Seafood, meat, grains, grain products
Boron	Bone development, cell membrane stability, immune system function, brain function	Impaired bone health, brain function, and immune response	Fruits, vegetables, legumes, nuts
Nickel	Possibly involved in hormonal membrane or enzyme activity	Depressed growth, impaired hematopoiesis	Nuts, legumes, grains, cocoa products (chocolate)
Silicon	Connective tissue, cartilage, and bone formation	Decreased collagen, long bone and skull abnormalities	Beer, unrefined grains, root vegetables
Vanadium	Mimics insulin action, inhibits Na^+/K^+-ATPase	Reduced survival and growth, metabolism changes	Shellfish, black pepper, parsley, mushrooms, dill seed

The fluoride content in most food groups is low, usually less than about 0.05 mg/100 g. However, a few foods contain higher amounts of fluoride, including some grains and cereal products, some fish (if consumed with the bones), and tea. Fish contain from ~0.01 to 0.17 mg/3.5 oz; canned sardines (with bones) have about 0.2 to 0.4 mg of fluoride/3.5 oz. Other seafood such as clams, lobster, crab, and shrimp are also good sources of fluoride. Tea, both caffeinated and decaffeinated, is rich in fluoride because tea leaves accumulate the element in fairly high amounts. Brewed tea contains from 1 to 6 mg of fluoride/L, with decaffeinated forms higher in fluoride than caffeinated. Table 14.2 provides the fluoride content of various food groups.

Most Americans obtain the majority of dietary fluoride from drinking water, which provides about 0.24 mg of fluoride/cup. Fluoridation of water continues to be recommended by various public health associations in amounts of about 0.7 to 1.2 mg of fluoride/L. Usual fluoride intake by Americans is up to about 3.4 mg/day. Sodium fluorosilicate is typically added to water, while sodium fluoride or monofluorophosphate is used in toothpaste or tablets. If swallowed, fluoride-containing toothpaste can be a significant source of the mineral; however, ingesting even small amounts of fluoride-containing toothpaste can result in ingestion of fluoride in amounts exceeding recommended intakes and thus can be dangerous, especially to young children. Consequently, many

Table 14.2 Fluoride Content of Selected Food Groups

Food Group	Fluoride Content Range (mg/100 g)
Dairy products	0.002–0.082
Meat and poultry	0.004–0.092
Grain products	0.008–0.201
Potatoes	0.008–0.084
Green leafy vegetables	0.008–0.070
Legumes	0.015–0.057
Root vegetables	0.009–0.048
Other vegetables	0.006–0.017
Fruits	0.002–0.013
Fats and oils	0.002–0.044

Source: Donald R. Taves, 'Dietary intake of fluoride ashed (total fluoride) v. unashed (inorganic fluoride) analysis of individual foods' in the British Journal of Nutrition, Vol. 49, Issue 03, May 1983, pp. 295–301. Reprinted with the permission of Cambridge University Press.

manufacturers recommend that toothpaste be kept out of reach of children and that only a "pea-sized" amount be used for tooth brushing.

Absorption, Transport, Storage, and Excretion

In foods, fluoride may be bound to proteins. Protein-bound fluoride must be hydrolyzed by pepsin or other proteases before absorption. Additionally, some minerals in foods, especially calcium and magnesium, are thought to form insoluble complexes with fluoride to decrease its absorption. Absorption of fluoride, which occurs by passive diffusion in the stomach, is nearly 100% and quite rapid (within 90 minutes of ingestion) when it is consumed as fluoridated water or toothpaste. Absorption diminishes to about 50% to 80% when fluoride is consumed as foods. Fluoride's rapid gastric absorption can be explained by the fact that it exists primarily as hydrogen fluoride, also called hydrofluoric acid, rather than as ionic fluoride, at the low pH of the stomach. Fluoride is also absorbed throughout the small intestine.

Fluoride is transported in the blood as ionic fluoride or hydrofluoric acid, as well as being bound to plasma proteins. Absorbed fluoride leaves the blood very quickly and is distributed rapidly throughout the body. Most fluoride is found in bones and teeth. Fluoride associated with bone is found in both an amorphous state (rapidly exchangeable pool) and a crystalline state (slowly exchangeable pool). In its more crystalline state, fluoride is sequestered in bones by apatite, a basic calcium phosphate with the theoretic formula $Ca_{10}(PO_4)_6(OH)_2$. Mineralized bone/teeth account for nearly 99% of total body fluoride. As the amount of absorbed fluoride increases, so does the quantity taken up by these tissues. However, the percentage retained at high absorption rates becomes lower because of accelerated urinary excretion. Skeletal growth rate influences fluoride balance, exemplified by the fact that young, growing people incorporate more fluoride into the skeleton than adults and excrete less in the urine.

Ionic fluoride is rapidly excreted in the urine, accounting for approximately 90% of total excretion. Some (about 35–45%) tubular reabsorption of hydrofluoric acid occurs by passive diffusion in the kidney. Urinary fluoride excretion normally ranges from about 0.2 to 1.1 mg of fluoride/L urine. Fecal elimination accounts for most of the remaining (up to about 10%) losses, with only minor losses occurring in sweat.

Functions and Deficiency

The major functions of fluoride are related to its effects on bone mineralization and the formation of dental enamels. Fluoride stimulates osteoblast proliferation and mineral deposition in bone; however, such effects are most apparent in children and have not been generally shown to be effective in the prevention or treatment of osteoporosis. In fact, the newly formed bone created in response to fluoride may lack normal structure and strength in adults. Some of the effects of fluoride appear to be mediated through changes in cell signaling pathways [1].

Fluoride increases the resistance of enamel to acid demineralization and increases tooth mineralization. To facilitate mineralization of the crystalline structure and to reduce enamel demineralization, fluoride replaces the hydroxide ions in hydroxyapatite. Ions can be replaced during initial crystal formation or by displacement from previously deposited mineral, according to the following equation: $Ca_{10}(PO_4)_6(OH)_2 + xF^- \longrightarrow Ca_{10}(PO_4)_6(OH)_2 - xF^-_x$. In bone and dental enamel, the ratio of substitution of F^- for OH^- is from about 1:20 to 1:40. With the deposition of fluoride in the hydroxyapatite, fluorohydroxyapatite is formed. Fluorohydroxyapatite is less acid soluble than hydroxyapatite and thus more resistant to cavity formation [2]. These benefits are more pronounced when fluoride is provided at pre-eruptive stages of tooth development. Additionally, fluoride inhibits acid production (by buffering the hydrogen ions) and dental plaque formation by oral bacteria. Topical fluoride also accelerates the growth of a new surface on partially demineralized subsurface crystals in dental cavities (lesions); such effects enhance remineralization [2]. Several meta-analyses of studies over the years have shown that water fluoridation helps to prevent dental caries (cavities).

Fluoride deficiency in test animals has been reported to result in curtailed growth, infertility, and anemia. However, these findings are not well documented and cannot be extrapolated to predict similar effects on humans. In humans, an optimal level of fluoride helps to reduce the incidence of dental caries and perhaps also to maintain the integrity of skeletal tissue.

Recommended Intake, Toxicity, and Assessment of Nutriture

With the goal of minimizing risk for dental caries in the population without causing side effects, the Food and Nutrition Board established Adequate Intakes of 4 and 3 mg of fluoride/day for adult males and females, respectively [3]. The inside front cover of the book provides additional AIs for fluoride for other age groups.

Acute toxicity (usually from accidental ingestion of fluoride supplements or excessive amounts of toothpaste) manifests as nausea, vomiting, diarrhea, acidosis, and cardiac arrhythmias. Death has been reported following ingestion of 5 to 10 g of sodium fluoride or about 32 to 64 mg of fluoride/kg body weight, although it may occur with an intake as low as 5 mg of fluoride/kg body weight [3,4]. Chronic toxicity of fluoride, called fluorosis, is characterized by changes in the teeth (dental fluorosis), the skeleton (including bone deformities, restricted joint movement, abnormal/excessive bone formation and mineralization, increased bone fracture risk), and nonskeletal tissues (including kidney dysfunction and impaired nerve and muscle function) [2]. Dental fluorosis is characterized by mottling of the tooth surface with white spots appearing on the teeth; however, more severe toxicity weakens the teeth and causes permanent brown spots to appear. With skeletal fluorosis, fluoride accumulates in the joints, making movement difficult. The Tolerable Upper Intake Levels for fluoride range from 1.3 mg/day for children age 1 to 3 years to 10 mg/day for children older than 8 years and adults [3]. Removal of excess fluoride from drinking water such that concentrations do not exceed 4.0 mg/L is required by the Environmental Protection Agency.

Plasma and urinary fluoride can be monitored to determine toxicity and fluoride exposure, respectively, but not the body's fluoride status. Normal plasma concentrations for ionic fluoride range from about 0.01 to 0.2 μg of fluoride/mL. Serum fluoride concentrations of 190 ng/mL have been associated with toxic effects on bone (abnormal bone formation and mineralization) [5]. Urinary fluoride excretion of 15 mg/L is associated with a fluoride exposure of about 20 to 30 mg; however, this level of exposure is likely to occur over one or more decades [5].

References Cited for Fluoride

1. Everett ET. Fluoride's effects on the formation of teeth and bones, and the influence of genetics. J Dent Res. 2011; 90:552–60.
2. Gazzano E, Bergandi L, Riganti C, et al. Fluoride effects: the two faces of Janus. Curr Med Chem. 2010; 17:2431–41.
3. Food and Nutrition Board, Institute of Medicine. Dietary Reference Intakes. Washington, DC: National Academy Press. 1997 pp. 288–313.
4. Whitford G. The physiological and toxicological characteristics of fluoride. J Dent Res. 1990; 69:539–49.
5. Nielsen FH. Micronutrients in parental nutrition: boron, silicon, and fluoride. Gastroenterology. 2009; 137:S55–60.

Suggested Readings

Bergman C, Gray-Scott D, Chen J, Meacham S. What is next for the dietary reference intakes for bone metabolism related to nutrients beyond calcium, phosphorus, magnesium, vitamin D and fluoride? Crit Rev Food Sci. 2009; 49:136–44.
Jha SK, Mishra VK, Sharma DK, Damodaran T. Fluoride in the environment and its metabolism in humans. Rev Environ Contam Tox. 2011; 211:121–42.
McGrady MG. Why fluoride? Dental Update 2010; 37:595–602.

Website providing information on fluoride in foods

http://www.nal.usda.gov/fnic/foodcomp/Data/Fluoride/Fluoride.html

ARSENIC

More than any other ultratrace mineral, arsenic, which is colorless and odorless, conjures an image of toxicity as a poison rather than of nutritional essentiality. The malevolent aspect of arsenic continues to attract attention because the majority of the arsenic literature addresses its toxicological rather than its nutritional properties. Nevertheless, evidence is accumulating that arsenic may be an essential element.

Sources

Arsenic is present throughout the earth's continental crust at an estimated concentration of 1.5 to 2.0 μg/g. It is present in water, rocks, and soils, although its concentration varies considerably among regions, based on the geological history of the soil as well as on pollution from unnatural sources. Fallout sources such as pesticides, smelters, and coal-fired power plants can, through aerosols and floating dust, enrich a particular area with arsenic, which then affects humans and animals when it is incorporated into water, foods, and foodstuffs. Seafood is rich in arsenic, with fish containing up to 80 μg/g and oysters up to 10 μg/g [1,2]. Arsenic is also present in meats (0.005–0.1 μg/g) and cereal and grain products (0.05–0.4 μg/g) as well as eggs and dairy products (milk, 0.01–0.05 μg/g; eggs, 0.01–0.1 μg/g), among other foods and beverages [2]. Relatively high amounts of arsenic are sometimes detected in samples of foods and/or beverages, such as apple and grape juices. In accordance with the U.S. Environmental Protection Agency, the U.S. Food and Drug Administration set a ≤10 parts per billion (ppb) standard for arsenic in bottled drinking water; however, at present, there are no federal limits for arsenic in foods or juices. Dietary intake of arsenic usually totals about 30 to 50 μg/day [1,2]. New standards limiting arsenic contamination of foods are likely to arise in the near future.

Arsenic is found in water and foods in organic and inorganic forms, and exists mostly in its trivalent [As^{3+}] and pentavalent [As^{5+}] states. The major inorganic forms of arsenic found in water and foods are pentavalent arsenate

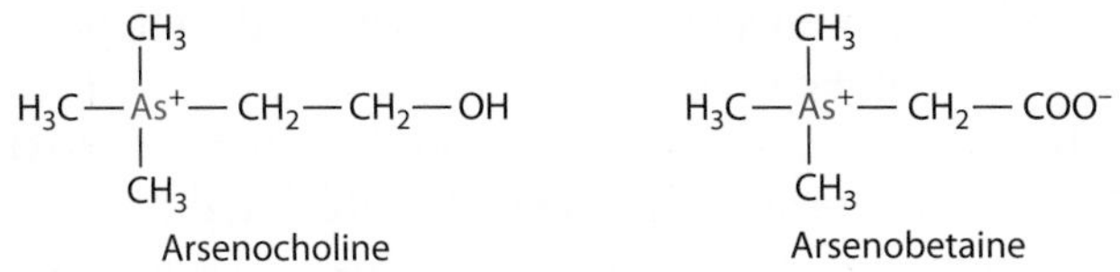

Figure 14.2 Two forms of arsenic commonly found in seafoods.

($H_2AsO_4^-$ or $HAsO_4^{2-}$) and trivalent arsenite (H_3AsO_3 and $H_2AsO_3^-$). Seafood contains mostly organic forms of arsenic: arsenobetaine and arsenocholine. Foods also may contain organic arsenic as arsenolipids and arsenosugars as well as some methylated forms of the element.

Absorption, Transport, Storage, and Excretion

Absorption of arsenic varies with its chemical form and solubility. Greater than 90% of arsenate and arsenite is absorbed from water, and between 60% and 75% of these inorganic forms of the element is absorbed with food. Of the organic forms, greater than 90% of arsenobetaine and between 70% and 80% of arsenocholine are absorbed.

Absorption of organic and inorganic arsenic is thought to occur by simple diffusion across the enterocyte membranes, although arsenate may be transported using an energy-dependent carrier. From the intestine, some arsenic is transported in the blood bound to transferrin. The liver takes up both inorganic and organic forms of the element from portal blood.

In the liver, the organic forms (Figure 14.2) arsenobetaine and arsenocholine undergo little metabolism, although some arsenocholine may be converted to arsenobetaine or may be incorporated into phospholipids similar to choline. In contrast to arsenocholine and arsenobetaine, inorganic arsenic is extensively metabolized—reduced and/or methylated—as shown in Figure 14.3; the reactions occur primarily in the liver. The

methylation reactions are dependent upon methyl groups generated mainly from the catabolism of choline and the amino acid methionine. From the chapter on proteins, you may remember that methionine catabolism produces S-adenosylmethionine (abbreviated SAM); SAM is thought to provide most of the methyl groups needed for arsenic methylation. The reduction reactions for arsenic's metabolism require glutathione or other thiols [3]. It has been estimated that 1 g of liver, which has about 70 million liver cells, can methylate up to 14.8 μmoles (1,108 μg) of inorganic trivalent arsenic in an hour [4]. In the liver, arsenate is reduced to arsenite, which is then methylated (using SAM) to become monomethylarsonic acid. The reaction is catalyzed by arsenite methyltransferase. In addition, another methyl group may be added to monomethylarsonic acid by monomethylarsonic acid methyltransferase to form dimethylarsinic acid. Dimethylarsinic acid represents the usual form of the mineral excreted in the urine; however, some of this compound may be reduced, forming dimethylarsenious acid, a relatively toxic form of the element. The general order of toxicity of other arsenicals is (mono)methylarsonous acid$^{(3+)}$ > arsenite^{3+} > arsenate^{5+} > (mono)methylarsonic acid$^{(5+)}$ = dimethylarsinic acid$^{(5+)}$ [5]. Arsenobetaine and arsenocholine are generally considered nontoxic.

Tissues that contain the most arsenic include the skin, hair, and nails. Within tissues, inorganic arsenic, especially As^{3+}, binds primarily to thiols (i.e., sulfhydryl [SH] groups) within proteins, such as metallothionein. Methylated organic (as opposed to unmethylated inorganic) forms of the element are less likely to bind to tissues.

Arsenic is excreted rapidly by the kidneys, which represent the major route of excretion. The main urinary metabolites of arsenic include monomethylarsonic acid, dimethylarsinic acid, and trimethylated arsenic; excretion of greater amounts of the monomethylated form of the mineral is associated with greater risk of cancer and other health problems [6,7]. Other organic forms of arsenic such

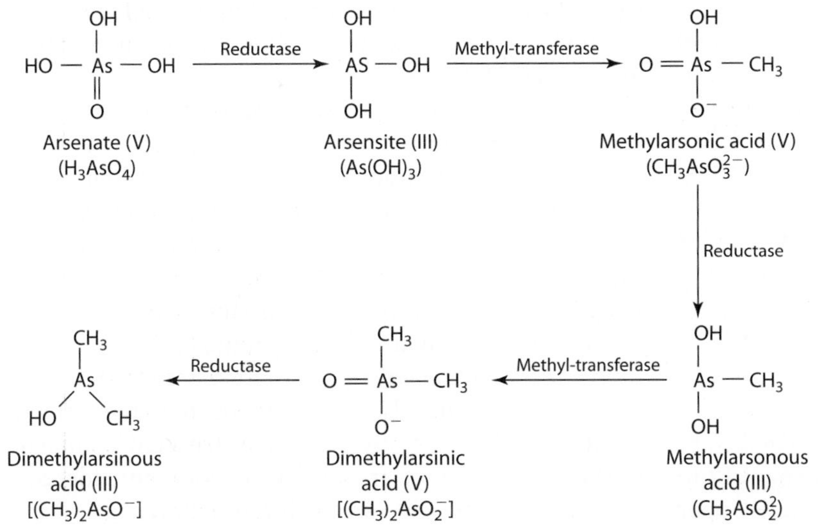

Figure 14.3 The metabolism (reductive methylations) of arsenic.

as arsenobetaine, arsenocholine, and arsenosugars are also excreted in the urine [8,9]. Typically, less than 50 μg arsenic is excreted in the urine of healthy adults each day.

Functions and Deficiency

Arsenic appears to facilitate the body's use of methyl groups, such as S-adenosylmethionine (SAM). SAM is one of the body's major methyl donors and provides for the methylation of several important compounds (such as DNA and histones). Decreased methylation of both histones and DNA results with arsenic deprivation [10]. In addition to influencing the use of methyl groups in the body, arsenic affects the regulation of cellular signal transduction pathways, including those involving insulin. Additionally, through activation of the G-protein-coupled receptor S1P1, arsenic influences cell proliferation and survival [11].

Arsenic deficiency in animals impairs the metabolism of methionine, resulting in decreased SAM concentrations, decreased S-adenosylmethionine decarboxylase activity, and decreased taurine production [12,13]. This reduction in SAM concentrations in turn diminishes the SAM-dependent production of creatine and polyamines. Other reported effects of arsenic deprivation in animals include diminished growth, reduced conception rate, abnormal reproduction, increased neonatal mortality, and altered lipid concentrations.

Arsenic and the Treatment of Cancer

A derivative of arsenic, arsenic trioxide (As_2O_3), has been approved by the U.S. Food and Drug Administration (FDA) for the treatment of acute promyelocytic leukemia. This form of arsenic exhibits potent antitumor activity and has been shown to promote complete remission in over 50% of patients with acute promyelocytic leukemia [7,14]. The use of arsenic trioxide, however, is not without side effects on the heart and blood cells.

Interactions with Other Nutrients

Arsenic seems to interact antagonistically with selenium and iodine. Because selenate and arsenate are both oxyanions with similar chemical properties, each may competitively inhibit the uptake and tissue retention of the other. The interaction of arsenic with iodine is exemplified by the observation that the ultratrace element is goitrogenic in mice. Arsenic is believed to antagonize iodine uptake by the thyroid gland, causing compensatory goiter.

Recommended Intake, Toxicity, and Assessment of Nutriture

Insufficient data are available to estimate a human dietary requirement for arsenic, although a requirement of 12 to 25 μg/day has been suggested [13]. No Tolerable Upper Intake Level for arsenic has been established by the Food and Nutrition Board [15].

Inorganic forms of arsenic tend to be more toxic than organic forms of the element; susceptibility to toxicity, however, appears to relate in part to nutritional status [16]. Acute toxicity results in gastrointestinal distress (leading to dehydration and electrolyte imbalance), encephalopathy, anemia, and liver damage. Chronic toxicity is associated with skin hyperpigmentation, hyperkeratosis, muscle weakness, peripheral neuropathy, excessive sweating, liver damage, delirium, encephalopathy, vascular changes, and cancers of the oral cavity, skin, lungs, prostate, colon, bladder, and kidneys [17–20]. It is the methylated intermediates monomethylarsonous acid and dimethylarsinous acid that appear to be the most carcinogenic [21]. In addition, the cardiovascular system is affected, often resulting in hypertension, cardiac arrhythmias, and death. Blackfoot disease, a peripheral vascular condition, has been associated with ingesting arsenic-contaminated drinking water in Taiwan [17,18].

Arsenic's toxicity relates in part to its interactions with sulfhydryl groups found in proteins (including enzymes); this interaction in turn disrupts normal function of the protein. Arsenic's inhibition of enzymes, for example, affects several metabolic pathways in the body and results in the formation of free radicals, which further damage cells. Pyruvate dehydrogenase, which converts pyruvate to the TCA cycle intermediate acetyl-CoA, is one example of an enzyme inhibited by trivalent arsenic; other metabolic pathways affected by arsenic include gluconeogenesis and fatty acid oxidation [21]. In blood vessels, arsenic reduces vasorelaxation through inhibition of endothelial nitric oxide synthase; it also increases platelet aggregation and reduces fibrinolysis, which enhance atherosclerosis [22]. Other toxic effects of arsenic result from its induction of oxidative stress in the body. The trivalent form of arsenic promotes cellular apoptosis. Further, the pentavalent forms of arsenic can substitute for phosphate in glycolysis and the electron transport chain; this substitution in the latter set of reactions uncouples oxidative phosphorylation and thus diminishes ATP formation [21].

Chronic or acute exposure to arsenic elevates blood, hair, and urine concentrations of the mineral. The usual range of arsenic is about 2 to 62 ng/mL in whole blood and 1 to 20 ng/mL in plasma or serum; however, blood levels are not a good indicator of long-term arsenic exposure. Arsenic levels in hair range from about 0.1 to 1.1 μg/g. Hair analysis is particularly useful in toxicity situations because hair arsenic content, unlike that of the fluids, represents an average content over an extended period and does not fluctuate if exposure to the element is intermittent. Because arsenic is excreted primarily in the urine, urinary arsenic excretion is considered a reliable marker of acute arsenic exposure [21].

References Cited for Arsenic

1. Eckhert CD. Other trace elements. In: Shils M, Shike M, Ross A, Caballero B, Cousins RJ, eds. Modern Nutrition in Health and Disease, 10th ed. Baltimore, MD: Williams and Wilkins. 2005 pp. 339–41.

2. Anke M. Arsenic. In: Mertz W, ed. Trace Elements in Human and Animal Nutrition. Orlando, FL: Academic Press. 1986, vol. 2, p. 360.

3. Gamble MV, Liu X, Ahsan H, et al. Folate, homocysteine, and arsenic metabolism in arsenic-exposed individuals in Bangladesh. Environ Hlth Perspectives. 2005; 113:1683–88.

4. Drobna Z, Walton FS, Paul DS, et al. Metabolism of arsenic in human liver: the role of membrane transporters. Arch Toxicol. 2010; 84:3–16.

5. Petrick JS, Ayala-Fierro F, Cullen W, et al. Monomethylarsonous acid (MMM^{III}) is more toxic than arsenite in Chang human hepatocytes. Toxicol Appl Pharmacol. 2000; 163:203–07.

6. Smith AH, Steinmaus CM. Health effects of arsenic and chromium in drinking water: recent human findings. Ann Rev Pub Health. 2009; 30:107–22.

7. Nicolis I, Curis E, Deschamps P, Benazeth S. Arsenite medicinal use, metabolism, pharmacokinetics and monitoring in human hair. Biochimie. 2009; 91:1260–67.

8. Sun G, Xu Y, Li X, et al. Urinary arsenic metabolites in children and adults exposed to arsenic in drinking water in inner Mongolia, China. Environ Hlth Perspectives. 2007; 115:648–52.

9. Agusa T, Kunito T, Kubota R, et al. Exposure, metabolism and health effects of arsenic in residents from arsenic-contaminated groundwater areas of Vietnam and Cambodia: a review. Rev Environ Health. 2010; 25:193–220.

10. Bernstam L, Nriagu J. Molecular aspects of arsenic stress. J Toxic Environ Hlth. 2000; 3:293–322.

11. Druwe IL, Vaillancourt RR. Influence of arsenate and arsenite on signal transduction pathways: an update. Arch Toxicol. 2010; 84:585–96.

12. Nielsen F. Ultratrace elements of possible importance for human health: an update. In: Prasad AS, ed. Essential and Toxic Trace Elements in Human Health. New York: Wiley-Liss. 1993 pp. 355–76.

13. Uthus E, Nielsen F. Determination of the possible requirement and reference dose level for arsenic in humans. Scand J Work Environ Health. 1993; 19(suppl 1):137–38.

14. Platanias LC. Biological responses to arsenic compounds. J Biol Chem. 2009; 284:18583–87.

15. Food and Nutrition Board. Dietary Reference Intakes for Vitamin A, Vitamin K, Arsenic, Boron, Chromium, Copper, Iodine, Iron, Manganese, Molybdenum, Nickel, Silicon, Vanadium, and Zinc. Washington, DC: National Academy Press. 2001 pp. 502–53.

16. Steinmaus C, Carrigan K, Kalman D, et al. Dietary intake and arsenic methylation in a U.S. population. Environ Hlth Perspectives. 2005; 113:1153–59.

17. Hall A. Chronic arsenic poisoning. Toxicol Letters. 2002; 128:69–72.

18. Weir E. Arsenic and drinking water. Can Med Assoc J. 2002; 166:69.

19. Abernathy C, Thomas D, Calderon R. Health effects and risk assessment of arsenic. J Nutr. 2003; 133:S1536–38.

20. Duker A, Carranza E, Hale M. Arsenic geochemistry and health. Environ Int. 2005; 31:631–41.

21. Jomova K, Jenisova Z, Feszterova M, et al. Arsenic: toxicity, oxidative stress, and human disease. J Appl Tox. 2011; 31:95–107.

22. Balakumar P, Kaur J. Arsenic exposure and cardiovascular disorders: an overview. Cardiovasc Toxicol. 2009; 9:169–76.

BORON

Boron, as boric acid and sodium borate ($Na_2B_4O_7 \cdot H_2O$, called borax), was used to preserve foods such as fish, meat, cream, butter, and margarine for over 50 years—that is, until the 1920s, when it was first considered dangerous for humans. Not until the 1980s did evidence for the essentiality of boron start mounting again.

Sources

Foods of plant origin including fruits, vegetables, nuts, and legumes represent good sources of boron. In addition, wine, cider, and beer contribute to dietary intake. Specific foods particularly rich in boron include avocados, peanuts, peanut butter, pecans, raisins, grapes, and wine [1,2]. Generally, raisins, legumes, nuts, and avocados provide about 1.0 to 4.5 mg of boron/100 g, and fruits and vegetables contain 0.1 to 0.6 mg of boron/100 g [1,4]. Meat, fish, and dairy products are poor sources of the element, usually providing less than about 0.6 mg of boron/100 g [3]. Drinking water and water-based beverages vary considerably in boron content based upon geographic location. Boron also is a contaminant or a major ingredient in some antibiotics, gastric antacids, lipsticks, lotions, creams, and soaps. Boron appears in foods as sodium borate or as organic borate esters [2,4]. Dietary boron intake is estimated at 0.8 to 1.5 mg/day [1,4].

Absorption, Transport, Storage, and Excretion

Greater than 85% of ingested boron is absorbed as boric acid (also called orthoboric acid; $[B(OH)_3]$) by passive diffusion from the gastrointestinal tract [4]. Boron is found in the blood as boric acid and the borate monovalent anion $B(OH)_4^-$. A sodium-dependent borate transporter appears to actively transport $B(OH)_4^-$ into cells [5]. Boron is found mainly in bones, teeth, nails, and hair. The body is thought to contain about 3 to 20 mg of boron. The element is excreted primarily (greater than 70%) in the urine, with less than 13% usually lost in the feces and only small amounts lost in sweat [4]. Urinary boron appears as boric acid [4].

Functions and Deficiency

Boron promotes health but has not been shown to have clear biochemical functions in humans. Beneficial effects of the element on bones, cell membranes, and immune system and possibly brain functions have been observed. The composition, structure, and strength of bones are influenced by boron, possibly through modulation of osteoblast and/or osteoclast activity as well as extracellular matrix turnover [6–8]. Boron may play a role in cell membrane stability and/or function through modulating cellular calcium uptake and/or the ability of hormones (including vitamin D, calcitonin, insulin, and estrogen) to bind to receptors and thus exert their actions [9]. Boron's effects on cell membrane function/stability may also result from its effects on transmembrane signaling pathways [6,9,10]. Boron also promotes anti-inflammatory actions in response to injury or infection [6]. Boron deprivation in animals is associated with diminished production of cytokines, antibodies, and blood cells, especially lymphocytes. Because of these effects, boron is purported to be beneficial in reducing the severity of rheumatoid arthritis (among other inflammatory conditions) [6]. Additionally, brain function may be negatively impacted by boron deprivation. Boron deprivation results in changes in electroencephalograms (EEG) and selected cognitive processes affecting attention and memory, among other skills [6,11]. Other reported effects of deficiency in some, but not all, animal species include depressed growth and embryonic and developmental defects, suggesting possible roles for the element in reproduction and/or development.

Recommended Intake, Toxicity, and Assessment of Nurture

Recommendations for intakes of boron have not been established. Intakes of 1 to 3 mg/day are thought to be beneficial for brain and bone health [6].

Acute boron toxicity results in nausea, vomiting, diarrhea, dermatitis, and lethargy. Chronic boron toxicity is associated with nausea, poor appetite, anemia, dermatitis, and seizures [10]. A Tolerable Upper Intake Level of 20 mg of boron per day has been established for adults, based on animal studies [12].

Urinary boron excretion is thought to be a good indicator of recent boron intake within an intake range of 0.35 to 10 mg of boron/day [4,6]. Plasma boron concentrations, which usually range from about 20 to 75 ng/mL, may be helpful in assessing boron status [11]. Plasma concentrations appear to rise in response to increased dietary intake of the element and may be representative of status if intake is low [11].

References Cited for Boron

1. Meacham S, Hunt C. Dietary boron intakes of selected populations in the United States. Biol Trace Elem Res. 1998; 66:65–78.
2. Rainey C, Nyquist L, Christensen R, et al. Daily boron intake from the American diet. J Am Diet Assoc. 1999; 99:335–40.
3. Devirian T, Volpe S. The physiological effects of dietary boron. Crit Rev Food Sci Nutr. 2003; 43:219–31.
4. Sutherland B, Woodhouse L, Strong P, King J. Boron balance in humans. J Trace Elem Exp Med. 1999; 12:271–84.
5. Park M, Li Q, Shcheynikov N, et al. NaBC1 is a ubiquitous electrogenic Na-coupled borate transporter essential for cellular boron homeostasis and cell growth and proliferation. Molec Cell. 2004; 16:331–41.
6. Nielsen FH. Is boron nutritionally relevant? Nutr Rev. 2008; 66:183–91.
7. Nzietchueng R, Dousset B, Franck P, et al. Mechanisms implicated in the effects of boron on wound healing. J Trace Elem Med Biol. 2002; 16:239–44.
8. Sheng M, Taper L, Veit H, et al. Dietary boron supplementation enhanced the action of estrogen, but not that of parathyroid hormone, to improve trabecular bone quality in ovariectomized rats. Biol Trace Elem Res. 2001; 82:109–23.
9. Nielsen F. The emergence of boron as nutritionally important throughout the life cycle. Nutrition. 2000; 16:512–14.
10. Nielsen FH. Micronutrients in parenteral nutrition: boron, silicon, and fluoride. Gastroenterol. 2009; 137:S55–60.
11. Penland JG. The importance of boron nutrition for brain and psychological function. Biol Trace Elem Res. 1998; 66:299–317.
12. Food and Nutrition Board. Dietary Reference Intakes for Vitamin A, Vitamin K, Arsenic, Boron, Chromium, Copper, Iodine, Iron, Manganese, Molybdenum, Nickel, Silicon, Vanadium, and Zinc. Washington, DC: National Academy Press. 2001 pp. 502–53.

NICKEL

Nickel is used industrially in various capacities, such as the production of stainless steel and nickel-cadmium batteries. Nickel is released into the environment when nickel-containing products are burned. Nickel's essentiality in human nutrition was first suggested in the 1930s; however, not until the mid-1970s did studies focus on its possible roles.

Sources

Foods of plant origin have a higher nickel content than foods of animal origin. Nuts, legumes, grains and grain products, and chocolate are particularly rich in the metal, providing up to ~228 μg/100 g [1]. Fruits and vegetables generally have intermediate nickel content, providing up to ~48 μg/100 g [1]. The nickel content of foods of animal origin, such as fish, milk, and eggs, generally is low. The total dietary intake of nickel by adults typically ranges from about 70 to 260 μg/day [2].

The chemical form of nickel in foods is unknown, but in plants it is probably largely inorganic and depends upon the nickel content of the soil. Dietary nickel derived from the contamination of processed foods is likely inorganic as well.

Absorption, Transport, Storage, and Excretion

Nickel absorption from foods is thought to be less than 10%. Absorption of nickel is higher (~20%, but it can be up to 50%) from water than from other beverages (such as coffee, tea, cow's milk, and orange juice) to which nickel has been added. Nickel absorption is not well characterized; it is thought to be absorbed across the enterocyte's brush border membrane by both a carrier and passive diffusion. Nickel competes with iron for carrier transport on divalent mineral transporter (DMT) 1 in the proximal small intestine; consequently, nickel absorption increases with iron deficiency. Transport across the basolateral membrane is thought to occur by diffusion or as part of a complex with an amino acid or other binding ligand.

In the blood, nickel binds mainly to albumin and to a lesser extent to amino acids, including histidine, cysteine, and aspartic acid. Other serum proteins, such as α-2 macroglobulin, also may transport nickel in the blood. Uptake of nickel into cells may occur with amino acids, with transferrin, or through a divalent cation channel such as Ca^{2+}.

Although nickel is widely distributed in the body (which is thought to contain about 10 mg), its concentration is extremely low, occurring at nanogram/gram levels [3]. The highest concentrations of nickel are found in the thyroid and adrenal glands as well as in hair, bones, and soft tissues such as lung, heart, kidney, and liver.

Most nickel is excreted in the urine in amounts less than about 13 μg/L [2]. Within the renal cells, nickel complexes with low-molecular-weight compounds such as uronic acid. In addition to urinary losses, small amounts (1.5–3.3 μg/day) of nickel are excreted in the bile [4]. Sweat nickel concentrations, however, can be fairly high (up to 69.9 μg/L) with active secretion of the element by sweat glands, even in acclimatized individuals [5].

Functions and Deficiency

No specific role for nickel in humans has been identified. Nickel may be involved with folate and vitamin B_{12} in the metabolism of methionine, either in the initial stages involving methionine's conversion to homocysteine or in the later stages, during which propionyl-CoA is converted to succinyl-CoA [6].

In most enzymes in which nickel can serve as a cofactor, the element can be substituted for other minerals, such as magnesium or zinc. An example of such a replacement is the formation of C3 convertase, an enzyme of the complement system, which classically requires Mg^{2+} for activity. The substitution of nickel for magnesium in this complex enhances both the stability and the activity of the enzyme, suggesting a possible physiological role for nickel in the complement system [7].

Signs of nickel deprivation in animals include decreased reproduction; depressed growth; and altered iron, carbohydrate, and lipid metabolism. Impaired hematopoiesis, probably caused by altered iron metabolism, along with effects on bone and thyroid hormone metabolism may also be present.

Interactions with Other Nutrients

Nickel, like many other metals, readily forms chelates with a wide variety of ligands. Consequently, it follows that nickel competes with other metals for ligand sites. The interactions of particular nutritional interest are those involving iron, copper, and zinc. As described in the section on absorption, nickel antagonizes iron absorption. Additionally, the replacement of iron, copper, or zinc by nickel as a cofactor in enzymes in turn typically negatively impacts enzymatic function.

Recommended Intake, Toxicity, and Assessment of Nutriture

Extrapolation from animal studies suggests that humans probably need less than 100 μg of nickel/day [2]. A Tolerable Upper Intake Level for adults for nickel is 1.0 mg/day in the form of soluble nickel salts (such as nickel sulfate, which may contaminate water) [2].

Signs of acute toxicity of nickel include headache, nausea, vomiting, insomnia, and irritability. Delayed symptoms, which may occur up to 5 days after ingestion, include tightness of the chest, cough, difficulty breathing, tachycardia (rapid heart rate), palpitations, sweating, weakness, and possibly death [3]. Chronic toxicity, which usually involves occupational exposure via inhalation of nickel dust or vapors, causes respiratory and other systemic disorders as well as cancer [3]. Nickel's carcinogenic effects target the body's DNA, causing hypermethylation of DNA, inhibition of acetylation of histones, condensation of chromatin, and gene silencing [8].

Serum or plasma nickel concentrations normally range from less than 1 to 23 ng/mL. However, the analysis of plasma or serum is not considered, at present, a valid method to assess nickel status [3].

References Cited for Nickel

1. Pennington J, Jones J. Molybdenum, nickel, cobalt, vanadium, and strontium in total diets. J Am Diet Assoc. 1987; 87:1644–50.
2. Food and Nutrition Board. Dietary Reference Intakes for Vitamin A, Vitamin K, Arsenic, Boron, Chromium, Copper, Iodine, Iron, Manganese, Molybdenum, Nickel, Silicon, Vanadium, and Zinc. Washington, DC: National Academy Press, 2001 pp. 502–53.
3. Das KK, Das SN, Dhundasi SA. Nickel: its adverse health effects and oxidative stress. Ind J Med Res. 2008; 128:412–25.
4. Rezuke W, Knight J, Sunderman F. Reference values for nickel concentrations in human tissue and bile. Am J Ind Med. 1987; 11:419–26.
5. Omokhodion F, Howard J. Trace elements in the sweat of acclimatized persons. Clin Chim Acta. 1994; 231:23–28.
6. Nielsen F. Nutritional requirements for boron, silicon, vanadium, nickel, and arsenic: current knowledge and speculation. FASEB J. 1991; 5:2661–67.
7. Fishelson Z, Muller-Eberhard H. C3 convertase of human complement: enhanced formation and stability of the enzyme generated with nickel instead of magnesium. J Immunol. 1982; 129:2603–07.
8. Cangul H, Broday L, Salnickow K, et al. Molecular mechanisms of nickel carcinogenesis. Toxicol Letters. 2002; 127:69–75.

SILICON

Silicon is second only to oxygen in earth-wide abundance. In fact, quartz, which is crystallized silica, is the most abundant mineral in the earth's crust. The element occurs naturally as silicon dioxide or silica, SiO_2, and as water-soluble ortho- or monosilicic acid, $Si(OH)_4$, formed by hydration of the oxide. In plants, silicon is deposited as the solid, hydrated oxide $SiO_2 \cdot nH_2O$, known as silica gel, following polymerization of silicic acid. Some other forms of silica include talc, clay, asbestos, and glass.

Whereas early investigations concentrated on silicon's toxic effects, such as silicon-related urolithiasis (stones in the urinary tract) and particularly silicosis (a respiratory condition caused by the inhalation of dust), since about the mid-1970s research has focused on the possible roles or functions of silicon in animals and humans.

Sources

Data on the silicon content of foods are sparse. It is known, however, that foods of plant origin normally are much richer in silicon than those of animal origin. Whole cereal grains and root vegetables appear to be especially rich sources of the element, providing about 14% and 8%, respectively, of intake [1,2]. Silica is also found in water, and thus beverages; it is also present in beer because of the hops and barley [1]. Silicon intakes by adults are thought to range from about 14 to 62 mg/day [1,3,4].

Absorption, Transport, Storage, and Excretion

The mechanism of silicon absorption is not well understood, and studies continue to be complicated by its diverse dietary forms. Silica, mono- or orthosilicic acid, phytolithic silica, and silicon found in organic combination (such as with pectin and mucopolysaccharides) are a few of its ingestible forms. In fluids, silicon is found as orthosilicic acid, $Si(OH)_4$. The most soluble form of silicon is metasilicate, which as sodium metasilicate has commonly been used in supplementation studies.

Overall estimates of silicon absorption range from 1% to greater than 70% depending upon the form of silicon ingested [5]. Consumption of fiber significantly impacts the mineral's absorption. For example, nearly 97% of dietary silicon contained in a high-fiber diet remained unabsorbed (lost in the feces), compared to a fecal excretion of only 60% when a low-fiber diet was consumed [2]. Silicon absorption from fluids is estimated at over 50%. In studies in animals, absorption also appears to be affected by age, sex, and various hormones [6].

Once orthosilicic acid is absorbed into the blood, it is almost entirely free (i.e., not bound to proteins), thus accounting for its rapid decrease in plasma concentration, its diffusion into tissue fluids, and its rapid urinary excretion [7]. After intravenous administration of ^{31}Si silicic acid, the label was most rapidly taken up by the liver, lungs, skin, and bones, with slower entry occurring in the heart, muscle, spleen, and testes. Negligible uptake into the brain was reported, indicating active exclusion by the blood-brain barrier. Generally, silicon concentrates in the body's connective tissues, such as bone, skin, blood vessels (such as the aorta), and tendons.

Most silicon is thought to be excreted in the urine as orthosilicic acid and as magnesium orthosilicate. Urinary silicon excretion is significantly correlated with silicon intake [4].

Functions and Deficiency

The physiological role of silicon centers on the normal formation, growth, and development of bones, connective tissues, and cartilage. Silicon is thought to play both metabolic and structural roles. In bones, silicon influences formation and growth processes, including bone mineralization and crystallization [7–12]. Silicon deficiency results in smaller, less flexible long bones and in skull deformation. In studies on chicks, the skull deformation was subsequently found to be caused by reduced collagen in the connective tissue matrix [7]. Decreases in femoral and vertebral calcium, copper, potassium, and zinc concentrations and increased plasma alkaline phosphatase activity have been reported with silicon deprivation in rats [9]. Moreover, silicon deprivation in rats diminished bone collagen formation (with decreased activity of ornithine aminotransferase, an enzyme required for collagen formation) and increased collagen breakdown [10]. In culture cells, orthosilicic acid stimulated collagen synthesis and bone cell differentiation [11]. Other studies suggest that silicon's effects on bone may be related to proton buffering [12].

Recommended Intake, Toxicity, and Assessment of Nutriture

The requirement for silicon is largely unknown, although estimates range from about 10 to 25 mg/day [13]. No Tolerable Upper Intake Level has been established for silicon, although a safe upper level of 1,750 mg/day has been suggested [14].

Toxicity from silicon has been associated with the formation of kidney stones; however, it is frequent, chronic (years) use of large amounts of silicon-containing antacids (e.g., magnesium trisilicate, which provides up to about 6.5 mg of elemental silicon per tablet) that appears to contribute to the rare development of kidney stones [3,14,15]. Toxicity of silicon also has been associated with diminished activities of several enzymes that prevent free radical damage, including glutathione peroxidase, superoxide dismutase, and catalase [16]. Silicosis occurs from the inhalation of dust high in silica; the condition is characterized by a progressive fibrosis of the lungs that leads to respiratory problems.

As in the case of most of the ultratrace elements, levels of silicon in biological fluids of healthy adults have been reported but may not accurately represent nutriture. Serum silicon concentrations usually range from about 11 to 31 µg/dL [14,17,18].

References Cited for Silicon

1. Pennington J. Silicon in foods and diet. Food Add Contam. 1991; 8:97–118.
2. Kelsay J, Behall K, Prather E. Effect of fiber from fruits and vegetables on metabolic responses of human subjects II: calcium, magnesium, iron, and silicon balances. Am J Clin Nutr. 1979; 32:1876–80.
3. Food and Nutrition Board. Dietary Reference Intakes for Vitamin A, Vitamin K, Arsenic, Boron, Chromium, Copper, Iodine, Iron, Manganese, Molybdenum, Nickel, Silicon, Vanadium, and Zinc. Washington, DC: National Academy Press. 2001 pp. 502–53.
4. Jugdaohsingh R, Anderson S, Tucker K, et al. Dietary silicon intake and absorption. Am J Clin Nutr. 2002; 75:887–93.
5. Benke G, Osborn T. Urinary silicon excretion by rats following oral administration of silicon compounds. Food Cosmet Toxicol. 1978; 17:123–27.
6. Charnot Y, Peres G. Silicon, endocrine balance and mineral metabolism. In: Bendz G, Lindquist I, eds. Biochemistry of Silicon and Related Problems. New York: Plenum Press. 1978 pp. 269–80.
7. Adler A, Etzion Z, Berlyne G. Uptake, distribution, and excretion of ^{31}silicon in normal rats. Am J Physiol. 1986; 251:E670–73.
8. Seaborn C, Nielsen F. Dietary silicon affects acid and alkaline phosphatase and ^{45}calcium uptake in bone of rats. J Trace Elem Exper Med. 1994; 7:11–18.
9. Seaborn C, Nielsen F. Dietary silicon and arginine affect mineral element composition of rat femur and vertebra. Biol Trace Elem Res. 2002; 89:239–50.
10. Seaborn C, Nielsen F. Silicon deprivation decreases collagen formation in wounds and bone, and ornithine transaminase enzyme activity in liver. Biol Trace Elem Res. 2002; 89:251–61.
11. Reffitt DM, Ogston N, Jugdaohsingh R, et al. Orthosilicic acid stimulates collagen type 1 synthesis and osteoblastic differentiation in human osteoblast-like cells in vitro. Bone. 2003; 32:127–35.
12. Eckhert CD. Other trace elements. In: Shils M, Shike M, Ross A, Caballerno B, Cousins RJ, eds. Modern Nutrition in Health and Disease, 10th ed. Baltimore, MD: Williams and Wilkins. 2005 pp. 346–47.
13. Carlisle EM. Silicon. In: O'Dell BL, Sunde RA, eds. Handbook of Nutritionally Essential Minerals. New York: Marcel Dekker. 1997 pp. 603–18.
14. Martin KR. The chemistry of silica and its potential health benefits. J Nutr Hlth & Aging. 2007; 11:94–98.
15. Haddad F, Kouyoumdjian A. Silica stones in humans. Urol Int. 1986; 41:70–76.
16. Najda J, Goss M, Gminski J, et al. The antioxidant enzyme activity in the conditions of systemic hypersilicemia. Biol Trace Elem Res. 1994; 42:63–70.
17. Nielsen FH. Micronutrients in parenteral nutrition: boron, silicon, and fluoride. Gastroenterol. 2009; 137:S55–60.
18. Bisse E, Epting T, Beil A. Reference values for serum silicon in adults. Anal Biochem. 2005; 337:130–35.

VANADIUM

Vanadium was first discovered in the early 1800s and named for a Swedish goddess, Vanadis [1]. The element occurs in several oxidation states from V^{2+} to V^{5+}, and in solution, vanadium produces a range of colors. In its pentavalent state it is yellowish orange, whereas in its divalent state it is blue [1]. V^{3+} has been shown to form complexes with amino acids such as alanine and aspartate [2]. In biological systems including the serum and body cells, vanadium is found primarily in its pentavalent V^{5+} state as vanadate or monovanadate (VO_3^-, VO_4^3, or $H_2VO_4^-$), or in its tetravalent V^{4+} state as vanadyl (VO^{2+}). The tetravalent state is less toxic than the pentavalent state.

Sources

The vanadium content of foods is very low and consequently so is the average dietary intake. Most fats and oils contain particularly low levels of the mineral, less than 0.3 µg/100 g [3]. A few items, including black pepper, parsley, dill seed, canned apple juice, fish sticks, and mushrooms, contain relatively high concentrations, and shellfish such as oysters are particularly rich in the element, with up to about 12 µg/100 g [3,4]. Cereals and grain products contribute fairly substantial amounts of vanadium (up to 15 µg/100 g) to the diet, as do sweeteners (up to 4.7 µg/100 g) [4]. Beer and wine also provide a source of vanadium [3,4]. Vanadium intake in the U.S. diet is thought to range from about 10 to 60 µg/day. Supplements providing vanadium as vanadyl sulfate, sodium metavanadate, and sodium orthovanadate are available.

Absorption, Transport, Storage, and Excretion

Absorption of vanadium varies with its oxidation states. For example, vanadate ($H_2VO_4^-$) may be reduced to vanadyl (VO^{2+}) in the stomach before being absorbed in the upper small intestine; however, vanadate may be absorbed directly using the same carrier system as used by phosphate. Compared to vanadyl, vanadate is three to five times more efficiently absorbed. Overall, vanadium absorption is generally less than 10%.

In blood cells, the plasma, and other body fluids, vanadium may be present as vanadate or it may be converted to vanadyl using glutathione, NADH, and ascorbic acid as reducing agents. In the plasma, vanadyl binds to albumin and iron-containing proteins such as transferrin and ferritin.

Vanadium is thought to enter cells as vanadate (HVO_4^{2-}) through transport systems used by phosphate. Similarly to its reduction in the plasma, intracellular vanadate is reduced primarily by glutathione to vanadyl, which is then almost exclusively bound to ligands, primarily phosphates and iron-containing proteins. Vanadyl may be converted back to vanadate by NADPH [5].

The total body pool of vanadium is about 100 to 200 µg, with most tissues containing less than 10 ng of vanadium/g [3,6]. Distribution studies indicate that although kidney cells retain most of the absorbed mineral soon after it is administered, accumulation later shifts principally to the bones and teeth, lungs, and thyroid gland, with somewhat lesser amounts in the spleen and liver.

Renal excretion is the major route for the elimination of absorbed vanadium [7]. Amounts of vanadium in the urine are generally less than 0.8 μg/L of urine. In addition to losses in the urine, small amounts of vanadium are excreted in the bile.

Functions and Deficiency

No specific biochemical function has been identified for vanadium. Further, many of vanadium's effects *in vivo* are predictable from a consideration of its aqueous chemistry. First, as vanadate, it competes with phosphate at the active sites of phosphate transport proteins, phosphohydrolases, and phosphotransferases. Because of this property, vanadate exhibits osteogenic action through incorporation into the amorphous hydroxyapatite lattice of bone in place of phosphate. Second, as vanadyl, it competes with other transition metals for binding sites on metalloproteins and for small ligands such as adenosine triphosphate (ATP). Third, it participates in redox reactions within the cell, particularly with substances that can reduce vanadate nonenzymatically, such as glutathione.

Vanadium is very active pharmacologically, exerting a broad assortment of effects. However, pharmacological activity is generally manifested only above a concentration threshold that is considerably greater than that required to fulfill the need for essentiality. A few of the more thoroughly investigated pharmacological effects of vanadium are described briefly. Vanadium inhibits Na^+/K^+-ATPase, an enzyme involved in the transport of ions against a concentration gradient. Vanadate is known to inhibit the enzyme by binding to its ATP hydrolysis site. In muscle, vanadate also has been shown to form ternary complexes with myosin and ADP and thus inhibit interactions with actin [8].

Vanadium, as vanadate, is believed to stimulate adenylate cyclase by promoting an association of an otherwise inactive guanine nucleotide regulatory protein (G protein) with the catalytic unit of the enzyme [9]. Adenylate cyclase catalyzes the formation of cyclic $3',5'$-adenosine monophosphate (cAMP) from ATP. Cyclic AMP then stimulates protein kinases, which catalyze the phosphorylation of various enzymes and other cellular proteins.

The effect of vanadate on the transport of amino acids across the intestinal mucosa exemplifies both its inhibitory effect on Na^+/K^+-ATPase and its stimulation of adenylate cyclase. At higher concentrations, vanadate inhibits the mucosal-to-serosal flux of alanine, commensurate with a decrease in Na^+/K^+-ATPase function. However, at a lower concentration (too low to affect Na^+/K^+-ATPase), it stimulates alanine transport; this

shift is attributable to an increase in adenylate cyclase activity and cAMP formation [10].

Vanadium, in pharmacological amounts as vanadate and vanadyl, mimics the action of insulin. Vanadium stimulates glucose uptake into cells, enhances glucose metabolism, and inhibits catecholamine-induced lipolysis in adipose tissue. The enhancement in glucose uptake occurs through improved translocation of the glucose transporter GLUT4 to cell membranes [11]. Vanadium also stimulates hepatic glycogen synthesis and inhibits gluconeogenesis. Notably, however, vanadate phosphorylates tyrosyl residues not in the insulin receptor, but in cytosolic and plasma membrane protein kinases. This activation of the cytosolic protein kinases affects glucose and lipid metabolism, while activation of the plasma membrane protein kinases triggers phosphatidylinositol-3-kinase, inhibits lipolysis, and stimulates glucose uptake [5]. Vanadate also has been shown to activate Akt signaling through inhibition of protein tyrosine phosphatase, thereby prolonging the activity of the phosphorylated enzymes and enhancing the insulin-signaling pathway (Akt is a protein involved in insulin signaling; see Chapter 7) [12]. Evidence also exists that vanadium inhibits the activity of other enzymes such as glucose-6-phosphatase, fructose-2,6-biphosphatase, and acidic and alkaline phosphatase. Moreover, vanadium's effects on protein tyrosine phosphatase have also been associated with cell cycle arrest and antitumoral properties [13]. Deficiency of vanadium in animals impairs survival, growth, and development.

Vanadium and Disease

Vanadium exerts cardioprotective effects in situations in which the heart or vascular system has been injured, such as with heart attack, heart failure, hypertension, and/or vascular diseases. Many of these beneficial effects are mediated through the Akt signaling pathway [12]. While most studies to date have been conducted in animals, the use of vanadium compounds to repair cardiomyocytes (heart muscle cells) is hoped to provide a novel approach in the treatment of heart damage in the near future [12].

Doses of 100 to 300 mg vanadyl sulfate or sodium metavanadate have been administered to people with type 2 diabetes in clinical trials. Vanadium improved insulin sensitivity and thereby reduced serum glucose concentrations and hemoglobin A1c. Gluconeogenesis and serum lipid concentrations were also reduced. A meta-analysis of studies examining the effectiveness of vanadium supplements on glycemic control in individuals with type 2 diabetes reported significant treatment effects including reductions in fasting blood glucose; however, because of the poor quality of most of the studies, the use of vanadium in the management of type 2 diabetes was not recommended [14]. See the articles by Thompson [15,16] for a review of the use of vanadium compounds in diabetes treatment.

In contrast to these possible benefits in those with type 2 diabetes and heart damage, vanadyl sulfate was found to be of no significant benefit in the management of impaired glucose tolerance, a risk factor for diabetes [17]. Similarly, data supporting the use of vanadyl sulfate (in doses up to about 60 mg daily) to enhance body weight and muscle mass are also limited.

Recommended Intake, Toxicity, and Assessment of Nutriture

The human requirement for vanadium is not established, although 10 μg/day has been suggested [18]. Intakes of up to 100 μg of vanadium/day are considered safe. A Tolerable Upper Intake Level of 1.8 mg of elemental vanadium per day has been established [19]. Side effects have been observed in humans with vanadium intakes above about 10 mg. Mild toxic manifestations include green tongue syndrome (from deposition of green-colored vanadium in the tongue), diarrhea, and gastrointestinal cramps [20]. Chronic toxicity of vanadium as seen in miners manifests in hypertension, neurological disorders, and hepatic, cardiac, and renal damage [20].

Methods to assess vanadium status have not been established. Blood vanadium concentrations typically range from about 0.4 to 2.8 ng/mL but may be greater than 500 ng/mL in those ingesting vanadium supplements [3,21]. Urinary excretion of vanadium averages about 8 μg/day [22].

References Cited for Vanadium

1. Harland B, Harden-Williams B. Is vanadium of human nutritional importance yet? J Am Diet Assoc. 1994; 94:891–94.
2. Bukietynska K, Podsiadly H, Karwecka Z. Complexes of vanadium (III) with L-alanine and L-aspartic acid. J Inorg Biochem. 2003; 94:317–25.
3. Byrne A, Kosta L. Vanadium in foods and in human body fluids and tissues. Sci Total Environ. 1978; 10:17–30.
4. Pennington J, Jones J. Molybdenum, nickel, cobalt, vanadium, and strontium in total diets. J Am Diet Assoc. 1987; 87:1644–50.
5. Goldwaser I, Gefel D, Gershonov E, et al. Insulinlike effects of vanadium: basic and clinical implications. J Inorg Biochem. 2000; 80:21–25.
6. Baran E. Oxovanadium (IV) and oxovanadium (V) complexes relevant to biological systems. J Inorganic Biochem. 2000; 80:1–10.
7. Heinemann G, Fichti B, Vogt W. Pharmacokinetics of vanadium in humans after intravenous administration of a vanadium containing albumin solution. Br J Clin Pharmacol. 2003; 55:231–45.
8. Aureliano M. Vanadate oligomer interactions with myosin. J Inorg Biochem. 2000; 80:141–43.
9. Krawietz W, Downs R, Spiegel A, Aurbach G. Vanadate stimulates adenylate cyclase via the guanine nucleotide regulatory protein by a mechanism differing from that of fluoride. Biochem Pharmacol. 1982; 31:843–48.
10. Hajjar J, Fucci J, Rowe W, Tomicic T. Effect of vanadate on amino acid transport in rat jejunum. Proc Soc Exp Biol Med. 1987; 184:403–09.
11. Srivastava A, Mehdi M. Insulino-mimetic and anti-diabetic effects of vanadium compounds. Diabet Med. 2005; 22:2–13.
12. Bhuiyan MS, Fukunaga K. Cardioprotection by vanadium compounds targeting Akt-mediated signaling. J Pharmacol Sci. 2009; 110:1–13.
13. Barrio DA, Etcheverry SB. Potential use of vanadium compounds in therapeutics. Curr Med Chem. 2010; 17:3632–42.
14. Smith DM, Pickering RM, Lewith GT. A systematic review of vanadium oral supplements for glycemic control in type 2 diabetes mellitus. Q J Med. 2008; 101:351–58.
15. Thompson KH, Orvig C. Vanadium in diabetes: 100 years from phase 0 to phase I. J Inorganic Biochem. 2006; 100:1925–35.
16. Thompson KH, Lichter J, LeBel C, et al. Vanadium treatment of type 2 diabetes: a view to the future. J Inorganic Biochem. 2009; 103:554–58.
17. Jacques-Camarena O, Gonzalez-Ortiz M, Martinez-Abundis E. Effect of vanadium on insulin sensitivity in patients with impaired glucose tolerance. Ann Nutr Metab. 2008; 53:195–98.
18. Nielsen F. Ultratrace elements in nutrition: current knowledge and speculation. J Trace Elem Exp Med. 1998; 11:251–74.
19. Food and Nutrition Board. Dietary Reference Intakes for Vitamin A, Vitamin K, Arsenic, Boron, Chromium, Copper, Iodine, Iron, Manganese, Molybdenum, Nickel, Silicon, Vanadium, and Zinc. Washington, DC: National Academy Press. 2001 pp. 502–53.
20. Baran EJ. Vanadium detoxification: chemical and biochemical aspects. Chem Biodiversity. 2008; 5:1475–84.
21. Goldfine AB, Patti M, Zuberi L, et al. Metabolic effects of vanadyl sulfate in humans with non-insulin-dependent diabetes mellitus: in vivo and in vitro studies. Metab. 2000; 49:400–10.
22. Tracey AS, Willsky GR, Takeuci ES. Vanadium Chemistry, Biochemistry, Pharmacology and Practical Applications. Boca Raton, FL: CRC Press. 2007 pp. 181–85.

COBALT

Little evidence exists that cobalt plays a role in human nutrition other than its being a part of vitamin B_{12} (cobalamin). Although ionic cobalt can substitute for other metals in metalloenzyme activity *in vitro*, no evidence exists that it acts in that capacity *in vivo*. In this respect, the metal is unique among the elements, in that the requirement in humans is not for an ionic form of the metal but for a preformed metallovitamin that cannot be synthesized from dietary metal. Therefore, it is the vitamin B_{12} content of foods and the diet, rather than the cobalt present, that is important in human nutrition.

NO, SILVER IS *NOT* ANOTHER ESSENTIAL ULTRATRACE MINERAL: TIPS TO IDENTIFYING BOGUS CLAIMS ABOUT DIETARY SUPPLEMENTS

Although found in the environment (and thus natural) and often worn as jewelry, the mineral silver is non-essential for human life. Silver has no known biochemical role or physiological function in the body. Yet, a quick search of "silver supplements" on the Internet will yield close to 20 million related Web sites. Many of these sites proclaim the benefits from ingesting supplements providing silver, either colloidal silver (a liquid suspension of tiny silver particles), ionic silver, native silver, or silver protein, among others forms of the element, as a cure for viral and bacterial infections, arthritis, gastrointestinal problems (such as gastroesophageal reflux), and various skin ailments including dry skin, rashes, and dermatitis. What the manufacturers of the oral silver supplements *do not* tell you is often more important—that is, the side effects or health hazards of silver supplements.

The 2009 television appearances (on the "Today Show," "Oprah," etc.) of the "man who turned blue" from the regular consumption of a liquid colloidal silver supplement provided visual proof of one of the supplement's detrimental effects—argyria. Argyria is a permanent (i.e., irreversible) bluish or grayish discoloration of skin, nails, gums, and conjunctiva (the membrane that covers the white part of the eye) that results from the ingestion of silver. The condition is not reversed upon discontinuation of the product or by medical interventions. The exact amount of silver that induces argyria is not clear; however, based on a review of cases of argyria associated with silver consumption, the Environmental Protection Agency established an oral reference dose of 5 μg of silver/kg body weight per day [1]. This corresponds to a daily intake of 341 μg of silver for a person weighing 150 lbs (68.2 kg). Other health hazards associated with consumption of silver—all unlikely to be disclosed by the manufacturer of the product—include brain, nerve, liver, and kidney damage and gastrointestinal problems, as well as headaches and seizures. Silver is a heavy metal; thus, with oral ingestion, the mineral accumulates in organs, causing destruction, and in arteries, which can lead to atherosclerosis (heart disease). Silver does, however, have a few approved medical uses. The mineral is used in topical ointments and in bandages/gauze dressings for the treatment of some burns, wounds, and infections of the skin; none of these silver-containing medical products, however, is ingested orally.

Silver supplements are just one example of the thousands of dietary supplements marketed to Americans to improve well-being and appearance, and to prevent or cure diseases or ailments. The advertisements for supplements appear in stores, newspapers, and magazines and on television; they also "pop up" on computers and other electronic devices while a user browses the Internet. Added to the harmful effects that many of these supplements have on the body is their economic impact: these products are not cheap. Health fraud is estimated to cost consumers over $25 billion each year.

The Dietary Supplement Health and Education Act (DSHEA) of 1994 considers dietary supplements, including minerals, vitamins, herbs or other botanicals, amino acids, dietary substances (such as enzymes), metabolites, constituents, and extracts, to be products ingested orally that contain dietary ingredient(s) intended to supplement the diet (not medications) [2]. As a consequence, the manufacturers of dietary supplements do not have to secure approval to sell products, nor do they have to demonstrate to any regulatory agency that the supplements are safe (unless they contain a dietary ingredient that was not sold prior to 1994). Moreover, manufacturers of supplements can list claims about their product on the label; specifically allowed are claims of general well-being, of structure/function (i.e., how the nutrient affects human body structure or function), and of benefit related to a classical nutrient deficiency disease [3]. Along with such claims, the supplement manufacturer must provide a disclaimer on the label stating that "this statement has not been evaluated by the Food and Drug Administration" and that "this product is not intended to diagnose, treat, cure, or prevent any disease." In addition, the manufacturer must have substantiation that the claim is truthful and not misleading, and must notify the U.S. Food and Drug Administration (FDA) that its product bears such a claim within 30 days of marketing the product [3].

Unfortunately, many consumers assume all dietary supplements are safe, and many fraudulent supplements remain on the market for a long time, causing injury or adverse reactions among users before the FDA accumulates enough evidence that a particular supplement is unsafe and removes it from the market. Consequently, the buyer must beware. Consumers must learn to identify bogus dietary supplement (as well as weight-loss diet) claims to avoid being scammed and potentially harmed. The Food and Nutrition Science Alliance (a coalition of four professional organizations: the Academy of Nutrition and Dietetics [formerly the American Dietetic Association], the American Society for Clinical Nutrition, the American Society for Nutritional Sciences, and the Institute of Food Technologists) developed "Ten Red Flags of Junk Science" to help consumers identify nutrition misinformation [4].

The Ten Red Flags of Junk Science [4] include:

1. Recommendations that promise a quick fix
2. Dire warnings of danger from a single product or regimen
3. Claims that sound too good to be true
4. Simplistic conclusions drawn from a single study
5. Recommendations based on a single study
6. Dramatic statements that are refuted by reputable scientific organizations
7. Lists of "good" and "bad" foods
8. Recommendations made to help sell a product
9. Recommendations based on studies published without peer review
10. Recommendations from studies that ignore individual or group differences

Many of these "red flags" are apparent in advertisements for dietary supplements, such as colloidal silver, which are frequently found on the Internet. (Remember: There are no rules to posting information on the Internet; anyone can create a Web site and post content.) Manufacturers' Web sites often guarantee a quick fix to problems, and it is not uncommon to see promises of dramatic or even miraculous results, with cures to one or more diseases (often those for which medical science has no cure). These claims, of course, are "too good to be true" and incorrectly suggest "one product can do it all." In addition, the products are often marketed as being "natural" (implying natural is "better," when in reality many "natural" substances are dangerous and many artificial or synthetic ones are not) and as containing "specialized formulas," making them superior to other products. Colloidal silver, for example, may be marketed as being better absorbed than other forms of silver because it contains nanoparticles (meaning it has a particle size between 1 and 100 nm) and because it is mined from secret (nondisclosed) natural sources. Finally, proof of the dietary supplement's effectiveness is usually provided by the manufacturer in the form of testimonials or anecdotes from satisfied consumers. Lacking are scientific data regarding the supplement's benefits provided by multiple well-designed, double-blind, placebo-controlled studies.

Each year hundreds of manufacturers of dietary supplements receive letters from the FDA warning against the promotion of products with unsubstantiated (false or misleading) claims. Products that present a direct health threat to consumers are usually targeted first by the FDA and Federal Trade Commission (which regulates the advertising of products), followed by those that present indirect health hazards. To facilitate the identification of harmful products, adverse events associated with the use of dietary supplements should be reported to the FDA's MedWatch program [5]. In addition, for reassurance that a product is of sufficient quality and potency, consumers can look for a U.S.P. (U.S. Pharmacopoeia) symbol or designation on the product's label. This designation indicates that the manufacturer followed established U.S.P. standards for quality, purity, strength, packaging, labeling, and storage. Nonetheless, the ultimate decision on whether to purchase and consume the supplement should be made with caution and considerable research. Remember the "Ten Red Flags of Junk Science," and remember to be skeptical and rely on reputable information sources in your evaluation of dietary supplements before spending your money.

References

1. FDA. Consumer advisory: dietary supplements containing silver may cause permanent discoloration of skin and mucous membranes (argyria). October 6, 2009. http://www.fda.gov/Food/DietarySupplements/Alerts/ucm184087.htm

2. Dietary Supplement Health and Education Act, 103–417, 3.(a). 1994 bill/resolution.

3. FDA. Dietary supplement safety act: how is FDA doing 10 years later. http://www.fda.gov/NewsEvents/Testimony/ucm113767.htm

4. Position of the American Dietetic Association: Food and Nutrition Misinformation. J Am Diet Assoc. 2006; 106:601–07.

5. FDA's MedWatch program. http://www.fda.gov/medwatch

Recommended Web Sites

National Council Against Health Fraud.
http://www.ncahf.org

National Institutes of Health, Office of Dietary Supplements.
http://dietary.supplements.info.nih.gov

Quackwatch: your guide to quackery, health fraud, and intelligent decisions.
http://www.quackwatch.org

U.S. Food and Drug Administration.
http://www.fda.gov

U. S. Food and Drug Administration. How to spot health fraud.
http://www.fda.gov/Drugs/EmergencyPreparedness/BioterrorismandDrugPreparedness/ucm137284.htm

GLOSSARY

Achlorhydria Lack of hydrochloric acid in gastric juice.

Activation energy Energy introduced into the reactant molecules to activate them to the transition state so that an exothermic reaction can take place.

Acute Having a rapid or sudden onset.

Adequate Intake (AI) A recommended daily dietary nutrient intake based on nutrient intake levels of healthy people; an AI is thought to exceed the requirement for a given nutrient.

Alkalosis A condition in which the pH of the blood is above about 7.45, the upper end of the normal range.

Alkoxyl radical (RO$^\bullet$ or LO$^\bullet$) A monovalent radical consisting of an alkyl group united with oxygen. Alkyl groups are derived from alkanes (a class of hydrocarbons in which the molecule contains only carbon and hydrogen atoms joined by single covalent bonds) by the removal of one hydrogen atom and have the general formula C_nH_{2n+1}.

Amenorrhea The absence of at least three consecutive menstrual cycles.

Amphibolic pathway A pathway that is involved in both the catabolism and the biosynthesis (anabolism) of carbohydrates, fatty acids, and/or amino acids.

Amphipathic Refers to a molecule that has a polar region at one location and a nonpolar region at another.

Amphoteric Capable of reacting as either an acid or a base.

Anaplerotic reaction A reaction that involves replenishing or restoring a substrate (e.g., the conversion of pyruvate to oxaloacetic acid).

Anomeric carbon The carbon that comprises the carbonyl function that is capable of forming a ring structure with the OH group on the highest-numbered chiral carbon of a monosaccharide.

Anorexigenic Capable of producing anorexia or diminishing appetite.

Anticodons Three-base sequences of nucleotides within transfer RNA (tRNA) molecules.

Antral Pertaining to the antrum, the lower or distal portion of the stomach.

Apical At or near the apex; pertaining to the intestinal lumen side of an enterocyte.

Apolipoprotein The protein component of a lipoprotein particle; also called *apoprotein*.

Apoptosis An organized series of events that, once triggered, leads to cell death.

Arcuate nucleus The subcortical region of the brain that secretes appetite-enhancing neuropeptide Y and appetite-suppressing melanocortins.

Aromatic compound An organic compound that contains a benzene ring.

Ataxia Impaired muscle coordination, especially when trying to perform voluntary muscular movements.

Atheroma A mass of plaque consisting of degenerated, thickened arterial intima, occurring in atherosclerosis.

Autolysis The digestion of intracellular components (including organelles) by lysosomes.

Autophagy The breakdown or digestion of the body's proteins, such as those found in the blood or within cells.

Beriberi A condition resulting from a thiamin deficiency.

Bile A body fluid made in the liver and stored in the gallbladder that participates in emulsifying fat and forming micelles for fat absorption.

Bitot's spots Small, white, foamy-looking accumulations of sloughed cells and secretions in the eye that are associated with a vitamin A deficiency.

Buffer A compound that ameliorates a change in pH.

Calpain A calcium-dependent protease involved in protein turnover in the body.

Caspases A family of cysteine proteases involved in the degradative events during apoptosis (cell death).

Carboxylation The addition of a carboxyl group to a molecule.

Catabolism The process by which organic molecules are broken down to produce energy.

Cathepsins A group of enzymes involved in breaking down or digesting the body's proteins.

Cells The basic units for all organisms that arise from preexisting cells.

Chaperones Soluble intracellular proteins that bind to and deliver minerals to specific intracellular locations.

Chelators Small organic compounds that form a complex with another compound, such as a mineral.

Chemiosmotic theory The theory that most ATP synthesis occurs in a process whereby protons move down an electrochemical gradient, and the energy generated is used to phosphorylate ADP to make ATP.

Chiral carbon A carbon atom with four different atoms or groups covalently attached to it.

Chronic Long and drawn out in duration or recurring over a long period of time.

Chylomicron A type of lipoprotein that transports lipids and lipid-soluble vitamins from the intestine into the lymph and then the blood for use by body cells.

Chylomicron remnant The portion of a chylomicron that is left after blood lipoprotein lipase removes part of its triglycerides.

Chyme Partially digested food.

Cobalophilins A group of proteins, sometimes called R proteins, that are found in digestive juices and bind to vitamin B$_{12}$ to facilitate absorption.

Codon A three-base sequence in a DNA or mRNA molecule that specifies the location of a single, particular amino acid in a polypeptide chain.

Cohort A group of individuals that share common characteristics.

Colloids Substances comprised of very small particles that are suspended uniformly in a medium.

Colorimetric titration A method of measuring the volume of one reagent required to react with a measured volume of another reagent, using an indicator that changes color.

Complementary base pairing The pairing of nucleotide bases in two strands of nucleic acids; A pairs with T or U, while G pairs with C.

Complete protein A protein that contains all the essential (indispensable) amino acids in the approximate amounts needed by humans.

Confounder A statistical term that denotes a third variable that can distort the relationship between the two variables under analysis.

Connexin A protein involved in forming junctions between cells.

Coulometric titration A method for determining the amount of a substance released during electrolysis by measuring the electrical charge. (*Note:* A coulomb is a unit of electrical charge.)

Cross-over study A longitudinal study in which subjects receive a sequence of different treatments. Each subject receives all treatments (including placebos), usually in a random order.

Cytochromes Heme-containing proteins that serve as electron carriers (e.g., in oxidative phosphorylation or the cytochrome P450 system).

Cytokines A generic term for nonantibody protein messengers released from a macrophage or lymphocyte that is part of an intracellular immune response.

Cytoplast A cell from which the nucleus has been removed.

Cytoskeleton Microtubules and microfilaments in the cell that provide internal reinforcement and communication.

Cytosol (cytoplasm) The continuous aqueous solution of the cell and the organelles contained in it.

Deamination The removal of an amino (NH_2) group from an amino acid.

Dehydrogenases Enzymes that catalyze reactions in which hydrogens and electrons are removed from a reactant.

Desaturation The process of converting a saturated compound to an unsaturated one.

Dietary fiber Nondigestible (by human digestive enzymes) carbohydrates and lignin that are intact and intrinsic in plants.

Dipeptidylaminopeptidase A protein-digesting enzyme that breaks apart dipeptides.

Diphosphatidylglycerol A phosphatidylglycerol esterified through the C-1 hydroxyl group of the glycerol moiety to the head phosphoryl group of another phosphatidic acid molecule; also called *cardiolipin*.

Direct calorimetry A method of measuring the dissipation of heat from the body.

Disaccharides Sugars formed by combining two monosaccharides through a glycosidic bond between the hydroxyl group of one monosaccharide and the hydroxyl group of another.

Double blind study An experiment in which neither the person administering the treatment nor the subject knows which treatment (placebo or experimental) the subject is receiving.

Dowager's hump A deformity of the spine characterized by a humpback or being bent forward; also called *kyphosis*.

Eicosanoids Biologically active substances derived from linoleic and α-linolenic (n-6 and n-3) essential fatty acids.

Electron transport chain The sequential transfer of electrons from reduced coenzymes to oxygen that is coupled with ATP formation and occurs within the mitochondria.

Elongation (1) The extension of the polypeptide chain of the protein product during protein synthesis. (2) The addition of carbons (in two-carbon increments) to a fatty acid chain.

Endocrine system All of the body's hormone-secreting glands.

Endocytosis Uptake of a substance into a cell through the formation of vesicles derived from the plasma membrane.

Endopeptidase An enzyme that hydrolyzes amino acids linked to other amino acids in the interior of a peptide or protein.

Endoplasmic reticulum (ER) A network of membranous channels pervading the cytosol and providing continuity between the nuclear envelope, the Golgi apparatus, and the plasma membrane.

Endothermic reaction A reaction in which the products have more free energy than the reactants; it therefore requires energy.

Enkephalins Peptides that bind to opioid receptors found in the brain and gastrointestinal tract.

Enterocyte An intestinal cell.

Enterohepatic circulation The movement of a substance, such as bile, from the liver to the intestine and then back to the liver.

Enzymes Protein catalysts that increase the rate of a chemical reaction in the body.

Epidemiology The science concerned with studying those factors that influence the frequency and distribution of disease in a defined human population.

Equivocal Uncertain or ambiguous.

Erythrocyte A red blood cell.

Estimated Average Requirement (EAR) The amount of a nutrient thought to meet the requirements of 50% of healthy individuals in a specified age and gender group.

Eukaryotic cells Cells with a defined nucleus surrounded by a nuclear membrane.

Exocytosis A process by which compounds may be released from cells.

Exons The segments of a gene that code for a sequence of nucleotides in a specific molecule of mRNA.

Exopeptidase An enzyme that hydrolyzes amino acids off the terminal end of a peptide or protein.

Exothermic reaction A reaction in which the reactants have more free energy than the products; it therefore gives off energy as heat.

Exudate Fluids that have exuded (been forced or pressed) out of a tissue or its capillaries.

Ferment To break down substrates anaerobically to yield reduced products and energy.

Fermentation An anaerobic breakdown of carbohydrates and protein by bacteria.

Fibrotic Pertaining to fibrosis, formation of fibrous tissue as a reactive or repair process.

Free energy The potential energy inherent in the chemical bonds of nutrients.

Free radical An atom or molecule that has one or more unpaired electrons.

Functional fiber Nondigestible carbohydrates that have been isolated, extracted, or manufactured and have been shown to have beneficial physiological effects in humans.

Gap junctions Channels between cells.

Gene A section of chromosomal DNA that codes for a single protein.

Genome The sum of all the chromosomal genes of a cell.

Ghrelin A hormone secreted by the stomach and duodenum that signals hunger.

Gluconeogenesis The formation of glucose by the liver or kidney from noncarbohydrate precursors.

Glucose tolerance factor (GTF) A chromium-containing compound whose structure has yet to be characterized but may potentiate the action of insulin in the body.

Glycocalyx The layer of glycoprotein and polysaccharide that surrounds many cells.

Glycogenesis The pathway by which glucose is converted to glycogen.

Glycogenolysis The pathway by which glycogen is enzymatically broken down to glucose.

Glycolysis The pathway by which glucose is converted to pyruvate.

Glycoproteins Proteins covalently bound to a carbohydrate.

Glycosaminoglycan An unbranched polysaccharide consisting of alternate units of two different sugars.

Glycosidases/carbohydrases Digestive enzymes that hydrolyze polysaccharides to their constituent monosaccharide units.

Golgi apparatus (network) The part of the cell responsible for modifying macromolecules synthesized in the endoplasmic reticulum and packaging them to be transported to the cell surface or cytosol.

Haptocorrins A group of proteins, sometimes called R proteins, that are found in digestive juices and bind to vitamin B_{12} to facilitate absorption.

Hartnup disease A hereditary disorder in which tryptophan absorption and excretion are abnormal.

Hemochromatosis An inherited disorder characterized by excessive iron absorption and iron overload in the body.

Heterodimers Complexes formed between two or more different receptors or molecules.

Hexose monophosphate shunt See *pentose phosphate pathway.*

Homeostasis The tendency to stability in the internal environment of an organism.

Homodimers Complexes formed between two of the same receptors or molecules.

Hormones Chemical messengers synthesized and secreted by endocrine tissue (glands) and transported in the blood to target tissues or organs.

Hydrolases Enzymes that catalyze cleavage of bonds between carbon atoms and some other kind of atom by the addition of water.

Hydroperoxyl (perhydroxyl) radical ($HO_2^{\bullet}$ or $H\!-\!O\!-\!O^{\bullet}$) A protonated superoxide radical.

Hydroxyapatite A crystal-lattice-like substance with the formula $Ca_{10}(PO_4)_6(OH)_2$, found in bones and teeth.

Hydroxyl radical ($^{\bullet}OH$) An oxygen-centered radical that can be generated in the body when it is exposed to γ rays, low-wavelength electromagnetic radiation.

Hypercalciuria Excessive urinary calcium excretion.

Hyperglycemia An above-normal blood glucose level.

Hyperinsulinemia An above-normal level of insulin in the blood.

Hyperkalemia High concentrations of potassium in the blood.

Hyperlipidemia A general term for an elevated blood level of any lipid.

Hyperphosphatemia High concentrations of phosphorus in the blood.

Hyperplasia Abnormal cell proliferation.

Hyperpnea An abnormal increase in the rate and depth of breathing.

Hypertrophied Grown larger or increased in size.

Hypertrophy Enlargement of the size of cells to increase the size of an organ or tissue.

Hypocalcemia Low concentrations of calcium in the blood.

Hypochondriasis Abnormal anxiety about one's own health.

Hypoglycemia A below-normal blood glucose level.

Hypokalemia Low concentrations of potassium in the blood.

Hyponatremia Low concentrations of sodium in the blood.

Immunoproteins Proteins made by plasma cells that help destroy foreign substances in the body; also called *immunoglobulins* or *antibodies.*

In vitro In a test tube or culture (outside the body).

In vivo Within the body.

Incomplete protein A dietary protein source that is missing or contains insufficient amounts of one or more indispensable amino acids needed for protein synthesis in the body. Incomplete proteins may also be called *low-quality proteins* and are generally derived from plants.

Indirect calorimetry Measurement of the consumption of oxygen and the expiration of carbon dioxide by the body, used to estimate metabolic rate.

Intermediate filaments Strong, ropelike cytoskeletal fibers that are made of protein and that function to provide mechanical stability for cells.

Intervention study A study testing a cause-effect relationship by intervening in a population, modifying a supposed causal factor, and measuring the effect of the change.

Introns Noncoding regions of a gene.

Ion An electrically charged atom or group of atoms; positively charged ions are called *cations,* and negatively charged ions are called *anions.*

Ischemia Deficiency of blood in a tissue.

Isomer One of two or more different chemical compounds that have the same molecular formula.

Isomerases Enzymes that catalyze the interconversion of optical or geometric isomers.

Isoprenoid Refers to the structure of the side chains of five-carbon units, as found in vitamins E and K.

Isotope infusion The direct introduction of an isotope (either radioactive or stable) into the bloodstream.

Keratinocytes Cells that produce the protein keratin.

Ketogenesis The process of producing ketone bodies.

Ketone bodies Compounds (acetoacetate, β-hydroxybutyrate, and acetone) formed during the oxidation of fatty acids in the absence of adequate four-carbon intermediates.

Krebs cycle See *tricarboxylic acid (TCA) cycle.*

Kyphosis A deformity of the spine characterized by a humpback or being bent forward; also called *dowager's hump.*

Lanugo Fine, soft, lightly pigmented hair that usually is found on a fetus toward the end of pregnancy but may appear on malnourished individuals.

Leptin A polypeptide hormone secreted by adipose tissue that reduces hunger through hypothalamic mechanisms.

Leukotrienes Biologically active compounds derived from linoleic or α-linolenic acids (n-6 and n-3 essential fatty acids).

Ligands Small molecules or minerals that bind to a larger molecule.

Ligases Enzymes that catalyze the formation of bonds between carbon and other atoms.

Limiting amino acid The amino acid within a protein with the lowest amino acid or chemical score; it is the amino acid present in a protein in the lowest amount, compared with a reference amount.

Lingual Pertaining to the tongue.

Lipophilicity The state of being attracted to lipids and thus repelled by water.

Lipoproteins Complexes of lipids and proteins that play a role in the transport and distribution of lipids.

Lyases Enzymes that catalyze cleavage of carbon-carbon, carbon-sulfur, and certain carbon-nitrogen bonds without hydrolysis or oxidation-reduction.

Lysosomes Cell organelles that contain digestive enzymes.

Macronutrients The dietary nutrients that supply energy, including fats, carbohydrates, and proteins.

Marasmus Malnutrition caused by prolonged intake of a diet deficient in energy (kcal).

Metabolic syndrome A clustering of risk factors for cardiovascular disease and type 2 diabetes, including elevated blood pressure and obesity.

Microfilament A solid cytoskeletal structure made of a double-helix polymer of the protein actin that plays a role in cell motility.

Microflora Bacteria adapted to living in a specific environment, such as the intestines.

Microtubules Hollow, cylindrical cytoskeletal structures composed of the protein tubulin that act to support the cell structure.

Microvilli Extensions of intestinal epithelial cells designed to present a large surface area for absorbing dietary nutrients.

Mitochondria Cellular organelles that are the site of energy production by oxidative phosphorylation and the site of the tricarboxylic acid (Krebs) cycle; they are surrounded by an outer membrane that is very permeable and an inner membrane that is only selectively permeable.

Monosaccharides The simplest form of carbohydrates, which cannot be reduced in size to smaller carbohydrate units.

Motility Movement.

Mucins Glycoproteins found in some body secretions, such as saliva.

Natriuresis The excretion of large amounts of sodium in the urine.

Nervous system The system of nervous tissue made up of neurons and glial cells.

Nitrogen dioxide radical ($^\bullet NO_2$ or $^\bullet ONO$) A nitrogen- and oxygen-containing radical, formed from a reaction between nitric oxide and molecular oxygen, in which one of the two oxygen atoms possesses an unpaired electron.

Nitrosation The substitution of a hydrogen atom in an organic compound with a nitroso group ($-N=O$)

Nitrosothiol (RSNO) A compound, which is typically organic, that contains a nitroso group ($-N=O$) attached to a sulfur atom of a thiol.

Nuclear envelope A set of two membranes that contain nuclear pores and surround the cell nucleus.

Nucleoli Regions of the nucleus containing condensed chromatin and sites for synthesizing ribosomal RNA.

Nucleotides A phosphate ester of the $5'$-phosphate of a purine or pyrimidine in N-glycosidic linkage with ribose or deoxyribose, occurring in nucleic acids.

Nystagmus Constant, involuntary movement of the eyeball.

Observational study An epidemiological study in which the assignments of subjects into control or treated groups is outside of the investigator's control. Inferences about the possible effects of the treatment are drawn from the differences between the two groups.

Oligomer Polypeptide chains joined to form a functional protein.

Oligosaccharides Short chains of monosaccharide units joined by covalent bonds.

Oncogenes Genes capable of causing a normal cell to convert to a cancerous cell.

Oncosis A prelethal pathway accompanied by cellular swelling, organelle swelling, and increased membrane permeability that lead to cell death.

Ophthalmoplegia Paralysis of the ocular muscles.

Orexigenic Pertaining to increasing or stimulating the appetite.

Oscilloscope An instrument that displays a visual representation of electrical variations on a cathode tube such as one used to visualize echoes as part of an ultrasound examination.

Osmosis The net movement of the solvent (such as water) from a solution of lesser to one of greater concentration when the two solutions are separated by a membrane that selectively prevents passage of solute molecules but is permeable to the solvent.

Osmotic pressure A property of a solution that is proportional to the nondiffusible solute concentration.

Osteoblasts Bone-forming cells.

Osteoclasts Cells that break down or resorb bone.

Osteomalacia A disorder characterized by bone mineralization defects that may occur in adults because of inadequate vitamin D intake.

Oxidation An enzymatic reaction in which oxygen is added to, or hydrogen and its electrons are removed from, the reactant.

Oxidative phosphorylation The pathway in the mitochondria that makes ATP from ADP and P_i.

Oxidoreductases Enzymes that catalyze all reactions in which one compound is oxidized and another is reduced.

Oxygenation reactions Reactions that involve the introduction of or require one or more oxygen atoms.

Parallel study A clinical trial that compares the results of a treatment on two separate groups of patients.

Parenchymal cells The functional cells of an organ such as the liver.

Pellagra A condition that results from niacin deficiency.

Pentose phosphate pathway The pathway that metabolizes glucose-6-phosphate to pentose phosphate, producing NADPH.

Peroxisomes Cell organelles containing enzymes that perform oxidative catabolic reactions.

Peroxyl radical (O_2^{2-}) A radical that contains a peroxyl ($-O-O-$) group.

Peroxynitrate ($O_2NOO^\bullet$) A nitrogen- and oxygen-containing radical that is generated from a reaction between nitrogen dioxide and a superoxide radical and that typically decomposes to form singlet oxygen and nitrogen dioxide.

Peroxynitrite ($ONOO^\bullet$) A nitrogen- and oxygen-containing radical, formed by a reaction between nitric oxide and superoxide radicals, that can decompose to generate hydroxyl and nitrogen dioxide radicals or react with carbon dioxide to produce carbonate and nitrogen dioxide radicals.

Petechiae Skin discolorations caused by ruptured small blood vessels.

Phagocytosis An endocytotic process in which material is engulfed into a cell.

Phospholipids Lipids that belong to a class of complex lipids containing phosphate and one or more fatty acid residues.

Phosphorolysis Cleavage of a chemical bond with the addition of phosphoric acid, analogous to hydrolysis (an example is the sequential release of individual glucose units from glycogen).

Phosphorylation The metabolic process of adding a phosphate group to an organic molecule.

Phytochemical A biologically active, nonnutritive substance that is found in plants.

Phytyl tail Refers to the structure of the side chains of vitamins E and K.

Pinocytosis Uptake of a substance into a cell through the formation of vesicles derived from the plasma membrane.

Plasma The liquid portion of blood that has been separated from the particulate portion (through the removal of cells and platelets).

Plasma membrane The membrane encapsulating a cell.

Polymer A substance with a high molecular weight, made up of a chain of repeating units.

Polysaccharides Long chains of monosaccharide units that may number from several into the hundreds or thousands.

Porphyrin The nitrogen- and iron-containing nonprotein portion of hemoglobin.

Postprandial Occurring after a meal.

Potentiometry A method using electrodes that enables direct measurement of various anions and cations such as potassium, sodium, and chloride.

Prebiotics Nondigestible food ingredients that serve as substrates to promote the colonic growth and/or activity of selected health-promoting species of bacteria.

Preprandial Occurring before a meal.

Probiotics Products that contain specific strains of microorganisms in sufficient numbers to alter the microflora of the gastrointestinal tract, ideally to exert beneficial health effects.

Prokaryotic cells Primitive cells that do not contain a defined nucleus.

Propagation The ongoing generation of free radicals following the initiation stage of free radical formation.

Prophylactic A substance or regime that helps to prevent disease or illness.

Prospective study An epidemiological study in which subjects are selected on the basis of factors that are to be examined in the future for possible effects on some outcome.

Prostaglandins Biologically active compounds derived from linoleic or α-linolenic acids (n-6 or n-3 essential fatty acids).

Proteases Enzymes that digest (break down) proteins.

Protein kinases A family of enzymes that transfers a phosphate group to another protein from ATP.

Proteoglycans Large molecules made up of proteins and glycosaminoglycans.

Proteolytic Pertaining to the breakdown of protein.

Quenching A process by which electronically excited molecules, such as singlet molecular oxygen, are inactivated.

Receptors Macromolecules (usually proteins) that bind a signal molecule with a high degree of specificity that triggers intracellular events.

Recommended Dietary Allowance (RDA) The average daily dietary intake level of a nutrient that is thought to be sufficient to meet the nutrient requirements of about 97% of healthy individuals.

Reflex An involuntary response to a stimulus.

Reperfusion The resupply of an organ or tissue with oxygen, nutrients, or both.

Replication The synthesis of a daughter duplex DNA molecule identical to the parental duplex DNA.

Resin A compound that is usually solid or semisolid and usually exists as a polymer.

Respiratory quotient (RQ) The ratio of the volume of CO_2 expired to the volume of O_2 consumed.

Retrospective study An epidemiological study in which participating individuals are classified as exhibiting some outcome or lacking that outcome.

Rhodopsin A vitamin A–containing protein found in the eye.

Rickets A condition in infants and children that results from vitamin D deficiency.

Ryanodine receptor A calcium channel in the sarcoplasmic reticulum of muscle that opens to permit the release of calcium.

Sarcoplasmic reticulum The smooth endoplasmic reticulum that is found in muscle cells and is the site of the calcium pump.

Scintillation counter An instrument used to measure concentrations of radioactive isotopes in a sample.

Scurvy A condition resulting from vitamin C deficiency.

Seborrheic dermatitis An inflammatory skin condition.

Secretagogue An agent that stimulates secretion of another compound.

Sense strand The strand of DNA that serves as a template for mRNA.

Serum The pale yellowish, clear fluid portion of blood from which the clotting factors (fibrinogen) have been removed.

Short-chain fatty acids Fatty acids typically containing two to four carbons.

Sideroblastic anemia An inherited disorder that affects red blood cell production and function.

Signal-lipidomics A branch of the emerging field of lipidomics, which studies the pathways and networks of cellular lipids. Signal-lipidomics studies the lipidomics of various signaling sites of cell membranes, which often involve polyunsaturated fatty acids such as docosahexaenoic acid.

Single blind study An experiment in which the subjects do not know which treatment (placebo or experimental) they are receiving, but the study investigators do know.

Singlet molecular oxygen An electronically excited radical in which one of oxygen's electrons is excited to an orbital above the one it normally occupies.

Sphingolipids Phospholipids that contain the amino alcohol sphingosine, rather than glycerol.

Splanchnic Pertaining to the internal organs (viscera), especially the intestines.

Standard reduction potential The tendency of a molecule to donate or receive electrons.

Steatorrhea The presence of an excessive amount of fat in the feces.

Stellate cells Storage cells of the liver.

Stereoisomers A group of compounds that have the same structure but different configurations.

Sterols A subclass of lipids that contain a cyclopentanoperhydrophenanthrene ring system, a hydroxyl group, and a side chain.

Substrate-level phosphorylation The process of transferring a phosphate group from one organic molecule to another.

Superoxide radical An oxygen-centered free radical, $O_2^{\bullet-}$.

Teratogenic Capable of causing birth defects in a fetus.

Tetany A condition resulting from inadequate blood calcium concentrations, characterized by prolonged muscle contraction.

Thalassemia A hereditary form of anemia associated with defective synthesis of hemoglobin.

Thermogenesis The production of heat within the body.

Thermoregulation The process whereby a regulatory mechanism keeps heat production and loss about equal.

Thiobarbituric acid reactive substances Compounds such as hexanal, pentanal, or pentane that react with thiobarbituric acid and suggest oxidative damage has occurred.

Thromboxanes Biologically active compounds derived from linoleic or α-linolenic acids (n-6 or n-3 essential fatty acids).

Tolerable Upper Intake Level The highest daily intake level that is likely to cause no risk of adverse health effects to most individuals in the general population.

Tonic Pertaining to or characterized by tension or contraction.

Transcaltachia Rapid intestinal calcium absorption stimulated by the active form of vitamin D.

Transcription The process by which the genetic information (base sequence) in a single strand of DNA is used to specify a complementary sequence of bases in an mRNA chain.

Transcription factors Auxiliary proteins that bind to specific sites in the DNA and alter the transcription of nearby genes.

Transducin A G-protein, found in the eye, that responds to changes in opsin and is involved in the visual cycle.

Transferases Enzymes that catalyze reactions not involving oxidation and reduction in which a functional group is transferred from one substrate to another.

Transition state Energy level at which reactant molecules have been activated and can undergo an exothermic reaction.

Translation The process by which genetic information in an mRNA molecule specifies the sequence of amino acids in the protein product.

Translocation Movement of a compound or agent across a cell membrane, such as the intestinal cell, and into the blood.

Transport proteins Proteins that transport nutrients in blood or into and out of cells or cell organelles.

Tricarboxylic acid cycle An aerobic metabolic cycle in the mitochondria that produces ATP; also called the *citric acid cycle* or *Krebs cycle*.

Tropical sprue A disease common in tropical regions and characterized by weakness, weight loss, poor nutrient digestion and absorption, and steatorrhea.

Tumor necrosis factor A cytokine released by immune cells and mast cells that causes destruction of tumors and migration of neutrophils toward the site of bacterial infections.

Ubiquinol The alcohol form of ubiquinone, a fat-soluble molecule that functions in electron transport and ultimately ATP generation; also called *coenzyme Q_{10}* or *CoQ_{10}*.

Ubiquitin A protein that attaches to other proteins within cells or tissues to promote the degradation of the protein.

Vascular system The circulatory pathway that delivers blood to and from organs.

VO_2 max The maximal uptake of oxygen, as measured during a test with increasing work intensity.

Ward's triangle A region within the pelvis (hip).

Xenobiotics Foreign chemicals such as drugs, carcinogens, pesticides, food additives, pollutants, or other noxious compounds.

Xerophthalmia Dryness of the conjunctiva and keratinization of the epithelium of the eye following inflammation of the conjunctiva associated with vitamin A deficiency.

Zwitterion A dipolar ion that has both negatively and positively charged regions, such as an amino acid. The ion has no net charge in solution.

Zymogen An inactive form of an enzyme, also referred to as a *proenzyme*.

INDEX

A

α1-acid glycoprotein, 214
α1-globulins, 214
α2-globulins, 214
α2 macroglobulin, 214, 247
α-aminolevulinic acid (ALA), 252, 362, 491
α-amylase, 40, 41, 65
abdomen, skin-fold measurement at, 280
abdominal obesity, 274
absorptiometry, 282–283
absorption
    of carbohydrates, 70–77
    of lipids, 148–151, 150*f*
    of protein, 189–192
Acceptable Macronutrient Distribution Range (AMDR), 244
accessory organs, **33,** 34*f,* 47–51
acetal bonds, 67
acetaldehyde toxicity, 177
acetic acid, 121–122
acetyl-ACP, 168
acetyl-CoA, 253
acetyl-CoA carboxylase, 168, 174
    biotin, 341
acetyl-CoA oxidation, 89
acetyl-CoA production, 168
achlorhydria, **359**
acid–base balance, 469–472, 505
acidic ash load, 243, 452
acidosis, **470,** 472
acinar exocrine cells, 47
aconitase activity, 488*f,* 490
acrodermatitis enteropathica, 501
activated fatty acid (acyl-CoA), 164
activation energy, 22*f,* **23**
active transport, 52*f,* 72
acute pancreatitis, 47
acute phase reactant proteins, 214
acyl carrier protein (ACP), 337
acyl-CoA dehydrogenase, 164
acyl-CoA retinol acyl transferase (ARAT), 376
acyl-CoA synthetase, 164
acylglycerols, 141
adapted starvation, 247*f*
adaptive thermogenesis, 289–290
adenine, 222*f*
adenosine diphosphate ribose (ADP-ribose), 332, 494

adenosine triphosphate (ATP), 5, 6, 21*f,* 66, 441
    formation of, 90
    generation of, 25*f*
    phosphorylation of ADP to form, 95*f*
adenosylcobalamin, 356
Adequate Intake (AI), 126, 242–244, **308**
adiponectin, 296
adipose tissue, 155
adipose tissue lipolysis, 246
adrenocortical hormones, 58, 142, 146, 174, 212
adrenocorticotropic hormone (ACTH), 174, 212
adventitia, 33, 34
aerobic glycolysis, 89–90
aerobic metabolism, 268, 269
agouti-related protein (AGRP), 58
α-helix, 74, 209
air-displacement plethysmography, 282
alanine, 193, 196, 228
alanine–glucose cycle, 229*f*
albumin, 49, 130, 141, 149, 213, 214
alcohol consumption, hypertension and, 476
alcohol dehydrogenase, 176, 506
alcohol dehydrogenase (ADH) pathway, 175–176
alcoholism, 177–178
aldehyde oxidase, 494, 540
aldolase reaction, 24, 97
aldolases, 18
aldoses, 64
aldosterone, 247, 314, 327, 457, 461, 465
alkaline phosphatase, 193, 505
alkalosis, **470**
alkaptonuria, 199
alkoxyl radical, 315
allosteric activation, 82–83
allosteric enzyme modulation, 17, 101, 174
allracemic (all-rac) α-tocopheryl acetate, 401
all-*trans* retinol, 371, 382. *See also* vitamin A and carotenoids
α-melanocyte-stimulating hormone (α-MSH), 58
amenorrhea, 301, 451

amidases, 18
amidation, 194, 516
amidoxime reductase, 540–541, 541*f*
amine oxidases, 515
amino acids
    absorption, 189, 190
    aromatic, 197–198, 199
    branched-chain, 203–204, 229, 230*f*
    carbon skeletons of, 196
    classification, 183–186, 184*t*
    deamination of, 194
    dicarboxylic, 185
    disposal of, 194
    essentiality of, 186
    exhibiting net change, 185*t*
    glutamyl cycle for transport of, 193*f*
    metabolic roles of, 235
    metabolism, 192–207, 225–226, 232*f,* 537
    net electrical charge, 185
    neutral, 185*t*
    organ interaction in, 259–261
    and pH balance, 213*f*
    polar and nonpolar, 185*t*
    polarity, 185
    recommended intakes, 242–244
    sodium (Na⁺) dependent transport, 190*f*
    sources of, 186–187
    Tolerable Upper Intake Level (UL), 243
    transamination reactions, 192
amino acid score, 240
amino and acid derivatives, 67
aminobutyric acid (GABA), 362
aminolevulinic acid dehydratase, 506
aminopeptidases, 48, 189, 506
aminotransferases, 193, 235
ammonia, 223
AMP-activated protein kinase (AMPK), 252–253
amphibolic intermediates, 251–252
amphibolic pathway, 252–253
amphoteric substances, **470**
ampulla of Vater, 47
amylase inhibitors, 70
amylin, 57
amylopectin, structure of, 69*f*
anabolism, 207–208
anaerobic glycolysis, 83–86
anaerobic metabolism, 258